£125.00

£3.00

Evidence-based Gastroenterology and Hepatology

Second edition

Updates for *Evidence Based Gastroenterology and Hepatology* will be regularly posted to the following website. These updates give the latest trial data and recommendations for implementation in practice.

www.evidbasedgastro.com

Evidence-based Gastroenterology and Child Health

Second edition

Edited by

John WD McDonald

Professor of Medicine, University of Western Ontario
Gastroenterology Service
London Health Sciences Centre
London, Ontario, Canada

Andrew K Burroughs

Consultant Physician/Hepatologist
Royal Free Hospital
London, UK

Brian G Feagan

Professor of Medicine, University of Western Ontario
Gastroenterology Service
London Health Sciences Centre
London, Ontario, Canada

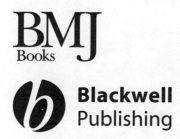

BMJ
Books

Blackwell
Publishing

© 2004 by Blackwell Publishing Ltd
BMJ Books is an imprint of the BMJ Publishing Group

Blackwell Publishing, Inc., 350 Main Street, Malden, Massachusetts 02148-5020, USA
Blackwell Publishing Ltd, 9600 Garsington Road, Oxford OX4 2DQ, UK
Blackwell Publishing Asia Pty Ltd, 550 Swanston Street, Carlton, Victoria 3053, Australia

First published in 2000
by BMJ Books, BMA House, Tavistock Square, London WC1H 9JR

First Edition 1999
Second Edition 2004

Library of Congress Cataloging-in-Publication Data

Evidence-based gastroenterology and hepatology.— 2nd ed.
    p. ; cm.
  Includes bibliographical references and index.
  ISBN 0-7279-1751-X
  1. Gastrointestinal system—Diseases. 2. Liver—Diseases. 3. Evidence-based medicine.
[DNLM: 1. Gastrointestinal Diseases—therapy. 2. Evidence-Based Medicine—methods.
3. Liver Diseases—therapy. WI 140 E927 2004]

  RC816.E85 2004
  610.3'3—dc22   2004017089

ISBN 0 7279 1751 X

A catalogue record for this book is available from the British Library

Set in India by Siva Math Setters, Chennai
Printed and bound in India by Gopsons Papers Limited, New Delhi

Commissioning Editor: Mary Banks
Development Editor: Nic Ulyatt
Production Controller: Kate Charman

www.evidbasedgastro.com

For further information on Blackwell Publishing, visit our website:
http://www.blackwellpublishing.com

The publisher's policy is to use permanent paper from mills that operate a sustainable forestry policy, and which has been manufactured from pulp processed using acid-free and elementary chlorine-free practices. Furthermore, the publisher ensures that the text paper and cover board used have met acceptable environmental accreditation standards.

Contents

Contributors

Paul C Adams

Diamond Sherin Alidina

Piero Almasio

Vicente Arroyo

Mark Bradette

Andrew K Burroughs

Calogero Cammà

Laura Cecilioni

Roger Chapman

Naoki Chiba

Nicholas Church

Massimo Colombo

Ann Cranney

Antonia Craxi

Sue Cullen

Lucy Dagher

Chris Day

Douglas A Drossman

Catherine Dube

Carlo A Fallone

Brian G Feagan

Peter Ferenci

Peter Ginès

Marco Giunta

John Goulis

James Gregor

Albena Halpert

Jenny Heathcote

Gary Jeffrey

Derek P Jewell

Michael B Kimmey

Jarol Knowles

Bret A Lashner

Calvin HL Law

Bernard Levin

Robert Lofberg

Andreas Maetzel

Michael Peter Manns

Patrick Marcellin

Philippe Mathurin

Lynne V McFarland

Dana McKay

John WD McDonald

Christian Müller

Nick Murphy

Kelvin Palmer

George Papath

Thierry Poynard

Joel E Richter

Juan Rodés

Nancy Rolando

Alaa Rostom

William J Sandborn

Michael D Saunders

Andreas Schüler

Jonathon Springer

Hillary Steinhart

Christian M Surawicz

Lloyd R Sutherland

Ved R Tandan

Rosangela Texeira

Peter Tugwell

Sander JO Van Zanten

Marcelo F Vela

Jim J Wade

Alastair JM Watson

George Wells

Julia Wendon

Grading of recommendations and levels of evidence used in *Evidence-based Gastroenterology and Hepatology*

Grade A

Level 1a   Evidence from large randomized clinical trials (RCTs) or systematic reviews (including meta-analyses) of multiple randomized trials which collectively has at least as much data as one single well-defined trial.

Level 1b   Evidence from at least one "All or None" high quality cohort study; in which ALL patients died/ failed with conventional therapy and some survived/ succeeded with the new therapy (for example, chemotherapy for tuberculosis, meningitis, or defibrillation for ventricular fibrillation); or in which many died/failed with conventional therapy and NONE died/failed with the new therapy (for example, penicillin for pneumococcal infections).

Level 1c   Evidence from at least one moderate-sized RCT or a meta-analysis of small trials which collectively only has a moderate number of patients.

Level 1d   Evidence from at least one RCT.

Grade B

Level 2   Evidence from at least one high quality study of non-randomized cohorts who did and did not receive the new therapy.

Level 3   Evidence from at least one high quality case–control study.

Level 4   Evidence from at least one high quality case series.

Grade C

Level 5   Opinions from experts without reference or access to any of the foregoing (for example, argument from physiology, bench research or first principles).

A comprehensive approach would incorporate many different types of evidence (for example, RCTs, non-RCTs, epidemiologic studies, and experimental data), and examine the architecture of the information for consistency, coherence and clarity. Occasionally the evidence does not completely fit into neat compartments. For example, there is strong (A-1a) evidence through very large randomized trials that fecal occult blood testing on an annual or semi-annual basis modestly reduces mortality from colon cancer in a population at average risk for this disease. The evidence that direct examination of the colon at intervals of 5 to 10 years results in even greater benefit has been derived only from case control studies (B-3). Physicians, patients and policy advisers should have both levels of evidence available to make informed decisions.

Recommendation grades appear either within the text, for example, **Grade A** and **Grade A1a** or within a table in the chapter.

The grading system clearly is only applicable to preventive or therapeutic interventions. It is not applicable to many other types of data such as descriptive, genetic or pathophysiologic.

Evidence-based Gastroenterology and Hepatology, Second edition CD Rom

Features

Evidence-based Gastroenterology and Hepatology, Second edition PDF eBook

- Bookmarked and hyperlinked for instant access to all headings and topics
- Fully indexed and searchable text – just click the 'Search Text' button

Website BMJ Books

- Instant access to the BMJ Books website, including a full catalogue of related books.

Also included – a direct link to the Evidence-based Gastroenterology and Hepatology update website

Instructions for use

The CD Rom should start automatically upon insertion, on all Windows systems. The menu screen will appear and you can then navigate by clicking on the headings. If the CD Rom does not start automatically upon insertion, please browse using "Windows Explorer" and double-click the file "BMJ_Books.exe".

Tips

The viewable area of the PDF ebook can be expanded to fill the full screen width by hiding the bookmarks. To do this, click and hold on the divider in between the bookmark window and the main window, then drag it to the left as required.

By clicking once on a page in the PDF ebook window, you 'activate' the window. You can now scroll through pages using the scroll-wheel on your mouse, or by using the cursor keys on your keyboard.

Note: the Evidence-based Gastroenterology and Hepatology PDF eBook is for search and reference only and, aside from the free consumers sections and faces figures, cannot be printed.

Troubleshooting

If any problems are experienced with use of the CD Rom, further information and updates can be found at: http://www.evidbasedgastro.com

Glossary

5-ALA	5-aminolevulinic acid
AAD	antibiotic associated diarrhea
ACPO	acute colonic pseudo-obstruction
ACS	American Cancer Society
AFP	α-fetoprotein
AGA	antigliadin antibodies
AIH	autoimmune hepatitis
ALD	alcoholic liver disease
ALT	alanine aminotransferase(transaminase)
ANCA	anti-neutrophil cytoplasmic antibodies
APC	antigen-presenting cells
ApoA-I	apolipoprotein A-I
ARA	antireticulin antibodies
ARR	absolute risk reduction
AST	aspartate aminotransferase (transaminase)
BCAA	branched chain amino acids
BMD	bone mineral density
BMI	body mass index
CBT	cognitive behavior therapy
CD	Crohn's disease
cGMP	cyclic guanosine monophosphate
CI	confidence interval
CLD	chronic liver disease
CMV Ig	CMV hyperimmune globulins
CNS	central nervous system
COX-2	cyclo-oxygenase-2
CPP	cerebral perfusion pressure
CRC	colorectal cancer
CRP	C-reactive protein
CSOP	corticosteroid-induced osteoporosis
CT	computed tomography
CVP	central venous pressure
DALM	dysplasia-associated lesion or mass
DCBE	double contrast barium enema
DES	diffuse esophageal spasm
DM	diabetes mellitus
DSRS	selective distal splenorenal shunt
DXA	dual energy x ray absorptiometry
EASL	European Association for the Study of the Liver
EATL	enteropathy-associated T cell lymphoma
EGD	esophagogastroduodenoscopy
EIA	enzyme immunoassay
ELISA	enzyme-linked immunosorbent assay
EMA	anti-endomysial antibody
ERCP	endoscopic retrograde cholangiopancreatography
FAP	familial adenomatous polyposis
FDA	Food and Drug Administration
FFA	free fatty acids
FFP	fresh frozen plasma
FHF	fulminant hepatic failure
FOBT	fecal occult blood testing
GABA	γ-amino butyric acid
G-CSF	granulocyte-colony stimulating factor
GERD	gastroesophageal reflux disease
GGT	γ-glutamyl transpeptidase
H₂-RA	H$_2$-receptor antagonists
HBIG	hepatitis B immune globulin
HBsAg	Hepatitis B s antigen
HCC	hepatocellular carcinoma
HCV	hepatitis C virus
HLA	human leukocyte antigen
HN Ig	human normal immunoglobulin
HNPCC	hereditary non-polyposis colorectal cancer (syndrome)
HVPG	hepatic venous pressure gradient
IBD	inflammatory bowel disease
IBS	Irritable bowel syndrome
ICAM	serum intercellular adhesion molecule
ICP	intracranial pressure
ICU	intensive care unit
IEL	intraepithelial lymphocyte (count)
IFN	interferon
iNOS	inducible nitric oxide synthase
IPAA	ileal pouch–anal anastomosis
LCBDE	laparoscopic common bile duct exploration
LES	lower esophageal sphincter
LR	likelihood ratio
MELD	Mayo End-stage Liver Disease (score)
MHC	major histocompatibility complex
MRCP	magnetic resonance cholangiopancreatography
MRI	magnetic resonance imaging
MRSA	methicillin-resistant *Staphylococcus aureus*
NAC	*N*-acetylcysteine
NAFLD	non-alcoholic fatty liver disease
NASH	non-alcoholic steatohepatitis
NCT	number connection test
Nd:YAG	neodymium:yttrium-aluminum-garnet
NE	nutcracker esophagus
NERD	non-erosive reflux disease
NNT	number needed to treat
NO	nitric oxide
OCBDE	open common bile duct exploration
OLT	orthotopic liver transplantation
OR	odds ratio
PAF	platelet activating factor

PAOP	pulmonary artery occlusion pressure	RATG	rabbit antithymocyte globulin
PBC	primary biliary cirrhosis	RR	relative risk
PCR	polymerase chain reaction	RRR	relative risk reduction
PCS	portacaval shunt	SBD	selective bowel decontamination
PDAI	pouchitis disease activity index	SCFA	short chain fatty acids
PDT	Photodynamic therapy	SIRS	systemic inflammatory response syndrome
PEG	polyethylene glycol	SSBE	short segment Barrett's esophagus
PEI	percutaneous ethanol injection	SSRI	selective serotonin reuptake inhibitor
PET	positron emission tomography	TACE	transcatheter arterial chemoembolization
PIIIP	procollagen III propeptide	TCE	total colon examination
PPAR	peroxisome proliferator activated receptor	TIPS	transjugular intrahepatic portosystemic shunt
PPI	proton pump inhibitors	TLESRs	transient lower esophageal sphincter relaxations
PSC	primary sclerosing cholangitis	TPN	total parenteral nutrition
PSE	portal–systemic encephalopathy	tTG	tissue transglutaminase
PTH	parathyroid hormone	UC	ulcerative colitis
PUD	peptic ulcer disease	UDCA	ursodeoxycholic acid
RAI	Rejection Activity Index	VRE	vancomycin-resistant *Enterococcus*

1 Introduction

John WD McDonald, Brian G Feagan, Andrew K Burroughs

Over the past three decades the emergence of evidence-based medicine (EBM) has had a substantial impact on clinical practice. In the first half of the twentieth century, diagnostic tests or treatments, usually based on a strong scientific rationale and experimental work in animals, were routinely introduced into clinical care without good scientific proof of efficacy in people. Some of these interventions, such as gastric freezing for the treatment of ulcers and penicillamine therapy for primary biliary cirrhosis, were ultimately shown to be ineffective[1,2] and harmful. There is little doubt that the widespread acceptance by physicians of unproved treatments has been detrimental to the well-being of many patients.

Fortunately, the need for a more critical approach to medical practice was recognized. In 1948 the first randomized controlled trial (RCT) in humans was carried out under the direction of the British Medical Research Council.[3] Epidemiologists and statisticians, notably Sir Richard Doll and Sir Bradford Hill, provided scientific leadership to the medical community, which responded with improvements in the quality of clinical research. The use of randomized allocation to control for confounding variables and to minimize bias was recognized as invaluable for conducting valid studies of treatments. The initiation of these landmark experiments defined a new era in clinical research; the RCT soon became the benchmark for the evaluation of medical and surgical interventions. Gastroenterologists played an important part in these early days. In 1955 Professor Sidney Truelove conducted the first randomized trial in the discipline of gastroenterology.[4] He and his colleagues proved that cortisone was more effective than a placebo for the treatment of ulcerative colitis. As noted in Chapter 11, this treatment has stood the test of time. The ascendancy of the RCT was accompanied by a call for greater scientific rigor in the usual practice of clinical medicine. Strong advocates of the application of epidemiological principles to patient care emerged and found a growing body of support among clinicians.

As the number of randomized trials grew to the point of becoming unmanageable, it was recognized that there was a the need to provide summaries of the evidence provided by these trials for the use of practitioners, who frequently lack both time and expertise to consult the primary research. Busy clinicians may consult local experts, with the tacit assumption that they will make recommendations based on evidence. Liberati and colleagues[5] provided evidence that this approach led to inappropriate care for many women with breast cancer. Subsequently, convincing evidence became available through the work of Antman *et al.*[6] and of Mulrow[7] that the conventional review article and the traditional textbook chapter are seldom comprehensive, and are frequently biased. More recently, Jefferson[8] reinforced this conclusion on the basis of a survey concerning recommendations for vaccination for cholera, which appeared in editorials and review articles. He pointed out that authors of editorials and reviews frequently resort to the "desk drawer" technique, pulling out evidence with which they are very familiar, but failing to assemble and review all of the evidence in a systematic way.

In the UK Archie Cochrane, as early as 1979, made a compelling case that there was a need to prepare and maintain summaries of all randomized trials.[9] Cochrane's challenge to the medical community to use scientific methods to identify, evaluate, and systematically summarize the world's medical literature pertaining to all health care interventions is now being met. From its inception in 1993, the electronic database prepared by the volunteer members of the Cochrane Collaboration and published as the *Cochrane Library*[10] has grown exponentially. Systematic reviews and especially Cochrane reviews are now widely used by clinicians in the daily practice of medicine, by researchers and by the public. Accordingly, data from systematic reviews published in the *Cochrane Library* are featured prominently in several chapters in *Evidence-based Gastroenterology and Hepatology*. Unfortunately, coverage in the *Cochrane Library* of topics in gastroenterology and hepatology is still far from complete.

Several other clinical epidemiologists played important roles in the evolution of evidence-based medicine. Beginning in the 1970s, David Sackett encouraged practicing physicians to become familiar with the basic principles of critical appraisal. Criteria developed by Sackett and others for the evaluation of clinical studies assessing therapy, causation, prognosis, and other clinical topics were widely published.[11,12] His text *Clinical epidemiology: a basic science for clinical medicine*, co-authored by colleagues Gordon

Guyatt, Brian Haynes and Peter Tugwell, introduced many physicians to the concepts of EBM.[13] In the USA, Alvin Feinstein called attention to the need for increased rigor in the design and interpretation of observational studies and explored the scientific principles of diagnostic testing.[14,15] Among gastroenterologists, Thomas Chalmers, a strong, early advocate for the RCT,[16] was responsible for introducing gastroenterologists and others to the importance of randomized trials in gastroenterology and hepatology[17] and to the concept of systematic reviews and meta-analysis as means of summarizing data from these studies.[18]

Despite the opposition of some,[19] the popularity of EBM continues to grow. Although the explanations for this phenomenon are complex, one factor is that many practitioners recognize that ethical patient care should be based on the best possible evidence. For this, and other reasons, the fundamental concept behind EBM – the use of the scientific method in the practice of clinical medicine – has been widely endorsed by medical opinion leaders, patients and governments.

What is evidence-based gastroenterology and hepatology?

Evidence-based gastroenterology and hepatology is the application of the most valid scientific information to the care of patients with gastrointestinal and hepatic diseases. Physicians who treat patients with digestive diseases must provide their patients with the most appropriate diagnostic tests, the most accurate prognosis and the most effective and safe therapy. To meet this high standard individual clinicians must have access to and be able to evaluate scientific evidence. Although many practitioners argue that this has always been the standard of care in clinical medicine, a great deal of evidence exists to the contrary. Wide variations in practice patterns among physicians have been documented for many treatments, despite the presence of good data from widely publicized RCTs and the promotion of practice guidelines by content experts. For example, Scholefield *et al.* carried out a survey of British surgeons who were questioned regarding the performance of screening colonoscopy for colon cancer.[20] Although this study was done in 1998 (after publication of the results of the RCTs described in Chapter 16 which demonstrated a benefit of this practice), many of these physicians failed to make appropriate recommendations for screening patients at risk. What is the explanation for this finding? One possibility is that many clinicians rely for information on their colleagues, on local experts, or on review articles or textbook chapters that are not written-based on the principles of EBM.

Two important points about EBM should be emphasized. First, use of the principles of EBM in the management of

patients is complementary to traditional clinical skills and will never supersede the recognized virtues of careful observation, sound judgment and compassion for the patient. It is noteworthy that many good doctors have intuitively used the basic principles of EBM; hence, the promotion of such well known clinical aphorisms as "go where the money is" and "do the last test first". Knowledge of EBM enables physicians to understand why these basic rules of clinical medicine are valid through the use of a quantitative approach to decision making. This paradigm can in no way be considered detrimental to the doctor–patient relationship.

Second, although RCTs are the most valuable source of data for evaluating healthcare interventions, other kinds of evidence must frequently be used. In some instances, most obviously in studies of causation, it is neither possible nor ethical to conduct RCTs. Here, data from methodologically rigorous observational studies are extremely valuable. A dramatic example was the demonstration by several authors (quoted in Chapter 24) that the relative risk of hepatocellular carcinoma in chronic carriers of the hepatitis B virus is dramatically higher than in persons who are not infected. Although these data are observational, the strength of the association is such that it is exceedingly unlikely that a cause other than hepatitis B virus is responsible for the development of cancer in these people. Case–control studies are especially useful for studying rare diseases and for the initial development of scientific hypotheses regarding causation. The etiological role of non-steroidal anti-inflammatory drugs in the development of gastric ulcer[21] was recognized using this methodology. Finally, case series can provide compelling evidence for the adoption of a new therapy in the absence of data from RCTs, if the natural history of the disease is both well characterized and severe. An example is the identification of orthotopic liver transplantation as a dramatically effective intervention for patients with advanced liver disease.

Box 1.1 shows a generally agreed approach to ranking the strength of evidence that arises from various types of studies of healthcare interventions, and this system is used throughout the book. This ranking of evidence has appeared in a number of publications; we have chosen to reproduce it from *Evidence-based Cardiology,*[22] along with the system used by its editors, Yusuf *et al.*, for making recommendations on the basis of these levels of evidence. As mentioned in Box 1.1, throughout this book recommendation grades appear as Grade A or Grade A1a .

Clinical decision making in gastroenterology and hepatology

Clinical decision making by gastroenterologists usually falls into one of the following categories:

Box 1.1   Grading of recommendations and levels of evidence used in *Evidence-based Gastroenterology and Hepatology*

GRADE A
- Evidence from large randomized clinical trials (RCTs) or systematic reviews (including meta-analyses) of multiple randomized trials which collectively have at least as much data as one single well-defined trial
- Evidence from at least one "All or None" high quality cohort study; in which ALL patients died/failed with conventional therapy and some survived/succeeded with the new therapy (for example, chemotherapy for tuberculosis, meningitis, or defibrillation for ventricular fibrillation): or in which many died/failed with conventional therapy and NONE died/failed with the new therapy (for example, penicillin for pneumococcal infections)
- Evidence from at least one moderate sized RCT or a meta-analysis of small trials which collectively only has a moderate number of patients.
- Evidence from at least one RCT

GRADE B
- Evidence from at least one high quality study of non-randomized cohorts who did and did not receive the new therapy
- Evidence from at least one high quality case control study
- Evidence from at least one high quality case series

GRADE C
- Opinions from experts without reference or access to any of the foregoing (for example, argument from physiology, bench research or first principles)

A comprehensive approach would incorporate many different types of evidence (for example, RCTs, non-RCTs, epidemiologic studies and experimental data), and examine the architecture of the information for consistency, coherence and clarity. Occasionally the evidence does not completely fit into neat compartments. For example, there may not be an RCT that demonstrates a reduction in mortality in individuals with stable angina with the use of β-blockers, but there is overwhelming evidence that mortality is reduced following myocardial infarction (MI). In such cases, some may recommend use of β-blockers in angina patients with the expectation that some extrapolation from post-MI trials is warranted. This could be expressed as Grade A/C. In other instances (for example, smoking cessation or a pacemaker for complete heart block), the non-randomized data are so overwhelmingly clear and biologically plausible that it would be reasonable to consider these interventions as Grade A.

Recommendation grades appear either within the text, for example, Grade A and Grade A1a or within a table in the chapter.

- Deciding whether to apply a specific diagnostic test in arriving at an explanation of a patient's problem, or determining the status of the patient's disease.
- Offering a prognosis to a patient.
- Deciding among a number of interventions available for managing a patient's problem. In this category, the first question is "Does a given intervention do more good than harm?" The second is "Does it do more good than other effective interventions?" The third is "Is it more or less cost effective than other interventions?"

Application of a diagnostic test

Example   A 4-year-old child is experiencing diarrhea and has a positive family history of celiac disease. Should a serological test for antiendomysial antibody (EMA) be done?

Chapter 9 includes an extensive treatment of this topic with a summary of studies (see Table 9.1) that included various groups of patients with a greater or lesser probability of having celiac disease (ranging from patients with gastrointestinal symptoms to patients in whom celiac disease was suspected on clinical grounds). At least one of the studies in Table 9.1, that of Cataldo *et al.*,[23] is relevant to this patient.

When evaluating this test the reader may wish to adopt the approach of Kitching *et al.*[24] for deciding on the clinical usefulness of a diagnostic test (Figure 1.1).

The criteria listed in Figure 1.1 for validity of a diagnostic test were clearly met in Cataldo's study. In Chapter 9 Gregor and Alidina explores the utility of the test and points out that tests with high positive likelihood ratios (LR > 10) and low negative likelihood ratios (LR < 0·1) are generally considered to be clinically useful. The EMA test clearly falls into this category. The authors draws attention to the fact that the probability that a specific patient actually has celiac disease (based on a positive test), or does not have it (based on a negative test), also depends on the *pretest odds* of the patient having the disease (see Table 1.1).

If the child in question, whose pretest likelihood of celiac disease is estimated to be 8%, has a negative test it may be concluded that the child almost certainly does not have celiac disease; on the other hand, if the child has a positive test, the likelihood of him or her having celiac disease is still only 65%.

As Gregor and Alidina point out, the implications of misdiagnosis must be considered carefully. In the circumstance of a positive test in the child with non-specific symptoms the physician and the child's parents should consider whether it is now reasonable to proceed to intestinal

- **Are the study results valid?**
1 Was there an independent blind comparison (or unbiased comparison) with a reference ("gold") standard of diagnosis?
2 Was the diagnostic test evaluated in an appropriate spectrum of patients (like those seen in the reader's practice)?
3 Was the reference standard applied regardless of the diagnostic test result?

- **What are the results?**
Cataldo F, Ventura A, Lazzari R *et al*. Antiendomysium antibodies and celiac disease: solved and unsolved questions. An Italian multicentre study. *Acta Paediatr* 1995;**84**:1125–31.
A study of IgA endomysium antibodies (EMA) in 1485 children with gastrointestinal disease (688 with celiac disease confirmed by intestinal biopsy)

Results for antiendomysial antibody (EMA) test

| | No. of patients with biopsy proven celiac disease | | |
	Present	Absent	Totals
EMA positive	645	20	665
	a	b	a+b
EMA negative	c	d	c+d
	43	777	810
	a+c	b+d	a+b+c+d
Totals	688	797	1485

Sensitivity = a/(a + c) = 645/688 = 0·94
Specificity = d/(b + d) = 777/797 = 0·97
Likelihood ratio (positive result) = sensitivity/(1–specificity) = 0·94/(1–0·97) = 31
Likelihood ratio (negative result) = (1–sensitivity)/specificity = (1–0·94)/0·97 = 0·06
Positive predictive value = a/(a + b) = 645/665 = 0·97
Negative predictive value = d/c + d = 777/810 = 0·96

Figure 1.1 Approaches to evaluating evidence about diagnosis

Table 1.1 The anti-endomysial antibody (EMA) test for celiac disease. Dependence of post-test likelihood of celiac disease on pretest likelihood, assuming positive LR = 31, negative LR = 0.06

Pretest likelihood of celiac disease	Post-test likelihood with a positive EMA test (%)	Post-test likelihood with a negative EMA test (%)
8% (non-specific symptoms, positive family history)	65	0·5
50% (more specific symptoms)	97	6
0·25% (population screen)	8	0·02

Data from Chapter 9

biopsy to confirm the diagnosis, rather than recommending a gluten-free diet, presumably for life. If a search for other clinical or laboratory clues reveals that celiac disease is very likely to be the correct diagnosis, the pretest likelihood may be as high as 50%. This would raise the post-test likelihood to 97%. The physician and parents may be comfortable accepting the diagnosis and proceed to a trial of a gluten-free diet, rather than subjecting a young child to intestinal biopsy. This is an excellent example of how a skilled clinician must integrate the principles of evidence-based medicine with traditional clinical skills and judgment.

Offering a prognosis

Example A 50-year-old woman with recently diagnosed celiac disease has learned at a meeting of the local celiac society that patients with celiac disease have a substantial increase in the risk of developing a number of cancers and

Table 1.2   Cancer mortality in 210 patients with celiac disease at the end of 1985

Site of cancer	ICD8	O	E	O/E	P
All sites	140–208	31	15·48	2·0	**
Mouth and pharynx	141–147	3	0·31	9·7	*
Esophagus	150	3	0·24	12·3	*
Non-Hodgkin's lymphoma	200, 202	9	0·21	42·7	**
Gastrointestinal tract	151–154	3	3·07	1·0	NS
Remainder		13	11·65	1·1	NS

*P<0·01.
**P<0·001.
O, observed numbers; E, expected numbers
Source: Holmes GKT *et al. Gut* 1989;**30**:333–8.[25]

Table 1.3   Cancer morbidity by diet group

Site of cancer	Diet group[a]	No.	O	E	O/E	P
All sites	1	108	14	9·06	1·5	
	2	102	17	6·42	2·6	**
Mouth, pharynx,	1	108	1	0·33	3·0	
esophagus	2	102	5	0·22	22·7	**
Non-Hodgkin's	1	108	2	0·12	16·7	*
lymphoma	2	102	7	0·09	77·8	**
Remainder	1	108	11	8·61	1·3	
	2	102	5	6·11	0·8	

*P<0·01.
**P<0.001.
[a]Diet group 1, strict adherence to gluten-free diet; group 2, reduced gluten diet or normal diet.
Source: Holmes GKT *et al. Gut* 1989;**30**:333–8.[25]

that this cancer risk is reduced by strict adherence to a gluten-free diet.

Chapter 9 describes the types of study which are relevant to determination of prognosis and discusses the strengths and weaknesses of case–control and cohort studies.

Gregor and Alidina point out that certain case–control studies which reported very high mortality and malignancy rates may have been subject to selection bias (inclusion of particularly ill or refractory patients) and measurement bias (patients with abdominal symptoms being more likely to undergo investigations such as small bowel biopsy which may lead to a diagnosis of celiac disease). They refer to a British study in which a cohort of patients with celiac disease was assembled and followed for 10 years. This design attempts to minimize the biases that are inherent in the case–control studies. Table 1.2 shows that the risk of certain cancers is increased compared to the risk in the general population. Table 1.3 shows that strict adherence to a gluten-free diet significantly reduced this risk and may have eliminated the excess risk for several of the identified cancers. .

On the basis of this evidence it is reasonable to advise the patient that her disease does carry with it an increased risk of certain relatively uncommon cancers and that adherence to a strict gluten-free diet appears to minimize this increased risk.

Recommendations concerning therapy

We have provided examples of how evidence concerning the use of diagnostic tests and prognosis can be analyzed and incorporated into clinical practice. Most chapters in this book deal more extensively with evidence concerning therapy and rely heavily on data from randomized trials and meta-analyses.

Example   Should a 28-year-old woman who has had an uncomplicated resection of the terminal ileum for Crohn's disease receive maintenance therapy with a 5-aminosalicylate (ASA) product? Prior to the surgery she had had steroid-dependent disease and had failed treatment with both azathioprine and methotrexate.

- **Are the results valid?**
1 Was the assignment of patients to treatment really randomized (and the randomization code concealed)?
2 Were all patients who entered the study accounted for at its conclusion?
3 Were the clinical outcomes measured blindly?

- **Is the therapeutic effect important?**
1 Were both statistical and clinical significance considered?
2 Were all clinically important outcomes reported?

- **What are the results?**
  McLeod RS, Wolff BG, Steinhart AH *et al.* Prophylactic mesalamine treatment decreases postoperative recurrence of Crohn's disease. *Gastroenterology* 1995;**109**:404–13.

  Randomized controlled trial in which 163 patients with Crohn's disease who had all visible disease resected were randomized to receive mesalamine (Pentasa) 3 g daily or a placebo for a median period of 34 months. Primary outcome was recurrent Crohn's disease defined by recurrence of symptoms and radiographic or endoscopic documentation of recurrence.

	Recurrent Crohn's disease		Risk (%)	ARR (%)	RRR (%)
	Yes	No			
5-ASA	27	60	31	10	24
Placebo	31	45	41	–	–

  ARR, absolute risk reduction; RRR, relative risk reduction.

- **Are the results relevant to my patient?**
1 Were the study patients recognizably similar to my own?
2 Is the therapeutic maneuver feasible in my practice?

Figure 1.2 Elements of a valid and useful randomized trial

A search of the literature for placebo-controlled randomized trials of 5-ASA for maintenance of remission in patients with a surgically induced remission of disease would reveal several trials. The largest published trial is that of McLeod and colleagues,[26] who randomized 163 adult patients to receive either 3 g/day of 5-ASA or a placebo following surgery. The primary outcome of interest was the recurrence of active Crohn's disease as defined by the recurrence of symptoms and the documentation of active disease either radiologically or endoscopically. At the end of the follow up period (maximum duration 72 months, median duration 34 months), 31% of patients who received active treatment remained in remission compared with 41% of those who received a placebo ($P = 0.031$). 5-ASA was well tolerated. A low proportion of patients developed adverse reactions in the control and active treatment groups. One patient treated with 5-ASA developed pancreatitis that was attributed to the study drug. The results of this study can be evaluated using the guidelines described in Figure 1.2, which is modeled after the approach of Kitching *et al.*[24]

Are the results of this study valid?

A review of the methods section of the article[26] confirms that an appropriate method of randomization was employed (computer-generated in permutated blocks), which insured concealment of the randomization code. Furthermore, inspection of the baseline characteristics of the treatment and control groups shows that they are well balanced with respect to such confounding variables as the time from surgery to randomization. This information further supports the legitimacy of the randomization process. Assessment of the method of randomization is important, because non-randomized designs are especially vulnerable to the effects of bias. Studies which employ "quasi-randomization" schemes such as allocation to treatment according to the day of the week or alphabetically by the patient's surname have been shown to consistently overestimate the treatment effect identified by RCTs that employ a valid randomization scheme.[27,28] However, it may be noted that 87 patients were randomized to 5-ASA, compared with only 76 patients in the control group. This observation raises the concern that the analysis might not have been done according to the "intent to treat" principle which specifies that patients are analyzed in the group to which they were originally assigned, irrespective of the treatment that was ultimately received. The use of this strategy reduces the possibility of bias, which might occur if investigators selectively withdrew from the analysis patients who had done poorly or experienced toxicity. For this reason, the intent to treat principle yields a conservative estimate of the true benefit of the treatment. However, detailed review shows that in this study the discrepancy in patient numbers occurred because five patients who were randomized to the active treatment group withdrew consent prior to receiving the study medication and were not included. Thus it appears that the analysis was based on the intent to treat principle.

Approximately 10% of patients in both treatment groups had incomplete follow up. Methodologically rigorous studies have a very low proportion of patients for whom data are missing. This issue is important, since patients who are lost to follow up usually have a different prognosis than those for whom complete information is available. If there is incomplete follow up data for a substantial proportion of patients the results are uninterpretable.[29]

Turning to an assessment of the outcomes in this study, both the patients and investigators were unaware of the treatment allocation. Blinding is used to reduce bias in the interpretation of outcomes. This is especially important when a subjective outcome is evaluated.[30] In this study objective demonstration of recurrent disease (endoscopy and/or radiology) was required in addition to the more subjective measure of the introduction of treatment for recurrent symptoms. Thus the reader can be satisfied that the primary outcome measure was both clinically meaningful and objectively assessed.

Finally, the data analysis and results should be examined. A great deal of useful information can be obtained by reviewing the assumptions that were used in the sample size calculation. In this study, which analyzes a difference in proportions, the investigators had to define four variables: the alpha (type 1) error rate, the beta (type 2) error rate, the expected proportion of patients who would be expected to relapse in the placebo group, and the minimum difference in the rate of relapse which the investigator wished to detect. In this publication these parameters are easily identified. The rate of symptomatic recurrence was estimated to be 12·5% per year and it was anticipated that treatment with 5-ASA would reduce this rate by 50% to an absolute value of 6·25% per year. In contrast to the expected 50% relative risk reduction which was anticipated, the 3-year *actuarial* risk of recurrence was 26% in the treatment group compared to 45% in the group that received 5-ASA ($P = 0.039$). Therefore, the relative risk reduction ([45%–26%]/45% = 42%) is slightly lower than the figure which the investigators considered to be clinically meaningful. Furthermore, the probability of a type 1

error is described as a one-tailed value of $P = 0.05$. This implies that one-tailed statistical testing was used to derive the P value of 0·039. The use of one-sided statistical testing raises legitimate concerns regarding the statistical inferences made in the study.[31] It is inappropriate to hypothesize that 5-ASA therapy could *only* be beneficial, given that the drug can cause diarrhea and colitis.[32] For these reasons, uncertainty exists regarding both the clinical and statistical interpretation of these data.

Are the results of this valid study important?

To assess the importance of this result it is necessary to quantify the magnitude of the treatment effect. How the evidence is presented may influence both physicians and patients in making choices. The most basic means of expressing the magnitude of a treatment of fact is the absolute risk reduction (ARR), which is defined as the proportion of patients in the experimental group with a treatment success minus the proportion of patients with this outcome in the control group. In this instance the annual rate of relapse in the placebo-treated patients was 15% (success rate of 85%) compared with 8·7% (success rate of 91·3%) in those who received the active treatment. This yields an ARR of 6·3%. The number needed to treat (NNT), the number of patients with Crohn's disease who would have to be treated with 3 g/day of 5-ASA to maintain remission over a year, can be calculated as the reciprocal of this number, and is 16. Alternative ways of describing effectiveness include calculating the observed relative risk reduction (RRR = 6·3/15) of 42%, or even stating that about 90% of patients respond to maintenance therapy, ignoring the substantial placebo effect which is evident. The evidence presented as the ARR or NNT, rather than the numbers which show the treatment in a more favorable light, may still lead the physician to recommend this form of treatment and cause the patient to choose to accept this strategy over no intervention. However, the expectations of the physician and patients are likely to be more realistic[33] than they may be if the physician accepts and promotes in an uncritical way the information that 90% of patients who receive 5-ASA maintenance therapy will remain in remission over 1 year.

Are these results applicable to my patient?

Following an assessment of the validity of the evidence using the criteria described in the preceding paragraphs it is necessary to decide whether the conclusions of the study are relevant and important to the individual patient. An initial step is to evaluate the demographic characteristics of the patients in the RCT and compare them to those of the patient in question. If the patient for whom maintenance therapy is being considered is similar to the patients who were evaluated in the trial, it is reasonable to assume that she will experience the same benefit of therapy and is at no greater risk for the development of adverse drug reactions. Alternatively, this patient may have characteristics that make it unlikely that a benefit from 5-ASA will be realized. For example, if the patient had residual active Crohn's disease it would be difficult to generalize the results of the study of McLeod *et al.*,[26] since the patients in this trial had resection of all visible disease prior to study entry.

At this point, if we accept that the results are generalizable to our patient example, the relative risks and benefits of the therapy must be weighed and the patient's preferences should be considered. Evaluation of the data reveals that the trial was methodologically rigorous and evaluated an important outcome. However, it is doubtful whether conventional statistical significance was demonstrated. This raises the question of whether the observed differences between the treatment groups might have occurred by chance. Furthermore, the magnitude of the treatment effect is relatively small. In presenting to the patient the benefit of an annual reduction in the risk of recurrence of 6·3% it is also necessary to consider the cost and inconvenience of taking medication for an asymptomatic condition. One observation in favor of recommending the treatment is that the risk of serious toxicity with 5-ASA appears to be low.

Because there is a degree of uncertainty concerning the true benefit of 5-ASA maintenance therapy based on analysis of this single RCT, it would be prudent to review additional published data. A meta-analysis of 5-ASA therapy has been published.[34] Meta-analysis, the process of combining the results of multiple RCTs using quantitative methods, is an important tool for the practitioner of EBM. Pooling the results of multiple RCTs increases statistical power and thus may resolve the contradictory results of individual studies. Combining data from RCTs statistically also increases the precision of the estimate of a treatment effect. Moreover, the greater statistical power afforded by meta-analysis may allow insight into the benefits of treatment for specific subgroups of patients. These properties are particularly relevant to the case under consideration, given the previously identified concerns.

The meta-analysis summarized data from 15 RCTs which evaluated the efficacy of 5-ASA maintenance therapy in 1371 patients with quiescent Crohn's disease. Patients were randomly assigned to receive either 5-ASA or placebo for treatment periods of 4–48 months. Although 5-ASA was superior to placebo in 13 of the 15 studies, the results of only two trials were statistically significant. Separate analyses were done using data from the four trials that included patients with a surgically induced remission (Figure 1.3) in distinction to those that evaluated patients after a medically induced remission. Sensitivity analyses assessed the response to

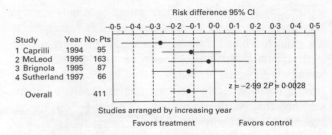

Figure 1.3 Meta-analysis of the four RCTs of mesalamine for prevention of clinical relapse in quiescent Crohn's disease after surgically induced remission. Cumulative risk difference and the respective 95% CIs are shown. (Reproduced with permission from Camma C *et al. Gastroenterology* 1997;**113**:1469[34])

therapy in specific subgroups of patients. The overall analysis concluded that 5-ASA has a statistically significant benefit; the risk of symptomatic relapse in patients who received 5-ASA was reduced by 6·3% (95% confidence interval −10·4% to −2·1%, $2P = 0·0028$), which corresponds to an NNT of 16. Importantly, the greatest benefit was observed in the four trials that evaluated patients following a surgical resection. In these studies there was a 13·1% reduction in the risk of a relapse (95% CI −21·8% to −4·5%, $2P = 0·0028$), which corresponds to an NNT of 8. No statistically significant effect was demonstrable in the analysis, which was restricted to the patients with medically induced remission.

Are the results of this meta-analysis valid and reliable?

Figure 1.4 provides some useful guidelines for the interpretation of overview analyses. It is important that a comprehensive search strategy be adopted since publication bias, the selective publication of studies with positive results, is an important threat to the validity of meta-analysis.[35] This criterion was met. Camma and colleagues' review of the literature was extensive and not limited to English language publications. The investigators also searched review articles, primary studies and abstracts by hand. Quality scores were used to evaluate the validity of the individual studies and a sensitivity analysis was done which assessed the effect of trial quality on the result. No important change in the overall result was noted when studies of lower quality were excluded from consideration. However this type of analysis was not carried out in the analysis of the subgroups of four trials (411 patients) which evaluated 5-ASA after a surgically induced remission.

One of the included studies, that of Caprilli *et al.*,[36] which involved 95 patients, showed a greater benefit for 5-ASA than

---

- Are the results of this overview valid and reliable?
1 Is it an overview of randomized trials of treatments?
2 Does it include a methods section that describes:
    (a) finding and including all the relevant trials?
    (b) assessing their individual validity?
    (c) using valid statistical methods that compare "like with like" stratified by study?

3 Were the results consistent from study to study?
4 Are the conclusions based on sufficiently large amounts of data to exclude a spurious difference (type 1 error) or missing a real difference (type II error).

- Are these applicable to your patient?
Differences between subgroups should only be believed if you can say "yes" to all of the following:
1 Was it hypothesized before the study began (rather than the product of dredging the data), and has it been confirmed in other, independent studies?
2 Was it one of just a few subgroups analyses carried out in this study?
3 Is the difference both clinically (beneficial for some but useless or harmful for others) and statistically significant?
4 Does it really make biologic and clinical sense?

Figure 1.4 Approaches to evaluating evidence concerning overviews. (Reproduced from Yusuf S *et al.*, eds. *Evidence-based Cardiology*. London: BMJ Books, 1998[22])

any other trial, medical or surgical, which has been performed. An important methodological deficiency of this RCT was the failure to conceal the treatment allocation from the investigators. Since these physicians were aware of the treatment assignment, and the definition of relapse used required clinical interpretation, it is possible that the 27% reduction in the risk of relapse identified is an overestimation of the true treatment effect. Accordingly, the inclusion of the results of this study in the subgroup analysis of the surgical studies may overestimate the true benefit of 5-ASA. Furthermore, Camma *et al.* did not include an additional trial by Lochs[37] which was only available as a preliminary report at the time the meta-analysis was done. This study, which is the largest RCT to evaluate 5-ASA following surgery, assigned 318 patients to receive either 4 g of active drug or a placebo for 18 months. Although Camma and colleagues described this study as "confirming" a benefit of 5-ASA after surgery, the results are not impressive. Only a 6·9% reduction in the rate of relapse was observed in patients who received the active treatment (24·5% 5-ASA compared with 31·4% placebo). This difference was *not* statistically significant.

This example underscores the importance of updating systematic reviews as new information becomes available, which is the approach of the Cochrane Collaboration, but not of reviews in conventional publications. When the data provided by Lochs *et al.* were aggregated with those of the other trials, the overall estimate of benefit for 5-ASA was less (ARR 4%, NNT 25).[38] On the basis of these data it can be concluded that 5-ASA may be an effective maintenance therapy following surgery, but if it is the magnitude of the treatment effect is modest at best.

Are these results applicable to our patient example?

The meta-analysis of surgical trials by Camma *et al.* provides important information to the clinician who must decide whether or not to offer patients 5-ASA for maintenance therapy. The concern regarding statistical significance raised by the critique of the McLeod study has been reduced. It seems likely that the beneficial effect of 5-ASA following surgery is real. However, although the majority of the criteria outlined in Figure 1.4 have been met, the issue of clinical relevance remains. The most optimistic estimate of the size of the treatment effect, derived from the meta-analysis, is an NNT of 8. However, given the possibility of bias in the study of Caprilli *et al.*, a more conservative estimate could be based on the data of Lochs and colleagues from the single large randomized trial which yielded an NNT of 15 or from the revision by Sutherland of Camma's meta-analysis that yielded an ARR of only 4%, and an NNT of 25.

In presenting this information to the patient the following points should be emphasized.

- The existing data suggest that 5-ASA is not effective, or at the most, very marginally effective.
- The annual risk of relapse following surgery is relatively low without treatment.
- 5-ASA therapy is safe.
- The cost of 5-ASA therapy is approximately US$70 per month.
- To derive a benefit from the treatment the medication must be taken on a regular basis. This requires the patient to take six pills each day.

Patients undoubtedly will react in different ways to this information. Our patient chose not to accept this therapy.

Rationale for a book on evidence-based gastroenterology and hepatology

Gastroenterologists, hepatologists and general surgeons are fortunate to have many excellent textbooks that provide a wealth of information regarding digestive diseases. Such traditional textbooks concentrate on the pathophysiology of disease and are comprehensive in their scope. *Evidence-based Gastroenterology and Hepatology* is not intended to replace these texts, since its focus is on clinical evidence.

Excellent electronic databases are available, and many traditional publications contain relevant research evidence and important summaries and reviews to support evidence-based practice. However, Cumbers and Donald[39] have found that physicians in clinical practice find the acquisition of data from these sources time consuming. Their study revealed that even locating relevant articles required on average 3 days for practitioners with an onsite library and a week for those without such a facility. This book has been written for the purpose of saving valuable time for busy practitioners of gastroenterology and hepatology, and for general internists and general surgeons who deal with substantial numbers of patients with disorders ranging from gastroesophageal reflux disease to liver transplantation. It has been extensively revised since the first edition was published in 1999 in order to provide more recent evidence that serve as the basis for recommendations. For example strong evidence that infliximab is beneficial in Crohn's disease is presented in this edition along with a careful consideration of its adverse effect profile.

The book cannot claim to be comprehensive; for example, the reader will not find chapters on the management of traveler's diarrhea, infectious enterocolidities or acute diverticulitis. However, since the first edition of this book was published, chapters have been added on antibiotic-associated diarrhea, microscopic and collagenous colitis, esophageal motility disorder, management of Barrett's metaplasia of the esophagus, Ogilvie's syndrome, management of obesity, management of hepatitis B and C after liver transplantation and non-alcoholic steatohepatitis. These chapters have been added to provide the reader with more complete coverage of topics. Nevertheless, in arriving at the composition of the book for the second edition, we have had to establish a list of priority areas where we felt that there was important evidence to be reviewed and summarized on one hand and available authors with the required expertise on the other. We hope that future editions will expand further the number of topics that are included.

A limitation of any textbook is the timeliness of the information that it is possible to provide in print form. New evidence accumulates rapidly in clinical medicine and it is impossible to include the most up-to-date information in a textbook because of the time required for production. To meet the needs of our readers for the most timely information the editors have endeavored to include, where possible, new evidence that became available during the editorial process. It is also planned to produce electronic updates of chapters at regular intervals. These updates, like those for the companion book *Evidence-based Cardiology*, will appear on the BMJ website (www.bmj.com).

References

1   Ruffin JM, Grizzle JE, Hightower NC, McHardy G, Shull H, Kirsner JB. A co-operative double blind evaluation of gastric "freezing" in the treatment of duodenal ulcer. *N Engl J Med* 1969;**281**:16–19.

2   Dickson ER, Fleming TR, Wiesner RH *et al.* Trial of penicillamine in advanced primary biliary cirrhosis. *N Engl J Med* 1985;**312**:1011–15.

3   A Medical Research Council Investigation. Streptomycin treatment of pulmonary tuberculosis. *BMJ* 1948:770–82.

4   Truelove SC, Witts LJ. Cortisone in ulcerative colitis. Final report on a therapeutic trial. *BMJ* 1955:1041–8.

5   Liberati A, Apolone G, Nicolucci A *et al.* The role of attitudes, beliefs, and personal characteristics of italian physicians in the surgical treatment of early breast cancer. *Am J Public Health* 1990;**81**:38–41.

6   Antman EM, Lau J, Kupelnick B, Mosteller F, Chalmers TC. A comparison of results of meta-analyses of randomized control trials and recommendations of clinical experts. Treatments for myocardial infarction. *JAMA* 1992;**268**:240–8.

7   Mulrow CD. The medical review article: state of the science. *Ann Intern Med* 1987;**106**:485–8.

8   Jefferson T. What are the benefits of editorials and non-systematic reviews? *BMJ* 1999;**318**:135.

9   Cochrane AL. Archie Cochrane in his own words. Selections arranged from his 1972 introduction to "Effectiveness and efficiency: random reflections on the health services" 1972. *Control Clin Trials* 1989;**10**:428–33.

10 The Cochrane Collaboration. *Cochrane Library.* 1999; www.cochrane.org

11 Sackett DL. Clinical epidemiology. *Am J Epidemiol* 1969; **89**:125–8.

12 Sackett DL. Interpretation of diagnostic data: 1. How to do it with pictures. *Can Med Assoc J* 1983;**129**:429–32.

13 Sackett D, Haynes RB, Tugwell P, Guyatt GH. *Clinical epidemiology: a basic science for clinical medicine*, 2nd edn. Boston, MA: Little,Brown and Company, 1991.

14 Reid MC, Lachs MS, Feinstein AR. Use of methodological standards in diagnostic test research. getting better but still not good. *JAMA* 1995;**274**:645–51.

15 Ransohoff DF, Feinstein AR. Problems of spectrum and bias in evaluating the efficacy of diagnostic tests. *N Engl J Med* 1978;**299**:926–30.

16 Chalmers TC. Randomization of the first patient. *Med Clin North Am* 1975;**59**:1035–8.

17 Resnick RH, Iber FL, Ishihara AM, Chalmers TC, Zimmerman H. A controlled study of the therapeutic portacaval shunt. *Gastroenterology* 1974;**67**:843–57.

18 Sacks HS, Berrier J, Reitman D, Ancona-Berk VA, Chalmers TC. Meta-analyses of randomized controlled trials. *N Engl J Med* 1987;**316**:450–5.

19 Kernick D. Lies, damned lies, and evidence-based medicine. Jabs and jibes. *Lancet* 1998;**351**:1824.

20 Scholefield JH, Johnson AG, Shorthouse AJ. Current Surgical Practice in Screening for Colorectal Cancer Based on Family History Criteria. *Br J Surg* 1998;**85**:1543–6.

21 Gabriel SE, Jaakkimainen L, Bombardier C. Risk for serious gastrointestinal complications related to use of nonsteroidal anti-inflammatory drugs. A Meta-Analysis. *Ann Intern Med* 1991;**115**:787–96.

22 Yusuf S, Cairns JA, Camm AJ, Fallen EL, Gersh BJ. *Evidence-based Cardiology*, 2nd edn. London: BMJ Books, 2003.

23 Cataldo F, Ventura A, Lazzari R. Anti-endomysium antibodies and celiac disease: solved and unsolved questions. An Italian mulitcentre study. *Acta Paediatr* 1995;**84**: 1125–31.

24 Kitching A, Sackett D, Yusuf S. *Approaches to Evaluating Evidence. Evidence-based Cardiology*. London: BMJ Books, 1998.

25 Holmes GKT, Prior R, Lane MR *et al.* Malignancy in celiac disease: effect of a gluten-free diet. *Gut* 1989;**30**:333–8.

26 McLeod RS, Wolff BG, Steinhart AH *et al.* Prophylactic mesalamine treatment decreases postoperative recurrence of Crohn's disease. *Gastroenterology* 1995;**109**:404–13.

27 Chalmers TC, Celano P, Sacks HS, Smith H Jr. Bias in treatment assignment in controlled clinical trials. *N Engl J Med* 1983;**309**:1358–61.

28 Schulz KF, Chalmers I, Hayes RJ, Altman DG. Empirical evidence of bias. Dimensions of methodological quality associated with estimates of treatment effects in controlled trials. *JAMA* 1995;**273**:408–12.

29 ICH Steering Committee. ICH Harmonised Tripartite Guideline. *Statistical Principles for Clinical Trials.* Section 5.3–Missing Values and Outliers. Geneva: International Conference on Harmonisation of Technical Requirements for Registration of Pharmaceuticals for Human Use, 1998.

30 Feagan BG, McDonald JWD, Koval JJ. Therapeutics and inflammatory bowel disease: a guide to the interpretation of randomized controlled trials. *Gastroenterology* 1996;**110**: 275–83.

31 Koch GG. One-sided and two-sided tests and p values. *J Biopharm Stat* 1991;**1**:161–70.

32 Kapur KC, Williams GT, Allison MC. Mesalazine induced exacerbation of ulcerative colitis. *Gut* 1995;**37**:838–9.

33 Naylor CD, Chen E, Strauss B. Measured enthusiasm: does the method of reporting trial results alter perceptions of therapeutic effectiveness? *Ann Intern Med* 1992;**117**: 916–21.

34 Camma C, Giunta M, Rosselli M, Cottone M. Mesalamine in the maintenance treatment of Crohn's disease: a meta-analysis adjusted for confounding variables. *Gastroenterology* 1997;**113**:1465–73.

35 Oxman AD, Cook DJ, Guyatt GH. User's guides to the medical literature. VI How to use an overview. Evidence-Based Medicine Working Group. *JAMA* 1994;**272**:1367–71.

36 Caprilli R, Andreoli A, Capurso L *et al.* Oral mesalazine (5-aminosalicylic acid; asacol) for the prevention of post-operative recurrence of Crohn's disease. *Aliment Pharmacol Ther* 1994;**8**:35–43.

37 Lochs H, Mayer M, Fleig WE *et al.* Prophylaxis of postoperative relapse in Crohn's disease with mesalazine (Pentasa) in comparison to placebo. *Gastroenterology* 2000; **119**:264–73.

38 Sutherland LR. Mesalamine for the prevention of postoperative recurrence: is nearly there the same as being there? *Gastroenterology* 2000;**118**:264–73.

39 Cumbers B, Donald A. Evidence-Based Practice. Data Day. *Health Serv J* 1999;**109**:30–1.

2 Gastroesophageal reflux disease

Naoki Chiba

Introduction

Heartburn is a very common symptom in clinical practice. Most patients with gastroesophageal reflux disease (GERD) have heartburn, but patients with heartburn don't necessarily have GERD. Earlier studies focused on diagnosis-based management of patients with predominant heartburn. Endoscoped patients either have erosive esophagitis or non-erosive reflux disease (NERD). Healing the mucosa is an easy objective endpoint compared to assessing symptom responses. It is now apparent that symptom severity does not predict endoscopic mucosal damage, and patients with NERD, as well as patients with erosive esophagitis, experience decrements in quality of life (QOL). In treating both groups of patients, as well as those patients with uninvestigated symptomatic heartburn, proton pump inhibitors (PPIs) offer better healing and symptom relief than any other class of medication. The available PPIs are generally considered to be equally effective, with the exception that there is some evidence that esomeprazole heals esophagitis better than omeprazole or lansoprazole. For patients with documented erosive esophagitis and those with uninvestigated heartburn, maintenance therapy with standard dose PPI is recommended. For patients with documented NERD, half dose PPI therapy is probably adequate, and treatment can be given on-demand. The PPIs are safe and offer excellent long-term control of symptoms. Anti-reflux surgery is an available option, especially since the laparoscopic alternative has now become well established. The choice for surgery should be based on patient preference rather than enforced because of perceived cost effectiveness.

The definition of gastroesophageal reflux disease is controversial

Gastroesophageal reflux occurs physiologically in all persons, when gastric contents reflux into the esophagus. However, due to acid neutralization by saliva and prompt esophageal clearance of refluxate, symptoms occur in a minority of people. The typical symptoms of GERD are heartburn, acid regurgitation and dysphagia. It is difficult to determine at what point reflux results in disease. Many patients may regard some degree of heartburn as normal and

only a small proportion of patients seek medical care, conceptually outlined in Castell's "iceberg".[1] Reflux also may result in extraesophageal manifestations such as asthma, non-cardiac chest pain, and posterior laryngitis and hoarseness. A discussion of these manifestations is beyond the scope of this chapter.

Early literature often incorrectly used the terms hiatus hernia and gastroesophageal reflux synonymously. Hiatus hernia is a structural abnormality and reflux is a functional or mechanical event. Subsequently, reflux disease was considered to be present when abnormally prolonged acid refluxate resulted in esophageal damage, either macroscopic (endoscopic esophagitis and/or Barrett's esophagus) or microscopic (histological esophagitis). However, more recently, it has been recognized that symptomatic gastroesophageal reflux without obvious damage, otherwise known as "endoscopy negative reflux disease" (ENRD) or "non-erosive reflux disease" is an important part of the spectrum of reflux disease.[2] Another term, symptomatic GERD has been used to refer to NERD. This term is imprecise and should be applied only to patients with uninvestigated reflux-like symptoms. Moreover, patients will often present not only with reflux symptoms but also with epigastric pain and/or discomfort, symptoms associated with "dyspepsia" rather than GERD.[3,4]

It is now evident that GERD is really a spectrum of diseases. Attention has been focused on the typical symptoms of heartburn and acid regurgitation which are often not accompanied by any pathological findings. Even without endoscopic esophagitis, these patients have reduced health-related QOL comparable with that experienced by patients with esophagitis.[5–7] Awareness of this fact has led some experts to erroneously equate the symptoms of dominant heartburn with a diagnosis of GERD.[8,9] Patients with these symptoms have only a little better than chance probability of having GERD as defined by 24-hour esophageal pH studies.[10] Almost all (96%) patients with endoscopic esophagitis will complain of heartburn,[11] and even if heartburn is not the predominant symptom, endoscopic esophagitis can be identified in up to 36% of patients.[12] Thus, it is clear that heartburn by itself is an insufficient criterion to diagnose GERD. Fortunately for the patient, the focus has shifted to symptomatic treatment as opposed to trying to make a diagnosis, since the treatment is generally the same.

Despite the lack of identity of GERD and heartburn, some experts continue to mix symptoms and damage in the same definition. The American College of Gastroenterology definition of GERD is, "chronic symptoms *or* mucosal damage produced by the abnormal reflux of gastric contents into the esophagus".[13] Experts from the Genval Workshop further expanded this definition to include the patient-centered perspective that gastroesophageal reflux causes "clinically significant impairment of health-related well-being (quality of life) due to reflux-related symptoms".[9]

What are the symptoms of gastroesophageal reflux disease?

The typical symptoms of GERD include heartburn (a rising retrosternal burning discomfort), acid regurgitation and dysphagia. Many investigators consider that the diagnosis of GERD is based primarily on typical symptoms with the specificity of heartburn and acid regurgitation being 89% and 95%, respectively.[14] Indeed 96% of patients with documented erosive or worse esophagitis have heartburn.[11] An early study reported that when heartburn or regurgitation occurred daily, there was a positive predictive value of 59% and 66%, respectively, for the diagnosis of GERD.[15] When an abnormal pH-metry is the gold standard, symptoms have 72% sensitivity and 63% specificity.[16] Many patients have other symptoms but according to recent concepts, these patients are probably more correctly classified as having dyspepsia rather than GERD.[17]

Epidemiology

With inconsistency of definitions and methods of diagnosis, it is difficult to determine the current prevalence of GERD in the general population. Do we mean the prevalence of the symptoms of heartburn or acid regurgitation or do we mean the prevalence of endoscopic esophagitis? The prevalence varies between surveys of the general population and studies of symptomatic patients that present to the family practitioner. Heartburn is experienced by 4–7% of the population on a daily basis and by 34–44% of the population at least once a month (Table 2.1).[4,18–21] Similarly high rates have been observed in New Zealand.[28] Recent data suggest that Asian patients have a lower prevalence of GERD symptoms than Western populations,[23,29] as well as a very low prevalence of esophagitis.[30]

The overall prevalence of reflux esophagitis in Western countries has been estimated to be about 2%.[31] Twenty-seven percent of adults self-treat with antacids more than twice a month, and 84% of this group have objective evidence of reflux esophagitis if investigated.[32]

The incidence of GERD is estimated to be 4·5 per 100 000 with a dramatic increase in persons over the age of 40 years.[33] A Canadian study found that heartburn occurred at least once a week in 19% of persons > 60 years old, compared with 4·8% of persons < 27 years old.[22] A large American retrospective cohort study in VA patients also identified older age along with being a white male as the group associated with the most severe forms of GERD.[34]

Nebel *et al.* in 1976[24] studied the point prevalence and precipitating factors associated with symptomatic gastroesophageal reflux using a questionnaire in 446 hospitalized and 558 outpatients (see Table 2.1). Age, sex or hospitalization did not significantly affect prevalence. Fried or "spicy" foods and alcohol were the most common precipitating factors. In a Finnish study of 1700 adults, only 16% of symptomatic patients reported taking medications and only 5% had sought medical care.[25]

In clinical practice, the relevant population is the group of patients that present with symptomatic heartburn. In this population, it has been estimated that about 50–70% of patients have normal endoscopies and thus, 30–50% have endoscopic esophagitis.[35] In a recently reported Canadian study of prompt endoscopy in patients with uninvestigated dyspepsia, the overall prevalence of endoscopic esophagitis was 43%, and in those with dominant heartburn, the prevalence of esophagitis was 55%.[12] Thus in this population, NERD was seen in less than half of the patients (45%).

Table 2.1 Population-based questionnaire studies of heartburn prevalence

Authors	Daily (%)	At least once weekly (%)	At least once a month (%)	Total at least once/month (%)
Nebel *et al.* (1976)[24]	7	14	15	36
Thompson and Heaton (1982)[22]	4	10	21	34
Gallup Organization (1988)[26]	–	–	–	44
Isolauri and Laippala (1995)[25]	5	15	21	41
Lock *et al.* (1997)[21]	–	18	–	42
Wong *et al.* (2000)[23]	–	2·5	8·9	–
Diaz-Rubio *et al.* (2004)[27]	–	9·8	–	–

Pathophysiology

GERD is primarily a motility disorder of the esophagus that allows abnormal reflux of injurious gastric refluxate. Reflux occurs as a failure of the anti-reflux barrier provided primarily by the lower esophageal sphincter (LES) and crural diaphragm. The two key abnormalities are thought to be abnormal transient lower esophageal sphincter relaxations (TLESRs),[36,37] precipitated by gastric distension in the post-prandial period[38] and poor basal LES tone.[36] The result is prolonged dwell time of gastric refluxate and increasing damage when the pH of the refluxate is below 3, which is optimal for pepsin activation.[39,40] A hiatus hernia may act as a reservoir for acid refluxate that can reflux freely up the esophagus.[41,42] Patients with hiatus hernia have been found to have greater esophageal acid exposure and more reflux episodes.[43]

Pathophysiology in non-erosive reflux disease

Further support for the concept that patients can have typical symptoms of reflux with a normal endoscopy comes from studies in which 6–15% of patients with symptomatic reflux had normal 24-hour esophageal pH-metry.[44–46] Pathological reflux has been identified in 21–61% of endoscopy negative patients.[47–49] A recent study identified abnormal acid reflux in 84% of patients with either erosive esophagitis or NERD, a much higher proportion that previously reported.[50] The reason for these variable results is unknown. In contrast, 71–91% of patients with endoscopic erosive esophagitis have pathological reflux.[47–49] The proportion of time below pH 4 increases over the spectrum from NERD to worsening grades of esophagitis.[51]

Of 96 patients with normal 24-hour esophageal acid exposure, 12·5% were found to have a statistically significant association between symptoms and reflux episodes.[45] In these patients, the duration of reflux episodes was shorter and the pH of reflux episodes was lower than in patients with typical GERD, suggesting that esophageal hypersensitivity is a cause for their symptoms. This work has led to the concept of an acid-sensitive esophagus.

An esophageal balloon distension study provided further experimental evidence of esophageal hypersensitivity in patients with normal acid exposure times with value for symptom index (SI) > 50%.[44] These patients had significantly lower thresholds for initial perception and discomfort from esophageal balloon distension, compared with both normal controls and patients with confirmed reflux. In contrast, Fass *et al.* studied patients with GERD and controls without GERD and determined that patients showed enhanced perception of acid perfusion but not of esophageal distension.[52] They concluded that chronic acid reflux by itself was not the cause of esophageal hypersensitivity to distension in patients with non-cardiac chest pain.

Carlsson *et al.*[53] demonstrated an impaired esophageal mucosal barrier in symptomatic GERD patients by measuring the transmucosal epithelial potential difference.

An interesting study examined differences in spatio-temporal reflux characteristics between symptomatic and asymptomatic reflux episodes.[54] They used a pH sensor positioned 3, 6, 9, 12, and 15 cm above the LES and found the duration of acid exposure was longer and the proximal extent was higher in symptomatic than in asymptomatic reflux episodes. A similar study also determined that patients with NERD compared with healthy controls, had a higher, intraesophageal proximal reflux of acid.[55] Even NERD patients with normal acid exposure time, seemed to perceive proximal reflux very readily, implying that their proximal esophageal mucosa is more sensitive to short duration refluxes than that of patients with esophagitis.

What role does a hiatus hernia play?

The mere presence of a hiatus hernia bears no relationship to the diagnosis of esophagitis and is frequently seen in those without esophagitis. Up to half the healthy population has a hiatus hernia.[56] Moreover, only half of the patients with symptoms of heartburn and regurgitation have a hiatus hernia.[57] Some studies have suggested that patients with a hiatus hernia have greater esophageal acid exposure and more reflux episodes[43] and more severe reflux esophagitis than patients without.[58,59] A large hiatus hernia may act as a reservoir for acid that regurgitates readily when a swallow is initiated.[41,42]

A study in patients with pathologic reflux (pH < 4 for more than 5% of a 24-hour intraesophageal pH-metry study) identified hiatus hernia in 71% of patients with mild esophagitis, compared with 39% of those without esophagitis.[60] Patients with a hiatus hernia also had higher 24-hour intraesophageal acid exposure compared with those without, particularly during the night. However, there were no differences in symptoms of heartburn or regurgitation, whether or not patients had a hiatus hernia or esophagitis.

Another study identified that the presence of hiatus hernia correlated with more severe manifestations of GERD.[61] Hiatus hernia was seen in 29% of symptomatic patients, 71% with erosive esophagitis, and 96% with long segment Barrett's esophagus.

Although TLESRs are thought to be a key mechanism for pathological reflux, van Herwaarden *et al.*[43] did not find differences in LES pressure, and the incidence of TLESRs, and the proportion of TLESRs associated with acid reflux were comparable in those with and without hiatus hernia. They felt that the excess reflux in GERD patients with hiatus hernia was caused by malfunction of the gastroesophageal barrier during low LES pressure, swallow-associated normal LES relaxations, deep inspiration and straining.

What is the natural history of gastroesophageal reflux disease?

There are few data about this important topic, and existing studies are somewhat difficult to interpret as they usually include heterogeneous populations. In a Swedish population-based survey of over a 1000 citizens conducted over 7 years, the prevalence of GERD remained stable over time at about 17–19%.[62]

A small retrospective study published in 1991 identified patients with symptoms of GERD but with a normal endoscopy and 24-hour pH study.[63] All patients received antacids or prokinetic drugs or both for 3–6 months. Thus this was not a study of untreated patients but a study that employed weak treatments. However, 19 of the 33 patients still had symptoms at the end of 6 months and of these, 5 (26%) developed erosive esophagitis. The remainder of the patients remained asymptomatic. There was no difference in baseline pH-metry between those that went on to develop esophagitis and those that did not.

Another study reported data on patients with objectively proven GERD conservatively managed without treatment over a 17–22-year follow up.[64] The authors reported on 60 patients from an initial cohort of 87 patients. While 10 of the patients had an antireflux procedure, of the remaining 50, 36 (72%) were less symptomatic at follow up. Of the latter group, only six became symptom free. However, the majority[34] no longer used antireflux medications. Only five patients remained unchanged and nine became worse. The prevalence of erosive esophagitis fell from 40% at referral to 27% at follow up endoscopy, and six new cases of Barrett's metaplasia developed. At follow up, 66% of the patients had objective evidence of GERD with either esophagitis, a pathological pH study or newly recognized Barrett's metaplasia. Neither the presence of esophagitis or of hiatal hernia, nor the severity of symptoms at baseline predicted the course of the disease at follow up. The authors concluded that the severity of reflux symptoms declined in the long-term, but pathological reflux persisted in the majority of the conservatively treated patients.

For patients with mild esophagitis, the course of the disease may be benign with only 23% progressing to more severe esophagitis, while 31% improve and 46% spontaneously heal with no further episodes.[65] Patients with endoscopic esophagitis diagnosed more than 10 years earlier were contacted by postal questionnaire and phone interview.[66] Of the respondents, over 70% continued to have significant symptoms of reflux, and 40–50% were still taking acid suppressive medications regularly and had reduced QOL (lower Short Form (SF)-36, physical and social function domain scores). Thus, GERD is a chronic disease with significant morbidity and it impacts negatively on QOL.

Despite frequent symptoms, even severe reflux disease has little effect on life expectancy, with almost no deaths directly due to GERD reported in long-term follow up.[33,64,66] However, a recent population-based study, identified GERD as a strong risk factor for esophageal adenocarcinoma, but not squamous cell carcinoma.[67]

Esophageal complications of gastroesophageal reflux disease

Complications of GERD include bleeding (< 2%), ulceration (around 5%), and strictures (from 1·2% to 20%).[66,68,69] Patients with strictures are older and more frequently have a hiatus hernia.[68] Barrett's esophagus has been identified in 10–20% of GERD patients.[70] Six of 50 patients (12%) developed Barrett's esophagus during approximately 20 years of follow up, a crude incidence of 0·6% per year.[64]

Heading estimated that GERD patients would require 10 operations per 100 000 persons/year and that 5–10% of patients seen by gastroenterologists would require fundoplication.[69] However, this observation was made before the introduction of PPIs that have dramatically changed the approach to medical therapy for GERD.

Effects of gastroesophageal reflux disease on quality of life

Increased attention is being paid to patient QOL assessments as opposed to pathology of the esophagus. Several general health status and disease-specific QOL instruments have been developed, validated and used. These include: Medical Outcomes Study SF-36,[71] Psychological General well-being (PGWB) index,[72] the Gastrointestinal Symptom Rating Scale (GSRS),[73–75] and the Quality of Life in Reflux and Dyspepsia questionnaire (QOLRAD).[76] More recently, there has been an increase in validated GERD-specific instruments focusing more on assessing patient satisfaction and QOL.[76–83]

Patients with gastrointestinal disorders have decreased functional status and well-being.[84] Recently, a study assessing heartburn with multiple assessments using the GSRS, QOLRAD, SF-36 and the Hospital Anxiety and Depression (HAD) scale determined that heartburn substantially impairs all aspects of health-related QOL.[85]

Those patients with chronic gastrointestinal disorders and congestive heart failure have the poorest health perceptions. These perceptions are worse than those that characterize some other chronic conditions such as hypertension and arthritis.[73,84,86] Studies have shown that successful treatment of GERD is associated with improvements in QOL.[87] Patients with reflux esophagitis are generally considered to have equally impaired QOL to those with non-erosive disease,[6] but those with very severe reflux esophagitis may have more impairment.[87] NERD patients do not necessarily have objective markers such as endoscopic esophagitis or abnormal esophageal 24-hour pH-metry results that can be used to define treatment success. Symptom reduction to a level that does not cause significant impairment of health-related QOL is essential. Both the PGWB and GSRS scores show good discriminative ability to reflect the severity of impairments in quality of life in NERD patients.[88] Improvements in health-related QOL with treatment of NERD and of erosive esophagitis have also been documented.[6,89] These improvements are greatest with PPIs compared to ranitidine[6] or cisapride.[90]

Diagnosis of gastroesophageal reflux disease

The diagnosis of GERD depends on the definition of "pathological" in diagnostic tests. Problems of definition have been recognized for more than two decades.[56] Methods of diagnosing GERD are outlined in Table 2.2. These tests evaluate different features of GERD, and none of them measures all aspects of the disease. Tests such as barium studies, scintigraphy and 24-hour esophageal pH studies show whether reflux occurs; endoscopy allows for the diagnosis of mucosal changes and assessments of complications; 24-hour pH studies can quantify the amount of acid exposure; mucosal sensitivity can be assessed by the Bernstein test. The interpretation of tests is also important. For example, a patient with documented endoscopic esophagitis with a negative Bernstein test should not be regarded as having a "false negative" Bernstein test, but rather an acid insensitive esophagus. With variable patient populations, and with differences in definitions, techniques and gold standards, it is impossible to compare sensitivity and specificity values.[91]

Manometry and lower esophageal pressure measurement

LES pressures alone are not of diagnostic value as there is considerable overlap of pressures in those with and without esophagitis. In a review[92] of six studies, LES pressure < 10 mmHg correlated with an abnormal acid exposure with a sensitivity of only 58% and specificity of 84%. However, there may be some utility in low LES pressures as a predictor for identifying patients with the most severe reflux.[56] Manometry prior to surgery has been advocated to document a mechanically defective lower esophageal sphincter,[94] but there is no good evidence that this affects outcome.

Radiological diagnosis

A variety of outcome measures have been used in studies of radiology in GERD. Some have measured gastroesophageal reflux (with and without reflux provoking maneuvers) and correlated this with other measures of reflux such as esophageal pH studies. Others have examined the ability of radiological studies to identify esophagitis.

The radiological diagnosis of reflux esophagitis is generally considered to be unreliable. The diagnostic accuracy of barium radiography compared with endoscopy is 0–53% for mild, 79–93% for moderate and 95–100% for severe esophagitis.[93,95] Many of the early studies[96] compared radiological techniques to endoscopy as a gold standard. By 1980, it was recognized that about half the patients with symptomatic reflux did not have endoscopic esophagitis.[48,56] Thus, many patients would be expected to have normal barium studies. From a technical perspective, the gastroesophageal junction is not well visualized in up to a third of patients due to inadequate distension.[96,97]

Measuring reflux alone does not determine whether patients have GERD nor does it correlate with patients' symptoms. With provocative tests, reflux is seen in not only 25–71% of symptomatic patients but also in 20% of controls.[95] Low density contrast media are no better than regular barium.[98] Radiological studies are frequently falsely negative in patients in whom endoscopy or esophageal pH-metry studies are abnormal.

Measurement of the internal diameter of the cardiac esophagus was shown to predict 89% of patients with mild endoscopic esophagitis.[99] However, this was not confirmed in a study that found that the gastroesophageal junction could not be adequately visualized in 29% of patients.[96]

Free, severe reflux as seen on barium studies may by a highly specific predictor of reflux as confirmed by 24-hour esophageal pH monitoring.[92,96,100,101] However, esophagitis is rarely diagnosed radiographically in patients with abnormal intraesophageal pH studies.[102]

Scintigraphy

Reflux is assessed following ingestion of a liquid containing a radiolabeled pharmaceutical such as sulfur colloid or ^{99m}Tc in an acidified liquid suspension. This procedure is similar to the assessment of reflux during radiology, although scintigraphy may be superior.[57] Graded abdominal compression to detect reflux is unreliable with variable sensitivity of 14–90%.[57,93,95,96,103] The biggest problem appears to be the short duration of the imaging test, as reflux occurs intermittently. With the availability of endoscopy and 24-hour intraesophageal pH monitoring, this test appears to have little value in the diagnosis of GERD.

Upper gastrointestinal endoscopy

Endoscopy provides the most accurate means of assessing mucosal detail of the esophagus, but is insensitive in diagnosing reflux. Definite endoscopic reflux esophagitis is

Table 2.2   Summary of diagnostic tests in gastroesophageal reflux disease

Test	What does it measure?	Comments
Esophageal manometry	Measures lower esophageal sphincter pressure only. Low (< 10 mmHg) LES pressure: 58% sensitivity and 84% specificity for abnormal acid exposure[92] Does not measure risk for reflux Does not assess esophagitis	• Too much overlap with normals to diagnose GERD • Does not detect transient LES relaxation • May be useful in pre/post-operative evaluation
Radiology	Shows morphological findings, for example stricture and may rule out other pathology, (for example ulcers). Best test for dysphagia Detects gastroesophageal reflux. Some use abdominal compression Can detect hiatus hernia Poor detection for mild esophagitis 0–53%[93] Does not assess symptoms	• Best test for this • In patients with GERD detects reflux in 10–50%[93] • Free reflux correlates best • Unclear role in most patients with GERD • Many with hiatus hernia have no symptoms • For moderate esophagitis, sensitivity 79–93%[93] • For severe esophagitis, sensitivity 95–100%[93]
Scintigraphy	Can show reflux	• Sensitivity 14–86%[93] • Limited utility as reflux is intermittent • Requires radioactivity exposure
Endoscopy	Detects esophagitis Detects Barrett's esophagus Allows biopsy, but esophageal histology has limited utility	• Lacks sensitivity
Bernstein (acid perfusion test)	• Measures esophageal acid sensitivity, not a test for esophagitis • Can be positive in patients with normal endoscopy and 24-hour pH studies • Determines esophageal origin of pain • May identify those with "acid sensitive esophagus"	• Sensitivity 42–100%, mean 77%[93] • Specificity 50–100%, mean 86%[93] • May be useful in patients with atypical symptoms and NCCP
24-hour esophageal pH monitoring	• Quantifies gastroesophageal reflux • Allows assessment of whether "pathological reflux" occurs • Does not detect mucosal damage	• Normal in 14–29% of those with esophagitis • Normal in 6–15% of patients with abnormal SI
SI with 24-hour esophageal pH monitoring	Correlates symptoms with reflux events	Bimodal predictive value Can be positive when pH study is normal
PPI test	Positive test detects acid reflux as probable cause of symptoms Tests reflux, acid damage, esophageal sensitivity	May be best overall test Simplicity, reduces cost

GERD, gastroesophageal reflux disease; LES, lower esophageal sphincter; SI, symptom index; NCCP, non-cardiac chest pain; PPI, proton pump inhibitor

unequivocal evidence that the patient suffers from GERD. Patients with an "acid sensitive" esophagus who experience symptoms in the absence of esophagitis cannot be diagnosed by endoscopy. The 24-hour intraesophageal pH study can be abnormal in 50% of patients with reflux symptoms and normal endoscopy.[48,104] Thus a negative endoscopy does not exclude GERD. Histological diagnosis may be difficult due to inadequate size of the biopsy,[105] patchy distribution of the histological findings[106] or minimal changes.[107]

Berstad and Hatlebakk[108] prospectively evaluated patients using their own unique endoscopic grading system. Those with true GERD had endoscopic findings according to their classification, but the presence of whitish exudate in the lesions and the width of the lesions were the only two endoscopic features that correlated with the severity of esophageal acid exposure as measured by 24-hour pH-metry.[109] Confirmatory data from other investigators using this classification are lacking.

The most widely applied esophagitis grading system had been the Savary–Miller classification in the original and modified forms. A newer classification[110] which measures metaplasia, ulcer, stricture and erosions (known as the MUSE classification), records the degree of severity of each as absent, mild, moderate and severe. This is now known as the Los Angeles (LA) classification and is the one that is most commonly used.[111] The key features are:

- Grade A: one (or more) mucosal break no longer than 5 mm, that does not extend between the tops of two mucosal folds
- Grade B: one (or more) mucosal break more than 5 mm long that does not extend between the tops of two mucosal folds
- Grade C: one (or more) mucosal break that is continuous between the tops of two or more mucosal folds but which involves less than 75% of the circumference
- Grade D: one (or more) mucosal break which involves at least 75% of the esophageal circumference.[112]

The LA classification was tested in a subsequent study that evaluated the circumferential extent of esophagitis by the criterion of whether mucosal breaks extended between the tops of mucosal folds, gave acceptable agreement (κ 0·4) among observers.[112] Severity of esophageal acid exposure was significantly ($P < 0·001$) related to the LA severity grade of esophagitis. The preteatment esophagitis grades A–C were related to heartburn severity ($P < 0·01$), outcomes of omeprazole treatment ($P < 0·01$), and the risk for symptom relapse off therapy ($P < 0·05$).

Bernstein test as a measure of esophageal acid sensitivity

This test was first described in 1958 to distinguish chest pain of esophageal from cardiac origin.[113] In an early 1978 prospective, comparative study of upper gastrointestinal endoscopy, upper gastrointestinal barium series, esophageal manometry and the Bernstein test in patients with suspected reflux esophagitis, the Bernstein test had the greatest sensitivity (85%) for diagnosing esophagitis. However, there were many false positives as half the patients without esophagitis also had a positive Bernstein test. The lack of specificity for esophagitis is not very surprising, since most of these patients are now considered to have an acid sensitive esophagus, consistent with NERD. Another study found the sensitivity of the Bernstein test to be 70% in patients with typical reflux symptoms. However, 97% of patients with a negative test had either endoscopic, histologic or scintigraphic evidence of GERD.[114] In a review of seven studies,[115] the overall sensitivity of this test was 77% and specificity 86%. Although the Bernstein test does not establish that there is mucosal damage (esophagitis), and patient acceptance is limited, a positive test result implies that the esophagus is likely to be the origin of the symptoms.

24-hour ambulatory esophageal pH monitoring

Many experts consider that an abnormal 24-hour intraesophageal pH study is the gold standard for diagnosing GERD.[48] In this context, GERD is considered erosive or worse esophagitis, i.e. evidence of mucosal damage. This test is useful in quantifying the amount and frequency of acid reflux that occurs. However, it is difficult to separate physiological from pathological reflux, and the threshold levels which separate "normal" from "abnormal" test results are not clear. Threshold levels suggested on the basis of separation from the mean by two standard deviations[48] or on the basis of receiver-operating-characteristic (ROC) analysis are listed in Table 2.3. ROC analysis correlates true and false positive rates for a series of cut-offs and is proposed as an alternative method of analysis to using means and standard deviations to define threshold abnormalities, since GERD parameters are not normally distributed.

The test may be useful for investigating patients with atypical reflux symptoms or non-cardiac chest pain in whom GERD is suspected to be the cause of symptoms. The predictive value of specific threshold levels is age dependent.[120] The technique has many other limitations including lack of availability, invasiveness, cost, lack of patient acceptability, debatable reproducibility, and technical problems such as improper placement of the pH probe, probe failures and recording device failures.[120]

A cutoff pH of 4 to define pathological reflux has been validated.[91,116] Furthermore, this pH threshold makes physiological sense as proteolytic activity of pepsin is low at a pH above 4, and high below pH 3.[40] Unfortunately, even this cut-off may miss up to 50% of reflux episodes.[121]

DeMeester studied a large series of patients using the normal values in Table 2.3. Both the sensitivity and specificity of 24-hour esophageal pH monitoring for acid reflux was 90%.[48] Other studies[91,122] using the same variables, reported sensitivity of 85–96% and specificity of 100%. However, another study using the same scoring system was able to distinguish only 41% of symptomatic patients from controls.[47] In these hospitalized patients, only 21% of those with a normal endoscopy had an abnormal intraesophageal pH, while in those with esophagitis, 71% had an abnormal study. A very important observation was that 93% of the endoscopy normal patients responded to anti-reflux therapy, and another explanation for the symptoms was found in only one patient.

Table 2.3   Summary of 24-hour esophageal pH study criteria

Author	Parameter to define thresholds	Normal value	Comments
DeMeester *et al.* (1980)[48]	No. of reflux episodes pH < 4	< 50	They had relatively few controls to establish normal values.
	Total time pH < 4	< 4·2%	
	Upright time pH < 4	< 6·3%	Abnormal score is placed 2 SD above the mean. This may not be valid as values do not follow a normal distribution
	Supine time pH < 4	< 1·2%	
	No reflux episodes ≥ 5 min duration	≤ 3	
	Duration of longest reflux episode	9·2 min	90% sensitivity and specificity
	Using these criteria they developed a composite scoring system		Others have not reported the same results with the same criteria[45]
Schindlbeck *et al.* (1987)[117]	Upright time pH < 4	< 10·5%	They assessed all the same factors as DeMeester above
	Supine time pH < 4	< 6·0%	They carried out ROC analysis
	One or both above threshold = abnormal		
Klauser *et al.* (1989)[16]	Upright time pH < 4	< 8·2%	Same group as Schindlbeck but larger reference sample gave lower threshold values
	Supine time pH < 4	< 3·0%	
	One or both above threshold = abnormal		
Johnsson *et al.* (1987)[116]	Total time pH < 4	< 3·4%	Complete separation between patients and controls with single determinant
			Sensitivity 87% specificity 97%
Masclee *et al.* (1990)[49]	Total time pH < 4	< 4·0%	Either equally predictive
	Number of reflux episodes	> 30 in 24 hours	
Jamieson, *et al.* (1992)[118]	Composite score as in DeMeester above		Used a combination of the composite score and ROC analysis.
	Total time pH < 4	< 4·5%	
Mattox and Richter (1990)[119]	Upright time pH < 4	< 6·7%	These are 95th percentile figures for asymptomatic controls
	Supine time pH < 4	< 2·4%	
	Total time pH < 4	< 4·7%	
	Any of above threshold = abnormal		

ROC, receiver operating characteristic

Thus, typical symptoms were important for predicting treatment response in spite of the endoscopic and esophageal pH findings.

A study of 45 outpatients with typical reflux symptoms and 42 asymptomatic controls[117] used ROC analysis to obtain maximum values for sensitivity of 93·3% and specificity of 92·9% using the following criteria:

- only percent of time with esophageal pH < 4
- both the upright and supine reflux values are below threshold to define a normal test
- threshold levels of pH < 4 for 10·5% of the time in upright position and 6% in the supine position.

A limitation of this retrospective study is that it was restricted to patients with typical symptoms.

When DeMeester's group refined their own analysis by using not only their composite score but also the ROC analysis they reported values for sensitivity of 96% and specificity of 100%.[91]

Values for sensitivity of 79–95% and for specificity of 85–100% for extended esophageal pH monitoring were described in a comprehensive review[120] and supported by several individual studies.[48,49,116,122–124] While esophageal 24-hour pH-metry is often considered to be the gold standard for diagnosing GERD, the false negative rate can be as high as 14–35% in patients with endoscopic esophagitis.[47,48,125–128] These data raise doubt whether the pH-metry should be considered to be the gold standard test.[129] There are virtually no recent reports that determine new thresholds to define abnormal reflux.

However, a new disposable miniature sensor probe has been developed whose *in vitro* response to acid exposure below pH 4 is linearly determined by the duration of the acid exposure and the degree of acidity.[130] A significant correlation was found between the exposure of the distal esophagus to acid and the acid exposure probe ($r = 0.85$; $P < 0.0001$). The sensitivity and specificity of the sensor to predict esophageal acid exposure > 5% of time was 91% and 93%, respectively. This new probe is less expensive, disposable, easier to apply than the 24-hour pH probe and does not require recording equipment to be carried. Thus, there is the potential for this new method to greatly simplify esophageal pH measurements.

Symptoms as diagnostic predictors

An important study of patients with reflux-like symptoms was reported by Joelsson and Johnsson.[131] Erosive esophagitis (Savary–Miller grade 1 or worse) was identified in a third of patients with symptoms. Whether the patient had erosive disease or not, the frequency of heartburn and acid regurgitation correlated with median esophageal acid exposure time measured by 24-hour pH monitoring. Although patients with an endoscopically normal esophagus had lower overall median acid exposure, there was a trend towards more acid exposure in those with more severe symptoms. Figure 2.1 shows the relationship between severity of symptoms and acid exposure time. The authors concluded that reflux-like dyspepsia is accompanied by increased esophageal acid exposure, a concept that is supported by others.[49,126] Unfortunately severity of symptoms is a poor predictor of mucosal damage.[48,132,133]

Johannessen *et al.*[134] determined that heartburn showed the best discrimination for patients with esophagitis. Typical symptoms of GERD correlate with abnormal intraesophageal pH exposure in 56–73% of patients.[16,48]

In an effort to improve the diagnostic value of the history, investigators have applied structured questionnaires.[135–140] Using the questionnaire developed by Johnsson,[135] a positive response to all four questions is required to achieve a high positive predictive value, thus limiting its usefulness. The description of symptoms as opposed to using the term heartburn, may be a factor which improves the predictive value of this questionnaire.

DeMeester reported a retrospective review of 100 consecutive patients with symptoms of GERD.[48] The combination of the presence of grade 2 or 3 symptoms on the standardized questionnaire and endoscopic esophagitis, predicted increased acid exposure on 24-hour intraesophageal pH monitoring with a specificity of 97% and a positive predictive value of 98%.

The Carlsson–Dent questionnaire that is intended to identify responders to PPI therapy has been extensively validated for reflux esophagitis detected at endoscopy and abnormal 24-hour intraesophageal pH-metry.[136] The

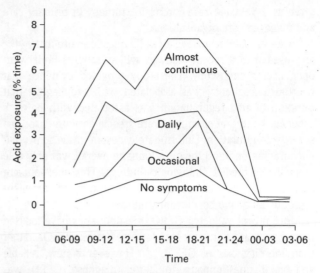

Figure 2.1 Acid exposure of the distal part of the esophagus during eight 3-hour periods expressed as median % time spent with pH < 4 in 190 patients with different degrees of heartburn and acid regurgitation and 50 asymptomatic endoscopically normal subjects. Reproduced with permission from Joelsson B *et al. Gut* 1989;**30**:1523–5.[131]

questionnaire has a maximum score of 18. In the endoscopic comparison, using a threshold of 4, the questionnaire had 70% sensitivity but only 46% specificity for diagnosis of esophagitis. When used in dyspeptic patients, the questionnaire had a sensitivity of 92% but a specificity of only 19% for diagnosis of GERD when compared with abnormal 24-hour intraesophageal pH monitoring. The mean score of 11 for GERD patients was higher than that observed in the dyspepsia cohort (mean 4.6). Symptom relief during treatment with omeprazole was predicted by the presence of heartburn, described as "a burning feeling rising from the stomach or lower chest up towards the neck" (odds ratio 4) and by "relief from antacids" (odds ratio 2.2). Even in a non-ulcer dyspepsia study from which patients with predominant heartburn were excluded, 42% of the patients indicated that they had a "rising burning feeling", a description that defines heartburn in the Carlsson–Dent questionnaire. Even in this group of presumed non-GERD patients, those patients who answered positively to this key question had the best symptom relief with omeprazole. One prospective validation of this questionnaire in a primary care population did not find that the questionnaire was better able to discriminate omeprazole responders than the physician's provisional diagnosis.[141] The utility of this questionnaire as a clinical practice tool appears to be limited, although it remains important for research purposes.

Similar in its goal to the Carlsson–Dent questionnaire, the 12-item "GERD Screener" demonstrated construct, convergent and predictive validity. This instrument was practical, short, and easily administered and was intended to serve as a valuable case-finding instrument in primary care and managed care organizations.[140]

Locke *et al.*[142] developed a GERD questionnaire in 1994[138] and used it in a recent study in which patients underwent open access endoscopy. The study provided evidence that heartburn frequency was associated with esophagitis, that duration of acid regurgitation was associated with Barrett's esophagus and that strictures were associated with dysphagia severity and duration. Unfortunately, despite these somewhat encouraging findings, the questionnaire overall was only able to modestly predict endoscopic findings. This questionnaire was adapted to the Spanish population with excellent reproducibility and concurrent validity.[143]

More recent validated GERD questionnaires have focused more on creating instruments for assessment of QOL rather than for diagnosis of GERD.[76-82] However a new, reliable and valid questionnaire to better diagnose GERD was developed[139] and the internal consistency, interobserver reliability, criteria validity using 24-h esophageal pH monitoring, construct validity, and extreme group validation were assessed using patients with pathologic GERD. This questionnaire had sensitivity, specificity and positive predictive values of over 90% while the negative predictive value was 79%.[139] A new Chinese GERD questionnaire was found to discriminate between controls and GERD patients with a sensitivity of 82% and a specificity of 84%.[144]

Symptom index

A quantitative method for correlating symptoms and esophageal acid reflux events was developed in 1986 and called the "symptom index". This index is calculated as the number of times the symptom occurred when the pH is < 4, divided by the total number of symptoms, multiplied by 100. Initial validation studies in 100 patients found the SI to be distributed in a bimodal fashion. Of patients with SI above 75%, 97·5% had an abnormal esophageal pH study.[145] If the SI was less than 25%, the proportion of patients with a normal esophageal pH study was 81%, and 90% of this group had a normal endoscopy.[146] Endoscopy was normal in nearly 30% of patients with a high SI. Thus, if endoscopy is found to be normal in the course of evaluating patients suspected of having GERD, an esophageal pH study measuring SI may be useful. There was very poor correlation between results of the Bernstein test and the SI. The negative predictive value of a low SI is useful. A limitation of the SI is that it does not take into account the reflux episodes that were symptom free. More recently, the SI was not found to be useful for diagnosing non-cardiac chest pain.[147]

The symptom association probability (SAP) is another method that has been developed with the intent to reduce the shortcomings of the SI.[148] This method correlates pH data

during both symptomatic and asymptomatic reflux episodes and requires further validation.

Therapeutic trial of acid suppression as a diagnostic test

All of the diagnostic tests described above are cumbersome or invasive and detect different features of reflux. PPIs such as omeprazole are the most effective intervention for all grades of esophagitis and for treatment of symptoms such as heartburn. A therapeutic trial with a PPI may be useful in diagnosing GERD in a variety of patient populations including patients with typical symptoms of GERD, patients with non-cardiac chest pain, and in those with positive and negative findings on endoscopy or pH monitoring. The variation of patients studied makes direct comparisons between studies impossible.

In a double blind, placebo-controlled study of patients with reflux symptoms (92% had heartburn) and only minor or no esophagitis at endoscopy, patients were randomized to receive omeprazole 40 mg once daily or a placebo for 14 days.[127] A 75% reduction in heartburn was considered to be a positive omeprazole test. There was a significant ($P = 0·04$) correlation between response to omeprazole and the results of the pH-metry. A response to omeprazole occurred in 68% of patients with abnormal reflux and in only 37% of patients with a normal pH study. Only 13% of patients responded to placebo.

A randomized trial of omeprazole 20 mg twice daily or placebo for 1 week tested the efficacy of omeprazole to determine reflux disease among dyspeptic patients.[149] A diagnosis of GERD was made on the basis of either grade II–III esophagitis or esophageal reflux with pH < 4 for more than 4% of the esophageal pH monitoring time. Using this definition, 135 of 160 (84%) patients were found to have GERD. Of those patients with presumed NERD, 63% had an abnormal pH study. Twenty percent (18/92) of patients with esophagitis had normal pH studies. Using symptom improvement of at least one grade for the definition of a positive test, the "omeprazole test" had a sensitivity of 71–81% for diagnosing GERD, compared with the sensitivity of placebo of 36–47%. With a more stringent definition for a positive test of total symptom relief, the sensitivity of omeprazole to diagnose reflux was lower at 48–59%, compared with 6–19% for placebo. Thus the difference became greater between omeprazole and placebo. However, the specificity of the test was low, and actually was higher with placebo than with omeprazole. Thus the test may be more useful for ruling out the diagnosis than ruling it in. Even patients who did not have GERD by definition had better symptom relief with omeprazole than with placebo. These may be patients with an acid sensitive esophagus who respond well to acid suppression despite their esophageal pH being within normal limits.

A recent UK study of 90 patients with dyspeptic symptoms suggestive of GERD evaluated the cost effectiveness of an open course of treatment with omeprazole 40 g daily for 14 days as a diagnostic test.[150] There was no significant correlation between endoscopic and pH monitoring findings. The cost per correct diagnosis was £47 for omeprazole (95% CI £40 to 59) compared with £480 for endoscopy (95% CI £396 to 608). The authors concluded that an empirical trial of omeprazole was cost effective both for symptom relief and for diagnosing GERD in patients with typical symptoms.

In a small, 4-week, randomized placebo-controlled crossover study[125] in patients with normal endoscopy and esophageal pH-metry, but with an SI of > 50, 10 of 12 (83%) of patients with a positive SI showed improvement on omeprazole 20 mg twice daily for decreased symptom frequency, severity and consumption of antacids ($P < 0.01$). The SF-36, QOL parameters for bodily pain and vitality also significantly improved. In the group with a negative SI only one patient clearly improved.

Thirty-three consecutive patients with symptoms of reflux, abnormal pH studies, but normal endoscopies[151] were sequentially allocated to receive ranitidine 150 mg twice daily, omeprazole 40 mg once daily, or omeprazole 40 mg twice daily for 7–10 days. On the last day of treatment an esophageal pH study was repeated and the results were correlated with symptoms. Both doses of omeprazole were superior to ranitidine and this benefit was correlated with reduction in mean acidity. Using a 75% reduction in symptoms as a positive test, and the pH test as the gold standard, the sensitivity of the omeprazole test using a dose of 40 mg twice daily was 83·3% while the sensitivity with omeprazole 40 mg once daily was only 27·2%. The authors concluded that the diagnosis of GERD could be practically ruled out if a patient failed to respond to a short course of high dose PPI.

Fass *et al.*[152] also used an omeprazole 60 mg daily test versus placebo in GERD positive (35/42, 83%) and GERD negative patients (17%). Twenty-eight GERD positive and three GERD-negative patients responded to the omeprazole test, providing sensitivity of 80·0% and specificity of 57·1%. Economic analysis revealed that the omeprazole test saved US$348 per average patient evaluated, with 64% reduction in the number of upper endoscopies and a 53% reduction in the use of pH testing.

Most studies have used omeprazole in the "PPI test". However, a study using 60 mg of lansoprazole once daily versus placebo for 5 days found that 85% tested positive during active treatment compared with 9% with placebo.[153] The PPI test sensitivity was 85% and specificity was 73%.

Esomeprazole is more potent than omeprazole and it has now been evaluated as a diagnostic tool.[154] Patients ($n = 440$) were randomized to receive esomeprazole 40 mg once daily, esomeprazole 20 mg twice daily or a placebo for 14 days.

Endoscopy and 24-hour esophageal pH-monitoring were carried out to determine the presence of gastroesophageal reflux disease (GERD). The esomeprazole treatment test had sensitivity in confirming the diagnosis of GERD of between 79% and 86% (for the two doses of PPI) after 5 days, while the corresponding value for placebo was 36%.

In a small, 8-week, placebo-controlled study of 36 patients with non-cardiac chest pain and abnormal esophageal 24-hour pH-metry, overall pain improvement was reported by 81% of omeprazole and 6% of placebo-treated patients.[155] Similar results were reported in another small study of 39 patients.[128] The omeprazole test correctly classified 78% of patients considered GERD patients by 24-hour esophageal monitoring and/or endoscopy and was positive in only 14% of GERD negative patients. Thus, a therapeutic trial may be useful in conditions other than typical GERD such as non-cardiac chest pain, an observation that is further supported by more recent studies.156,157

These lines of evidence indicate that a therapeutic trial of a PPI for 1–2 weeks may be a reasonable approach for the diagnosis of GERD. The advantages of this approach include simplicity, non-invasiveness, ease of prescription and consumption, tolerability, and savings in terms of direct costs and time lost by the patient. The therapeutic trial also predicts therapeutic response. These studies also support the notion that a symptom-based treatment is reasonable for most patients with reflux disease without a specific diagnosis.

Treatment of gastroesophageal reflux disease

Symptoms of gastroesophageal reflux are common and have a significant adverse impact on QOL. The costs of disease include both drug acquisition costs, and indirect costs such as physician visits and time off work. Because of the difficulty in make a definitive diagnosis of GERD through investigations, the physician must make a presumptive diagnosis and initiate a management plan. The goals of therapy are to provide adequate symptom relief, heal esophagitis and prevent complications. Since initial studies in GERD have focused on mucosal healing, healing of erosive esophagitis will be discussed first, followed by discussions on NERD, and finally on symptomatic treatments.

Acid suppression therapy for gastroesophageal reflux disease

While transient relaxations of the LES and defective basal LES tone are thought to be primary determinants of reflux, damage to the esophagus and symptoms result from acidic reflux.[37] Thus, the focus of treatment has been on acid suppression.

Acid secretion can be controlled by various drug classes. Antimuscarinic agents are weak inhibitors of the parietal cell M_3 cholinergic receptors and clinical use is limited by anticholinergic side effects. H_2-receptor antagonists (H_2-RAs) inhibit parietal cell histamine receptors and thus acid inhibition can be partially overcome by stimulation of gastrin and cholinergic receptors, as occurs when food is eaten.[158] Tolerance to H_2-RAs develops and reduces their efficacy over time.[159] PPIs provide the most potent acid inhibition through covalent binding to the H^+, K^+-ATPase (acid or proton pump) located in the secretory canaliculus of the parietal cell. Inhibiting the proton pump, which is the final common pathway, blocks acid secretion to all known stimuli. The PPIs have a long duration of action that depends on the rate of synthesis of new proton pumps by the parietal cell. These pharmacological differences predict that PPIs should be more effective than H_2-RAs.

Studies of 24-hour intragastric acidity have been used extensively to assess the degree and duration of acid inhibition with anti-secretory drugs.[160,161] These studies have confirmed that PPIs are superior to H_2-RAs in their ability to suppress food stimulated, daytime and total 24-hour acid secretion. Bell *et al.*[160] have shown by meta-analysis, that the healing rate of erosive esophagitis correlated directly with the duration of acid suppression over the 24-hour period. The primary determinants of healing were the length of treatment, the degree of acid suppression and the duration of acid suppression over the 24-hour period. There was also a highly significant correlation between the time that the pH in the esophagus was below 4 (i.e. below the threshold considered "normal") and the ability to heal erosive esophagitis. This work concluded that if intragastric acidity could be maintained above pH 4 for 20–22 hours of the day, 90% of patients with erosive esophagitis would be healed by 8 weeks. Thus, the superiority of PPIs over H_2-RAs was predicted, based on their pharmacologic ability to effectively suppress acid secretion.

Lifestyle modifications

Although lifestyle modifications are recommended frequently, there is little evidence that these are of benefit (Box 2.1). One study assessed patients with 24-hour esophageal pH testing and found no difference in lifestyle alteration and anxiety between those with positive and negative pH profiles.[162] Meining and Classen reviewed this topic in detail and determined that for many of the recommendations, the data are conflicting, weak, and at best equivocally supportive.[163] However, the data that white wine (*v* red wine) induces reflux is reasonably robust.[164,165] There are several mechanisms identified, including reduced LES pressure,[165] disturbed esophageal clearance due to increased simultaneous contractions and failed peristalsis.[166,167] The most recently identified mechanism is the occurrence of repeated reflux events into the esophagus when pH is still acidic from a previous reflux episode, the so-called "re-reflux" phenomenon.[168] Although caffeine itself is thought to be associated with reflux, one study has proposed that it is something in coffee other than caffeine, that is responsible.[168] Smoking is also often implicated (Box 2.1) but results concerning its role are controversial. One 24-hour pH study has shown an association with smoking[169] while another has not.[170] Vigorous exercise has also been implicated, with emphasis on running,[171–176] but also on weightlifting and cycling.[172,176] Thus, there is some rationale for "mother's advice" not to exercise right after eating. In one study, ranitidine 300 mg given 1 hour before running reduced esophageal acid exposure.[175] While there is some evidence that elevating the head of the bed is beneficial, not all investigators agree.[177] Lastly, posture is interesting, as more acid reflux seems to occur in the right lateral position. Thus the left lateral position is recommended for sleeping.[178–180]

Changing dietary habits and lifestyle modifications are generally considered useful by physicians.[208,209] However, when patients were asked about advice they had received from physicians, lifestyle changes were only modestly recommended.[210] If a patient is under the age of 50, and has no serious "alarm symptoms" such as unexplained weight loss, dysphagia or hematemesis, it is reasonable to start empirical therapy[151] as the most cost effective approach.[211]

Box 2.1   Recommended lifestyle modifications in gastroesophageal reflux disease

- Avoid precipitating foods and drinks: fat[181,182] (two studies found no effect of fat,[183,184] another found no effect of caloric density[185]), chocolate,[186,187] peppermint,[188] spices,[189] raw onions,[190] carbonated beverages,[163,191] caffeine,[1,168,192–194] coffee,[168] orange juice and tomato drink[191,195]
- Avoid alcohol[1,191,196–198]
- Avoid cigarette smoking[1,169,197–199]
- Avoid large meals and gastric distension[38,200]
- Avoid lying down within 3–4 hours of a meal[201]
- Aggravating factors to be avoided: posture,[201] physical exertion especially running,[166–171] weightlifting and cycling[172,176]
- Raising the head of the bed has some efficacy[201–204]
- Sleeping on the left lateral position reduces reflux[178–180]
- Avoid tight clothes[1]
- Obesity: may be a risk factor,[1,27,197] weight reduction helps symptoms,[205] weight reduction does not help[206,207]
- Avoid certain drugs if possible: β-blockers, anticholinergics including certain antidepressants, theophylline, calcium antagonists, nitrates[1]

Antacids and alginate

A small randomized placebo-controlled trial of Maalox TC at a full dose of 15 ml seven times daily for 4 weeks in 32 patients showed no significant symptom relief.[212] There appears to be marginal if any benefit of antacids and alginates over placebo, and antacids do not heal esophagitis.[213–215] Ald

In an uncontrolled study of patients with grade I to III esophagitis healed with either an H_2-RA or omeprazole, patients were given alginate for symptomatic maintenance treatment.[216] At 6 months, 76% were in remission. Those with more severe baseline esophagitis relapsed more frequently. In a randomized controlled trial, sodium alginate 10 ml four times daily was slightly more effective than cisapride 5 mg four times daily for reducing both symptoms measured on a visual analog scale (0–100) (alginate 29 ± 22, cisapride 35 ± 25, $P = 0.01$) and the number of reflux episodes in a 4-week period (alginate 2 ± 2, cisapride 3 ± 4, $P = 0.001$).[217] Conservative symptomatic therapy with alginate may be useful in some patients. Ald

Collings *et al.*[218] recently demonstrated that a calcium carbonate gum decreased heartburn and intraesophageal acidity more than chewable antacids, with effects that lasted for a couple of hours. This observation suggests that such a gum may be useful for intermittent therapy.

Placebo healing rates

Because healing of moderate to severe esophagitis with placebo therapy occurs in about 28% of patients,[11,219] the use of placebo controls has been important especially for the less effective drugs, such as H_2-RAs and prokinetics. For PPIs, the therapeutic gain is so large that placebo-controlled trials are less necessary.[11]

H_2-receptor antagonists

H_2-RAs are not very effective in the treatment of GERD but maintain a minor role in symptomatic therapy and are discussed here for completeness.

Intermittent/on-demand therapy for heartburn relief

Acid suppressive therapy with H_2-RAs has been the mainstay of treatment for acid-related disorders and in many countries these agents are available for over-the-counter (OTC) use.[220] This availability permits intermittent, on-demand use by the patient. A blinded crossover trial of famotidine 5, 10 and 20 mg versus placebo showed that all famotidine doses were more effective than placebo for the prevention of meal-induced heartburn and other dyspeptic symptoms.[221] This study established that heartburn severity peaked 1–2 hours after a meal. Thus, a small dose of H2-RA taken before eating may be useful to reduce symptoms induced by meals.

A unique formulation of a readily dissolving famotidine wafer (20 mg) was compared with standard dose (150 mg) ranitidine.[222] With both treatments, about half the patients had some symptom relief within 3 hours. A similar randomized trial found trivial but statistically significant differences between ranitidine and famotidine for time to adequate symptom relief (ranitidine 15 minutes, famotidine 18.5 minutes, $P = 0.005$) and for the proportion of patients with symptom relief at one hour (ranitidine 92%, famotidine 84%; $P = 0.02$).[223] Thus, for mild reflux symptoms, use of H_2-RA on an as needed basis is useful. Ald However, an observational study reported in abstract form,[224] of ranitidine effervescent tablets used on-demand for 1 year in patients with grade I and II esophagitis revealed that the grade of esophagitis did not improve in spite of reporting satisfaction with treatment by 84% of patients. Patients may be satisfied with their relief of symptoms, although damage to the esophagus continues.

High dose H_2-receptor antagonists

While standard doses of H_2-RAs heal more severe, (grade II to IV esophagitis) in about 52% of patients,[11] higher doses of H_2-RA (150–300 mg four times daily) are more effective, healing 74–80% of patients in 12 weeks, under conditions in which the healing rate with placebo is 40–58%.[225,226] Silver *et al.*[227] compared regimens of ranitidine 300 mg twice daily and 150 mg four times daily for treatment of erosive esophagitis. At 12 weeks, the healing proportion observed for the four times daily regimen was 77% and for the twice daily regimen, 66% (absolute risk reduction (ARR) 11%, number needed to treat (NNT) 9). Ranitidine 150 mg four times daily was superior to standard dose (150 mg twice daily) ranitidine or cimetidine (800 mg twice daily) in patients with erosive esophagitis.[228] In another randomized trial in patients with erosive esophagitis,[229] healing with ranitidine 150 mg twice daily the proportion of patients healed was 54% at 8 weeks compared with 75% with 300 mg four times daily (ARR 21%, NNT 5). Ald Famotidine is pharmacologically more potent than ranitidine and a large dose of 40 mg twice daily was superior to standard dose 20 mg twice daily or ranitidine 150 mg twice daily in patients with erosive or worse esophagitis.[230] Ald

Prokinetic drugs

In a randomized, placebo-controlled trial, metoclopramide and domperidone did not improve esophageal motility, duration of acid exposure or esophageal clearance, although both agents significantly increased LES pressure.[231] Cisapride is the only prokinetic drug that increases both esophageal clearance and enhances LES tone.[233-234] However, one study has reported that cisapride increased acid reflux in comparison with omeprazole and famotidine.[235]

Placebo-controlled trials show marginal benefit for cisapride in healing esophagitis and improving symptoms.[234,236-238] Ald

For mild grades of esophagitis, cisapride is as effective as H_2-RA for healing and symptom relief with comparable tolerability.[238-243] Unfortunately, this drug requires prolonged use for up to 12 weeks before clinical benefit is seen.[237,238,240,242,244-246]

In one randomized trial in patients with milder GERD, omeprazole 10 or 20 mg daily was significantly more effective than cisapride 10 mg four times daily for relief of heartburn, regurgitation and epigastric pain.[90] This and other studies suggest that for symptomatic GERD, the degree of acid suppression is a more important determinant of symptom relief than prokinetic activity. Ald

In healing grades I and II esophagitis, adding cisapride to omeprazole did not significantly increase efficacy over omeprazole alone.[247] In another study of healing grades II and III esophagitis, cisapride 20 mg twice daily added to pantoprazole 40 mg once daily did not improve healing over pantoprazole alone.[248] Thus, these two studies provide strong evidence that the addition of cisapride does not add any clinical benefit to treating with PPIs alone. Ald

Cisapride has shown some benefit for maintenance therapy for mild esophagitis.[246,247,249,250] However, in patients with more severe erosive esophagitis initially healed with antisecretory therapy, cisapride was not effective for maintenance treatment[238,240,251,252] and was not more effective than placebo.[253] Ald

Cisapride has been associated with the development of serious cardiac arrhythmias including torsades de pointes, when used with other drugs that inhibit cytochrome P450 3A4. These include fluconazole, itraconazole, ketoconazole, erythromycin, clarithromycin, ritonavir, indinavir, nefazodone, tricyclic antidepressants and certain tetracyclic antidepressants, certain antipsychotics, astemizole, terfenadine, and class 1A and III anti-arrhythmics.[254] Thus, cisapride is not recommended because its potential for producing significant adverse events is greater than that for other more effective agents, and in many jurisdictions, the drug is not readily available.

Sucralfate in gastroesophageal reflux disease

For grade I–III GERD, there have been four small, randomized trials of sucralfate 1 g four times daily compared with standard dose H_2-RA which did not show significant differences with respect to symptom resolution and healing.[255-258] However, none of these studies showed very large benefits from either intervention, with low rates of heartburn relief (34–62%) and healing (31–64%). Combining

sucralfate and cimetidine was not better than monotherapy with either drug.[259,260] The Chiba et al.'s meta-analysis of randomized trials for grade II–IV esophagitis yielded a pooled value for healing proportion of 39·2% for sucralfate compared with 28% for placebo.[11] However, the 95% CI was wide (3·6 to 74·8%). A1c

In a 6-month study of grade I–II GERD, sucralfate was effective for preventing relapse compared with placebo (sucralfate 31%, placebo 65%; ARR 34, NNT 3, $P < 0.001$).[261] Ald

It is interesting that sucralfate, which does not lower acid output, reduce esophageal acid exposure or improve esophageal transit time[262] has any efficacy given our understanding of the pathophysiology of this condition. The adverse effect of constipation, the need for four times daily dosing and the modest observed benefit make sucralfate an unattractive choice for most patients.

Erosive gastroesophageal reflux disease

Meta-analysis of healing and symptom relief with proton-pump inhibitors and H_2-receptor antagonists

An early meta-analysis of randomized trials of patients with more severe esophagitis (grade II in 61·8%, grade III in 31·7% and grade IV in 6·5%) established the clinical efficacy of PPIs.[11] Subsequent published studies support the conclusions derived from this meta-analysis.[14,19,228,230,263-279] Ald

In the meta-analysis,[11] the rate of healing, expressed as "percent healed per week", was significantly superior with PPI therapy compared with H_2-RA, particularly early in the course of treatment (weekly healing rate in first 2 weeks: PPI 32%, H_2-RA 15%). The rate of healing slowed with increasing duration of treatment as fewer patients remained unhealed, but PPI remained superior to H_2-RA. The overall healing proportions during 12 weeks, using pooled results irrespective of dose and duration were: PPI 84% (95% CI 79 to 88), H_2-RA 52% (95% CI 47 to 57), sucralfate 39% (95% CI 4 to 75) and placebo 28% (95% CI 19 to 37). These data were used to plot rate of healing against time on a "healing time curve" (Figure 2.2). By the end of the second week, PPI had healed 63·4 ± 6·6% of patients, while H_2-RA required 12 weeks to achieve healing in a similar proportion of patients (60·2 ± 5·9%). Linear regression analysis of individual study results showed that PPI heal at an overall rate of 11·7% per week (95% CI 10·7 to 12·6), twice as rapidly as H_2-RA (5·9% per week, 95% CI 5·5 to 6·3) and four times more rapidly than placebo (2·9, 95% CI 2·4 to 3·4).

Heartburn was present in all but 3·8% (95% CI 2·1 to 5·5) of patients at baseline. Overall heartburn relief was seen in 77·4 ± 10·4% of patients treated with PPI and in 47·6 ± 15·5% treated with H_2-RA. Data for heartburn relief

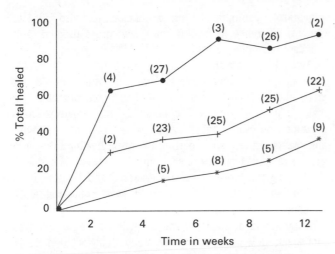

Figure 2.2 Healing-time curve expressed as the mean total healing for each drug class per evaluation time in weeks. By week 4, PPIs (proton pump inhibitors) heal more patients than any other drug class, even after a much longer duration of treatment (12 weeks), implying a substantial therapeutic gain despite the fact that all drug classes achieve higher healing with longer durations of therapy. The number of studies is shown in parentheses. •, PPI; +, H_2-RA, *, placebo. Reproduced with permission from Chiba N *et al. Gastroenterology* 1997;**112**:1798–1810[11]

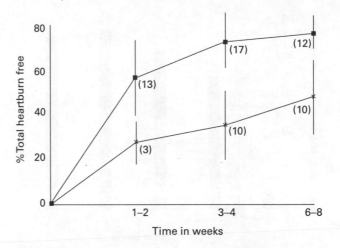

Figure 2.3 Symptom relief–time curve expressed as the mean total heartburn relief for each drug class corrected for patients free of heartburn at baseline at 1–2, 3–4, and 6–8 weeks. By week 2, more patients treated with PPIs (proton pump inhibitors) are asymptomatic compared with H_2-RA (H_2-receptor antagonists) even after a much longer duration of treatment (8 weeks), implying a substantial therapeutic gain despite the fact that both drug classes achieve greater symptom relief with longer durations of treatment. The number of studies is shown in parentheses. ■, PPI; x, H_2-RA. Reproduced with permission from Chiba N *et al. Gastroenterology* 1997;**112**:1798–1810[11]

were plotted against time to create a "symptom relief time curve" (Figure 2.3). Linear regression analysis of the data yielded an overall heartburn relief rate of 11·5% per week for PPI (95% CI 9·9 to 13·0) and 6·4% per week for H_2-RA (95% CI 5·4 to 7·4).

Some studies measured heartburn in categories of none, mild, moderate or severe and reported the shift in heartburn relief with treatment (Figures 2.4 and 2.5). The proportion of patients with residual mild to moderate symptoms after 8 weeks of therapy was 11·1% for PPI and 57·4% for H_2-RAs.

This meta-analysis provided evidence that PPI are significantly better than H_2-RA for both healing esophagitis and relieving symptoms in patients with moderately severe esophagitis. There was also evidence in one RCT that PPI therapy is effective for healing persistent grade II–IV esophagitis after treatment failure with 12 weeks standard dose H2-RA.280 Ald

Are there differences between proton pump inhibitors?

There are now five proton-pump inhibitors available in North America. These are omeprazole, lansoprazole, pantoprazole, rabeprazole and esomeprazole.

For symptom relief, esomeprazole was shown to be more rapidly effective than both omeprazole[19,274] and

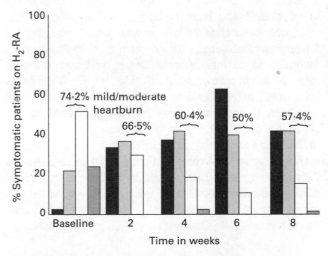

Figure 2.4 Shift in heartburn relief with H_2-RAs (H_2-receptor antagonists). From studies using a symptom scale of none, mild, moderate, or severe, the shift in symptom severity with duration of treatment can be observed. With H_2-RAs, although there is an increase in the number of patients completely heartburn free, at the end of the study, more than half of the patients still have mild to moderate symptoms. ■, None; ▨, mild; □, moderate; ■, severe. Reproduced with permission[118] from Chiba N *et al. Gastroenterology* 1997;**112**:1798–1810[11]

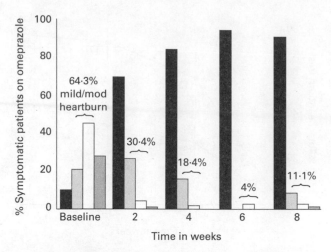

Figure 2.5 Shift in heartburn relief with PPIs. PPIs (omeprazole)-treated patients have a dramatic shift in the number of patients completely symptom free, particularly early in treatment, and at the end of the study, very few patients have any residual heartburn in contrast to patients treated with H₂-RAs, ■, None; ▨, mild; □, moderate; ▨, serve. Reproduced with permission from Chiba N *et al. Gastroenterology* 1997;**112**:798–1810[11]

lansoprazole.[268] In one study, lansoprazole was more rapidly effective than omeprazole.[20] However, differences in symptom relief were no longer apparent at the end of the study.[263,271,281] In another study, omeprazole and pantoprazole were found to be equivalent with each other but not with lansoprazole.[282] Similar results were found in a comparison of rabeprazole and omeprazole.[283] Low, half-doses of PPIs compared with standard doses were not found to be effective for healing esophagitis or for symptom relief.[132,263] However, for maintenance therapy some data suggest that low dose PPIs are as effective as standard doses.[32,284,285] While there were small differences between overall study results, the data from these studies were insufficient to establish the superiority of any one drug over all others.[286]

Vakil and Fennerty recently carried out a careful systematic review of randomized controlled trials that directly compared PPIs to determine whether there is a difference in clinical outcomes between any of these agents.[286] They restricted this review to more recent (1998–2002), better quality trials. *They found similar healing rates for the following comparisons:*

- lansoprazole 30 mg daily compared with omeprazole 20 mg[281] or 40 mg,[264] or pantoprazole 40 mg daily[275]
- pantoprazole 40 mg[287] or rabeprazole 20 mg[265,273] compared with omeprazole 20 mg daily.[286] Alc

They found that for esophagitis healing, esomeprazole was superior to omeprazole and lansoprazole.[19,268,274] Earlier randomized trials comparing two different PPIs (lansoprazole,

omeprazole, pantoprazole and rabeprazole) had also failed to show a difference in healing rates with drugs used at their standard recommended doses.[14,263,271,281,288–291] Ald

Two other meta-analyses also showed that esomeprazole was superior to omeprazole and that the other PPI did not have higher healing rates compared with omeprazole.[292,293] Alc Another review concluded that lansoprazole, pantoprazole and rabeprazole were comparable with omeprazole in terms of heartburn control, healing rates, and relapse rates.[294] Esomeprazole 40 mg daily was more effective for healing the more severe LA grades C and D esophagitis in randomized trials in which it was compared with omeprazole 20 mg daily[19,274] or lansoprazole 30 mg.[268] Ald One randomized trial that included 284 patients and was similar in design to the latter study that included 5241 patients showed no difference between esomeprazole 40 mg and lansoprazole 30 mg for healing of erosive (or worse) esophagitis in 4 or 8 weeks, but the smaller trial may have lacked statistical power. Alc

Esomeprazole is the first PPI shown to be more effective than any other PPI; all other direct comparisons have shown that healing rates are essentially the same for all agents in this class.[269] Esomeprazole is the (S)-isomer of omeprazole and as a result of increased systemic exposure and less interindividual variability, it produces potent acid suppression. In a review by Hatlebakk,[295] esomeprazole 40 mg daily was significantly more effective at controlling gastric acidity than lansoprazole 30 mg daily, pantoprazole 40 mg daily and rabeprazole 20 mg daily. Esomeprazole 20 mg daily was also significantly more effective than lansoprazole 15 mg daily. Thus, the improved clinical benefits are consistent with the pharmacological potency of this drug.

A study of the Food and Drug Administration database reported very few drug interactions for omeprazole, lansoprazole and pantoprazole.[296] Of the rare interactions, vitamin K antagonist reactions were most common but even these were seen in only 0·09–0·11 per million packages prescribed. This report concluded that the safety of the drugs was likely a class effect with no significant differences among the PPIs.

Is there a rationale for higher dose proton pump inhibitor therapy?

The standard doses of PPI are very effective for healing esophagitis, and it is clear that there is a correlation between the degree of acid suppression and healing.[160] In clinical practice, patients with persistent or recurrent symptoms are often told to double their dose of PPI, typically to take the doses on a twice daily regimen. There is no strong evidence for this approach from the following relevant studies.

Patients with complicated or atypical GERD were randomly assigned to receive 30 mg lansoprazole (*n* = 26) or 40 mg pantoprazole (*n* = 24) once daily.[297] Esophageal acid exposure was normalized in all lansoprazole patients (in 35% of cases with double dose), whereas 25% of the pantoprazole-treated patients did not have lowered or normalized esophageal acid exposure, even with the dose doubled ($P = 0.008$). A pantoprazole 40 mg versus 80 mg daily study in patients with stage II or III esophagitis showed healing proportions of 78% versus 72% at 4 weeks.[266] These data suggest that for pantoprazole, increasing the dose beyond the standard dose is not likely to be of any benefit.

Klinkenberg-Knol *et al.* have followed a cohort of GERD patients for many years and reported that doubling the dose of omeprazole to 40 mg daily was effective to treat relapses.[298] A longer-term report followed 230 patients for up to 11 years on continuous therapy.[299] Of those followed, a third each had grade II, III and IV disease. It was estimated that there was only one relapse for every 9 years of treatment and the median maintenance dose was 20 mg daily. Dose titration (range 20 mg every second day to 120 mg once daily) allowed most patients to remain in remission. Another study showed that titrating the dose of omeprazole to 40–60 mg daily was as effective for maintenance of remission as antireflux surgery.[300] B4

One trial compared rabeprazole 20 mg daily with a high dose of omeprazole (40 mg daily) in patients with erosive esophagitis for 4–8 weeks and found no significant differences between treatments for symptom relief or healing rates.[278] A1d This is a clinically relevant finding as doubling doses leads to greater costs.

There is concern about patients on multiple daily doses of PPIs, a practice that increases cost. Inadomi *et al.*[301] identified and recruited such patients through the use of pharmacy records of PPI prescriptions. Eligible subjects were stepped-down to single dose PPI (lansoprazole 30 mg or omeprazole 20 mg daily) and 80% did not report recurrent symptoms of heartburn or acid regurgitation. These authors concluded that "this intervention can decrease management costs without adversely affecting quality of life".[301] B4

Maintenance therapy for patients with documented healed esophagitis

For mild GERD, as seen at a community level, 46% of patients can heal spontaneously.[65] For moderately severe GERD, healing and symptom relief are readily obtained with PPI, but, within 6–12 months, irrespective of the initial healing agent, recurrences are reported in 36–82% of patients in the absence of maintenance therapy.[302–304]

After acute healing or stopping maintenance therapy, symptoms recur within a day, and erosive esophagitis can recur in most patients within 10 days[305] to one month.[306] Thus, maintenance therapy is required in most patients with GERD.

A meta-analysis of the rate of relapse of erosive esophagitis reported in five omeprazole trials that included 1154 patients

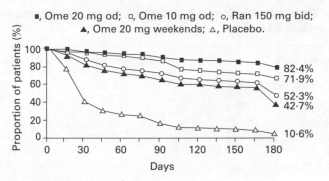

Figure 2.6 Actuarial life-table analysis. Estimated proportion of patients in endoscopic remission at the end of the 6-month follow up period with maintenance treatment. Reproduced with permission from Carlsson *et al. Aliment Pharmacol Ther* 1997;**11**:473–82[307]

in whom erosive GERD was initially healed by omeprazole 20–40 mg was carried out by Carlsson *et al.*[307] Figure 2.6 shows the effects of various regimens. Omeprazole 20 mg daily which maintained 82·4% of patients in remission for 6 months was significantly better than omeprazole 10 mg daily ($P = 0.04$). Both of these regimens were significantly better than ranitidine 150 mg twice daily and omeprazole 20 mg on weekends. Thus, omeprazole should be given continuously, and dosing intermittently for only three days per week is not adequate. A1a Two trials assessed maintenance over 12 months. Omeprazole 20 mg daily was superior to ranitidine 150 mg twice daily (omeprazole 80·2%, ranitidine 39·4%; ARR 40·8%, NNT 2). A1a The proportions of patients with asymptomatic endoscopic esophagitis relapse were: omeprazole 20 mg 4·5%, omeprazole 10 mg 12·5%, and ranitidine 14·6%. Regression analysis identified four risk factors for recurrence: pretreatment severity of esophagitis, younger age, non-smoking status and moderate to severe reflux pre-entry.

A previous systematic review of continuous maintenance therapy[308] in patients with initial grades II–IV esophagitis was updated from the previous edition of this book.[309] This review included only data from fully published papers.[32,284,285,310–316] The estimated results from each study are recorded in Table 2.4. For this review, the numbers of patients in remission/relapse were derived from the numbers given or estimated from the intention to treat analysis as much as possible, or from the all-evaluable patients in life-table analysis. Not all trials were homogeneous and some were only of 6 months' duration. The esomeprazole studies used the LA classification to grade esophagitis. LA grade A is not directly comparable to either the Hetzel–Dent or Savary–Miller grade I classifications. For some trials proportions had to be estimated for the life-table analyses. However, the crude pooled, cumulative, mean relapse rates are shown in Table 2.5. Readers are cautioned about

Table 2.4 **Randomized controlled trials of maintenance therapy in patients with erosive or worse gastroesophageal reflux disease**

Authors	Duration of treatment	Treatment regimens[d]	% relapse (*n* relapsed/*n* treated)
Simon *et al.* (1995)[321]	6 months	F 40 twice daily	11 (8/72)
		F 20 twice daily	22 (15/69)
		Placebo	61 (19/31)
Sontag *et al.* (1997)[323]	6 months	O 20 once daily	30 (41/138)
		O 20 once daily, 3 days/week	66 (90/137)
		Placebo	89 (116/131)
Bardhan *et al.* (1998)[317]	6 months	O 10 once daily	22 (28/130)
		Placebo	57 (76/133)
Lundell *et al.* (1991)[318]	12 months	O 20 once daily	32 (11/34)
		R 300 twice daily	88 (14/16)
Dent *et al.* (1994)[324]	12 months	O 20 once daily	12 (5/43)
		O 20 once daily, 3 days/week	71 (34/48)
		R 150 twice daily	79 (38/48)
Hallerback *et al.* (1994)[325]	12 months	O 20 once daily	28 (37/131)
		O 10 once daily	38 (51/133)
		R 150 twice daily	55 (70/128)
Bate *et al.* (1995)[326]	12 months	O 20 once daily	32 (22/68)
		O 10 once daily	50 (30/60)
		Placebo	90 (56/62)
Vigneri *et al.* (1995)[250]	12 months	O 20 once daily	20 (7/35)
		R 150 thrice daily	51 (18/35)
		C 10 thrice daily	46 (16/35)
		R+C	34 (12/35)
		O+C	11 (4/35)
Gough *et al.* (1996)[319]	12 months	L 30 once daily	20 (15/75)
		L 15 once daily	31 (27/86)
		R 300 twice daily	68 (50/74)
Robinson *et al.* (1996)[322]	12 months	L 30 once daily	11 (6/56)
		L 15 once daily	22 (13/59)
		Placebo	76 (42/55)
Sontag *et al.* (1996)[306]	12 months	L 30 once daily	45 (22/49)
		L 15 once daily	34 (17/50)
		Placebo	87 (41/47)
Hatlebakk *et al.* (1997)[327b]	12 months	L 30 once daily	18 (4/22)
		L 15 once daily	44 (8/18)
Bardhan *et al.* (1998)[317a]	12 months	O 10 once daily	38 (49/130)
		Placebo	78 (104/133)
Carling *et al.* (1998)[320]	12 months	O 20 once daily	9 (11/122)
		L 30 once daily	10 (12/126)
Escourrou *et al.* (1999)[310]	12 months	P 20 once daily	24 (49/203)
		P 40 once daily	16 (30/193)
Plein *et al.* (2000)[311]	6 months	P 20 once daily	13 (25/192)
		P 40 once daily	9 (16/185)
	12 months	P 20 once daily	26 (45/174)
		P 40 once daily	22 (39/174)

(Continued)

Table 2.4 (Continued)

Authors	Duration of treatment	Treatment regimens[d]	% relapse (*n* relapsed/*n* treated)
Caos *et al.* (2000)[312]	12 months	Rab 10 once daily Rab 20 once daily Placebo	27 (19/70) 10 (7/69) 71 (50/70)
Birbara *et al.* (2000)[313]	12 months	Rab 10 once daily Rab 20 once daily Placebo	23 (22/95) 14 (11/94) 71 (70/99)
Thjodleifsson *et al.* (2000)[284]	12 months	Rab 10 once daily Rab 20 once daily O 20 once daily	5 (4/82) 4 (3/78) 5 (4/83)
Vakil *et al.* (2001)[285]	6 months	E 40 once daily E 20 once daily E 10 once daily Placebo	12 (11/92) 21 (21/98) 46 (42/91) 71 (67/94)[c]
Johnson *et al.* (2001)[32]	6 months	E 40 once daily E 20 once daily E 10 once daily Placebo	6 (5/82) 7 (6/82) 43 (33/77) 71 (55/77)[c]
Lauritsen *et al.* (2003)[314]	6 months	E20 once daily L15 once daily	16 (84/522) 24 (117/489)[c]
Pilotto *et al.* (2003)[315]	6 months	P20 once daily Placebo	20 (10/49) 70 (39/56)
Metz and Bochenck (2003)[316]	12 months	P 10 once daily P 20 once daily P 40 once daily R 150 twice daily	60 (53/89) 32 (30/93) 18 (17/94) 67 (64/95)[c]

[a]Bardhan study is the only one with 6 and 12-month relapse data
[b]Data given for patients who had initial grade 2 esophagitis
[c]Estimated *n* from intention to treat life-table percentages given in the paper
[d]All drug doses given in mg
F, famotidine; O, omeprazole; R, ranitidine; C, cisapride; L, lansoprazole; Rab, rabeprazole; E, esomeprazole

interpreting these pooled data between studies as there are few observations in each treatment arm and the confidence intervals are very wide.

Only two studies provided relapse data at 6 and 12 months and in both studies, the relapse rate was higher at 12 months.[311,317] Within individual dose-finding studies, the highest dose of PPI given was associated with the lowest relapse rate. Alc The pooled data also show the trend toward better maintenance of remission with standard doses of the PPIs than with the lower doses. Not surprisingly, the placebo relapse rate was the highest at nearly 80% and the H_2-RAs were only slightly more effective, despite the fact that relatively high doses of the latter were used in some trials.[250,318,319] Alc Only three trials directly compared more than one PPI. One trial compared lansoprazole 30 mg and omeprazole 20 mg once daily and found the same healing and symptom relief.[320] Another used low dose lansoprazole 15 mg and esomeprazole 20 mg and found that esomeprazole was significantly better.[314] Lastly, the study by Thjodleifsson[284] was somewhat of an anomaly as the relapse rates with rabeprazole 10 mg or 20 mg and omeprazole 20 mg daily were all comparable but all very low at about 5%. It is thus difficult to conclude that any one PPI is better than another from this review and further randomized trials that directly compare agents are needed.

One study was done specifically in the elderly population aged 65 years and over.[315] Patients with grade I–III esophagitis were treated with pantoprazole 40 mg once daily for 8 weeks, then with pantoprazole 20 mg daily for 6 months. Thereafter they were randomized to receive pantoprazole 20 mg once daily or a placebo for a further 6 months. After 8 weeks, esophagitis healing was 81·1%

Table 2.5 Summary of pooled gastroesophageal reflux disease relapse rates in patients on maintenance therapy

Drug regimen	6 month relapse			12 month relapse		
	No. of trials	Relapse % (n/total)	95% CI	No. of trials	Relapse % (n/total)	95% CI
Placebo	6	71 (372/522)	59 to 81	6	78 (363/466)	71 to 88
H$_2$-RA	2	16 (23/141)	–	6	64 (254/396)	53 to 82
Low dose proton pump inhibitors						
Omeprazole 10 mg once daily	1	22 (28/130)	–	3	40 (130/323)	25 to 59
Lansoprazole 15 mg once daily	1	24 (117/489)	–	4	31 (65/213)	18 to 48
Pantoprazole 10 mg once daily	–	–	–	1	60 (53/89)	–
Pantoprazole 20 mg once daily	2	15 (35/241)	–	3	26 (124/470)	17 to 38
Rabeprazole 10 mg once daily	–	–	–	3	18 (45/247)	–11 to 48
Esomeprazole 10 mg once daily	2	45 (75/168)	–	–	–	–
Esomeprazole 20 mg once daily	3	16 (111/702)	–3 to 33	–	–	–
Standard dose proton pump inhibitors						
Omeprazole 20 mg once daily	1	30 (41/138)	–	7	19 (97/516)	9 to 30
Lansoprazole 30 mg once daily	–	–	–	5	18 (59/328)	3 to 38
Pantoprazole 40 mg once daily	1	9 (16/185)	–	3	19 (86/461)	10 to 27
Rabeprazole 20 mg once daily	–	–	–	3	9 (21/241)	–2 to 19
Esomeprazole 40 mg once daily	2	14 (127/876)	–	–	–	–

(95% CI 75·1–87·1%) by intention to treat analysis. After 12 months, the observed healing rates by intention to treat analysis were 79·6% (68·3–90·9%) with pantoprazole 20 mg once daily and 30·4% (18·3–42·4%) in the placebo group ($P = 0.0001$). Ald Thus, there is no reason to consider that the elderly will respond any differently from younger patients.

There are limited maintenance data from studies of greater than 1 year's duration. An observational maintenance study with pantoprazole 40 mg once daily in 157 patients with healed stage II or III reflux esophagitis (Savary–Miller classification) showed endoscopic remission of 87% after 1 year and 76% after 2 years.[328] B4 There has been one randomized trial of 5 years' duration in which patients with initially healed erosive or worse esophagitis were randomized to receive rabeprazole 20 mg once daily, rabeprazole 10 mg once daily or omeprazole 20 mg once daily.[329] Of the initial 243 patients, 123 completed the 5-year study. Relapse rates were 11·5%, 9·8% and 13·3%, respectively. All treatments were safe and well tolerated and these data provide evidence that remission can be effectively maintained over long time periods.

Low dose continuous proton pump inhibitors as maintenance therapy

The H$_2$-RAs are marginally superior to placebo when considering pooled data and data from the one trial in which a direct comparison of H2-RA (famotidine 20 mg or 40 mg twice daily) with placebo was made.[321] A small dose of lansoprazole (15 mg) daily was superior to a high dose of ranitidine (300 mg twice daily).[319] Smaller and intermittent doses of PPI were less effective (see Table 2.4) than standard doses.

Bardhan *et al.*[317] treated patients with erosive esophagitis with omeprazole to produce healing and then randomized them to receive omeprazole 10 mg daily or a placebo. The small dose of omeprazole was effective for maintenance of remission for 18 months in 60% of patients. Symptomatic failures were well controlled on omeprazole 20 mg daily with relapse in only 9% of patients over 2 years. Scheduled endoscopy detected erosive changes in asymptomatic patients, accounting for a quarter of the relapses. A full dose of PPI is probably necessary to maintain better quality endoscopic and symptomatic remission. Ald

A 6-month maintenance study[314] after healed esophagitis showed that even the low dose esomeprazole 20 mg once daily was better than lansoprazole 15 mg once daily with remission rates of 83% (95% CI 80 to 86%) compared with 74% (95% CI 70 to 78%) by life-table analysis. Ald The endoscopic esophagitis relapse rate with esomeprazole was 16% versus 24% with lansoprazole. With more severe LA grades of esophagitis, esomeprazole treatment provided a significantly longer time to relapse than was observed in the lansoprazole treated patients. One trial[32] suggested that esomeprazole 20 mg was as effective as 40 mg daily. Another suggested that rabeprazole 10 mg was as effective as 20 mg daily,[329] although this observation was not confirmed in two other similar trials.[312,313]

The problem of healing the more severe grades of esophagitis is well known. The proportion of patients who experience acute healing for grade II esophagitis ranges from 76–100%, for grade III from 63–95% and for grade IV from 56–75%.[308] Grade IV disease relapses more frequently than grade II and III disease.[306,322] In clinical practice, it is suggested that the dose of PPI can be titrated upwards to maintain healing in most patients[298] or alternatively, the most potent PPI be used. Since standard dose PPI fails to maintain remission in about 20% of patients, maintenance therapy in this population should be continuous and not on-demand or intermittent. AId C5

Intermittent therapy as a strategy for long-term management of mild/moderate gastroesophageal reflux disease

A group of 677 adults with moderate to severe heartburn, (primary care practices, 33% NERD, 67% LA grade A–C esophagitis) were randomized to receive ranitidine 150 mg twice daily, or omeprazole 10 mg or 20 mg daily for 2 weeks.[330] The proportion of patients completely free of heartburn at 2 weeks was significantly higher ($P < 0.001$) in the omeprazole groups (ranitidine 26%, omeprazole 10 mg 40%, omeprazole 20 mg 55%). Patients on ranitidine or 10 mg omeprazole who remained symptomatic received double doses of their medications for a further 2 weeks, while those on 20 mg of omeprazole continued at this dose. After the acute phase, patients were followed up for 12 months. During this period, a recurrence of symptoms was treated with the previously effective regimen for 2–4 weeks. This strategy was effective for most patients. These patients did not need drug treatment for about 6 months on average. B4 Overall, symptoms were not adequately controlled in 22% of the patients, and the strategy of intermittent therapy for relapses was unacceptable for 9% of patients, who were then offered open label omeprazole (20 mg daily). While the authors stated that the results were similar in patients with erosive and non-erosive disease, the data were not given in the paper.[330]

At baseline, PGWB scores of about 95 indicated impaired QOL compared with normal population values of 103.[6] Baseline GSRS scores indicated patient perception of their symptoms as being of moderate severity. With 4 weeks of treatment, PGWB scores had improved to a normal value of about 106, and the reflux dimension of GSRS scores also improved. In the follow up period, relapses were accompanied by a fall in QOL to baseline levels, and with treatment, scores again improved. No differences in QOL scores were seen between patients with erosive esophagitis and NERD at baseline, in response to therapy, at relapse or with subsequent treatment. This study provides important documentation that in patients with NERD, who are generally considered to have milder disease, the impairment of QOL is as great as in patients with erosive disease.

A prospective cost effectiveness analysis of this study[331] indicated that the patients who were started on omeprazole 20 mg once daily had more symptom free days and days without medication than those who were started on ranitidine, and omeprazole tended to be the more cost effective drug ($P = 0.1$). The interpretation offered by the authors is that a step-up approach, either from omeprazole 10 mg to omeprazole 20 mg or from ranitidine to omeprazole, would be cost effective. B4

On-demand therapy as a strategy for long-term management of mild/moderate gastroesophageal reflux disease

Lansoprazole (15 mg daily and 30 mg on alternate days) was studied for maintenance of endoscopic healing and symptom relief over a 6-month period after healing of Savary–Miller grades I–III reflux esophagitis.[332] After 6 months, recurrence of esophagitis was observed in 12% of the 15-mg once daily group and in 19% of the 30-mg alternate day group. This difference was not statistically significant. However, 12.1% of patients who received 15 mg daily and 28.6% of those who received alternate day higher dose therapy ($P = 0.007$) had heartburn. AId

In another study, patients with esophagitis were initially treated until symptom resolution. Thereafter, they took "on-demand" lansoprazole (30 mg) or omeprazole (20 mg) for 6 months only when reflux symptoms relapsed.[333] There was no difference in the number of doses between groups receiving lansoprazole (0.73 doses/day) and omeprazole (0.71 doses /day) and there was no difference in reflux symptoms. AId

"On demand" therapy is not recommended for patients with documented erosive esophagitis as patients must experience recurrent symptoms before treatment is taken, and these patients are thus left with unhealed lesions. C5

Cost effectiveness of maintenance therapy

It is clear that overall, PPIs are the most effective treatments available to treat GERD. However, PPI are also more costly than H_2-RAs. Therefore cost effectiveness analyses become important in decision making. There are two well conducted reviews of cost effectiveness of therapies for GERD.[334,335] Studies differ substantially with respect to methods, assumptions, interventions and outcomes being evaluated, the inclusiveness of cost items, and the jurisdiction to which the analyses are applied. No perfect cost effectiveness study exists, and new advances in therapy and changes in cost overtime tend to render the conclusions out of date rather quickly. However, despite these limitations, these modeling studies are useful to put into perspective the role of existing interventions.

Many studies indicate that PPIs are more cost effective than H_2-RAs.[336–343] Cost effectiveness data from Canada,[344]

Sweden[345] and the USA[346,347] arrived at similar conclusions. Maintenance PPI over a 1-year period is consistently the most effective but also the most costly intervention.[344–347] Intermittent omeprazole to treat symptomatic relapse was more cost effective than continuous omeprazole therapy, although there was an increase in the number of symptomatic weeks per year.[344] Maintenance therapy with ranitidine or cisapride was less effective for controlling symptoms, but was of intermediate cost.

High dose H_2-RA was more costly and less effective than PPI, with more frequent relapses that ultimately led to PPI maintenance therapy.[346] Harris *et al.*[346] reported that treatment with continuous PPI becomes more cost effective than H_2-RA if patients with active symptoms of GERD experience a 9% decrement in QOL. When considering three different PPI maintenance strategies, starting continuous PPI after the second recurrence was least costly and least effective.[347] Continuous PPI started after the first recurrence added only a small increment of cost per recurrence prevented, compared with continuous PPI from the outset, which was 10 times more costly.[347] However, for patients with a 22% decrement in QOL, continuous therapy became cost effective when compared with maintenance after first relapse. All these strategies are modeled for only one year and may not be generalizable to lifelong treatment.

A very recent paper using a Markov model compared low versus standard dose PPI therapy.[348] The standard dose PPI was found to be the more cost effective strategy on the strength of the highest number of symptom-free patient-years and the quality adjusted life years gained. However, this study did not derive estimates from studies of esomeprazole 20 mg or rabeprazole 10 mg daily, two effective lower dosing regimens that may have altered the results.

Treatment of non-erosive reflux disease

NERD or endoscopy-negative reflux disease (ENRD) is present in patients without endoscopic findings of whom 21–63% may have an abnormal 24-hour esophageal pH-metry result.[47,149] Other patients in this category may have a positive Bernstein test, or a positive symptom index and experience improvement with acid suppressive therapy. Basically these are patients without obvious abnormalities in the investigations undertaken.

One of the first studies in this group of patients was reported by Bate *et al.* in 1996.[349] Patients with NERD were randomized in a double blind trial to receive omeprazole 20 mg once daily ($n = 98$) or placebo ($n = 111$). At 4 weeks, omeprazole was more effective than placebo ($P < 0.0001$). with respect to patients with freedom from heartburn (omeprazole 57%, placebo 19%), or regurgitation (omeprazole 75%, placebo 47%) and complete relief of symptoms (omeprazole 43%, placebo 14%), Alc Patients in the omeprazole arm used less antacids and time to first heartburn-free day was more rapid with omeprazole.

Another randomized trial in 495 patients with NERD compared low dose omeprazole 10 mg or a placebo for 6 months.[350] Placebo-treated patients were nearly twice as likely to discontinue treatment before the end of 6 months. Life-table estimates for cumulative remission at 6 months, were 73% for omeprazole and 48% for placebo (ARR 25%, NNT 4, $P = 0.0001$). QOL assessments showed a more significant deterioration in the GSRS reflux domain for placebo patients ($P < 0.05$), but no significant differences were noted in PGWB. Thus, a continuous dose of omeprazole 10 mg daily is effective maintenance therapy for the majority of patients with heartburn but no esophagitis (NERD). However, a larger dose of omeprazole may be required for up to a quarter of patients.

A Cochrane review evaluating short-term treatment in NERD was updated in 2003,[351] but included only the studies reported by Bate *et al.* and by Venables *et al.*[132] as described above and concluded that PPI therapy was not more effective than H_2-RA therapy, since the 95% CI of the pooled estimates of the effects of the two interventions crossed 1.[352] However, the latest trial included in this review was published in 2000. Thus, this review requires further updating.

A randomized trial compared omeprazole in doses of 20 mg or 10 mg daily and placebo in 509 patients with NERD in whom heartburn was the predominant complaint.[74] Symptomatic remission of heartburn (no more than one day of mild symptoms in the week prior to the final visit) was significantly more frequent after 2–4 weeks of therapy with omeprazole in either dose, and the standard dose of omeprazole was more effective than the lower dose. Symptom relief occurred in most patients by the end of the second week. With 4 weeks of treatment the proportion of patients indicating sufficient control of heartburn was 66% and 57% for the standard and low doses of omeprazole and only 31% for the placebo group. Alc The more abnormal the initial pH study, the better the response to a greater degree of acid suppression. There was a significant correlation of response to therapy with acid reflux, age and the presence of a hiatus hernia. No correlation was identified between body mass index and degree of acid exposure, despite the widely held view that being overweight worsens reflux. A randomized trial of 4 weeks' duration in NERD patients in the USA[352] found omeprazole 20 mg once daily to be better than omeprazole 10 mg once daily or placebo for increasing the proportion of patients with no heartburn at both day 7 (omeprazole 20 mg 62%, 10 mg 41%, placebo 14%) or day 27 (omeprazole 20 mg 74%, 10 mg 49%, placebo 23%). Omeprazole was also significantly ($P = 0.003$) more effective than placebo for relief of acid regurgitation, dysphagia, epigastric pain, and nausea. Alc

In a randomized trial in primary care settings in Norway heartburn was adequately controlled in 71% of patients taking omeprazole 20 mg daily, 22% of patients receiving cisapride 20 mg twice daily and 18% of patients receiving placebo after 4 weeks of treatment.[353] Alc

Katz *et al.*[354] reported the results of two randomized, double blind, trials with identical methodology that compared esomeprazole 40 mg once daily or 20 mg once daily with placebo for 4 weeks in 717 NERD patients. Complete resolution of heartburn was achieved in 65% of patients treated with either esomeprazole dose compared with 40% of placebo patients ($P < 0.001$). Ala

Two studies of lansoprazole in NERD patients have been reported by Richter.[355,356] The first study[355] compared lansoprazole 15 mg, lansoprazole 30 mg or placebo for 8 weeks. Lansoprazole patients reported less daytime and night-time heartburn and antacid usage, compared with placebo patients. The second study[356] found lansoprazole to be more effective than ranitidine 150 mg twice daily or placebo. In this study, lansoprazole 15 mg and 30 mg daily were equally effective. Alc

A randomized trial compared pantoprazole 20 mg once daily versus omeprazole 20 mg once daily in patients with very mild grade 1 reflux esophagitis.[357] While these patients are not strictly a NERD population, grade 1 is considered by some investigators to be almost normal. The rates of symptom relief and healing were comparable at 4 and 8 weeks. Another trial of pantoprazole 20 mg once daily versus ranitidine 150 mg twice daily in a similar patient group with grades 0–1 GERD found pantoprazole to be superior to ranitidine.[358] Alc

This is an important study as it establishes that PPIs are superior to H_2-RAs not only in more severe erosive GERD but also in patients with virtually normal endoscopies.

A randomized trial comparing rabeprazole (10 mg or 20 mg once daily) with placebo in NERD patients with moderately severe symptoms found that rabeprazole, like other PPIs rapidly and effectively relieved heartburn.[359] Other symptoms such as regurgitation, belching, bloating, early satiety and nausea were also improved. There was no difference in efficacy between the two rabeprazole doses. Alc

Bytzer[360] has performed a comprehensive review of the studies dealing with symptomatic GERD.[74,132,349,350,352,353,355,356,359,361–364] The studies he included were not necessarily those that had NERD patients only; some of the studies also included patients with erosive esophagitis. Bytzer noted that the endpoint in many of these studies was that of complete heartburn relief, a result that most patients probably do not aim for in the long term. For example, in the "on-demand" studies, patients took their PPIs once every 2–3 days, that is patients seemed to accept that their symptoms would relapse before they took on-demand medication. Also, the lowest response rates were observed in the studies that evaluated complete symptom relief compared with those studies in which the endpoint was less rigorous and permitted continued therapy despite lack of complete symptom relief.

Long-term treatment of non-erosive reflux disease

Another approach in endoscopy negative heartburn patients is to allow patient controlled, on-demand therapy.

The first methodologically sound on-demand randomized trial in 424 NERD patients compared omeprazole 20 mg or 10 mg, with placebo[363] for the outcome of time to discontinuation of treatment (due to unwillingness to continue) over a 6-month period. With life-table analysis, the remission rates were omeprazole 20 mg 83% (95% CI 77 to 89%) omeprazole 10 mg 69% (61 to 77%) and placebo 56% (46 to 64%) ($P < 0.01$ for all intergroup differences). Alc The mean number of study medications used daily was between 0.43 to 0.47. Treatment failure was associated with more than a doubling of antacid use, and a deterioration in patient QOL.

Two "on-demand" trials with the newest PPI, esomeprazole have been published. The first compared esomeprazole 20 mg once daily with placebo in 342 NERD patients for 6 months after initial symptom relief with PPI.[364] The proportion of patients who discontinued treatment due to lack of heartburn relief were esomeprazole 14% and placebo 51% ($P < 0.0001$). Alc Most patients took the study medication for periods of 1–3 consecutive days (esomeprazole) or 4–13 consecutive days (placebo). Use of antacids was more than two-fold higher among placebo recipients. In the second study, patients who had achieved complete heartburn resolution after short-term esomeprazole or omeprazole treatment ($n = 721$) were randomized to esomeprazole 20 mg ($n = 282$), 40 mg ($n = 293$) or placebo ($n = 146$) on-demand (maximum one dose/day) for 6 months.[365] Treatment was discontinued (due to unwillingness to continue) less often by esomeprazole treated patients (esomeprazole 20 mg 8%, 40 mg 11%, placebo 42%). Alc Patients took an average of one esomeprazole tablet every 3 days.

Cost effectiveness analysis using a Markov model was designed to compare the following three strategies for 6 months: on-demand esomeprazole 20 mg daily, intermittent 4-week acute treatment courses of omeprazole 20 mg daily, and continuous omeprazole 20 mg daily treatment following acute treatment. The expected number of relapses per patient was estimated to be 0.10 for the on-demand esomeprazole strategy, 0.47–0.75 for continuous omeprazole treatment and 0.57–1.12 for the intermittent omeprazole strategy. The on-demand treatment with esomeprazole 20 mg was found to be cost effective compared with the other strategies.[366]

Treatment of mixed groups of patients: erosive esophagitis and non-erosive reflux disease (post-endoscopy studies)

The problem with these studies that combine erosive esophagitis healing and relief of NERD is that all patients needed to be endoscoped first in order to select patients for treatment. The first step in these trials was to subject all patients with the same symptoms to diagnostic endoscopy and to treat all the patients so that symptom relief could be compared. This approach would best represent the population of all patients that would present to the practitioner. This approach was used in a randomized trial in 221 patients[367] with heartburn as the predominant symptom (about half of whom had NERD and half grade II or III esophagitis). Omeprazole 20 mg daily produced significantly better heartburn relief than cimetidine 400 mg four times daily. The entry grade of esophagitis did not correlate with heartburn severity, and treatment benefit did not depend on presence or absence of esophagitis. Patients who were still symptomatic after the initial phase were treated for 4 weeks with omeprazole 20 mg daily and a further 67% of patients (54/81) improved.

Patients who improved in the acute study were randomized to receive maintenance therapy with omeprazole 10 mg daily or cimetidine 800 mg nocte for 6 months.[368] Omeprazole maintained control of heartburn in more patients at both 3 months (omeprazole 69%, cimetidine 27%) and 6 months (omeprazole 60%, cimetidine 24%; ARR 36, NNT 3; $P < 0.0001$). Seventy-six percent of omeprazole treated patients compared with 46% of the cimetidine group were also free of regurgitation ($P = 0.0002$). Alc

Another study conducted in general practice settings in the UK by Venables *et al.* in 994 patients with predominant heartburn was also reported in 1997.[132] All patients were endoscoped, and the grade of esophagitis was established, permitting symptom relief and mucosal healing assessments. Patients with ulcerative esophagitis were excluded. The majority of patients (68·2%) had NERD. Patients were randomized to therapy for 4 weeks with omeprazole 10 mg or 20 mg once daily or ranitidine 150 mg twice daily. Overall relief of heartburn was defined as no more than one day of mild heartburn out of the 7 days prior to the visit. Omeprazole 20 mg was the most effective therapy and the 10 mg omeprazole dose was also more effective than ranitidine (omeprazole 20 mg 61%, omeprazole 10 mg 49%, ranitidine 150 mg twice daily 40%, $P < 0.01$). Ala Subgroup analysis revealed that with omeprazole 20 mg daily, heartburn relief was achieved in 79% of patients with erosive esophagitis but in only 52% of patients with NERD. With omeprazole 10 mg daily, heartburn relief was 48% in erosive esophagitis patients and 50% in the NERD group. In the ranitidine arm, heartburn relief in patients with erosive esophagitis was less frequent

(33%) than in patients with NERD (44%). These results suggest that with more potent acid suppression, as occurs with omeprazole 20 mg, heartburn relief may occur as a result of mucosal healing, while ranitidine with its weaker degree of acid suppression was unable to heal the esophagitis and hence provide symptom relief. Similar findings were reported by Armstrong *et al.* in a study using pantoprazole 40 mg once daily versus nizatidine 150 mg twice daily for 4 weeks.[369] In this study, the majority of patients (57%) had erosive esophagitis. Complete heartburn relief was achieved in 63% pf pantoprazole patients at 4 weeks, compared with 36% of nizatidine patients. Complete heartburn relief was observed in the pantoprazole group more frequently in the subgroup of patients with erosive esophagitis, (70%) than in the group with NERD (53%), but in the nizatidine group, there was a trend toward less symptom relief in patients with erosive disease (34%) than in patients with NERD (43%).[369] Alc

In another primary care study, patients were screened with the Carlsson–Dent questionnaire,[136] and those with a score suggestive of GERD were included after initial endoscopy.[361] NERD patients (48·5%) were randomized to placebo, omeprazole 10 mg or 20 mg once daily for 4 weeks, and patients with erosive esophagitis (51·5%) were randomized to omeprazole 10 mg or 20 mg once daily for 4 weeks. Baseline heartburn was present in 83·5% of NERD patients and in 95% of patients with erosive GERD. Treatment benefit was greater in endoscopy positive than in endoscopy negative patients for all treatment arms. After the initial treatment phase, patients were followed for 6 months without therapy. Relapse rates were high (esophagitis 90%, NERD 75%). These results suggest that NERD patients were more heterogeneous than those with endoscopically documented disease. Patient QOL was also evaluated in this study. Baseline PGWB scores were reduced in all patients prior to treatment and the scores improved to a similar extent in all treatment arms. The GSRS reflux dimension improved significantly ($P < 0.01$) in NERD patients after treatment with omeprazole and in those with erosive disease. Omeprazole 20 mg was superior to the 10 mg dose. Alc

The newer esomeprazole 40 mg once daily was compared with esomeprazole 20 mg twice daily or placebo in a mixed population of patients with erosive and non-erosive GERD.[154] The sensitivity of an esomeprazole treatment test in confirming GERD increased during the first days of treatment and was 79–86% after 5 days (both esomeprazole arms) compared with the observed sensitivity with placebo of 36%. Subgroup analysis of heartburn relief for the erosive versus NERD patients was not done.

It appears that patients with NERD do not respond as well to PPIs as those with erosive esophagitis.[370] Part of the reason may be that patients who do not have esophagitis are relatively refractory to the pharmacodynamic effects of PPIs on post-prandial integrated gastric acidity.[371]

Symptomatic gastroesophageal reflux disease: empirical therapy (uninvestigated patients)

The most pragmatic situation is at the primary care level, where patients present with predominant reflux symptoms of heartburn or acid regurgitation. If these patients do not have alarm symptoms, there is a considerable degree of agreement that they should be treated empirically with antisecretory therapy without prior endoscopy. With this approach in mind there has been a trend towards trials in patients without initial investigations, that is treating uninvestigated patients with the predominant symptom of heartburn. This is a mixed group of patients, of whom many do not have esophagitis.

A randomized, 4-week trial that included 424 patients with a history of proved esophagitis enrolled from general practices in the UK[372] showed that omeprazole 20 mg once daily was more effective for relief of heartburn and regurgitation than ranitidine 150 mg twice daily (omeprazole 59%, ranitidine 27%, ARR 22%, NNT 5). Ala The prior history of esophagitis limits generalizability of this study to all patients in primary care practices, but the good relief of symptoms regardless of initial symptom severity is noteworthy.

In a trial in primary care settings in the USA, 590 patients with moderately severe symptomatic GERD were randomized without endoscopy to receive ranitidine 150 mg twice daily or a placebo.[373] Ranitidine rapidly and significantly improved heartburn severity scores, physician global assessment of the response to treatment, and the SF-36 score for physical functioning, bodily pain and vitality dimensions. Ala Using a heartburn specific questionnaire a significant improvement in all dimensions: physical, heartburn pain, sleep, diet, social functioning and mental health was observed for ranitidine-treated patients.

In another American trial uninvestigated heartburn patients were randomized to receive either ranitidine, lansoprazole or stepped up therapy from ranitidine to lansoprazole or stepped down therapy from lansoprazole to ranitidine.[374] The continuous lansoprazole treatment was better than the other strategies in terms of reducing heartburn severity and increasing the number of heartburn-free days, and there appeared to be little rationale to stepping down to ranitidine.

A randomized trial[375] of 307 patients with GERD symptoms in Australian primary care settings showed that even a low dose of pantoprazole (20 mg daily) was significantly more effective than ranitidine 300 mg daily for complete control of symptoms at 4 weeks (40% v 19%; $P < 0.001$), 8 weeks (55% v 33%; $P < 0.001$), 6 months (71% v 56%; $P = 0.007$) and 12 months (77% v 59%; $P = 0.001$).

In the CADET-HR randomized, double blind trial in Canadian primary care settings 390 patients with reflux-predominant symptoms were randomized to receive ranitidine 150 mg twice daily or omeprazole 20 mg daily.[376] Heartburn relief at 4 weeks was reported by 55% of omeprazole and 27% of ranitidine-treated patients. Ala Greater improvements in GSRS for indigestion, abdominal pain, and reflux ($P < 0.05$) and in the GASTROQoL health-related QOL scales ($P < 0.003$) were also observed in omeprazole patients. After 4 weeks, patients with inadequate symptom relief were stepped up every 4–8 weeks from ranitidine to omeprazole 20 mg once daily or from omeprazole 20 mg once to twice daily.[377] "Step up" occurred in 100 patients with ranitidine and 57 with omeprazole. With step up therapy, by 16-weeks, heartburn relief resulted in 88% of patients who started with omeprazole and in 87% of those who started with ranitidine. Ala In the first 8 weeks, omeprazole provided complete heartburn relief in 53% while it took 16 weeks to achieve similar degree of relief in the group who were treated with ranitidine first. Thus, starting with omeprazole therapy produced significantly faster symptom relief. Patient responders then had the medications stopped, and 50% of patients experienced symptomatic relapse within 9 days.[378] Only 10% of patients had no further relapse over a 6-month period of follow up.

In a Cochrane review evaluating short-term treatment in symptomatic, non-endoscoped patients updated in 2003,[351] van Pinxteren *et al.* observed that the relative risk for not experiencing heartburn remission in placebo-controlled trials for PPI was 0·35 for PPI, 0·77 for H_2-RAs and 0·86 for prokinetics. In direct comparative trials PPIs were significantly ($P < 0.05$) more effective than H2-RAs (three trials, RR 0·67, 95% CI 0·57 to 0·80) and prokinetics. Thus, PPIs were superior to H2-RAs in empirical treatment of typical GERD symptoms. Ala

A large, methodologically sound, double blind, randomized trial in 3034 patients in 360 sites in the USA, patients with symptomatic, uninvestigated GERD symptoms received lansoprazole 30 mg once daily or esomeprazole 40 mg once daily[379] and heartburn assessments were carried out at days 1, 3, 7 and 14. The study setting was unclear and was unlikely to be all primary care practices. No statistically significant difference in heartburn relief were observed.[379] Ala Patients indicated that they were very pleased with their treatment, experienced substantial benefit and would recommend the medication to others. However, nearly 40% of patients still had some degree of day or night heartburn at the end of 2 weeks.

An interesting study evaluated a patient's willingness to pay for complete symptom relief in GERD.[380] The authors found that patients were willing to pay up to US$182 to obtain completer and faster symptom relief without side effects. Older patients were less willing to pay than younger patients to obtain symptom relief.

Economic evaluation in uninvestigated symptomatic heartburn

The costs and effectiveness of each drug and of each management strategy need to be evaluated. However, there are many subtle variations between studies that render direct comparisons difficult. Furthermore, decision analyses suffer from the inherent weakness of having to rely on estimates of treatment outcomes. Ofman recently reviewed the cost effectiveness studies in symptomatic GERD.[381] He concluded that the most cost effective strategies are PPI based step-down or PPI on-demand strategies.[381] He noted that most decision analyses had been constructed around uninvestigated GERD symptoms.

Does symptom improvement predict healing of esophagitis?

There is evidence that relief of symptoms by H_2-RAs does not predict healing of mucosal damage. Patients with heartburn initially treated in a 4-week study with omeprazole or cimetidine[367] were randomized to receive maintenance therapy with either omeprazole 10 mg once daily or cimetidine 800 mg nocte for 24 weeks.[368] Symptomatic remission, defined as no more than mild heartburn on 1 out of the 7 previous days was significantly more frequent with omeprazole (omeprazole 60%, cimetidine 24%; ARR 36%, NNT 3). Erosive esophagitis was seen in only 10% of patients in symptomatic remission on omeprazole compared with 33% on cimetidine.

One third of patients with relapse of erosive esophagitis by endoscopy during maintenance therapy with famotidine 40 mg twice daily were completely asymptomatic.[382]

A meta-analysis[307] suggested that if heartburn resolved, only 4·5% of patients treated with omeprazole 20 mg once daily but 14·6% with ranitidine 150 mg twice daily experienced asymptomatic relapse of endoscopic erosive esophagitis. Alc

The more recent trials show that significantly fewer esomeprazole treated patients had persistent esophagitis despite symptom relief than is the case for omeprazole-reated patients.[19,274] In patients with heartburn resolution at 4 weeks, esophagitis remained unhealed in 14·8%[274] to 16·8%[19] of patients receiving esomeprazole 40 mg daily compared with 23·2%[274] to 26·9%[19] of those receiving omeprazole 20 mg daily. Ala A similar result was seen in a comparison of esomeprazole 40 mg daily and lansoprazole 30 mg daily, with unhealed esophagitis in spite of heartburn resolution in 17·3% and 20·5% of these patients.[383] In the most severe forms of esophagitis, the healing was 11% better for grade C and 17% for grade D disease in esomeprazole-treated patients. It is unclear why, despite effective symptom resolution, many patients still have esophagitis. The most likely explanation in these studies is that when patients were healed at 4 weeks, they came out of the studies and the healing and symptom resolution could not be assessed at 8 weeks. In all these studies, esophagitis healing was much better at 8 weeks than at 4 weeks and had the patients been endoscoped at that time

point, the proportion of healed patients among those with heartburn resolution would have been expected to be higher.

These data thus support the recommendation that the most effective therapy, the PPI that achieves most potent acid suppression should be prescribed, since healing is best with PPI and a majority of patients who become heartburn free will also have healed mucosa. Since healing improves with prolonged therapy, these patients should receive continuous therapy.[32,285] Intermittent and on-demand strategies are not recommended because they leave increased numbers of patients with unhealed esophagitis. Alc C5

Treatment of esophageal peptic stricture

Esophageal peptic stricture, the most severe GERD complication, is difficult to manage. The H_2-RA may be marginally more effective than a placebo for reducing the need for repeat dilatations.[384,385] One study found no benefit from ranitidine 300 mg daily compared with placebo.[386] There are two randomized trials comparing standard dose omeprazole 20 mg daily with H_2-RA[387,388] and one comparing lansoprazole with high dose ranitidine.[389]

In one small study,[388] 34 patients with strictures were randomized to receive omeprazole 20 mg once daily, or ranitidine 150 mg or famotidine 20 mg twice daily. After 3 months, if esophagitis remained unhealed, the dose of medication was doubled and the patient was re-endoscoped at 6 months. At 3 months, there was no significant difference between PPI and H_2-RA for esophagitis healing or relief of dysphagia, although there was a trend in favor of the PPI. By 6 months, omeprazole treatment resulted in significantly better healing of esophagitis (omeprazole 100%, H_2-RA 53%; ARR 47%, NNT 2; $P < 0.01$) and relief of dysphagia (omeprazole 94%, H_2-RA 40%; ARR 54%, NNT = 2; $P < 0.01$). Ald *Post hoc* analysis also showed a trend to fewer dilatations required in omeprazole-treated patients (omeprazole 41%, H_2-RA 73%; $P = 0.07$). The number of dilatations required was significantly less for the omeprazole-treated patients (11 *v* 31 dilatations, mean of 0·6 *v* 2·1 sessions per patient, $P < 0.01$). Cost effectiveness analysis for healing and relief of dysphagia, that included costs of drugs, endoscopy and dilatations, and management of perforations, showed that omeprazole was 40–50% more cost effective than H_2-RA.

A second adequately powered trial compared constant doses of omeprazole 20 mg once daily and ranitidine 150 mg twice daily for 1 year.[387] Endoscopy was done as required and at the end of the study. Repeat dilatation was required less frequently in omeprazole-treated patients (omeprazole 30%, ranitidine 46%; ARR 16%, NNT 6). Alc Fewer dilatation sessions were required in omeprazole-treated patients (omeprazole 0·48, ranitidine 1·08; $P < 0.01$). Omeprazole was also superior with respect to the number of patients without stricture at the end of the study, esophagitis healing and improved heartburn and dysphagia.

In a study of 158 patients over 6 months, lansoprazole 30 mg daily was more effective than ranitidine 300 mg twice daily for relieving dysphagia. There was a trend toward a reduction in the need for repeat dilatations (lansoprazole 30·8%, ranitidine 43·8%; $P = 0·09$) over 12 months.[389] Ald

In an observational study 30 of 36 patients with reflux esophagitis and stricture treated with dilatation and omeprazole 20 mg twice daily for 6–8 weeks experienced healing of esophagitis and relief of dysphagia.[390] These 30 patients were then randomized to receive omeprazole 20 mg twice daily, lansoprazole 30 mg twice daily or pantoprazole 40 mg twice daily ($n = 10$ each arm). After 4 weeks of treatment, significantly more omeprazole-treated patients remained healed, but no difference was seen with respect to the need to repeat dilatation of strictures. This small study may lack power to demonstrate differences between effects of these strategies. Ald

Endoscopic treatments

Several endoscopic techniques have now been described and show some promise.[391,392] None are ready to replace the more traditional methods of managing GERD but are mentioned here briefly to introduce the concepts. These methods attempt to bolster or "strengthen" the defective lower esophageal sphincter in order to improve the mechanical barrier or to "injure" the LES and diminish spontaneous sphincter relaxations. There are three major methods used: (i) folds of the gastric cardia are plicated with sutures deployed through the endoscope; (ii) thermal injury is applied to the muscle of the LES; and (iii) inert substances are placed/injected into the region of the LES. The major advantages of these techniques are that they are potentially minimally invasive, they are performed in an outpatient setting and they have the potential to remove the need for long-term, costly medical treatments. Large, properly designed randomized trials comparing these new techniques to medical therapy are lacking and 1-year follow up reports are just emerging from the observational studies.[391]

Endoscopic suturing

Filipi reported on 64 GERD patients with 6-month follow up.[393] The average procedure time was 68 minutes, 11 patients needed general anesthesia, and 11 patients needed more than one procedure. These data certainly do not begin to fulfill the promise of a straightforward, routine outpatient procedure. While heartburn improved, objective measures were less impressive. While 24-hour pH values improved, the values were still in the abnormal range, there was no change in LES pressures and esophagitis healed in only 25% of patients. B4 One patient sustained a suture perforation that was treated with antibiotics. PPI use was decreased in 62% of patients, a result that is similar to that reported by Mahmood in a similar study with 1-year follow up.[394] In this latter smaller series of 26 patients (four lost to follow up), complications included bleeding and a gastric tear. Rothstein[395] reviewed the available literature and concluded that the Endocinch procedure seemed safe and gave good short-term symptom relief. However, he noted that normalization of 24-hour total acid exposure rarely occurred and no significant healing of esophagitis was seen. B4

Radio-frequency energy (Stretta procedure)

Triadafilopoulos *et al.*[396] reported the first observational study of patients treated with radiofrequency energy application to create thermal lesions submucosally at the level of the gastroesophageal junction (the Stretta procedure). In contrast to the suturing methods above, there was 50% healing of grades I and II esophagitis at 6 months. These authors also reported[397] significant improvements in reflux symptoms, satisfaction, and mental and physical quality of life in a larger group followed for one year. Esophageal acid exposure significantly improved but was still in the abnormal range. The need for chronic PPI therapy fell from 88% to 30% but drug use could not be completely stopped. B4 Complications arose in 9% of patients. Vakil and Sharma reported that there were significant, serious complications such as hematemesis and perforations resulting in repeat surgeries and deaths.[392]

Injection therapies

An example of this approach is the use of Enteryx, a preparation of polyvinyl alcohol with tantalum that is injected into the muscle layer of the esophagus. Johnson *et al.* reported a 12-month follow up of a multicenter observational study in 85 patients.[398] This procedure took a mean time of 34 minutes to complete. Over 90% of patients suffered chest pain after the procedure with resolution of pain in only 83% of patients after 2 weeks. Dysphagia occurred in 20% of patients. At 3 months, implant volume had slipped to 75% of original as assessed radiographically. At 12 months, 77% of 81 evaluable patients were treatment responders and of these, 67% had stopped PPI use. B4 Nearly a quarter of patients required reimplantation, usually 1–3 months after the first procedure. Esophageal pH was normalized in 39% of patients at 12 months, a result that may be better than that reported in the observational studies of suturing or the radiofrequency procedures. There was worsening of esophagitis grade in 27% and improvement in 18% of patients and the rest were unchanged.

Antireflux surgery

Medical therapy versus surgical antireflux therapy

Two older randomized trials comparing antireflux surgery with medical therapy provided evidence that surgery was more effective.[399,400] Alc Unfortunately, these studies are no longer relevant, since they do not take into account present day optimal medical therapy with PPIs and laparoscopic surgery.

However, Spechler *et al.* have provided an update of the patients in the original study.[401] They were able to account for a remarkable 97% (239/247) of the original cohort, 79 of whom had died. After a mean of 9–10 years follow up, regular antireflux medications were taken by 92% of the medical patients and 62% of the surgical patients ($P < 0.001$). Survival was significantly decreased in the surgical treatment group, mostly because of excess deaths from heart disease. The nature of the association between surgery and these deaths is unclear. Patients with Barrett's esophagus at baseline developed esophageal adenocarcinomas at an annual rate of 0·4%, whereas these cancers developed in patients without Barrett's at an annual rate of 0·07%. This study suggests that antireflux surgery should not be advised with the expectation that patients with GERD will no longer need to take anti-secretory medications or that the procedure prevents esophageal cancer among those with GERD and Barrett metaplasia. Alc

There are remarkably few direct comparisons of a PPI versus antireflux surgery. There are limited data, from one study with 5-year follow up[300] and from one pharmacological study of shorter duration.[402]

The first is the large study by Lundell *et al.* with 5-year follow up.[300] Three hundred and ten patients were randomized to receive open surgical fundoplication or continuous omeprazole therapy and followed for up to 5 years. Only 11 of 155 patients randomized to surgery refused the treatment. Omeprazole-treated patients were allowed dose increases to 40–60 mg daily to control symptoms. No significant differences in efficacy were demonstrated and QOL assessments (PGWB and GSRS) improved in both groups. Thus, surgical therapy was as effective as continuous omeprazole therapy in this trial. Ala However, laparoscopic fundoplication, the technique that is now widely used, was not performed.

A more recent, short-term observational study compared the efficacy of laparoscopic fundoplication and lansoprazole in normalizing abnormal reflux in patients with GERD.[402] Post antireflux surgery, all 55 patients were heartburn free and esophageal pH-monitoring 3–6 months after surgery was normal in 85% of patients. Patients treated with lansoprazole were titrated upwards to 90 mg daily and esophageal acid exposure was normalized in 96% of cases. Patients who became heartburn free did not necessarily normalize their esophageal acid exposure. Thus, to achieve the results of this study, all patients would require follow up 24-hour pH studies, an impractical situation. The results suggest that either approach may be reasonable for any given patient. B4

The data above do not support the contention that antireflux surgery is superior to PPIs, which are safe and effective medical therapies.[403] Surgical protagonists argue that medical therapies do not correct the underlying anatomical abnormalities. However, there are no long-term data to support the view that surgery achieves this result permanently either. One small follow up observational study of patients after 20 years demonstrated that about 30% of the fundoplications were defective, and abnormal reflux on esophageal pH studies was also seen in about 30% of patients assessed.[404] B4 Another study of 441 patients after a mean follow up of 18 years following the Hill procedure for GERD, reported good and excellent subjective results in 80% of patients.[405] B4 Thus, the results of fundoplication are reasonable but not completely durable. Even after 1 year, 6% of patients will require PPI therapy.[406] There is no evidence that surgery prevents progression to Barrett's metaplasia or protects against esophageal cancer.[406]

One randomized trial of open versus laparoscopic fundoplication[407] found no difference between the two approaches and more than 85% of patients were satisfied with their results. The major advantage for laparoscopic fundoplication is a significant reduction in hospital stay from 8–9 days for an open procedure to 2–5 days,[408–410] and less time off work for the patient (laparoscopic 21·3 days, open surgery 38·2 days, $P = 0.02$).[409] Thus, the procedure of choice is laparoscopic fundoplication; however, data on long-term outcomes are lacking. Ald

Surgical results continue to depend on surgical expertise, and the issue of a learning curve remains.[409,411] An intraoperative complication rate of 8% has been reported.[411] The most frequent adverse effects are dysphagia, inability to belch or vomit, postprandial fullness, bloating, pain and flatus.[412] Also, laparoscopic fundoplication is not without serious complications such as esophageal perforation, paraesopheageal herniations, pneumothorax and splenic damage requiring splenectomy.[413]

For some patients, there may be incomplete symptom relief with PPI therapy. In one randomized trial of antireflux surgery and omeprazole, those patients who were not improved on omeprazole 40 mg daily were offered antireflux surgery and fared well.[406] B4 Thus some patients with a partial response to PPIs may improve with antireflux surgery. However, it is of concern that 6/178 (3%) of these patients experienced postoperative complications that necessitated reoperation.

The best results with ARS are obtained in the patient with typical reflux symptoms, an abnormal esophageal pH study and good symptomatic response to PPIs.[370] Thus, the best indication for surgery is a patient who responds well to PPI but does not wish to take continuous medications to control their reflux.[414,415] B4 C5 With the relative ease and safety of laparoscopic surgery, it has become a reasonable alternative for selected patients. As with all surgery, patient selection has improved through objective testing with pre-operative esophageal pH-metry and manometry. Even if cost-effectiveness modeling studies favor surgery, a decision to have surgery should not be imposed upon a patient. Ultimately, the final decision should rest on the preferences of an informed patient.

References

1 Kitchin LI, Castell DO. Rationale and efficacy of conservative therapy for gastroesophageal reflux disease. *Arch Intern Med* 1991;**151**:448–54.

2 Fass R, Ofman JJ. Gastroesophageal reflux disease – should we adopt a new conceptual framework? *Am J Gastroenterol* 2002;**97**:1901–9.

3 Chiba N. Definitions of dyspepsia: time for a reappraisal. *Eur J Surg* 1998;**Suppl 583**:14–23.

4 Veldhuyzen van Zanten SJ, Flook N, Chiba N *et al.* An evidence-based approach to the management of uninvestigated dyspepsia in the era of *Helicobacter pylori.* Canadian Dyspepsia Working Group. *Can Med Assoc J* 2000;**162(Suppl 12)**:S3–S23.

5 Eloubeidi MA, Provenzale D. Health-related quality of life and severity of symptoms in patients with Barrett's esophagus and gastroesophageal reflux disease patients without Barrett's esophagus. *Am J Gastroenterol* 2000;**95**: 1881–7.

6 Wiklund I, Bardhan KD, Müller LS *et al.* Quality of life during acute and intermittent treatment of gastro-oesophageal reflux disease with omeprazole compared with ranitidine. Results from a multicentre clinical trial. The European Study Group. *Ital J Gastroenterol Hepatol* 1998;**30**:19–27.

7 Glise H. Quality of life and cost of therapy in reflux disease. *Scand J Gastroenterol Suppl* 1995;**210**:38–42.

8 Talley NJ, Stanghellini V, Heading RC, Koch KL, Malagelada JR, Tytgat GN. Functional gastroduodenal disorders. *Gut* 1999;**45(Suppl 2)**:II37–II42.

9 Dent J, Brun J, Fendrick AM *et al*, on behalf of the Genval Workshop Group. An evidence-based appraisal of reflux disease management – the Genval Workshop Report. *Gut* 1999;**44(Suppl 2)**:S1–S16.

10 Moayyedi P, Axon AT. The usefulness of the likelihood ratio in the diagnosis of dyspepsia and gastroesophageal reflux disease. *Am J Gastroenterol* 1999;**94**:3122–5.

11 Chiba N, de Gara CJ, Wilkinson JM, Hunt RH. Speed of healing and symptom relief in grade II to IV gastro-esophageal reflux disease: a meta-analysis. *Gastroenterology* 1997;**112**:1798–810.

12 Thomson AB, Barkun AN, Armstrong D *et al.* The prevalence of clinically significant endoscopic findings in primary care patients with uninvestigated dyspepsia: the Canadian Adult Dyspepsia Empiric Treatment-Prompt Endoscopy (CADET-PE) study. *Aliment Pharmacol Ther* 2003;**17**:1481–91.

13 DeVault KR, Castell DO. Updated guidelines for the diagnosis and treatment of gastroesophageal reflux disease. The Practice Parameters Committee of the American College of Gastroenterology. *Am J Gastroenterol* 1999;**94**:1434–42.

14 Vcev A, Stimac D, Vceva A *et al.* Lansoprazole versus omeprazole in the treatment of reflux esophagitis. *Acta Med Croatica* 1997;**51**:171–4.

15 Johnsson F, Joelsson B, Gudmundsson K, Greiff L. Symptoms and endoscopic findings in the diagnosis of gastroesophageal reflux disease. *Scand J Gastroenterol* 1987;**22**:714–18.

16 Klauser AG, Heinrich C, Schindlbeck NE, Müller-Lissner SA. Is long-term esophageal pH monitoring of clinical value? *Am J Gastroenterol* 1989;**84**:362–6.

17 Talley NJ, Colin-Jones D, Koch KL, Koch M, Nyren O, Stanghellini V. Functional dyspepsia: a classification with guidelines for diagnosis and management. *Gastroenterol Int* 1991;**4**:145–60.

18 Dekkers CP, Beker JA, Thjodleifsson B, Gabryelewicz A, Bell NE, Humphries TJ. Double-blind comparison [correction of Double-blind, placebo-controlled comparison] of rabeprazole 20 mg vs. omeprazole 20 mg in the treatment of erosive or ulcerative gastrooesophageal reflux disease. The European Rabeprazole Study Group. *Aliment Pharmacol Ther* 1999; **13**:49–57.

19 Kahrilas PJ, Falk GW, Johnson DA *et al.* Esomeprazole improves healing and symptom resolution as compared with omeprazole in reflux oesophagitis patients: a randomized controlled trial. The Esomeprazole Study Investigators. *Aliment Pharmacol Ther* 2000;**14**:1249–58.

20 Richter JE, Kahrilas PJ, Sontag SJ, Kovacs TO, Huang B, Pencyla JL. Comparing lansoprazole and omeprazole in onset of heartburn relief: results of a randomized, controlled trial in erosive esophagitis patients. *Am J Gastroenterol* 2001; **96**:3089–98.

21 Locke GR, Talley NJ, Fett SL, Zinsmeister AR, Melton LJ. Prevalence and clinical spectrum of gastroesophageal reflux: a population-based study in Olmsted County, Minnesota. *Gastroenterology* 1997;**112**:1448–56.

22 Thompson WG, Heaton KW. Heartburn and globus in apparently healthy people. *Can Med Assoc J* 1982;**126**: 46–8.

23 Wong WM, Lai KC, Lam KF, Hui WM *et al.* Prevalence, clinical spectrum and health care utilization of gastro-oesophageal reflux disease in a Chinese population: a population-based study. *Aliment Pharmacol Ther* 2003;**18**: 595–604.

24 Nebel OT, Forbes MF, Castell DO. Symptomatic gastroesophageal reflux: incidence and precipitating factors. *Am J Dig Dis* 1976;**21**:953–6.

25 Isolauri J, Laippala P. Prevalence of symptoms suggestive of gastroesophageal reflux disease in an adult population. *Ann Med* 1995;**27**:67–70.

26 Anonymous. *Heartburn across America: A Gallup Organization national survey.* Princeton, NJ: Gallup Organization, 1988.

27 Diaz-Rubio M, Moreno-Elola-Olaso C, Rey E, Locke GR, Rodriguez-Artalejo F. Symptoms of gastro-oesophageal reflux: prevalence, severity, duration and associated factors in a Spanish population. *Aliment Pharmacol Ther* 2004;**19**: 95–105.

28 Haque M, Wyeth JW, Stace NH, Talley NJ, Green R. Prevalence, severity and associated features of gastro-oesophageal reflux and dyspepsia: a population-based study. *NZ Med J* 2000;**113**:178–81.

29 Ho KY, Kang JY, Seow A. Prevalence of gastrointestinal symptoms in a multiracial Asian population, with particular reference to reflux-type symptoms. *Am J Gastroenterol* 1998;**93**:1816–22.

30 Wong WM, Lam SK, Hui WM *et al.* Long-term prospective follow-up of endoscopic oesophagitis in southern Chinese – prevalence and spectrum of the disease. *Aliment Pharmacol Ther* 2002;**16**:2037–42.

31 Richter JE, Kahrilas PJ, Sontag SJ, Kovacs TO, Huang B, Pencyla JL. Comparing lansoprazole and omeprazole in onset of heartburn relief: results of a randomized, controlled trial in erosive esophagitis patients. *Am J Gastroenterol* 2001;**96**:3089–98.

32 Johnson DA, Benjamin SB, Vakil NB *et al.* Esomeprazole once daily for 6 months is effective therapy for maintaining healed erosive esophagitis and for controlling gastroesophageal reflux disease symptoms: a randomized, double-blind, placebo-controlled study of efficacy and safety. *Am J Gastroenterol* 2001;**96**:27–34.

33 Brunnen PL, Karmody AM, Needham CD. Severe peptic oesophagitis. *Gut* 1969;**10**:831–7.

34 el Serag HB, Sonnenberg A. Associations between different forms of gastro-oesophageal reflux disease. *Gut* 1997;**41**: 594–9.

35 Fass R. Epidemiology and pathophysiology of symptomatic gastroesophageal reflux disease. *Am J Gastroenterol* 2003;**98**:S2–S7.

36 Dent J, Holloway RH, Toouli J, Dodds WJ. Mechanisms of lower oesophageal sphincter incompetence in patients with symptomatic gastro-oesophageal reflux. *Gut* 1988;**29**: 120–8.

37 Dent J. Recent views on the pathogenesis of gastro-oesophageal reflux disease. *Baillieres Clin Gastroenterol* 1987;**1**:727–45.

38 Holloway RH, Hongo M, Berger K, McCallum RW. Gastric distension: a mechanism for postprandial gastroesophageal reflux. *Gastroenterology* 1985;**89**:779–84.

39 Venables CW. Mucus, pepsin and peptic ulcer. *Gut* 1986; **27**:233–8.

40 Goldberg HI, Dodds WJ, Gee S, Montgomery C, Zboralske FF. Role of acid and pepsin in acute experimental esophagitis. *Gastroenterology* 1969;**56**:223–30.

41 Mittal RK, Lange RC, McCallum RW. Identification and mechanism of delayed esophageal acid clearance in subjects with hiatus hernia. *Gastroenterology* 1987;**92**:130–5.

42 Sloan S, Kahrilas PJ. Impairment of esophageal emptying with hiatal hernia. *Gastroenterology* 1991;**100**:596–605.

43 van Herwaarden MA, Samsom M, Smout AJ. Excess gastroesophageal reflux in patients with hiatus hernia is caused by mechanisms other than transient LES relaxations. *Gastroenterology* 2000;**119**:1439–46.

44 Trimble KC, Pryde A, Heading RC. Lowered oesophageal sensory thresholds in patients with symptomatic but not excess gastro-oesophageal reflux: evidence for a spectrum of visceral sensitivity in GORD. *Gut* 1995;**37**:7–12.

45 Shi G, Bruley des Varannes S, Scarpignato C, Le Rhun M, Galmiche JP. Reflux related symptoms in patients with normal oesophageal exposure to acid. *Gut* 1995;**37**:457–64.

46 Eriksen CA, Cullen PT, Sutton D, Kennedy N, Cushieri A. Abnormal esophageal transit in patients with typical reflux symptoms but normal endoscopic and pH profiles. *Am J Surg* 1991;**161**:657–61.

47 Schlesinger PK, Donahue PE, Schmid B, Layden TJ. Limitations of 24-hour intraesophageal pH monitoring in the hospital setting. *Gastroenterology* 1985;**89**:797–804.

48 DeMeester TR, Wang CI, Wernly JA *et al.* Technique, indications, and clinical use of 24 hour esophageal pH monitoring. *J Thorac Cardiovasc Surg* 1980;**79**:656–70.

49 Masclee AAM, De Best ACAM, De Graaf R, Cluysenaer OJJ, Jansen JBMJ. Ambulatory 24-hour pH-metry in the diagnosis of gastroesophageal reflux disease. Determination of criteria and relation to endoscopy. *Scand J Gastroenterol* 1990;**25**: 225–30.

50 Zentilin P, Dulbecco P, Bilardi C *et al.* Circadian pattern of intragastric acidity in patients with non-erosive reflux disease (NERD). *Aliment Pharmacol Ther* 2003;**17**:353–9.

51 Fiorucci S, Santucci L, Chiucchiú S, Morelli A. Gastric acidity and gastroesophageal reflux patterns in patients with esophagitis. *Gastroenterology* 1992;**103**:855–61.

52 Fass R, Naliboff B, Higa L, Johnson C, Kodner A, Munakata J, Ngo J, Mayer EA. Differential effect of long-term esophageal acid exposure on mechanosensitivity and chemosensitivity in humans. *Gastroenterology* 1998;**115**:1363–73.

53 Carlsson R, Fandriks L, Jonsson C, Lundell L, Orlando RC. Is the esophageal squamous epithelial barrier function impaired in patients with gastroesophageal reflux disease? *Scand J Gastroenterol* 1999;**34**:454–8.

54 Weusten BL, Akkermans LM, vanBerge-Henegouwen GP, Smout AJ. Symptom perception in gastroesophageal reflux disease is dependent on spatiotemporal reflux characteristics. *Gastroenterology* 1995;**108**:1739–44.

55 Cicala M, Emerenziani S, Caviglia R *et al.* Intra-oesophageal distribution and perception of acid reflux in patients with non-erosive gastro-oesophageal reflux disease. *Aliment Pharmacol Ther* 2003;**18**:605–13.

56 Breen KJ, Whelan G. The diagnosis of reflux oesophagitis: an evaluation of five investigative procedures. *Aust NZ J Surg* 1978;**48**:156–61.

57 Kaul B, Petersen H, Grette K, Erichsen H, Myrvold HE. Scintigraphy, pH measurement, and radiography in the evaluation of gastoesophageal reflux. *Scand J Gastroenterol* 1985;**20**:289–94.

58 Kaul B, Petersen H, Myrvold HE. Hiatus hernia in gastro-esophageal reflux disease. *Scand J Gastroenterol* 1986; **21**:31–4.

59 Berstad A, Weberg R, Frøyshov Larsen I, Hoel B, Hauer Jensen M. Relationship of hiatus hernia to reflux esophagitis. A prospective study of coincidence, using endoscopy. *Scand J Gastroenterol* 1986;**21**:55–8.

60 Smout AJPM, Geus WP, Mulder PGH, Stockbrügger RW, Lamers CBHW. Gastro-oesophageal reflux disease in the Netherlands. Results of a multicentre pH study. *Scand J Gastroenterol* 1996;**31(Suppl 218)**:10–15.

61 Cameron AJ. Barrett's esophagus: prevalence and size of hiatal hernia. *Am J Gastroenterol* 1999;**94**:2054–9.

62 Agreus L, Svardsudd K, Talley NJ, Jones MP, Tibblin G. Natural history of gastroesophageal reflux disease and functional abdominal disorders: a population-based study. Am J Gastroenterol 2001;**96**:2905–14.

63 Pace F, Santalucia F, Bianchi Porro G. Natural history of gastroesophageal reflux disease without esophagitis. *Gut* 1991;**32**:845–8.

64 Isolauri J, Luostarinen M, Isolauri E, Reinikainen P, Viljakka M, Keyriläinen O. Natural course of gastroesophageal reflux disease: 17–22 year follow-up of 60 patients. *Am J Gastroenterol* 1997;**92**:37–41.

65 Ollyo JB, Monnier P, Fontolliet C, Savary M. The natural history, prevalence and incidence of reflux oesophagitis. *Gullet* 1993;**3(Suppl 3)**:3–10.

66 McDougall NI, Johnston BT, Kee F, Collins JSA, McFarland RJ, Love AHG. Natural history of reflux oesophagitis: a 10 year follow up of its effect on patient symptomatology and quality of life. *Gut* 1996;**38**:481–6.

67 Lagergren J, Bergstrom R, Lindgren A, Nyren O. Symptomatic gastroesophageal reflux as a risk factor for esophageal adenocarcinoma. *N Engl J Med* 1999;**340**:825–31.

68 Ben Rejeb M, Bouché O, Zeitoun P. Study of 47 consecutive patients with peptic esophageal stricture compared with 3880 cases of reflux esophagitis. *Dig Dis Sci* 1992;**37**:733–6.

69 Heading RC. Epidemiology of oesophageal reflux disease. *Scand J Gastroenterol* 1989;**24**:33–7.

70 Wienbeck M, Barnert J. Epidemiology of reflux disease and reflux esophagitis. *Scand J Gastroenterol* 1989;**24**:7–13.

71 Ware JEJ, Sherbourne CD. The MOS 36-item short-form health survey (SF-36). I. Conceptual framework and item selection. *Med Care* 1992;**30**:473–83.

72 Dupuy HJ. The Psychological General Well-Being (PGWB) index. In: Wenger NK, Mattson ME, Furberg CF, Elinson J eds. *Assessment of quality of life in clinical trials of cardiovascular therapies.* New York: Le Jacq Publishing Inc, 1984.

73 Dimenas E, Glise H, Hallerback B, Hernqvist H, Svedlund J, Wiklund I. Well-being and gastrointestinal symptoms among patients referred to endoscopy owing to suspected duodenal ulcer. *Scand J Gastroenterol* 1995;**30**:1046–52.

74 Lind T, Havelund T, Carlsson R *et al.* Heartburn without oesophagitis: efficacy of omeprazole therapy and features determining therapeutic response. *Scand J Gastroenterol* 1997;**32**:974–9.

75 Revicki DA, Wood M, Wiklund I, Crawley J. Reliability and validity of the Gastrointestinal Symptom Rating Scale in patients with gastroesophageal reflux disease. *Qual Life Res* 1998;**7**:75–83.

76 Wiklund IK, Junghard O, Grace E *et ali.* Quality of life in reflux and dyspepsia patients. Psychometric documentation of a new disease-specific questionnaire (QOLRAD). *Eur J Surg* 1998;**164**:41–9.

77 Schünemann HJ, Armstrong D, Degl'innocenti A *et al.* A randomized multi-center trial to evaluate simple utility elicitation techniques in patients with gastroesophageal reflux disease. *Med Care* 2004 (in press).

78 Rothman M, Farup C, Stewart W, Helbers L, Zeldis J. Symptoms associated with gastroesophageal reflux disease: development of a questionnaire for use in clinical trials. *Dig Dis Sci* 2001;**46**:1540–9.

79 Allen CJ, Parameswaran K, Belda J, Anvari M. Reproducibility, validity, and responsiveness of a disease-specific symptom questionnaire for gastroesophageal reflux disease. *Dis Esophagus* 2000;**13**:265–70.

80 Shaw MJ, Talley NJ, Beebe TJ *et al.* Initial validation of a diagnostic questionnaire for gastroesophageal reflux disease. *Am J Gastroenterol* 2001;**96**:52–7.

81 Colwell HH, Mathias SD, Pasta DJ, Henning JM, Hunt RH. Development of a health-related quality-of-life questionnaire for individuals with gastroesophageal reflux disease: a validation study. *Dig Dis Sci* 1999;**44**:1376–83.

82 Raymond JM, Marquis P, Bechade D *et al.* [Assessment of quality of life of patients with gastroesophageal reflux. Elaboration and validation of a specific questionnaire]. *Gastroenterol Clin Biol* 1999;**23**:32–9.

83 Coyne KS, Wiklund I, Schmier J, Halling K, Degl' Innocenti A, Revicki D. Development and validation of a disease-specific treatment satisfaction questionnaire for gastro-oesophageal reflux disease. *Aliment Pharmacol Ther* 2003;**18**:907–15.

84 Stewart AL, Greenfield S, Hays RD, *et al.* Functional status and well-being of patients with chronic conditions: results from the medical outcomes study. *JAMA* 1989;**262**:907–13.

85 Madisch A, Kulich KR, Malfertheiner P *et al.* Impact of reflux disease on general and disease-related quality of life – evidence from a recent comparative methodological study in Germany. *Z Gastroenterol* 2003;**41**:1137–43.

86 Dimenas E. Methodological aspects of evaluation of quality of life in upper gastrointestinal disease. *Scand J Gastroenterol* 1993;**28**:18–21.

87 Dimenas E, Glise H, Hallerback B, Hernqvist H, Svedlund J, Wiklund I. Quality of life in patients with upper gastrointestinal symptoms: an improved evaluation of treatment regimens? *Scand J Gastroenterol* 1993;**28**:681–7.

88 Dimenas E, Carlsson R, Glise H, Israelsson B, Wiklund I. Relevance of norm values as part of the documentation of quality of life instruments for use in upper gastrointestinal diseases. *Scand J Gastroenterol* 1996;**31(Suppl 221)**:8–13.

89 Mathias SD, Castell DO, Elkin EP, Matosian ML. Health-related quality of life of patients with acute erosive esophagitis. *Dig Dis Sci* 1996;**41**:2123–9.

90 Galmiche JP, Barthelemy P, Hamelin B. Treating the symptoms of gastro-oesophageal reflux disease: a double-blind comparison of omeprazole and ciaspride. *Aliment Pharmacol Ther* 1997;**11**:765–73.

91 Howard PJ, Maher L, Pryde A, Heading RC. Symptomatic gastro-oesophageal reflux, abnormal oesophageal acid exposure, and mucosal acid sensitivity are three separate, though related, aspects of gastro-oesophageal reflux disease. *Gut* 1991;**32**:128–32.

92 Richter JE, Castell DO. Gastroesophageal reflux; pathogenesis, diagnosis, and therapy. *Ann Intern Med* 1982;**97**:93–103.

93 Wu WC. Ancillary tests in the diagnosis of gastroesophageal reflux disease. *Gastroenterol Clin North Am* 1990;**19**:671–82.

94 Fuchs KH, DeMeester TR, Albertucci M. Specificity and sensitivity of objective diagnosis of gastroesophageal reflux disease. *Surgery* 1987;**102**:575–80.

95 DeVault KR, Castell DO. Guidelines for the diagnosis and treatment of gastroesophageal reflux disease. *Arch Intern Med* 1995;**155**:2165–73.

96 Sellar RJ, De Caestecker JS, Heading RC. Barium radiology: a sensitive test for gastro-oesophageal reflux. *Clin Radiol* 1987;**38**:303–7.

97 Chen YM, Ott DJ, Gelfand DW, Munitz HA. Multiphasic examination of the esophagogastric region for strictures, rings and hiatal hernia: evaluation of the individual techniques. *Gastrointest Radiol* 1985;**10**:311–16.

98 Fransson SG, Sökjer H, Johansson KE, Tibbling L. Radiologic diagnosis of gastro-oesophageal reflux. Comparison of barium and low-density contrast medium. *Acta Radiol* 1987;**28**:295–8.

99 Graziani L, De Nigris E, Pesaresi A, Baldelli S, Dini L, Montesi A. Reflux oesophagitis: radiographic-endoscopic correlation in 39 symptomatic cases. *Gastrointest Radiol* 1983;**8**:1–6.

100 Pope CE. Pathophysiology and diagnosis of reflux esophagitis. *Gastroenterology* 1976;**70**:445–4.

101 Ott DJ, Dodds WJ, Wu WC, Gelfand DW, Hogan WJ, Stewart ET. Current status of radiology in evaluating for gastroesophageal reflux disease. *J Clin Gastroenterol* 1982;**4**:365–75.

102 Chen MY, Ott DJ, Sinclair JW, Wu WC, Gelfand DW. Gastroesophageal reflux disease: correlation of esophageal pH testing and radiographic findings. *Radiology* 1992;**185**:483–6.

103 Jenkins AF, Cowan RJ, Richter JE. Gastroesophageal scintigaphy: is it a sensitive screening test for gastro-esophageal reflux disease? *J Clin Gastroenterol* 1985;**7**:127–31.

104 Spechler SJ. Epidemiology and natural history of gastro-oesophageal reflux disease. *Digestion* 1992; **51(Suppl 1)**:24–9.

105 Knuff TE, Benjamin SB, Worsham GF, Hancock J, Castell DO. Histologic examination of chronic gastroesophageal relux: an evaluation of biopsy methods and diagnostic criteria. *Dig Dis Sci* 1984;**29**:194–201.

106 Ismail-Beigi F, Pope CE. Distribution of the histological changes of gastroesophageal reflux in the distal esophagus of man. *Gastroenterology* 1974;**66**:1109–13.

107 Schindlbeck NE, Wiebecke B, Klauser AG, Voderholzer WA, Müller-Lissner SA. Diagnostic value of histology in non-erosive gastro-oesophageal reflux disease. *Gut* 1996;**39**:151–4.

108 Berstad A, Hatlebakk JG. The predictive value of symptoms in gastro-oesophageal reflux disease. *Scand J Gastroenterol* 1995;**30(Suppl 211)**:1–4.

109 Hatlebakk JG, Berstad A. Endoscopic grading of reflux oesophagitis: what observations corelate with gastro-oesophageal reflux? *Scand J Gastroenterol* 1997;**32**:760–5.

110 Armstrong D, Emde C, Inauen W, Blum AL. Diagnostic assessment of gastroesophageal reflux disease: what is possible vs what is practical? *Hepatogastroenterology* 1992;**39(Suppl 1)**:3–13.

111 Armstrong D, Bennett JR, Blum AL *et al.* The endoscopic assessment of esophagitis: a progress report on observer agreement. *Gastroenterology* 1996;**111**:85–92.

112 Lundell LR, Dent J, Bennett JR *et al.* Endoscopic assessment of oesophagitis: clinical and functional correlates and further validation of the Los Angeles classification. *Gut* 1999;**45**:172–80.

113 Bernstein LM, Baker LA. A clinical test for esophagitis. *Gastroenterology* 1958;**34**:760–81.

114 Kaul B, Petersen H, Grette K, Myrvold HE, Halvorsen T. The acid perfusion test in gastroesophageal reflux disease. *Scand J Gastroenterol* 1986;**21**:93–6.

115 Richter JE. Acid perfusion (Bernstein) test. In: Castell DO, Wu WC, and Ott DJ, eds. *Gastroesophageal Reflux Disease: Pathogenesis, Diagnosis and Therapy.* London: Futura Publishing Co Inc, 1985.

116 Johnsson F, Joelsson B, Isberg PE. Ambulatory 24 hour intraesophgeal pH-monitoring in the diagnosis of gastroesophageal reflux disease. *Gut* 1987;**28**:1145–50.

117 Schindlbeck NE, Heinrich C, König A, Dendorfer A, Pace F, Müller-Lissner SA. Optimal thresholds, sensitivity, and specificity of long-term pH-metry for the detection of gastroesophageal reflux disease. *Gastroenterology* 1987; **93**:85–90.

118 Jamieson JR, Stein HJ, DeMeester TR, Bonavina L, Schwizer W, Hinder RA, Albertucci M. Ambulatory 24-h esophageal pH monitoring: normal values, optimal thresholds, specificity, sensitivity, and reproducibility. *Am J Gastroenterol* 1992;**87**:1102–11.

119 Mattox HE, Richter JE. Prolonged ambulatory esophageal pH monitoring in the evaluation of gastroesophageal reflux disease. *Am J Med* 1990;**89**:345–56.

120 Rosen SN, Pope CE. Extended esophageal pH monitoring. An analysis of the literature and assessment of its role in the diagnosis and management of gastroesophageal reflux. *J Clin Gastroenterol* 1989;**11**:260–70.

121 Wyman JB, Dent J, Holloway RH. Changes in oesophageal pH associated with gastro-oesophageal reflux. Are traditional criteria sensitive for detection of reflux? *Scand J Gastroenterol* 1993;**28**:827–32.

122 Mattioli S, Pilotti V, Spangaro M *et al*. Reliability of 24-hour home esophageal pH monitoring in diagnosis of gastroesophageal reflux. *Dig Dis Sci* 1989;**34**:71–8.

123 Breedijk M, Akkermans LM. Twenty-four hour ambulatory pH recording with computerised analysis. *Med Biol Eng Comput* 1984;**22**:609–12.

124 Wiener GJ, Morgan TM, Copper JB *et al*. Ambulatory 24-hour esophageal pH monitoring. Reproducibility and variability of pH parameters. *Dig Dis Sci* 1988;**33**:1127–33.

125 Watson RG, Tham TC, Johnston BT, McDougall NI. Double blind cross-over placebo controlled study of omeprazole in the treatment of patients with reflux symptoms and physiological levels of acid reflux – the "sensitive oesophagus". *Gut* 1997;**40**:587–90.

126 Vitale GC, Cheadle WG, Sadek S, Michel ME, Cushieri A. Computerized 24-hour ambulatory esophageal pH monitoring and esophagogastroduodenoscopy in the reflux patient. *Ann Surg* 1984;**200**:724–8.

127 Schenk BE, Kuipers EJ, Klinkenberg Knol EC *et al*. Omeprazole as a diagnostic tool in gastroesophageal reflux disease. *Am J Gastroenterol* 1997;**92**:1997–2000.

128 Fass R, Fennerty MB, Ofman JJ *et al*. The clinical and economic value of a short course of omeprazole in patients with noncardiac chest pain. *Gastroenterology* 1998;**115**:42–9.

129 Quigley EM. 24-h pH monitoring for gastroesophageal reflux disease: already standard but not yet gold? *Am J Gastroenterol* 1992;**87**:1071–5.

130 Tack J, Vantrappen G, Huyberechts G, Sifrim D, Janssens J, Van Overstraeten R. Validation of a new method of measuring esophageal acid exposure: comparison with 24-hour pH monitoring. *Dig Dis Sci* 2003;**48**:16–21.

131 Joelsson B, Johnsson F. Heartburn – the acid test. *Gut* 1989;**30**:1523–5.

132 Venables TL, Newland RD, Patel AC, Hole J, Wilcock C, Turbitt ML. Omeprazole 10 milligrams once daily, omeprazole 20 milligrams once daily, or ranitidine 150 milligrams twice daily, evaluated as initial therapy for the relief of symptoms of gastro-oesophageal reflux disease in general practice. *Scand J Gastroenterol* 1997;**32**:965–73.

133 Galmiche JP, Bruley des Varannes S. Symptoms and disease severity in gastro-oesophageal reflux disease. *Scand J Gastroenterol* 1994;**29(Suppl 201)**:62–8.

134 Johannessen T, Petersen H, Kleveland PM, Dybdahl JH, Sandvik AK, Brenna E, Waldum H. The predictive value of history in dyspepsia. *Scand J Gastroenterol* 1990;**25**:689–97.

135 Johnsson F, Roth Y, Damgaard Pedersen NE, Joelsson B. Cimetidine improves GERD symptoms in patients selected by a validated GERD questionnaire. *Aliment Pharmacol Ther* 1993;**7**:81–6.

136 Carlsson R, Dent J, Bolling-Sternevald E *et al*. The usefulness of a structured questionnaire in the assessment of symptomatic gastroesophageal reflux disease. *Scand J Gastroenterol* 1998;**33**:1023–9.

137 Tefera L, Fein M, Ritter MP *et al*. Can the combination of symptoms and endoscopy confirm the presence of gastroesophageal reflux disease? *Am Surg* 1997;**63**:933–6.

138 Locke GR, Talley NJ, Weaver AL, Zinsmeister AR. A new questionnaire for gastroesophageal reflux disease. *Mayo Clin Proc* 1994;**69**:539–47.

139 Manterola C, Munoz S, Grande L, Bustos L. Initial validation of a questionnaire for detecting gastro-esophageal reflux disease in epidemiological settings. *J Clin Epidemiol* 2002;**55**:1041–5.

140 Ofman JJ, Shaw M, Sadik K *et al*. Identifying patients with gastroesophageal reflux disease: validation of a practical screening tool. *Dig Dis Sci* 2002;**47**:1863–9.

141 Numans ME, de Wit NJ. Reflux symptoms in general practice: diagnostic evaluation of the Carlsson-Dent gastro-oesophageal reflux disease questionnaire. *Aliment Pharmacol Ther* 2003;**17**:1049–55.

142 Locke GR, Zinsmeister AR, Talley NJ. Can symptoms predict endoscopic findings in GERD? *Gastrointest Endosc* 2003;**58**:661–70.

143 Moreno Elola-Olaso C, Rey E, Rodriguez-Artalejo F, Locke GR, III, Diaz-Rubio M. Adaptation and validation of a gastroesophageal reflux questionnaire for use on a Spanish population. *Rev Esp Enferm Dig* 2002;**94**:745–58.

144 Wong WM, Lam KF, Lai KC *et al*. A validated symptoms questionnaire (Chinese GERDQ) for the diagnosis of gastro-oesophageal reflux disease in the Chinese population. *Aliment Pharmacol Ther* 2003;**17**:1407–13.

145 Ward BW, Wu WC, Richter JE, Lui KW, Castell DO. Ambulatory 24-hour esophageal pH monitoring: technology seaching for a clinical application. *J Clin Gastroenterol* 1986;**8(Suppl 1)**:59–67.

146 Wiener GJ, Richter JE, Copper JB, Wu WC, Castell DO. The symptom index: a clinically important parameter of ambulatory 24-hour esophageal pH monitoring. *Am J Gastroenterol* 1988;**83**:358–61.

147 Dekel R, Martinez-Hawthorne SD, Guillen RJ, Fass R. Evaluation of symptom index in identifying gastro-esophageal reflux disease-related non-cardiac chest pain. *J Clin Gastroenterol* 2004;**38**:24–9.

148 Weusten BL, Roelofs JM, Akkermans LM, Berge-Henegouwen GP, Smout AJ. The symptom-association probability: an improved method for symptom analysis of 24-hour esophageal pH data. *Gastroenterology* 1994;**107**:1741–5.

149 Johnsson F, Weywadt L, Solhaug JH, Hernqvist H, Bengtsson L. One-week omeprazole treatment in the diagnosis of gastro-oesophageal reflux disease. *Scand J Gastroenterol* 1998;**33**:15–20.

150 Bate CM, Riley SA, Chapman RWG, Durnin AT, Taylor MD. Evaluation of omeprazole as a cost-effective diagnostic test for gastro-oesophageal reflux disease. *Aliment Pharmacol Ther* 1999;**13**:59–66.

151 Schindlbeck NE, Klauser AG, Voderholzer WA, Müller-Lissner SA. Empiric therapy for gastroesophageal reflux disease. *Arch Intern Med* 1995;**155**:1808–12.

152 Fass R, Ofman JJ, Gralnek IM *et al.* Clinical and economic assessment of the omeprazole test in patients with symptoms suggestive of gastroesophageal reflux disease. *Arch Intern Med* 1999;**159**:2161–8.

153 Juul-Hansen P, Rydning A, Jacobsen CD, Hansen T. High-dose proton-pump inhibitors as a diagnostic test of gastro-oesophageal reflux disease in endoscopic-negative patients. *Scand J Gastroenterol* 2001;**36**:806–10.

154 Johnsson F, Hatlebakk JG, Klintenberg AC *et al.* One-week esomeprazole treatment: an effective confirmatory test in patients with suspected gastroesophageal reflux disease. *Scand J Gastroenterol* 2003;**38**:354–9.

155 Achem SR, Kolts BE, MacMath T, Richter J, Mohr D, Burton L, Castell DO. Effects of omeprazole versus placebo in treatment of noncardiac chest pain and gastro-esophageal reflux. *Dig Dis Sci* 1997;**42**:2138–45.

156 Fass R, Fennerty MB, Johnson C, Camargo L, Sampliner RE. Correlation of ambulatory 24-hour esophageal pH monitoring results with symptom improvement in patients with noncardiac chest pain due to gastroesophageal reflux disease. *J Clin Gastroenterol* 1999;**28**:36–9.

157 Pandak WM, Arezo S, Everett S, Jesse R, DeCosta G, Crofts T, Gennings C, Siuta M, Zfass A. Short course of omeprazole: a better first diagnostic approach to noncardiac chest pain than endoscopy, manometry, or 24-hour esophageal pH monitoring. *J Clin Gastroenterol* 2002;**35**:307–14.

158 Hunt RH. The relationship between the control of pH and healing and symptom relief in gastro-oesophageal reflux disease. *Aliment Pharmacol Ther* 1995;**9**:3–7.

159 Hatlebakk JG, Berstad A. Gastro-oesophageal reflux during 3 months of therapy with ranitidine in reflux oesophagitis. *Scand J Gastroenterol* 1996;**31**:954–8.

160 Bell NJV, Burget D, Howden CW, Wilkinson J, Hunt RH. Appropriate acid suppression for the management of gastro-oesophageal reflux disase. *Digestion* 1992;**51**:59–67.

161 Bell NJV, Hunt RH. Role of gastric acid suppression in the treatment of gastro-oesophageal reflux disease. *Gut* 1992;**33**:118–24.

162 Lim PL, Gibbons MJ, Crawford EJ, Watson RG, Johnston BT. The effect of lifestyle changes on results of 24-h ambulatory oesophageal pH monitoring. *Eur J Gastroenterol Hepatol* 2000;**12**:655–6.

163 Meining A, Classen M. The role of diet and lifestyle measures in the pathogenesis and treatment of gastroesophageal reflux disease. *Am J Gastroenterol* 2000;**95**:2692–7.

164 Pehl C, Wendl B, Pfeiffer A, Schmidt T, Kaess H. Low-proof alcoholic beverages and gastroesophageal reflux. *Dig Dis Sci* 1993;**38**:93–6.

165 Pehl C, Pfeiffer A, Wendl B, Kaess H. Different effects of white and red wine on lower esophageal sphincter pressure and gastroesophageal reflux. *Scand J Gastroenterol* 1998;**33**:118–22.

166 Pehl C, Frommherz M, Wendl B, Schmidt T, Pfeiffer A. Effect of white wine on esophageal peristalsis and acid clearance. *Scand J Gastroenterol* 2000;**35**:1255–9.

167 Pehl C, Frommherz M, Wendl B, Pfeiffer A. Gastroesophageal reflux induced by white wine: the role of acid clearance and "rereflux". *Am J Gastroenterol* 2002;**97**:561–7.

168 Wendl B, Pfeiffer A, Pehl C, Schmidt T, Kaess H. Effect of decaffeination of coffee or tea on gastro-oesophageal reflux. *Aliment Pharmacol Ther* 1994;**8**:283–7.

169 Kadakia SC, Kikendall JW, Maydonovitch C, Johnson LF. Effect of cigarette smoking on gastroesophageal reflux measured by 24-h ambulatory esophageal pH monitoring. *Am J Gastroenterol* 1995;**90**:1785–90.

170 Pehl C, Pfeiffer A, Wendl B, Nagy I, Kaess H. Effect of smoking on the results of esophageal pH measurement in clinical routine. *J Clin Gastroenterol* 1997;**25**:503–6.

171 Van Nieuwenhoven MA, Brouns F, Brummer RJ. Gastrointestinal profile of symptomatic athletes at rest and during physical exercise. *Eur J Appl Physiol* 2003: Nov 22 [Epub ahead of print].

172 Collings KL, Pierce PF, Rodriguez-Stanley S, Bemben M, Miner PB. Esophageal reflux in conditioned runners, cyclists, and weightlifters. *Med Sci Sports Exerc* 2003;**35**:730–5.

173 Choi SC, Yoo KH, Kim TH, Kim SH, Choi SJ, Nah YH. Effect of graded running on esophageal motility and gastroesophageal reflux in fed volunteers. *J Korean Med Sci* 2001;**16**:183–7.

174 Yazaki E, Shawdon A, Beasley I, Evans DF. The effect of different types of exercise on gastrooesophageal reflux. *Aust J Sci Med Sport* 1996;**28**:93–6.

175 Kraus BB, Sinclair JW, Castell DO. Gastroesophageal reflux in runners. Characteristics and treatment. *Ann Intern Med* 1990;**112**:429–33.

176 Clark CS, Kraus BB, Sinclair J, Castell DO. Gastro-esophageal reflux-induced by exercise in healthy volunteers. *JAMA* 1989;**261**:3599–601.

177 Pollmann H, Zillessen E, Pohl J *et al.* [Effect of elevated head position in bed in therapy of gastroesophageal reflux]. *Z Gastroenterol* 1996;**34(Suppl 2)**:93–9.

178 Shay SS, Conwell DL, Mehindru V, Hertz B. The effect of posture on gastroesophageal reflux event frequency and composition during fasting. *Am J Gastroenterol* 1996;**91**:54–60.

179 Tobin JM, McCloud P, Cameron DJ. Posture and gastro-oesophageal reflux: a case for left lateral positioning. *Arch Dis Child* 1997;**76**:254–8.

180 Katz LC, Just R, Castell DO. Body position affects recumbent postprandial reflux. *J Clin Gastroenterol* 1994;**18**:280–3.

181 Becker DJ, Sinclair J, Castell DO, Wu WC. A comparison of high and low fat meals on postprandial esophageal acid exposure. *Am J Gastroenterol* 1989;**84**:782–6.

182 Nebel OT, Castell DO. Lower esophageal sphincter pressure changes after food ingestion. *Gastroenterology* 1972;**63**:778–83.

183 Pehl C, Waizenhoefer A, Wendl B, Schmidt T, Schepp W, Pfeiffer A. Effect of low and high fat meals on lower esophageal sphincter motility and gastroesophageal reflux in healthy subjects. *Am J Gastroenterol* 1999;**94**:1192–6.

184 Penagini R, Mangano M, Bianchi PA. Effect of increasing the fat content but not the energy load of a meal on gastro-oesophageal reflux and lower oesophageal sphincter motor function. *Gut* 1998;**42**:330–3.

185 Pehl C, Pfeiffer A, Waizenhoefer A, Wendl B, Schepp W. Effect of caloric density of a meal on lower oesophageal sphincter motility and gastro-oesophageal reflux in healthy subjects. *Aliment Pharmacol Ther* 2001;**15**:233–9.

186 Wright LE, Castell DO. The adverse effect of chocolate on lower esophageal sphincter pressure. *Am J Dig Dis* 1975;**20**:703–7.

187 Murphy DW, Castell DO. Chocolate and heartburn: evidence of increased esophageal acid exposure after chocolate ingestion. *Am J Gastroenterol* 1988;**93**:633–6.

188 Sigmund CJ, McNally EF. The action of a carminative on the lower esophageal sphincter. *Gastroenterology* 1969;**56**:13–18.

189 Babka JC, Castell DO. On the genesis of heartburn. The effects of specific foods on the lower esophageal sphincter. *Am J Dig Dis* 1973;**18**:391–7.

190 Allen ML, Mellow MH, Robinson MG, Orr WC. The effect of raw onions on acid reflux and reflux symptoms. *Am J Gastroenterol* 1990;**85**:377–80.

191 Feldman M, Barnett C. Relationships between the acidity and osmolality of popular beverages and reported postprandial heartburn. *Gastroenterology* 1995;**108**:125–31.

192 Thomas FB, Steinbaugh JT, Fromkes JJ, Mekhjian HS, Caldwell JH. Inhibitory effect of coffee on lower esophageal sphincter pressure. *Gastroenterology* 1980;**79**:1262–6.

193 McArthur K, Hogan D, Isenberg JI. Relative stimulatory effects of commonly ingested beverages on gastric acid secretion in humans. *Gastroenterology* 1982;**83**:199–203.

194 Pehl C, Pfeiffer A, Wendl B, Kaess H. The effect of decaffeination of coffee on gastro-oesophageal reflux in patients with reflux disease. *Aliment Pharmacol Ther* 1997;**11**:483–6.

195 Price SF, Smithson KW, Castell DO. Food sensitivity in reflux esophagitis. *Gastroenterology* 1978;**75**:240–3.

196 Vitale GC, Cheadle WG, Patel B, Sadek SA, Michel ME, Cushieri A. The effect of alcohol on nocturnal gastroesophageal reflux. *JAMA* 1987;**258**:2077–9.

197 Locke GR III, Talley NJ, Fett SL, Zinsmeister AR, Melton LJ III. Risk factors associated with symptoms of gastroesophageal reflux. *Am J Med* 1999;**106**:642–9.

198 Watanabe Y, Fujiwara Y, Shiba M *et al.* Cigarette smoking and alcohol consumption associated with gastro-oesophageal reflux disease in Japanese men. *Scand J Gastroenterol* 2003;**38**:807–11.

199 Waring JP, Eastwood TF, Austin JM, Sanowski RA. The immediate efects of cessation of cigarette smoking on gastroesophageal reflux. *Am J Gastroenterol* 1989;**84**:1076–8.

200 Dodds WJ, Dent J, Hogan WJ, Helm JF, Hauser R, Patel GK, Egide MS. Mechanisms of gastroesophageal reflux in patients with reflux esophagitis. *N Engl J Med* 1982;**307**:1547–52.

201 Stanciu C, Bennett JR. Effects of posture on gastro-oesophageal reflux. *Digestion* 1977;**15**:104–9.

202 Harvey RF, Gordon PC, Hadley N *et al.* Effects of sleeping with the bed-head raised and of ranitidine in patients with severe peptic oesophagitis. *Lancet* 1987;**ii**:1200–3.

203 Johnson LF, DeMeester TR. Evaluation of elevation of the head of the bed, bethanecol, and antacid foam tablets on gastroesophageal reflux. *Dig Dis Sci* 1981;**26**:673–80.

204 Hamilton JW, Boisen RJ, Yamamoto DT, Wagner JL, Reichelderfer M. Sleeping on a wedge diminishes exposure of the esophagus to refluxed acid. *Dig Dis Sci* 1988;**33**:518–22.

205 Fraser-Moodie CA, Norton B, Gornall C, Magnago S, Weale AR, Holmes GK. Weight loss has an independent beneficial effect on symptoms of gastro-oesophageal reflux in patients who are overweight. *Scand J Gastroenterol* 1999;**34**:337–40.

206 Kjellin A, Ramel S, Rossner S, Thor K. Gastroesophageal reflux in obese patients is not reduced by weight reduction. *Scand J Gastroenterol* 1996;**31**:1047–51.

207 Mathus-Vliegen LM, Tytgat GN. Twenty-four-hour pH measurements in morbid obesity: effects of massive overweight, weight loss and gastric distension. *Eur J Gastroenterology Hepatol* 1996;**8**:635–40.

208 Chiba N, Bernard L, O'Brien BJ, Goeree R, Hunt RH. A Canadian physician survey of dyspepsia management. *Can J Gastroenterology* 1998;**12**:83–90.

209 Meining A, Driesnack U, Classen M, Rosch T. Management of gastroesophageal reflux disease in primary care: results of a survey in 2 areas in Germany. *Z Gastroenterol* 2002;**40**:15–20.

210 Blair DI, Kaplan B, Spiegler J. Patient characteristics and lifestyle recommendations in the treatment of gastro-esophageal reflux disease. *J Fam Pract* 1997;**44**:266–72.

211 Sonnenberg A, Delco F, El-Serag HB. Empirical therapy versus diagnostic tests in gastroesophageal reflux disease. A medical decision analysis. *Dig Dis Sci* 1998;**43**:1001–8.

212 Graham DY, Patterson DJ. Double-blind comparison of liquid antacid and placebo in the treatment of symptomatic reflux esophagitis. *Dig Dis Sci* 1983;**28**:559–63.

213 Farup PG, Weberg R, Berstad A *et al.* Low-dose antacids versus 400 mg cimetidine twice daily for reflux oesophagitis. A comparative, placebo-controlled, multicentre study. *Scand J Gastroenterol* 1990;**25**:315–20.

214 Grove O, Bekker C, Jeppe-Hansen MG *et al.* Ranitidine and high-dose antacid in reflux oesophagitis. A randomized, placebo-controlled trial. *Scand J Gastroenterol* 1985;**20**:457–61.

215 Koelz HR. Treatment of reflux esophagitis with H$_2$-blockers, antacids and prokinetic drugs. An analysis of randomized clinical trials. *Scand J Gastroenterol* 1989;**24(Suppl 156)**:25–36.

216 Poynard T, and a French Co-operative Study Group. Relapse rate of patients after healing of esophagitis – a prospective study of alginate as self-care treatment for 6 months. *Aliment Pharmacol Ther* 1993;**7**:385–92.

217 Poynard T, Vernisse B, Agostini H, for a multicentre group. Randomized, multicentre comparison of sodium alginate

and cisapride in the symptomatic treatment of uncomplicated gastro-oesophageal reflux. *Aliment Pharmacol Ther* 1998;**12**:159–65.

218 Collings KL, Rodriguez-Stanley S, Proskin HM, Robinson M, Miner PB, Jr. Clinical effectiveness of a new antacid chewing gum on heartburn and oesophageal pH control. *Aliment Pharmacol Ther* 2002;**16**:2029–35.

219 Pace F, Maconi G, Molteni P, Minguzzi M, Bianchi Porro G. Meta-analysis of the effect of placebo on the outcome of medically treated reflux esophagitis. *Scand J Gastroenterol* 1995;**30**:101–5.

220 Hunt RH. Habit, prejudice, power and politics: issues in the conversion of H2-receptor antagonists to over-the-counter use. *Can Med Assoc J* 1996;**154**:49–53.

221 Gottlieb S, Decktor DL, Eckert JM, Simon TJ, Stauffer L, Ciccone PE. Efficacy and tolerability of famotidine in preventing heartburn and related symptoms of upper gastrointestinal discomfort. *Am J Ther* 1995;**2**:314–19.

222 Johannessen T, Kristensen P. On-demand therapy in gastroesophageal relux disease: a comparison of the early effects of single doses of fast-dissolving famotidine wafers and ranitidine tablets. *Clin Ther* 1997;**19**:73–81.

223 Engzelius JM, Solhaug JH, Knapstad LJ, Kjærsgaard P. Ranitidine effervescent and famotidine wafer in the relief of episodic symptoms of gastro-oesophageal reflux disease. *Scand J Gastroenterol* 1997;**32**:513–18.

224 Wilhelmsen I, Hatlebakk JG, Olaffson S, Berstad A. On demand therapy of reflux oesophagitis: a study of symptoms, patient satisfaction, and quality of life. *Gastroenterology* 1998;**114**:A331.

225 Euler AR, Murdock RH Jr, Wilson TH, Silver MT, Parker SE, Powers L. Ranitidine is effective therapy for erosive esophagitis. *Am J Gastroenterol* 1993;**88**:520–4.

226 Roufail W, Belsito A, Robinson M, Barish C, Rubin A. Ranitidine for erosive oesophagitis: a double-blind, placebo- controlled study. Glaxo Erosive Esophagitis Study Group. *Aliment Pharmacol Ther* 1992;**6**:597–607.

227 Silver MT, Murdock RH Jr, Morrill BB, Sue SO. Ranitidine 300mg twice daily and 150 mg four-times daily are efffective in healing erosive esophagitis. *Aliment Pharmacol Ther* 1996;**10**:373–80.

228 McCarty-Dawson D, Sue SO, Morrill B, Murdock RH Jr. Ranitidine versus cimetidine in the healing of erosive esophagitis. *Clin Ther* 1996;**18**:1150–60.

229 Johnson NJ, Boyd EJS, Mills JG, Wood JR. Acute treatment of reflux oesophagitis: a multi-centre trial to compare 150 mg ranitidine b.d. with 300 mg ranitidine q.d.s. *Aliment Pharmacol Ther* 1989;**3**:259–66.

230 Simon TJ, Berlin RG, Tipping R, Gilde L. Efficacy of twice daily doses of 40 or 20 milligrams famotidine or 150 milligrams ranitidine for treatment of patients with moderate to severe erosive esophagitis. Famotidine Erosive Esophagitis Study Group. *Scand J Gastroenterol* 1993;**28**:375–80.

231 Grande L, Lacima G, Ros E *et al.* Lack of effect of metoclopramide and domperidone on esophageal peristalsis and esophageal acid clearance in reflux esophagitis. A randomized, double-blind study. *Dig Dis Sci* 1992;**37**:583–8.

232 Ceccatelli P, Janssens J, Vantrappen G, Cucchiara S. Cisapride restores the decreased lower oesophageal sphincter pressure in reflux patients. *Gut* 1988;**29**:631–5.

233 Collins BJ, Spence RAJ, Ferguson R, Laird J, Love AHG. Cisapride: Influence on oesophageal and gastric emptying and gastro-oesoghageal reflux in patients with reflux oesophagitis. *Hepatogastroenterology* 1987;**34**:113–16.

234 Robertson CS, Evans DF, Ledingham SJ, Atkinson M. Cisapride in the treatment of gastro-oesophageal reflux disease. *Aliment Pharmacol Ther* 1993;**7**:181–90.

235 Sekiguchi T, Nishioka T, Matsuzaki T *et al.* Comparative efficacy of acid inhibition by drug therapy in reflux esophagitis. *Gastroenterologia* 1991;**26**:137–44.

236 Castell DO, Sigmund CJr, Patterson D *et al.*, and the CIS-USA-52 investigator group. Cisapride 20mg b.i.d. provides symptomatic relief of heartburn and-related symptoms of chronic mild to moderate gastroesophageal reflux disease. *Am J Gastroenterol* 1998;**93**:547–52.

237 Richter JE, Long JF. Cisapride for gastroesophageal reflux disease: a placebo- controlled, double-blind study. *Am J Gastroenterol* 1995;**90**:423–30.

238 Geldof H, Hazelhoff B, Otten MH. Two different dose regimens of cisapride in the treatment of reflux oesophagitis: a double-blind comparison with ranitidine. *Aliment Pharmacol Ther* 1993;**7**:409–15.

239 Dakkak M, Jones BP, Scott MG, Tooley PJ, Bennett JR. Comparing the efficacy of cisapride and ranitidine in oesophagitis: a double-blind, parallel group study in general practice. *Br J Clin Pract* 1994;**48**:10–14.

240 Galmiche JP, Fraitag B, Filoche B *et al.* Double-blind comparison of cisapride and cimetidine in treatment of reflux esophagitis. *Dig Dis Sci* 1990;**35**:649–55.

241 Janisch HD, Hüttemann W, Bouzo MH. Cisapride versus ranitidine in the treatment of reflux esophagitis. *Hepatogastroenterology* 1988;**35**:125–7.

242 Maleev A, Mendizova A, Popov P *et al.* Cisapride and cimetidine in the treatment of erosive esophagitis. *Hepatogastroenterology* 1990;**37**:403–7.

243 Arvanitakis C, Nikopoulos A, Theoharidis A *et al.* Cisapride and ranitidine in the treatment of gastro-oesophageal reflux disease – a comparative randomized double-blind trial. *Aliment Pharmacol Ther* 1993;**7**:635–41.

244 Baldi F, Bianchi PG, Dobrilla G *et al.* Cisapride versus placebo in reflux esophagitis. A multicenter double-blind trial. *J Clin Gastroenterol* 1988;**10**:614–18.

245 Lepoutre L, VanDerSpek P, Vanderlinden I, Bollen J, Laukens P, Van der Spek P. Healing of grade-II and III oesophagitis through motility stimulation with cisapride. *Digestion* 1990;**45**:109–14.

246 Toussaint J, Gossuin A, Deruyttere M, Huble F, Devis G. Healing and prevention of relapse of reflux oesophagitis by cisapride. *Gut* 1991;**32**:1280–5.

247 Kimmig JM. Treatment and prevention of relapse of mild oesophagitis with omeprazole and cisapride: a comparison of two strategies. *Aliment Pharmacol Ther* 1995;**9**:281–6.

248 van Rensburg CJ, Bardhan KD. No clinical benefit of adding cisapride to pantoprazole for treatment of gastro-oesophageal reflux disease. *Eur J Gastroenterol Hepatol* 2001;**13**:909–14.

249 Blum AL, Adami B, Bouzo MH *et al.* Effect of cisapride on relapse of esophagitis. A multinational, placebo-controlled trial in patients healed with an anti-secretory drug. The Italian Eurocis Trialists. *Dig Dis Sci* 1993;**38**:551–60.

250 Vigneri S, Termini R, Leandro G *et al.* A comparison of five maintenance therapies for reflux esophagitis. *N Engl J Med* 1995;**333**:1106–10.

251 Tytgat GN, Anker-Hansen O, Carling L *et al.* Effect of cisapride on relapse of reflux oesophagitis, healed with antisecretory drugs. *Scand J Gastroenterol* 1992;**27**: 175–83.

252 McDougall NI, Watson RGP, Collins JSA, McFarland RJ, Love AHG. Maintenance therapy with cisapride after healing of erosive oesophagitis: a double-blind placebo-controlled trial. *Aliment Pharmacol Ther* 1997;**11**: 487–95.

253 Hatlebakk JG, Johnsson F, Vilien M, Carling L, Wetterhus S, Thøgersen T. The effect of cisapride in maintaining symptomatic remission in patients with gastro-oesophageal reflux disease. *Scand J Gastroenterol* 1997;**32**:1100–6.

254 Wysowski DE, Bacsanyi J. Cisapride and fatal arrhythmia. *N Engl J Med* 1996;**335**:290–1.

255 Hameeteman W, v d Boomgaard DM, Dekker W, Schrijver M, Wesdorp ICE, Tytgat GNJ. Sucralfate versus cimetidine in reflux esophagitis. A single-blind multicentre study. *J Clin Gastroenterol* 1987;**9**:390–4.

256 Chopra BK, Kazal HL, Mittal PK, Sibia SS. A comparison of the clinical efficacy of ranitidine and sucralfate in reflux esophagitis. *J Assoc Phys Ind* 1992;**40**:439–41.

257 Bremner CG, Marks IN, Segal I, Simjee A. Reflux esophagitis therapy: sucralfate versus ranitidine in a double blind multicenter trial. *Am J Med* 1991;**91**:119S–122S.

258 Simon B, Mueller P. Comparison of the effect of sucralfate and ranitidine in reflux esophagitis. *Am J Med* 1987;**83**:43–7.

259 Schotborgh RH, Hameeteman W, Dekker W *et al.* Combination therapy of sucralfate and cimetidine, compared with sucralfate monotherapy, in patients with peptic reflux esophagitis. *Am J Med* 1989;**86**:77–80.

260 Herrera JL, Shay SS, McCabe M, Peura DA, Johnson LF. Sucralfate used as adjunctive therapy in patients with severe erosive peptic esophagitis resulting from gastroesophageal reflux. *Am J Gastroenterol* 1990;**85**: 1335–8.

261 Tytgat GNJ, Koelz HR, Vosmaer GDC, and the Sucralfate Investigational Working Team. Sucralfate maintenance therapy in reflux esophagitis. *Am J Gastroenterol* 1995; **90**:1233–7.

262 Jorgensen F, Elsborg L. Sucralfate versus cimetidine in the treatment of reflux esophagitis, with special reference to the esophageal motor function. *Am J Med* 1991;**91**: 114S–118S.

263 Castell DO, Richter JE, Robinson M, Sontag S, Haber MM, and the Lansoprazole Group. Efficacy and safety of lansoprazole in the treatment of erosive reflux esophagitis. *Am J Gastroenterol* 1996;**91**:1749–57.

264 Mulder CJ, Dekker W, Gerretsen M, on behalf of the Dutch Study Group. Lansoprazole 30mg versus omeprazole 40mg in the treatment of reflux oesophagitis grade II, III and IVa (a Dutch multicentre trial). *Eur J Gastroenterology Hepatol* 1996;**8**:1101–6.

265 Dekkers CP, Beker JA, Thjodleifsson B, Gabryelewicz A, Bell NE, Humphries TJ. Double-blind comparison [correction of Double-blind, placebo-controlled comparison] of rabeprazole 20 mg vs. omeprazole 20 mg in the treatment of erosive or ulcerative gastro-oesophageal reflux disease. The European Rabeprazole Study Group [published erratum appears in *Aliment Pharmacol Ther* 1999 Apr;**134**:567]. *Aliment Pharmacol Ther* 1999;**13**:49–57.

266 van Rensburg CJ, Honiball PJ, Grundling HD *et al.* Efficacy and tolerability of pantoprazole 40 mg versus 80 mg in patients with reflux oesophagitis. *Aliment Pharmacol Ther* 1996;**10**:397–401.

267 Earnest DL, Dorsch E, Jones J, Jennings DE, Greski Rose PA. A placebo-controlled dose-ranging study of lansoprazole in the management of reflux esophagitis. *Am J Gastroenterol* 1998;**93**:238–43.

268 Castell DO, Kahrilas PJ, Richter JE *et al.* Esomeprazole (40 mg) compared with lansoprazole (30 mg) in the treatment of erosive esophagitis. *Am J Gastroenterol* 2002;**97**: 575–83.

269 Howden CW, Ballard EDII, Robieson W. Evidence for therapeutic equivalence of lansoprazole 30mg and esomeprazole 40mg in the treatment of erosive oesophagitis. *Clin Drug Invest* 2002;**22**:99–109.

270 Vcev A, Stimac D, Vceva A *et al.* Pantoprazole versus omeprazole in the treatment of reflux esophagitis. *Acta Med Croatica* 1999;**53**:79–82.

271 Mee AS, Rowley JL, and the Lansoprazole clinical research goup. Rapid symptom relief in reflux oesophagitis: a comparison of lansoprazole and omeprazole. *Aliment Pharmacol Ther* 1996;**10**:757–63.

272 Farley A, Wruble LD, Humphries TJ. Rabeprazole versus ranitidine for the treatment of erosive gastroesophageal reflux disease: a double-blind, randomized clinical trial. Raberprazole Study Group. *Am J Gastroenterol* 2000; **95**:1894–9.

273 Delchier JC, Cohen G, Humphries TJ. Rabeprazole, 20 mg once daily or 10 mg twice daily, is equivalent to omeprazole, 20 mg once daily, in the healing of erosive gastrooesophageal reflux disease. *Scand J Gastroenterol* 2000;**35**:1245–50.

274 Richter JE, Kahrilas PJ, Johanson J *et al.* Efficacy and safety of esomeprazole compared with omeprazole in GERD patients with erosive esophagitis: a randomized controlled trial. *Am J Gastroenterol* 2001;**96**:656–65.

275 Dupas JL, Houcke P, Samoyeau R. Pantoprazole versus lansoprazole in French patients with reflux esophagitis. *Gastroenterol Clin Biol* 2001;**25**:245–50.

276 Korner T, Schutze K, Van Leendert RJ *et al.* Comparable efficacy of pantoprazole and omeprazole in patients with moderate to severe reflux esophagitis. Results of a multinational study. *Digestion* 2003;**67**:6–13.

277 Meneghelli UG, Boaventura S, Moraes-Filho JP *et al.* Efficacy and tolerability of pantoprazole versus ranitidine in the treatment of reflux esophagitis and the influence of *Helicobacter pylori* infection on healing rate. *Dis Esophagus* 2002;**15**:50–6.

278 Holtmann G, Bytzer P, Metz M, Loeffler V, Blum AL. A randomized, double-blind, comparative study of standard-dose rabeprazole and high-dose omeprazole in gastro-oesophageal reflux disease. *Aliment Pharmacol Ther* 2002;**16**:479–85.

279 Richter JE, Bochenek W. Oral pantoprazole for erosive esophagitis: a placebo-controlled, randomized clinical trial. Pantoprazole US GERD Study Group. *Am J Gastroenterol* 2000;**95**:3071–80.

280 Sontag SJ, KoGut DG, Fleischmann R *et al.* Lansoprazole heals erosive reflux esophagitis resistant to histamine H2-receptor antagonist therapy. *Am J Gastroenterol* 1997; **92**:429–37.

281 Hatlebakk JG, Berstad A, Carling L *et al.* Lansoprazole versus omeprazole in short-term treatment of reflux oesophagitis. Results of a Scandinavian multicentre trial. *Scand J Gastroenterol* 1993;**28**:224–8.

282 Mulder CJ, Westerveld BD, Smit JM *et al.* A double-blind, randomized comparison of omeprazole Multiple Unit Pellet System (MUPS) 20 mg, lansoprazole 30 mg and pantoprazole 40 mg in symptomatic reflux oesophagitis followed by 3 months of omeprazole MUPS maintenance treatment: a Dutch multicentre trial. *Eur J Gastroenterology Hepatol* 2002;**14**:649–56.

283 Holtmann G, Bytzer P, Metz M, Loeffler V, Blum AL. A randomized, double-blind, comparative study of standard-dose rabeprazole and high-dose omeprazole in gastro-oesophageal reflux disease. *Aliment Pharmacol Ther* 2002;**16**:479–85.

284 Thjodleifsson B, Beker JA, Dekkers C, Bjaaland T, Finnegan V, Humphries TJ. Rabeprazole versus omeprazole in preventing relapse of erosive or ulcerative gastro-esophageal reflux disease: a double-blind, multicenter, European trial. The European Rabeprazole Study Group. *Dig Dis Sci* 2000;**45**:845–53.

285 Vakil NB, Shaker R, Johnson DA *et al.* The new proton pump inhibitor esomeprazole is effective as a maintenance therapy in GERD patients with healed erosive oesophagitis: a 6-month, randomized, double-blind, placebo-controlled study of efficacy and safety. *Aliment Pharmacol Ther* 2001;**15**:927–35.

286 Vakil N, Fennerty MB. Direct comparative trials of the efficacy of proton pump inhibitors in the management of gastro-oesophageal reflux disease and peptic ulcer disease. *Aliment Pharmacol Ther* 2003;**18**:559–68.

287 Mossner J, Holscher AH, Herz R, Schneider A. A double-blind study of pantoprazole and omeprazole in the treatment of reflux oesophagitis: a multicentre trial. *Aliment Pharmacol Ther* 1995;**9**:321–6.

288 Mulder CJ, Dekker W, Gerretsen M. Lansoprazole 30 mg versus omeprazole 40 mg in the treatment of reflux oesophagitis grade II, III and IVa (a Dutch multicentre trial). Dutch Study Group. *Eur J Gastroenterology Hepatol* 1996;**8**:1101–6.

289 Dekkers CPM, Beker JA, Thjodleifsson B, Gabryelewicz A, Bell NE, Humphries TJ, and the European Rabeprazole Study Group. Double-blind, placebo-controlled comparison of rabeprazole 20mg vs omeprazole 20mg in the treatment of erosive or ulcerative gastro-oesophageal reflux disease. *Aliment Pharmacol Ther* 1999;**13**:49–57.

290 Corinaldesi R, Valentini M, Belaiche J, Colin R, Geldof H, Maier C, The European Pantoprazole Study Group. Pantoprazole and omeprazole in the treatment of reflux oesophagitis: a European multicentre study. *Aliment Pharmacol Ther* 1995;**9**:667–71.

291 Mossner J, Holscher AH, Herz R, Schneider A. A double-blind study of pantoprazole and omeprazole in the treatment of reflux oesophagitis: a multicentre trial. *Aliment Pharmacol Ther* 1995;**9**:321–6.

292 Edwards SJ, Lind T, Lundell L. Systematic review of proton pump inhibitors for the acute treatment of reflux oesophagitis. *Aliment Pharmacol Ther* 2001;**15**:1729–36.

293 Klok RM, Postma MJ, van Hout BA, Brouwers JR. Meta-analysis: comparing the efficacy of proton pump inhibitors in short-term use. *Aliment Pharmacol Ther* 2003;**17**:1237–45.

294 Caro JJ, Salas M, Ward A. Healing and relapse rates in gastroesophageal reflux disease treated with the newer proton-pump inhibitors lansoprazole, rabeprazole, and pantoprazole compared with omeprazole, ranitidine, and placebo: evidence from randomized clinical trials. *Clin Ther* 2001;**23**:998–1017.

295 Hatlebakk JG. Review article: gastric acidity – comparison of esomeprazole with other proton pump inhibitors. *Aliment Pharmacol Ther* 2003;**17(Suppl 1)**:10–15.

296 Labenz J, Petersen KU, Rosch W, Koelz HR. A summary of Food and Drug Administration-reported adverse events and drug interactions occurring during therapy with omeprazole, lansoprazole and pantoprazole. *Aliment Pharmacol Ther* 2003;**17**:1015–19.

297 Frazzoni M, De Micheli E, Grisendi A, Savarino V. Effective intra-oesophageal acid suppression in patients with gastro-oesophageal reflux disease: lansoprazole vs. pantoprazole. *Aliment Pharmacol Ther* 2003;**17**:235–41.

298 Klinkenberg-Knol EC, Festen HPM, Jansen JBMJ *et al.* Long-term treatment with omeprazole for refractory reflux esophagitis: efficacy and safety. *Ann Intern Med* 1994;**121**:161–7.

299 Klinkenberg-Knol EC, Nelis F, Dent J *et al.* Long-term omeprazole treatment in resistant gastroesophageal reflux disease: efficacy, safety, and influence on gastric mucosa. *Gastroenterology* 2000;**118**:661–9.

300 Lundell L, Miettinen P, Myrvold HE *et al* Continued (5-year) follow up of a randomized clinical study comparing antireflux surgery and omeprazole in gastroesophageal reflux disease. *J Am Coll Surg* 2001;**192**:172–9.

301 Inadomi JM, McIntyre L, Bernard L, Fendrick AM. Step-down from multiple- to single-dose proton pump inhibitors (PPIs): a prospective study of patients with heartburn or acid regurgitation completely relieved with PPIs. *Am J Gastroenterol* 2003;**98**:1940–4.

302 Koelz HR, Birchler R, Bretholz A *et al.* Healing and relapse of reflux esophagitis during treatment with ranitidine. *Gastroenterology* 1986;**91**:1198–205.

303 Hetzel DJ, Dent J, Reed WD *et al.* Healing and relapse of severe peptic esophagitis after treatment with omeprazole. *Gastroenterology* 1988;**95**:903–12.

304 Olbe L, Lundell L. Medical treatment of reflux esophagitis. *Hepatogastroenterology* 1992;**39**:322–4.

305 Klinkenberg-Knol EC, Jansen JBMJ, Lamers CBHW, Nelis F, Meuwissen SGM. Temporary cessation of long-term maintenance treatment with omeprazole in patients with H2-receptor-antagonist-resistant reflux oesophagitis. Effects on symptoms, endoscopy, serum gastrin, and gastric acid output. *Scand J Gastroenterol* 1990;**25**:1144–50.

306 Sontag SJ, KoGut DG, Fleischmann R, Campbell DR, Richter J, Haber M, and the Lansoprazole Maintenance Study Group. Lansoprazole prevents recurrence of erosive reflux esophagitis previously-resistant to H2-RA therapy. *Am J Gastroenterol* 1996;**91**:1758–65.

307 Carlsson R, Galmiche JP, Dent J, Lundell L, Frison L. Prognostic factors influencing relapse of oesophagitis during maintenance therapy with anti-secretory drugs: a meta-analysis of long-term omeprazole trials. *Aliment Pharmacol Ther* 1997;**11**:473–82.

308 Chiba N. Proton pump inhibitors in acute healing and maintenance of erosive or worse esophagitis: a systematic overview. Can J *Gastroenterology* 1997;**11(Suppl B)**:66B–73B.

309 Chiba N, Hunt RH. Gastroesophageal Reflux Disease. In: McDonald J, Burroughs A, Feagan B, eds. *Evidence-Based Gastroenterology and Hepatology*. London: BMJ Books, 1999.

310 Escourrou J, Deprez P, Saggioro A, Geldof H, Fischer R, Maier C. Maintenance therapy with pantoprazole 20 mg prevents relapse of reflux oesophagitis. *Aliment Pharmacol Ther* 1999;**13**:1481–91.

311 Plein K, Hotz J, Wurzer H, Fumagalli I, Luhmann R, Schneider A. Pantoprazole 20 mg is an effective maintenance therapy for patients with gastro-oesophageal reflux disease. *Eur J Gastroenterology Hepatol* 2000;**12**:425–32.

312 Caos A, Moskovitz M, Dayal Y, Perdomo C, Niecestro R, Barth J. Rabeprazole for the prevention of pathologic and symptomatic relapse of erosive or ulcerative gastro-esophageal reflux disease. Rebeprazole Study Group. *Am J Gastroenterol* 2000;**95**:3081–8.

313 Birbara C, Breiter J, Perdomo C, Hahne W. Rabeprazole for the prevention of recurrent erosive or ulcerative gastro-oesophageal reflux disease. Rabeprazole Study Group. *Eur J Gastroenterology Hepatol* 2000;**12**:889–97.

314 Lauritsen K, Deviere J, Bigard MA *et al.* Esomeprazole 20 mg and lansoprazole 15 mg in maintaining healed reflux oesophagitis: Metropole study results. *Aliment Pharmacol Ther* 2003;**17**:333–41.

315 Pilotto A, Leandro G, Franceschi M. Short- and long-term therapy for reflux oesophagitis in the elderly: a multi-centre, placebo-controlled study with pantoprazole. *Aliment Pharmacol Ther* 2003;**17**:1399–406.

316 Metz DC, Bochenek WJ. Pantoprazole maintenance therapy prevents relapse of erosive oesophagitis. *Aliment Pharmacol Ther* 2003;**17**:155–64.

317 Bardhan KD, Cherian P, Vaishnavi A *et al.* Erosive oesophagitis: outcome of repeated long-term maintenance treatment with low dose omeprazole 10 mg or placebo. *Gut* 1998;**43**:458–64.

318 Lundell L, Backman L, Ekstrom P *et al.* Prevention of relapse of reflux esophagitis after endoscopic healing: the efficacy and safety of omeprazole compared with ranitidine. *Scand J Gastroenterol* 1991;**26**:248–56.

319 Gough AL, Long RG, Cooper BT, Foster CN, Garrett AD, Langworthy CH. Lansoprazole versus ranitidine in the maintenance treatment of reflux oesophagitis. *Aliment Pharmacol Ther* 1996;**10**:529–39.

320 Carling L, Axelsson CK, Forssell H *et al.* Lansoprazole and omeprazole in the prevention of relapse of reflux oesophagitis: a long-term comparative study. *Aliment Pharmacol Ther* 1998;**12**:985–90.

321 Simon TJ, Roberts WG, Berlin RG, Hayden LJ, Berman RS, Reagan JE. Acid suppression by famotidine 20mg twice daily or 40mg twice daily in preventing relapse of endoscopic recurrence of erosive esophagitis. *Clin Ther* 1995;**17**:1147–56.

322 Robinson M, Lanza F, Avner D, Haber M. Effective maintenance treatment of reflux esophagitis with low-dose lansoprazole. A randomized, double-blind, placebo-controlled trial. *Ann Intern Med* 1996;**124**:859–67.

323 Sontag SJ, Robinson M, Roufail W *et al.* Daily omeprazole surpasses intermittent dosing in preventing relapse of oesophagitis: a US multi-centre double blind study. *Aliment Pharmacol Ther* 1997;**11**:373–80.

324 Dent J, Yeomans ND, MacKinnon M *et al.* Omeprazole v ranitidine for prevention of relapse in reflux oesophagitis. A controlled double blind trial of their efficacy and safety [See comments]. *Gut* 1994;**35**:590–8.

325 Hallerback B, Unge P, Carling L *et al* Omeprazole or ranitidine in long-term treatment of reflux esophagitis. The Scandinavian Clinics for United Research Group. *Gastroenterology* 1994;**107**:1305–11.

326 Bate CM, Booth SN, Crowe JP *et al.*, and the Solo Investigator Group. Omeprazole 10 mg or 20 mg once daily in the prevention of recurrence of reflux oesophagitis. *Gut* 1995;**36**:492–8.

327 Hatlebakk JG, Berstad A. Lansoprazole 15 and 30 mg daily in maintaining healing and symptom relief in paitents with reflux oesophagitis. *Aliment Pharmacol Ther* 1997;**11**:365–72.

328 van Rensburg CJ, Honiball PJ, van Zyl JH *et al.* Safety and efficacy of pantoprazole 40 mg daily as relapse prophylaxis in patients with healed reflux oesophagitis-a 2-year follow-up. *Aliment Pharmacol Ther* 1999;**13**:1023–8.

329 Thjodleifsson B, Rindi G, Fiocca R, Humphries TJ, Morocutti A, Miller N, Bardhan KD. A randomized, double-blind trial of the efficacy and safety of 10 or 20 mg rabeprazole compared with 20 mg omeprazole in the maintenance of gastrooesophageal reflux disease over 5 years. *Aliment Pharmacol Ther* 2003;**17**:343–51.

330 Bardhan KD, Muller-Lissner S, Bigard MA *et al.* Symptomatic gastro-oesophageal reflux disease: double blind controlled study of intermittent treatment with omeprazole or ranitidine. The European Study Group. *BMJ* 1999;**318**:502–7.

331 Stalhammar NO, Carlsson J, Peacock R *et al.* Cost effectiveness of omeprazole and ranitidine in intermittent treatment of symptomatic gastrooesophageal reflux disease. *Pharmacoeconomics* 1999;**16**:483–97.

332 Baldi F, Morselli-Labate AM, Cappiello R, Ghersi S. Daily low-dose versus alternate day full-dose lansoprazole in the maintenance treatment of reflux esophagitis. *Am J Gastroenterol* 2002;**97**:1357–64.

333 Johnsson F, Moum B, Vilien M, Grove O, Simren M, Thoring M. On-demand treatment in patients with oesophagitis and reflux symptoms: comparison of lansoprazole and omeprazole. *Scand J Gastroenterol* 2002;**37**:642–7.

334 Sridhar S, Huang JQ, O'Brien BJ, Hunt RH. Clinical economics review: cost-effectiveness of treatment alternatives for gastooesophageal reflux disease. *Aliment Pharmacol Ther* 1996;**10**:865–73.

335 Sadowski D, Champion M, Goeree R *et al.* Health economics of gastroesophageal reflux disease. *Can J Gastroenterol* 1997;**11(Suppl B)**:108B–112B.

336 Bate CM. Cost-effectiveness of omeprazole in the treatment of reflux oesophagitis. *Br J Med Econ* 1991;**1**:53–61.

337 Bate CM, Richardson PDI. A one year model for the cost-effectiveness of treating reflux oesophagitis. *Br J Med Econ* 1992;**2**:5–11.

338 Bate CM, Richardson PDI. Symptomatic assessment and cost effectiveness of treatments for reflux oesophagitis: comparisons of omperazole and histamine H2-receptor antagonists. *Br J Med Econ* 1992;**2**:37–48.

339 Bate CM. Omeprazole vs Ranitidine and cimetidine in reflux oesophagitis: The British perspective. *Pharmacoeconomics* 1994;**5**:35–43.

340 Hillman AL, Bloom BS, Fendrick AM, Schwartz JS. Cost and quality effects of alternative treatments for persistent gastroesophageal reflux disease. *Arch Intern Med* 1992;**152**:1467–72.

341 Bloom BS. Cost and quality effects of treating erosive esophagitis: a re-evaluation. *Pharmacoeconomics* 1995;**8**:139–46.

342 Jones RH, Bosanquet N, Johnson NJ, Chong SL. Cost-effective management strategies for acid-peptic disorders. *Br J Med Econ* 1994;**7**:99–114.

343 Zagari M, Villa KF, Freston JW. Proton pump inhibitors versus H2-receptor antagonists for the treatment of erosive gastroesophageal reflux disease: a cost-comparative study. *Am J Man Care* 1995;**1**:247–55.

344 O'Brien BJ, Goeree R, Hunt R, Wilkinson J, Levine M, Willan A. Economic evaluation of alternative therapies in the long-term management of peptic ulcer disease and gastroesophageal relux disease. 1996. McMaster University. Canadian Coordinating Office of Health Technology Assessment (CCOHTA) report. 1996.

345 Jönsson B, Stålhammar NO. The cost-effectiveness of omeprazole and ranitidine in intermittent and maintenance treatment of reflux oesophagitis – the case of Sweden. *Br J Med Econ* 1993;**6**:111–26.

346 Harris RA, Kuppermann M, Richter JE. Proton pump inhibitors or histamine-2 receptor antagonists for the prevention of recurrences of erosive reflux esophagitis: a cost-effectiveness analysis. *Am J Gastroenterol* 1997;**92**:2179–87.

347 Harris RA, Kuppermann M, Richter JE. Prevention of recurrences of erosive reflux esophagitis: a cost-effectiveness analysis of maintenance proton pump inhibition. *Am J Med* 1997;**102**:78–88.

348 You JH, Lee AC, Wong SC, Chan FK. Low-dose or standard-dose proton pump inhibitors for maintenance therapy of gastrooesophageal reflux disease: a cost-effectiveness analysis. *Aliment Pharmacol Ther* 2003;**17**:785–92.

349 Bate CM, Griffin SM, Keeling PW *et al.* Reflux symptom relief with omeprazole in patients without unequivocal oesophagitis. *Aliment Pharmacol Ther* 1996;**10**:547–55.

350 Venables TL, Newland RD, Patel AC, Hole J, Copeman MB, Turbitt ML. Maintenance treatment for gastro-oesophageal reflux disease. A placebo-controlled evaluation of 10 milligrams omeprazole once daily in general practice. *Scand J Gastroenterol* 1997;**32**:627–32.

351 van Pinxteren B, Numans ME, Bonis PA, Lau J. Short-term treatment with proton pump inhibitors, H2-receptor antagonists and prokinetics for gastrooesophageal reflux disease-like symptoms and endoscopy negative reflux disease (Cochrane Review). In: Cochrane Collaboration. *Cochrane Library* 2003:**4**. Chichester, UK, John Wiley & Sons, Ltd.

352 Richter JE, Peura D, Benjamin SB, Joelsson B, Whipple J. Efficacy of omeprazole for the treatment of symptomatic acid reflux disease without esophagitis. *Arch Intern Med* 2000;**160**:1810–16.

353 Hatlebakk JG, Hyggen A, Madsen PH *et al.* Heartburn treatment in primary care: randomised, double blind study for 8 weeks. *BMJ* 1999;**319**:550–3.

354 Katz PO, Castell DO, Levine D. Esomeprazole resolves chronic heartburn in patients without erosive oesophagitis. *Aliment Pharmacol Ther* 2003;**18**:875–82.

355 Richter JE, Kovacs TO, Greski-Rose PA, Huang section sign B, Fisher R. Lansoprazole in the treatment of heartburn in patients without erosive oesophagitis. *Aliment Pharmacol Ther* 1999;**13**:795–804.

356 Richter JE, Campbell DR, Kahrilas PJ, Huang B, Fludas C. Lansoprazole compared with ranitidine for the treatment of non-erosive gastroesophageal reflux disease. *Arch Intern Med* 2000;**160**:1803–9.

357 Bardhan KD, van Rensburg C. Comparable clinical efficacy and tolerability of 20 mg pantoprazole and 20 mg omeprazole in patients with grade I reflux oesophagitis. *Aliment Pharmacol Ther* 2001;**15**:1585–91.

358 Kaspari S, Biedermann A, Mey J. Comparison of pantoprazole 20 mg to ranitidine 150 mg b.i.d. in the treatment of mild gastroesophageal reflux disease. *Digestion* 2001;**63**:163–70.

359 Miner P Jr, Orr W, Filippone J, Jokubaitis L, Sloan S. Rabeprazole in non-erosive gastroesophageal reflux

disease: a randomized placebo-controlled trial. *Am J Gastroenterol* 2002;**97**:1332–9.

360 Bytzer P. Goals of therapy and guidelines for treatment success in symptomatic gastroesophageal reflux disease patients. *Am J Gastroenterol* 2003;**98**:S31–S39.

361 Carlsson R, Dent J, Watts R *et al.*, and the International GORD Study Group. Gastrooesophageal reflux disease in primary care: an international study of different treatment strategies with omeprazole. *Eur J Gastroenterology Hepatol* 1998;**10**:119–24.

362 Havelund T, Aalykke C. The efficacy of a pectin-based raft-forming anti-reflux agent in endoscopy-negative reflux disease. *Scand J Gastroenterol* 1997;**32**:773–7.

363 Lind T, Havelund T, Lundell L *et al.* On demand therapy with omeprazole for the long-term management of patients with heartburn without oesophagitis – a placebo-controlled randomized trial. *Aliment Pharmacol Ther* 1999;**13**:907–14.

364 Talley NJ, Lauritsen K, Tunturi-Hihnala H *et al.* Esomeprazole 20 mg maintains symptom control in endoscopy-negative gastrooesophageal reflux disease: a controlled trial of "on-demand" therapy for 6 months. *Aliment Pharmacol Ther* 2001;**15**:347–54.

365 Talley NJ, Venables TL, Green JR *et al.* Esomeprazole 40 mg and 20 mg is efficacious in the long-term management of patients with endoscopy-negative gastrooesophageal reflux disease: a placebo-controlled trial of on-demand therapy for 6 months. *Eur J Gastroenterology Hepatol* 2002;**14**:857–63.

366 Wahlqvist P, Junghard O, Higgins A, Green J. Cost effectiveness of proton pump inhibitors in gastrooesophageal reflux disease without oesophagitis: comparison of on-demand esomeprazole with conventional omeprazole strategies. *Pharmacoeconomics* 2002;**20**:267–77.

367 Bate CM, Green JR, Axon AT *et al.* Omeprazole is more effective than cimetidine for the relief of all grades of gastrooesophageal reflux disease-associated heartburn, irrespective of the presence or absence of endoscopic oesophagitis. *Aliment Pharmacol Ther* 1997;**11**:755–63.

368 Bate CM, Green JR, Axon AT *et al.* Omeprazole is more effective than cimetidine in the prevention of recurrence of GERD-associated heartburn and the occurrence of underlying oesophagitis. *Aliment Pharmacol Ther* 1998;**12**:41–7.

369 Armstrong D, Pare P, Pericak D, Pyzyk M. Symptom relief in gastroesophageal reflux disease: a randomized, controlled comparison of pantoprazole and nizatidine in a mixed patient population with erosive esophagitis or endoscopy-negative reflux disease. *Am J Gastroenterol* 2001;**96**:2849–57.

370 Quigley EM. Factors that influence therapeutic outcomes in symptomatic gastroesophageal reflux disease. *Am J Gastroenterol* 2003;**98**:S24–S30.

371 Gardner JD, Gallo-Torres H, Sloan S, Robinson M, Miner PB. The basis for the decreased response to proton pump inhibitors in gastrooesophageal reflux disease patients without erosive oesophagitis. *Aliment Pharmacol Ther* 2003;**18**:891–905.

372 Hungin APS, Gunn SD, Bate CM, Turbitt ML, Wilcock C, Richardson PDI. A comparison of the efficacy of omeprazole 20 mg once daily with ranitidine 150 mg bd in the relief of symptomatic gastrooesophageal reflux disease in general practice. *Br J Clin Res* 1993;**4**:73–88.

373 Rush DR, Stelmach WJ, Young TL *et al.* Clinical effectiveness and quality of life with ranitidine vs placebo in gastroesophageal reflux disease patients: a clinical experience network (CEN) study. *J Fam Pract* 1995;**41**:126–36.

374 Howden CW, Henning JM, Huang B, Lukasik N, Freston JW. Management of heartburn in a large, randomized, community-based study: comparison of four therapeutic strategies. *Am J Gastroenterol* 2001;**96**:1704–10.

375 Talley NJ, Moore MG, Sprogis A, Katelaris P. Randomised controlled trial of pantoprazole versus ranitidine for the treatment of uninvestigated heartburn in primary care. *Med J Aust* 2002;**177**:423–7.

376 Armstrong D, Barkun AN, Chiba N *et al.*, and CADET HR investigators. Initial PPI therapy is most effective in the management of heartburn-dominant uninvestigated dyspepsia (UD) in primary care practice (PCP) – The CADET-HR study. *Can J Gastroenterol* 2002; **16(Suppl A)**:97A.

377 Armstrong D, Barkun AN, Chiba N *et al.*, and CADET HR investigators. "Start high – a better acid suppression strategy for heartburn-dominant uninvestigated dyspepsia (UD) in primary care practice – the CADET-HR study. *Can J Gastroenterol* 2002;**16 (Suppl A)**:97A–98A.

378 Armstrong D, Barkun AN, Chiba N *et al.*, and CADET HR investigators. Symptom relapse after acute therapy for heartburn-dominant uninvestigated dyspepsia (UD) in primary care practice (PCP)–The CADET-HR study. *Can J Gastroenterol* 2002;**16(Suppl A)**:98A.

379 Chey W, Huang B, Jackson RL. Lansoprazole and esomperazole in symptomatic GERD: A double-blind, randomised, multicentre trial in 3000 patients confirms comparable symptom relief. *Clin Drug Invest* 2003;**23**:69–84.

380 Kleinman L, McIntosh E, Ryan M, Schmier J, Crawley J, Locke GR, III, De Lissovoy G. Willingness to pay for complete symptom relief of gastroesophageal reflux disease. *Arch Intern Med* 2002;**162**:1361–6.

381 Ofman JJ. The economic and quality-of-life impact of symptomatic gastroesophageal reflux disease. *Am J Gastroenterol* 2003;**98**:S8–S14.

382 Bianchi Porro G, Pace F, Sangaletti O *et al.* High-dose famotidine in the maintenance treatment of refractory esophagitis: results of a medium-term open study. *Am J Gastroenterol* 1991;**86**:1585–7.

383 Castell DO, Kahrilas PJ, Richter JE *et al.* Esomeprazole (40 mg) compared with lansoprazole (30 mg) in the treatment of erosive esophagitis. *Am J Gastroenterol* 2002;**97**:575–83.

384 Starlinger M, Appel WH, Schemper M, Schiessel R. Long-term treatment of peptic esophageal stenosis with dilation and cimetidine: factors influencing clinical results. *Eur Surg Res* 1985;**17**:207–14.

385 Ferguson R, Dronfield MW, Atkinson M. Cimetidine in treatment of reflux esophagitis with peptic stricture. *BMJ* 1979;**2**:472–4.

386 Farup PG, Modalsli B, Tholfsen JK. Long-term treatment with 300 mg ranitidine once daily after dilatation of peptic oesophageal strictures. *Scand J Gastroenterol* 1992;**27**: 594–8.

387 Smith PM, Kerr GD, Cockel R *et al.* A comparison of omeprazole and ranitidine in the prevention of recurrence of benign esophageal stricture. The RESTORE Investigator Group. *Gastroenterology* 1994;**107**:1312–18.

388 Marks RD, Richter JE, Rizzo J, Koehler RE, Spenney JG, Mills TP, Champion G. Omeprazole versus H$_2$-receptor antagonists in treating patients with peptic stricture and esophagitis. *Gastroenterology* 1994;**106**:907–15.

389 Swarbrick ET, Gough AL, Foster CS, Christian J, Garrett AD, Langworthy CH. Prevention of recurrence of oesophageal stricture, a comparison of lansoprazole and high-dose ranitidine. *Eur J Gastroenterology Hepatol* 1996; **8**:431–8.

390 Jaspersen D, Diehl KL, Schoeppner H, Geyer P, Martens E. A comparison of omeprazole, lansoprazole, and pantoprazole in the maintenance treatment of severe reflux oesophagitis. *Aliment Pharmacol Ther* 1998;**12**:49–52.

391 Galmiche JP, Bruley des Varannes S. Endoluminal therapies for gastrooesophageal reflux disease. *Lancet* 2003;**361**: 1119–21.

392 Vakil N, Sharma P. Review article: endoscopic treatments for gastrooesophageal reflux disease. *Aliment Pharmacol Ther* 2003;**17**:1427–34.

393 Filipi CJ, Lehman GA, Rothstein RI *et al.* Transoral, flexible endoscopic suturing for treatment of GERD: a multicenter trial. *Gastrointest Endosc* 2001;**53**:416–22.

394 Mahmood Z, McMahon BP, Arfin Q *et al.* Endocinch therapy for gastrooesophageal reflux disease: a one year prospective follow up. *Gut* 2003;**52**:34–9.

395 Rothstein RI, Filipi CJ. Endoscopic suturing for gastroesophageal reflux disease: clinical outcome with the Bard EndoCinch. *Gastrointest Endosc Clin North Am* 2003;**13**:89–101.

396 Triadafilopoulos G, DiBaise JK, Nostrant TT *et al.* Radiofrequency energy delivery to the gastroesophageal junction for the treatment of GERD. *Gastrointest Endosc* 2001;**53**:407–15.

397 Triadafilopoulos G, DiBaise JK, Nostrant TT *et al.* The Stretta procedure for the treatment of GERD: 6 and 12 month follow-up of the U.S. open label trial. *Gastrointest Endosc* 2002;**55**:149–56.

398 Johnson DA, Ganz R, Aisenberg J *et al.* Endoscopic implantation of enteryx for treatment of GERD: 12-month results of a prospective, multicenter trial. *Am J Gastroenterol* 2003;**98**:1921–30.

399 Behar J, Sheahan DG, Biancani P, Spiro HM, Storer EH. Medical and surgical management of reflux esophagitis. A 38-month report of a prospective clinical trial. *N Engl J Med* 1975;**293**:263–8.

400 Spechler SJ. Comparison of medical and surgical therapy for complicated gastroesophageal reflux disease in veterans. The Department of Veterans Affairs Gastroesophageal Reflux Disease Study Group. *N Engl J Med* 1992;**326**: 786–92.

401 Spechler SJ, Lee E, Ahnen D *et al.* Long-term outcome of medical and surgical therapies for gastroesophageal reflux disease: follow up of a randomized controlled trial. *JAMA* 2001;**285**:2331–8.

402 Frazzoni M, Grisendi A, Lanzani A, Melotti G, De Micheli E. Laparoscopic fundoplication versus lansoprazole for gastrooesophageal reflux disease. A pH-metric comparison. *Dig Liver Dis* 2002;**34**:99–104.

403 Moss SF, Armstrong D, Arnold R *et al.* GERD 2003 – a consensus on the way ahead. *Digestion* 2003;**67**:111–17.

404 Luostarinen M, Isolauri J, Laitinen J *et al.* Fate of Nissen fundoplication after 20 years. A clinical, endoscopical, and functional analysis. *Gut* 1993;**34**:1015–20.

405 Low DE, Anderson RP, Ilves R, Ricciardelli E, Hill LD. Fifteen- to twenty-year results after the Hill antireflux operation. *J Thorac Cardiovasc Surg* 1989;**98**:444–9.

406 Lundell L, Dalenbäck J, Hattlebakk J *et al.* Outcome of open antireflux surgery as assessed in a Nordic multicentre prospective clinical trial. Nordic GORD-Study Group. *Eur J Surg* 1998;**164**:751–7.

407 Laine S, Rantala A, Gullichsen R, Ovaska J. Laparoscopic vs conventional Nissen fundoplication. A prospective randomized study. *Surg Endosc* 1997;**11**:441–4.

408 Blomqvist AM, Lönroth H, Dalenbäck J, Lundell L. Laparoscopic or open fundoplication? A complete cost analysis. *Surg Endosc* 1998;**12**:1209–12.

409 Champault G, Volter F, Rizk N, Boutelier P. Gastroesophageal reflux: conventional surgical treatment versus laparoscopy. A prospective study of 61 cases. *Surg Laparosc Endosc* 1996;**6**:434–40.

410 Peters JH, Heimbucher J, Kauer WK, Incarbone R, Bremner CG, DeMeester TR. Clinical and physiologic comparison of laparoscopic and open Nissen fundoplication [See comments]. *J Am Coll Surg* 1995;**180**:385–93.

411 Eshraghi N, Farahmand M, Soot SJ, Rand LL, Deveney CW, Sheppard BC. Comparison of outcomes of open versus laparoscopic Nissen fundoplication performed in a single practice. *Am J Surg* 1998;**175**:371–4.

412 Lundell L. Laparoscopic fundoplication is the treatment of choice for gastrooesophageal reflux disease. Protagonist. *Gut* 2002;**51**:468–71.

413 Watson DI, Jamieson GG. Anti-reflux surgery in the laparoscopic era. *Br J Surg* 1998;**85**:1173–84.

414 Galmiche JP, Zerbib F. Laparoscopic fundoplication is the treatment of choice for gastrooesophageal reflux disease. Antagonist. *Gut* 2002;**51**:472–4.

415 Anvari M, Allen CJ. Prospective evaluation of dysphagia before and after laparoscopic Nissen fundoplication without routine division of short gastrics. *Surg Laparosc Endosc* 1996;**6**:424–9.

3 Barrett's esophagus

Carlo A Fallone, Marc Bradette, Naoki Chiba

Introduction

Attention was first focused on what was later to be called Barrett's esophagus in the 1950s by Norman Barrett.[1] This is a condition in which the normally squamous mucosa of the esophagus is replaced by metaplastic columnar epithelium due to injury from gastroesophageal reflux. Hence, Barrett's esophagus is one of the complications of gastroesophageal reflux disease (GERD), whose importance is based entirely on its association with esophageal adenocarcinoma. The latter develops in approximately 0·5% of patients with Barrett's esophagus per year.[2]

Definition

The definition of Barrett's esophagus has changed over the past few years. From its original description as a columnar lined lower esophagus,[1,3] to one requiring at least 3 cm of circumferential columnar lining or intestinal metaplasia,[4] it has evolved most recently to the absolute requirement for histologically confirmed intestinal metaplasia in the esophagus but without any specified minimal length.[5,6] The Practice Parameters Committee of the American College of Gastroenterology has most recently agreed to continue to define this entity as "a change in the esophageal epithelium of any length that can be recognized at endoscopy and is confirmed to have intestinal metaplasia by biopsy of the tubular esophagus and excludes intestinal metaplasia of the cardia".[6]

There are three important components to this definition that are worth highlighting. First, intestinal metaplasia must be present. Gastric metaplasia without intestinal metaplasia does not constitute Barrett's esophagus, as it is the specialized intestinal epithelium that is associated with adenocarcinoma.[6,7] Second, this definition encompasses not only the classical Barrett's esophagus (≥ 3 cm columnar lined mucosa of distal esophagus with intestinal metaplasia) but also the short segment Barrett's esophagus (SSBE) defined as specialized columnar epithelium lining < 3 cm of the distal esophagus.[8] This is because the risk for developing dysplasia and esophageal cancer with SSBE is not substantially lower than it is with classical Barrett's esophagus.[9–14] Finally, intestinal metaplasia of the gastric cardia is not included, as this entity does not have the same implications as intestinal metaplasia of the tubular esophagus. The risk of esophageal cancer with intestinal metaplasia of the cardia is unclear, and no recommendation for cancer surveillance is established. This point underlines the importance of identification of appropriate landmarks such as the gastroesophageal junction at endoscopy.

Epidemiology

Incidence and prevalence

The prevalence of Barrett's esophagus has been established by both endoscopic and autopsy studies. The figures vary according to the population studied and the definition used. Approximately 6–12% of patients undergoing endoscopy for symptoms of GERD had Barrett's esophagus, with the majority having SSBE (6–10% SSBE *v* 5% classical Barrett's).[9,15–17] In a group of Canadian patients with dyspeptic symptoms (as opposed to only GERD symptoms), in whom prompt endoscopy was carried out, the prevalence of Barrett's esophagus was 2·4%.[18] Another study on dyspeptic patients obtained a rate of only 0·3%, but this estimate excluded patients with alarm symptoms and those over 45 years of age.[19] Other studies have also obtained an estimate of ≤ 1% in unselected patient populations undergoing endoscopy.[9,20,21] Autopsy studies, on the other hand, suggest that the actual prevalence of Barrett's esophagus is about 21 times higher than that detected endoscopically, and that the vast majority of patients with Barrett's esophagus remain unrecognized.[22]

The reported incidence of Barrett's esophagus has increased since the 1970s in parallel with the increased use of gastroscopy. There are approximately 10 new diagnoses of Barrett's per 100 000 persons per year.[23] The median age of development and of diagnosis of the condition have been estimated to be 40 and 63 years, respectively.[20]

Risk factors

Barrett's esophagus appears to be found predominately in white males.[6,15] However, rates similar to whites have been found in Hispanics[24,25], and in some Asians.[26] In addition, one would expect that as lifestyle and dietary habits change in developing countries to approximate those of the Western world, the prevalence of Barrett's esophagus would increase. The decreasing prevalence of *Helicobacter pylori* infection has been suggested to play a role in the simultaneous increase of Barrett's, but this is controversial.[27–29]

In addition to age, sex and race, longer duration of GERD is a risk factor for Barrett's esophagus.[15,30,31] Compared with patients with reflux symptoms for < 1 year, Barrett's esophagus was three times more common if reflux symptoms were present for 1–5 years, five times more common for symptoms present for 5–10 years or 6·4 times more common if reflux symptoms were present longer than 10 years.[31] Increased severity of nocturnal reflux symptoms[30–32] and increased complications of GERD such as esophagitis, ulceration and bleeding are also associated with Barrett's esophagus,[30] but the evidence regarding peptic strictures is conflicting.[30,33,34] There is also a higher incidence of hiatal hernia with Barrett's esophagus.[35,36] Although these factors are associated with Barrett's esophagus, many patients with this condition have symptoms that are no different from those experienced by other GERD patients. Many patients have no significant symptoms, possibly due to reduced esophageal sensitivity to acid.[22,37]

Natural history

The survival of a patient with Barrett's esophagus is very similar to that of patients with benign esophageal disorders such as achalasia or Schatzki's ring.[38] The overwhelming majority of patients with Barrett's esophagus will never experience the complication feared in this condition, esophageal adenocarcinoma. Yet, if it were not for this association, Barrett's esophagus would not have any clinical importance.

Original studies estimated the incidence of esophageal adenocarcinoma in Barrett's esophagus at 1–2%, but more recent analysis of epidemiologic studies have suggested an incidence closer to 0·5%.[38–42] The original overestimation was due to publication bias of the more positive results. This was demonstrated by Shaheen *et al.*[2] who showed that the smaller study size of reports examining cancer in Barrett's esophagus correlated with increased risk (Figure 3·1). In addition, the risk ratios from the different studies were skewed to the right (stronger association) of the median rather then evenly distributed to both sides, as would be expected if there were no publication bias. In addition some patients with Barrett's esophagus who develop cancer present

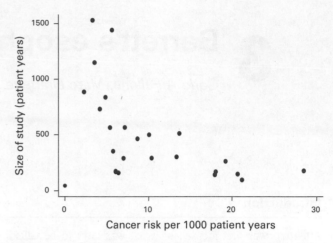

Figure 3.1 Reported cancer risk in Barrett's esophagus versus size of the study. The higher values for small studies suggest a bias against publishing small studies with low risks. (Reproduced from Shaheen NJ *et al. Gastroenterology* 2000;**119**:333–8 with permission from Elsevier[2])

simultaneously with both findings, a factor that increases the apparent strength of association.[43]

Nevertheless, Barrett's esophagus is definitely associated with esophageal carcinoma, and this cancer is increasing in incidence in Western societies. Since the mid 1970s, the incidence in white men from the USA rose from 0·7/100 000 to an estimated 3·7/100 000 in 2001.[9] This rise is not felt to be due to the previous misclassification of gastroesophageal junction esophageal carcinomas as gastric cancer, as there has not been a concomitant decrease of gastric cardia cancers.[9] The proportion of esophageal cancer due to adenocarcinoma has also increased substantially in the same period, but the absolute number of all esophageal cancers is still quite low in comparison to colorectal cancer, which is 10 times more common.[9,44] In Canada, it appears that the overall prevalence of esophageal cancer did not increase substantially for either men or women. It is still a rare cancer, ranked fourteenth for males and eighteenth for females in estimated new cancer cases in Canada in 2002.[45]

The length (extent) of Barrett's esophagus may be a risk factor for esophageal adenocarcinoma. A 5-cm difference in segment length was associated with a trend toward increased cancer risk.[14] However, a statistically significant association was not demonstrated in this study that may have lacked statistical power (relative risk 1·7, 95% CI 0·8 to 3·8). Other reported risk factors for esophageal adenocarcinoma include severity, frequency and duration of reflux symptoms,[46–48] size of hiatal hernia,[49] obesity,[50] smoking,[51] and diet low in raw fruit content.[52] Medications that lower the lower esophageal sphincter pressure have also been found to be associated with esophageal cancer, but not in all studies.[53,54] Also controversial is the possibility that *H. pylori* and in particular those with the *cagA* gene protects against esophageal cancer.[29,55] One study found the prevalence of *H. pylori* infection with *cagA*+ strains to be inversely associated with GERD complications (non-erosive GERD 41% *cagA*+, erosive GERD 31%, Barrett's esophagus 13%, Barrett's with dysplasia or adenocarcinoma 0%).[29]

The presence and degree of dysplasia associated with Barrett's esophagus is also a risk factor for the subsequent development of esophageal adenocarcinoma. Dysplasia is a histologic diagnosis usually expressed as "not present, indefinite, low grade or high grade". There is significant interobserver variability (< 50% agreement) with low grade dysplasia and there are few prospective studies.[56,57] Estimates of progression to high grade dysplasia or adenocarcinoma range from 10% to 28% within 5 years.[57] Patients with high grade dysplasia, however, have been shown clearly to have a substantially increased risk of cancer. Reid *et al.*[58] found that cancer developed in 33 of 76 patients (43%) with high grade dysplasia compared to 9 of 251 (4%) with negative, indefinite or low grade dysplasia during 5 years of observation. The results from different studies vary substantially, with 5–7-year cumulative cancer incidence estimates of 16–59%.[56,59,60] Preliminary studies have suggested that flow cytometry can also be used to predict outcome. For patients without flow cytometric abnormalities and no definite or low grade dysplasia on histology, the 5-year incidence of cancer was 0%, whereas aneuploidy, increased 4N fractions or high grade dysplasia were present in all of the 35 patients who developed cancer in the 5 years of follow up.[58]

Pathogenesis

Barrett's esophagus is felt to result from severe mucosal injury of the distal esophagus in conjunction with reflux of either acid alone or acid and bile. This perception is based on animal studies that demonstrated that excision of the esophageal mucosa results in re-epithelialization of the esophagus with columnar epithelium only if done in conjunction with acid reflux or acid and bile reflux.[61,62] Bile reflux alone did not cause columnar re-epithelialization, and excision alone resulted in re-epithelialization with primarily squamous epithelium. Although there is no direct human experimental evidence that reflux causes Barrett's esophagus, this theory is supported by human 24-hour pH monitoring studies that demonstrated a larger esophageal acid exposure in patients with Barrett's esophagus than in GERD patients without Barrett's esophagus.[63,64] In addition, the duration of esophageal acid exposure correlates with the length of Barrett's esophagus.[65] A hiatal hernia is almost always present with Barrett's esophagus. The lower pressures in the lower esophagus in these patients compared to other GERD

patients,[36,63] is a possible mechanism for the increased reflux for Barrett's metaplasia. The increased acid reflux does not appear to be due to increased acid production, since no difference is present in terms of basal or peak acid outputs.[66]

A current conceptual approach to GERD is that it represents a spectrum of disease from non-endoscopic reflux disease (NERD) to esophagitis, Barrett's esophagus, dysplasia and esophageal adenocarcinoma (Figure 3.2a). Acid reflux is felt to contribute to esophagitis and to development of Barrett's metaplasia, but the cause of progression to dysplasia in Barrett's patients is unknown. Patients with NERD, however, uncommonly develop erosive esophagitis,[67] and Barrett's esophagus is almost always diagnosed on first endoscopy.[68] It is for this reason that Fass and Ofman[69] have suggested a new conceptual model that considers GERD as three distinct groups of patients: NERD, erosive esophagitis, and Barrett's esophagus (Figure 3.2b). They suggested that patients from each group have little chance to move to other groups, but each has its own potential complications that are listed in Figure 3.2b.

Diagnosis

The diagnosis of Barrett's esophagus requires the demonstration of intestinal metaplasia on biopsy sampling of abnormally appearing esophageal mucosa.[6] This diagnosis is difficult for several reasons. There are no symptoms specific for this condition. For the most part, the symptoms are identical to those of GERD and some, if not most[22] patients are asymptomatic. In addition, the identification of the location of the gastroesophageal junction is required in order to determine if the squamocolumnar junction is displaced proximally, as this displacement is what alerts the endoscopist to the possibility of the diagnosis and leads to biopsy. The position of the junction can be very difficult to determine endoscopically because of the presence of a hiatal hernia, esophagitis and the constant movement of the area. This difficulty was highlighted by a multicenter study in which only 72% of the endoscopists correctly recorded endoscopic landmarks in the diagnosis of Barrett's esophagus.[70] SSBE can thus be particularly difficult to identify and distinguish from an irregular Z line. This distinction is very important because intestinal metaplasia in the gastric cardia does not have the same implications as intestinal metaplasia of the esophagus. Erythema or erosive esophagitis can also impair the visual recognition of Barrett's esophagus, and re-endoscopy after treatment with acid suppression may be necessary to make the diagnosis of Barrett's.[71]

Intestinal metaplasia must be present in order to make the diagnosis of Barrett's esophagus. This fact, however, seems not to be fully understood as many pathologists continue to

(a)

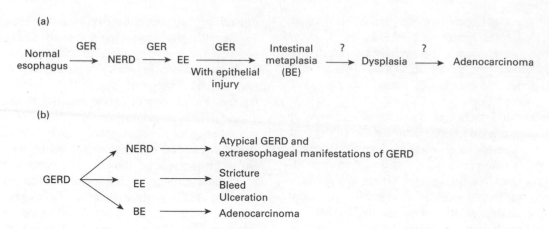

(b)

Figure 3.2 (a) Conventional concept for GERD. (b) Fass and Ofman's new concept of GERD as three distinct entities and complications associated with each.[69] GER, gastroesophageal reflux; NERD, non-endoscopic reflux disease; EE, erosive esophagitis; BE, Barrett's esophagus

classify patients without intestinal metaplasia as Barrett's esophagus.[72] The hematoxylin and eosin stain combined with alcian blue at pH 2·5 is usually used in order to identify the acid mucin-containing goblet cells characteristic of intestinal metaplasia.[5] In one study, intestinal metaplasia without dysplasia was correctly identified by only 35% of 20 community-based pathologists.[72]

A further difficulty with diagnosis is sampling error i.e. failing to biopsy the area with metaplasia. This problem introduces the important unresolved issue of the number of biopsies required. A larger number of biopsies taken and biopsy samples of greater size (i.e. jumbo forceps *v* standard) result in more accurate diagnosis, but no optimal number of biopsies has been established. It has been suggested that chromoendoscopy may help in targeting biopsies. Methylene blue, toluene blue, indigo carmine, and Lugol's iodine have all been used.[73–76] Methylene blue may be the most promising technique.[6] It is sprayed over the esophageal mucosa at the time of endoscopy. The areas of intestinal metaplasia are thought to stain preferentially. However, staining may be tedious and the results are not necessarily reproducible.[77] Magnification endoscopy has also been proposed as a means to target biopsies, but the results are preliminary.[78]

Dysplasia is only detectable histologically. It represents a change in architecture of the metaplastic glands and is the next step in the neoplastic process. The histology is thought to progress from no dysplasia to low grade dysplasia, high grade dysplasia and adenocarcinoma, although the time course of this progression is highly variable and not inevitable. Dysplasia is not detectable endoscopically and is focal, rendering the targeting of biopsy sampling difficult. In addition, there is significant interobserver variation in the diagnosis of and the grading of dysplasia by both

non-academic and academic pathologists.[9] Reactive change due to esophagitis can also be difficult to distinguish from dysplasia.

Although the diagnosis of Barrett's esophagus can be difficult, if the endoscopist suspects that the level of the squamocolumnar junction is above the esophagogastric junction (the proximal margin of the gastric fold), biopsies are required. If intestinal metaplasia is present, then the diagnosis of Barrett's esophagus has been established.

Treatment

The goals of treatment for Barrett's esophagus are the same as for GERD: the control of symptoms and maintenance of healed mucosa.[6]

Acid control

Lifestyle modifications including dietary adjustment may help control GERD symptoms somewhat, but these measures are unlikely to have an effect on the regression of Barrett's metaplasia. Some individuals with Barrett's esophagus are asymptomatic to begin with possibly due to the replacement of the normal squamous epithelium with the acid-resistant Barrett's epithelium. Nevertheless, these patients may benefit from acid suppression, given the potential regression of Barrett's metaplasia discussed below.[6]

Histamine H_2-receptor antagonists (H_2-RA) can control GERD symptoms but they do not cause regression of Barrett's metaplasia.[79,80] B4, A1c As mentioned in Chapter 2, proton pump inhibitors (PPI) are the most effective antisecretory agents, and are superior to H_2-RA in the treatment of symptoms and the healing of esophagitis.[81] A1a In Barrett's

Table 3.1 Randomized clinical trials for the treatment of Barrett's esophagus[a]

Interventions compared	No. of patients	Outcome	Reference
Omeprazole 40 mg twice daily *v* Ranitidine 150 mg twice daily	26 27	Regression in Barrett's length (*P* = 0.06) and area (*P* = 0.02) with omeprazole compared to ranitidine	Peters *et al.*[80] Alc
Medical (ranitidine or omeprazole) *v* Antireflux surgery	27 32	Length of Barrett's esophagus decreased in 8/27, (increased in 3) in the surgical group and in 2/32 (increased in 11) in the medical group (*P* < 0.01). Dysplasia appeared in 6 medically treated patients (mild in 5, severe in 1) and in 1 surgically treated patient (severe)	Ortiz *et al.*[88] Alc
Medical (ranitidine 150 mg twice daily) *v* Surgical therapy	91[b] 38[b]	No difference in incidence of adenocarcinoma between groups, but there may have been insufficient power to detect such a difference	Spechler *et al.*[89] Alc
PDT with photophrin and omeprazole *v* Omeprazole 20 mg twice daily	138 70	Ablation of all high grade dysplasia in 80% of PDT group and in 40% in omeprazole group (*P* < 0.0001). Cancer in 9.2% *v* 18.6%, respectively (*P* = 0.076)	Overholt *et al.*[90c] Alc
PDT + 5-ALA *v* Placebo + ALA	18 16	16/18 of the PDT group had some response compared to 2/18 of the placebo group (*P* < 0.001)	Ackroyd *et al.*[91] Alc

[a]This list is not an exhaustive list of all randomized clinical trials in the literature.
[b]This includes all GERD patients, not just those with Barrett's esophagus.
[c]Results are available in abstract form only.
PDT, photodynamic therapy; ALA, aminolevulinic acid

esophagus, these same endpoints are well controlled with PPIs.[82–84] Some studies have also suggested a modest regression of Barrett's esophagus, although these studies usually used a high dose PPI.[80,82,85–87] In a randomized controlled trial, Peters *et al.*[80] demonstrated that omeprazole 40 mg twice daily resulted in an 8% reduction of surface area of Barrett's esophagus and a 6% decrease in length, superior to the comparator, ranitidine 150 mg twice daily (Table 3.1). There is also evidence that normalization of intraesophageal acid exposure decreases cellular proliferation rates.[92] It is noteworthy that despite adequate symptom control, even high dose PPI may not normalize acid exposure.[93–96] However, there is no evidence that normalization of pH leads to less cancer. Hence it is not rational to routinely perform pH-metry to determine the level of acid suppression. What is often seen with acid suppression is an increase in islands of squamous epithelium within the Barrett's segment. Unfortunately this may lead to a false sense of security, as biopsies of such islands have often shown underlying intestinal metaplasia,[97] and no study has shown a reduction of esophageal adenocarcinoma or mortality.

Nevertheless, PPIs are the best pharmacological treatment for Barrett's presently available.

Given that even high dose PPI may fail to normalize esophageal pH,[93–96,98–100] some have considered antireflux surgery as an alternative. Surgery does provide excellent control of symptoms and squamous islands also develop after surgery, suggesting possible regression. One randomized trial comparing medical therapy with antireflux surgery with follow up of 1–11 years (Table 3.1) showed a 25% rate of some regression in the surgically treated (9% progression, 3/32) compared to 7% regression (41% progression, 11/27) in the medical group.[88] Alc However, complete regression of Barrett's metaplasia with surgery is very uncommon and may in fact reflect "pseudoregression" due to surgical repositioning of the esophagus.[9] Some studies have also reported a reduced risk of progression of low grade dysplasia.[101] B4 Another study demonstrated that cancers occur within the first 39 months following surgery, suggesting that these may have been cancers present but missed at the time of surgery.[102] Others have reported that both dysplasia and cancer continue to occur after surgery.[89,103–105] B4

Csendes *et al.*[105] found that dysplasia developed in 17 (10·5%) and adenocarcinoma in 4 (2·5%) of 161 patients who had undergone surgery at late (7–21 years) follow up. In a randomized controlled study comparing medical to surgical antireflux therapy, there was no significant difference between groups in incidence of esophageal cancer (Table 3.1).[89] Alc Hence surgery does not prevent dysplasia or cancer and therefore, does not remove the need for surveillance.

Ablative therapies

Given the theory that Barrett's esophagus develops after healing of injured esophageal epithelium in an acid environment, reinjuring of the metaplastic epithelium with ablative therapy in an environment lower in acid, is theorized to result in re-epithelialization with normal squamous epithelium. This would then decrease the risk for dysplasia and esophageal adenocarcinoma. The ablation can be achieved by thermal techniques (electrocoagulator, heater probe, argon plasma coagulator, laser including Nd:YAG, etc.), photodynamic therapy or endoscopic mucosal resection.

Reports using different thermal techniques have suggested both complete or incomplete histological regression in Barrett's esophagus, but complications are not uncommon.[9] Multipolar electrocoagulation has resulted in a fibrotic and friable esophagus with adhesions to the pleura in one patient.[106] Argon plasma coagulation has caused significant complications including chest pain and odynophagia (58%), fever and pleural effusion (15%), strictures (9%), pneumomediastinum (3%) and perforation.[107,108] In addition, one study using heater probe reported buried islands of intestinal metaplasia in 23% of patients.[109] Thermal techniques have also been used in patients with dysplasia or early cancer. Most reports are small case series but results are interesting, with reversal of abnormalities in some cases.[9] Further studies are required.

Photodynamic therapy (PDT) is a process in which a light-sensitive agent, which concentrates in metaplastic or dysplastic tissue, is administered and subsequently activated by light of an appropriate wavelength. This results in selective damage of the abnormal tissues. The agents used include porfimer sodium, a hematoporphyrin derivative or 5-aminolevulinic acid (5-ALA). Reports describe regression of dysplasia and even early cancers, but complete regression did not occur in the majority.[110] A randomized trial compared PDT using sodium porfimer to omeprazole in 208 patients (Table 3.1) with high grade dysplasia.[90] At 12-month follow up, 9·2% of the PDT group developed cancer compared to 18·6% of the omeprazole group (NS), but strictures developed in 38% of the patients who underwent PDT.[90] Alc Another randomized study compared PDT with 5-ALA to placebo in low grade dysplasia patients and achieved regression of dysplasia in 89% (16/18) versus 11% (2/18) of patients in the placebo group (Table 3.1), but only 30% of the surface area

was reduced in the 5-ALA group.[91] Alc Hence, the risk of progression for this residual tissue still remains. In fact, adenocarcinoma has been reported to develop underneath a new squamous epithelium after treatment for high grade dysplasia with PDT using sodium porfimer.[9]

Endoscopic mucosal resection has also been performed in patients with visible lesions within Barrett's esophagus. In one study, this resulted in complete local remission of 97% (34/35) of patients with low risk lesions characterized by diameter < 20 mm, well or moderately differentiated histology, lesion limited to mucosa, or non-ulcerated lesion compared to only 59% (13/22) of patients with high risk lesions characterized by diameter > 20 mm, poorly differentiated histology, lesion extending into submucosa, or ulcerated lesions.[111] However metachronous lesions or recurrent high grade dysplasia or cancer was detected in the subsequent year in 17% of the low risk and 14% of the high risk group. Larger studies with longer follow up are required.

Hence with all ablative therapies, even if all of the Barrett's epithelium is eliminated, some residual intestinal metaplasia may be present underneath the neosquamous epithelium along with its inherent risk of cancer development. In addition, these techniques are associated with significant risk for stricture and perforation. They are for the most part costly and the methods have not yet been standardized. In addition, the need for surveillance is still present but may be more difficult given that the endoscopic landmarks may be less easily identified after ablative therapy.[9] Hence ablative therapy is perhaps most appealing in the non-operative patient with high grade dysplasia or superficial adenocarcinoma.

Prevention of esophageal adenocarcinoma with anti-inflammatory agents

The use of aspirin (ASA) or non-steroidal anti-inflammatory drugs (NSAIDs) has been found to be associated with a reduced risk of developing esophageal adenocarcinoma.[112,113] Cyclooxygenase-2 (COX-2) expression is also increased in Barrett's epithelium[114] and COX-2 inhibition reduces cell growth in esophageal adenocarcinoma cell lines.[115] To determine whether COX-2 inhibitors decrease the risk of esophageal cancer in patients with Barrett's epithelium, would require a very large number of patients and long follow up.[9,116]

Screening and surveillance

Screening for the detection of Barrett's esophagus is currently recommended in patients with chronic GERD symptoms.[6] This is based on the finding that patients with longer duration of symptoms have a higher prevalence of

Barrett's esophagus.[31,47] B3 Given that GERD patients who are white, male or have more severe acid reflux also have a higher prevalence of Barrett's esophagus,[6,63,64] these patients should perhaps be more aggressively sought. It has been suggested that a "once in a lifetime" endoscopy should be performed in all GERD patients, and this approach was favored by 76% of Canadian gastroenterologists, although the timing at which this should be carried out is still unclear.[117,118] Although the asymptomatic Barrett's esophagus patient would not be identified with this case finding approach, the application of a screening endoscopy to the general population is not recommended. All individuals undergoing gastroscopy for any reason should have the distal esophagus well examined.

The aim of the "once in a lifetime" gastroscopy in GERD patients is to detect Barrett's esophagus, as this entity increases the risk of developing esophageal adenocarcinoma. Cancer surveillance, once Barrett's is discovered, is costly. Assuming a cancer incidence of 0·5% per year in patients with Barrett's esophagus, a recent analysis showed that surveillance of Barrett's esophagus for the prevention of cancer would cost almost US$98 000 per quality-adjusted life year saved.[39] It is, however, the only method currently available to identify the high risk patients with dysplasia who may benefit from new ablative therapies.

Arguments in support of a screening and surveillance strategy

The rationale for screening for and surveying Barrett's esophagus is based on the fact that GERD is a risk factor for esophageal adenocarcinoma,[47] that Barrett's esophagus represents an intermediate step between esophagitis and adenocarcinoma and in fact is the only known precursor of esophageal adenocarcinoma,[6] that the rate of esophageal adenocarcinoma is steadily increasing in Western societies[119] and the prognosis for esophageal adenocarcinoma is very poor unless detected early.[120] Over 50% of all esophageal tumors on the National Cancer Database (USA) for 1988 were stage III or IV at the time of detection with poor 5-year disease specific survivals of 15% and 3%, respectively.[121] It is argued that surveillance programs will detect cancers at an earlier stage when the outlook is much better. In stage I or II cases the 5-year disease specific survival rates were 42% and 29%, respectively.[121] In addition small retrospective studies suggest that surveillance may improve survival. A comparison was made between patients who initially presented with esophageal adenocarcinoma ($n = 54$) and those in whom the cancer had been detected during surveillance ($n = 16$) of Barrett's esophagus.[122] B4 Surveyed patients had significantly earlier stages than non-surveyed patients (75% had stage 0 or I, 25% stage II and 0% stage III compared to 26%, 25%, and 56%, respectively for non-surveyed patients). Survival was

also significantly superior in the surveyed group, with a 2-year survival of 86% versus 43%. Similar results were found by an earlier retrospective study comparing 17 adenocarcinoma patients identified during surveillance programs to 35 patients who had not been in a program.[123] Again, the cancers in the surveyed group were at an earlier stage and survival was significantly greater in the surveyed group than in the group that had not been surveyed prior to diagnosis. B4 A third study obtained similar results with 5-year survival at 62% in those who underwent surveillance compared to 20% in those who did not.[124] B4

Arguments against a surveillance strategy

Although the incidence of esophageal adenocarcinoma is on the rise, the absolute prevalence of this condition remains relatively low. In addition, the benefits of screening and surveying patients with Barrett's esophagus are not as clear-cut as they are with colonic polyps and colon cancer. Furthermore, 93–98% of esophageal adenocarcinomas occur in patients without prior diagnosis of Barrett's esophagus.[23,125–127] Most patients with Barrett's esophagus do not die from esophageal cancer.[128–130] GERD is very common and close to 90% of GERD patients do not have Barrett's esophagus.[17] Surveillance is expensive, time consuming (prevents endoscopists from carrying out other tasks), and not error free; sampling error is a problem as is interobserver variation in endoscopic and histological diagnosis. In addition most patients with Barrett's esophagus are asymptomatic. The prevalence of Barrett's esophagus at autopsy was 20 times higher than the estimate from endoscopic diagnosis.[22] Thus, for each case of Barrett's, another 20 cases go unrecognized. Considering that the true prevalence of Barrett's esophagus in the community is much higher than previously thought, the observed incidence of adenocarcinoma of the esophagus is very small in relation to the community prevalence of Barrett's epithelium.[131]

One hundred and sixty-six patients with Barrett's esophagus who deliberately did not undergo a surveillance program were re-examined a mean of 9·3 years later.[130] B4 The authors were able to obtain follow up information in 93% of the patients. They determined the incidence of esophageal cancer was 1 in 180 patient years, a 40-fold increased risk compared to an age and sex matched group from the general population. All eight patients with cancer were symptomatic and the cancer was detected at diagnostic endoscopy. Of interest is that only two of these patients died because of their esophageal cancer, one of postoperative complications and the other died 4 years postoperatively with liver metastases. Three had successful surgery, and three died of unrelated illness (pancreatitis, myocardial infarction, asthma). During the follow up period, there were 77 other unrelated deaths at

Table 3.2   World Health Organization's principles for early disease detection

Principles	Are the principles met in Barrett's esophagus?
1. The target health problem is important	Yes
2. There should be an accepted treatment for the target problem	Unclear
3. Facilities for diagnosis and treatment should be available	Yes
4. There should be a recognized latent or early symptomatic stage	Unclear
5. There should exist a suitable screening test or examination	Yes
6. The test should be acceptable to the population to be screened	Yes
7. The natural history and development of the condition should be adequately understood	Unclear
8. There should be an agreed policy on whom to treat	Unclear
9. The process of case finding should be cost effective	Possibly
10. Case finding should be a continuing process	Possibly

Modified from Gudlaugsdottir S *et al. Eur J Gastroenterol Hepatol* 2001;**13**:639–45[136] and Chiba N. *Can J Gastroenterol* 2002;**16**:541–5.[137]

a mean age of 75 years. The authors concluded that a surveillance program would have had marginal benefit, as so few actually died of esophageal cancer.[130] A Danish study, also found that only 1·3% of the patients had a diagnosis of Barrett's esophagus more than 1 year before cancer was identified.[125] B4 Thus, most cancers were detected in patients who would not have entered into a surveillance program and this strategy would be unlikely to reduce the death rate from esophageal cancer in the general population.

Cost effectiveness

Unfortunately, there are no randomized controlled trials of surveillance strategies. A cost-effectiveness study examining the screening of patients with Barrett's esophagus assumed that GERD patients underwent a one-time gastroscopy at age 60 years with biopsies targeting abnormal mucosa.[132] Screening in this model cost US$24 700 per life year saved, a reasonable amount. However, the results were based on a relatively high prevalence of Barrett's esophagus, high grade dysplasia and adenocarcinoma, a high sensitivity and specificity of endoscopy and minor reduction in quality of life after esophagectomy. Any variation in these parameters easily altered the cost effectiveness of this strategy.

Another report estimated the cost of detecting one esophageal cancer at US$23 000 (£14 868) for male and US$65 000 (£42 084) for female patients with Barrett's esophagus.[133] Another found the cost was lower than the cost of surveillance mammography.[134] Sonnenberg *et al.*[135] found that the incremental cost effectiveness of biennial surveillance was approximately US$16 700 per year of life saved. Provenzale *et al.*[39] concluded that surveillance every 5 years was the preferred strategy with a cost of US$98 000 per quality adjusted life year gained.

Putting it all together

At this time, the question of whether surveillance should be undertaken cannot be easily answered. Applying the World Health Organization's 10 principles of early disease detection helps determine whether screening for Barrett's esophagus is beneficial.[136,137] Although some of these criteria are met, most are not (Table 3.2). In the absence of a definitive study, there are arguments to support both sides of the controversy. However, recognizing that Barrett's mucosa is a risk factor for esophageal adenocarcinoma, it is difficult to disregard present recommendations for surveillance endoscopy until evidence to the contrary is available.

How to perform surveillance

Screening is currently recommended in patients with chronic GERD symptoms.[6] Some patients are at greater risk of Barrett's metaplasia and a screening strategy could target more aggressively this group, that includes white men aged over 60 years with a longer history of reflux symptoms. This suggestion does not mean that younger patients with chronic GERD symptoms should not be screened. Once Barrett's metaplasia is established by endoscopy and histology, the patient should enter a surveillance program. Patients who have comorbid illness that would exclude them from esophagectomy or ablative therapy would not benefit from surveillance.

The surveillance intervals are determined by the grade of dysplasia.[6] These intervals have been arbitrarily determined. More recent suggestions have taken into account the previous overestimates of rates of progression to cancer and cost effectiveness studies mentioned above. Two to three years is recommended for patients without dysplasia, every 6 months for 1 year and then yearly, for low grade dysplasia, and every

Table 3.3 Current practice guidelines for surveillance of Barrett's *esophagus*[a]

Source	Date published	Surveillance intervals[b]			Biopsy sampling[a]
		No dysplasia	Low grade dysplasia	High grade dysplasia[c]	
ACG[6]	2002	3 years after 2 normal EGD with biopsy	1 year until no dysplasia	Focal – 3 months (jumbo biopsies) Multifocal – intervention Mucosal irregularity – EMR	4 quadrants every 2 cm and mucosal abnormalities
SFED[141]	2000	CBE – 2 years SSBE – 3 years	6 months–1 year	Surgery or alternative therapy	4 quadrants CBE – every 2 cm SSBE – every 1 cm
ASGE[142]	2000	Periodic (interval not specified)	More frequent than if no dysplasia	Consider surgery	4 quadrants every 1–2 cm
CAG[140]	1997	2 years	3–6 months	Surgery or esophageal mucosal ablation for poor risk patients	4 quadrants every 2 cm

[a]Modified from MacNeil-Covin L *et al. Can J Gastroenterol* 2003;17:313–17.[118]
[b]Interval at which surveillance endoscopy should be performed.
[c]Requires confirmation.
[d]Protocol to be followed for biopsy sampling.
ACG, American College of Gastroenterology; CAG, Canadian Association of Gastroenterology; EMR, endoscopic mucosal resection; SSBE, short segment Barrett's esophagus (length < 3 cm); SFED, French Society of Digestive Endoscopy; EGD, esophagogastroduodenoscopy; CBE, classical Barrett's esophagus (length > 3cm)

3 months after confirmation with expert pathologist review for high grade dysplasia if no surgical intervention is undertaken.[6,9]

During the surveillance gastroscopy, four quadrant biopsy specimens should be obtained at least every 2 cm along the entire length of Barrett's epithelium. C5 The endoscopy should be performed on acid suppression so that esophagitis and reactive change do not confound the diagnosis. In addition, any mucosal abnormalities detected at endoscopy should be biopsied.[9] It has been suggested that the use of 1-cm intervals and jumbo biopsy forceps is more accurate,[138,139] but this approach is more labor intensive and would require endoscopy with a therapeutic gastroscopy. Hence it may not be feasible in community practice.

Summary of practice guidelines

Guidelines for diagnosis, surveillance and treatment of Barrett's esophagus have been established and updated.[5,6,140–142] Table 3.3 summarizes the most recent recommendations. Essentially, the guidelines offered by several expert groups are very similar. The American Society of Gastrointestinal Endoscopy guidelines (which were generated together with the Society for Surgery of the Alimentary Tract and the American Gastroenterological Association) are similar to those of the American College of Gastroenterology and the Canadian Association of Gastroenterology. For patients without dysplasia, surveillance endoscopy can be performed every two to three years (Table 3.3). C5 For patients with low grade dysplasia, surveillance endoscopy should be performed at 6 and 12 months after discovery. If there is no progression of dysplasia, patients can then resume a standard surveillance program. Finally, for patients with high grade dysplasia, management should be individualized. The recommendations of the French Society of Digestive Endoscopy differ slightly from the other guidelines. C5 The suggested surveillance interval and biopsy protocol vary depending upon the length of Barrett's esophagus. In the case of Barrett's esophagus extending more than 3 cm, four biopsies (one in each quadrant) obtained every 2 cm from the gastroesophageal junction is recommended.[141] In the case of Barrett's esophagus of less than 3 cm, two to four biopsies obtained every 1 cm is recommended. In the absence of dysplasia, endoscopy is recommended every 2 years for Barrett's esophagus > 3 cm, and every 3 years for Barrett's esophagus < 3 cm. In the case of low grade dysplasia (confirmed during two subsequent examinations and by two independent pathologists), endoscopy is recommended every 6–12 months. In the case of doubtful low grade dysplasia, repeat examination should take place after 2 months of treatment with double-dose PPI. Finally, in the case of severe dysplasia, endoscopy should be repeated after 1 month of treatment with a double-dose PPI with four-quadrant biopsies obtained every 1 cm and if confirmed, surgery or alternative therapy considered.

Conclusion

Barrett's esophagus is a well recognized complication of chronic gastroesophageal reflux and a definite risk factor for esophageal adenocarcinoma. It should, however, be realized that esophageal cancer is uncommon and most patients with esophageal cancer do not have clinically recognized Barrett's esophagus before cancer is diagnosed. Also, no randomized trials have convincingly demonstrated that a screening strategy prolongs survival or improves quality of life for these patients. However, for some patients, surveillance of Barrett's esophagus may permit detection of cancer at an earlier stage, and therefore improve survival. Therefore, endoscopic screening for Barrett's esophagus should be considered for patients with chronic symptoms of gastroesophageal reflux disease and particularly in certain high risk patients such as white males over the age of 50 years.

There is insufficient scientific evidence to conclude that aggressive anti-reflux therapy with either high dose PPI or surgery will cause Barrett's esophagus to revert to normal squamous mucosa or that it will reduce the risk of developing cancer. There are insufficient data to support the routine use of the various ablative therapies. This modality remains experimental until proved effective in randomized trials.

At present, patients with clinically recognized Barrett's esophagus should be offered participation in a surveillance program as recommended by the American College of Gastroenterology. Surveillance should be undertaken every 3 years for patients without dysplasia (after two normal examinations) and every year for patients with low grade dysplasia. For patients with high grade dysplasia, surgical intervention should be considered once confirmed by expert gastrointestinal pathologists in centers carrying out a high volume of esophagectomies.

References

1 Barrett NR. The lower esophagus lined by columnar epithelium. *Surgery* 1957;**41**:881–94.

2 Shaheen NJ, Crosby MA, Bozymski EM, Sandler RS. Is there publication bias in the reporting of cancer risk in Barrett's esophagus? *Gastroenterology* 2000;**119**:333–8.

3 Naef AP, Savary M, Ozzello L. Columnar-lined lower esophagus: an acquired lesion with malignant predisposition. Report on 140 cases of Barrett's esophagus with 12 adenocarcinomas. *J Thorac Cardiovasc Surg* 1975;**70**:826–35.

4 Spechler SJ. Comparison of medical and surgical therapy for complicated gastroesophageal reflux disease in veterans. The Department of Veterans Affairs Gastroesophageal Reflux Disease Study Group. *N Engl J Med* 1992;**326**:786–92.

5 Sampliner RE, The Practice Parameters Committee of the American College of Gastroenterology. Practice guidelines on the diagnosis, surveillance, and therapy of Barrett's esophagus. *Am J Gastroenterol* 1998;**93**:1028–32.

6 Sampliner RE, The Practice Parameters Committee of the American College of Gastroenterology. Updated guidelines for the diagnosis, surveillance, and therapy of Barrett's esophagus. *Am J Gastroenterol* 2002;**97**:1888–95.

7 Hamilton SR, Smith RR. The relationship between columnar epithelial dysplasia and invasive adenocarcinoma arising in Barrett's esophagus. *Am J Clin Pathol* 1987;**87**:301–12.

8 Sharma P, Morales TG, Sampliner RE. Short segment Barrett's esophagus – the need for standardization of the definition and of endoscopic criteria. *Am J Gastroenterol* 1998;**93**:1033–6.

9 Falk GW. Barrett's esophagus. *Gastroenterology* 2002;**122**: 1569–91.

10 Sharma P, Morales TG, Bhattacharyya A, Garewal HS, Sampliner RE. Dysplasia in short-segment Barrett's esophagus: a prospective 3-year follow-up. *Am J Gastroenterol* 1997;**92**: 2012–16.

11 Schnell TG, Sontag SJ, Chejfec G. Adenocarcinomas arising in tongues or short segments of Barrett's esophagus. *Dig Dis Sci* 1992;**37**:137–43.

12 Nandurkar S, Martin CJ, Talley NJ, Wyatt JM. Curable cancer in a short segment Barrett's esophagus. *Dis Esophagus* 1998;**11**:284–7.

13 Weston AP, Krmpotich PT, Cherian R, Dixon A, Topalosvki M. Prospective long-term endoscopic and histological follow-up of short segment Barrett's esophagus: comparison with traditional long segment Barrett's esophagus. *Am J Gastroenterol* 1997;**92**:407–13.

14 Rudolph RE, Vaughan TL, Storer BE, Haggitt RC, Rabinovitch PS, Levine DS, Reid BJ. Effect of segment length on risk for neoplastic progression in patients with Barrett esophagus. *Ann Intern Med* 2000;**132**:612–20.

15 Hirota WK, Loughney TM, Lazas DJ, Maydonovitch CL, Rholl V, Wong RK. Specialized intestinal metaplasia, dysplasia, and cancer of the esophagus and esophagogastric junction: prevalence and clinical data. *Gastroenterology* 1999;**116**:277–85.

16 Johnston MH, Hammond AS, Laskin W, Jones DM. The prevalence and clinical characteristics of short segments of specialized intestinal metaplasia in the distal esophagus on routine endoscopy. *Am J Gastroenterol* 1996;**91**:1507–11.

17 Winters C Jr, Spurling TJ, Chobanian SJ *et al.* Barrett's esophagus. A prevalent, occult complication of gastroesophageal reflux disease. *Gastroenterology* 1987;**92**: 118–24.

18 Velduyzen van Zanten S, Thomson ABR, Barkun AN *et al.*, CADET-PE Study Group. The prevalence of Barrett's

esophagus (BE) in primary care patients with uninvestigated dyspepsia. (CADET-PE study). *Can J Gastroenterol* 2003; **17**(Suppl A):127A.

19 Breslin NP, Thomson ABR, Bailey RJ *et al.* Gastric cancer and other endoscopic diagnoses in patients with benign dyspepsia. *Gut* 2000;**46**:93–7.

20 Cameron AJ, Lomboy CT. Barrett's esophagus: age, prevalence, and extent of columnar epithelium. *Gastroenterology* 1992;**103**:1241–5.

21 Gruppo Operativo per lo Studio delle Precancerosi dell Esofago (GOSPE). Barrett's esophagus: Epidemiological and clinical results of a multicentric survey. *Int J Cancer* 1991;**48**:364–8.

22 Cameron AJ, Zinsmeister AR, Ballard DJ, Carney JA. Prevalence of columnar-lined (Barrett's) esophagus. Comparison of population-based clinical and autopsy findings. *Gastroenterology* 1990;**99**:918–22.

23 Conio M, Cameron AJ, Romero Y *et al.* Secular trends in the epidemiology and outcome of Barrett's oesophagus in Olmsted County, Minnesota. *Gut* 2001;**48**:304–9.

24 Bersentes K, Fass R, Padda S, Johnson C, Sampliner RE. Prevalence of Barrett's esophagus in Hispanics is similar to Caucasians. *Dig Dis Sci* 1998;**43**:1038–41.

25 Fass R. Barrett's esophagus: are Caucasians the only ethnic group at risk? *Cancer Detect Prev* 1999;**23**:177–8.

26 Yeh C, Hsu CT, Ho AS, Sampliner RE, Fass R. Erosive esophagitis and Barrett's esophagus in Taiwan: a higher frequency than expected. *Dig Dis Sci* 1997;**42**:702–6.

27 El-Serag HB, Sonnenberg A. Opposing time trends of peptic ulcer and reflux disease. *Gut* 1998;**43**:327–33.

28 Fallone CA, Barkun AN, Friedman G *et al.* Is *Helicobacter pylori* eradication associated with gastroesophageal reflux disease? *Am J Gastroenterol* 2000;**95**:914–20.

29 Vicari JJ, Peek RM, Falk GW *et al.* The seroprevalence of *cagA*-positive *Helicobacter pylori* strains in the spectrum of gastroesophageal reflux disease. *Gastroenterology* 1998; **115**:50–7.

30 Eisen GM, Sandler RS, Murray S, Gottfried M. The relationship between gastroesophageal reflux disease and its complications with Barrett's esophagus. *Am J Gastroenterol* 1997;**92**:27–31.

31 Leiberman DA, Oehlke M, Helfand M. Risk factors for Barrett's esophagus in community-based practice. GORGE consortium. Gastroenterology Outcomes Research Group in Endoscopy. *Am J Gastroenterol* 1997;**92**:1293–7.

32 Avidan B, Sonnenberg A, Schnell TG, Sontag SJ. There are no reliable symptoms for erosive oesphagitis and Barrett's oesophagus: endoscopic diagnosis is still essential. *Aliment Pharmacol Ther* 2002;**16**:735–42.

33 Spechler SJ, Sperber H, Doos WG, Schimmel EM. The prevalence of Barrett's esophagus in patients with chronic peptic esophageal strictures. *Dig Dis Sci* 1983;**28**:769–74.

34 Kim SL, Wo JM, Hunter JG, Davis LP, Waring JP. The prevalence of intestinal metaplasia in patients with and without peptic strictures. *Am J Gastroenterol* 1998;**93**: 53–5.

35 Avidan B, Sonnenberg A, Schnell TG, Sontag SJ. Hiatal hernia and acid reflux frequency predict presence and length of Barrett's esophagus. *Dig Dis Sci* 2002;**47**:256–64.

36 Cameron AJ. Barrett's esophagus: prevalence and size of hiatal hernia. *Am J Gastroenterol* 1999;**94**:2054–9.

37 Johnson DA, Winters C, Spruling TJ, Chobanian SJ, Cattau El Jr. Esophageal acid sensitivity in Barrett's esophagus. *J Clin Gastroenterol* 1987;**9**:23–7.

38 Eckardt VF, Kanzler G, Bernhard G. Life expectancy and cancer risk in patients with Barrett's esophagus: a prospective controlled investigation. *Am J Med* 2001;**111**:33–7.

39 Provenzale D, Schmitt C, Wong JB. Barrett's esophagus: a new look at surveillance based on emerging estimates of cancer risk. *Am J Gastroenterol* 1999;**94**:2043–53.

40 Katz D, Rothstein R, Schned A, Dunn J, Seaver K, Antonioli D. The development of dysplasia and adenocarcinoma during endoscopic surveillance of Barrett's esophagus. *Am J Gastroenterol* 1998;**93**:536–41.

41 O'Conner JB, Falk GW, Richter JE. The incidence of adenocarcinoma and dysplasia in Barrett's esophagus: report on the Cleveland Clinic Barrett's Esophagus Registry. *Am J Gastroenterol* 1999;**94**:2037–42.

42 Drewitz DJ, Sampliner RE, Garewal HS. The incidence of adenocarcinoma in Barrett's esophagus: a prospective study of 170 patients followed 4·8 years. *Am J Gastroenterol* 1997;**92**:212–15.

43 Katzka DA, Rustgi AK. Gastroesophageal reflux disease and Barrett's esophagus. *Med Clin North Am* 2000;**84**:1137–61.

44 Cancer Facts and Figures 2001. Atlanta: American Cancer Society, 2001.

45 National Cancer Institute of Canada: Canadian Cancer Statistics 2002, Toronto, Canada, 2002.

46 Shaheen N, Ransohoff DF. Gastroesophageal reflux, Barrett's esophagus and esophageal cancer: scientific review. *JAMA* 2002;**287**:1972–81.

47 Lagergren J, Bergstrom R, Lindgren A, Nyren O. Symptomatic gastroesophageal reflux as a risk factor for esophageal adenocarcinoma. *N Engl J Med* 1999;**340**:825–31.

48 Farrow DC, Vaughan TL, Sweeney C *et al.* Gastroesophageal reflux disease, use of H2 receptor antagonists, and risk of esophageal and gastric cancer. *Cancer Causes Control* 2000;**11**:231–8.

49 Avidan B, Sonnenberg A, Schnell TG, Chejfec G, Metz A, Sontag SJ. Hiatal hernia size, Barrett's length, and severity of acid reflux are all risk factors for esophageal adenocarcinoma. *Am J Gastroenterol* 2002;**97**:1930–6.

50 Lagergren J, Bergstrom R, Nyren O. Association between body mass and adenocarcinoma of the esophagus and gastric cardia. *Ann Intern Med* 1999;**130**:883–90.

51 Gammon MD, Schoenberg JB, Ahsan H *et al.* Tobacco, alcohol, and socioeconomic status and adenocarcinomas of the esophagus and gastric cardia. *J Natl Cancer Inst* 1997;**89**:1277–84.

52 Brown LM, Swanson CA, Gridley G *et al.* Adenocarcinoma of the esophagus: role of obesity and diet. *J Natl Cancer Inst* 1995;**87**:104–9.

53 Lagergren J, Bergstrom R, Adami HO, Nyren O. Association between medications that relax the lower esophageal sphincter and risk for esophageal adenocarcinoma. *Ann Intern Med* 2000;**133**:165–75.

54 Vaughan TL, Farrow DC, Hansten PD *et al.* Risk of esophageal and gastric adenocarcinomas in relation to use

of calcium channel blockers, asthma drugs, and other medications that promote gastroesophageal reflux. *Cancer Epidemiol Biomarkers Prev* 1998;**7**:749–56.

55 Chow WH, Blaser MJ, Blot WJ *et al.* An inverse relation between *cagA*+ strains of *Helicobacter pylori* infection and risk of esophageal and gastric cardia adenocarcinoma. *Cancer Res* 1998;**58**:588–90.

56 Peterson WL, American Gastroenterological Association Consensus Development Panel. Improving the management of GERD; evidence-based therapeutic strategies. *AGA Press* 2002:1–21.

57 Spechler SJ. Clinical practice. Barrett's esophagus. *N Engl J Med* 2002;**346**:836–42.

58 Reid BJ, Levine DS, Longton G, Blount PL, Rabinovitch PS. Predictors of progression to cancer in Barrett's esophagus: baseline histology and flow cytometry identify low- and high-risk patient subsets. *Am J Gastroenterol* 2000;**95**:1669–76.

59 Buttar NS, Wang KK, Sebo TJ *et al.* Extent of high-grade dysplasia in Barrett's esophagus correlates with risk of adenocarcinoma. *Gastroenterology* 2001;**120**:1630–39.

60 Schnell TG, Sontag SJ, Chejfec G *et al.* Long-term nonsurgical management of Barrett's esophagus with high-grade dysplasia. *Gastroenterology* 2001;**120**:1607–19.

61 Bremner CG, Lynch VP, Ellis FH Jr. Barrett's esophagus: congenital or acquired? An experimental study of esophageal mucosal regeneration in the dog. *Surgery* 1970;**68**:209–16.

62 Gillen P, Keeling P, Byrne PJ, West AB, Hennessy TPJ. Experimental columnar metaplasia in the canine oesophagus. *Br J Surg* 1988;**75**:113–15.

63 Singh P, Taylor RH, Colin-Jones DG. Esophageal motor dysfunction and acid exposure in reflux esophagitis are more severe if Barrett's metaplasia is present. *Am J Gastroenterol* 1994;**89**:349–56.

64 Oberg S, DeMeester TR, Peters JH *et al.* The extent of Barrett's esophagus depends on the status of the lower esophageal sphincter and the degree of esophageal acid exposure. *J Thorac Cardiovasc Surg* 1999;**117**:572–80.

65 Fass R, Hell RW, Garewal HS *et al.* Correlation of oesophageal acid exposure with Barrett's oesophagus length. *Gut* 2001;**48**:310–13.

66 Hirschowitz BI. Gastric acid and pepsin secretion in patients with Barrett's esophagus and appropriate controls. *Dig Dis Sci* 1996;**41**:1384–91.

67 Pace F, Santalucia F, Bianchi Porro G. Natural history of gastro-oesophageal reflux disease without oesophagitis. *Gut* 1991;**32**:845–8.

68 Freston JW, Malagelada JR, Petersen H, McCloy RF. Critical issues in the management of gastroesophageal reflux disease. *Eur J Gastroenterol Hepatol* 1995;**7**:577–86.

69 Fass R, Ofman JJ. Gastroesophageal reflux disease – should we adopt a new conceptual framework? *Am J Gastroenterol* 2002;**97**:1901–9.

70 Ofman JJ, Shaheen NJ, Desai AA, Moody B, Bozymski EM, Weinstein WM. The quality of care in Barrett's esophagus: endoscopist and pathologist practices. *Am J Gastroenterol* 2001;**96**:876–81.

71 Weinstein WM, Lee S, Lewin K, Dasen S, Rosenberger S, Miska D. Erosive esophagitis impairs accurate detection of Barrett's esophagus: a prospective randomized double blind study. *Gastroentrology* 1999;**116**:A352 (G1538).

72 Alikhan M, Rex D, Khan A, Rahmani E, Cummings O, Ulbright TM. Variable pathologic interpretation of columnar lined esophagus by general pathologists in community practice. *Gastrointest Endosc* 1999;**50**:23–6.

73 Canto MI, Setrakian S, Willis J *et al.* Methylene blue-directed biopsies improve detection of intestinal metaplasia and dysplasia in Barrett's esophagus. *Gastrointest Endosc* 2000;**51**:560–8.

74 Chobanian SJ, Cattau EL Jr, Winters C Jr *et al.* In vivo staining with toluidine blue as an adjunct to the endoscopic detection of Barrett's esophagus. *Gastrointest Endosc* 1987;**33**:99–101.

75 Stevens PD, Lightdale CJ, Green PH, Siegel LM, Garcia-Carrasquillo RJ, Rotterdam H. Combined magnification endoscopy with chromoendoscopy for the evaluation of Barrett's esophagus. *Gastrointest Endosc* 1994;**40**:747–9.

76 Woolf GM, Riddell RH, Irvine EJ, Hunt RH. A study to examine agreement between endoscopy and histology for the diagnosis of columnar lined (Barrett's) esophagus. *Gastrointest Endosc* 1989;**35**:541–4.

77 Wo JM, Ray MB, Mayfield-Stokes S *et al.* Comparison of methylene blue-directed biopsies and conventional biopsies in the detection of intestinal metaplasia and dysplasia in Barrett's esophagus: a preliminary study. *Gastrointest Endosc* 2001;**54**:294–301.

78 Guelrud M, Herrera I, Essenfeld H, Castro J. Enhanced magnification endoscopy: a new technique to identify specialized intestinal metaplasia in Barrett's esophagus. *Gastrointest Endosc* 2001;**53**:559–65.

79 Sampliner RE, Garewal HS, Fennerty MB, Aickin M. Lack of impact of therapy on extent of Barrett's esophagus in 67 patients. *Dig Dis Sci* 1990;**35**:93–6.

80 Peters FT, Ganesh S, Kuipers EJ *et al.* Endoscopic regression of Barrett's oesophagus during omeprazole treatment; a randomised double blind study. *Gut* 1999;**45**:489–94.

81 Chiba N, De Gara CJ, Wilkinson JM, Hunt RH. Speed of healing and symptom relief in grade II to IV gastroesophageal reflux disease: a meta-analysis. *Gastroenterology* 1997;**112**:1798–810.

82 Sampliner RE. Effect of up to 3 years of high-dose lansoprazole on Barrett's esophagus. *Am J Gastroenterol* 1994;**89**:1844–8.

83 Neumann CS, Iqbal TH, Cooper BT. Long term continuous omeprazole treatment of patients with Barrett's oesophagus. *Aliment Pharmacol Ther* 1995;**9**:451–4.

84 Cooper BT, Neumann CS, Cox MA, Iqbal TH. Continuous treatment with omeprazole 20 mg daily for up to 6 years in Barrett's oesophagus. *Aliment Pharmacol Ther* 1998;**12**:893–7.

85 Gore S, Healey CJ, Sutton R *et al.* Regression of columnar lined (Barrett's) oesophagus with continuous omeprazole therapy. *Aliment Pharmacol Ther* 1993;**7**:623–8.

86 Malesci A, Savarino V, Zentilin P *et al.* Partial regression of Barrett's esophagus by long-term therapy with high-dose omeprazole. *Gastrointest Endosc* 1996;**44**:700–5.

87 Wilkinson SP, Biddlestone L, Gore S, Shepherd NA. Regression of columnar-lined (Barrett's) oesophagus with omeprazole 40 mg daily: results of 5 years of continuous therapy. *Aliment Pharmacol Ther* 1999;**13**:1205–9.

88 Ortiz A, Martinez de Haro LF, Parrilla P *et al.* Conservative treatment versus antireflux surgery in Barrett's oesophagus: long term results of a prospective study. *Br J Surg* 1996;**83**:274–8.

89 Spechler SJ, Lee E, Ahnen D *et al.* Long-term outcome of medical and surgical therapies for gastroesophageal reflux disease: follow-up of a randomized controlled trial. *JAMA* 2001;**285**:2331–8.

90 Overholt BF, Haggitt RC, Bronner MP *et al.,* on behalf of 30 investigators. A multicenter, partially blinded randomized study of the efficacy of photodynamic therapy (PDT) using porfimer sodium (POR) for the ablation of high grade dysplasia (HGD) in Barrett's esophagus (BE): results of a 6 month follow-up. *Gastroenterology* 2001;**120**:A79.

91 Ackroyd R, Brown NJ, Davis MF *et al.* Photodynamic therapy for dysplastic Barrett's oesophagus: a prospective, double blind, randomised, placebo controlled trial. *Gut* 2000;**47**:612–17.

92 Ouatu-Lascar R, Fitzgerald RC, Triadafilopoulos G. Differentiation and proliferation in Barrett's esophagus and the effects of acid suppression. *Gastroenterology* 1999; **117**:327–35.

93 Ouatu-Lascar R, Triadafilopoulos G. Complete elimination of reflux symptoms does not guarantee normalization of intraesophageal acid reflux in patients with Barrett's esophagus. *Am J Gastroenterol* 1998;**93**:711–16.

94 Fass R, Sampliner RE, Malagon IB *et al.* Failure of oesophageal acid control in candidates for Barrett's oesophagus reversal on a very high dose of proton pump inhibitor. *Aliment Pharmacol Ther* 2000;**14**:597–602.

95 Ortiz A, Martinez de Haro LF, Parrilla P, Molina J, Bermejo J, Munitiz V. 24-h pH monitoring is necessary to assess acid reflux suppression in patients with Barrett's oesophagus undergoing treatment with proton pump inhibitors. *Br J Surg* 1999;**86**:1472–4.

96 Katzka DA, Castell DO. Successful elimination of reflux symptoms does not insure adequate control of acid reflux in patients with Barrett's esophagus. *Am J Gastroenterol* 1994;**89**:989–91.

97 Sharma P, Morales TG, Bhattacharyya A, Garewal HS, Sampliner RE. Squamous islands in Barrett's esophagus: What lies underneath? *Am J Gastroenterol* 1998;**93**: 332–5.

98 Fiorucci S, Santucci L, Farroni F, Pelli MA, Morelli A. Effect of omeprazole on gastroesophageal reflux in Barrett's esophagus. *Am J Gastroenterol* 1989;**84**:1263–7.

99 Kovacs BJ, Chen YK, Lewis TD, DeGuzman LJ, Thompson KS. Successful reversal of Barrett's esophagus with multipolar electrocoagulation despite inadequate acid suppression. *Gastrointest Endosc* 1999;**49**:547–53.

100 Katz PO, Anderson C, Khoury R, Castell DO. Gastro-oesophageal reflux associated with nocturnal gastric acid breakthrough on proton pump inhibitors. *Aliment Pharmacol Ther* 1998;**12**:1231–4.

101 Low DE, Levine DS, Dail DH, Kozarek RA. Histological and anatomic changes in Barrett's esophagus after antireflux surgery. *Am J Gastroenterol* 1999;**94**:80–5.

102 McDonald ML, Trastek VF, Allen MS, Deschamps C, Pairolero PC, Pairolero PC. Barretts's esophagus: does an antireflux procedure reduce the need for endoscopic surveillance? *J Thorac Cardiovasc Surg* 1996;**111**:1135–8.

103 Yau P, Watson DI, Devitt PG, Game PA, Jamieson GG. Laparoscopic antireflux surgery in the treatment of gastroesophageal reflux in patients with Barrett esophagus. *Arch Surg* 2000;**135**:801–5.

104 Csendes A, Braghetto I, Burdiles P *et al.* Long-term results of classic antireflux surgery in 152 patients with Barrett's esophagus: clinical, radiologic, endoscopic, manometric, and acid reflux test analysis before and late after operation. *Surgery* 1998;**123**:645–57.

105 Csendes A, Burdiles P, Braghetto I, Smok G, Castro C, Korn O, Henriquez A. Dysplasia and adenocarcinoma after classic antireflux surgery in patients with Barrett's esophagus: the need for long-term subjective and objective follow-up. *Ann Surg* 2002;**235**:178–85.

106 Fennerty MB, Coreless CL, Sheppard B, Faigel DO, Lieberman DA, Sampliner RE. Pathological documentation of complete elimination of Barrett's metaplasia following endoscopic multipolar electrocoagulation therapy. *Gut* 2001;**49**:142–4.

107 Pereira-Lima JC, Busnello JV, Saul C *et al.* High power setting argon plasma coagulation for the eradication of Barrett's esophagus. *Am J Gastroenterol* 2000;**95**:1661–8.

108 Byrne JP, Armstrong GR, Attwood SE. Restoration of the normal squamous lining in Barrett's esophagus by argon beam plasma coagulation. *Am J Gastroenterol* 1998;**93**: 1810–15.

109 Michopoulos S, Tsibouris P, Bouzakis H, Sotiropoulou M, Kralios N. Complete regression of Barrett's esophagus with heat probe thermocoagulation: mid-term results. *Gastrointest Endosc* 1999;**50**:165–72.

110 Overholt BF, Panjehpour M, Haydek JM. Photodynamic therapy for Barrett's esophagus: follow-up in 100 patients. *Gastrointest Endosc* 1999;**49**:1–7.

111 Ell C, May A, Gossner L *et al.* Endoscopic mucosal resection of early cancer and high-grade dysplasia in Barrett's esophagus. *Gastroenterology* 2000;**118**:670–7.

112 Farrow DC, Vaughan TL, Hansten PD *et al.* Use of aspirin and other nonsteroidal anti-inflammatory drugs and risk of esophageal and gastric cancer. *Cancer Epidemiol Biomarkers Prev* 1998;**7**:97–102.

113 Langman MJ, Cheng KK, Gilman EA, Lancashire RJ. Effect of anti-inflammatory drugs on overall risk of common cancer: case–control study in general practice research database. *BMJ* 2000;**320**:1642–6.

114 Shirvani VN, Ouatu-Lascar R, Kaur BS, Omary M, Triadafilopoulos G. Cyclooxygenase 2 expression in Barrett's esophagus and adenocarcinoma: *Ex vivo* induction by bile salts and acid exposure. *Gastroenterology* 2000;**118**: 487–96.

115 Souza RF, Shewmake K, Beer DG, Cryer B, Spechler SJ. Selective inhibition of cyclooxygenase-2 suppresses

growth and induces apoptosis in human esophageal adenocarcinoma cells. *Cancer Res* 2000;**60**:5767–72.

116 Fennerty MB, Triadafilopoulos G. Barrett's-related esophageal adenocarcinoma: is chemoprevention a potential option? *Am J Gastroenterol* 2001;**96**:2302–5.

117 Armstrong D. Motion – All patients with GERD should be offered once in a lifetime endoscopy: Arguments for the motion. *Can J Gastroenterol* 2002;**16**:549–51.

118 MacNeil-Covin L, Casson AG, Malatjalian D, Veldhuyzen van Zanten S. A survey of Canadian gastroenterologists about management of Barrett's esophagus. *Can J Gastroenterol* 2003;17:313–17.

119 Devesa SS, Blot WJ, Fraumeni JF Jr. Changing patterns in the incidence of esophageal and gastric carcinoma in the United States. *Cancer* 1998;**83**:2049–53.

120 Farrow DC, Vaughan TL. Determinants of survival following the diagnosis of esophageal adenocarcinoma (United States). *Cancer Causes Control* 1996;**7**:322–7.

121 Daly JM, Karnell LH, Menck HR. National Cancer Data Base report on esophageal carcinoma. *Cancer* 1996;**78**:1820–8.

122 van Sandick JW, van Lanschot JJB, Kuiken BW, Tytgat GNJ, Offerhaus GJA, Obertop H. Impact of endoscopic biopsy surveillance of Barrett's oesophagus on pathological stage and clinical outcome of Barrett's carcinoma. *Gut* 1998;**43**:216–22.

123 Peters JH, Clark GWB, Ireland AP, Chandrasoma P, Smyrk TC, DeMeester TR. Outcome of adenocarcinoma arising in Barrett's esophagus in endoscopically surveyed and nonsurveyed patients. *J Thorac Cardiovasc Surg* 1994;**108**:813–21.

124 Streitz JM Jr, Andrews CW Jr, Ellis FH Jr. Endoscopic surveillance of Barrett's esophagus: does it help? *J Thorac Cardiovasc Surg* 1993;**105**:383–8.

125 Bytzer P, Christensen PB, Damkier P, Vinding K, Seersholm N. Adenocarcinoma of the esophagus and Barrett's esophagus: a population-based study. *Am J Gastroenterol* 1999;**94**:86–91.

126 Brown CM, Jones R, Shirazi T, Codling B, Valori RM. Prior diagnosis of Barrett's esophagus is rare in patients with esophageal adenocarcinoma. *Gut* 1996;**381**(Suppl 1):A23.

127 Menke-Pluymers MB, Schoute NW, Mulder AH, Hop WC, van Blankenstein M, Tilanus HW. Outcome of surgical treatment of adenocarcinoma in Barrett's oesophagus. *Gut* 1992;**33**:1454–8.

128 Van der Veen AH, Dees J, Blankensteijn JD, Van Blankenstein M. Adenocarcinoma in Barrett's oesophagus: an overrated risk. *Gut* 1989;**30**:14–18.

129 Macdonald CE, Wicks AC, Playford RJ. Final results from 10 year cohort of patients undergoing surveillance for Barrett's oesophagus: observational study. *BMJ* 2000;**321**:1252–5.

130 van der Burgh A, Dees J, Hop WC, van Blankenstein M. Oesophageal cancer is an uncommon cause of death in patients with Barrett's oesophagus. *Gut* 1996;**39**:5–8.

131 Nandurkar S, Talley NJ. Barrett's esophagus: the long and the short of it. *Am J Gastroenterol* 1999;**94**:30–40.

132 Soni A, Sampliner RE, Sonnenberg A. Screening for high-grade dyplasia in gastroesophageal reflux disease: is it cost-effective? *Am J Gastroenterol* 2000;**95**:2086–93.

133 Wright TA, Gray MR, Morris AI, Gilmore IT, Ellis A, Smart HL, Myskow M, Nash J, Donnelly RJ, Kingsnorth AN. Cost effectiveness of detecting Barrett's cancer. *Gut* 1996;**39**:574–9.

134 Streitz JM Jr, Ellis FH Jr, Tilden RL, Erickson RV. Endoscopic surveillance of Barrett's esophagus: a cost-effectiveness comparison with mammographic surveillance for breast cancer. *Am J Gastroenterol* 1998;**93**:911–15.

135 Sonnenberg A, Soni A, Sampliner RE. Medical decision analysis of endoscopic surveillance of Barrett's oesophagus to prevent oesophageal adenocarcinoma. *Aliment Pharmacol Ther* 2002;**16**:41–50.

136 Gudlaugsdottir S, van Blankenstein M, Dees J, Wilson JHP. A majority of patients with Barrett's oesophagus are unlikely to benefit from endoscopic cancer surveillance. *Eur J Gastroenterol Hepatol* 2001;**13**:639–45.

137 Chiba N. Motion – Screening and surveillance of Barrett's epithelium is practical and cost effective: Arguments against the motion. *Can J Gastroenterol* 2002;**16**:541–5.

138 Levine DS, Haggitt RC, Blount PL, Rabinovitch PS, Rusch VW, Reid BJ. An endoscopic biopsy protocol can differentiate high-grade dysplasia from early adenocarcinoma in Barrett's esophagus. *Gastroenterology* 1993;**105**:40–50.

139 Reid BJ, Blount PL, Feng Z, Levine DS. Optimizing endoscopic biopsy detection of early cancers in Barrett's high-grade dysplasia. *Am J Gastroenterol* 2000;**95**:3089–96.

140 Beck IT, Champion MC, Lemire S, Thomson ABR, contibuting participants. The second Canadian Consensus Conference on the management of patients with gastroesophageal reflux disease. *Can J Gastroenterol* 1997;**11**(Suppl B):7B–20B.

141 Boyer J, Robaszkiewicz M, The Council of the French Society of Digestive Endoscopy (SFED). Guidelines of the French Society of Digestive Endoscopy: monitoring of Barrett's esophagus. *Endoscopy* 2000;**32**:498–9.

142 SSAT, AGA, ASGE Consensus Panel. Management of Barrett's esophagus. *J Gastrointest Surg* 2000;**4**:115–16.

4 Esophageal motility disorders: achalasia and spastic motor disorders

Marcelo F Vela, Joel E Richter

Esophageal motility disorders present with dysphagia and chest pain as the main symptoms, accompanied by abnormalities on manometric studies. The best characterized esophageal motility disorders are achalasia and diffuse esophageal spasm. The treatment options for these disorders, which range from non-invasive medical therapy to surgery, are presented in this chapter.

Achalasia

Achalasia is a primary esophageal motor disorder characterized by abnormal relaxation of the lower esophageal sphincter (LES) and absent esophageal peristalsis. With an estimated incidence of approximately 1/100 000 and a prevalence of close to 10/100 000,[1] this uncommon disease stands out among the esophageal motility disorders as the most clearly defined (clinically, manometrically and radiographically) and the most successfully treated.

The exact etiology of achalasia remains unknown, but autoimmune, infectious, degenerative and hereditary processes, whether alone or in combination, lead to a chronic inflammatory response in the myenteric plexus that results in selective loss of inhibitory neurons.[2] Manometrically this is manifested by high LES pressure, abnormal LES relaxation and aperistalsis.[3] The combination of an atonic esophageal body with a functional obstruction at the gastroesophageal junction produce esophageal dilatation that can, over a prolonged period of time, lead to the development of a megaesophagus.

The most common symptoms of achalasia are dysphagia for solids and liquids in over 90% of patients, and regurgitation of undigested food and saliva in approximately 75%. Chest pain is present in 40–50% of patients, weight loss in nearly 60%, and heartburn in approximately 40% of subjects.[4,5] The presence of the disease is strongly supported by a barium esophagram showing a dilated esophagus that tapers into a "bird-beak" at the gastroesophageal junction with fluoroscopy revealing lack of normal peristalsis, usually with to-and-fro disordered bolus movement. The manometric features described above, the most important of which is abnormal LES relaxation, confirm the diagnosis.

Treatment of achalasia

Overview

Currently, there is no available treatment that can correct the underlying neuropathology of achalasia; LES function and peristalsis cannot be restored. Therefore, therapy is based on reduction of the resting LES pressure to allow esophageal emptying by gravity. The goals of treatment are three-fold: relieve symptoms, improve esophageal emptying and prevent the development of megaesophagus. In assessing response to a therapeutic intervention, useful endpoints are symptom relief and physiologic evaluation, the latter through manometric determination of LES pressure and measurement of esophageal emptying by barium examination or nuclear scintigraphy.

Reduction of the LES pressure can be achieved through different therapeutic modalities including pharmacologic therapy, endoscopic injection of botulinum toxin, pneumatic dilatation and surgical myotomy[6]; the last two being the most effective treatments available.[4,7] "Endstage" cases presenting with a markedly dilated and sometimes sigmoid esophagus may require esophagectomy.[8] The choice of therapy depends on patient characteristics (age, comorbid illnesses and disease stage), patient's preference, degree of expertise and available modalities in the medical center, and a careful balance between risks and benefits.

Pharmacologic treatment

Pharmacological reduction of the LES basal pressure through smooth muscle relaxants has been attempted with several medications. The most studied classes include nitrates, calcium channel blockers and, more recently, sildenafil.

Nitrates activate guanylate cyclase, leading to production of a protein kinase that inhibits smooth muscle contraction through dephosphorylation of the myosin light chain.

Table 4.1 Nitrates and calcium channel blockers in the treatment of achalasia

Authors	No. of patients	Treatment	% Symptom improvement
Bortolotti and Labo[16]	20	Nifedipine	70
Traube et al.[15]	10	Nifedipine	53
Coccia et al.[17]	14	Nifedipine	77
Gelfond et al.[12]	15	Nifedipine	53
	15	ISDN	87
Gelfond et al.[13]	24	ISDN	83
Rozen et al.[14]	15	ISDN	58
Eherer et al.[19]	3	Sildenafil	0

ISDN isosorbide dinitrate.
Modified from Vaezi M, Richter JE. *J Clin Gastroenterol* 1998;**27**:21–35.

Additionally, nitrates liberate nitric oxide (NO), an inhibitory neurotransmitter mediated by cyclic guanosine monophosphate (cGMP). Significant reduction of LES pressure has been demonstrated 10 minutes after sublingual administration of a 5 mg dose of isosorbide dinitrate.[9] Very few randomized controlled trials have evaluated the effect of nitrates on achalasia. Wong et al.[10] found a significant decrease in LES pressure and significant improvement in esophageal emptying 30 minutes after a single dose (0·4 mg) of sublingual nitroglycerin in a randomized crossover study. In several other small studies,[11–14] nitrates have decreased LES pressure by 30–65%, with symptom improvement in 58–87% of patients (Table 4.1), but these were uncontrolled studies that traditionally tend to overemphasize the benefits of interventions. Calcium channel blockers produce smooth muscle relaxation by decreasing entry of calcium, necessary for contraction, into smooth muscle cells. In a double blind randomized controlled trial in 10 achalasia patients,[15] sublingual nifedipine (10–30 mg dose, titrated according to patient tolerance) given before meals achieved a significant reduction in LES pressures 30 minutes after administration. However, despite this reduction, LES pressures were still substantial after treatment (mean LES pressure of 30 mmHg). These investigators also reported a modest improvement of dysphagia with nifedipine, with a reduction in the average number of meals per day with dysphagia from 1·9 to 0·9. Ald Other uncontrolled studies suggest that calcium channel blockers decrease LES pressure by 13–49% and improve symptoms in 53–77% of patients.[11,12,15–17] B4

A small randomized controlled trial comparing calcium channel blockers and nitrates in 15 patients[12] found sublingual isosorbide dinitrate (5 mg) to be superior to sublingual nifedipine (20 mg) for the treatment of achalasia. Ald In comparison to nifedipine, isosorbide dinitrate achieved a more pronounced reduction in basal LES pressure (47% v 64%). Additionally, more patients receiving isosorbide dinitrate experienced complete radionuclide meal clearance at 10 minutes (53% v 15%) and relief of dysphagia (87% v 53%).

Sildenafil (Viagra) inhibits smooth muscle contraction by promoting accumulation of NO stimulated cGMP (NO-cGMP) through inhibition of NO phosphodiesterase type 5, an enzyme that degrades NO-cGMP. Recently, in a placebo-controlled randomized trial of sildenafil (50 mg) in 14 achalasia patients, Bortolotti et al.[18] showed that sildenafil by direct intragastric infusion significantly reduced basal LES pressure, postdeglutitive LES residual pressure and esophageal body contraction amplitude. Peak effect was reached 15–20 minutes after infusion and lasted less than 1 hour. Eherer et al.[19] administered sildenafil orally (50 mg) to 11 patients with esophageal motor disorders, three of whom had a diagnosis of achalasia. LES pressure decreased in two of these patients, but none had relief of symptoms.

Overall, nitrates and calcium channel blockers can reduce LES pressure. effect on symptoms is variable, short-lived, and usually suboptimal. Ald Additionally, adverse effects such as headache, hypotension, and pedal edema may limit their use and tachyphilaxis is frequent.[11] Therefore, these agents should be reserved for the short-term relief of achalasia symptoms, either as a temporizing measure while awaiting more definitive therapy or in patients who are too sick or unwilling to undergo other treatments. Sildenafil merits further study in randomized controlled trials.

Botulinum toxin

Endoscopic injection of botulinum toxin into the LES is a relatively recent addition to the treatment options for achalasia. It produces reduction in LES pressure by inhibiting acetylcholine release from nerve endings, thereby counterbalancing the effect of the selective loss of inhibitory neurotransmitters (nitrous oxide and vasoactive intestinal peptide) in achalasia. It is safe, easy to administer and provides symptom relief initially in approximately 85% of patients; however, the effect of a single injection is usually limited to 6 months or less in over 50% of patients.[3] B4

Table 4.2 Botulinum toxin injection for the treatment of achalasia

Authors	No. of patients	% Symptomatic improvement after one injection				% Responding to repeat injections
		<1 mo	6 mo	12 mo	24 mo	
Pasricha et al.[20,21]	31	90	55			27
Cuillere et al.[23]	55	75	50			33
Rollan et al.[24]	3	100	66			
Fishman et al.[25]	60	70		36		86
Annese et al.[26]	8	100	13			100
Gordon and Eaker[27]	16	75	44			
Muehldorfer et al.[28]	12	75	50	25	10	
Vaezi et al.[29]	22	63	36	32		
Annese et al.[30]	118	82		64		100
Kolbasnik et al.[31]	30	77	57	39	25	100
Mikaeli et al.[32]	20	65	25	15		60
Allescher et al.[33]	23	74		45	30	
Neubrand et al.[34]	25	65			36	0

Modified from Hoogerwerf WA *et al. Gastrointest. Endosc Clin North Am* 2001;**11**:311–23.[22]
mo, months

In a 6-month randomized controlled trial of 21 patients, the administration of botulinum toxin (100 units) resulted in significant symptom score improvement (from $7·1 ± 1·2$ to $1·6 ± 2·2$), compared to placebo (from $5·9 ± 1·6$ to $5·4 ± 2·0$) ($P = 0·001$) at 1 week. By 6 months the proportion of patients in remission had declined from 82% to 66%.[20] Ald A subsequent study by the same group[21] evaluated the efficacy of botulinum toxin over a 2–3-year period and found that 65% (20/31) of patients had good symptom improvement at 6 months. However, 19 of these 20 responders eventually relapsed, requiring repeat injections and two-thirds of the patients eventually chose a more definitive form of therapy. In the analysis of subgoups in this small study the response rate appeared to be higher for patients over the age of 50 years and those with the "vigorous" form of achalasia. Subsequent studies[20–33] have confirmed that botulinum toxin is initially effective but the benefit of a single injection lasts less than 1 year in the majority of patients, with all patients requiring repeat injections or other forms of therapy for their achalasia (Table 4.2). Ald, B4 Botulinum toxin is extremely safe, with 25% of patients presenting with transient, mild, postprocedural chest pain, and 5% developing symptomatic gastroesophageal reflux disease (GERD).[6]

Botulinum toxin is an effective and safe option for the short-term treatment of achalasia. Symptoms are relieved on average for 6 months with repeat treatments being required to keep patients in long-term remission. Botulinum toxin is inferior to pneumatic dilatation or surgery (see comparative studies below), but it can be particularly useful in the elderly who may have a higher response rate than younger patients (under age 50 years) and who may not tolerate more aggressive therapies.

Pneumatic dilatation

Disruption of the muscle fibers of the LES through forceful dilatation has been used as treatment of achalasia for many years. The first description of dilatation dates from 1674 when a patient with achalasia was treated by passing a piece of carved whalebone with a sponge affixed to the distal end down the esophagus into the stomach.[7] The first pneumatic (i.e. air filled) dilators were introduced in the late 1930s, and both the equipment and technique have evolved over the years. Not only are the dilators and techniques varied, but the definitions of success differ across studies. However, there is sufficient experience with the currently used balloon dilators to comment on their efficacy and safety.

Kadakia and Wong calculated the pooled effect of the older dilators (Brown-McHardy, Mosher and Hurst-Tucker balloons) among a total of 235 patients studied in five prospective studies. Symptomatic response was excellent or good in 61–100% of patients who were followed for a mean of 2·7 years.[35] B4 Currently, the most widely used dilator in the USA is the Rigiflex polyethylene balloon (Boston Scientific, Boston, MA), which is available in three different diameters (30, 35 and 40 mm).[11] The current technique consists of endoscopy to determine landmarks, followed by placement of a balloon across the LES under fluoroscopic guidance. The balloon is then inflated to sufficient pressure (usually 7–12 psi; 48·3–82·7 kPa) for up to 60 seconds to disrupt the muscle fibers of the LES.

There are no clinical trials that compare pneumatic dilatation to placebo (i.e. sham dilatation). In three recent randomized controlled trials comparing pneumatic dilatation

Table 4.3 **Rigiflex balloon dilatation for the treatment of achalasia**

Authors	No. of patients	Study design[a]	% With exc/ good response	Follow up in months (mean)	Perforation rate (%)
Cox et al.[37]	7	P	86	9	0
Gelfand and Kozarek[38]	24	P	93	NR	0
Barkin et al.[39]	50	P	90	20	2
Stark et al.[40]	10	P	74	6	0
Makela et al.[41]	17	R	75	6	5·9
Levine et al.[42]	62	R	85	NR	0
Kim et al.[43]	14	P	75	4	0
Lee et al.[44]	28	P	87	NR	0
Abid et al.[45]	36	P	88	27	6·6
Wehrmann et al.[46]	40	R	87	NR	2·5
Lambroza and Schuman[47]	27	P	89	21	0
Muehldorfer et al.[48]	12	R	83	18	8·3
Bhatnager et al.[49]	15	R	84	14	0
Gideon et al.[50]	24	R	NR	6	4
Khan et al.[51]	9	P	85	NR	0
Kadakia and Wong[35,52]	56	P	88	59	0
Vela and Richter[5]	100	P	82	24	2

[a]P, prospective; R, retrospective.
Modified and updated from Vaezi MF and Richter JE. *J Clin Gastroenterol* 1998;**27**:21–35[11] and Gelfand MD and Kozarek RA. *Am J Gastroenterol* 1989;**84**:924–7.[38]
NR, not reported

to botulinum injection, symptom improvement rates for dilatation at 12 months ranged between 53% and 70%.[28,29,32] A1d Table 4.3 summarizes the results of 17 uncontrolled studies of Rigiflex pneumatic dilatation for the treatment of achalasia,[5,35,37–52] the degree of heterogeneity of these studies is not known. The pooled results of 597 patients followed for a mean of 17 months yield an excellent to good response in 82% of patients. B4 However, it should be emphasized that uncontrolled studies tend to exaggerate the benefits of interventions. Very little is known about the long-term outcome of pneumatic dilatation. In the only randomized controlled trial with follow up extending beyond 12 months, 50% of patients treated with pneumatic dilatation had relapse of dysphagia at 30 months.[28] A1d Recently, West et al.[53] reported on the success of pneumatic dilatation in patients followed for more than 5 years. Although this study presents serious methodological limitations–dilatations were carried out with different types of balloons and therapeutic success was defined based on a symptom questionnaire – it is the only study with extended follow up. The overall therapeutic success rate was 50% in 81 patients followed for more than 5 years and the mean number of dilatations per patient was four. Success rate decreased in patients with longer follow up; it was 60% in patients followed between 5 and 9 years, 50% for those followed between 10 and 14 years, and 40% in the group followed for more than 15 years. B4

The perforation rate associated with pneumatic dilatation is approximately 2%.[11] Mortality from the procedure is estimated to be 0·2%.[6] Gastroesophageal reflux after pneumatic dilatation occurs in 15–33% of patients.[5,35]

A1d, B4 Overall, pneumatic dilatation results in good to excellent symptom relief in approximately 80% of patients. Limited data suggest that over 50% of patients will require repeat dilation after 2 years. Pneumatic dilatation is the most effective non-surgical treatment available for achalasia and has a success rate comparable with that of surgery (see comparative studies below). It should be considered an acceptable alternative to surgery for treatment of achalasia.

Heller myotomy

Surgical myotomy was originally described by Ernest Heller in 1914 and involved cutting the anterior and posterior aspects of the LES through a thoracotomy.[54] The surgical technique has evolved and with the advent of minimally invasive surgery in the 1990s, laparoscopic myotomy has become the preferred operation. Whether an antireflux procedure should be performed (to prevent reflux) or not (to avoid postoperative dysphagia) remains a matter of controversy.[3,7]

The only randomized controlled trial that evaluated Heller myotomy compared it to pneumatic dilatation finding that myotomy via a laparotomy resulted in symptom resolution in 95% of patients compared with 65% of patients treated with an older pneumatic balloon (the Mosher bag).[55] A1c More details of this comparison are given in the following section.

Table 4.4 Thoracoscopic myotomy for the treatment of achalasia

Authors	No. of patients	Anti-reflux procedure	% Symptom good/excellent	Follow up months (mean)	% Complication GERD
Patti et al.[56]	30	No	87	NR*	NR
Cade and Martin[57]	12	No	92	3	18
Raiser et al.[58]	10	Yes	62	15	57
Pellegrini et al.[59]	35	No	87	12	60
Ramacciato et al.[60]	16	No	63	35	31

Modified and updated from Vaezi MF and Richter JE. *J Clin Gastroenterol* 1998;**27**:21–35.[11] NR, not reported; GERD, gastroesophageal reflux disease

Table 4.5 Laparoscopic myotomy for the treatment of achalasia

Author	No. of patients	Anti-reflux procedure	% Symptom improvement good/excellent	Follow up in months (mean)	% Complication GERD
Rosati et al.[61]	25	Yes	96	12	NR
Ancona et al.[62]	17	Yes (D[a])	100	8	6
Mitchell et al.[63]	14	Yes (D)	86	NR	7
Swanstrom and Pennings[64]	12	Yes (T[b])	100	16	16
Raiser et al.[58]	39	Yes (D/T)	63	26	27
Morino et al.[65]	18	Yes (D)	100	8	6
Robertson et al.[66]	10	No	88	14	13
Bonovina et al.[67]	33	Yes (D)	97	12	NR
Delgado et al.[68]	12	Yes (D)	83	4	NR
Hunter et al.[69]	40	Yes (D/T)	90	13	18
Kjellin et al.[70]	21	No	52	22	38
Ackroyd et al.[71]	82	Yes (D)	87	24	5
Yamamura et al.[72]	24	Yes (D)	88	17	0
Patti et al.[73]	102	Yes (D)	89	25	NR
Pechlivanides et al.[74]	29	Yes (D)	90	12	10
Sharp et al.[75]	100	No	87	10	14
Donahue et al.[76]	81	Yes (D)	84	45	26
Zaninotto et al.[77]	113	Yes (D)	92	12	5
Ramacciato et al.[60]	17	Yes (D)	94	18	6
Luketich et al.[78]	62	Yes (T/D)	92	19	9
Dccker et al.[79]	73	Yes (T/D)	83	31	11

[a]D, Dorr
[b]T, Toupet
Modified from Vaezi MF and Richter JE. *J Clin Gastroenterol* 1998;**27**:21–35[11] for abbreviations see Table 4.4

Minimally invasive surgery and especially laparoscopy, has become the standard approach to perform myotomy. No randomized controlled trial has examined laparoscopic Heller myotomy for the treatment of achalasia. Uncontrolled studies of the thoracoscopic[11,56–60] and laparoscopic[11,56,60–79] techniques are summarized in Tables 4.4 and 4.5, respectively. Pooled results of 103 patients in 5 studies of thoracoscopy yield good to excellent symptom response in 82% of patients with a mean follow up of 16 months, GERD developed in 42%.[20] The pooled symptom response rate was 88% in 924 patients undergoing laparoscopic Heller myotomy in 21 uncontrolled trials; 13% of these patients developed GERD.[20] B4 The degree of benefit may be overestimated in these uncontrolled studies.

While there are no randomized controlled trials of myotomy performed with the modern and most widely used techniques, the success rate appears to be approximately 85%, which is similar to that observed with pneumatic dilatation. Heller myotomy, preferably through the laparoscopic approach, should be considered as effective as pneumatic dilatation and should be offered to patients who present an acceptable surgical risk. It can also be offered to those who have failed pneumatic dilatation.

Table 4.6 Randomized trials comparing symptomatic response 12 months after pneumatic dilatation or botulinum toxin injection for treatment of achalasia

| Authors | No. of patients | No. (%) of patients with symptomatic remission | | P value |
		Pneumatic dilatation	Botulinum toxin injection	
Vaezi *et al.*[29]	42	14/20 (70)	7/22 (32)	0·017
Mikaeli *et al.*[32]	39	10/19 (53)	3/20 (15)	<0·01
Muehldorfer *et al.*[28]	24	8/12 (67)	3/12 (25)	<0·05

Comparisons of different treatment modalities

Pneumatic dilatation versus botulinum toxin: These two therapeutic approaches have been compared in three randomized controlled trials (Table 4.6). Ald Vaezi *et al.*[29] treated 42 patients who were randomized to botulinum toxin injection or graded pneumatic dilatation with 30 and 35 mm Rigiflex balloons and found success at 12 months (defined as improvement in symptom score greater than 50%) to be 70% for dilatation and 32% for botulinum toxin. Using a similar design and criteria for symptom response, Mikaeli *et al.*[32] found the response rate at 12 months was 53% with single pneumatic dilatation compared with 15% with a single botulinum toxin injection. Success after repeat dilation or repeat injection was observed, respectively, in 100% and 60% of patients at 12 months. Muehldorfer *et al.*[28] randomized 24 patients to botulinum toxin or dilatation with a 40 mm latex balloon; symptomatic response was superior with pneumatic dilatation compared with botulinum toxin at 12 months (67% *v* 25%) and at 30 months (50% *v* 0%). Identification of predictors of response was not possible in any of these three small randomized trials. Although randomization codes were concealed, patients and investigators were not blinded as to the treatments received.

Pneumatic dilatation versus Heller myotomy: As previously described, the only randomized controlled trial that compared pneumatic dilatation to myotomy[55] found that myotomy via laparotomy had a success rate of 95% compared with 65% for pneumatic dilatation with the Mosher bag. Ald Neither of these techniques is used today and the results may not be generalizable to other techniques. Spiess and Kahrilas[7] pooled all uncontrolled series of 10 or more patients undergoing pneumatic dilatation or surgery with follow up greater than a year performed between 1966 and 1997. They reported response rates as weighted means and found good to excellent symptom response in 80 ± 42% of participants with pneumatic dilatation. Response rates for surgery were 84 ± 20% with thoracotomy, 85 ± 42% with laparotomy, and 92 ± 18% with laparoscopy. However, criteria for including or excluding reports were not stated, and these uncontrolled studies may tend to overestimate the benefits of treatment. B4

From these data and the uncontrolled studies summarized in Tables 4.4, 4.5 and 4.6 we conclude that Heller myotomy and pneumatic dilatation have similar success rates. B4

Esophagectomy

A small number of patients develop "endstage" achalasia, characterized by progressive dilatation and tortuosity of the esophagus.[8] This may be seen in cases that are refractory to treatment or in patients with longstanding untreated disease. If these patients do not respond to Heller myotomy, esophageal resection is frequently required.

There are few studies that assess the effectiveness of the two approaches to resection of the esophagus, i.e. the use of colonic interposition or a gastric pull-up. No randomized controlled trials have been carried out in this area. The available uncontrolled data show symptom improvement in over 80% of endstage cases of achalasia with mortality rates between 0% and 5·4%, and development of GERD in 8–36% of patients (Table 4.7).[8,80–87] The studies performed are insufficient to determine whether there are advantages of colonic interposition compared with gastric pull-through. B4

Summary

Several options are available for the treatment of achalasia, ranging from medications to esophagectomy. Unfortunately, there have been very few controlled trials to guide our approach to these patients. Techniques and outcome measures vary over time and between studies. The outcomes of symptom resolution and objective improvement in esophageal emptying are not always correlated. This problem was demonstrated in a study by Vaezi *et al.*,[88] who performed timed studies of barium emptying (measuring the column of barium in the esophagus 1 and 5 minutes after a bolus) in patients treated with pneumatic dilatation. They found that 31% of patients who reported near complete symptom resolution had less than 50% improvement in barium emptying after treatment. With these limitations in mind, the available evidence is sufficient to make the following recommendations. Pharmacologic therapy has variable and limited response and is hindered by adverse effects. Calcium

Table 4.7 Esophagectomy in the treatment of refractory achalasia

Authors	No. of patients	% Symptom improvement	Follow up in months (mean)	GERD	% Complication Post-op dilation	Mortality
Pinotti et al.[81]	122	83	93	36	17	4.1
Watson et al.[82]	104	98	NR	20	30	2
Orringer and Stirling[83]	26	100	30	15	39	3.9
Cecconello et al.[84]	64	94	81	16	NR	NR
Miller et al.[85]	37	91	76	8	14	5.4
Banbury et al.[8]	32	87	43	31	60	0
Peters et al.[86]	19	80	72	NR	28	0
Devaney et al.[87]	93	95	38	NR	46	2.1

Modified and updated from Khazanchi A and Katz PO. *Gastrointest Endosc Clin North Am* 2001;**11**:325–45[80]
For abbreviations see Table 4.4

channel blockers and nitrates should be used in patients who cannot tolerate or are unwilling to receive other treatments. The use of sildenafil should be restricted to research protocols. Botulinum toxin is safe and effective but generally lasts less than 6 months–1 year. It should be used in elderly or frail individuals in whom more aggressive treatments pose a high risk. Pneumatic dilatation and laparoscopic Heller myotomy have similar efficacy and should be offered as first-line treatments to all patients who can tolerate these procedures. Pneumatic dilatation appears to be the most cost-effective therapeutic approach over a 5-year horizon, but whether this holds true with longer follow up is not known.[89,90] Although some patient characteristics and patients' preferences should be taken into consideration, we currently have no way of predicting which patient will respond better to pneumatic dilatation or surgery. The risks and benefits of the intervention need to be carefully weighed in each case. Esophagectomy may be necessary in patients with endstage achalasia. The algorithm in Figure 4.1 depicts a general approach to the treatment of achalasia supported by a guideline paper by the American College of Gastroenterology.[4] A randomized controlled trial of pneumatic dilatation versus laparoscopic Heller myotomy to compare efficacy and safety, and identify predictors of response is greatly needed.

Complicated patients, including those who are refractory to initial treatment, may benefit from evaluation and treatment at a tertiary center that can offer expertise in all the treatments available for this disorder. A multi-modality approach is often necessary in this group.

Spastic motility disorders

Spastic motor abnormalities of the esophagus include diffuse esophageal spasm (DES), the nutcracker esophagus (NE), and hypertensive lower esophageal sphincter. These abnormal manometric patterns have been described in association with chest pain and dysphagia. However, whether these abnormal motility patterns represent true diseases as opposed to manometric findings present in, but not responsible for, dysphagia and chest pain remains controversial. Therefore, in contrast to achalasia, the clinical importance of these abnormalities is less clear.

Diffuse esophageal spasm is characterized by normal peristalsis with intermittent simultaneous contractions that can lead to chest pain and dysphagia. The manometric description requires 20% or more simultaneous contractions during water swallows. Adhering to these criteria DES is rare, with an estimated incidence of 0·2/100 000.[91] This motility disorder is seen in 3–5% of patients who undergo manometry for non-cardiac chest pain or dysphagia.[92] NE, which may be considered a variant of DES, is a manometric abnormality characterized by an average distal esophageal contraction amplitude of 180 mmHg or greater during swallows. Symptom presentation, i.e. dysphagia and chest pain, is similar for DES and NE. Furthermore, manometric findings may show fluctuation across these disorders, with periods of return to normal peristalsis and, rarely, progression to achalasia.

The etiology of DES and its spastic variants remains unknown. Proposed theories include a malfunction in endogenous NO synthesis and degradation[93] and defects in cholinergic mechanisms.[91] Other studies suggest that DES can be caused by gastroesophageal reflux[94] and stressful events.[95]

The most common presenting symptoms are chest pain, which can occur in association with swallowing or spontaneously, and dysphagia. The chest pain may be clinically indistinguishable from angina of cardiac origin. Dysphagia occurs with both solids and liquids and is transitory and non-progressive.

The diagnosis of a spastic motility disorder is made based on the presence of dysphagia or chest pain, accompanied by an abnormal manometry. Chest pain may be stimulated during provocative testing with edrophonium.[3] The diagnosis should only be made after cardiac causes have been

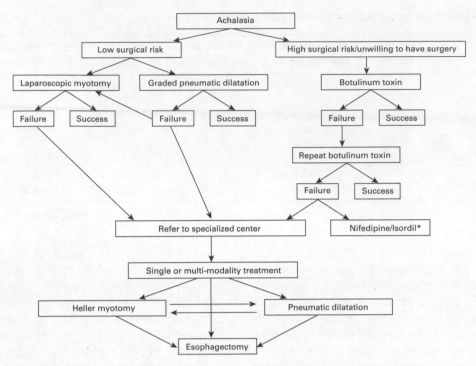

Figure 4.1 Algorithm for the treatment of achalasia. *Isosorbide dinitrate. (Modified from Vaezi MF and Richter JE. *Am J Gastroenterol* 1999;**94**:3406–12[4])

thoroughly ruled out. It is important to determine whether gastroesophageal reflux is present by 24-hour pH monitoring because acid reflux can be a cause of chest pain. If GERD is found, it should be aggressively treated with acid suppression.

Treatment of spastic motility disorders

Overview

Therapeutic trials for spastic motility disorders are scarce, and most of them are uncontrolled studies with small numbers of patients. The unknown etiology and pathophysiology, the controversies surrounding the clinical importance of DES and NE, which make development of therapies challenging, and the rarity of these disorders have interfered with design and performance of large randomized trials. Furthermore, a high association with psychiatric diseases (depression, anxiety, panic disorder) and issues of heightened visceral sensation pose additional problems.[95,96] The main goal of therapy is symptomatic relief. An important component in the treatment of DES and NE consists of educating and reassuring the patient about the non-progressive and benign nature of the disease. Many of the treatments used for achalasia have also been used in spastic motility disorders; these include medications such as calcium channel blockers and nitrates, endoscopic botulinum toxin injection, pneumatic dilatation and surgical myotomy.

Additionally, psychotropic agents have been shown to be useful in patients with chest pain of esophageal origin. Observational studies of a number of interventions for these disorders have been carried out[19,97–107] and the results of a small number of randomized trials are summarized in Table 4.8.

Medications

Treatment aimed at reducing muscle contractility has been attempted with nitrates or calcium channel blockers. Intravenous nitroglycerin (100–200 micrograms/kg) was shown to decrease the duration of contractions and relieve symptoms in five patients with DES.[93] There are no randomized controlled trials evaluating the efficacy of nitrates in the treatment of esophageal spasm. A randomized controlled trial of diltiazem (60 mg three times daily for 2 weeks) found that chest pain and dysphagia were not improved after therapy with this calcium channel antagonist.[97] Ald In another randomized controlled trial of 14 patients with chest pain, nine of them with manometric diagnosis of NE, diltiazem (60 mg PO four times daily for 8 weeks) resulted in a significant decrease in mean chest pain scores.[98] Ald However, the symptomatic improvement occurred regardless of whether manometry showed NE. In uncontrolled studies, nifedipine resulted in relief of dysphagia in five of six patients with DES[99] and improved

Table 4.8 Randomized controlled trials of treatment for spastic disorders of esophageal motality

Authors	No. of patients	Treatment	Design	Duration	% Symptom improvement
Drenth et al.[97]	8	Diltiazem 60 mg three times daily	Crossover	4 weeks	0
Richter et al.[101]	20	Nifedipine 10–30 mg three times daily	Crossover	6 weeks	10
Clouse et al.[102]	29	Trazadone 100–150 mg/day	Double blind Parallel	6 weeks	Trazadone 50 Placebo 10 ($P = 0.02$)
Cannon et al.[96]	49	Imipramine 50 mg at bed time	Double blind Parallel	3 weeks	Imipramine 52 ± 25 Placebo 1 ± 86 ($P = 0.03$)

chest pain in four of six patients with DES or NE.[100] However, in a 14-week, double blind crossover study of patients with non-cardiac chest pain and NE, nifedipine (10–30 mg PO three times daily for 14 weeks) decreased the distal esophageal contraction amplitude but did not reduce the frequency or severity of chest pain compared to placebo.[101] Ald Although other small studies or anecdotal reports describe manometric improvement with nitrates or calcium channel blockers, these were not always accompanied by a good clinical response and adverse effects such as headache, hypotension or lower extremity edema are frequent. More recently, a small uncontrolled study of sildenafil (50 mg PO every day) for the treatment of four patients with NE and one patient with DES, found a symptom relief rate of 60%.[19] C5

The use of psychotropic drugs for DES is aimed at altering visceral sensation and targeting stress as a potential cause of spasm. In a randomized controlled trial of 29 patients with chest pain treated with the serotonin reuptake inhibitor trazodone (100–150 mg/day for 6 weeks), distress over esophageal symptoms was significantly reduced, with no effect on the manometric abnormalities.[102] In a second randomized controlled trial, the tricyclic antidepressant imipramine (50 mg at bedtime) in patients with chest pain and normal cardiac evaluation achieved a 52 ± 25% reduction in episodes of chest pain compared with only 1 ± 86% in placebo-treated patients ($P = 0.03$).[96] Ald Abnormal manometry was present in only half of the patients and did not predict the response to treatment.

In summary, there are no good data showing improvement of chest pain or dysphagia with nitrates or calcium channel blockers. However, given the lack of established treatments, and since symptoms may be alleviated in some subjects, a therapeutic trial with these agents is reasonable. Therapeutic trials with trazodone or imipramine are recommended for treating chest pain of esophageal origin, although their effect on dysphagia has not been studied. As in the treatment of achalasia, controlled trials with sildenafil are needed.

Botulinum toxin

Inhibition of esophageal contraction after botulinum toxin injection has been recently introduced as a treatment of spastic motility disorders. Miller et al.[103] used botulinum toxin to treat chest pain in patients with a diagnosis of non-reflux, non-cardiac, non-achalasia spastic esophageal motility disorder (including DES, hypertensive LES or NE). This uncontrolled study of 29 patients receiving botulinum toxin injection at the esophagogastric junction into the LES muscle (the esophageal body was not injected), found 50% or greater reduction in chest pain in 70% of patients and complete relief in 48%. Mean duration of symptom relief was 7 months. B4 Storrs et al.[104] injected botulinum toxin in 1·5-cm intervals into the esophageal body of nine patients with DES, finding 50% or greater improvement in dysphagia and chest pain in 89% of patients at 6 months. There are no randomized controlled trials evaluating the use of botulinum toxin for the treatment of DES or NE. Uncontrolled studies tend to overestimate the benefits of treatment. However, this agent has a remarkable safety profile and can be tried in patients who fail medical therapy. B4

Pneumatic dilatation and Heller myotomy

In an uncontrolled study, Ebert et al.[105] found that pneumatic dilatation improved symptoms in eight of nine (89%) patients with DES and manometry showing high LES pressure in addition to spasm. The procedure, however, did not result in correction of the abnormal esophageal body contractions. Irving et al.[106] used dilatation with Rigiflex balloon to treat 20 DES patients with severe symptoms that were refractory to conservative management; symptom response was reported to be good in 70% of patients. B4

Patti et al.[107], using thoracoscopic myotomy in 10 patients with DES and NE, found that this minimally invasive approach improved symptoms in 80% of patients. Ellis et al.[108] reported an overall symptomatic improvement rate of 70% in 42 patients with esophageal motor disorders

(32 had a diagnosis of esophageal spasm) treated with long esophagomyotomy performed through a thoracotomy.

There are no randomized controlled trials evaluating pneumatic dilatation or esophageal myotomy as treatment of DES. The uncontrolled studies may overestimate the benefit of these treatments. Given the morbidity associated with these invasive procedures, they should be reserved for patients with severe symptoms who are refractory to other forms of treatment. These procedures should only be carried out after careful discussion of risks and benefits with the patient. B4

Summary

Diffuse esophageal spasm and its spastic variants are rare disorders. It is critical that a cardiac etiology is ruled out before making the diagnosis of a spastic motility disorder as a cause of chest pain. Gastroesophageal reflux should be investigated and treated when present. Randomized controlled trials in large populations evaluating treatment for these disorders are lacking. The available data suggest that therapeutic trials of muscle relaxants, such as nitrates and calcium channel blockers, may be warranted in some patients. Psychotropic medications, like trazodone or imipramine, are recommended as symptomatic treatment for chest pain associated with a motility disorder but have no proven role in the treatment of dysphagia. Botulinum toxin has resulted in symptom improvement in uncontrolled trials; this agent warrants further study in randomized controlled trials and is attractive because of its excellent adverse effect profile. Finally, pneumatic dilatation and myotomy should be reserved for patients with severe, refractory symptoms after careful consideration of the risks associated with these procedures.

References

1 Mayberry JF. Epidemiology and demographics of achalasia. *Gastrointest Endosc Clin North Am* 2001;**11**:235–47.

2 Wong RKH, Maydonovitch CL. Achalasia. In: Castell DO, Richter JE, eds. *The Esophagus, 3rd edn.* Philadelphia: Lippincott Williams & Wilkins, 1999:185–213.

3 Richter JE. Oesophageal motility disorders. *Lancet* 2001;**358**: 823–828.

4 Vaezi MF, Richter JE. Diagnosis and management of achalasia. *Am J Gastroenterol* 1999;**94**:3406–12.

5 Vela MF, Richter JE. Management of achalasia at a tertiary center – a complicated disease. *Gastroenterology* 2003;**124**: A236.

6 Spechler SJ. AGA technical review on treatment of patients with dysphagia caused by benign disorders of the distal esophagus. *Gastroenterology* 1999;**117**:223–54.

7 Spiess AE, Kahrilas PJ. Treating achalasia: from whalebone to laparoscope. *JAMA* 1998;**280**:638–42.

8 Banbury MK, Rice TW, Goldblum JR *et al.* Esophagectomy with gastric reconstruction for achalasia. *J Thorac Cardiovasc Surg* 1999;**117**:1077–85.

9 Gelfond M, Rozen P, Gilat T. Effect of nitrates on LOS pressure in achalasia: a potential therapeutic aid. *Gut* 1981;**22**:312–18.

10 Wong RK, Maydonovitch C, Garcia JE, Johnson LF, Castell DO. The effect of terbutaline sulfate, nitroglycerin, and aminophylline on lower esophageal sphincter pressure and radionuclide esophageal emptying in patients with achalasia. *J Clin Gastroenterol* 1987;**9**:386–9.

11 Vaezi MF, Richter JE. Current therapies for achalasia: comparison and efficacy. *J Clin Gastroenterol* 1998;**27**: 21–35.

12 Gelfond M, Rozen P, Gilat T. Isosorbide dinitrate and nifedipine treatment of achalasia: a clinical, manometric and radionuclide evaluation. *Gastroenterology* 1982;**83**:963–9.

13 Gelfond M, Rozen P, Keren S, Gilat T. Effect of nitrates on LOS pressure in achalasia: a potential therapeutic aid. *Gut* 1981;**22**:312–18.

14 Rozen P, Gelfond M, Salzman S *et al.* Radionuclide confirmation of the therapeutic value of isosorbide dinitrate in relieving the dysphasia in achalasia. *J Clin Gastroenterol* 1982;**4**:17–22.

15 Traube M, Dubovik S, Lange RC, McCallum RW. The role of nifedipine therapy in achalasia: results of a randomized, double-blind, placebo-controlled study. *Am J Gastroenterol* 1989;**84**:1259–62.

16 Bortolotti M, Labo G. Clinical and manometric effects of nifedipine in patients with esophageal achalasia. *Gastroenterology* 1981;**80**:39–44

17 Coccia G, Bortolotti M, Michetti P, Dodero M. Prospective clinical and manometric comparing pneumatic dilation and sublingual nifedipine in the treatment of esophageal achalasia. *Gut* 1991;**32**:604–6.

18 Bortolotti M, Mari C, Lopilato C *et al.* Effects of sildenafil on esophageal motility of patients with idiopathic achalasia. *Gastroenterology* 2000;**118**:253–7.

19 Eherer AJ, Schwetz I, Hammer HF, *et al.* Effect of sildenafil on oesophageal motor function in healthy subjects and patients with oesophageal motor disorders. *Gut* 2002;**50**:758–64.

20 Pasricha PJ, Ravich WJ, Hendrix TR *et al.* Intrasphincteric botulinum toxin for the treatment of achalasia. *N Engl J Med* 1995;**332**:774–8.

21 Pasricha PJ, Rudra R, Ravich WJ *et al.* Botulinum toxin for achalasia: long-term outcome and predictors of response. *Gastroenterology* 1996;**110**:1410–15.

22 Hoogerwerf WA, Pasricha PJ. Pharmacologic therapy in treating achalasia. *Gastrointest Endosc Clin North Am* 2001;**11**:311–23.

23 Cuilliere C, Ducrotte P, Zerbib F *et al.* Achalasia: outcome of patients treated with intrasphincteric injection of botulinum toxin. *Gut* 1997;**41**:87–92.

24 Rollan A, Gonzales R, Carvajal S *et al.* Endoscopic intrasphincteric injection of botulinum toxin for the treatment of achalasia. *J Clin Gastroenterol* 1995;**20**: 189–91.

25 Fishman VM, Parkman HP, Schiano TD *et al.* Symptomatic improvement in achalasia after botulinum toxin injection of the lower esophageal sphincter. *Am J Gastroenterol* 1996; **91**:1724–30.

26 Annese V, Basciani M, Perri F *et al.* Controlled trial of botulinum toxin injection versus placebo and pneumatic dilation in achalasia. *Gastroenterology* 1996;**111**:1418–24.

27 Gordon JM, Eaker EY. Prospective study of esophageal botulinum toxin injection in high-risk achalasia patients. *Am J Gastroenterol* 1997;**92**:1812–16.

28 Muehldorfer SM, Schneider TH, Hochberger J *et al.* Esophageal achalasia: intrasphincteric injection of botulinum toxin versus balloon dilation. *Endoscopy* 1999; **31**:517–21.

29 Vaezi MJ, Richter JE, Wilcox CM *et al.* Botulinum toxin versus pneumatic dilation in the treatment of achalasia: a randomized trial. *Gut* 1999;**44**:231–9.

30 Annese V, Bassotti G, Coccia G *et al.* A multicenter randomized study of intrasphincteric botulinum toxin in patients with oesophageal achalasia. *Gut* 2000;**46**:597–600.

31 Kolbasnik J, Waterfall WE, Fachnie B *et al.* Long-term efficacy of botulinum toxin in classical achalasia; a prospective study. *Am J Gastroenterol* 1999;**94**:3434–9.

32 Mikaeli J, Fazel A, Montazeri G *et al.* Randomized controlled trial comparing botulinum toxin injection to pneumatic dilatation for the treatment of achalasia. *Aliment Pharmacol Ther* 2001;**15**:1389–96.

33 Allescher HD, Storr M, Seige M *et al.* Treatment of achalasia: botulinum toxin injection vs pneumatic balloon dilation. A prospective study with long-term follow-up. *Endoscopy* 2001;**33**:1007–17.

34 Neubrand M, Scheurlen C, Schepke M, Sauerbach T. Long-term results and prognostic factors in the treatment of achalasia with botulinum toxin. *Endoscopy* 2002;**34**: 519–23.

35 Kadakia SC, Wong RKH. Pneumatic balloon dilation for esophageal achalasia. *Gastrointest Endosc Clin North Am* 2001;**11**:325–45.

36 Wong RKH, Maydonovitch C. Utility of parameters measured during pneumatic dilation as predictors of successful dilation. *Am J Gastroenterol* 1996;**91**:1126–9.

37 Cox J, Buckton GK, Bennett JR. Balloon dilatation in achalasia: a new dilator. *Gut* 1986;**27**:986–9.

38 Gelfand MD, Kozarek RA. An experience with polyethylene balloon for pneumatic dilation for achalasia. *Am J Gastroenterol* 1989;**84**:924–7.

39 Barkin JS, Guelrud M, Reiner DK *et al.* Forceful balloon dilation: An outpatient procedure for achalasia. *Gastrointest Endosc* 1990;**36**:123–5.

40 Stark GA, Castell DO, Richter JE *et al.* Prospective randomized comparison of Browne-McHardy and Microvasive balloon dilator in the treatment of achalasia. *Am J Gastroenterol* 1990;**85**:1322–6.

41 Makela J, Kiviniemi H, Laitinen S. Heller's cardiomyotomy compared with pneumatic dilation for the treatment of oesophageal achalasia. *Eur J Surg* 1991;**157**:411–14.

42 Levine ML, Moskowitz GW, Dorf BS *et al.* Pneumatic dilation in patients with achalasia with a modified Gruntzig dilator (Levine) under direct endoscopic control. Results after 5 years. *Am J Gastroenterol* 1991;**86**:1581–4.

43 Kim CH, Cameron AJ, Hsu JJ *et al.* Achalasia: prospective evaluation of relationship between lower esophageal sphincter pressure, esophageal transit, and esophageal diameter and symptoms in response to pneumatic dilation. *Mayo Clin Proc* 1993;**68**:1067–73.

44 Lee JD, Cecil BD, Brown PE *et al.* The Cohen test does not predict outcome in achalasia after pneumatic dilation. *Gastrointest Endosc* 1992;**39**:157–60.

45 Abid S, Champion G, Richter JE *et al.* Treatment of achalasia: The best of both worlds. *Am J Gastroenterol* 1993;**89**:979–85.

46 Wehrmann T, Jacobi V, Jung M *et al.* Pneumatic dilation in achalasia with a low-compliance balloon. Results of a 5-year prospective evaluation. *Gastrointest Endosc* 1995;**42**:31–6.

47 Lambroza A, Schuman RW. Pneumatic dilation for achalasia without fluoroscopic guidance: Safety and efficacy. *Am J Gastroenterol* 1995;**90**:1226–9.

48 Muehldorfer SM, Hahn EG, Eli C. High- and low-compliance balloon dilators in patients with achalasia: a randomized prospective comparison trial. *Gastrointest Endosc* 1996;**44**:398–403.

49 Bhatnager MS, Nanivadekar SA, Sawant P *et al.* Achalasia cardia dilation using polyethylene balloon (Rigiflex) dilator. *Indian J Gastroenterol* 1996;**15**:49–51.

50 Gideon RM, Castell DO, Yarze J. Prospective randomized comparison of pneumatic dilation techniques in patients with idiopathic achalasia. *Dig Dis Sci* 1999;**44**:1853–7.

51 Khan AA, Shah WH, Alam A *et al.* Massively dilated esophagus in achalasia: response to pneumatic balloon dilation. *Am J Gastroenterol* 1999;**94**:2363–6.

52 Kadakia SC, Wong RKH. Graded pneumatic dilation using Rigiflex achalasia dilators in patients with primary esophageal achalasia. *Am J Gastroenterol* 1993;**88**:34–8.

53 West RL, Hirsch DP, Batelsman JFWM *et al.* Long term results of pneumatic dilatation in achalasia followed for more than 5 years. *Am J Gastroenterol* 2002;**97**:1346–51.

54 Amjad A, Pellegrini CA. Laparoscopic myotomy: technique and efficacy in treating achalasia. *Gastrointest Endosc Clin North Am* 2001;**11**:347–57.

55 Csendes A, Braghetto I, Heriquez A *et al.* Late results of a prospective randomized study comparing forceful dilatation and esophagomyotomy in patients with achalasia. *Gut* 1989;**30**:299–304.

56 Patti MG, Pelligrini CA, Arcerito M *et al.* Comparison of medical and minimally invasive surgical therapy for achalasia. *Arch Surg* 1997;**132**:233–40.

57 Cade RJ, Martin CJ. Thoracoscopic cardiomyotomy for achalasia. *Aust NZ J Surg* 1996;**66**:107–9.

58 Raiser F, Perdikis G, Hinder RA *et al.* Heller myotomy via minimal access surgery: an evaluation of anti-reflux procedure. *Am J Surg* 1995;**169**:424–7.

59 Pellegrini CA, Leichter R, Patti M, *et al.* Thoracoscopic esophageal myotomy in the treatment of achalasia. *Ann Thorac Surg* 1993;**56**:680–2.

60 Ramacciato G, Mercantini P, Amodio PM *et al.* The laparoscopic approach with antireflux surgery is superior to

the thoracoscopic approach for the treatment of esophageal achalasia. *Surg Endosc* 2002;**16**:1431–7.

61 Rosati R, Fumagalli U, Bonavina L *et al*. Laparoscopic approach to esophageal achalasia. *Am J Surg* 1995;**169**: 424–7.

62 Ancona E, Anselmino M, Zaninotto G *et al*. Esophageal achalasia: laparoscopic vs conventional open Heller-Dor operation. *Am J Surg* 1995;**170**:265–70.

63 Mitchell PC, Watson DI, Devitt PG *et al*. Laparoscopic cardiomyotomy with a Dor patch for achalasia. *J Am Coll Cardiol* 1995;**38**:445–9.

64 Swanstrom LL, Pennings J. Laparoscopic esophagomyotomy for achalasia. *Surg Endosc* 1995;**9**:286–72.

65 Morino M, Rebecchi F, Festa V, Garrone C. Laparoscopic Heller cardiomyotomy with intraoperative manometry in the management of oesophageal achalasia. *Int Surg* 1995; **80**:332–5.

66 Robertson GSM, Lloyd DM, Wicks ACB *et al*. Laparoscopic Heller's cardiomyotomy without an antireflux procedure. *Br J Surg* 1995;**82**:957–9.

67 Bonovina L, Rosati P, Segalin A, Peracchia A. Laparoscopic Heller-Dor operation for the treatment of oesophageal achalasia: technique and early results. *Ann Chir Gynaecol* 1995;**84**:165–8.

68 Delgado F, Bolufer JM, Martinex-Abad M *et al*. Laparoscopic treatment of esophageal achalasia. *Surg Laparosc Endosc* 1996;**2**:83–90.

69 Hunter JG, Trus TL, Branum GD, Waring JP. Laparoscopic Heller myotomy and fundoplication for achalasia. *Ann Surg* 1997;**225**:655–65.

70 Kjellin AP, Granquist S, Ramel S, Thor KBA. Laparoscopic myotomy without fundoplication in patients with achalasia. *Eur J Surg* 1999;**165**:1162–6.

71 Ackroyd R, Watson DI, Devitt PG, Jamieson GG. Laparoscopic cardiomyotomy and anterior partial fundoplication for achalasia. *Surg Endosc* 2001;**15**:683–6.

72 Yamamura MS, Gilster JC, Myers BS *et al*. Laparoscopic Heller myotomy and anterior fundoplication for achalasia results in a high degree of patient satisfaction. *Arch Surg* 2000;**135**:902–6.

73 Patti MG, Molena D, Fisichella PM *et al*. Laparoscopic Heller myotomy and Dor fundoplication for achalasia. Analysis of successes and failures. *Arch Surg* 2001;**136**: 870–7.

74 Pechlivanides G, Chryos E, Athanasakis E *et al*. Laparoscopic Heller cardiomyotomy and Dor fundoplication for esophageal achalasia. *Arch Surg* 2001;**136**:1240–3.

75 Sharp KW, Khaitan L, Scholz S *et al*. 100 consecutive minimally invasive Heller myotomies: lessons learned. *Ann Surg* 2002;**235**:631–9.

76 Donahue PE, Horgan S, Liu KJM, Madura JA. Floppy Dor fundoplication after esophagocardiomyotomy for achalasia. *Surgery* 2002;**132**:716–22.

77 Zaninotto G, Costantini M, Portale G *et al*. Etiology, diagnosis and treatment of failures after laparoscopic Heller myotomy for achalasia. *Ann Surg* 2002;**235**:186–192.

78 Luketich JD, Fernando HC, Christie NA *et al*. Outcome after minimally invasive esophagomyotomy. *Ann Thorac Surg* 2001;**72**:1909–13.

79 Decker G, Borie F, Bouamirrene D *et al*. Gastrointestinal quality of life before and after laparoscopic Heller myotomy with partial posterior fundoplication. *Surgery* 2002;**236**: 750–8.

80 Khazanchi A, Katz PO. Strategies for treating severe refractory dysphagia. *Gastrointest Endosc Clin North Am* 2001;**11**:325–45.

81 Pinotti HW, Cecconcello I, Da Rocha JM *et al*. Resection for achalasia of the esophagus. *Hepatogastroenterology* 1991;**38**:470–3.

82 Watson TJ, DeMeester TR, Kauer WKH *et al*. Esophageal replacement for end-stage benign esophageal disease. *J Thorac Cardiovasc Surg* 1998;**115**:1241–7.

83 Orringer MB, Stirling MC. Esophageal resection for achalasia: Indications and results. *Ann Thorac Surg* 1989; **47**:340–5.

84 Cecconcello I, Da Rocha JM, Pollara W *et al*. Long-term evaluation of gastroplasty in achalasia. In: Siewert JR, Holscher AH (eds). *Diseases of the Esophagus*. Berlin, Springer Verlag, 1998:975.

85 Miller DL, Allen MS, Trastek VF *et al*. Esophageal resection for recurrent achalasia. *Ann Thorac Surg* 1995;**60**:922–5.

86 Peters JH, Kauer WKH, Crookes PF *et al*. Esophageal resection with colon interposition for end-stage achalasia. *Arch Surg* 1995;**130**:632–6.

87 Devaney EJ, Lannettoni MD, Orringer MB, Marshall B. Esophagectomy for achalasia: patient selection and clinical experience. *Ann Thorac Surg* 2001;**72**:854–8.

88 Vaezi MF, Baker ME, Richter JE. Assessment of esophageal emptying post-pneumatic dilation: use of the timed barium esophagram. *Am J Gastroenterol* 1999;**94**:1802–7.

89 Imperiale TF, O'Connor JB, Vaezi MF *et al*. A cost analysis of alternative treatment strategies for achalasia. *Am J Gastroenterol* 2000;**85**:2737–45.

90 O'Connor JB, Singer ME, Imperiale TF, Vaezi MF, Richter JE. *Dig Dis Sci* 2002;**47**:1516–25.

91 Storr M, Allescher HD, Classen M. Current concepts on pathophysiology, diagnosis and treatment of diffuse oesophageal spasm. *Drugs* 2001;**61**:579–91.

92 Katz PO, Dalton CB, Richter JE. Esophageal testing of patients with non-cardiac chest pain or dysphagia. *Ann Intern Med* 1987;**106**:593–7.

93 Konturec JW, Gillesen A, Domschke W. Diffuse esophageal spasm: a malfunction that involves nitric oxide? *Scand J Gastroenterol* 1995;**30**:1041–5.

94 Peters LJ, Maas LC, Petti D *et al*. Spontaneous non-cardiac chest pain: evaluation by 24-hour ambulatory esophageal motility and pH monitoring. *Gastroenterology* 1988;**94**: 878–6.

95 Anderson KO, Dalton CB, Bradley LA *et al*. Stress induces alterations of esophageal pressures in healthy volunteers and non-cardiac chest pain patients. *Dig Dis Sci* 1989;**34**: 83–91.

96 Cannon RO, Quyyumi AA, Mincemoyer R *et al*. Imipramine in patients with chest pain despite normal coronary angiograms. *N Engl J Med* 1994;**330**:1411–17.

97 Drenth JPH, Bos LP, Engels LGJ. Efficacy of diltiazem in the treatment of diffuse oesophageal spasm. *Aliment Pharmacol Ther* 1990;**4**:411–16.

98 Cattau EL, Castell DO, Johnson DA *et al.* Diltiazem therapy for symptoms associated with nutcracker esophagus. *Am J Gastroenterol* 1991;**86**:272–6.

99 Thomas E, Witt P, Willis M, Morse J. Nifedipine therapy for diffuse esophageal spasm. *South Med J* 1986;**79**:847–9.

100 Nasrallah SM, Tommaso CL, Singleton RT, Backhaus EA. Primary esophageal motor disorders: clinical response to nifedipine. *South Med J* 1985;**78**:312–15.

101 Richter JE, Dalton CB, Bradley L, Castell DO. Oral nifedipine in the treatment of noncardiac chest pain in patients with the nutcracker esophagus. *Gastroenterology* 1987;**93**:21–8.

102 Clouse RE, Lustman PJ, Eckert TC *et al.* Low-dose trazodone for symptomatic patients with esophageal contraction abnormalities. A double-blind, placebo-controlled trial. *Gastroenterology* 1987;**92**:1027–36.

103 Miller LS, Pullela SV, Parkman HP *et al.* Treatment of chest pain in patients with noncardiac, nonreflux, nonachalasia spastic esophageal motor disorders using botulinum toxin injection into the gastroesophageal junction. *Am J Gastroenterol* 2002;**97**:1640–6.

104 Storr M, Allescher HD, Rosch T *et al.* Treatment of symptomatic diffuse esophageal spasm by endoscopic injections of botulinum toxin: a prospective study with long-term follow-up. *Gastrointest Endosc* 2001;**54**:754–9.

105 Ebert EC, Ouyang E, Wright SH *et al.* Pneumatic dilatation in patients with symptomatic diffuse esophageal spasm and lower esophageal sphincter dysfunction. *Dig Dis Sci* 1983;**28**:481–5.

106 Irving JD, Owen WJ, Linsell J, Mc Cullagh M *et al.* Management of diffuse esophageal spasm with balloon dilatation. *Gastrointest Radiol* 1992;**17**:189–92.

107 Patti MG, Pellegrini CA, Arcerito M *et al.* Comparison of medical and minimally invasive surgical therapy for primary esophageal disorders. *Arch Surg* 1995;**130**:615–16.

108 Ellis FH. Esophagomyotomy for noncardiac chest pain resulting from diffuse esophageal spasm and related disorders. *Am J Med* 1992;**5A**:129S-131S.

5 Ulcer disease and *Helicobacter pylori*

Naoki Chiba

Introduction

Peptic ulcer disease, particularly duodenal ulcer disease, was thought to result from gastric acid hypersecretion and pepsin damage. Indeed Schwarz's dictum,[1] "no acid, no ulcer" is still relevant. Peptic ulcers were thought to be caused by a variety of factors such as smoking, stress and non-steroidal anti-inflammatory drugs (NSAIDs) including aspirin. Therapy was directed primarily against lowering acid production in the stomach to permit healing of ulceration. However, the discovery and characterization of intragastric infection with *Helicobacter pylori* has revolutionized our concepts of pathogenesis and ulcer therapy. As duodenal ulcer has long been thought to result from an imbalance between protective and aggressive factors in the mucosa, *H. pylori* can be considered an "aggressive" factor which may tip the balance toward mucosal damage and result in ulceration. Thus, the assignment of an etiologic role to *H. pylori* does not contradict the traditional concepts, but rather extends them.

Warren and Marshall's seminal paper in 1983 first identified the spiral bacterium that is now known as *H. pylori,* associated with active chronic gastritis.[2] Their subsequent paper[3] demonstrated an association between the gastric infection and peptic ulcer, particularly duodenal ulcer. *H. pylori* was present in antral biopsies of 100% of their duodenal ulcer patients.

Evidence has dispelled initial skepticism of the role of this infection as an important gastroduodenal pathogen. This chapter reviews and presents the evidence for the etiological role of *H. pylori* in peptic ulcer disease. Causes of ulcers by agents other than *H. pylori* will be discussed. Lastly, treatment of ulcer disease with an emphasis on *H. pylori* eradication will be reviewed.

What is the evidence for the role of *H. pylori* in peptic ulcer disease?

One approach is to determine whether "Koch's postulates", which link an infectious agent with disease(s) are fulfilled. The postulates state that the "agent (i) must be found in patients with the disease only; (ii) must be grown outside of the body; (iii) when inoculated into a susceptible animal, must cause the same disease; and (iv) must be grown from the lesions observed".[4] Many of the organisms currently accepted as pathogens do not necessarily fit all of Koch's postulates. Furthermore, there is limited applicability to chronic disease such as that caused by *H. pylori* infection.[5] A more applicable approach[5] is to use the criteria for assessing epidemiological evidence, as outlined by Hill.[6]

An early methodological review,[5] concluded that there was insufficient evidence in 1990 to establish *H. pylori* as a cause of duodenal ulcer. Since then, new evidence has accumulated and is summarized in Box 5.1.

Association of *H. pylori* with ulcer disease (strength, consistency and specificity)

In this section the prevalence of *H. pylori* in both duodenal and gastric ulcer patients is considered.

Duodenal ulcer

The prevalence of *H. pylori* in ulcer disease had been well reviewed by Kuipers *et al.,*[9] who identified relevant studies published since the discovery of *H. pylori* in 1983. In the decade to 1993 they found that infection with *H. pylori* was present in 94·9% (95% CI 94 to 96%) of 1695 duodenal ulcer patients studied. Borody *et al.* found *H. pylori* in 94% of 302 duodenal ulcer patients in Australia.[10] Of the 14 patients who were negative for *H. pylori* at the time of endoscopy, four had taken antibiotics shortly before endoscopy and may have had falsely negative results, and eight had NSAID-induced ulcers. Overall, in only one of 302 patients was no cause for duodenal ulcer identified. Thus, almost all duodenal ulcers which were not caused by NSAIDs were attributable to *H. pylori.*

A strong association by itself, does not prove causality.[4,5] While the association of *H. pylori* with duodenal ulcer is strong and consistent, it is not specific, since *H. pylori* is also found in many patients without ulcer disease. The reasons

---

Box 5.1   Evidence for role of *H. pylori* in peptic ulcer disease (PUD) according to Hill's criteria

Association (strength, consistency, specificity) of *H. pylori* with PUD

- prevalence of *H. pylori* in DU ~90%, GU ~80%
- *strength* and *consistency* of association is high
- *specificity* is low as *H. pylori* seen in many without ulcers
- *overall, data are supportive*

Temporal relationship: does *H. pylori* infection precede PUD?

- self-administration of *H. pylori* shown to cause active chronic gastritis – fulfills one of Koch's postulates
- but, no direct evidence that PUD is caused
- case–control study (Nomura *et al.*[7]) shows preceding *H. pylori* infection increases risk of DU, GU and gastric cancer
- cohort study (Sipponen *et al.*[8]), >10% *H. pylori* positives developed DU over 10 years but < 1% if *H. pylori* negative
- *thus, data are supportive*

Biological gradient

- no consistent data to support higher levels of bacterial load correlate with PUD

Biological plausibility: numerous plausible pathophysiological alterations (see text) that include:

- *vacA* causing epithelial cell damage – not consistent
- *cagA* associations with disease states such as DU, gastric cancer and MALTomas – not consistent or universally seen
- elevated gastrin and acid secretion that revert to normal after *H. pylori* eradication
- numerous alterations in mucosal cytokines
- *thus, data are supportive*

Effects of interventions: outcomes following *H. pylori* eradication. Alterations in natural history of PUD disease with *H. pylori* eradication provide the strongest evidence that *H. pylori* is a true pathogen. Randomized controlled trials' data of *H. pylori* eradication shows:

- DU and GU relapse effectively prevented
- DU heal with eradication of *H. pylori* infection alone without ulcer healing drugs
- DU heal faster when *H. pylori* eradicated than with ulcer healing drugs alone
- DU refractory to ulcer healing drugs can heal if *H. pylori* eradicated
- Re-bleeding from ulcers can be prevented
- *thus, data are strongly supportive*

Coherence of *H. pylori* data with previous epidemiological data

- consistent historical correlations between presumed *H. pylori* prevalence, ulcer disease prevalence, death rates and perforations from ulcer disease
- improvements in hygiene and sanitation in industrialized nations have resulted in declining prevalence of both *H. pylori* and ulcer disease
- prevalence of *H. pylori* infection and ulcer disease have become the same in males/females
- *thus, data are supportive*

---

why *H. pylori* causes disease in a minority of patients infected with the organism are not yet known. This question remains the subject of intense ongoing research.

Duodenal ulcers not related to *H. pylori* and NSAIDs

The new millennium has seen an increase in *H. pylori* negative duodenal ulcers, perhaps related to successful treatment of *H. pylori*.[11] Quan and Talley[11] concluded that it was difficult to accurately determine the true prevalence of *H. pylori* negative ulcers because of the cross-sectional nature of the studies. Patients could be misclassified as being *H. pylori* negative if there had been recent antibiotic or bismuth use and also if proton pump inhibitor (PPI) use had not been

stopped at least two weeks prior to testing, especially by the urea breath test. Also, as the presence of *H. pylori* in the gastric mucosa could be patchy, mucosal biopsy methods required adequate biopsy sampling and preferably, the use of multiple methods of *H. pylori* determination. Retrospective series suffer from the inability to accurately determine surreptitious NSAID use.

A meta-analysis of seven rigorously designed North American duodenal ulcer studies identified that 20% of patients in these studies had ulcer recurrence within 6 months, despite successful cure of infection and no reported use of NSAIDs.[11] In a review of similar studies, Ciociola *et al.*[13] estimated that the prevalence of *H. pylori* and NSAID negative duodenal ulcers was 22%. One American study identified *H. pylori* infection in only 62% of duodenal ulcer and 44% of gastric ulcer patients.[14] No reason for these low *H. pylori* prevalence rates was offered. There may be ethnic differences in the proportion of ulcers related to *H. pylori*. For example in Japan, the *H. pylori* negative peptic ulcer prevalence appears to be less than 5%.[11] Despite these reports that 20% or more are non-*H. pylori*, non-NSAID ulcers, a report from Italy suggested that of their patients, after careful review of *H. pylori* status, NSAID ingestion and recent antibiotic use, only 0·8% (6/774) could be truly considered idiopathic.[15]

In an interesting, prospective population survey of 2416 Danish subjects that assessed risk factors for peptic ulcer disease, the *H. pylori* negative duodenal ulcer prevalence was 13%.[16] The causes of these ulcers could not be adequately ascertained as there were so few ulcers but there were suggestions that smoking, minor tranquilizer use and tea consumption were possibly related.

Most duodenal ulcer recurrences after eradication of *H. pylori* are related to NSAIDs[17] and the role of pentagastrin-stimulated peak acid output is unclear.[18,19] Smoking has been implicated as an important additional risk factor to *H. pylori* and NSAIDs.[20]

Gastric ulcer

There are fewer studies on the role of *H. pylori* in gastric ulcer and NSAIDs play an important role in its etiology. *H. pylori* infection is diagnosed in 60–100% of gastric ulcer patients (mean about 70%).[9,21] As Thijs *et al.* point out,[16,21] many of the earlier studies suffered methodological problems that probably led to an underestimate of the prevalence of *H. pylori* in gastric ulcer disease. Most gastric ulcers are associated with *H. pylori*-related active chronic gastritis whether or not NSAIDs are involved.[21–23] However, up to 11% may have no identifiable cause.[22] The study by Nomura *et al.*[7] also showed that prior infection with *H. pylori* increased the risk that the patient may develop gastric ulcer subsequently.

Other newer drugs such as bisphosphonates [24,25] have been found to cause gastric ulcers and there may be a synergistic effect with naprosyn.[26] Potassium supplements and chemotherapeutic drugs such as floxuridine have also been identified as causative agents.[11]

Thus, *H. pylori* remains an important cause of duodenal and gastric ulcers.[27] *H. pylori* negative ulcers are commonly caused by NSAIDs.[21] Furthermore, the proportion of *H. pylori* negative ulcers increases as the overall prevalence of *H. pylori* infection falls.[14,28]

Temporal relationship

Whether *H. pylori* infection precedes the development of ulcer disease cannot be assessed by retrospective, point prevalence studies, since it is impossible to assess retrospectively when these patients were infected.[5]

Marshall [29] described three "self-administration" experiments in humans. In these cases active chronic gastritis ensued, fulfilling one of Koch's postulates for at least the first step in the development of peptic ulceration, although actual ulcer disease did not develop.

The temporal relationship between infection with *H. pylori* and the development of duodenal ulcer has been best proved in a cohort study reported by Sipponen *et al.*[8] Of the 321 patients with *H. pylori* at study entry, 34 developed a duodenal ulcer over the next 10 years while only one of 133 *H. pylori* negative patients developed an ulcer.

An IgG serological nested case–control study of a group of 5443 Japanese-American men with stored sera obtained between 1967 to 1970 demonstrated that pre-existing *H. pylori* infection increased the subsequent risk of developing either duodenal or gastric ulcer disease over a surveillance period of greater than 20 years.[7] The odds ratio (OR) for development of ulcer was 4.0 (95% CI 1·1 to 14.2) for duodenal ulcer and 3·2 (1·6 to 6·5) for gastric ulcer. The relationship was statistically significant even when the ulcer diagnosis was first made 10 or more years after the serum sample had been obtained. A further analysis of this Hawaiian cohort[30] identified that *H. pylori* infected men of higher birth order had an increased risk of gastric (OR 1·64) but not duodenal ulcer. Those *H. pylori* infected men from larger sibships (OR 2·06) and higher birth order (OR 1·67) were at increased risk of developing gastric cancer. These data are consistent with the hypothesis that early infection with *H. pylori* increases the risk of developing gastric ulcer and cancer.

Biological gradient

Showing a higher bacterial load in the stomach of patients with ulcers versus those without an ulcer would be good evidence supporting a causative role.[4] In biopsy studies, there has been insufficient gastric mucosal sampling to assess whether there was a biologic gradient present.[5] It is problematic to rely on biopsy specimens due to sampling error. A test such as a urea breath test (UBT) may be more useful in this regard. Ingested urea is digested by bacterial urease activity with the labeled CO_2 breakdown product being excreted in the breath. Significant correlation has been observed between labeled CO_2 excretion in the breath and intragastric bacterial load [31,32] and mucosal inflammation.[31–33] However, there has not been consistent correlation with endoscopic findings.[31] Most of the available literature did not find a correlation between endoscopic findings and higher urea breath test values, and authors did not report whether the finding of higher test results predicted the finding of a duodenal ulcer.[34–36] Thus, data supporting a relationship between a higher load of *H. pylori* and ulcer development are limited.

Biological plausibility

H. pylori is an unique bacterium that has evolved ecologically to survive and persist in the harsh acidic environment of the stomach. Bacterial urease, flagellar motility and surface adhesins appear necessary for colonization.[37] Despite the high prevalence of infection, not all infected persons develop disease, and most remain asymptomatic. Are there more virulent strains that predispose to disease states? The vacuolating cytotoxin (*vacA*) which causes surface epithelial cell damage and vacuolation of epithelial cells, has not been found consistently to correlate with disease states.[37] The *cagA* protein is a marker of the *cag* pathogenicity island of *H. pylori* and several studies have determined that in developed countries, duodenal ulcers, intestinal metaplasia, gastric carcinoma and mucosa-associated lymphoid tissue (MALT) lymphoma are more commonly seen in patients infected with a *cagA* positive strains.[37] However, this relationship is not universally seen in patients of all ethnic origins.

If *H. pylori* is primarily an *intragastric* infection, how does it cause ulcers in the duodenal bulb? Observations prior to and after the discovery of *H. pylori* identified that patients with duodenal ulcers had gastric metaplasia in the duodenal bulb.[38–43] This change is thought to arise as a result of hypersecretion of acid as observed in duodenal ulcer patients. The gastric metaplasia may [44–46] or may not[47] improve after *H. pylori* eradication. Patients infected with *H. pylori* have increased basal and stimulated gastrin release irrespective of whether they have duodenal ulcer disease or not.[48–50] The elevated gastric acid secretion also results in increased postprandial duodenal acid load.[51] Furthermore, *H. pylori* eradication[52,53] or suppression[54] results in normalization of these gastrin levels in most subjects, with lowering of acid secretion.[48,52] However, a subset of patients with recurrent duodenal ulcer have persistently high acid secretion despite *H. pylori* eradication.[55] *H. pylori* can colonize islands of gastric metaplasia in the duodenum. Numerous toxigenic factors have been identified by which *H. pylori* might cause mucosal damage, although there is no one pathophysiological factor accepted as being pathognomonic. Adhesion of *H. pylori* to epithelial cells results in elevated levels of mucosal cytokines such as interleukin (IL)-8 which is increased in the mucosa of *H. pylori* infected patients.[56] *CagA* positive strains have higher levels of tumor necrosis factor (TNF)-α, IL-1β, IL-6, IL-8 and are associated with more severe inflammation (active chronic gastritis) in the gastric mucosa.[57] This T-helper subtype 1 (Th1) proinflammatory cytokine response may predominate in ulcer disease whereas a mixed Th1/Th2 pattern predominates in those with chronic gastritis but no ulcer.[58] There may be a link between increased IL-8 and gastrin release that is potentiated by *H. pylori* sonicates.[59] Thus, there are plausible multifactorial mechanisms by which *H. pylori* may cause pathogenic effects.

Effects of interventions: outcomes following *H. pylori* eradication

In the days before recognition of *H. pylori*, ulcers could be healed but inevitably relapsed over the next year.[60–65] The most clinically relevant evidence for the role of *H. pylori* comes from intervention trials in which *H. pylori* was eradicated and recurrence of ulcer disease prevented.[66]

The first reported randomized trial in 1987[67] showed that the risk of recurrent duodenal ulcer could be reduced to virtually zero when *H. pylori* eradication therapy was given. In 1988, Marshall *et al.*[68] reported a randomized double blind trial in duodenal ulcer patients in which more ulcers healed and fewer ulcers recurred over 12 months with *H. pylori* eradication therapy. Other important early contributions supported these observations.[69–73] Alc

Reviews of studies from 1987 to 1994 agree that the recurrence rate for duodenal ulcer at 1 year ranges from 0 to 9% when *H. pylori* infection is successfully eradicated.[21,74,75] There are fewer data on ulcer recurrence after periods longer than 1 year after *H. pylori* eradication, but reported recurrence rates range from 0 to 18%.[75] Labenz and Börsch reported that at 1 year, infection with *H. pylori* and duodenal ulcer recurred in 2·4% and 0·8 % of treated patients, respectively.[76] Longer follow up showed no further *H. pylori* or ulcer recurrence at 3 and 4 years.[76] Another study reported that 92% of patients remained free of *H. pylori* after 7 years of follow up while those who were *H. pylori* positive remained persistently positive.[77] B4 In 15 randomized trials in which *H. pylori* eradication was compared with no eradication, the ulcer recurrence rate was 7% in patients in whom *H. pylori* was eradicated versus 67% in those who remained infected.[75] A systematic review[78] has shown that the median 12-month duodenal ulcer recurrence rate is 67% if *H. pylori* infection persists but is reduced to 6% if *H. pylori* is eradicated. Ala Comparable results for gastric ulcer recurrence are 59% and 4%, respectively. A more recent meta-analysis examined studies that directly compared gastric and duodenal ulcers and identified that for duodenal ulcer the 1-year ulcer recurrence rate was 2% and for gastric ulcer 3% if *H. pylori* was eradicated but if the infection persisted, the ulcer relapse rate was 42% for duodenal ulcer and 39% for gastric ulcer.[79] Ala Thus, regardless of whether the patient suffers from duodenal ulcer or gastric ulcer, successful eradication results in cure for most patients.

Other strongly supportive data include the observations that duodenal ulcer healed without ulcer healing drugs if *H. pylori* was eradicated and that the rate of healing was faster with *H. pylori* eradication. Eradication of *H. pylori* has been shown to prevent re-bleeding from ulcers as well. These important data will be expanded in the sections below.

Coherence of the data with earlier epidemiological information

The presumed prevalence of *H. pylori* infection parallels data showing that there was a peak in ulcer disease at the end of the nineteenth century.[4] This is consistent with epidemiological data that show that the death rate of duodenal ulcer patients was highest in those born around 1890.[80] The highest risk for ulcer perforation risks was identified in a cohort of men born between 1900 and 1920.[81] This is also the generation with the highest *H. pylori* prevalence in an *H. pylori* seropositivity study carried out in the UK.[82] This relationship is consistent with the hypothesis that *H. pylori* plays an important role in ulcer complications.

Improvements in hygiene and sanitation are associated with a declining risk of infection, as is the case today in industrialized nations compared with less developed countries which still endure a poor socioeconomic status. The number of admissions for ulcer disease has steadily declined since the middle of the twentieth century which infers a declining severity and prevalence of duodenal ulcer.[83] This decline parallels a declining prevalence of *H. pylori* infection.

While duodenal ulcer disease has long been thought to be a disease of men, data since 1979 have shown that the prevalence of duodenal ulcer and the death rate for men and women have become similar.[84] This is consistent with the prevalence of *H. pylori* infection which is the same in both sexes.[85]

Treatment of duodenal ulcer

Healing of duodenal ulcer with acid suppressive therapy

A meta-analysis[86] has shown a close linear relationship between the degree of suppression of intragastric acidity and duodenal ulcer healing. A more complex meta-analysis of this relationship between the duration of acid suppression and healing led to the definition of three primary determinants of the benefits of anti-secretory drugs: (i) the degree of suppression of acidity; (ii) the duration of suppression of acidity over the 24-hour period; and (iii) the duration of the treatment.[87] For duodenal ulcer, the duration of time the intragastric acidity can be maintained at or above pH 3·0 is the most important factor. This model identified that maintaining intragastric pH at or above the threshold pH of 3·0 for 18–20 hours of the day predicts a 100% healing of duodenal ulcer.[87] Lesser degrees of acid suppression were found to prolong the duration of time needed to achieve optimal healing. Thus, these models of degree of acid suppression help explain the results of controlled trials of agents for healing ulcers.

Treatment of duodenal ulcer in the pre-*H. pylori* era was revolutionized by H_2-receptor antagonists (H_2-RAs), and subsequently, PPIs whose effects were proved in placebo-controlled trials. Numerous methodologically sound, double blind, randomized controlled trials using comparative healing rates of endoscopically proven ulcers as the outcome measure, have established that PPIs heal ulcers faster than H_2-blockers and also provide more rapid symptom relief.[61,88–93] In the chapter in the first edition of this textbook,[94] a summary of the results of 21 such randomized controlled trials[60–62,88–93,95–106] was presented. Since that time, additional new studies with similar results have been added to the literature.[14,107–112] Ala

There is no proved difference in ulcer healing rates and safety between different PPIs.[109,113,114] There are direct comparative trials of lansoprazole versus omeprazole,[107,108] pantoprazole versus omeprazole[109] and rabeprazole versus omeprazole[110] which showed equivalent duodenal ulcer healing. Alc

Maintenance therapy for prevention of recurrence of duodenal ulcer

Although ulcers were healed effectively by acid suppressive therapy, ulcer recurrence was almost inevitable with about 80% recurrence at 1 year once treatment was stopped.[60–65] Thus, in an effort to prevent recurrent ulcers, patients were given maintenance therapy with H_2-RAs. In a large ($n = 399$) 2-year maintenance study of ranitidine 150 mg daily versus placebo, ulcer symptoms remained controlled in only about half the patients but ulcer recurrence was prevented in 83% of patients.[115] This study also identified significantly ($P < 0·002$) more complications such as bleeding in the placebo arm. Ala After a long-term follow up of 464 patients on maintenance ranitidine, 81% remained free of symptomatic duodenal ulcer recurrence over 9 years.[64] A 1-year relapse rate of between 20% and 30% has been identified consistently through meta-analyses[116,117] and reviews.[63] Most of the maintenance studies used suboptimal half doses of the H_2-RAs, and full ulcer healing doses were more effective in preventing relapse.[63,118,119] Alc Ulcers treated with tripotassium dicitrato bismuthate appeared to prolong remission beyond that seen with H_2-RAs. It has since been suggested that this effect is, in part, due to the suppressive effects of bismuth on *H. pylori* infection and its ability as a single agent to eradicate *H. pylori* in around 20% of patients.[120]

For duodenal ulcers resistant to healing with H_2RAs, lansoprazole was more effective than placebo in maintaining healing over 1 year when used in doses of 15 mg (70% remission) or 30 mg (85% remission).[121] Ald The sample size was inadequate to determine whether the larger dose was more effective.

Influence of *H. pylori* eradication on healing of duodenal ulcer

The interval between *H. pylori* eradication therapy and reassessment may influence ulcer healing data. In a cohort study of patients given *H. pylori* eradication therapy it was observed that at 1 month, 22/212 (10·4%) had persistent duodenal ulcer. These patients were followed for another 2 months without additional ulcer healing treatment, and ultimately only three ulcers remained unhealed for a total healing success rate of 98·1%.[122]

Furthermore, duodenal ulcers heal faster when *H. pylori* infection is eradicated than with acid suppressive therapy alone using either H_2-RAs[68,71,73] or omeprazole.[123] Ulcers refractory to healing with conventional acid suppressive therapy may heal with *H. pylori* eradication therapy[69,124–127] Alc and remain healed over a 4-year follow up period.[76] B4 In the pre-*H. pylori* era, it was shown that ulcers could be healed with antibiotics alone.[128–130] Similar results have been shown in subsequent studies that aimed to heal ulcers with anti-*H. pylori* antibiotic treatment alone without the need for additional ulcer healing drugs.[131–135] These findings further emphasize the important role of *H. pylori* as a bacterial pathogen.

Acid suppressive therapy need not be continued beyond the duration of eradication treatment

There is good evidence[132,136–139] that uncomplicated, active duodenal ulcers heal without the need to continue ulcer healing drugs beyond the duration of eradication therapy. Alc

There are several methodologically sound trials in which patients all received the same eradication therapy and were randomized to either placebo or an ulcer healing drug for a further 2–3 weeks to test the hypothesis that continued ulcer healing drugs were not required after the eradication period.[137,140–144] In all these studies, the ulcer healing proportions at 4 weeks were the same regardless of whether an antisecretory drug was continued or not. In one study, the trend towards ulcer healing at 2 weeks was higher in patients who continued antisecretory therapy (continued therapy 91%, placebo 76%; $P = 0.14$) but at four weeks all ulcers had healed in both treatment groups.[137] In another study, by 3 weeks the healing rates were 89% in the continued omeprazole arm and 81% in the placebo arm and by 8 weeks, the healing rates were the same.[142]

Duodenal ulcer complications and effects of *H. pylori*

Gastroduodenal ulcer disease causes serious complications such as bleeding in 15–20%, perforation in about 5% and obstruction in up to 2% of affected patients.[145]

Bleeding

A natural history study of duodenal ulcer before the *H. pylori* era provided interesting data from 2119 patients.[146] Of these patients, 13·5% presented with hemorrhage as the first indication of ulcer disease. The overall mortality was 4·5% in those patients who bled and only 1% in those without bleeding. Most deaths not due to bleeding were due to perforation. The rebleeding rate was 13% overall versus 2% for patients who continued on therapy with an H_2-RA. B4

As the rate of recurrent bleeding in the past was high, strategies for prevention of rebleeding were necessary. Two randomized placebo-controlled trials have evaluated a maintenance dose of ranitidine 150 mg. One trial did not show that ranitidine reduced rebleeding. However, the study lacked statistical power.[147] The other trial[148] showed a significantly reduced risk of rebleeding, (ranitidine 9%, placebo 36%; absolute risk reduction (ARR) 27%, number needed to treat (NNT) 4). Ald However, the maintenance H_2-blocker arm still carried a rebleeding risk of nearly 10% and half the episodes were asymptomatic. The risk of rebleeding did not diminish over time, as those patients on placebo were at continuous risk of rebleeding over the 3-year follow up period.

The prevalence of *H. pylori* infection in bleeding duodenal ulcers appears to be lower than in non-bleeding ulcers.[149,150] For bleeding gastric ulcers, 10% of patients were neither infected with *H. pylori* nor taking NSAIDs.[145]

Currently, it is accepted that eradication of *H. pylori* leads to a reduction in ulcer recurrence and hence prevents recurrent bleeding. In observational and cohort studies, patients with *H. pylori* eradication had a rebleeding rate of less than 3·5% per year, while those with persistent *H. pylori* infection exhibited re-bleeding rates of 50% at 1 year[151] and 82% at 4 years.[152] There was also evidence from randomized placebo-controlled trials that eradication of *H. pylori* prevented the risk of recurrent duodenal ulcer bleeding. In patients with a bleeding duodenal ulcer and persistent *H. pylori* infection, the rate of ulcer rebleeding ranged from 7% to 37% per year. However, if *H. pylori* was eradicated, the rebleeding risk was very low (Table 5.1). Alc The trial reported by Lai *et al.*[150] did not show a significant reduction of rebleeding when the data were analyzed according to the study arm, perhaps because therapeutic endocopy was carried out in all patients. However, only 5% of the patients who were *H. pylori* negative post-treatment had rebleeding, compared with 29% of patients who remained *H. pylori* positive ($P = 0.003$). In the recent study reported by Arkkila *et al.*[153] 223 patients were randomized to receive eradication therapy in the form of quadruple therapy ($n = 88$) or dual therapy ($n = 88$) or to omeprazole only ($n = 47$). The authors presented the rebleeding data over the 1-year follow up according to whether the patient was *H. pylori* positive or negative after acute treatment and not according to the initial

Table 5.1 Summary of *Helicobacter pylori* eradication and ulcer bleeding recurrence rates

Bleeding ulcer recurrence rate (%) after *H. pylori* eradication *v* no maintenance therapy

Reference	*H. pylori* eradication	No therapy	Follow up (months)	*P* value	ARR (%)	NNT
Open/cohort studies						
Jaspersen *et al.*[151]	3·4 (*n*=29)	50 (*n*=4)[a]	12	–	47 ·	2
Macri *et al.*[152]	0 (*n*=21)	81·8 (*n*=11)[b]	48	<0·002	82	1
Randomized controlled trials						
Graham *et al.*[154]	0 (*n*=17)	28·6 (*n*=14)	12	0·031	29	3
Jaspersen *et al.*[158]	0 (*n*=29)	27·3 (*n*=22)	12	<0·01	27	3
Labenz *et al.*[159]	0 (*n*=42)	37·5 (*n*=24)	12	0·01	38	3
Rokkas *et al.*[160]	0 (*n*=16)	33 (*n*=15)	12	0·018	33	3
Lai *et al.*[150]	10 (*n*=60)	20 (*n*=60)	60	0·2	10	10
Arkkila *et al.*[153]	1 (*n*=167)[c]	7 (*n*=43)[c]	12	0·03	6	17

Bleeding ulcer recurrence rate after *H. pylori* eradication *v* ranitidine maintenance therapy

Reference	*H. pylori* eradication	Ranitidine maintenance[d]	Follow up (months)	*P* value
Non-randomized controlled trial				
Santander *et al.*[155]	2·3 (*n*=84)[e]	12·1 (*n*=41)	12	<0·001
Randomized controlled trials				
Riemann *et al.*[156]	4·2 (*n*=47)[f]	8·3 (*n*=48)	24	0·29
Sung *et al.*[157]	0 (*n*=97)	3·0 (*n*=99)	12	0·08

[a]Open study with one rebleed after successful eradication and 50% rebleeding with persistent infection.
[b]Cohort study of patients given eradication therapy, then *H. pylori* positive and negative followed for 48 months.
[c]Three arm study, two different eradication arms *v* omeprazole, rebleeding data given only for whether *H. pylori* negative or positive at study end.
[d]Maintenance therapy with ranitidine 150 mg daily.
[e]These two patients who rebled were reinfected with *H. pylori.*
[f]Both patients that rebled were *H. pylori* negative but were on NSAIDs.
ARR, absolute risk reduction; NNT, number needed to treat

arm of randomization. Ala Thus in Table 5.1, the data under "*H. pylori* eradication" corresponds to those that were *H. pylori* negative after treatment and the 'no therapy' arm to those who were still *H. pylori* positive. The overall rebleeding rate in this study was lower than in the other studies.

A Cochrane review of this topic has recently been published.[161] In this meta-analysis the mean percentage of rebleeding in the *H. pylori* eradication group was 4·5% and in the non-eradication group without subsequent long-term maintenance antisecretory therapy 23·7% (odds ratio (OR) 0·18, 95% CI 0·09 to 0·37). Ala

There are three controlled trials that compared *H. pylori* eradication with maintenance acid suppressive therapy. In one of these the allocation of patients to the two interventions was not randomized[155]; the other two were randomized trials.[156,157] Although these trials were generally better designed than the placebo-controlled trials, and included larger numbers of patients, the rebleeding rates were nevertheless low in all studies, and they did not show

statistically significant differences between the treatment groups. There is the possibility of a type II error. However, all studies agreed that if *H. pylori* infection was eradicated, recurrent bleeding was not seen even without maintenance therapy. The pooled rebleeding rate in the ranitidine arms of the three trials was 5·6%.[155–157] In the Cochrane review of these studies,[161] the mean percentage of rebleeding in the *H. pylori* eradication group was 1·6%, and in the non-eradication group with long-term maintenance antisecretory therapy it was 5·6% (OR 0·25, 95% CI 0·08 to 0·76). Ala

In a study of a somewhat different design, Liu *et al.* investigated the role of different long-term maintenance therapies after healing of bleeding ulcers and successful *H. pylori* eradication.[162] Patients were assigned to 16-week maintenance treatment with: (i) 15 ml antacid four times daily; (ii) colloidal bismuth subcitrate 300 mg four times daily; (iii) famotidine 20 mg twice daily; or (iv) placebo twice daily. During the mean follow up of 56 months, there was no ulcer recurrence and no *H. pylori* reinfection. Thus, after

H. pylori eradication is achieved, there is no need for any maintenance therapy.

All studies agree that *H. pylori* eradication significantly reduces the rebleeding rate and hence *H. pylori* should be looked for and eradicated if identified.

Perforation

There are few data available concerning the role of *H. pylori* infection in other complications such as ulcer perforation. A controlled trial involving 60 patients undergoing simple closure of perforated duodenal ulcer demonstrated a significant ($P < 0.05$) benefit for decreasing complications of peptic ulcer disease with postoperative cimetidine treatment.[163] Ald This study did not consider the role of *H. pylori* infection. NSAID use increases the risk of ulcer perforation by a factor of 5 to 8.[164] Separate relative risks for duodenal and gastric ulcers are not known. In 80 patients presenting with acute perforated duodenal ulcer, the prevalence of *H. pylori* infection by serology was only about 50%, approximately equal to that in a control group, and NSAIDs were frequently the cause of the perforation.[165] More recent studies using biopsy-based methods of *H. pylori* detection have shown a higher *H. pylori* prevalence of 73%[166,167] to 80% or more in perforated duodenal ulcer patients.[168-170]

A case series of *H. pylori* positive patients with perforated peptic ulcer demonstrated that after *H. pylori* eradication, there was no need for re-operation and no mortality after a median 44 month follow up.[167] Ald

There are two randomized trials of *H. pylori* eradication in patients with perforated peptic ulcer.[166,171] In a Hong Kong study, patients with perforated duodenal ulcer were initially treated with simple closure.[171] The prevalence of *H. pylori* was 81% and these 99 patients were randomized to receive eradication therapy or 4 weeks of PPI alone. After 1 year, the rate of ulcer relapse was 38% in patients treated with omeprazole alone and 5% in those who received anti-*Helicobacter* therapy.[171] Ald Kate *et al.* followed 202 patients for 2 years after simple closure of a perforated duodenal ulcer and also retrospectively reviewed the records of 60 patients.[166] In the prospective study, patients were randomized to receive ranitidine alone or ranitidine quadruple eradication therapy. In patients in whom *H. pylori* was eradicated, the risk of recurrent ulcer was between 4% and 28% and the authors did not report any subsequent perforations. Alc Thus, there is now good evidence to recommend the use of *H. pylori* eradication in infected patients with a perforated ulcer. Alc

Obstruction

The prevalence of this complication may be as low as 0.5%, and the strength of evidence for this rare complication is restricted to case reports[172,173] and observational studies.[174,175] The prevalence of *H. pylori* in patients with pyloric obstruction ranges from 45% to 90%,[176] with a mean value of 69% reported in one review.[176] Gastric outlet obstruction seems to improve following *H. pylori* eradication in most reports,[172,173,174] B4 and in combination with balloon dilatation of the pylorus in some reports.[174]

Treatment of gastric ulcer

Healing of gastric ulcer with acid suppressive therapy

Gastric ulcer healing rates with H_2-RAs in the pre-*H. pylori* era were 3–43% at 2 weeks, 54–70% at 4 weeks, 82–92% at 8 weeks and 89–94% at 12 weeks.[177] Thus gastric ulcer take 4–8 weeks longer to heal than duodenal ulcer. There are no important differences in healing rates between various H_2-RAs. However, PPIs have been shown to produce higher healing rates than H_2-RAs in several randomized trials.[177-180] An early meta-analysis[177] demonstrated that the most important determinant of healing was duration of treatment. A later meta-analysis, comparing omeprazole and ranitidine in healing gastric ulcers demonstrated more rapid and complete healing with more potent acid suppression.[178] Alc Another meta-analysis in which the rates of gastric ulcer healing were expressed as ulcers healed per week, showed that PPI (represented by omeprazole) healed gastric ulcers 24% faster than other agents.[181] Alc A more recent update suggested that rabeprazole, pantoprazole or lansoprazole showed better improvement in the clinical symptoms when compared with omeprazole.[182] Alc However, healing of gastric ulcer with pantoprazole[183] and rabeprazole[184] was comparable to that with omeprazole.

Maintenance therapy for prevention of recurrence of gastric ulcer

Maintenance therapy with H_2-RAs (cimetidine, ranitidine, famotidine, nizatidine) in half standard dose at night, has been shown to reduce the risk of symptomatic recurrence in 1 year to 6.7–36% compared with a rate of 49–76% without therapy.[63] A PPI (omeprazole, lansoprazole, pantoprazole) in standard dose once daily reduced the recurrence of gastric ulcer to only 4.5% over 6 months.[185]

A randomized trial demonstrated that lansoprazole in doses of 15 mg and 30 mg prevented recurrence of healed gastric ulcer in 83% and 93% of patients over a 12-month period ($P < 0.001$).[186] Alc

Effect of *H. pylori* eradication on healing and recurrence of gastric ulcer

Eradication of *H. pylori* speeds gastric ulcer healing in 6 weeks to 84.9% compared with a rate of 60% in patients with persistent *H. pylori* infection ($P = 0.0148$).[187] A larger more recent study has shown that almost all gastric ulcers can be healed if *H. pylori* is eradicated compared with 60–70% healing if the infection persists.[188]

Eradication of *H. pylori* infection has been shown in randomized controlled trials to reduce the recurrence rate of gastric ulcers, although there are fewer available data than is the case for duodenal ulcer.[21,72,75,189–193] Alc Two studies are particularly noteworthy in which gastric ulcers were healed by *H. pylori* eradication therapy alone, without the continued administration of an antisecretory drug for ulcer healing.[191,194] *H. pylori* eradication almost eliminates gastric ulcer recurrence, while persistently infected patients have a relapse rate of about 50%.[74,75] Alc Labenz and Börsch reported that at 1 year, *H. pylori* recurred in 3·4% of patients, while gastric ulcer recurrence was not observed.[76] Longer follow up showed no additional *H. pylori* infection or ulcer recurrence at 3 and 4 years.[76] B4

H. pylori eradication therapy

Antibiotic regimens

The evolution of *H. pylori* eradication treatment has been rapid. It was determined early on that this infection was easy to suppress but difficult to cure. Thus, if the patient were tested too early following completion of a course of an eradication treatment, the organism would be "cleared" but be falsely identified as having been eradicated. A time interval of at least 4 weeks after the end of eradication treatment was identified as the minimum necessary to define eradication.[120,195]

The first meta-analysis of *H. pylori* eradication regimens[120] established that single antimicrobial agents were insufficient to eradicate *H. pylori*. A later review identified clarithromycin as a drug that can eradicate *H. pylori* infection in up to 54% of patients when given alone. However, resistance can rapidly develop, and its use as a single agent is not recommended.[196] Combinations of two antimicrobials were found to result in improved eradication rates but the best regimens were "bismuth triple therapies".[120] The best regimen in 1992 was triple therapy with bismuth, metronidazole and tetracycline (BMT) which was superior to triple therapy with bismuth, metronidazole and amoxicillin.[75,120,197] However, this combination was felt to be too cumbersome, and more "user friendly" PPI-based therapies emerged.

Because the literature is extensive, background materials and reviews will be summarized and only very recent data about effects of new therapies and treatment of eradication failures will be discussed.

Proton pump inhibitor-based combination therapies

The PPIs are potent acid suppressing agents that effectively heal duodenal and gastric ulcers and provide prompt symptom relief. They may have a synergistic effect with antimicrobials by providing an optimal intragastric pH milieu.[198,199] They also have some direct suppressive effects on *H. pylori*.[200] Thus, there is good rationale to use these agents as part of an *H. pylori* eradication regimen.

PPI dual therapy

PPI plus amoxicillin A dual therapy with omeprazole and amoxicillin enjoyed a brief period of popularity. Overall efficacy in several reviews and meta-analyses was of the order of 60% and results were not consistent. Therefore this regimen was not recommended as standard therapy.[75,196,197,201–204] Alc However, one potential advantage with an amoxicillin regimen is that *H.pylori* rarely becomes resistant to amoxicillin. Thus, this dual regimen could be administered more than once. Some experts suggest that high doses of PPI with amoxicillin may be effective in treatment failures. This does not appear to be dependent on the presence of CYP-2C19 genetic polymorphisms.[205] Results though are not consistent – in an American study, Malaty *et al.* found that even very high doses of omeprazole (40 mg thrice daily) or lansoprazole (60 mg thrice daily) with amoxicillin 750 mg thrice daily for 14 days was ineffective.[206] Another study comparing omeprazole 20 mg twice daily plus amoxicillin 750 mg thrice daily versus omeprazole 40 mg thrice daily with amoxicillin 750 mg thrice daily for 2 weeks found that the higher doses were not more effective than the standard doses.[207] Present data do not suggest that higher doses of PPI with amoxicillin would be more effective.

Gisbert *et al.* carried out a meta-analysis of rabeprazole-based therapies in *H. pylori* eradication.[208] Results with rabeprazole and amoxicillin were similar to those reported for omeprazole and amoxicillin. Alc

PPI plus clarithromycin With the identification of clarithromycin as the most effective single therapy,[209] Alc it came to be used in dual therapy regimen with omeprazole. This combination gave more consistent and reliable results than omeprazole and amoxicillin dual therapy. However, the eradication rate with this regimen was only about 70%.[197,201,204] Two weeks of therapy with relatively high doses of clarithromycin 500 mg twice daily to thrice daily were required. The increased cost of this regimen detracted from its usefulness.[197] More importantly, the high rate of development of clarithromycin resistance in patients with treatment failure may preclude its re-use as part of an *H. pylori* eradication regimen.[210] Thus, any regimen that uses clarithromycin should have the best possible efficacy for eradication to prevent development of secondary clarithromycin resistance.[210] C5

Other PPI dual therapies

One study used rabeprazole with levofloxacin for either 5, 7 or 10 days and found low eradication rates of 50–70%

while the eradication rate with triple therapy with rabeprazole, amoxicillin and levofloxacin was 90%.[211]

PPI triple therapy

Better eradication rates were achieved with regimens which combined a PPI with two anti-microbials. The first regimen known as the Bazzoli regimen,[212] used omeprazole 20 mg once daily, clarithromycin 250 mg twice daily and tinidazole 500 mg twice daily for 1 week and achieved 100% efficacy. A meta-analysis of relevant trials suggested that this was the most effective therapy.[197] Ala Many subsequent trials using omeprazole, lansoprazole or pantoprazole have demonstrated that the PPI-based triple therapies are consistently superior to dual therapies.[197] Meta-analyses of rabeprazole triple therapies show similar efficacy.[208] Patients in whom treatment failed with omeprazole and amoxicillin dual therapy can be effectively treated with triple combinations of omeprazole, amoxicillin and either metronidazole or clarithromycin with eradication rates of 84–94%.[213] The first large randomized placebo-controlled eradicaton trial was the Metronidazole, Amoxicillin, Clarithromycin, *H. pylori*, 1-week therapy (MACH 1) study.[214] While this study was criticized for having only one test of *H. pylori* eradication after treatment, the regimens identified as being the most effective have stood the test of time and are recommended by most consensus conferences as first-line therapy.[215–218] The most effective 1 week, twice daily regimens in the MACH 1 study were: (i) omeprazole 20 mg, clarithromycin 500 mg and amoxicillin 1 g or (ii) omeprazole 20 mg, clarithromycin 250 mg and metronidazole 400 mg.[218] Ala Studies with similar efficacy for analogous regimens were reported using lansoprazole[219–227] or pantoprazole-based triple therapies.[197,228–231] Ala Laine reviewed triple therapy with esomeprazole, clarithromycin and amoxicillin and identified that a 7-day regimen yielded 86–90% eradication rates in duodenal ulcer patients in studies in Europe and Canada but in the USA, even 10 days appeared to be slightly less successful (77–78%).[231] Alc Thus, overall, esomeprazole triple therapies were considered to have comparable success to other PPI triple therapies.

Rabeprazole-based triple therapies were exhaustively reviewed in a meta-analysis by Gisbert *et al.* and comparable regimens gave similar results.[208] This held true for similar regimens using different PPI in head-to-head comparisons.[208,232] Alc A subsequent head-to-head randomized trial compared rabeprazole or omeprazole with clarithromycin and metronidazole or amoxicillin (RCM, OCM, RCA, OCA – four arms) and found that the choice of PPI did not materially influence the overall eradication rate.[233] Alc Another direct comparative study of rabeprazole or lansoprazole with clarithromycin and amoxicillin found that the rabeprazole triple therapy was significantly more effective (88%) than the lansoprazole (78%) in intention to treat analysis, and the

eradication rate of clarithromycin resistant strains was low for both therapies.[234] Ald

A meta-analysis designed to determine whether there are differences in eradication rates among PPIs in PPI triple therapies [235] yielded the following observations: cure rates were similar for omeprazole and lansoprazole (75% v 76%), omeprazole and rabeprazole (78% v 81%), omeprazole and esomeprazole (88% v 89%), and lansoprazole and rabeprazole (81% v 86%). Ald They concluded that the various PPI had similar effectiveness when used for *H. pylori* eradication in standard triple therapy. Similar results were reported in another systematic review.[236] Another review reported that rabeprazole, omeprazole and lansoprazole triple therapies all gave comparable results.[208]

Most experts recommend that one of the PPI, clarithromycin and amoxicillin (PPI-CA) regimens be used as first-line therapy rather than a PPI, clarithromycin and a nitroimidazole regimen because of the higher prevalence of *H. pylori* imidazole resistance compared with clarithromycin resistance. However, in comprehensive meta-analyses, no difference in efficacy between these two regimens was found.[237,238] Ald Also, one study found that the PPI-CA regimen gave slightly lower eradication with more frequent adverse effects (38%) compared with PPI, clarithromycin and metronidazole (PPI-CM) (20%, $P < 0.05$).[239]

These twice daily, 1-week regimens are well tolerated with few patients discontinuing therapy due to drug intolerance. A meta-analysis did not show any difference in efficacy between a lower dose of clarithromycin (250 mg twice daily) versus the conventional 500 mg twice daily dose in combination with a PPI and metronidazole.[240] Patients treated with the lower dose had only half the incidence of adverse effects.[241] Alc While the smaller dose of clarithromycin may be adequate for many patients, consensus groups have advocated the 500 mg twice daily dose for consistency and to avoid possible confusion and prescribing errors. C5 For PPI-CA combinations, the larger clarithromycin dose of 500 mg twice daily was found to be superior to the 250 mg twice daily dose.[240]

Another triple therapy regimen with PPI, amoxicillin and metronidazole was generally less effective than the PPI, clarithromycin and amoxicillin (PPI-CA) and PPI-CM regimens in head-to-head trials.[188,214,227] Alc

Some declining efficacy In the new millennium, data show that these PPI-based triple therapies are not quite as effective as some years ago. For example a randomized trial in Canada in 2003 compared esomeprazole versus omeprazole with metronidazole and clarithromycin for 7 days and found that eradication rates were now only 76% and 72%, respectively [242] whereas in the 1996 MACH 1 study, the observed eradication rate for the same regimen was 90%.[243] Unfortunately, this study did not assess *H. pylori* antibiotic resistance.

Optimum duration of PPI triple therapy Original recommendations were for a 1-week treatment course. American data suggested that longer 10–14 day therapy was necessary, however a recent study using rabeprazole, amoxicillin and clarithromycin found equivalent eradication rates with 7-day and 10-day treatment regimens.[244] Ald More recently with the apparent decline in treatment success, even the Maastricht 2 consensus guidelines recommend that treatment should be given for *a minimum* of 7 days.[215] In one study that used lansoprazole, clarithromycin and amoxicillin to eradicate *H. pylori* the eradication rate was 75% with 1 week and 86% with 2 weeks of therapy but this difference was not statistically significant.[245] Ald

Calvet *et al.*[246] carried out a meta-analysis of 13 randomized studies that directly compared different durations of treatment to determine the optimal treatment duration for triple therapy. They found that 10–14 day therapies were better than 7-day therapies and when direct comparisons were made in randomized trials 14 days was better than 7 days with a therapeutic gain of 7–9%. Ala Cost effectiveness analysis of the different durations of treatment was carried out in relation to two basic strategies: UBT carried out in all patients post-treatment or UBT carried out only if symptoms relapsed.[247] The costs in Spain (low cost model) and USA (high cost) were estimated. For either follow up strategy, the 7-day regimen had lower costs. In sensitivity analyses, the 10-day regimens would have to be 10–12%, and the 14-day regimen 25–35% more effective than 7-day regimens for the longer duration therapies to become cost effective in Spain. For the USA, the corresponding figures were 3–5% and 8–11%, respectively. Thus, even though the longer durations are more effective, in terms of economic evaluation, the shorter duration appear to be more cost effective.

Influence of antibiotic resistance on PPI triple therapies

Nitroimidazole (i.e. metronidazole, tinidazole) A meta-analysis in 1997 of *H. pylori* eradication rates with a variety of regimens in nitroimidazole-resistant and sensitive strains[248] revealed that the efficacy of PPI with nitroimidazole and amoxicillin or clarithromycin, was significantly reduced from 93% in sensitive strains to 69% in resistant strains. A regimen of PPI, nitroimidazole and amoxicillin was less effective (64%) than the corresponding regimen with clarithromycin (76%) for nitroimidazole-resistant stains. Alc For sensitive strains, both regimens were very effective with eradication rates of 92–93% and the duration of therapy did not influence eradication success.

The MACH 2 study, published after this meta-analysis was carried out, carefully evaluated antibiotic resistance and determined that baseline metronidazole resistance reduced the efficacy of the omeprazole, clarithromycin, metronidazole (OCM) triple therapy from 95% to 76%.[249,250] A similar reduction in efficacy of about 15% was reported in a lansoprazole study.[227] Importantly, the MACH 2 study also showed that the addition of omeprazole, with its potent acid suppression helped partially to overcome metronidazole resistance. When baseline metronidazole resistance was present, clarithromycin and metronidazole alone was successful in only 43% of cases, but with the addition of omeprazole the efficacy improved to 76%. For metronidazole-sensitive strains, the eradication rate with the antibiotics alone was 86% and the addition of omeprazole improved the eradication rate only slightly to 95%.[249] Alc In the MACH studies, the dose of metronidazole was 400 mg twice daily, slightly lower than the 500 mg twice daily available in Canada. However, a meta-analysis has shown these two doses are similar in effectiveness.[251] Alc The higher metronidazole dose may be better on theoretical grounds, since higher doses may be more effective against resistant *H. pylori* strains.[252] C5

Amoxicillin allergy is common and a contraindication for the use of the PPI-CA regimen. Since this regimen does not contain metronidazole, there is rationale for using it in patients with suspected or documented metronidazole-resistant strains.[253]

Resistance to clarithromycin There is no doubt that the primary determinant of treatment failure is resistance to clarithromycin (macrolides). Laine *et al.* summarized the data for esomeprazole, amoxicillin and clarithromycin and determined that for clarithromycin-sensitive strains, the eradication rate was 89% but for clarithromycin-resistant *H. pylori*, the eradication rate was much reduced to 45%.[254] After treatment with this triple therapy, clarithromycin resistance developed in 33% (2/6) of patients, compared with 85% (23/27) after treatment with esomeprazole and clarithromycin dual therapy. Even worse eradication success for clarithromycin-resistant strains was reported by Murakami *et al.*[234] In patients treated with rabeprazole or lansoprazole with amoxicillin and clarithromycin, the eradication success for clarithromycin-sensitive strains was 98% and 89%, respectively, but for clarithromycin-resistant strains, the eradication rates were 8·1% and 0%, respectively.[234] Alc Other studies have also shown that PPI triple therapies containing clarithromycin are ineffective in the presence of clarithromycin resistance.[255]

For patients treated with PPI-CA triple therapy, the primary determinant of treatment failure has been found to be clarithromycin resistance with minor if any influence of CPY-2C19 genetic polymorphism.[256,257] For clarithromycin-sensitive strains, the eradication rate was 97% versus 6% (1/16) for resistant strains[256] in one study and in another, the corresponding rates were 86% versus 24%, respectively.[257] Alc

The rate of acquired clarithromycin resistance was found to be 88·9% (8/9) in patients treated with PPI clarithromycin dual therapy while with PPI-CA or PPI-CM triple therapies these rates were 38·7% (12/31) and 90·0% (9/10), respectively (*P* < 0·01).[258] Murakami *et al.* suggested that amoxicillin-containing regimens may help prevent acquired clarithromycin resistance.[258]

Other factors affecting success of eradication

Wermeille *et al.*[259] treated 78 patients with 1 week lansoprazole, clarithromycin, amoxicillin (LCA) and overall eradication success by intention to treat analysis was only 65·4% (95% CI 54.8 to 76·0%). The eradication rate in "good compliers" was 69·6% (95% CI 58·7 to 80·5%). B4 They found that presence of an ulcer, age, sex and smoking habits did not differ significantly between the patients in the eradicated and non-eradicated groups. They concluded that while poor compliance and bacterial resistance were important factors in determining treatment success, these reasons only explained 40% of failures.

Broutet and colleagues reported a retrospective analysis using individual patient data from triple therapy eradication studies carried out prior to 1999 in France in order to identify risk factors for *H. pylori* eradication failure.[260] The key finding was that failure of eradication was more frequent in patients diagnosed with functional dyspepsia than in those with duodenal ulcer (34% *v* 22% failure: *P* < 0·01). This result is consistent with another literature review.[261] B4 However, in another review, for PPI-CA triple therapy, the same eradication rate was seen in peptic ulcer and functional dyspepsia patients.[262] Broutet found that for duodenal ulcer patients, eradication failed more often in smokers and 10-day was more effective than 7-day therapy.[260] Better eradication rates were observed in patients over 60 years of age.

A very comprehensive meta-analysis by Fischbach *et al.* showed differences in success of eradication among patients of different ethnic origins[263] with the highest success observed in patients in northeast Asia. Populations where there was a high prevalence of childhood *H. pylori* infection and with high drug resistance were characterized by lower treatment success.

Proton pump inhibitor is an essential component of triple therapy regimens

There is evidence to support the view that the PPI is a necessary component of triple therapies to achieve optimal eradication rates.[250,264,265] In one such study, all patients were given 1 week clarithromycin 250 mg and tinidazole 500 mg twice daily and were randomized to receive either no omeprazole, omeprazole 20 mg once daily or omeprazole 20 mg twice daily. The eradication rates were higher in the omeprazole groups (omeprazole once daily 88%, twice daily 89%, placebo 64%; ARR for twice daily omeprazole *v* antibiotics alone 0·25, NNT 4).[264] Alc In the omeprazole groups, 33 patients who harbored metronidazole-resistant strains of

H. pylori were cured by the omeprazole regimen, providing further evidence that the addition of the PPI may help overcome metronidazole resistance. Another study treated ulcer patients with once daily clarithromycin 500 mg, tinidazole 1 g and either placebo or lansoprazole 60 mg and found that the antibiotics alone eradicated *H. pylori* in 39% of patients, but the addition of the PPI increased the eradication success to 72%.[135] Laine pooled results from three American studies of duodenal ulcer patients treated with amoxicillin, clarithromycin and either placebo or omeprazole and showed that eradication with antibiotics alone was achieved in 39% of patients, but if omeprazole was added, the eradication rate was improved to 84%.[134] Alc In another study, the cure rate was significantly higher for omeprazole, clarithromycin and amoxicillin (82%) than for clarithromycin and amoxicillin without the PPI (18%) and for omeprazole, clarithromycin and metronidazole the cure rate was 67%, only slightly better than the 59% cure rate observed with clarithromycin and metronidazole alone.[266] This study showed that the impact of the PPI was much more significant in improving the eradication efficiency with clarithromycin and amoxicillin triple therapy.

Proton pump inhibitor twice daily dosing is recommended

A meta-analysis found that the eradication rates with double doses of PPI were 83·9% compared with 77·7% with single doses of PPI (OR 1·51, 95% CI 1·23 to 1·85; *P* < 0·01).[267] Alc An earlier study that compared once daily omeprazole, metronidazole and amoxicillin (35% success), omeprazole, metronidazole and azithromycin (65%) and omeprazole, metronidazole and clarithromycin found that 78% could be eradicated with the last regimen.[268] A more recent trial comparing lansoprazole, clarithromycin and tinidazole either as standard doses twice daily or double doses once daily, found that the once daily dosing was less effective.[135] Thus, there is little evidence to suggest that PPI triple therapy should be given less than twice daily. Alc

Comparison of H₂-receptor antagonists with proton pump inhibitors in triple therapies

Graham *et al.* carried out a meta-analysis of studies that directly compared an H_2-RA with a PPI and two antibiotics.[269] They identified a total of 12 studies with 1415 patients. The pooled estimate of efficacy was similar for the two strategies: (H_2-RAs 78%, PPIs 81%; OR 0·86, 95% CI 0·66 to 1·12). The PPI and H_2-RA appeared to be similarly effective adjuvants for *H. pylori* triple eradication therapy.[269] Ala However, another meta-analysis led to the conclusion that PPI-based triple therapies were more effective than H_2-RA-based regimens.[270] This systematic review included more studies[22] with 2374 patients. The pooled estimate of efficacy was 74% (95%

CI 71 to 76%) for the PPIs and 69% (95% CI 66 to 71%) for the H_2-RA triples (OR 1·31, 95% CI 1·09 to 1·58). With these data, it seems reasonable to continue using the PPIs rather than H_2-RAs as the antisecretory drugs in combination regimens. A1a

Triple and quadruple bismuth-based therapies

In the first meta-analysis published in 1992, triple therapy with BMT was more effective than triple therapy with bismuth, metronidazole and amoxicillin.[75,120,197] A1c However, the large number of pills required and relatively long 2-week duration of treatment affected compliance adversely. Poor compliance (< 60% of pills) led to only 69% eradication success compared with 96% in patients who take > 60% of pills.[271] Later meta-analyses demonstrated that 1 week of therapy was as effective as 2 weeks.[75,193,204] The greater number of adverse effects suffered with bismuth triple therapies leads to more treatment discontinuation than is observed with PPI triple therapies[193] or PPI-BMT quadruple therapy.[272] In patients who harbor a metronidazole-resistant *H. pylori* infection, eradication efficacy was reduced to 58–64% compared with 86–89% for metronidazole-sensitive strains.[193,248] A1c

PPIs have been used in combination with the traditional bismuth triple therapy. This quadruple regimen resulted in high eradication rates (80–90%) with 1 week of treatment[197,204,273,274] and was superior to bismuth triple therapy without a PPI. A1c There have been studies using omeprazole,[255, 275–278] lansoprazole,[279,280] pantoprazole[272,281–283] and rabeprazole[284,285] as the PPI in these quadruple therapies. Most of the regimens were given four times daily.

PPI-BMT versus PPI-CA

Published studies that have directly compared these regimens are summarized in Table 5.2. A variety of different PPIs have been used, and the trials showed that the PPI-BMT regimens were as effective as the PPI-CA triple therapies.[255,272,277,278,279] A1c There appeared to be no real difference in adverse events with the PPI-BMT quadruple therapy compared with the gold-standard PPI-triples. Also the proportions of patients who discontinued drugs due to adverse effects was very small with both regimens. Thus, PPI-BMT should be considered an alternative first-line therapy.

Attempts to improve compliance

New triple BMT capsule The major drawback of this quadruple regimen is that it generally requires four times daily dosing with at least 18 pills. One recent trial using a three times daily regimen showed that this approach may be efective.[277] Adverse events are generally mild, but frequent enough that they may impair compliance. Most patients can complete the treatment if counseled about possible adverse effects, and treatment discontinuation is infrequent (see Table 5.2).

Recognizing the difficulty of taking so many pills, an unique capsule has been developed that contains bismuth biskalcitrate 140 mg (as 40 mg Bi_2O_3 equivalent), metronidazole 125 mg and tetracycline 125 mg (Helizide; Axcan Pharma, Mont Saint-Hilaire, Quebec, Canada). In an observational study, three of these capsules taken four times daily with omeprazole 20 mg twice daily for 10 days was successful for eradication in 93% of patients by intention to treat analsysis and 97% by per protocol analysis.[286] B4 The eradication rate of metronidazole-resistant and metronidazole-sensitive strains was 93% and 95%, respectively. This capsule was also evaluated in a quadruple therapy regimen and compared with the gold standard PPI-CA triple therapy in a randomized controlled trial; this therapy was well tolerated with an adverse event rate comparable with PPI-CA and eradication results were equal.[255] A1c

Is twice daily dosing with PPI-BMT effective? Another attempt to improve compliance and tolerability has been to use the PPI-BMT regimen twice daily. Earlier pilot studies reported modest eradication rates of 71–78% using 1 week of omeprazole-BMT twice daily[287,288] and 70% with 10 days of lansoprazole-BMT (LBMT).[289] The latter study showed that this LBMT regimen was 90% effective for metronidazole-sensitive strains, and 41% for resistant strains.[289] These three studies all used bismuth subsalicylate as the bismuth compound.

More recently, two Italian studies reported excellent results [290,291] with a regimen consisting of omeprazole 20 mg, tetracycline 500 mg, metronidazole 500 mg and colloidal bismuth subcitrate caplets 240 mg all twice daily with the noontime and evening meals for 14 days. This regimen differs from others described above in the bismuth compound used, the dosing at lunch and supper and the longer 14-day duration. In the first study, in 118 dyspeptic patients of whom 76 were treated for the first time (naive) and 42 had experienced two or more treatment failures (salvage) the regimen was well tolerated, with 95% compliance and 3% dropout due to side effects. The eradication rates were 95% and 98% by intention to treat analysis and per protocol analysis, respectively.[290] A1d There was no difference in the eradication rates between naive and salvage patients. The second study using the same drug regimen included data from the first 42 patients in a total of 71 patients who had failed at least two prior attempts at eradication with a PPI triple regimen.[291] In this study, the eradication rates were 93% and 97% by intention to treat and per protocol analyses.[291] The regimen was well tolerated with trivial adverse effects. B4

A slightly different quadruple therapy was also evaluated in a twice daily regimen.[292] Treatment with omeprazole 20 mg, amoxicillin 1 g, tinidazole 500 mg and bismuth subcitrate

Table 5.2 Randomized controlled trials of PPI-triple v PPI-BMT

Study	Diagnosis	Days	Triple therapy	ITT	PP	Quadruple therapy	ITT	PP	AE (%) Tr, Qu	Discontinuations (%) Tr, Qu
Calvet et al.[277] Spain	Peptic ulcer	7	O 20 mg twice daily A 1 g twice daily C 500 mg twice daily	132/171 (77%)	132/153 (86%)	O 20 mg twice-daily B subcitrate 120 mg thrice daily M 500 mg thrice daily twice day T 500 mg thrice daily	139/168 (83%)	139/157 (89%)	33, 30	NS, NS
Katelaris et al.[272] Australia, NZ[a]	NUD	7	P 40 mg twice daily A 1 g twice daily C 500 mg twice daily	104/134 (78%)	94/114 (82%)	P 40 mg twice daily B subcitrate 108 mg four times daily M 200 mg thrice daily + 400 mg at bed time T 500 mg four times daily	110/134 (82%)	92/105 (88%)	75, 78	2, 3
Laine et al.[255] North America	DU	10	O 20 mg twice daily A 1 g twice daily C 500 mg twice daily	114/137 (83%)	108/124 (87%)	O 20 mg twice daily B biskalcitrate 420 mg four times daily M 375 mg four times daily T 375 mg four times daily	121/138 (88%)	111/120 (92%)	59, 59	0·7, 0
Mantzaris et al.[278] Greece	DU	10	O 20 mg twice dail A 1 g twice daily C 500 mg twice daily	61/78 (78%)	61/69 (88%)	O 20 mg twice daily CBS 120 mg four times daily M 500 mg thrice daily T 500 mg four times daily	46/71 (65%)	46/59 (78%)y	NS, NS[b]	4, 7
Pai et al.[280] India	Peptic ulcer	10	L 30 mg twice daily A 500 mg four times daily C 500 mg twice daily	29/35 (83%)	29/33 (88%)	L 30 mg twice daily CBS 120 mg four times daily M 400 mg thrice daily T 500 mg four times daily	24/33 (73%)	24/28 (86%)	12, 18	0, 6

[a]In this study there was a third arm with bismuth, metronidazole, tetracycline triple therapy for 14 days. ITT eradication rate 69%, PP 74%, significantly lower than PBMT, P<0·01.

[b]The number of side effects not given, but reported that OBMT had higher incidence of side effects than OAC (P<0·01).

ITT, intention to treat; PP, per protocol analysis; NUD, non-ulcer dyspepsia; DU, duodenal ulcer; A, amoxicillin; C, clarithromycin; B, bismuth; CBS, colloidal bismuth subcitrate, M, metronidazole; T, tetracycline; O, omeprazole; P, pantoprazole; L, lansoprazole; AE, adverse event or side effects; NS, not specified; Tr, triple; Qu, quadruple; PPI, proton

240 mg all twice daily (OATinB) for 7 days was slightly less effective than the PPI-ACM regimen described below in the promising regimens section, with observed eradication rates in 43 patients of 84% and 86% by intention to treat and per protocol analysis.

Quadruple (PPI-BMT) therapy is effective even with nitroimidazole resistance PPI-BMT therapy may be effective for treatment failures, and even metronidazole-resistant strains may be successfully eradicated.[255,272,293] In van der Wouden *et al.*'s meta-analysis, the only regimen that was not affected by metronidazole resistance was PPI, bismuth, nitroimidazole and tetracycline for at least 7 days.[248] C4 Adding a PPI is responsible for this effectiveness in metronidazole-resistant strains. In the trial reported by by Katelaris *et al.*,[272] patients were treated with pantoprazole with BMT (PBMT) for 7 days or BMT without a PPI for 14 days. In this trial, the eradication of metronidazole-resistant strains was more frequent with PBMT than with BMT (PBMT 81%, BMT 55%; *P* < 0·02). A1c Futhermore, the drugs were discontinued by 9% of patients receiving the BMT 14-day regimen compared with 3% for the PBMT 7-day regimen.

As clarithromycin resistance significantly reduces the efficacy of clarithromycin-containing triple therapies, it is noteworthy that OBMT eradication rates were not significantly different between clarithromycin-sensitive and resistant strains.[255]

PPI-BMT in treatment failures

Observational studies

Patients in whom triple therapy with PPI, clarithromycin and amoxicillin had failed were treated with pantoprazole 40 mg twice daily, colloidal bismuth sulfate (CBS) 120 mg four times daily, tetracycline 500 mg four times daily, and metronidazole 500 mg thrice daily for 7 days.[281] The *H. pylori* eradication rate was 82% (95% CI 75 to 88%), treatment was well tolerated and major adverse effects were not observed. No differences in eradication success were observed in relation to underlying disease, i.e. whether the patient had peptic ulcer or functional dyspepsia.[281] B4

Patients in whom ranitidine bismuth citrate (RBC)-based regimens had failed were treated with OCA for a week and eradication success was 68%.[294] B4 Those who failed to respond to OCA were given quadruple therapy (omeprazole 20 mg twice daily, bismuth subcitrate 120 mg, tetracycline 500 mg and metronidazole 400 mg four times daily) with 71% (5/7) success. Of those treated previously with clarithromycin containing regimens, OCA was 58% (11/19) successful, while quadruple therapy was 83% (5/6) successful. The numbers of patients are too small to permit definite conclusions, but quadruple therapy appears to be somewhat effective despite repeated failures of clarithromycin-based therapies. B4

Direct comparative trials/systematic reviews (Table 5.3)

The study by Peitz *et al.*[295] compared second-line therapy with OCA and OBMT. While neither regimen was particulary effective, OBMT was superior (68% eradication) to OCA (43%) as second-line therapy. When failures of the second line treatment were treated with the alternative agent, the observed eradication rates were 50% for OBMT and 16% for OCA. Thus, while overall treatment success was only modest, OBMT had limited efficacy.

Two systematic reviews concluded that PPI-BMT was superior to an alternative PPI-based triple therapy for second-line therapy and thus remained the treatment regimen of choice.[296,297] A1c

Ranitidine bismuth citrate regimens

Ranitidine bismuth citrate plus clarithromycin dual therapy

RBC is a new chemical entity, which incorporates bismuth and citrate into the ranitidine molecule and has been specifically developed for *H. pylori* eradication. RBC combination therapies have recently been comprehensively reviewed.[299] When combined with clarithromycin, eradication rates were 55–96% by intention to treat analysis.[299] The optimal dose of clarithromycin was found to be 500 mg twice daily.[299] Although the twice-daily regimen is convenient, the longer 2 week duration of therapy makes this treatment more costly than some others. A randomized trial comparing 1 week and 2 weeks of therapy with RBC did not show a statistically significant difference in effectiveness between these regimens.[300] A1d Bardhan *et al.* treated patients with RBC, clarithromycin and either metronidazole (triple) or placebo (dual therapy) and observed eradication rates of 93% and 84%.[301] In a recent randomized trial 1-week ranitidine bismuth citrate-clarithromycin (RBC-C) eradication was observed in 66% of patients compared to 78% of patients treated with OCA triple therapy.[302] A1d The dual combination of RBC with clarithromycin was not effective against clarithromycin-resistant *H. pylori*.[303]

RBC triple regimens

A triple regimen with RBC, clarithromycin and a nitroimidazole (either metronidazole or tinidazole) and triple therapy with RBC, clarithromycin and amoxicillin were equally effective in 71–94% (mean 82–84%) of patients.[299] One week was as effective as 2 weeks for either treatment.[299] B4 There was a slight trend towards more adverse effects with longer duration of treatment.[304]

Some head-to-head trials of RBC versus PPI triple therapies have also been done, and good results with both regimens have been reported[299,304–311] for both *H. pylori* eradication and ulcer

Table 5.3 PPI-triple v PPI-BMT studies in treatment failures

Study	Failed regimen	Days treated	Triple therapy	ITT	PP	Quadruple therapy	ITT	PP	AE (%) Tr, Qu	Discontinuations (%) Tr, Qu
Peitz et al.[295] Germany	AS, macrolide, nitroimidazole.	7 days	O 40 mg twice daily A 1 g twice daily C 500 mg twice daily	19/44 (43%)	19/38 (50%)	O 20 mg twice daily BSS 600 mg four times daily M 400 mg thrice daily T 500 mg four times daily	27/40 (68%)	27/39 (69%)	66, 45	NS, NS
Magaret et al.[298] USA	PPI triple, LBMT, dual therapy	14 days	L 30 mg twice daily A 1 g twice daily C 500 mg twice daily	15/20 (75%)	– (82%)	L 30 mg twice daily BSS 2 tabs four times daily M 250 mg four times daily T 250 mg four times daily	20/28 (71%)	– (80%)	84, 82	0, 0

AS, acid suppressive drug, either an H_2-RA or PPI; O, omeprazole; L, lansoprazole; A, amoxicillin; C, clarithromycin; BSS, bismuth subsalicylate; M, metronidazole, T, tetracyline, AE, adverse event or side effects, NS, not specified, Tr, triple, Qu, quadruple. For other abbreviations see Table 5.2

healing.[299,304] Two meta-analyses suggested that for RBC or PPI with clarithromycin and amoxicillin the efficacy was comparable, but the RBC triple therapy appeared to be more effective when combined with clarithromycin and a nitroimidazole.[238,312] Alc Randomized trials directly comparing RBC-CM and PPI-CM have shown that the RBC-CM regimen is better,[309,313] particularly for metronidazole resistant strains.[313] Ald

When patients who failed treatment with a PPI, clarithromycin and amoxicillin were treated with RBC, tetracycline and tinidazole for 2 weeks eradication was achieved in 82% of patients.[314] In another study patients who failed first-line treatment with PPI-CA were randomized to receive one of three RBC regimens.[315] RBC, amoxicillin and tinidazole was more effective than RBC, clarithromycin and tinidazole, and RBC, amoxicillin and clarithromycin (eradication rates 81%, 62% and 43%, respectively). Ald

RBC may overcome antibiotic resistance

RBC *in vitro* appears to act synergistically in combination with other antibiotics against metronidazole[316,317] and clarithromycin-resistant *H. pylori* strains.[318] In addition, RBC may decrease the emergence of metronidazole resistance.[316] In clinical trials of RBC, clarithromycin and metronidazole[301,319,320] and RBC, clarithromycin and amoxicillin,[321] baseline metronidazole resistance did not appear to impair treatment efficacy. The impact of metronidazole resistance is less clear for RBC, tetracycline and metronidazole triple therapy. Lower efficacy in the presence of metronidazole resistance was reported in one trial (eradication rate: metronidazole-sensitive 97%, metronidazole-resistant 57%) [321] but not in two other trials from Hong Kong.[320,322] Unfortunately, sales of this drug were low, and it has been withdrawn from almost all markets worldwide. Thus, while an effective drug, it is for practical purposes, unavailable.

New regimens

Numerous new regimens have been explored and are summarized in Table 5.4.

Promising regimens

Furazolidone Furazolidone is an older, inexpensive antibiotic that may be effective in areas of high metronidazole resistance, although it may not be available in all markets. A large scale Chinese trial has shown that when furazolidone 100 mg twice daily was used in triple therapy with omeprazole and amoxicillin, eradication can be achieved in 86% of patients.[323] Ala Two other furazolidone regimens were slightly less effective. RBC in combination with furazolidone 100 mg twice daily and either amoxicillin or tetracycline was also very effective (eradication rates of 82–85%).[324] In Iran where baseline metronidazole resistance is said to be high, a

quadruple regimen of omeprazole, amoxicillin, bismuth subcitrate and furazolidone or clarithromycin also produced high eradication rates of 84% and 85%, respectively.[325] In a study[326] in which relatives of patients with gastric cancer were screened and offered treatment for *H. pylori* if found, the enrolled patients were randomized to receive once daily doses of lansoprazole 30 mg, clarithromycin 500 mg and furazolidone 200 mg or 400 mg for 1 week. The eradication rate observed with the triple therapy regimen that used the 400 mg dose of furazolidone was 87%. Ald This once daily regimen was well-tolerated and relatively inexpensive.

Fluoroquinolones Levofloxacin regimens appear to be promising. The first report by Cammarota *et al.* showed that levofloxacin, amoxicillin and rabeprazole, and levofloxacin, tinidazole and rabeprazole triple therapies were both very effective with observed eradication rates greater than 90%.[327] A subsequent randomized controlled trial confirmed this high rate with levofloxacin, amoxicillin and rabeprazole triple therapy for 1 week.[211] Ald

A fluoroquinolone, moxifloxacin used by itself or with lansoprazole was not effective, but a regimen consisting of lansoprazole 30 mg once daily, clarithromycin 500 mg twice daily and moxifloxacin 400 mg once daily, produced an eradication rate of 90% in an observational study in 40 Italian patients.[328] B4 Further confirmatory data are required.

Sequential therapy Zullo *et al.* carried out a randomized controlled trial in 1049 dyspeptic Italian patients[331] who were randomized to receive either sequential therapy for a total of 10 days, (5 days with rabeprazole 40 mg once daily and amoxicillin 1 g twice daily followed by 5 days with rabeprazole 20 mg, clarithromycin 500 mg and tinidazole 500 mg twice daily) or triple therapy with rabeprazole 20 mg, clarithromycin 500 mg and amoxicillin 1 g twice daily for 1 week. Sequential therapy was more effective than the standard therapy regimen (eradication rates: sequential 92%, standard 74%; $P < 0.0001$). Ala A subsequent study of the same sequential therapy regimen compared two different doses of clarithromycin, 250 mg (low dose) versus 500 mg (high dose). Both doses were very effective with eradication rates of 92–95%.[332] Ala

PPI or RBC with amoxicillin, clarithromycin and metronidazole for 5 days A 5-day regimen of rabeprazole 20 mg, amoxicillin 750 mg, clarithromycin 200 mg and metronidazole 250 mg (RACM) all twice daily was more effective than the control RCA, 1-week triple therapy in a RCT in 80 Japanese patients (eradication rates: RACM 93%, RAC 81%).[329] Ald Serious adverse events were not observed and compliance was excellent. An earlier study by the same group used the same regimens for 5 days and the observed eradication rates were 94% for RACM and 80% for RAC.[333]

Table 5.4 "New" *H. pylori* eradication regimens: what's hot in the new millenium!

Reference	N	Diagnosis	Treatment/duration	Eradication rate (%)		Comments
				ITT	PP	
PPI-BMT (See also Table 5.3 for PPI-triple v PPI-BMT studies)						
Laine et al.[255]	138	DU	OBMT 10 days	88	93	RCT, North America
	137	DU	OAC 7 days	83	87	"Single triple" capsule of BMT
Other quadruple therapies						
Nagahara et al.[329]	80	GU, DU or	RACM 5 days	93	95	RCT, Japan
	80	NUD	RCA 7 days	81	82	
Treiber et al.[330]	83	Mixed	LACM 5 days	89	94	RCT, Germany
	80		RanACM 5 days	89	90	
	80		L 5 days + ACM day 3–5	81	86	
Furazolidone						
Xiao et al.[323]	219	NUD or	OMC 7 days	65	66	RCT, China
	229	healed DU	OFuraC 7 days	69	69	
	225		OFuraA 7 days	86	87	
	219		BFuraC 7 days	78	80	
Lu et al.[324]	60	NUD or	RbcFuraA 7 days	82	85	RCT, China
	60	healed DU	RbcFuraT 7 days	85	91	
Fakheri et al.[325]	55	DU	OABC 14 days	85	90	RCT, Iran
	63		OABFura 14 days	84	90	
Coelho et al.[326]	40	Asymptomatic	LCFura400 7 days	87	87	Relatives of gastric cancer
	39	relatives	LCFura200 7 days	61	61	patients, once daily doses
Fluoroquinolone regimens (levofloxacin and moxifloxacin)						
Cammarota et al.[327]	50	Mixed	LevoAR 7 days	92	92	RCT, Italy
	50		LevoTR 7 days	90	90	
Di Caro et al.[211]	40	Mixed	LevoAR 7 days	90	90	RCT, Italy
	40		LevoR 5 days	50	50	Dual therapy no good
	40		LevoR 7 days	70	70	
	40		LevoR 10 days	65	65	
Di Caro et al.[328]	40	Mixed	Moxi 7 days	22	22	RCT, Italy
	40		MoxiL 7 days	33	33	
	40		MoxiCL 7 days	90	90	
Sequential therapy						
Zullo et al.[331]	522	Mixed	RA 5 days then RCTin 5 days	92	95	Sequential therapy, total 10 days
	527		RAC 7 days	74	77	Multicenter Italian study
Hassan et al.[332]	75	DU	RA 5 days then RC500Tin 5 days	95	97	RCT, Italy, total 10 days treatment
	77		RA 5 days then RC250Tin 5 days	92	96	Arms differed in C dose

ITT, intention-to-treat; PP, per protocol; analysis; RCT, randomized controlled trial; GU, gastric ulcer; DU, duodenal ulcer patients; NUD, non-ulcer dyspepsia; Mixed, *H. pylori* positive patient of any diagnosis; L, lansoprazole; R, rabeprazole; O, omeprazole; Rbc, ranitidine bismuth citrate; Ran, ranitidine; A, amoxicillin; C, clarithromycin; Tin, tinidazole; B, bismuth compound; M, metronidazole; T, tetracycline; Levo, levofloxacin; Moxi, moxifloxacin; Fura, furazolidone

The results with a similar regimen used for a short duration was reported from Germany.[330] Patients were randomized to receive quadruple therapy with lansoprazole 30 mg twice daily, amoxicillin 1 g twice daily, clarithromycin 250 mg twice daily and metronidazole 400 mg twice daily for 5 days (LACM5), ranitidine 300 mg twice daily with the same antibiotics (RanACM), or lansoprazole for 5 days but the antibiotics for the 3-day period from the third to the fifth day (LACM3). The observed eradication rates were excellent and not statistically significantly different (89%, 89% and 81%, respectively). Ald In the original trial of this regimen reported in 1998 in which omeprazole with the same antibiotics (OACM) for 5 days was compared with OCM for 7 days eradication rates of 90% were observed with each regimen.[334]

Earlier reports with similar regimens have yielded remarkably consistent results. With lansoprazole Neville *et al.* observed a better eradication rate with LACM (88%) than with LCM (81%) or LCA (59%) triple therapy regimens.[335] In this study, the baseline metronidazole resistance rate was 52%. Catalano randomized patients to receive a regimen consisting of either omeprazole or RBC as the anti-secretory drug for 5 days and and the ACM antibiotic combination for only the three days period from days 3 to 5 or to one of the standard triple therapy regimens of OCA and RBC-CA.[336] The observed eradication rates with these regimens were OACM 89%, OAC 82%, RBC-ACM 95% and RBC-CA 78%. Ald An observational study of a similar regimen using omeprazole, amoxicillin, clarithromycin and tinidazole all twice daily for 4 days eradicated *H. pylori* in 88% of patients (91% by per protocol analysis).[337] Another observational study of this regimen in which roxithromycin was substituted for clarithromycin and treatment was given for 7 days reported a 92% eradication rate in 169 patients.[338] B4

This PPI-ACM regimen for 5 days consistently has resulted in eradication rates of 89–95% compared with rates of 59–90% for the control 1-week triple therapies. Further trials of this regimen are clearly warranted, especially as a strategy for treatment failures.

Less promising regimens

Azithromycin does not appear to be a very useful drug for *H. pylori* eradication. When it was used in place of clarithromycin as part of a quadruple therapy regimen, a lower eradication rate was observed.[339] Azithromycin is usually given for 5 days even when the other drugs are given for 7 days. The combination of omeprazole, amoxicillin and azithromycin in France, yielded an eradication rate of only 38%, substantially less than the observed OCA rate of 72% or OCM rate of 61%.[340] Ald In other studies where azithromycin was used for only 3 days, eradication success was suboptimal.[341–343]

Alternative agents

Fish oil (eicosapen) contains ω-3-fatty acids which have been shown to have anti-*H. pylori* bacteriostatic effects. However, replacing metronidazole with eicosapen is ineffective.[344] C5

Pronase, a mucolytic agent with no antibacterial effect on *H. pylori*, added to lansoprazole, amoxicillin and metronidazole significantly improved the eradication rate to 94% compared with 77% ($P = 0.004$) observed with the LAM triple therapy alone.[345] Ald Regimens adding pronase deserve further study.

A few studies have evaluated the effects of probiotics such as *Lactobacillus GG*,[346,347] *Saccharomyces boulardii*[347] or a combination of *Lactobacillus* and bifidobacteria[347,348] as adjuvant therapies for *H. pylori* treatment. Two studies[346,347] showed no difference in *H. pylori* eradication rates when the probiotic was used, but adverse effects of eradication therapy such as diarrhea and taste disturbances were reduced. Ald Only one study using *Lactobacillus* and bifidobacteria showed that the addition of the probiotics improved the eradication rate.[348]

Second-line/eradication failure treatments

There are now numerous regimens summarized in Table 5.5 that have shown efficacy for treatment failures.

In patients who have failed initial therapy, successive therapies are always more difficult. The most studied and consistently effective regimen is quadruple therapy with PPI, bismuth compound, nitroimidazole and tetracycline for 7–14 days as discussed above. One drawback is that in some countries bismuth compounds are not available. Such is the case in Japan. However, rabeprazole, amoxicillin and metronidazole triple therapies may be an effective rescue regimen in that country.[349,350] Some of the RBC triple regimens have been found to be very effective, but as the drug is essentially unavailable, this information is of little practical use.

Rifabutin regimens

Rifabutin containing regimens have emerged as strong contenders for treating eradication failures. The regimen has been studied in Italy where a randomized trial has shown that a larger dose of rifabutin 300 mg daily is more effective than 150 mg daily when used in combination with pantoprazole and amoxicillin for 10 days.[282] This triple regimen was more effective (87%) than pantoprazole-BMT quadruple therapy (67%), the most commonly recommended salvage therapy. Ald This observed eradication rate was apparently better than the 71% eradication rate observed in 41 patients treated in the pilot study.[351] This regimen requires further study. In another small pilot study of a triple therapy regimen of rifabutin 150 mg, amoxicillin 1 g, and lansoprazole 30 mg all twice daily for 1 week a relatively low eradication rate of 72% (86% by per protocol analysis) was observed.[352] B4 In an observational study in only 14 patients who had failed two

Table 5.5   Regimens for treatment failures

Reference	N	Design	Failed regimen(s)	Treatment/duration	Eradication rate (%)		Comments
					ITT	PP	
PPI-BMT (See also Table 5.3 for PPI-triple v PPI-BMT studies)							
Dore et al.[291]	71	Open	2 or more PPI triples	OBMT twice daily 14 days	93	97	Dosed at lunch and supper
Other quadruples							
Chi et al.[355]	50	RCT	OAC	OBAT 7 days	78	89	RCT
	50			OBAM 7 days	58	67	
Georgopoulos et al.[356]	49	RCT	OAC	OBMT 7 days	84	89	RCT
	46			OBMC 7 days	59	64	
Perri et al.[282]	45	RCT	PPI triples or RbcC	PARifa150od 10 days	67	68	Fewer AE than PBMT (9–11% v 47%)
	45			PARifa300od 10 days	87	87	
	45			PBMT 10 days	67	73	Effective in both MR and CR
Wong et al.[285]	56	RCT	PPI or Rbc triple(s)	LevoRifaR 7 days	91	91	
	53			RBMT 7 days	91	92	
Perri et al.[283]	59	RCT	OCA	RbcAT 7 days	85	86	PPI-BMT remains good
	58			LevoAP 7 days	63	66	
	55			PBMT 7 days	83	91	
Nista et al.[284]	70	RCT	RCA	LevoAR 10 days	94	94	Levofloxacin triple therapies better than RBMT quadruple
	70			LevoTinR 10 days	90	90	
	70			RBMT 7 days	63	69	
	70			RBMT 14 days	69	80	
Lin et al.[357]	78	Open	Bismuth triple	LBAC 7 days	83	84	
Isakov et al.[358]	35	RCT	Not given	BTFura 7 days	86	91	All had MR strains
	35			OBMT 7 days	74	90	
PPI triples							
Isomoto et al.[349]	63	RCT	LAC	RA 14 days	59	66	RCT
	60			RAM 7 days	82	88	
Murakami et al.[350]	92	Open	PPI-AC	RAM 7 days	88	91	Better if MS 97%, MR 82%
Zullo et al.[354]	36	Open	2 or more failures	LevoAR 10 days	83	88	
Wong et al.[359]	50	Open	PPI or Rbc triple(s)	OFuraA 7 days	52	53	Overall poor, if MS and CS eradication was 88%

ITT, intention-to-treat; PP, per protocol; O, omeprazole; L, lansoprazole; P, pantoprazole; R, rabeprazole; Rbc, ranitidine bismuth citrate; B, bismuth compound; M, metronidazole; T, tetracycline; A, amoxicillin; C, clarithromycin; Levo, levofloxacin; Rifa, rifabutin; Fura, furazolidone; Tin, tinidazole; MR, metronidazole resistant; MS, metronidazole sensitive; CR, clarithromycin resistant; CS, clarithromycin sensitive; AE, adverse events; RCT, randomized controlled trial

courses of therapy, the first with PPI-CA and the second with either PPI or RBC-BMT, third-line therapy with omeprazole, amoxicillin and rifabutin 150 mg twice daily for 14 days was successful in 79% of patients.[353] B4 A drawback to rifabutin is that it is an expensive drug and not readily available.

In a randomized trial in China rifabutin combined with levofloxacin (another promising new drug) and rabeprazole was compared with rabeprazole-BMT quadruple therapy for 7 days.[285] This triple therapy regimen is very simple, as both levofloxacin and rifabutin are given only once daily. The eradication rate was 91% with both regimens. Ala Even in patients-resistant to both metronidazole and clarithromycin, the observed eradication rates were 85% (17/20) with the triple therapy and 87% (13/15) with the quadruple therapy regimen.[285] Thus, these are both promising regimens for treatment failures.

Box 5.2 *H. pylori* eradication treatment recommendations 2004

Recommended first line therapies

PPI or RBC triples
- PPI or RBC twice daily + clarithromycin 500 mg twice daily + amoxicillin 1 g twice daily for 7 days
- PPI or RBC twice daily + clarithromycin 500 mg twice daily + metronidazole 500 mg twice daily for 7 days

PPI–BMT
- PPI twice daily + colloidal bismuth citrate or bismuth subsalicylate 2 tabs four times daily, metronidazole 250–500 mg four times daily, tetracycline 500 mg four times daily for 7 days
- *PPI–BMT twice daily: PPI twice daily + colloidal bismuth subcitrate 2 tabs twice daily, metronidazole 500 mg twice daily and tetracycline 500 mg twice daily, at noon and supper with the meal for 14 days*

Promising first-line therapies (Table 5.4)

Levofloxacin triples
- LAR: Levofloxacin 500 mg once daily, amoxicillin 1 g twice daily and rabeprazole 20 mg once daily for 7 days
- LTR: Levofloxacin 500 mg once daily, tinidazole 500 mg twice daily and rabeprazole 20 mg once daily for 7 days

Sequential therapy
- RA+RCT: Rabeprazole 40 mg once daily and amoxicillin 1 g twice daily for first 5 days, then rabeprazole 20 mg, clarithromycin 500 mg and tinidazole 500 mg twice daily for 5 more days

PPI–ACM for 5 days
- PPI twice daily, amoxicillin 750 mg to 1 g twice daily, clarithromycin 250 mg twice daily and metronidazole 500 mg twice daily

Recommended for treatment failures

PPI–BMT: PPI twice daily + colloidal bismuth citrate or bismuth subsalicylate 2 tabs four times daily, metronidazole 250–500 mg four times daily, tetracycline 500 mg four times daily for 14 days

Promising (Table 5.5)

- PPI–BMT twice daily: PPI twice daily + colloidal bismuth subcitrate 2 tabs twice daily, metronidazole 500 mg twice daily and tetracycline 500 mg twice daily, at noon and supper with the meal for 14 days
- BTFura: Colloidal bismuth subcitrate 240 mg twice daily, tetracycline 750 mg twice daily and furazolidone 200 mg twice daily for 7 days
- LevoRifaR: Levofloxacin 500 mg once daily, Rifabutin 300 mg once daily, Rabeprazole 20 mg twice daily for 7 days
- PARifa: Pantoprazole 40 mg twice daily, amoxicillin 1 g twice daily, and rifabutin 300 mg once daily for 10 days
- LevoAR: Levofloxacin 500 mg once daily, amoxicillin 1 g twice daily and rabeprazole 20 mg twice daily for 10 days
- LevoTinR: Levofloxacin 500 mg once daily, tinidazole 500 mg twice daily and rabeprazole 20 mg twice daily for 10 days

PPI, proton pump inhibitor: omeprazole 20 mg, lansoprazole 30 mg, pantoprazole 40 mg, esomeprazole 40 mg or rabeprazole 20 mg. In regimens where a specific PPI is given, this reflects the study data although in practice, all could probably be used interchangeably. RBC, ranitidine bismuth citrate

---

Levofloxacin regimens

The combination of levofloxacin, amoxicillin and rabeprazole was identified as a promising regimen above. Indeed this regimen, as well as a similar, levofloxacin, tinidazole and rabeprazole triple therapy were both very effective in treatment failures with observed eradication rates of 90% or more.[284] When these new triple therapies were compared against the present standard rabeprazole quadruple therapy (RBMT) treatment failure regimen for either 7 to 14 days, the observed eradication rates for the quadruple therapies were only 63–69%.[284] Ald Not only were the triple therapies more effective, the adverse effects were significantly less frequent than were observed in the RBMT 14 day group. In another study, even after patients had failed 2 or more previous standard regimens, the levofloxacin, amoxicillin and rabeprazole triple therapy regimen for 10 days was effective in 83% of patients.[354] B4 In a similar study in which pantoprazole was used instead of rabeprazole with levofloxacin and amoxicillin for one week the observed rate of eradication was only 63%.[283] While the choice of PPI does not seem to make much difference for other regimens, the consistent better performance of the rabeprazole regimens is interesting and randomized trials comparing PPIs in combination with levofloxacin and amoxicillin are needed.

Furazolidone regimens

A regimen combining omeprazole, amoxicillin and furazolidone was largely ineffective with an observed eradication rate of only 52%. If antibiotic sensitivity testing can be done, this regimen is 88% effective against strains that are still sensitive to metronidazole and clarithromycin.[359] However, in clinical practice, antibiotic sensitivity testing after the first failure is impractical. Also, the probablity that *H. pylori* would still be susceptible to both antibiotics after treatment failure is fairly small. However, another small observational study with furazolidone quadruple therapy did show some promise. Patients who failed on an initial regimen of clarithromycin, metronidazole, and acid suppression with or without amoxicillin were treated with a quadruple therapy regimen of lansoprazole, bismuth, metronidazole and tetracycline with only 39% success.[360] These treatment failures were next treated with lansoprazole, bismuth, tetracycline and furazolidone 200 mg twice daily for 1-week and surprisingly, eradication was observed in nine of 10 patients. B4

When patients who had metronidazole-resistant *H. pylori* by agar dilution[358] were randomized to receive bismuth, tetracycline and furazolidone 200 mg twice daily (BTF), or OBMT the observed eradication rates were 86% versus 74% ($P = $ NS). However, the study may have lacked power to show a significant difference if one existed. Patients treated with the BTF regimen experienced fewer adverse effects than those treated with OBMT (31 v 0%; $P = 0.03$). Thus, furazolidone may be an excellent substitute for metronidazole.

Summary

Helicobacter pylori is an important cause of ulcer disease and is accepted as a definite pathogen that fulfills almost all of Hill's criteria for causation. In the new millennium, ulcers not caused by *H. pylori* or non-steroidal anti-inflammatory drugs appears to be on the increase. The older data from the pre-*H. pylori* era have become important again as there may be little to offer these patients for ulcer healing and prevention of recurrence other than continuous acid-suppressive therapy. For those with *H. pylori* infection, eradication is important to facilitate ulcer healing, reduce ulcer relapse and prevent complications such as recurrent hemorrhage. Eradication of *H. pylori* heals ulcers without the need to continue ulcer healing drugs, heals refractory ulcers and also results in faster ulcer healing than occurs with traditional acid-suppressive therapy. The presently recommended first-line therapies include triple therapy with either PPIs, or RBC with clarithromycin and amoxicillin or metronidazole, or quadruple therapy with a PPI, bismuth compound, metronidazole and tetracycline (Box 5.2). First-line therapy should be for 7–10 days, and for treatment failures, 10–14 days of treatment are recommended. With emerging antimicrobial resistance, first line therapies may not be quite as effective as in the recent past. Many promising new regimens are continuing to be developed to treat these eradication failures (see Box 5.2).

References

1   Schwarz K. Uber penetrierende Magen und Jejunalgeschwure. *Beiträge Zur Klinische Chirurgie* 1910;**67**:96–128.

2   Warren JR, Marshall BJ. Unidentified curved bacillus on gastric epithelium in active chronic gastritis. *Lancet* 1983; **1**:1273–5.

3   Marshall BJ, Warren JR. Unidentified curved bacilli in the stomach of patients with gastritis and peptic ulceration. *Lancet* 1984;**i**:1311–15.

4   Mégraud F, Lamouliatte H. *Helicobacter pylori* and duodenal ulcer. Evidence suggesting causation. *Dig Dis Sci* 1992;**37**:769–72.

5   Rabeneck L, Ransohoff DF. Is *Helicobacter pylori* a cause of duodenal ulcer? A methodologic critique of current evidence. *Am J Med* 1991;**91**:566–72.

6   Hill BA. The environment and disease: association or causation? *Proc R Soc Med* 1965;**58**:295–300.

7   Nomura A, Stemmerman GN, Chyou P-H, Perez-Perez GI, Blaser MJ. *Helicobacer pylori* infection and the risk for duodenal and gastric ulceration. *Ann Intern Med* 1994; **120**:977–81.

8   Sipponen P, Varis K, Fraki O, Korri UM, Seppala K, Siurala M. Cumulative 10-year risk of symptomatic duodenal and gastric ulcer disease in people with or without chronic gastritis: a clinical follow up study of 454 outpatients. *Scand J Gastroenterol* 1990;**25**:966–73.

9   Kuipers EJ, Thijs JC, Festen HPM. The prevalence of *Helicobacter pylori* in peptic ulcer disease. *Aliment Pharmacol Ther* 1995;**9(Suppl 2)**:59–69.

10 Borody TJ, George LL, Brandl S *et al*. *Helicobacter pylori* negative duodenal ulcer. *Am J Gastroenterol* 1991;**86**:1154–7.

11 Quan C, Talley NJ. Management of peptic ulcer disease not related to *Helicobacter pylori* or NSAIDs. *Am J Gastroenterol* 2002;**97**:2950–61.

12 Laine L, Hopkins RJ, Girardi LS. Has the impact of *Helicobacter pylori* therapy on ulcer recurrence in the United States been overstated? A meta-analysis of rigorously designed trials. *Am J Gastroenterol* 1998;**93**:1409–15.

13 Ciociola AA, McSorley DJ, Turner K, Sykes D, Palmer JB. *Helicobacter pylori* infection rates in duodenal ulcer patients in the United States may be lower than previously estimated. *Am J Gastroenterol* 1999;**94**:1834–40.

14 Cloud ML, Enas N, Humphries TJ, Bassion S. Rabeprazole in treatment of acid peptic diseases: results of three placebo-controlled dose-response clinical trials in duodenal ulcer, gastric ulcer, and gastroesophageal reflux disease (GERD). The Rabeprazole Study Group. *Dig Dis Sci* 1998;**43**:993–1000.

15 Gisbert JP, Blanco M, Mateos JM *et al*. *H. pylori*-negative duodenal ulcer prevalence and causes in 774 patients. *Dig Dis Sci* 1999;**44**:2295–302.

16 Rosenstock S, Jorgensen T, Bonnevie O, Andersen L. Risk factors for peptic ulcer disease: a population based prospective cohort study comprising 2416 Danish adults. *Gut* 2003;**52**:186–93.

17 Hyvärinen H, Salmenkylä S, Sipponen P. *Helicobacter pylori*-negative duodenal and pyloric ulcer: role of NSAIDs. *Digestion* 1996;**57**:305–9.

18 Harris AW, Gummett PA, Phull PS, Jacyna MR, Misiewicz JJ, Baron JH. Recurrence of duodenal ulcer after *Helicobacter pylori* eradication is related to high acid output. *Aliment Pharmacol Ther* 1997;**11**:331–4.

19 McColl KEL, El-Nujumi AM, Chittajallu RS *et al.* A study of the pathogenesis of *Helicobacter pylori* negative chronic duodenal ulceration. *Gut* 1993;**34**:762–8.

20 Kurata JH, Nogawa AN. Meta-analysis of risk factors for peptic ulcer. Nonsteroidal antiinflammatory drugs, *Helicobacter pylori*, and smoking. *J Clin Gastroenterol* 1997; **24**:2–17.

21 Thijs JC, Kuipers EJ, van ZA, Pena AS, de GJ. Treatment of *Helicobacter pylori* infections. *QJM* 1995;**88**:369–89.

22 Borody TJ, Brandl S, Andrews P, Jankiewicz E, Ostapowicz N. *Helicobacter pylori* negative gastric ulcer. *Am J Gastroenterol* 1992;**87**:1403–6.

23 Rauws EAJ, Langenberg W, Houthoff HJ, Zanen HC, Tytgat GNJ. *Campylobacter pyloridis*-associated chronic active antral gastritis. *Gastroenterology* 1988;**94**:33–40.

24 Graham DY, Malaty HM. Alendronate gastric ulcers. *Aliment Pharmacol Ther* 1999;**13**:515–19.

25 Thomson AB, Marshall JK, Hunt RH *et al.* 14 day endoscopy study comparing risedronate and alendronate in postmenopausal women stratified by *Helicobacter pylori* status. *J Rheumatol* 2002;**29**:1965–74.

26 Graham DY, Malaty HM. Alendronate and naproxen are synergistic for development of gastric ulcers. *Arch Intern Med* 2001;**161**:107–10.

27 Walsh JH, Peterson WL. The treatment of *Helicobacter pylori* infection in the management of peptic ulcer disease. *N Engl J Med* 1995;**333**:984–91.

28 Jyotheeswaran S, Shah AN, Jin HO, Potter GD, Ona FV, Chey WY. Prevalence of *Helicobacter pylori* in peptic ulcer patients in greater Rochester, NY: is empirical triple therapy justified? *Am J Gastroenterol* 1998;**93**:574–8.

29 Marshall BJ. *Helicobacter pylori* in peptic ulcer: have Koch's postulates been fulfilled? *Ann Med* 1995;**27**:565–8.

30 Blaser MJ, Chyou P-H, Nomura A. Age at establishment of *Helicobacter pylori* infection and gastric carcinoma, gastric ulcer, and duodenal ulcer risk. *Cancer Res* 1995;**55**:562–5.

31 Perri F, Clemente R, Pastore M *et al.* The 13C-urea breath test as a predictor of intragastric bacterial load and severity of *Helicobacter pylori* gastritis. *Scand J Clin Lab Invest* 1998;**58**:19–27.

32 Labenz J, Börsch G, Peitz U *et al.* Validity of a novel biopsy urease test (HUT) and a simplified 13C-urea breath test for diagnosis of *Helicobacter pylori* infection and estimation of the severity of gastritis. *Digestion* 1996;**57**:391–7.

33 Hilker E, Domschke W, Stoll R. 13C-urea breath test for detection of *Helicobacter pylori* and its correlation with endoscopic and histologic findings. *J Physiol Pharmacol* 1996; **47**:79–90.

34 Moshkowitz M, Konikoff FM, Peled Y *et al.* High *Helicobacter pylori* numbers are associated with low eradication rate after triple therapy. *Gut* 1995;**36**:845–7.

35 Sharma TK, Prasad VM, Cutler AF. Quantitative non-invasive testing for *Helicobacter pylori* does not predict gastroduodenal ulcer disease. *Gastrointest Endosc* 1996;**44**:679–82.

36 Lewis JD, Kroser J, Bevan J, Furth EE, Metz DC. Urease-based tests for *Helicobacter pylori* gastritis. Accurate for diagnosis but poor correlation with disease severity. *J Clin Gastroenterol* 1997;**25**:415–20.

37 Moran AP, Wadström T. Pathogenesis of *Helicobacter pylori*. *Curr Opin Gastroenterol* 1998;**14(Suppl 1)**:S9–S14.

38 Yang H, Dixon MF, Zuo J *et al. Helicobacter pylori* infection and gastric metaplasia in the duodenum in China. *J Clin Gastroenterol* 1995;**20**:110–12.

39 Harris AW, Gummett PA, Walker MM, Misiewicz JJ, Baron JH. Relation between gastric acid output, *Helicobacter pylori*, and gastric metaplasia in the duodenal bulb. *Gut* 1996;**39**:513–20.

40 Walker MM, Dixon MF. Gastric metaplasia: its role in duodenal ulceration. *Aliment Pharmacol Ther* 1996; **10(Suppl 1)**:119–28.

41 Madsen JE, Vetvik K, Aase S. *Helicobacter*-associated duodenitis and gastric metaplasia in duodenal ulcer patients. *APMIS* 1991;**99**:997–1000.

42 Steer HW. Surface morphology of the gastroduodenal mucosa in duodenal ulceration. *Gut* 1984;**25**:1203–10.

43 Carrick J, Lee A, Hazell S, Ralston M, Daskalopoulos G. *Campylobacter pylori*, duodenal ulcer, and gastric metaplasia: possible role of functional heterotopic tissue in ulcerogenesis. *Gut* 1989;**30**:790–7.

44 Khulusi S, Mendall MA, Badve S, Patel P, Finlayson C, Northfield TC. Effect of *Helicobacter pylori* eradication on gastric metaplasia of the duodenum. *Gut* 1995;**36**: 193–7.

45 Rudnicka L, Bobrzynski A, Stachura J. Short-term eradication therapy for *Helicobacter pylori* does not reduce the incidence of gastric metaplasia in duodenal ulcer patients. *Pol J Pathol* 1997;**48**:103–6.

46 Khulusi S, Badve S, Patel P *et al.* Pathogenesis of gastric metaplasia of the human duodenum: role of *Helicobacter pylori*, gastric acid, and ulceration. *Gastroenterology* 1996; **110**:452–8.

47 Urakami Y, Kimura M, Seki H. Gastric metaplasia and *Helicobacter pylori*. *Am J Gastroenterol* 1997;**92**:795–9.

48 el-Omar E, Penman I, Dorrian CA, Ardill JE, McColl KE. Eradicating *Helicobacter pylori* infection lowers gastrin mediated acid secretion by two thirds in patients with duodenal ulcer. *Gut* 1993;**34**:1060–5.

49 Gillen D, el-Omar EM, Wirz AA, Ardill JES, McColl KEL. The acid response to gastrin distinguishes duodenal ulcer patients from *Helicobacter pylori*-infected healthy subjects. *Gastroenterology* 1998;**114**:50–7.

50 Graham DY, Opekun A, Lew GM, Klein PD, Walsh JH. *Helicobacter pylori*-associated exaggerated gastrin release in duodenal ulcer patients. The effect of bombesin infusion and urea ingestion. *Gastroenterology* 1991;**100**:1571–5.

51 Hamlet A, Olbe L. The influence of *Helicobacter pylori* infection on postprandial duodenal acid load and duodenal bulb pH in humans. *Gastroenterology* 1996;**111**:391–400.

52 el Omar EM, Penman ID, Ardill JE, Chittajallu RS, Howie C, McColl KE. *Helicobacter pylori* infection and abnormalities of acid secretion in patients with duodenal ulcer disease. *Gastroenterology* 1995;**109**:681–91.

53 Harris AW, Gummett PA, Misiewicz JJ, Baron JH. Eradication of *Helicobacter pylori* in patients with duodenal ulcers lowers basal and peak acid outputs in response to gastrin releasing peptide and pentagastrin. *Gut* 1996;**38**:663–7.

54 Beardshall K, Moss S, Gill J, Levi S, Ghosh P, Playford RJ, Calam J. Suppression of *Helicobacter pylori* reduces gastrin releasing peptide stimulated gastrin release in duodenal ulcer patients. *Gut* 1992;**33**:601–3.

55 Harris AW, Gummett PA, Phull PS, Jacyna MR, Misiewicz JJ, Baron JH. Recurrence of duodenal ulcer after *Helicobacter pylori* eradication is related to high acid output. *Aliment Pharmacol Ther* 1997;**11**:331–4.

56 Rieder G, Hatz RA, Moran AP, Walz A, Stolte M, Enders G. Role of adherence in interleukin-8 induction induction in *Helicobacter pylori*-associated gastritis. *Infect Immun* 1997;**65**:3622–30.

57 Yamaoka Y, Kita M, Kodama T, Sawi N, Kashima K, Imanishi J. Induction of various cytokines and development of severe mucosal inflammation by *cagA* gene positive *Helicobacter pylori* strains. *Gut* 1997;**41**:442–51.

58 D'Elios MM, Manghetti M, Almerigogna F *et al.* Different cytokine profile and antigen-specificity repertoire in *Helicobacter pylori*-specific T cell clones from the antrum of chronic gastritis patients with or without peptic ulcer. *Eur J Immunol* 1997;**27**:1751–5.

59 Beales I, Blaser MJ, Srinivasan S *et al.* Effect of *Helicobacter pylori* products and recombinant cytokines on gastrin release from cultured canine G cells. *Gastroenterology* 1997;**113**:465–71.

60 Londong W, Barth H, Dammann HG *et al.* Dose-related healing of duodenal ulcer with the proton pump inhibitor lansoprazole. *Aliment Pharmacol Ther* 1991;245–54.

61 Bardhan KD, Bianchi Porro G, Bose K *et al.* A comparison of two different doses of omeprazole versus ranitidine in treatment of duodenal ulcers. *J Clin Gastroenterol* 1986;**8**:408–13.

62 Misra SC, Dasarathy S, Sharma MP. Omeprazole versus famotidine in the healing and relapse of duodenal ulcer. *Aliment Pharmacol Ther* 1993;**7**:443–9.

63 Dammann HG, Walter TA. Efficacy of continuous therapy for peptic ulcer in controlled clinical trials. *Aliment Pharmacol Ther* 1993;**7(Suppl 2)**:17–25.

64 Penston JG, Wormsley KG. Nine years of maintenance treatment with ranitidine for patients with duodenal ulcer disease. *Aliment Pharmacol Ther* 1992;**6**:629–45.

65 O'Brien BJ, Goeree R, Hunt R, Wilkinson J, Levine M, Willan A. Economic evaluation of alternative therapies in the long term management of peptic ulcer disease and gastroesophageal relux disease. Canadian Coordinating Office of Health Technology Assessment (CCOHTA) report Hamilton, Ontario: McMaster University, 1996.

66 Veldhuyzen van Zanten SJO, Bradette M, Farley A *et al.* The DU-MACH study: eradication of *Helicobacter pylori* and ulcer healing in patients with acute duodenal ulcer using omeprazole based triple therapy. *Aliment Pharmacol Ther* 1999;**13**:289–95.

67 Coghlan JG, Humphries H, Dooley C *et al.* *Campylobacter pylori* and recurrence of duodenal ulcer – a 12 month follow up study. *Lancet* 1987;**ii**:1109–11.

68 Marshall BJ, Goodwin CS, Warren JR *et al.* Prospective double-blind trial of duodenal ulcer relapse after eradication of *Campylobacter pylori*. *Lancet* 1988;**ii**:1437–42.

69 Rauws EAJ, Tytgat GNJ. Cure of duodenal ulcer associated with eradication of *Helicobacter pylori*. *Lancet* 1990;**335**:1233–5.

70 George LL, Borody TJ, Andrews P *et al.* Cure of duodenal ulcer after eradication of *Helicobacter pylori*. *Med J Aust* 1990;**153**:145–9.

71 Graham DY, Lem GM, Evans DG, Evans DJ Jr, Klein PD. Effect of triple therapy (anti-biotics plus bismuth) on duodenal ulcer healing. A randomized controlled trial. *Ann Intern Med* 1991;**115**:266–9.

72 Graham DY, Lew GM, Klein PD *et al.* Effect of treatment of *Helicobacter pylori* infection on the long-term recurrence of gastric or duodenal ulcer. A randomized, controlled study. *Ann Intern Med* 1992;**116**:705–8.

73 Hentschel E, Brandstatter G, Dragosics B *et al.* Effect of ranitidine and amoxicillin plus metronidazole on the eradication of *Helicobacter pylori* and the recurrence of duodenal ulcer. *N Engl J Med* 1993;**328**:308–12.

74 Tytgat GNJ. Review article: treatments that impact favourably upon the eradication of *Helicobacter pylori* and ulcer recurrence. *Aliment Pharmacol Ther* 1994;**8**:359–68.

75 Penston JG. *Helicobacter pylori* eradication – understandable caution but no excuse for inertia. *Aliment Pharmacol Ther* 1994;**8**:369–89.

76 Labenz J, Börsch G. Highly significant change of the clinical course of relapsing and complicated peptic ulcer disease after cure of *Helicobacter pylori* infection. *Am J Gastroenterol* 1994;**89**:1785–8.

77 Forbes GM, Glaser ME, Cullen DJE *et al.* Duodenal ulcer treated with *Helicobacter pylori* eradication: seven year follow-up. *Lancet* 1994;**343**:258–60.

78 Hopkins RJ, Girardi LS, Turney EA. Relationship between *Helicobacter pylori* eradication and reduced duodenal and gastric ulcer recurrence: a review. *Gastroenterology* 1997;**110**:1244–52.

79 Leodolter A, Kulig M, Brasch H, Meyer-Sabellek W, Willich SN, Malfertheiner P. A meta-analysis comparing eradication, healing and relapse rates in patients with *Helicobacter pylori*-associated gastric or duodenal ulcer. *Aliment Pharmacol Ther* 2001;**15**:1949–58.

80 Susser M. Civilization and peptic ulcer. *Lancet* 1962;**1**:115–19.

81 Svanes C, Lie RT, Kvåle G, Svanes K, Søreide O. Incidence of perforated ulcer in Western Norway 1935–1990: cohort or period dependent time trends? *Am J Epidemiol* 1995;**141**:836–44.

82 Banatvala N, Mayo K, Mégraud F, Jennings R, Deeks JJ, Feldman RA. The cohort effect and *Helicobacter pylori*. *J Infect Dis* 1993;**168**:219–21.

83 Coggon D, Lambert P, Langman MJS. 20 years of hospital admissions for peptic ulcer in England and Wales. *Lancet* 1981;**1**:1302–4.

84 Kurata JH. Ulcer epidemiology: an overview and proposed research framework. *Gastroenterology* 1989;**96**:569–80.

85 Mégraud F, Brassens-Rabbé MP, Denis F, Belbouri A, Hoa DQ. Seroepidemiology of *Campylobacter pylori* in various populations. *J Clin Microbiol* 1989;**27**:1870–3.

86 Jones DB, Howden CW, Burget DW, Kerr GD, Hunt RH. Acid suppression in duodenal ulcer: a meta-analysis to define optimal dosing with anti-secretory drugs. *Gut* 1987;**28**:1120–7.

87 Burget DW, Chiverton SG, Hunt RH. Is there an optimal degree of acid suppression for healing of duodenal ulcers? A model of the relationship between ulcer healing and acid suppression. *Gastroenterology* 1990;**99**:345–51.

88 Wilairatana S, Kurathong S, Atthapaisalsarudee C, Saowaros V, Leethochawalit M. Omeprazole or cimetidine once daily for the treatment of duodenal ulcers? *J Gastroenterol Hepatol* 1989;**4**:45–52.

89 Archambault AP, Pare P, Bailey RJ *et al.* Omeprazole (20mg daily) versus cimetidine (1200mg daily) in duodenal ulcer healing and pain relief. *Gastroenterology* 1988;**94**:1130–4.

90 Hawkey CJ, Long RG, Bardhan KD *et al.* Improved symptom relief and duodenal ulcer healing with lansoprazole, a new proton pump inhibitor, compared with ranitidine. *Gut* 1993;**34**:1458–62.

91 Judmaier G, Koelz HR and pantopazole duodenal ulcer study group. Comparison of pantoprazole and ranitidine in the treatment of acute duodenal ulcer. *Aliment Pharmacol Ther* 1994;**8**:81–6.

92 McFarland RJ, Bateson MC, Green JRB, O'Donogue DP, Dronfield MW. Omeprazole provides quicker symptom relief and duodenal ulcer healing than ranitidine. *Gastroenterology* 1990;**98**:278–83.

93 van Rensburg CJ, van Eeden PJ, Marks IN *et al.* Improved duodenal ulcer healing with pantoprazole compared with ranitidine: a multicentre study. *Eur J Gastroenterol Hepatol* 1994;**6**:739–43.

94 Chiba N, Hunt RH. Ulcer disease and *Helicobacter pylori* infection: etiology and treatment. In: McDonald J, Burroughs A, and Feagan B, eds. *Evidence-based Gastroenterology and Hepatology.* London: BMJ Books, 1999.

95 Arber N, Avni Y, Eliakim R, Swissa A, Melzer E, Rachmilewitz D, Konikoff F. A multicenter, double blind, randomized controlled study of omeprazole versus ranitidine in the treatment of duodenal ulcer in Israel. *Isr J Med Sci* 1994;**30**:757–61.

96 Barbara L, Blasi A, Cheli R *et al.* Omeprazole vs. ranitidine in the short-term treatment of duodenal ulcer: an Italian Multicenter study. *Hepatogastroenterology* 1987;**34**:229–32.

97 Classen M, Dammann HG, Domschke W *et al.* Omeprazole heals duodenal, but not gastric ulcers more rapidly than ranitidine. Results of two German multicentre trials. *Hepatogastroenterology* 1985;**32**:243–45.

98 Cremer M, Lambert R, Lamers CBHW, Delle Fave G, Maier C, and the European Pantoprazole study group. A double-blind study of pantoprazole and ranitidine in treatment of acute duodenal ulcer. A multicentre study. *Dig Dis Sci* 1995;**40**:1360–4.

99 Crowe JP, Wilkinson SP, Bate CM, Willoughby CP, Peers EM, Richardson PDI and the OPUS (Omeprazole Peptic Ulcer Study) Research Group. Symptom relief and duodenal ulcer healing with omeprazole or cimetidine. *Aliment Pharmacol Ther* 1989;**3**:83–91.

100 Hui WM, Lam SK, Lau WY, Branicki FJ, Lok ASF, Ng MMT, Lai CL, Poon GP. Omeprazole and ranitidine in duodenal ulcer healing and subsequent relapse: a randomized double-blind study with weekly endoscopic assessment. *J Gastroenterol Hepatol* 1989;**4**:35–43.

101 Hotz J, Kleiner R, Grymbowski T, Hennig U, Schwarz JA. Lansoprazole versus famotidine: efficacy and tolerance in the acute management of duodenal ulceration. *Aliment Pharmacol Ther* 1992;**6**:87–95.

102 Lanza F, Goff J, Scowcroft C, Jennings D, Greski RP. Double-blind comparison of lansoprazole, ranitidine, and placebo in the treatment of acute duodenal ulcer. Lansoprazole Study Group. *Am J Gastroenterol* 1994;**89**:1191–200.

103 Mulder CJJ, Tijtgat GNJ, Cluysenaer OJJ *et al.* Omeprazole (20 mg o.m.) versus ranitidine (150 mg b.d.) in duodenal ulcer healing and pain relief. *Aliment Pharmacol Ther* 1989;**3**:445–51.

104 Schepp W, Classen M. Pantoprazole and ranitidine in the treatment of acute duodenal ulce. A multicentre study. *Scand J Gastroenterol* 1995;**30**:511–14.

105 Wang CY, Wang TH, Lai KH *et al.* Alimentary tract and pancreas. Double-blind comparison of omeprazole 20 mg OM and ranitidine 300 mg NOCTE in duodenal ulcer: A Taiwan multi-centre study. *J Gastroenterol Hepatol* 1992;**7**:572–6.

106 Valenzuela JE, Berlin RG, Snape WJ *et al.* US experience with omeprazole in duodenal ulcer. Multicenter double-blind comparative study with ranitidine. *Dig Dis Sci* 1991;**36**:761–8.

107 Ekstrom P, Carling L, Unge P, Anker-Hansen O, Sjostedt S, Sellstrom H. Lansoprazole versus omeprazole in active duodenal ulcer. A double-blind, randomized, comparative study. *Scand J Gastroenterol* 1995;**30**:210–15.

108 Dobrilla G, Piazzi L, Fiocca R. Lansoprazole versus omeprazole for duodenal ulcer healing and prevention of relapse: a randomized, multicenter, double-masked trial. *Clin Ther* 1999;**21**:1321–2.

109 Rehner M, Rohner HG, Schepp W. Comparison of pantoprazole versus omeprazole in the treatment of acute duodenal ulceration – a multicentre study. *Aliment Pharmacol Ther* 1995;**9**:411–16.

110 Dekkers CP, Beker JA, Thjodleifsson B, Gabryelewicz A, Bell NE, Humphries TJ. Comparison of rabeprazole 20 mg versus omeprazole 20 mg in the treatment of active duodenal ulcer: a European multicentre study. *Aliment Pharmacol Ther* 1999;**13**:179–86.

111 Meneghelli UG, Zaterka S, de Paula CL, Malafaia O, Lyra LG. Pantoprazole versus ranitidine in the treatment of duodenal ulcer: a multicenter study in Brazil. *Am J Gastroenterol* 2000;**95**:62–6.

112 Breiter JR, Riff D, Humphries TJ. Rabeprazole is superior to ranitidine in the management of active duodenal ulcer disease: results of a double-blind, randomized North American study. *Am J Gastroenterol* 2000;**95**:936–42.

113 Ekstrom P, Carling L, Unge P, Anker-Hansen O, Sjostedt S, Sellstrom H. Lansoprazole versus omeprazole in active

duodenal ulcer. A double-blind, randomized, comparative study. *Scand J Gastroenterol* 1995;**30**:210–15.

114 Beker J, Bianchi Porro G, Bigard M *et al.* Double-blind comparison of pantoprazole and omeprazole for the treatment of acute duodenal ulcer. *Eur J Gastroenterol Hepatol* 1995;**7**:407–10.

115 Ruszniewski Ph, Slama A, Pappo M, Mignon M, GEMUD. Two year maintenance treatment of duodenal ulcer disease with ranitidine 150mg: a prospective multicentre randomised study. *Gut* 1993;**34**:1662–5.

116 Palmer RH, Frank WO, Karlstadt R. Maintenance therapy of duodenal ulcer with H₂-receptor antagonists – a meta-analysis. *Aliment Pharmacol Ther* 1990;**4**:283–94.

117 Kurata JH, Koch GG, Nogawa AN. Comparison of ranitidine and cimetidine ulcer maintenance therapy. *J Clin Gastroenterol* 1987;**9**:644–50.

118 Penston JG, Wormsley KG. Review article: maintenance treatment with H₂-receptor antagonists for peptic ulcer disease. *Aliment Pharmacol Ther* 1992;**6**:3–29.

119 Lee FI, Hardman M, Jaderberg ME. Maintenance treatment of duodenal ulceration: ranitidine 300 mg at night is better than 150mg in cigarette smokers. *Gut* 1991;**32**:151–53.

120 Chiba N, Rao BV, Rademaker JW, Hunt RH. Meta-analysis of the efficacy of anti-biotic therapy in eradicating *Helicobacter pylori*. *Am J Gastroenterol* 1992;**87**:1716–27.

121 Kovacs TO, Campbell D, Richter J, Haber M, Jennings DE, Rose P. Double-blind comparison of lansoprazole 15 mg, lansoprazole 30 mg and placebo as maintenance therapy in patients with healed duodenal ulcers resistant to H2-receptor antagonists. *Aliment Pharmacol Ther* 1999;**13**: 959–67.

122 Gisbert JP, Boixeda D, Martín De Argila C, Álvarez Baleriola I, Abraira V, García Plaza A. Unhealed duodenal ulcers despite *Helicobacter pylori* eradication. *Scand J Gastroenterol* 1997;**32**:643–50.

123 Hosking SW, Ling TK, Yung MY, Cheng A, Chung SC, Leung JW, Li AK. Randomised controlled trial of short term treatment to eradicate *Helicobacter pylori* in patients with duodenal ulcer. *BMJ* 1992;**305**:502–4.

124 Avsar E, Kalayci C, Tözün N *et al.* Refractory duodenal ulcer healing and relapse: comparison of omeprazole with *Helicobacter pylori* eradication. *Eur J Gastroenterol Hepatol* 1996;**8**:449–52.

125 Bianchi Porro G, Parente F, Lazzaroni M. Short and long term outcome of *Helicobacter pylori* positive resistant duodenal ulcers treated with colloidal bismuth subcitrate plus antibiotics or sucralphate alone. *Gut* 1993;**34**:466–9.

126 Mantzaris GJ, Hatzis A, Tamvakologos G, Petraki K, Spiliadis C, Triadaphyllou G. Prospective, randomized, investigator-blind trial of *Helicobacter pylori* infection treatment in patients with refractory duodenal ulcers. Healing and long-term relapse rates. *Dig Dis Sci* 1993;**38**:1132–6.

127 Wagner S, Gebel M, Haruma K *et al.* Bismuth subsalicylate in the treatment of H2-blocker resistant duodenal ulcers: role of *Helicobacter pylori*. *Gut* 1992;**33**:179–83.

128 Zheng ZT, Wang ZY, Chu YX, Li YN, Li QF, Lin SR, Xu SR. Double-blind short-term trial of furazolidone in peptc ulcer. *Lancet* 1985;**i**:1048–9.

129 Zhao HY, Li G, Guo J, Yan Z, Sun S, Li L, Duan Y, Yue F. Furazolidone in peptic ulcer. *Lancet* 1985;**ii**:276–7.

130 Quintero Diaz M, Sotto Eschobar A. Metronidazole versus cimetidine in the treatment of gastroduodenal ulcer. *Lancet* 1986;**i**:907.

131 Lam SK, Ching CK, Lai KC, Wong BC, Lai CL, Chan CK, Ong L. Does treatment of *Helicobacter pylori* with antibiotics alone heal duodenal ulcer? A randomised double blind placebo controlled study. *Gut* 1997;**41**:43–8.

132 Hosking SW, Ling TKW, Chung SCS *et al.* Duodenal ulcer healing by eradication of *Helicobacter pylori* without anti-acid treatment: randomized controlled trial. *Lancet* 1994;**343**:508–10.

133 Logan RPH, Gummett PA, Misiewicz JJ, Karim QN, Walker MM, Baron JH. One week's anti-*Helicobacter pylori* treatment for duodenal ulcer. *Gut* 1994;**35**:15–18.

134 Laine L, Suchower L, Frantz J, Connors A, Neil G. Twice-daily, 10-day triple therapy with omeprazole, amoxicillin, and clarithromycin for *Helicobacter pylori* eradication in duodenal ulcer disease: results of three multicenter, double-blind, United States trials. *Am J Gastroenterol* 1998;**93**:2106–12.

135 Wheeldon TU, Hoang TT, Phung DC, Bjorkman A, Granstrom M, Sorberg M. *Helicobacter pylori* eradication and peptic ulcer healing: the impact of deleting the proton pump inhibitor and using a once-daily treatment. *Aliment Pharmacol Ther* 2003;**18**:93–100.

136 Harris AW, Misiewicz JJ, Bardhan KD *et al.* Incidence of duodenal ulcer healing after 1 week of proton pump inhibitor triple therapy for eradication of *Helicobacter pylori*. The Lansoprazole Helicobacter Study Group. *Aliment Pharmacol Ther* 1998;**12**:741–5.

137 Labenz J, Idstrom JP, Tillenburg B, Peitz U, Adamek RJ, Borsch G. One-week low-dose triple therapy for *Helicobacter pylori* is sufficient for relief from symptoms and healing of duodenal ulcers. *Aliment Pharmacol Ther* 1997;**11**:89–93.

138 Goh KL, Navaratnam P, Peh SC *et al.* *Helicobacter pylori* eradication with short-term therapy leads to duodenal ulcer healing without the need for continued acid suppression therapy. *Eur J Gastroenterol Hepatol* 1996;**8**:421–3.

139 Gisbert JP, Boixeda D, Martín DA *et al.* [New one-week triple therapies with metronidazole for the eradication of *Helicobacter pylori*: clarithromycin or amoxycillin as the second antibiotic). *Med Clin (Barc)* 1998;**110**:1–5.

140 Tulassay Z, Kryszewski A, Dite P *et al.* One week of treatment with esomeprazole-based triple therapy eradicates *Helicobacter pylori* and heals patients with duodenal ulcer disease. *Eur J Gastroenterol Hepatol* 2001;**13**:1457–65.

141 Marchi S, Costa F, Bellini M *et al.* Ranitidine bismuth citrate-based triple therapy for seven days, with or without further anti-secretory therapy, is highly effective in patients with duodenal ulcer and *Helicobacter pylori* infection. *Eur J Gastroenterol Hepatol* 2001;**13**:547–50.

142 Tepes B, Krizman I, Gorensek M, Gubina M, Orel I. Is a one-week course of triple anti-*Helicobacter pylori* therapy sufficient to control active duodenal ulcer? *Aliment Pharmacol Ther* 2001;**15**:1037–45.

143 Colin R. Duodenal ulcer healing with 1-week eradication triple therapy followed, or not, by anti-secretory treatment: a multicentre double-blind placebo-controlled trial. *Aliment Pharmacol Ther* 2002;**16**:1157–62.

144 Marzio L, Cellini L, Angelucci D. Triple therapy for 7 days vs. triple therapy for 7 days plus omeprazole for 21 days in treatment of active duodenal ulcer with *Helicobacter pylori* infection. A double blind placebo controlled trial. *Dig Liver Dis* 2003;**35**:20–3.

145 Laine L. *Helicobacter pylori* and complicated ulcer disease. *Am J Med* 1996;**100**:52S–59S.

146 Bardhan KD, Nayyar AK, Royston C. The outcome of bleeding duodenal ulcer in the era of H_2 receptor antagonist therapy. *QJM* 1998;**91**:231–7.

147 Murray WR, Cooper G, Laferla G, Rogers P, Archibald M. Maintenance ranitidine treatment after haemorrhage from a duodenal ulcer: a 3 year follow up study. *Scand J Gastroenterol* 1988;**23**:183–7.

148 Jensen DM, Cheng S, Kovacs TOG *et al.* A controlled study of ranitidine for the prevention of recurrent hemorrhage from duodenal ulcer. *N Engl J Med* 1994;**330**:382–6.

149 Hosking SW, Yung MY, Chung SC, Li AKC. Differing prevalence of *Helicobacter* in bleeding and nonbleeding ulcers. *Gastroenterology* 1992;**102**:A85.

150 Lai KC, Hui WM, Wong WM, Wong BC, Hu WH, Ching CK, Lam SK. Treatment of *Helicobacter pylori* in patients with duodenal ulcer hemorrhage – a long-term randomized, controlled study. *Am J Gastroenterol* 2000;**95**: 2225–32.

151 Jaspersen D, Körner T, Schorr W, Brennenstuhl M, Hammar CH. Omeprazole-amoxycillin therapy for eradication of *Helicobacter pylori* in duodenal ulcer bleeding: preliminary results of a pilot study. *J Gastroenterology* 1995;**30**: 319–321.

152 Macri G, Milani S, Surrenti E, Passaleva MT, Salvadori G, Surrenti C. Eradication of *Helicobacter pylori* reduces the rate of duodenal ulcer rebleeding: a long-term follow-up study. *Am J Gastroenterol* 1998;**93**:925–7.

153 Arkkila PE, Seppala K, Kosunen TU *et al.* Eradication of *Helicobacter pylori* improves the healing rate and reduces the relapse rate of non-bleeding ulcers in patients with bleeding peptic ulcer. *Am J Gastroenterol* 2003;**98**: 2149–56.

154 Graham DY, Hepps KS, Ramirez FC, Lew GM, Saeed ZA. Treatment of *Helicobacter pylori* reduces the rate of re-bleeding in peptic ulcer disease. *Scand J Gastroenterol* 1993;**28**:939–42.

155 Santander C, Grávalos RG, Gómez-Cedenilla A, Cantero J, Pajares JM. Antimicrobial therapy for *Helicobacter pylori* infection versus long-term maintenance antisecretion treatment in the prevention of recurrent hemorrhage from peptic ulcer: prospective nonrandomized trial on 125 patients. *Am J Gastroenterol* 1996;**91**:1549–52.

156 Riemann JF, Schilling D, Schauwecker P, Wehlen G, Dorlars D, Kohler B, Maier M. Cure with omeprazole plus amoxicillin versus long-term ranitidine therapy in *Helicobacter pylori*-associated peptic ulcer bleeding. *Gastrointest Endosc* 1997;**46**:299–304.

157 Sung JJY, Leung WK, Suen R *et al.* One-week antibiotics versus maintenance acid suppression therapy for *Helicobacter pylori*-associated peptic ulcer bleeding. *Dig Dis Sci* 1997;**42**:2524–8.

158 Jaspersen D, Koerner T, Schorr W, Brennenstuhl M, Raschka C, Hammar CH. *Helicobacter pylori* eradication reduces the rate of rebleeding in ulcer hemorrhage. *Gastrointest Endosc* 1995;**41**:5–7.

159 Labenz J, Borsch G. Role of *Helicobacter pylori* eradication in the prevention of peptic ulcer bleeding relapse. *Digestion* 1994;**55**:19–23.

160 Rokkas T, Karameris A, Mavrogeorgis A, Rallis E, Giannikos N. Eradication of *Helicobacter pylori* reduces the possibility of rebleeding in peptic ulcer disease. *Gastrointest Endosc* 1995;**41**:1–4.

161 Gisbert J, Khorrami S, Carballo F, Calvet X, Gene E, Dominguez-Munoz J. *H. pylori* eradication therapy vs. antisecretory non-eradication therapy (with or without long-term maintenance antisecretory therapy) for the prevention of recurrent bleeding from peptic ulcer. *Cochrane Database Syst Rev* 2003;**4**:CD004062.

162 Liu CC, Lee CL, Chan CC *et al.* Maintenance treatment is not necessary after *Helicobacter pylori* eradication and healing of bleeding peptic ulcer: a 5-year prospective, randomized, controlled study. *Arch Intern Med* 2003;**163**: 2020–4.

163 Simpson CJ, Lamont G, Macdonald I, Smith IS. Effect of cimetidine on prognosis after simple closure of perforated duodenal ulcer. *Br J Surg* 1987;**74**:104–5.

164 Svanes C, Øvrebø K, Søreide O. Ulcer bleeding and perforation: non-steroidal anti-inflammatory drugs or *Helicobacter pylori*. *Scand J Gastroenterol* 1996; **31(Suppl 220)**:128–31.

165 Reinbach DH, Cruickshank G, McColl KE. Acute perforated duodenal ulcer is not associated with *Helicobacter pylori* infection. *Gut* 1993;**34**:1344–7.

166 Kate V, Ananthakrishnan N, Badrinath S. Effect of *Helicobacter pylori* eradication on the ulcer recurrence rate after simple closure of perforated duodenal ulcer: retrospective and prospective randomized controlled studies. *Br J Surg* 2001;**88**:1054–8.

167 Metzger J, Styger S, Sieber C, von Flue M, Vogelbach P, Harder F. Prevalence of *Helicobacter pylori* infection in peptic ulcer perforations. *Swiss Med Wkly* 2001;**131**: 99–103.

168 Sebastian M, Chandran VP, Elashaal YI, Sim AJ. *Helicobacter pylori* infection in perforated peptic ulcer disease. *Br J Surg* 1995;**82**:360–2.

169 Ng EK, Chung SC, Sung JJ *et al.* High prevalence of *Helicobacter pylori* infection in duodenal ulcer perforations not caused by non-steroidal anti-inflammatory drugs. *Br J Surg* 1996;**83**:1779–1781.

170 Matsukura N, Onda M, Tokunaga A *et al.* Role of *Helicobacter pylori* infection in perforation of peptic ulcer: an age- and gender-matched case-control study. *J Clin Gastroenterol* 1997;**25(Suppl 1)**:S235–S239.

171 Ng EK, Lam YH, Sung JJ *et al.* Eradication of *Helicobacter pylori* prevents recurrence of ulcer after simple closure of

duodenal ulcer perforation: randomized controlled trial. *Ann Surg* 2000;**231**:153–8.

172 De Boer WA, Driessen WM. Resolution of gastric outlet obstruction after eradication of *Helicobacter pylori*. *J Clin Gastroenterol* 1995;**21**:329–30.

173 Annibale B, Marignani M, Luzzi I, Delle FG. Peptic ulcer and duodenal stenosis: role of *Helicobacter pylori* infection. *Ital J Gastroenterol* 1995;**27**:26–8.

174 Lam Y, Lau JY, Law KB, Sung JJ, Chung SS. Endoscopic balloon dilation and *Helicobacter pylori* eradication in the treatment of gastric outlet obstruction. *Gastrointest Endosc* 1997;**46**:379–80.

175 Taskin V, Gurer I, Ozyilkan E, Sare M, Hilmioglu F. Effect of *Helicobacter pylori* eradication on peptic ulcer disease complicated with outlet obstruction. *Helicobacter* 2000;**5**:38–40.

176 Gisbert JP, Pajares JM. Review article: *Helicobacter pylori* infection and gastric outlet obstruction – prevalence of the infection and role of antimicrobial treatment. *Aliment Pharmacol Ther* 2002;**16**:1203–8.

177 Howden CW, Jones DB, Peace KE, Burget DW, Hunt RH. The treatment of gastric ulcer with antisecretory drugs. Relationship of pharmacological effect to healing rates. *Dig Dis Sci* 1988;**33**:619–24.

178 Holt S, Howden CW. Omeprazole: overview and opinion. *Dig Dis Sci* 1991;**36**:385–93.

179 Howden CW, Hunt RH. The relationship between suppression of acidity and gastric ulcer healing rates. *Aliment Pharmacol Ther* 1990;**4**:25–33.

180 Howden CW, Burget DW, Hunt RH. A meta-analysis to predict gastric ulcer healing from acid suppression. *Gastroenterology* 1991;**100**:A13.

181 Howden CW, Burget DW, Hunt RH. A comparison of different drug classes with respect to rapidity of healing of gastric ulcer (GU). *Gastroenterology* 1993;**104**:A105.

182 Salas M, Ward A, Caro J. Are proton pump inhibitors the first choice for acute treatment of gastric ulcers? A meta analysis of randomized clinical trials. *BMC Gastroenterol* 2002;**2**:17.

183 Witzel L, Gutz H, Huttemann W, Schepp W. Pantoprazole versus omeprazole in the treatment of acute gastric ulcers. *Aliment Pharmacol Ther* 1995;**9**:19–24.

184 Dekkers CP, Beker JA, Thjodleifsson B, Gabryelewicz A, Bell NE, Humphries TJ. Comparison of rabeprazole 20 mg vs. omeprazole 20 mg in the treatment of active gastric ulcer – a European multicentre study. The European Rabeprazole Study Group. *Aliment Pharmacol Ther* 1998;**12**:789–95.

185 Pilotto A, Di Mario F, Battaglia G *et al.* The efficacy of two doses of omeprazole for short-and long-term peptic ulcer treatment in the elderly. *Clin Ther* 1994;**16**:935–41.

186 Kovacs TO, Campbell D, Haber M, Rose P, Jennings DE, Richter J. Double-blind comparison of lansoprazole 15 mg, lansoprazole 30 mg, and placebo in the maintenance of healed gastric ulcer. *Dig Dis Sci* 1998;**43**:779–85.

187 Labenz J, Börsch G. Evidence for the essential role of *Helicobacter pylori* in gastric ulcer disease. *Gut* 1994;**35**:19–22.

188 Malfertheiner P, Kirchner T, Kist M *et al. Helicobacter pylori* eradication and gastric ulcer healing – comparison of three pantoprazole-based triple therapies. *Aliment Pharmacol Ther* 2003;**17**:1125–35.

189 Tatsuta M, Ishikawa H, Iishi H, Okuda S, Yokota Y. Reduction of gastric ulcer recurrence after suppression of *Helicobacter pylori* by cefixime. *Gut* 1990;**31**:973–6.

190 Asaka M, Ohtaki T, Kato M *et al.* Causal role of *Helicobacter pylori* in peptic ulcer relapse. *J Gastroenterol* 1994;**29(Suppl 7)**:134–8.

191 Sung JJY, Chung SCS, Ling TKW *et al.* Antibacterial treatment of gastric ulcers associated with *Helicobacter pylori*. *N Engl J Med* 1995;**332**:139–42.

192 Bayerdörffer E, Miehlke S, Lehn N *et al.* Cure of gastric ulcer disease after cure of *Helicobacter pylori* infection – German Gastric Ulcer Study. *Eur J Gastroenterol Hepatol* 1996;**8**:343–9.

193 Malfertheiner P, Bayerdorffer E, Diete U *et al.* The GU-MACH study: the effect of 1-week omeprazole triple therapy on *Helicobacter pylori* infection in patients with gastric ulcer. *Aliment Pharmacol Ther* 1999;**13**:703–12.

194 Higuchi K, Fujiwara Y, Tominaga K *et al.* Is eradication sufficient to heal gastric ulcers in patients infected with *Helicobacter pylori*? A randomized, controlled, prospective study. *Aliment Pharmacol Ther* 2003;**17**:111–17.

195 Hopkins RJ, Girardi LS, Turney EA. *Helicobacter pylori* eradication as a surrogate for reduced peptic ulcer recurrence: a literature-based meta-analysis. *Gut* 1995;**37 (Suppl 1)**:A46(181).

196 Huang JQ, Hunt RH. Review: eradication of *Helicobacter pylori*. Problems and recommendations. *J Gastroenterol Hepatol* 1997;**12**:590–8.

197 Penston JG, McColl KEL. Eradication of *Helicobacter pylori*: an objective assessment of current therapies. *Br J Clin Pharmacol* 1997;**43**:223–43.

198 Hunt RH. Hp and pH: implications for the eradication of *Helicobacter pylori*. *Scand J Gastroenterol Suppl* 1993;**196**:12–16.

199 Hunt RH. pH and Hp – gastric acid secretion and *Helicobacter pylori*: implications for ulcer healing and eradication of the organism. *Am J Gastroenterol* 1993;**88**:481–3.

200 Gatta L, Perna F, Figura N *et al.* Antimicrobial activity of esomeprazole versus omeprazole against *Helicobacter pylori*. *J Antimicrob Chemother* 2003;**51**:439–42.

201 Chiba N, Wilkinson JM, Hunt RH. Clarithromycin (C) or amoxicillin (A) dual and triple therapies in H.pylori (Hp) eradication: A meta-analysis. *Gut* 1995;**37(Suppl 2)**:A31(T124).

202 Unge P, Berstad A. Pooled analysis of anti-*Helicobacter pylori* treatment regimens. *Scand J Gastroenterol* 1996;**31**:27–40.

203 Unge P. What other regimens are under investigation to treat *Helicobacter pylori* infection? *Gastroenterology* 1997;**113**:S131–S148.

204 Chiba N, Hunt RH. Drug therapy of *H.pylori* infection: a meta-analysis. In: Bianchi Porro G, Scarpignato C, eds. *Clinical Pharmacology and Therapy of* H. pylori *Infection*. Basel: Karger, 1999.

205 Miyoshi M, Mizuno M, Ishiki K *et al.* A randomized open trial for comparison of proton pump inhibitors, omeprazole versus rabeprazole, in dual therapy for *Helicobacter pylori* infection in relation to CYP2C19 genetic polymorphism. *J Gastroenterol Hepatol* 2001;**16**:723–8.

206 Malaty HM, El-Zimaity HMT, Genta RM, Cole RA, Graham DY. High-dose proton pump inhibitor plus amoxycillin for the treatment or retreatment of *Helicobacter pylori* infection. *Aliment Pharmacol Ther* 1996;**10**:1001–4.

207 van der Hulst RW, Weel JF *et al.* Treatment of *Helicobacter pylori* infection with low or high dose omeprazole combined with amoxycillin and the effect of early re-treatment. *Aliment Pharmacol Ther* 1996;**10**:165–71.

208 Gisbert JP, Khorrami S, Calvet X, Pajares JM. Systematic review: Rabeprazole-based therapies in *Helicobacter pylori* eradication. *Aliment Pharmacol Ther* 2003;**17**:751–64.

209 Peterson WL, Graham DY, Marshall BJ *et al.* Clarithromycin as monotherapy for eradication of *Helicobacter pylori*: a randomized, double-blind trial. *Am J Gastroenterol* 1993;**88**:1860–4.

210 Hoshiya S, Watanabe K, Tokunaga K *et al.* Relationship between eradication therapy and clarithromycin-resistant *Helicobacter pylori* in Japan. *J Gastroenterology* 2000;**35**:10–14.

211 Di Caro S, Assunta ZM, Cremonini F *et al.* Levofloxacin-based regimens for the eradication of *Helicobacter pylori*. *Eur J Gastroenterol Hepatol* 2002;**14**:1309–12.

212 Bazzoli F, Zagari RM, Fossi S, Pozzato P, Roda A, Roda E. Efficacy and tolerability of a short term, low dose triple therapy for eradication of *Helicobacter pylori*. *Gastroenterology* 1993;**104**:A40.

213 Sheu BS, Wu JJ, Yang HB, Huang AH, Lin XZ. One-week proton pump inhibitor-based triple therapy eradicates residual *Helicobacter pylori* after failed dual therapy. *J Formos Med Assoc* 1998;**97**:266–70.

214 Lind T, Veldhuyzen van Zanten SJO, Unge P *et al.* Eradication of *Helicobacter pylori* using one week triple therapies combining omeprazole with two antimicrobials – the MACH 1 study. *Helicobacter* 1996;**1**:138–44.

215 Malfertheiner P, Megraud F, O'Morain C *et al.* Current concepts in the management of *Helicobacter pylori* infection – the Maastricht 2–2000 Consensus Report. *Aliment Pharmacol Ther* 2002;**16**:167–80.

216 Hunt RH, Fallone C, Veldhuyzen van Zanten SJO, Sherman P, Smaill F, Thomson ABR, Canadian Helicobacter Study Group. Risks and benefits of *Helicobacter pylori* eradication: current status. *Can J Gastroenterology* 2002;**16**:57–62.

217 Peura DA. The report of the Digestive Health Initiative (SM) International Update Conference on *Helicobacter pylori*. *Gastroenterology* 1997;**113**:S4–S8.

218 Lam SK, Talley NJ. Report of the 1997 Asia Pacific Consensus Conference on the management of *Helicobacter pylori* infection. *J Gastroenterol Hepatol* 1998;**13**:1–12.

219 Schwartz H, Krause R, Sahba B *et al.* Triple versus dual therapy for eradicating *Helicobacter pylori* and preventing ulcer recurrence: a randomized, double- blind, multicenter study of lansoprazole, clarithromycin, and/or amoxicillin in different dosing regimens. *Am J Gastroenterol* 1998;**93**:584–90.

220 Lamouliatte H, Cayla R, Zerbib F *et al.* Dual therapy using a double dose of lansoprazole with amoxicillin versus triple therapy using a double dose of lansoprazole, amoxicillin, and clarithromycin to eradicate *Helicobacter pylori* infection: results of a prospective randomized open study. *Am J Gastroenterol* 1998;**93**:1531–4.

221 Spinzi GC, Bierti L, Bortoli A *et al.* Comparison of omeprazole and lansoprazole in short-term triple therapy for *Helicobacter pylori* infection. *Aliment Pharmacol Ther* 1998;**12**:433–8.

222 Fennerty MB, Kovacs TO, Krause R *et al.* A comparison of 10 and 14 days of lansoprazole triple therapy for eradication of *Helicobacter pylori*. *Arch Intern Med* 1998;**158**:1651–6.

223 Cammarota G, Tursi A, Papa A *et al.* Helicobacter pylori eradication using one-week low-dose lansoprazole plus amoxycillin and either clarithromycin or azithromycin. *Aliment Pharmacol Ther* 1996;**10**:997–1000.

224 Takimoto T, Satoh K, Taniguchi Y *et al.* The efficacy and safety of one-week triple therapy with lansoprazole, clarithromycin, and metronidazole for the treatment of *Helicobacter pylori* infection in Japanese patients. *Helicobacter* 1997;**2**:86–91.

225 Lazzaroni M, Bargiggia S, Porro GB. Triple therapy with ranitidine or lansoprazole in the treatment of *Helicobacter pylori*-associated duodenal ulcer. *Am J Gastroenterol* 1997;**92**:649–52.

226 Chey WD, Fisher L, Elta GH *et al.* Bismuth subsalicylate instead of metronidazole with lansoprazole and clarithromycin for *Helicobacter pylori* infection: a randomized trial. *Am J Gastroenterol* 1997;**92**:1483–6.

227 Misiewicz JJ, Harris AW, Bardhan KD *et al.* One week triple therapy for *Helicobacter pylori*: a multicentre comparative study. Lansoprazole Helicobacter Study Group. *Gut* 1997;**41**:735–9.

228 Adamek RJ, Szymanski C, Pfaffenbach B. Pantoprazole vs omeprazole in one-week low-dose triple therapy for cure of *H. pylori* infection. *Gastroenterology* 1997;**112**:A53.

229 Labenz J, Tillenburg B, Weismüller J, Lütke A, Stolte M. Efficacy and tolerability of a one-week triple therapy consisting of pantoprazole, clarithromycin and amoxicillin for cure of *Helicobacter pylori* infection in patients with duodenal ulcer. *Aliment Pharmacol Ther* 1997;**11**:95–100.

230 Frevel M, Daake H, Janisch HD, Kellner HU, Krezdorn HG, Tanneberger D, Wack R. Eradication of *Helicobacter pylori* with pantoprazole and two anti-biotics: a comparison of two short-term regimens. *Aliment Pharmacol Ther* 2000;**14**:1151–7.

231 Laine L. Review article: esomeprazole in the treatment of *Helicobacter pylori*. *Aliment Pharmacol Ther* 2002;**16(Suppl 4)**:115–18.

232 Catalano F, Terminella C, Branciforte G, Bentivegna C, Brogna A, Scalia A. Eradication therapy with rabeprazole versus omeprazole in the treatment of active duodenal ulcer. *Digestion* 2002;**66**:154–9.

233 Hawkey CJ, Atherton JC, Treichel HC, Thjodleifsson B, Ravic M. Safety and efficacy of 7-day rabeprazole- and omeprazole-based triple therapy regimens for the

eradication of *Helicobacter pylori* in patients with documented peptic ulcer disease. *Aliment Pharmacol Ther* 2003;**17**:1065–74.

234 Murakami K, Sato R, Okimoto T *et al.* Eradication rates of clarithromycin-resistant *Helicobacter pylori* using either rabeprazole or lansoprazole plus amoxicillin and clarithromycin. *Aliment Pharmacol Ther* 2002;**16**: 1933–8.

235 Vergara M, Vallve M, Gisbert JP, Calvet X. Meta-analysis: comparative efficacy of different proton-pump inhibitors in triple therapy for *Helicobacter pylori* eradication. *Aliment Pharmacol Ther* 2003;**18**:647–54.

236 Ulmer HJ, Beckerling A, Gatz G. Recent use of proton pump inhibitor-based triple therapies for the eradication of *H. pylori*: a broad data review. *Helicobacter* 2003;**8**:95–104.

237 Gisbert JP, Gonzalez L, Calvet X *et al.* Proton pump inhibitor, clarithromycin and either amoxycillin or nitroimidazole: a meta-analysis of eradication of helicobacter pylori [In Process Citation]. *Aliment Pharmacol Ther* 2000;**14**:1319–28.

238 Janssen MJ, Van Oijen AH, Verbeek AL, Jansen JB, De Boer WA. A systematic comparison of triple therapies for treatment of *Helicobacter pylori* infection with proton pump inhibitor/ranitidine bismuth citrate plus clarithromycin and either amoxicillin or a nitroimidazole. *Aliment Pharmacol Ther* 2001;**15**:613–24.

239 Bazzoli F, Zagari RM, Pozzato P *et al.* Low-dose lansoprazole and clarithromycin plus metronidazole vs. full-dose lansoprazole and clarithromycin plus amoxicillin for eradication of *Helicobacter pylori* infection. *Aliment Pharmacol Ther* 2002;**16**:153–8.

240 Huang JQ, Hunt RH. The importance of clarithromycin dose in the management of *Helicobacter pylori* infection: a meta-analysis of triple therapies with a proton pump inhibitor, clarithromycin and amoxicillin or metronidazole. *Aliment Pharmacol Ther* 1999;**13**:719–29.

241 Ellenrieder V, Fensterer H, Waurick M, Adler G, Glasbrenner B. Influence of clarithromycin dosage on pantoprazole combined triple therapy for eradication of *Helicobacter pylori*. *Aliment Pharmacol Ther* 1998;**12**:613–18.

242 Veldhuyzen vZ, Machado S, Lee J. One-week triple therapy with esomeprazole, clarithromycin and metronidazole provides effective eradication of *Helicobacter pylori* infection. *Aliment Pharmacol Ther* 2003;**17**:1381–7.

243 Lind T, Veldhuyzen vZ, Unge P *et al.* Eradication of *Helicobacter pylori* using one-week triple therapies combining omeprazole with two antimicrobials: the MACH I Study. *Helicobacter* 1996;**1**:138–44.

244 Vakil N, Schwartz HJ, Lanza FL, Nardi L, Hahne W, Barth J. A prospective, controlled, randomized trial of 3-, 7-, and 10-day rabeprazole-based triple therapy for *H. pylori* eradication in the USA. *Gastroenterology* 2002; **122(Suppl 1)**: A65(551).

245 Maconi G, Parente F, Russo A, Vago L, Imbesi V, Porro GB. Do some patients with *Helicobacter pylori* infection benefit from an extension to 2 weeks of a proton pump inhibitor-based triple eradication therapy? *Am J Gastroenterol* 2001;**96**:359–66.

246 Calvet X, Garcia N, Lopez T, Gisbert JP, Gene E, Roque M. A meta-analysis of short versus long therapy with a proton pump inhibitor, clarithromycin and either metronidazole or amoxycillin for treating *Helicobacter pylori* infection. *Aliment Pharmacol Ther* 2000;**14**:603–9.

247 Calvet X, Gene E, Lopez T, Gisbert JP. What is the optimal length of proton pump inhibitor-based triple therapies for *H. pylori*? A cost-effectiveness analysis. *Aliment Pharmacol Ther* 2001;**15**:1067–76.

248 van der Wouden EJ, Thijs JC, Van Zwet AA, Sluiter WJ, Kleibeuker JH. The influence of *in vitro* nitroimidazole resistance on the efficacy of nitroimidazole-containing anti-*Helicobacter pylori* regimens: a meta-analysis. *Am J Gastroenterol* 1999;**94**:1751–9.

249 Lind T, Mégraud F, Unge P *et al.* The MACH 2 study: role of omeprazole in eradication of *Helicobacter pylori* with 1-week triple therapies. *Gastroenterology* 1999;**116**:248–53.

250 Megraud F, Lehn N, Lind T *et al.* Antimicrobial susceptibility testing of *Helicobacter pylori* in a large multicenter trial: the MACH 2 study. *Antimicrob Agents Chemother* 1999;**43**:2747–52.

251 Chiba N, Sinclair P. Metronidazole 500 mg is as effective as metronidazole 400 mg in the MACH 1 regimen for *H. pylori* eradication: a meta-analysis. *Can J Gastroenterology* 1998;**12(Suppl A)**:91A.

252 Bardhan K, Bayerdorffer E, Veldhuyzen van Zanten SJ *et al.* The HOMER Study: the effect of increasing the dose of metronidazole when given with omeprazole and amoxicillin to cure *Helicobacter* pylori infection. *Helicobacter* 2000;**5**: 196-201.

253 Lerang F, Moum B, Haug JB, Berge T. Highly effective triple therapy with omeprazole, amoxicillin and clarithromycin in previous *H. pylori* treatment failures. *Gut* 1996; **39(Suppl 2)**:A36(4A:25).

254 Laine L, Fennerty MB, Osato M *et al.* Esomeprazole-based *Helicobacter pylori* eradication therapy and the effect of antibiotic resistance: results of three US multicenter, double-blind trials. *Am J Gastroenterol* 2000;**95**:3393–8.

255 Laine L, Hunt R, El Zimaity H, Nguyen B, Osato M, Spenard J, on behalf of the other 45 investigators. Bismuth-based quadruple therapy using a single capsule of bismuth biskalcitrate, metronidazole, and tetracycline given with omeprazole versus omeprazole, amoxicillin, and clarithromycin for eradication of *Helicobacter pylori* in duodenal ulcer patients: a prospective, randomized, multicenter, North American trial. *Am J Gastroenterol* 2003;**98**:562–7.

256 Miki I, Aoyama N, Sakai T *et al.* Impact of clarithromycin resistance and CYP2C19 genetic polymorphism on treatment efficacy of *Helicobacter pylori* infection with lansoprazole- or rabeprazole-based triple therapy in Japan. *Eur J Gastroenterol Hepatol* 2003;**15**:27–33.

257 Kawabata H, Habu Y, Tomioka H *et al.* Effect of different proton pump inhibitors, differences in CYP2C19 genotype and antibiotic resistance on the eradication rate of *Helicobacter pylori* infection by a 1-week regimen of proton pump inhibitor, amoxicillin and clarithromycin. *Aliment Pharmacol Ther* 2003;**17**:259–64.

258 Murakami K, Fujioka T, Okimoto T, Sato R, Kodama M, Nasu M. Drug combinations with amoxycillin reduce selection of clarithromycin resistance during *Helicobacter pylori* eradication therapy. *Int J Antimicrob Agents* 2002; **19**:67–70.

259 Wermeille J, Cunningham M, Dederding JP *et al.* Failure of *Helicobacter pylori* eradication: is poor compliance the main cause? *Gastroenterology Clin Biol* 2002;**26**:216–19.

260 Broutet N, Tchamgoue S, Pereira E, Lamouliatte H, Salamon R, Megraud F. Risk factors for failure of *Helicobacter pylori* therapy – results of an individual data analysis of 2751 patients. *Aliment Pharmacol Ther* 2003;**17**:99–109.

261 De Boer WA. Eradication therapy should be different for dyspeptic patients than for ulcer patients. *Can J Gastroenterology* 2003;**17(Suppl B)**:41B–45B.

262 Boixeda D, Martin DA, Bermejo F, Lopez SA, Hernandez RF, Garcia PA. Seven-day proton pump inhibitor, amoxicillin and clarithromycin triple therapy. factors that influence *Helicobacter pylori* eradications success. *Rev Esp Enferm Dig* 2003;**95**:206–9, 202.

263 Fischbach LA, Goodman KJ, Feldman M, Aragaki C. Sources of variation of *Helicobacter pylori* treatment success in adults worldwide: a meta-analysis. *Int J Epidemiol* 2002;**31**:128–39.

264 Moayyedi P, Sahay P, Tompkins DS, Axon AT. Efficacy and optimum dose of omeprazole in a new 1-week triple therapy regimen to eradicate *Helicobacter pylori*. *Eur J Gastroenterol Hepatol* 1995;**7**:835–40.

265 Bazzoli F, Zagari M, Pozzato P *et al.* Evaluation of short-term low-dose triple therapy for the eradication of *Helicobacter pylori* by factorial design in a randomized, double-blind, controlled study. *Aliment Pharmacol Ther* 1998;**12**:439–45.

266 Laine L, Frantz JE, Baker A, Neil GA. A United States multicentre trial of dual and proton pump inhibitor-based triple therapies for *Helicobacter pylori*. *Aliment Pharmacol Ther* 1997;**11**:913–17.

267 Vallve M, Vergara M, Gisbert JP, Calvet X. Single vs. double dose of a proton pump inhibitor in triple therapy for *Helicobacter pylori* eradication: a meta-analysis. *Aliment Pharmacol Ther* 2002;**16**:1149–56.

268 Laine L, Estrada R, Trujillo M *et al.* Once-daily therapy for H. pylori infection: a randomized comparison of four regimens. *Am J Gastroenterol* 1999;**94**:962–6.

269 Graham DY, Hammoud F, el Zimaity HM, Kim JG, Osato MS, el Serag HB. Meta-analysis: proton pump inhibitor or H2-receptor antagonist for *Helicobacter pylori* eradication. *Aliment Pharmacol Ther* 2003;**17**:1229–36.

270 Gisbert JP, Khorrami S, Calvet X, Gabriel R, Carballo F, Pajares JM. Meta-analysis: proton pump inhibitors vs. H2-receptor antagonists – their efficacy with anti-biotics in *Helicobacter pylori* eradication. *Aliment Pharmacol Ther* 2003;**18**:757–66.

271 Graham DY, Lew GM, Malaty HM *et al.* Factors influencing the eradication of *Helicobacter pylori* with triple therapy. *Gastroenterology* 1992;**102**:493–6.

272 Katelaris PH, Forbes GM, Talley NJ, Crotty B. A randomized comparison of quadruple and triple therapies for *Helicobacter pylori* eradication: The QUADRATE Study. *Gastroenterology* 2002;**123**:1763–9.

273 Chiba N, Hunt RH. Bismuth, metronidazole and tetracycline (BMT) +/− acid suppression in *H. pylori* eradication: a meta-analysis. *Gut* 1996;**39(Suppl 2)**:A36(4A:27).

274 Huang JQ, Chiba N, Wilkinson J, Hunt RH. Attempt by meta-analysis to define the optimal treatment regimen for eradicating *Helicobacter pylori* (*H. pylori*) infection. *Can J Gastroenterology* 1997;**11(Suppl A)**:44A(S14).

275 de Boer W, Driessen W, Jansz A, Tytgat G. Effect of acid suppression on efficacy of treatment for *Helicobacter pylori* infection. *Lancet* 1995;**345**:817–20.

276 De Boer WA, Driessen WMM, Potters HVPJ, Tytgat GNJ. Randomized study comparing 1 with 2 weeks of quadruple therapy for eradicating *Helicobacter pylori*. *Am J Gastroenterol* 1994;**89**:1993–7.

277 Calvet X, Ducons J, Guardiola J, Tito L, Andreu V, Bory F, Guirao R. One-week triple vs. quadruple therapy for *Helicobacter pylori* infection – a randomized trial. *Aliment Pharmacol Ther* 2002;**16**:1261–7.

278 Mantzaris GJ, Petraki K, Archavlis E *et al.* Omeprazole triple therapy versus omeprazole quadruple therapy for healing duodenal ulcer and eradication of *Helicobacter pylori* infection: a 24-month follow-up study. *Eur J Gastroenterol Hepatol* 2002;**14**:1237–43.

279 De Boer WA, van Etten RJXM, Lai JYL, Schneeberger PM, van de Wouw BAM, Driessen WMM. Effectiveness of quadruple therapy using lansoprazole, instead of omeprazole, in curing *Helicobacter pylori* infection. *Helicobacter* 1996;**1**:145–50.

280 Pai CG, Thomas CP, Biswas A, Rao S, Ramnarayan K. Quadruple therapy for initial eradication of *Helicobacter pylori* In peptic ulcer: comparison with triple therapy. Indian J *Gastroenterology* 2003;**22**:85–7.

281 Boixeda D, Bermejo F, Martin-de-Argila C, Lopez-Sanroman A, Defarges V, Hernandez-Ranz F, Milicua JM, Garcia-Plaza A. Efficacy of quadruple therapy with pantoprazole, bismuth, tetracycline and metronidazole as rescue treatment for *Helicobacter pylori* infection. *Aliment Pharmacol Ther* 2002;**16**:1457–1460.

282 Perri F, Festa V, Clemente R, Villani MR, Quitadamo M, Caruso N, Bergoli ML, Andriulli A. Randomized study of two "rescue" therapies for *Helicobacter pylori*-infected patients after failure of standard triple therapies. *Am J Gastroenterol* 2001;**96**:58–62.

283 Perri F, Festa V, Merla A, Barberani F, Pilotto A, Andriulli A. Randomized study of different 'second-line' therapies for *Helicobacter pylori* infection after failure of the standard 'Maastricht triple therapy'. *Aliment Pharmacol Ther* 2003;**18**:815–820.

284 Nista EC, Candelli M, Cremonini F, Cazzato IA, Di Caro S, Gabrielli M, Santarelli L, Zocco MA, Ojetti V, Carloni E, Cammarota G, Gasbarrini G, Gasbarrini A. Levofloxacin-based triple therapy vs. quadruple therapy in second-line *Helicobacter pylori* treatment: a randomized trial. *Aliment Pharmacol Ther* 2003;**18**:627–633.

285 Wong WM, Gu Q, Lam SK, Fung FM, Lai KC, Hu WH, Yee YK, Chan CK, Xia HH, Yuen MF, Wong BC. Randomized

controlled study of rabeprazole, levofloxacin and rifabutin triple therapy vs. quadruple therapy as second-line treatment for *Helicobacter pylori* infection. *Aliment Pharmacol Ther* 2003;**17**:553–60.

286 O'Morain C, Borody T, Farley A *et al.* Efficacy and safety of single-triple capsules of bismuth biskalcitrate, metronidazole and tetracycline, given with omeprazole, for the eradication of *Helicobacter pylori*: an international multicentre study. *Aliment Pharmacol Ther* 2003;**17**:415–20.

287 Lahaie RG, Chiba N, Farley A. Efficacy of OBMT, in a twice daily (bid) dosage, for the eradication of *H. pylori*: a preliminary study. *Can J Gastroenterology* 1998; **12(Suppl A):**134A(S162).

288 Chiba N, Marshall C. Omeprazole, bismuth, metronidazole and tetracycline (OBMT) quadruple therapy given twice daily for *H. pylori* eradication in a community gastroenterology practice. *Gastroenterology* 1998;**114**:A91.

289 Graham DY, Hoffman J, el Zimaity HM, Graham DP, Osato M. Twice a day quadruple therapy (bismuth subsalicylate, tetracycline, metronidazole plus lansoprazole) for treatment of *Helicobacter pylori* infection. *Aliment Pharmacol Ther* 1997;**11**:935–8.

290 Dore MP, Graham DY, Mele R, Marras L, Nieddu S, Manca A, Realdi G. Colloidal bismuth subcitrate-based twice-a-day quadruple therapy as primary or salvage therapy for *Helicobacter pylori* infection. *Am J Gastroenterol* 2002; **97**:857–60.

291 Dore MP, Marras L, Maragkoudakis E *et al.* Salvage therapy after two or more prior *Helicobacter pylori* treatment failures: the super salvage regimen. *Helicobacter* 2003;**8**:307–9.

292 Garcia N, Calvet X, Gene E, Campo R, Brullet E. Limited usefulness of a seven-day twice-a-day quadruple therapy. *Eur J Gastroenterol Hepatol* 2000;**12**:1315–18.

293 Tytgat GNJ. Aspects of anti-*Helicobacter pylori* eradication therapy. In: Hunt RH and Tytgat GNJ, eds. *Helicobacter pylori: Basic Mechanisms to Clinical Cure.* Lancaster, UK: Kluwer Academic Publishers, 1996.

294 Chan FK, Sung JJ, Suen R, Wu JC, Ling TK, Chung SC. Salvage therapies after failure of *Helicobacter pylori* eradication with ranitidine bismuth citrate-based therapies. *Aliment Pharmacol Ther* 2000;**14**:91–5.

295 Peitz U, Sulliga M, Wolle K *et al.* High rate of post-therapeutic resistance after failure of macrolide-nitroimidazole triple therapy to cure *Helicobacter pylori* infection: impact of two second-line therapies in a randomized study. *Aliment Pharmacol Ther* 2002;**16**:315–24.

296 Hojo M, Miwa H, Nagahara A, Sato N. Pooled analysis on the efficacy of the second-line treatment regimens for *Helicobacter pylori* infection. *Scand J Gastroenterol* 2001;**36**:690–700.

297 Nash C, Fischbach L, Veldhuyzen vZ. What are the global response rates to *Helicobacter pylori* eradication therapy? *Can J Gastroenterology* 2003;**17(Suppl B):**25B–29B.

298 Magaret N, Burm M, Faigel D, Kelly C, Peterson W, Fennerty MB. A randomized trial of lansoprazole, amoxycillin, and clarithromycin versus lansoprazole, bismuth, metronidazole and tetracycline in the treatment of patients failing initial *Helicobacter pylori* therapy. *Dig Dis* 2001;**19**:174–8.

299 Chiba N, Hunt RH, Thomson AB. Ranitidine bismuth citrate. *Can J Gastroenterology* 2001;**15**:389–98.

300 Pozzato P, Zagari M, Cardelli A *et al.* Ranitidine bismuth citrate plus clarithromycin 7-day regimen is effective in eradicating *Helicobacter pylori* in patients with duodenal ulcer. *Aliment Pharmacol Ther* 1998;**12**:447–51.

301 Bardhan KD, Morton D, Perry MJ *et al.* Ranitidine bismuth citrate with clarithromycin alone or with metronidazole for the eradication of *Helicobacter pylori*. *Aliment Pharmacol Ther* 2001;**15**:1199–204.

302 Veldhuyzen van Zanten SJO, Chiba N, Barkun A *et al.* A randomized trial comparing seven-day ranitidine bismuth citrate and clarithromycin dual therapy to seven-day omeprazole, clarithromycin and amoxicillin triple therapy for the eradication of *Helicobacter pylori*. *Can J Gastroenterology* 2003;**17**:533–8.

303 Perschy TB, McSorley DJ, Sorrells SC, Webb DD. Ranitidine bismuth citrate in combination with clarithromycin is effective against H. pylori strains with susceptible or intermediate clarithromycin sensitivity. *Gastroenterology* 2997;**112**:A257.

304 Savarino V, Zentilin P, Bisso G *et al.* Optimal duration of therapy combining ranitidine bismuth citrate with clarithromycin and metronidazole in the eradication of *Helicobacter pylori* infection. *Aliment Pharmacol Ther* 1999;**13**:43–7.

305 Spadaccini A, De Fanis C, Sciampa G *et al.* Triple regimens using lansoprazole or ranitidine bismuth citrate for *Helicobacter pylori* eradication. *Aliment Pharmacol Ther* 1998;**12**:997–1001.

306 Catalano F, Catanzaro R, Bentivegna C, Brogna A, Condorelli G, Cipolla R. Ranitidine bismuth citrate versus omeprazole triple therapy for the eradication of *Helicobacter pylori* and healing of duodenal ulcer. *Aliment Pharmacol Ther* 1998;**12**:59–62.

307 Sung JJY, Leung WK, Ling TKW *et al.* One-week use of ranitidine bismuth citrate, amoxycillin and clarithromycin for the treatment of *Helicobacter pylori*-related duodenal ulcer. *Aliment Pharmacol Ther* 1998;**12**:725–30.

308 Chuang CH, Sheu BS, Yang HB, Wu JJ, Lin XZ. Ranitidine bismuth citrate or omeprazole-based triple therapy for *Helicobacter pylori* eradication in *Helicobacter pylori*-infected non-ulcer dyspepsia. *Dig Liver Dis* 2001;**33**:125–30.

309 Farup PG, Tholfsen J, Wetternus S, Torp R, Hoie O, Lange OJ. Comparison of three triple regimens with omeprazole or ranitidine bismuth citrate for *Helicobacter pylori* eradication. *Scand J Gastroenterol* 2002;**37**:1374–9.

310 Bago J, Halle ZB, Strinic D, Kucisec N, Jandric D, Bevanda M, Tomic M, Bilic A. The impact of primary antibiotic resistance on the efficacy of ranitidine bismuth citrate- vs. omeprazole-based one-week triple therapies in H. pylori eradication – a randomised controlled trial. *Wien Klin Wochenschr* 2002;**114**:448–53.

311 Hung WK, Wong WM, Wong GS *et al.* One-week ranitidine bismuth citrate, amoxicillin and metronidazole

triple therapy for the treatment of *Helicobacter pylori* infection in Chinese. *Aliment Pharmacol Ther* 2002;**16**: 2067–72.

312 Gisbert JP, Gonzalez L, Calvet X, Roque M, Gabriel R, Pajares JM. *Helicobacter pylori* eradication: proton pump inhibitor vs. ranitidine bismuth citrate plus two antibiotics for 1 week-a meta-analysis of efficacy. *Aliment Pharmacol Ther* 2000;**14**:1141–50.

313 Wong BC, Wong WM, Wang WH *et al.* One-week ranitidine bismuth citrate-based triple therapy for the eradication of *Helicobacter pylori* in Hong Kong with high prevalence of metronidazole resistance. *Aliment Pharmacol Ther* 2001;**15**:403–9.

314 Rinaldi V, Zullo A, Francesco VD *et al. Helicobacter pylori* eradication with proton pump inhibitor-based triple therapies and re-treatment with ranitidine bismuth citrate-based triple therapy [In Process Citation]. *Aliment Pharmacol Ther* 1999;**13**:163–8.

315 Perri F, Villani MR, Quitadamo M, Annese V, Niro GA, Andriulli A. Ranitidine bismuth citrate-based triple therapies after failure of the standard "Maastricht triple therapy": a promising alternative to the quadruple therapy? *Aliment Pharmacol Ther* 2001;**15**:1017–22.

316 McLaren A, Donnelly C, McDowell S, Williamson R. The role of ranitidine bismuth citrate in significantly reducing the emergence of *Helicobacter pylori* strains resistant to antibiotics. *Helicobacter* 1997;**2**:21–6.

317 López-Brea M, Domingo D, Sánchez I, Alarcón T. Synergism study of ranitidine bismuth citrate and metronidazole against metronidazole resistant *H. pylori* clinical isolates. *Gastroenterology* 1997;**112**:A201.

318 Osato MS, Graham DY. Ranitidine bismuth citrate enhances clarithromycin activity against clinical isolates of *H. pylori. Gastroenterology* 1997;**112**:A1057.

319 van den Wouden EJ, Thijs JC, Van Zwet AA, Kooy A, Kleibeuker JH. Metronidazole resistance does not influence the efficacy of triple therapy with ranitidine bismuth citrate (RBC), clarithromycin (CLA) and metronidazole (MET) for *H. pylori (Hp)* infection. *Gastroenterology* 1998;**114**:A323(G1321).

320 Sung JJ, Chan FK, Wu JC *et al.* One-week ranitidine bismuth citrate in combinations with metronidazole, amoxycillin and clarithromycin in the treatment of *Helicobacter pylori* infection: the RBC-MACH study. *Aliment Pharmacol Ther* 1999;**13**:1079–84.

321 De Boer WA, Haeck PWE, Otten MH, Mulder CJJ. Optimal treatment of *Helicobacter pylori* with ranitidine bismuth citrate (RBC): a randomized comparison between two 7-day triple therapies and a 14-day dual therapy. *Am J Gastroenterol* 1998;**93**:1101–7.

322 Kung NN, Sung JJ, Yuen NW *et al.* One-week ranitidine bismuth citrate versus colloidal bismuth subcitrate-based anti-*Helicobacter* triple therapy: a prospective randomized controlled trial. *Am J Gastroenterol* 1999;**94**:721–4.

323 Xiao SD, Liu WZ, Hu PJ, Ouyang Q, Wang JL, Zhou LY, Cheng NN. A multicentre study on eradication of *Helicobacter pylori* using four 1-week triple therapies in China. *Aliment Pharmacol Ther* 2001;**15**:81–6.

324 Lu H, Zhang DZ, Hu PJ, Li ZS, Lu XH, Fang XC, Xiao SD. One-week regimens containing ranitidine bismuth citrate, furazolidone and either amoxicillin or tetracycline effectively eradicate *Helicobacter pylori*: a multicentre, randomized, double-blind study. *Aliment Pharmacol Ther* 2001;**15**:1975–79.

325 Fakheri H, Malekzadeh R, Merat S *et al.* Clarithromycin vs. furazolidone in quadruple therapy regimens for the treatment of *Helicobacter pylori* in a population with a high metronidazole resistance rate. *Aliment Pharmacol Ther* 2001;**15**:411–16.

326 Coelho LG, Martins GM, Passos MC *et al.* Once-daily, low-cost, highly effective *Helicobacter pylori* treatment to family members of gastric cancer patients. *Aliment Pharmacol Ther* 2003;**17**:131–6.

327 Cammarota G, Cianci R, Cannizzaro O *et al.* Efficacy of two one-week rabeprazole/levofloxacin-based triple therapies for *Helicobacter pylori* infection. *Aliment Pharmacol Ther* 2000;**14**:1339–43.

328 Di Caro S, Ojetti V, Zocco MA *et al.* Mono, dual and triple moxifloxacin-based therapies for *Helicobacter pylori* eradication. *Aliment Pharmacol Ther* 2002;**16**:527–32.

329 Nagahara A, Miwa H, Yamada T, Kurosawa A, Ohkura R, Sato N. Five-day proton pump inhibitor-based quadruple therapy regimen is more effective than 7-day triple therapy regimen for *Helicobacter pylori* infection. *Aliment Pharmacol Ther* 2001;**15**:417–21.

330 Treiber G, Wittig J, Ammon S, Walker S, van Doorn LJ, Klotz U. Clinical outcome and influencing factors of a new short-term quadruple therapy for *Helicobacter pylori* eradication: a randomized controlled trial (MACLOR study). *Arch Intern Med* 2002;**162**:153–60.

331 Zullo A, Vaira D, Vakil N *et al.* High eradication rates of *Helicobacter pylori* with a new sequential treatment. *Aliment Pharmacol Ther* 2003;**17**:719–26.

332 Hassan C, de Francesco V, Zullo A *et al.* Sequential treatment for *Helicobacter pylori* eradication in duodenal ulcer patients: improving the cost of pharmacotherapy. *Aliment Pharmacol Ther* 2003;**18**:641–6.

333 Nagahara A, Miwa H, Ogawa K, Kurosawa A, Ohkura R, Iida N, Sato N. Addition of metronidazole to rabeprazole-amoxicillin-clarithromycin regimen for *Helicobacter pylori* infection provides an excellent cure rate with five-day therapy. *Helicobacter* 2000;**5**:88–93.

334 Treiber G, Ammon S, Schneider E, Klotz U. Amoxicillin/metronidazole/omeprazole/clarithromycin: a new, short quadruple therapy for *Helicobacter pylori* eradication. *Helicobacter* 1998;**3**:54–58.

335 Neville PM, Everett S, Langworthy H *et al.* The optimal antibiotic combination in a 5-day *Helicobacter pylori* eradication regimen. *Aliment Pharmacol Ther* 1999;**13**: 497–501.

336 Catalano F, Branciforte G, Catanzaro R, Cipolla R, Bentivegna C, Brogna A. *Helicobacter pylori*-positive duodenal ulcer: three-day antibiotic eradication regimen. *Aliment Pharmacol Ther* 2000;**14**:1329–34.

337 Calvet X, Tito L, Comet R, Garcia N, Campo R, Brullet E. Four-day, twice daily, quadruple therapy with amoxicillin,

clarithromycin, tinidazole and omeprazole to cure *Helicobacter pylori* infection: a pilot study. *Helicobacter* 2000;**5**:52–6.

338 Okada M, Nishimura H, Kawashima M *et al.* A new quadruple therapy for *Helicobacter pylori*: influence of resistant strains on treatment outcome. *Aliment Pharmacol Ther* 1999;**13**:769–74.

339 Sullivan B, Coyle W, Nemec R, Dunteman T. Comparison of azithromycin and clarithromycin in triple therapy regimens for the eradication of *Helicobacter pylori*. *Am J Gastroenterol* 2002;**97**:2536–9.

340 Laurent J, Megraud F, Flejou JF, Caekaert A, Barthelemy P. A randomized comparison of four omeprazole-based triple therapy regimens for the eradication of *Helicobacter pylori* in patients with non-ulcer dyspepsia. *Aliment Pharmacol Ther* 2001;**15**:1787–93.

341 Anagnostopoulos GK, Kostopoulos P, Margantinis G, Tsiakos S, Arvanitidis D. Omeprazole plus azithromycin and either amoxicillin or tinidazole for eradication of *Helicobacter pylori* infection. *J Clin Gastroenterol* 2003;**36**:325–8.

342 Silva FM, Eisig JN, Chehter EZ, da Silva JJ, Laudanna AA. Low efficacy of an ultra-short term, once-daily dose triple therapy with omeprazole, azithromycin, and secnidazole for *Helicobacter pylori* eradication in peptic ulcer. *Rev Hosp Clin Fac Med Sao Paulo* 2002;**57**:9–14.

343 Ivashkin VT, Lapina TL, Bondarenko OY *et al.* Azithromycin in a triple therapy for *H.pylori* eradication in active duodenal ulcer. *World J Gastroenterology* 2002;**8**:879–82.

344 Meier R, Wettstein A, Drewe J, Geiser HR. Fish oil (Eicosapen) is less effective than metronidazole, in combination with pantoprazole and clarithromycin, for *Helicobacter pylori* eradication. *Aliment Pharmacol Ther* 2001;**15**:851–5.

345 Gotoh A, Akamatsu T, Shimizu T *et al.* Additive effect of pronase on the efficacy of eradication therapy against *Helicobacter pylori*. *Helicobacter* 2002;**7**:183–91.

346 Armuzzi A, Cremonini F, Bartolozzi F *et al.* The effect of oral administration of *Lactobacillus GG* on antibiotic-associated gastrointestinal side-effects during *Helicobacter pylori* eradication therapy. *Aliment Pharmacol Ther* 2001;**15**:163–9.

347 Cremonini F, Di Caro S, Covino M *et al.* Effect of different probiotic preparations on anti-*Helicobacter pylori* therapy-related side effects: a parallel group, triple blind, placebo-controlled study. *Am J Gastroenterol* 2002;**97**:2744–9.

348 Sheu BS, Wu JJ, Lo CY, Wu HW, Chen JH, Lin YS, Lin MD. Impact of supplement with *Lactobacillus-* and *Bifidobacterium*-containing yogurt on triple therapy for *Helicobacter pylori* eradication. *Aliment Pharmacol Ther* 2002;**16**:1669–75.

349 Isomoto H, Inoue K, Furusu H *et al.* High-dose rabeprazole-amoxicillin versus rabeprazole-amoxicillin-metronidazole as second-line treatment after failure of the Japanese standard regimen for *Helicobacter pylori* infection. *Aliment Pharmacol Ther* 2003;**18**:101–7.

350 Murakami K, Sato R, Okimoto T *et al.* Efficacy of triple therapy comprising rabeprazole, amoxicillin and metronidazole for second-line *Helicobacter pylori* eradication in Japan, and the influence of metronidazole resistance. *Aliment Pharmacol Ther* 2003;**17**:119–23.

351 Perri F, Festa V, Clemente R, Quitadamo M, Andriulli A. Rifabutin-based "rescue therapy" for *Helicobacter pylori* infected patients after failure of standard regimens. *Aliment Pharmacol Ther* 2000;**14**:311–16.

352 Bock H, Koop H, Lehn N, Heep M. Rifabutin-based triple therapy after failure of *Helicobacter pylori* eradication treatment: preliminary experience. *J Clin Gastroenterol* 2000;**31**:222–5.

353 Gisbert JP, Calvet X, Bujanda L, Marcos S, Gisbert JL, Pajares JM. "Rescue" therapy with rifabutin after multiple *Helicobacter pylori* treatment failures. *Helicobacter* 2003;**8**:90–4.

354 Zullo A, Hassan C, de Francesco V *et al.* A third-line levofloxacin-based rescue therapy for *Helicobacter pylori* eradication. *Dig Liver Dis* 2003;**35**:232–6.

355 Chi CH, Lin CY, Sheu BS, Yang HB, Huang AH, Wu JJ. Quadruple therapy containing amoxicillin and tetracycline is an effective regimen to rescue failed triple therapy by overcoming the antimicrobial resistance of *Helicobacter pylori*. *Aliment Pharmacol Ther* 2003;**18**:347–53.

356 Georgopoulos SD, Ladas SD, Karatapanis S *et al.* Effectiveness of two quadruple, tetracycline- or clarithromycin-containing, second-line, *Helicobacter pylori* eradication therapies. *Aliment Pharmacol Ther* 2002;**16**:569–75.

357 Lin CK, Hsu PI, Lai KH *et al* One-week quadruple therapy is an effective salvage regimen for *Helicobacter pylori* infection in patients after failure of standard triple therapy. *J Clin Gastroenterol* 2002;**34**:547–51.

358 Isakov V, Domareva I, Koudryavtseva L, Maev I, Ganskaya Z. Furazolidone-based triple "rescue therapy" vs. quadruple "rescue therapy" for the eradication of *Helicobacter pylori* resistant to metronidazole. *Aliment Pharmacol Ther* 2002;**16**:1277–82.

359 Wong WM, Wong BC, Lu H *et al.* One-week omeprazole, furazolidone and amoxicillin rescue therapy after failure of *Helicobacter pylori* eradication with standard triple therapies. *Aliment Pharmacol Ther* 2002;**16**:793–8.

360 Treiber G, Ammon S, Malfertheiner P, Klotz U. Impact of furazolidone-based quadruple therapy for eradication of *Helicobacter pylori* after previous treatment failures. *Helicobacter* 2002;**7**:225–31.

6 Non-steroidal anti-inflammatory drug-induced gastroduodenal toxicity

Alaa Rostom, Andreas Maetzel, Peter Tugwell, George Wells

Introduction

In 1999, when the first edition of this textbook was published, evidence from non-clinical and early clinical trials suggested that the gastrointestinal safety of the newer cyclo-oxygenase-2 (COX-2) selective non-steriodal anti-inflammatory drugs (NSAIDs) may be such that a fundamental change in the clinician's choice from the use of standard NSAIDs with a gastroprotective agent to monotherapy with a COX-2 selective NSAID (COX-2 inhibitors) was on the horizon. Indeed in Canada alone the number of NSAID prescriptions overall rose from 9·8 million in 1999 to 13·1 million in 2001. This increase was predominantly due to a rise in the number of prescriptions of COX-2 inhibitors from 1·9 million in 1999 to 7·7 million in 2001. Over the same time period the number of standard NSAID prescriptions fell from 7·9 million to 5·4 million suggesting that the rise in the use of COX-2 inhibitors was not only due to clinicians switching patients from standard NSAIDs to COX-2 inhibitors, but also due to the use of COX-2 inhibitors in patients who were previously not receiving conventional NSAIDs. Overall, the cost of these COX-2 inhibitor prescriptions rose from one-third to three-quarters of the annual cost of NSAID prescriptions, which in 2001 amounted to Can$467 million out of Can$620 million (Canadian Compuscript, IMS Health).

Background

NSAIDs including aspirin (ASA) are important agents in the management of patients with a variety of arthritic and inflammatory conditions.[1] Additionally, ASA is important in the treatment and prevention of both myocardial infarction and stroke.[2–5] The efficacy of these agents is well described, making NSAIDs among the most frequently used medications with an estimated world market in excess of US$6 billion annually.[6]

NSAIDs including ASA cause a variety of gastrointestinal adverse effects, which are associated with excess use of healthcare resources at a substantial cost.[7] Minor adverse effects such as nausea and dyspepsia are relatively common, but these clinical symptoms correlate poorly with serious adverse events.[8,9] Although, endoscopic ulcers, occurring with or without symptoms, can be documented in as many as 40% of chronic NSAID users,[10] serious NSAID-induced gastrointestinal toxicities are much less common.[9] Due to the vast numbers of individuals using these drugs, however, they have been linked directly to over 70 000 hospitalizations and over 7000 deaths annually in the USA alone.[11] NSAID use can also add significantly to the morbidity and mortality of chronic arthritic conditions. Among rheumatoid arthritis patients who are chronically using NSAIDs, the chance of hospitalization or death due to a gastrointestinal event is about 1·3–1·6% per year,[11] accounting for about 2600 deaths and 20 000 hospitalizations each year.[1] These figures have led some to suggest that NSAID toxicity is among the "deadliest" of rheumatic disorders.[11]

The serious gastrointestinal adverse effects such as hemorrhage, perforation or death occur collectively with an incidence of about 2% per year in an average patient population.[9] The relative risk of upper gastrointestinal hemorrhage or perforation with NSAID use varies in the literature from 4·7 in hospital-based case–control studies to 2·0 in cohort studies.[12–14] Gabriel et al. in a meta-analysis of 16 studies found that non-ASA NSAIDs were associated with a 2·7-fold increased risk of serious gastrointestinal events resulting in hospitalization.[15] Similarly, Langman et al. found that ASA and non-ASA NSAID use increased the risk of bleeding peptic ulcer 3·1-fold and 3·5-fold, respectively.[16] In a recent large prospective cohort study of 126 000 patients conducted over 3 years, MacDonald et al. found that NSAIDs increased the risk of any adverse gastrointestinal event 3·9-fold, similar to the findings above. However, NSAIDs appeared to raise the risk eight-fold, when only hemorrhage or perforation were considered,[17] a level which is sufficiently high as to imply causation. Armstrong *et al.* found that 60% of 235 consecutive patients presenting with a significant peptic ulcer complication were taking NSAIDs, and nearly 80% of all ulcer-related deaths occurred in NSAIDs users.[18]

NSAIDs have also been linked to a variety of other gastrointestinal adverse effects including pyloric stenosis, small bowel ulcerations, strictures, lower gastrointestinal bleeds, and the exacerbation of colitis.[6,19–21] Some experts suggest that the most effective means to prevent NSAID-induced gastrointestinal toxicity is to discontinue the use of the NSAID, or to substitute an analgesic which does not exert gastrointestinal adverse effects in its stead.[22] This approach is clearly not always feasible, since a large proportion of NSAID users rely heavily on these medications, and a delicate balance exists between the therapeutic benefits and the risks of these drugs.[23]

NSAIDs inhibit the enzyme cyclo-oxygenase (COX). This enzyme exists in two isoforms: COX-1 and COX-2. It is felt that NSAIDs exert their therapeutic anti-inflammatory and analgesic effects through the inhibition of inducible COX-2, whereas their gastric and renal adverse effects arise from the inhibition of the constitutive COX-1 isoform.[24,25] The antiplatelet effect of NSAIDs including ASA is mediated through inhibition of the COX-1 isoform. It has been recognized for some time that different NSAIDs have differing propensities toward gastroduodenal toxicity,[17] and recently it has been proposed that those NSAIDs with the greatest affinity for COX-1 are associated with the highest risk of gastrointestinal toxicity. As a result of these observations, there has been a rapid development of new NSAIDs with increasing COX-2 selectivity, with claims of retained anti-inflammatory and analgesic activity, but with little gastrointestinal toxicity.

A great deal of variability exists in the literature regarding the criteria by which an NSAID is classified as COX-2 selective and for the techniques used to make this determination. The most accepted technique involves determination of the COX-2 IC50 to COX-1 IC50 ratio (a ratio of the concentrations of the drug that results in 50% inhibition of the COX-2 and COX-1 iso-enzymes) through a whole blood assay. A value below one indicates greater affinity for COX-2 inhibition than COX-1 inhibition. The lower the value, the greater the COX-2 selectivity. However, a ratio below one does not guarantee COX-2 selectivity in clinical practice, since other factors are at play such as the COX-2 selectivity at target tissue like the gastric mucosa, and the effect of clinically used dosages of the drug on its COX-2 selectivity (i.e. an agent may be COX-2 selective only at subtherapeutic doses). Also, the reported COX-2 to COX-1 IC50 ratios for the available COX-2 selective NSAIDs differ from one report to another.

In this chapter the results of the original Cochrane Collaboration systematic review of NSAID prophylaxis,[26,27]

and the recently completed COX-2 inhibitor gastrointestinal safety meta-analysis performed for the Canadian Coordinating Office for Health Technology Assessment (CCOHTA) will be summarized.[28] We will discuss the risk factors for NSAID-induced gastrointestinal toxicity, including the current evidence for the role of *Helicobacter pylori* as a possible coexistent risk factor. We will then compare the possible strategies for the prevention of NSAID-related gastrointestinal toxicity among patients who require chronic NSAID use.

Risk factors for NSAID-related gastrointestinal toxicity

Several studies, meta-analyses and reviews have addressed the issue of risk factors for NSAID-induced gastrointestinal toxicity. Increasing age (> 65 years), previous peptic ulcer disease (PUD) with or without previous hemorrhage, and comorbid medical illnesses, particularly heart disease, have been consistently shown to increase the risk of an adverse gastrointestinal event among patients on long-term NSAID therapy.[9,11,13,15,29–33] Using multiple logistic regression to adjusts for risk factors simultaneously, Silverstein *et al.* found that among patients on chronic NSAIDs with none of these risk factors, only 0·4% developed a serious adverse gastrointestinal event at 6 months, whereas 9% of patients with all three risk factors experienced such an event.[9] Other risk factors have also been identified (Box 6.1). High doses of NSAIDs and the use of multiple NSAIDs increase the risk of adverse outcomes, as do the combined use of NSAIDs with corticosteroids, ASA, or warfarin.[32,34] Specific NSAIDs (Table 6.1), and in some studies female sex are also associated with an increased risk of gastrointestinal toxicity.[30–32,35–38] The newer COX-2 specific NSAIDs, are reported to cause gastrointestinal toxicity less frequently, and will be discussed at the end of this chapter.

Box 6.1   Risk factors for NSAID gastrointestinal toxicity

- Age > 60 years
- Previous peptic ulcer disease
- Underlying medical conditions
- Concomitant corticosteroid use
- Concomitant anticoagulant therapy or ASA
- High dose of NSAID or multiple NSAIDs
- Type of NSAID
- Duration of NSAID use/compliance
- *Helicobacter pylori*? See text

ASA, aspirin; NSAID, non-steroidal anti-inflammatory drug

Table 6.1   Individual NSAIDs and the risk of gastrointestinal events (relative to ibuprofen)

Drug	Relative risk
Azopropazone	9·2
Ketoprofen	4·2
Piroxicam	3·8
Tolmetin	3·0
Indomethacin	2·4
Naproxen	2·2
Diflunisal	2·2
Sulindac	2·1
Diclofenac	1·8
Aspirin	1·6
Fenoprofen	1·6
Ibuprofen	1·00
Dose: (ibuprofen)	
Low	1·6
High	4·2

Adapted from Henry D *et al. BMJ* 1996;**312**:1563–6.[37]
NSAID, non-steroidal anti-inflammatory drug

The duration of NSAID use has been reported as a risk factor for gastrointestinal adverse effects, with most studies suggesting that the risk is highest within the first month of use.[12,16,36,39,40] However, there is increasing evidence to suggest that the risk of significant NSAID toxicity does not diminish with prolonged use beyond 1 month. Silverstein *et al.*, in their prospective study of misoprostol for the prevention of serious NSAID-related gastrointestinal events, did not find a decreased risk with continued NSAID use.[9] Furthermore, in a large prospective cohort study of NSAID-related gastrointestinal toxicity, MacDonald *et al.* found that there was a four-fold relative risk increase associated with the use of NSAIDs and that this risk was nearly constant over the 3-year follow up period.[17] Additionally these investigators found that a two-fold relative risk of gastrointestinal toxicity persisted for at least 1 year after the last exposure to NSAIDs.

Compliance with NSAID use also appears to be a risk factor for gastrointestinal toxicity. Wynne *et al.* in a study of patient awareness of adverse effects and symptoms associated with NSAIDs, found that patients suffering an adverse gastrointestinal event had a higher rate of compliance (96%) with their NSAID use than those not suffering an event (70%).[41] Similarly, Griffin *et al.* found that patients suffering a terminal NSAID-related gastrointestinal event were more likely to have filled a prescription for an NSAID in the preceding month.[12] Symptoms, however, correlate quite poorly with the occurrence of endoscopic ulceration and adverse gastrointestinal events, and thus cannot be considered predictors of adverse gastrointestinal events.[8,9,18,34,42]

The role of *H. pylori* infection as a risk factor for NSAID-related gastrointestinal toxicity is controversial and is discussed below.

Do endoscopically diagnosed ulcers predict clinical events?

Gastrointestinal ulcers are established as the pathophysiologic correlate of clinical gastrointestinal adverse events resulting from the chronic use of NSAIDs. For this reason endoscopically confirmed ulcers have been used as surrogate outcomes for clinical gastrointestinal events resulting from NSAID use. Endoscopic definitions of gastroduodenal ulcers are controversial,[43] and do not equate with the pathological definition, which defines an ulcer as a loss of mucosal surface of sufficient depth to penetrate the muscularis mucosa.[44] In most clinical trials of NSAID prophylaxis, an endoscopic ulcer is defined as a break in the mucosal surface, usually greater than 3 mm in diameter with some appreciable depth. The strictness of these criteria has varied from study to study, with some authors requiring the use of an endoscopic measuring tool, or an estimation based on the size of an open biopsy forceps to measure the ulcer diameter. Formal estimates of interobserver variability among the endoscopists are often not presented, particularly in the larger multicenter trials. Some authors define an ulcer as the loss of mucosal surface of 5 mm or greater in diameter to better differentiate them from erosions and to achieving closer agreement with clinical events.[43] Varying definitions of endoscopic ulcers and the occasional use of composite endpoints all complicate comparison of results across studies.

Unfortunately, endoscopic ulcers are not ideal surrogate outcomes for clinical gastrointestinal events such as bleeding or perforation of an ulcer. In fact, the proportion of endoscopic ulcers that never become clinically symptomatic, is estimated to be as high as 85%.[9,45] From a theoretical perspective, Wittes *et al.*[46] point out that if a surrogate (in this case an endoscopic ulcer) is a marker for a variety of processes, then an intervention that alters the risk of the surrogate by a mechanism unrelated to the risk of the real endpoint (clinical gastrointestinal event), will appear effective in a surrogate endpoint trial, but will not be effective in practice (Figure 6.1).

With the publication of several large randomized controlled trials (RCTs) that used actual clinical endpoints to measure the safety of COX-2 inhibitors and of misoprostol prophylaxis,[9,47,48] it became possible to compare the reduction in clinical events with the reduction in endoscopic ulcers from the endoscopic studies.[26,27] *Although these indirect comparisons should be interpreted with caution, we have found in our systematic reviews that the standard NSAID arms of both the NSAID prophylaxis trials and the COX-2 trials were quite similar clinically, and demonstrated nearly identical NSAID ulcer and complication rates.*

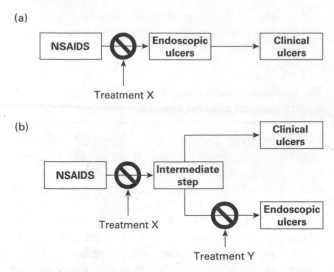

Figure 6.1 (a) If the mechanism of clinical ulcers goes through endoscopic ulcers, then treatment X will prevent both endoscopic and clinical ulcers. (b) However, if NSAIDs cause endoscopic ulcers and clinical ulcers by two different mechanisms then treatment X will still be effective in preventing both but treatment Y will only be effective in preventing endoscopic ulcers

The relative risk reduction in endoscopic gastric ulcers with misoprostol prophylaxis and with COX-2 inhibitors is about 80%. In the clinical endpoint studies, the relative risk reductions in NSAID ulcer-related perforations, obstructions and bleeding is about 50% with both these strategies. The consistency suggests that there is a relationship between the endoscopic and clinical endpoints. The relationship does not have to be 1:1. In fact based on our results, prophylactic agents, and COX-2 inhibitors are 1·5–2·0 times more effective at reducing the risk of endoscopic ulcers as they are at reducing the risk of clinical endpoints. Unfortunately, the studies using clinical gastrointestinal events as the primary outcome measure were not designed to look at the relationship of clinical events to endoscopic ulcers, and we used indirect comparisons to arrive at this result.[9] Nevertheless, while observing caution as recommended above, the reader can estimate what the expected reduction in clinical events would be, based on the results of an endoscopic endpoint study, assuming that the control groups are average risk arthritic patients requiring long-term NSAID use.

The role of *Helicobacter pylori* in NSAID-associated ulcers

The causal role of *H. pylori* in the development of gastroduodenal ulcers has added a new perspective to the management of patients with gastrointestinal complaints.[49–51]

NSAIDs are now thought to cause approximately 25% of gastroduodenal ulcers,[52] and do so in the absence of *H. pylori*.[53–56] The study of the potential interaction between *H. pylori* and NSAIDs has been complicated by the following facts: (i) NSAID use is most frequent among elderly patients, the same group with the highest *H. pylori* prevalence in Western populations[57,58]; (ii) in the presence of both factors, it has been difficult to determine whether an ulcer is caused by NSAIDs with incidental *H. pylori*, or caused by *H. pylori* with incidental or exacerbating NSAIDs[59,60]; and (iii) whereas one would expect, based on conventional thinking, an increased incidence of ulcers in the presence of these two well established risk factors, some clinical and observational studies found that infection with *H. pylori* decreased the likelihood of ulcers or gastroduodenal injury in NSAID users.[61–64] Still other studies have found no effect of *H. pylori* infection on NSAID-induced gastroduodenal injury.[62,65]

A meta-analysis published in 2002 has shed some light on our understanding of the clinical impact of the coexistence of *H. pylori* infection and NSAIDs use.[66] This systematic review of observational studies of PUD in adult patients taking NSAIDs used strict diagnostic criteria for the documentation of *H. pylori* infection and endoscopic ulcers. Twenty-five studies were included out of 61 potentially relevant publications. Sixteen studies with a total of 1625 patients assessed the effect of *H. pylori* infection on the risk of uncomplicated PUD in adult NSAID users. In these patients, *H. pylori* infection increased the risk of uncomplicated PUD 2·12-fold (95% CI 1·68 to 2·67).

The interaction between *H. pylori* infection and NSAID exposure was derived from five age-matched controlled studies of chronic (> 4 weeks) NSAID exposure. In the presence of *H. pylori* infection, the use of NSAIDs increased the risk of uncomplicated PUD 3·55-fold (95% CI 1·26 to 9·96); while in the presence of NSAIDs, *H. pylori* infection increased the risk of PUD 3·53-fold (95% CI 2·16 to 5·75). Compared with controls without either NSAID or *H. pylori* exposure, the combined exposure to both factors increased the risk of uncomplicated PUD 6.36-fold (95% CI 2·21 to 18·31) after correction for a zero event rate in *H. pylori* negative controls.

Nine case–control studies with 893 patients and 1002 controls assessed the effects of *H. pylori* infection and NSAID exposure on the risk of ulcer bleeding. *H. pylori* infection conferred a marginally increased risk of PUD bleed (odds ratio (OR) 1·67, 95% CI 1·02 to 2·72), which was more pronounced when the analysis was limited to studies using serology for diagnosis of *H. pylori* infection (OR 2·16, 95% CI 1·54 to 3·04). Studies using patients with non-bleeding ulcers as controls (as opposed to either healthy or hospitalized non-ulcer controls) tended to be negative, but the results of a sensitivity analysis based on the type of controls were not presented. NSAID exposure, which was principally short term in these studies (< 1 week and < 1 month in six and two out of nine studies, respectively), conferred an increased risk of ulcer bleeding (OR 4·79, 95% CI 3·78 to 6.06), whereas the combined exposure to NSAIDs and *H. pylori* led to an increased risk of PUD bleed of 6.13 (95% CI 3·93 to 9·56). The later findings are in keeping with the hypothesis that short-term NSAID exposure renders "silent" *H. pylori*-related ulcers clinically manifest, a notion which has been suggested by others.[67–69]

The authors of this systematic review support the conventional thinking that, in peptic ulcer disease, two sources of injuries are worse than one. However, the outcome of combined exposure to NSAIDs and *H. pylori* infection differs depending on the patient population (prior history of PUD or not), the type of NSAID exposure (first-time or not, short-term or long-term; ASA or non-ASA NSAID), the study outcome (ulcer healing, ulcer bleeding, ulcer prevention), and the co-administration of ulcer prophylaxis. Several recent prospective trials have addressed some of these issues, and will be reviewed in the paragraphs that follow.

Ulcer healing

Ulcer healing with omeprazole or ranitidine occurs more readily in the presence of *H. pylori* infection.[70,71] As well, the presence of *H. pylori* enhances the ability of omeprazole to raise gastric pH among patients with duodenal ulcer.[72] However, Porro *et al.* found that the presence of *H. pylori* did not statistically significantly affect the healing rates at either 4 or 8 weeks in a study of 100 chronic NSAID users with peptic ulcers.[73]

In a group of 81 *H. pylori* positive ulcer patients with ongoing requirement for NSAIDs, Hawkey *et al.* observed that the addition of *H. pylori* eradication to a 1-month course of omeprazole led to a significantly lower healing rate for gastric ulcers (50% v 88% healing at 4 weeks and 72% v 100% healing at 8 weeks, for the *H. pylori*-treated and omeprazole alone groups, respectively; *P* = 0·006), while the rates of duodenal ulcer healing were similar in both groups.[74]

Ulcer prevention in NSAID-naive patients

Chan *et al.* randomized 100 *H. pylori* positive, NSAID-naive patients with no prior history of peptic ulcer, to receive either naproxen alone or *H. pylori* eradication (bismuth, tetracycline and metronidazole) followed by naproxen for 8 weeks.[75] At 8 weeks, the ulcer recurrence was statistically significantly less frequent in the triple therapy group compared with the naproxen alone group in the intention-to-treat analysis (7% v 26%; *P* = 0·01), for a 74% relative risk reduction with *H. pylori* eradication. The importance of co-existent risk factors was highlighted by the fact that 73% of

ulcer patients were older than 60 years and that 73% of them also had comorbidity. A1c

In a more recent study, the same group enrolled 100 *H. pylori* positive, NSAID-naive patients with either a prior history of peptic ulcer (16% of the patients) or dyspepsia, to receive *H. pylori* eradication or omeprazole plus placebo for 1 week, followed by diclofenac 100 mg daily for 6 months.[76] Once again, in the NSAID-naive patients, *H. pylori* eradication conferred a protective effect, leading to a significantly reduced incidence of both endoscopic ulcers (12·1% (95% CI 3·1 to 21·1) v 34·4% (95% CI 21·1 to 47·7) in the eradication versus omeprazole alone groups, respectively) and of clinical ulcers (4·2% (95% CI 1·3 to 9·7) v 27·1% (95% CI 14·7 to 39·5) in the eradication versus omeprazole alone group, respectively) at 6 months. A1c It may be noted that 17% of these patients had received low-dose ASA prior to enrollment.

Secondary ulcer prevention in patients on continuous NSAID therapy

The role of *H. pylori* eradication for the prevention of recurrent upper gastrointestinal bleeding was studied by Chan *et al.*[77] Four hundred *H. pylori* positive, chronic users of ASA or other NSAIDs, presenting with a bleeding peptic ulcer, were randomized to receive either *H. pylori* eradication or ulcer prophylaxis with omeprazole and followed up for 6 months for the recurrence of clinical events. In the group of patients on low dose (80 mg daily) ASA, the probability of ulcer recurrence was similar among *H. pylori* treated patients and those on PPI prophylaxis. However, in patients on a non-ASA NSAID (naproxen 500 mg twice daily), *H. pylori* eradication did not confer the same magnitude of ulcer protection as omeprazole, so that the trial was terminated after the second interim analysis (probability of recurrence 18·8% v 4·4% for the *H. pylori* eradication and omeprazole groups, respectively (*P* = 0·005) at that point). A1a

Hawkey *et al.* studied the role of *H. pylori* eradication in a group of 285 *H. pylori* positive patients with a history of ulcer or dyspepsia and ongoing requirement for NSAIDs,[74] who were randomized to a 1-week course of either *H. pylori* eradication or omeprazole plus placebo. All patients went on to receive a 3-week course of omeprazole for ulcer healing. During the follow up period, patients received continuous NSAIDs without ulcer prophylaxis. The probability of ulcer recurrence at 6 months was similar in both groups, and the study concluded that in chronic NSAID (non-ASA) users, *H. pylori* eradication did not confer a protective effect on ulcer recurrence. A1a

In summary, we can conclude based on these recent RCTs, that *H. pylori* contributes to an excess ulcer risk in NSAID-naive patients, whereas ulcers occurring in long-term NSAID users are probably largely caused by NSAIDs themselves, irrespective of *H. pylori* status. Therefore, the impact of *H. pylori* is likely to be manifest early in the course of NSAID exposure, either because these patients are prone to early ulcer complications with NSAIDs, or because the administration of NSAIDs has precipitated complications in pre-existing *H. pylori* ulcers. We can also conclude that the impact of *H. pylori* eradication is related to the presence of coexisting ulcerogenic factors: while its benefits are more obvious in conjunction with low dose ASA administration, they are not significant in comparison to the ulcerogenic effects of "regular" NSAIDs and are less marked in the elderly or in the presence of comorbidity.

Based on this evidence, it is appropriate to eradicate *H. pylori* in NSAID-naive patients prior to starting chronic ASA or NSAID therapy. A1c However, *H. pylori* eradication alone appears to be insufficient for ulcer prophylaxis in chronic non-ASA NSAID users.

Definition of terms

In the discussion that follows, we use the relative risk (RR) to indicate the likelihood of an outcome for subjects on treatment as compared with those on placebo.[78,79] For example a RR of 0·25, would mean that the treatment is associated with only 25% or one-fourth the probability of the outcome as compared with placebo. Said in another way a RR of 0·25 means that the treatment reduces the "risk" of an event by 75% relative to placebo $(1 - 0·25 = 0·75$ or 75%). This relative risk reduction (RRR) differs from the absolute risk reduction (ARR), which is simply the arithmetic difference in the proportion of patients with the outcome between the placebo and treatment groups. If the stated 95% confidence interval overlaps with 1, then the observed risk is not statistically significant.

Misoprostol

Misoprostol is a synthetic prostaglandin E_1 analog.[80–83] It reduces basal and stimulated gastric acid secretion through a direct effect on parietal cells,[83] and reduces gastric damage caused by a variety of aggressive factors including bile salts and NSAIDs.[84] Misoprostol's protective effects are felt to be related to its ability to stimulate gastric bicarbonate and mucus secretion, and to maintain mucosal blood flow and the mucosal permeability barrier. Misoprostol also promotes epithelial proliferation in response to injury.[80] It appears that at doses of misoprostol sufficient to protect gastric mucosa, suppression of acid secretion also occurs.[82] However, since standard doses of H_2-receptor antagonists inhibit gastric acid secretion at least as effectively as misoprostol, and yet have not been shown to protect the gastric mucosa against NSAID-induced ulceration (see next section), it is likely that

mechanisms other than acid suppression are important for the prevention of gastric ulcers. Additionally, it has recently been suggested that misoprostol may be superior to proton pump inhibitors (PPIs) for the prevention of NSAID-induced gastric ulcers and gastroduodenal erosions.[85,86]

Misoprostol appears to be effective in preventing acute gastroduodenal injury induced by short courses of ASA and NSAIDs as measured by mucosal, or fecal blood loss, and by endoscopic injury scores.[87–91] However the clinical relevance of this effect is unclear, given the adaptation of gastroduodenal mucosa to acute injury with continued NSAID use.[65,92,93]

Long-term efficacy of misoprostol

In our meta-analysis,[26] we found 22 studies that assessed the long-term effect of misoprostol on the prevention of NSAID ulcers.[9,85,86,94–112] The dosage of misoprostol varied from 200 micrograms to 800 micrograms daily, and follow up ranged between 4 and 48 weeks. Although these studies considered erosions and ulcers in their analysis, the data we present below refers only to endoscopic ulcers ≥ 3 mm in diameter.

Eleven studies with 3641 patients compared the incidence of endoscopic ulcers after at least 3 months of misoprostol compared with placebo.[85,86,95,97,98,101,102,105,108,109,112] In these trials the proportions of patients receiving placebo medication who developed gastric and duodenal ulcers were 15% and 6%, respectively.

Endoscopic ulcers

Misoprostol significantly reduced the relative risk of gastric and duodenal ulcers by 74% (RR 0·26, 95%CI 0·17 to 0·39), and 53% (RR 0·47, 95% CI 0·33 to 0·69). These relative risks correspond to ARRs of 10·7% (from 14·9% to 4·2%), and 2·4% (from 6·0% to 3·6%) for gastric and duodenal ulcers, respectively. Interestingly, misoprostol was significantly more effective at reducing the relative risk of gastric than of duodenal ulcers, which is a pattern that was not seen with the H_2-receptor antagonists and the PPIs. A1a

Although all the studied doses of misoprostol were effective, misoprostol 800 micrograms daily was associated with the lowest risk (RR 0·17, 95% CI 0·11 to 0·24, ARR 13%) of endoscopic gastric ulcers when compared with placebo. Misoprostol 400 micrograms daily was associated with an RR of 0·39 (95% CI 0·3 to 0·51). This difference between high and low dose misoprostol reached statistical significance $(P = 0·0055)$. The pooled RRR of 78% (RR 0·21, 95% CI 0·09 to 0·49, ARR 4·7%) for duodenal ulcers with misoprostol 800 micrograms daily was not statistically significantly different from those of the lower daily misoprostol dosages. A1a

Shorter-term studies of less than 3 months duration tended to demonstrate slightly higher risk reductions. The pooling of these studies revealed 81% RRR of gastric ulcers with misoprostol (RR 0·17, 95% CI 0·09 to 0·31) and

72% RRR of duodenal ulcers (RR 0·28, 95% CI 0·14 to 0·56).[100,101,103,104,106,110,111,113] Ala

Head-to-head comparison

Two trials with 600 patients compared misoprostol with ranitidine 150 mg twice daily for NSAID ulcer prevention.[98,99] Misoprostol appears superior to standard dose ranitidine for the prevention of NSAID-induced gastric ulcers (RR 0·12, 95% CI 0·03 to 0·51) but not for duodenal ulcers (RR 1·00, 95% CI 0·14 to 7·14). The 0·12 RR in gastric ulcers corresponds to 5% absolute risk difference. Ala

In the combined analysis of two head-to-head studies of misoprostol versus PPIs in patients with a previously healed NSAID ulcer,[85,86] there was no statistically significant difference between PPIs and misoprostol for the prevention of NSAID-induced gastric ulcers. However, the study by Graham *et al.*[86] found that misoprostol was more effective than PPIs for gastric ulcer prevention. Likewise, Graham[114] recently reanalyzed the original Omeprazole versus Misoprostol for NSAID-induced Ulcer Management (OMNIUM)[71] and Acid Suppression Trial: Ranitidine versus Omeprazole for NSAID-associated Ulcer Treatment (ASTRONAUT)[85] study data, and found that these studies may have overestimated the effect of PPIs at reducing NSAID-induced gastric ulcers. In this reanalysis, misoprostol 400 micrograms/day was more effective than omeprazole 20 mg/day at reducing gastric ulcers (8·2% v 16·6% for misoprostol and omeprazole, respectively; $P < 0.05$), and PPIs were no better than misoprostol at preventing gastric ulcers in *H. pylori* positive subjects. PPIs were however more effective at reducing duodenal ulcers than gastric ulcers as our own meta-analysis has shown. Ala

Overall, these studies show that misoprostol is of clear benefit for the prevention of both endoscopically defined gastric and duodenal ulcers, with an RRR of over 70%, and an ARR of nearly 10%, compared with placebo. It also appears that higher doses of misoprostol are more effective than lower doses.

NSAID-induced clinical events

Silverstein *et al.* in 1995 published the landmark Misoprostol Ulcer Complication Study Outcomes Safety Assessment (MUCOSA) study, the first prospective study to evaluate the efficacy of misoprostol for the prevention of clinically important NSAID-induced adverse upper gastrointestinal events.[9] In this 6-month study, 8843 rheumatoid arthritis patients with a mean age of 68 years who were receiving continuous NSAID therapy were randomized to receive misoprostol 800 micrograms daily ($n = 4404$), or placebo ($n = 4439$). The patients were followed for the development of any suspicious gastrointestinal events. These events were reviewed by a blinded external committee and categorized as definite gastrointestinal complications if they fell into one of eight criteria (Box 6.2). Three other

criteria, such as melena without other supporting evidence, were classified as suggestive of possible or previous but not active bleeding. Of a total of 242 suspected gastrointestinal events, 67 were identified as definite as defined by categories 1–8, with 49 patients having "serious" gastrointestinal events (categories 1–6). Overall there was a combined event incidence of 0·76% over 6 months or about 1·5% per year. Considering all definite gastrointestinal events, 25 (0·57%) of 4404 of patients receiving misoprostol experienced events, compared with 42 (0·95%) of 4439 patients receiving the placebo (OR 0·60, representing an RR of 40%, $P = 0.049$). Ala The absolute risk difference was 0·38% (from 0·95% to 0·57%). If only perforation or obstruction (categories 1–2) were considered, then 1 of 4404 of subjects receiving misoprostol compared with 10 of 4439 of those receiving placebo suffered an event, (OR 0·101, RR 90% in these events, $P = 0.012$). However, the observed difference in occurrence of endoscopically proved gastrointestinal hemorrhage (categories 3–6) was not statistically significant (placebo 23 of 4439, misoprostol 15 of 4404, $P > 0.20$).

The wealth of data provided in this study has allowed clinicians and researchers alike to choose among the categories they feel are important and to derive widely differing estimates of the risk reductions associated with misoprostol therapy. For example, Maiden and Madhok in an editorial,[115] calculated that 1480 patients would need to be treated to prevent one case of gastric outlet obstruction (number needed to treat (NNT) = 1/absolute risk difference). However, these authors chose the rarest event and expressed there findings based on a 6 month observation period. If the NNT is calculated for prevention of obstruction or perforation (categories 1–2) for one year, the NNT is 264. If any definite gastrointestinal complication is chosen as the outcome measure (categories 1–8), the NNT is 132. Ala Clearly these choices would have considerable impact on the interpretation of this study's results, and on the calculated cost effectiveness of this therapy.

Box 6.2   Definite gastrointestinal events[9]

- Surgery proved perforated ulcer
- Endoscopy proved gastric outlet obstruction caused by ulceration and stricture
- Hematemesis, with endoscopically proved gastric or duodenal ulcer or erosion
- Active or recent visualized bleeding from endoscopically proved ulceration or erosion
- Melena with endoscopically proved ulceration or erosion
- Heme-positive stool with endoscopically proved ulceration or erosion, plus either a decrease hematocrit or an orthostatic change in blood pressure or pulse
- Hematemesis without endoscopically proved ulceration or erosion
- Melena, with heme-positive stool and without endoscopically proved ulceration or erosion

Table 6.2 Meta analysis of misoprostol-induced adverse effects in randomized placebo controlled trials of misopostol for prevention of NSAID-induced ulcers

Dose	Outcome	RR	95% CI	RD	Hetero
All	D/O adverse effects overall	1·41[a]	1·31–1·51	7·0	No
	D/O nausea	1·26[a]	1·07–1·48	1·1	No
	D/O diarrhea	2·36[a]	2·01–2·77	4·6	No
400 micrograms/day	D/O A/E overall	1·15	0·89–1·49	1·2	No
	D/O diarrhea	1·38	0·67–2·84	0·6	No
	D/O abdominal pain	1·53	0·90–2·59	1·3	No
	Diarrhea	1·92[a]	1·64–2·26	0·6	No
800 micrograms/day	D/O A/E overall	1·14	0·31–1·51	7·1	No
	D/O diarrhea	2·45[a]	2·09–2·88	5·2	No
	D/O abdominal pain	1·38[a]	1·17–1·63	1·7	No
	Diarrhea	3·05[a,b]	2·42–3·83	5·2	No

[a]denotes statistically significantly different from placebo.
[b]denotes statistically significantly different from the lower dose.
D/O, dropouts due to the outcome stated; A/E, adverse effects; RD, risk difference expressed as a percent; Hetero, heterogeneity; CI, confidence interval, NSAID, non-steroidal anti-inflammatory drug.

Adverse effects

The most frequently reported adverse effects with misoprostol therapy are diarrhea and abdominal pain. Additionally, misoprostol is an abortifacient and it must be used cautiously in women of childbearing age. In the study by Silverstein *et al.*, 732 of 4404 patients on misoprostol experienced diarrhea or abdominal pain, compared with 399 of 4439 patients on placebo (RR 1·82 associated with misoprostol, *P* < 0·001). Overall 27% of patients on misoprostol experienced one or more adverse effects.[9] In our review of the misoprostol trials (Table 6.2), misoprostol was associated with a small but statistically significant 1·4-fold excess risk of drop out due to drug-induced adverse effects, and an excess risk of dropouts due to nausea (RR 1·26), and diarrhea (RR 2·36). When analyzed by dose, misoprostol 800 micrograms daily, showed a statistically significant excess risk of dropouts due to diarrhea (RR 2·45), and abdominal pain (RR 1·38). Both misoprostol doses were associated with a statistically significant risk of diarrhea. However, the risk of diarrhea with 800 micrograms/day (RR 3·05) was significantly higher than that seen with 400 micrograms/day (RR 1·92, *P* = 0·0012). Ala

Cost effectiveness

The cost effectiveness of misoprostol for the prophylaxis of NSAID-related endoscopically defined ulcers has been evaluated in eight studies.[116–123] Misoprostol was found to be either cost saving or cost effective when calculations were based on the estimate of 80% for prevention of endoscopically defined ulcers. Misoprostol was later shown to reduce clinically serious gastrointestinal events by only 40%.[9] By relying on studies with endoscopically defined ulcers as the outcomes, authors of earlier economic evaluations overestimated the reduction in downstream events, such as outpatient endoscopy and hospitalizations. Furthermore, the MUCOSA study also showed that approximately 85% of endoscopic ulcers are asymptomatic and never get investigated.[45] A revision of the cost-effectiveness of misoprostol, based on this new evidence, showed that misoprostol is not cost effective when prescribed to all patients, but becomes cost effective if patients are selected who are at higher risk of a clinically serious gastrointestinal event,[45] such as older patients and those with a positive history of peptic ulcer disease.

In conclusion, misoprostol prophylaxis significantly reduces the risk of ulcers as well as serious gastrointestinal events in patients on long-term NSAID therapy. Misoprostol is more effective at reducing the risk of gastric than duodenal ulcers, and may be more effective than PPIs at reducing the risk of gastric ulcers. The use of misoprostol, particularly at higher doses, is associated with more frequent gastrointestinal adverse effects often resulting in the patient discontinuing the medication, which is an important consideration, given the symptoms associated with NSAID use alone. The effectiveness outside of clinical trials of misoprostol for prevention of ulcer may be lower than figures which have been presented above. However, since misoprostol is the only prophylactic agent that has been directly shown to reduce serious NSAID-related gastrointestinal complications, it should be considered to be the first-line agent in the primary prophylaxis of NSAID complications particularly in high risk groups. Ala

H_2-receptor antagonists

Treatment of NSAID-induced ulcers

The efficacy of H_2-receptor antagonists in the treatment and prevention of NSAID-related upper gastrointestinal toxicity has been exclusively evaluated in studies in which ulcers were defined endoscopically. In several early open label studies of cimetidine for healing of ulcers associated with the use of NSAIDs, it was shown that greater than 75% of gastric and duodenal ulcers could be healed with 12 weeks of therapy despite continued use of NSAIDs.[124–128] B4 There was a trend toward improved efficacy with higher doses. However, in a randomized trial in which patients with NSAID-induced ulcers were randomized to receive standard dose ranitidine, or the more potent acid suppressor omeprazole, omeprazole was nearly twice as effective,[129] although ranitidine was still effective.[129,130] A1c O'Laughlin *et al.* found that ulcer size correlated inversely with healing rates.[128] At 8 weeks, ulcers with a diameter < 5 mm were healed in greater than 90% of patients compared with 35% healing for ulcers > 5 mm.[131] Hudson *et al.* reported similar observations.[132] The potency of acid suppression and initial ulcer size are important determinants of the rapidity of ulcer healing, and that continued use of NSAIDs in the presence of gastric acid may slow ulcer healing.

Prevention of NSAID-induced ulcers

Standard doses of H_2-receptor antagonists have been consistently shown to be effective for prevention of endoscopically defined duodenal ulcers, but not of gastric ulcers.[96,133–142] Koch *et al.*[143] in a meta-analysis of randomized trials which employed standard doses of H_2-receptor antagonists[133–135,137,139,140] and Stalnikowicz *et al.*[10] were also unable to show a benefit for the prevention of gastric ulcers. A1a Similarly, our meta-analysis of the standard dose H_2-receptor antagonist trials confirms that there is no statistically significant reduction in the relative risk of endoscopically defined gastric ulcers.[26,27] A1a

Seven trials with 1188 patients assessed the effect of standard dose H_2-receptor antagonists on the prevention of endoscopic NSAID ulcers at 1 month,[133–136,139,140,144] and five trials with 1005 patients assessed these outcomes at 3 months or longer.[133,136,137,142,145] Standard dose H_2-receptor antagonists are effective at reducing the risk of duodenal ulcers (RR 0·24, 95% CI 0·10 to 0·57 and RR 0·36, 95% CI 0·18 to 0·74 at 1 and 3 or more months, respectively), but not of risk of gastric ulcers (not significant).[26,27] A1a One study did not have a placebo comparator and was not included in the pooled estimate.[142]

Although achlorhydria has been reported not to prevent early NSAID-induced gastric lesions,[146] there is accumulating evidence that profound acid suppression can reduce acute NSAID and ASA-induced gastric mucosal injury.[147–149] Based on these observations, several investigators have tested the hypothesis that higher doses of H_2-receptor antagonists may achieve more consistent acid suppression and may therefore be effective for the prevention of gastric ulcer among chronic NSAID users. We identified three RCTs with 298 patients that assessed the efficacy of double dose H_2-receptor antagonists for the prevention of NSAID-induced upper gastrointestinal toxicity.[132,136,150] Double dose H_2-receptor antagonists when compared with placebo were associated with a statistically significant reduction in the risk of both duodenal (RR 0·26, 95% CI 0·11 to 0·65) and gastric ulcers (RR 0·44, 95% CI 0·26 to 0·74). This 56% RRR in gastric ulcers corresponds to a 14·6% ARR (from 25·9% to 11·3%). A1c Analysis of the secondary prophylaxis studies alone yielded similar results.

H_2-receptor antagonists were generally quite well tolerated in the presented studies. Standard doses of these agents appear to be effective in preventing NSAID-induced duodenal but not gastric ulcers. However, double dose H_2-receptor antagonists appear to be effective for healing and prevention of both gastric and duodenal ulcers in patients taking NSAIDs chronically. However the clinical use of this class of drugs for the prevention of gastroduodenal ulceration may be questioned for several reasons. In terms of the trial results, the ulcer rates in the placebo groups of the famotidine studies are higher than are generally reported. Furthermore, since H_2-receptor antagonists are associated with tolerance to their acid suppression effects,[151–153] the long-term efficacy of these drugs must be questioned. Finally, even if effective for ulcer prevention, there is no economic or therapeutic advantage to using double doses of these drugs rather than standard doses of PPIs which produce more potent and reliable acid suppression.

Proton pump inhibitors

PPIs block the final step of gastric acid secretion by inhibiting parietal cell $H + K + ATPase$. Direct evidence for the efficacy of PPIs in the primary or secondary prevention of clinically important NSAID-induced upper gastrointestinal toxicity is lacking. Several factors have prompted interest in the use of PPIs for prophylaxis against NSAID-induced ulcers: (i) dissatisfaction with the adverse effects of misoprostol; (ii) the apparent efficacy of PPIs in healing NSAID ulcers; (iii) the proved efficacy of PPIs in other acid–peptic disorders; (iv) the attractive tolerability profile of PPIs.

PPIs appear to be effective for the prevention of early NSAID-induced upper gastrointestinal injury assessed either endoscopically or through the detection of mucosal blood loss in healthy volunteers given ASA or naproxen.[147–149,154]

However, as discussed previously the clinical relevance of these early lesions is in question.

Healing of ulcers with continued NSAID use

Omeprazole has been shown to heal both gastric and duodenal ulcers irrespective of continued NSAID use.[71,85,129,155–157] Walan *et al.* in a double blind trial, assessed the healing rates of benign gastric and prepyloric ulcers in 602 patients randomized to receive either omeprazole (40 mg or 20 mg) or ranitidine 150 mg twice daily.[129] In a subset of 58 patients with endoscopically documented ulcers who continued to take NSAIDs, the proportions of patients whose ulcers healed at 8 weeks were: omeprazole 40 mg 95% (similar to results for patients with non-NSAID ulcers), omeprazole 20 mg 82% and ranitidine 53% ($P < 0.05$). These data suggest that selected patients with endoscopically documented NSAID ulcers can experience ulcer healing with omeprazole despite continued NSAID use. Ala However, caution should be exercised in extrapolating these results to patients presenting with NSAID-induced upper gastrointestinal hemorrhage. In these patients the decision to continue the NSAID must be individualized, since the safety and efficacy of omeprazole in this setting has not been assessed.

NSAID ulcer prevention

In our meta analysis[26] we identified eight RCTs with a total of 2181 patients that assessed the effect of PPIs on the prevention of NSAID-induced upper gastrointestinal toxicity.[71,85,86,158–162]

Three of these studies compared omeprazole to placebo.[161,162] Of the two studies that compared a PPI to placebo and to misoprostol, one used lansoprazole[86] while the other used omeprazole as prophylaxis.[85] Chan *et al.* compared omeprazole with diclofenac to celecoxib,[158] while Jensen *et al.* compared omeprazole with misoprostol.[160] Another compared pantoprazole to placebo,[159] while the last compared omeprazole with ranitidine.[71]

Overall, PPIs significantly reduced the relative risk of endoscopic duodenal ulcers by 81% (RR 0.19, 95% CI 0.09 to 0.37) and gastric ulcers by 60% (RR 0.40, 95% CI 0.32 to 0.51) compared with placebo in both primary and secondary (studies that enrolled patients that had NSAIDs ulcers that were healed in an initial healing phase) prophylaxis trials. These RRs correspond to ARRs of 8.2% (from 10.1% to 1.9%) and 14.0% (from 26.7% to 12.7%) for duodenal and gastric ulcers, respectively. Ala Although PPIs appear to reduce the relative risk of duodenal ulcers more than of gastric ulcers, this difference did not reach statistical significance ($P = 0.068$).

The OMNIUM and ASTRONAUT studies deserve a more detailed discussion.[71,85] These two trials were of nearly identical design, and included an 8-week healing phase,

followed by a 26-week secondary prophylaxis phase. The results of the healing phase will be addressed first.

Healing phase

A total of 935 patients with a mean age of 62 ears, were enrolled into the OMNIUM study.[85] Thirty-five percent of these patients had erosions only, 40% had gastric ulcers, 20% had duodenal ulcers, with the remainder having combinations of these lesions. The patients were randomized to receive omeprazole 20 mg daily ($n = 308$), omeprazole 40 mg daily ($n = 315$), or misoprostol 800 micrograms daily ($n = 298$). Overall treatment success was defined as ulcer healing, the presence of less than five erosions and the presence of not more than mild dyspeptic symptoms. At 8 weeks the healing rates for gastric ulcers were 87%, 80% and 73%, for the omeprazole 20 mg, omeprazole 40 mg, and the misoprostol groups, respectively. The difference between the omeprazole 20 mg and misoprostol groups was statistically significant ($P = 0.004$). Ala Duodenal ulcer healing rates were significantly higher with omeprazole 20 mg (93%) and 40 mg (89%) than with misoprostol (77%) ($P < 0.001$). Ala In contrast, misoprostol produced significantly higher healing rates of gastroduodenal erosions than either omeprazole doses (87% *v* 77% and 79% respectively, $P = 0.01$). Ala The authors identified that the presence of duodenal ulcer, or erosions in contrast to gastric ulcers, and the presence of *H. pylori* were significant favorable prognostic factors predicting ulcer healing.

In the healing phase of the ASTRONAUT study 541 slightly younger patients, (mean age 57 years), were randomized to receive omeprazole 20 mg ($n = 174$), omeprazole 40 mg ($n = 187$) or ranitidine 150 mg twice daily ($n = 174$) for 8 weeks.[71] The baseline characteristics and ulcer distributions were similar to those of the OMNIUM study. Omeprazole at either dose was more effective than ranitidine for healing of gastric ulcer (omeprazole 20 mg 84%, omeprazole 40 mg 87%, ranitidine 64%, $P < 0.001$). Ala Omeprazole was also more effective than ranitidine for healing duodenal ulcer (omeprazole 20 mg 92%, omeprazole 40 mg 88%, ranitidine 81%, $P = 0.03$ for comparison of omeprazole 20 mg and ranitidine). Both doses of omeprazole were more effective than ranitidine for healing erosions (omeprazole 20 mg 89%, omeprazole 40 mg 86%, ranitidine 77%, $P = 0.008$ for the comparison of omeprazole 20 mg and ranitidine). At 4 weeks but not at 8 weeks omeprazole 20 mg daily was superior to ranitidine for the relief of moderate to severe dyspeptic symptoms. The same favorable prognostic factors identified in the OMNIUM study were found.

Secondary prophylaxis

Patients who experienced healing of their ulcers during the initial phase of these two studies were re-randomized to maintenance treatment without consideration for the treatment they initially received for purposes of ulcer healing. The patients were followed for a total of 6 months with endoscopic evaluations made at 1, 3, and 6 months or if troublesome symptoms arose. Patients were considered to be in remission if they were free of ulcers, had < 10 gastric or duodenal erosions, and had not more than mild dyspeptic symptoms.

The OMNIUM maintenance study randomized 732 chronic NSAID users whose ulcer/erosions were healed during the healing phase study, to receive maintenance therapy with omeprazole 20 mg daily, misoprostol 200 micrograms twice daily, or placebo.[85] At 6 months 61%, 48% and 27% of patients were in remission as defined above for the omeprazole, misoprostol and placebo groups, respectively. The results reached statistical significance for omeprazole versus misoprostol ($P = 0.001$) and for omeprazole versus placebo ($P < 0.001$). Ala When only erosions were considered, fewer patients relapsed on misoprostol than on omeprazole or placebo (7% v 12% and 14%, respectively).

The ASTRONAUT maintenance study randomized 432 patients who achieved treatment success during the healing phase study.[71] This study compared maintenance omeprazole 20 mg daily to standard dose ranitidine (150 mg twice daily). At 6 months 72% of patients on omeprazole versus 59% on ranitidine were in remission ($P = 0.004$). Ala Again, in both these maintenance phase studies the presence of *H. pylori* was associated with a significantly higher likelihood of remaining in remission. It would have been interesting to compare omeprazole to higher doses of misoprostol or double dose ranitidine. Clearly, the investigators chose a dose of misoprostol that they felt would be most tolerable. However, it is clear, as discussed in the previous sections, that standard doses of H$_2$-receptor antagonists are ineffective at preventing NSAID-induced gastric ulcers.

Although PPIs appear to be effective agents, the findings of the OMNIUM study suggesting that misoprostol may be more effective at preventing gastroduodenal erosions raises some concerns which seem to be echoed in more recent trials. The combined analysis of the OMNIUM and Graham studies of PPIs versus misoprostol showed that the two interventions were equally effective at reducing gastric ulcers. The Graham study however, individually showed that misoprostol was more effective at reducing gastric ulcers than lansoprazole.[86] Furthermore, Graham re-analyzed the OMNIUM study results and found that the effectiveness of omeprazole at reducing NSAID-related gastric ulcers may have been overestimated.[114] This potentially important finding needs to be confirmed since gastric ulcers account for the majority (75%) of NSAID ulcers and our own meta-analysis results showed that PPIs demonstrated a trend toward greater effectiveness at reducing the relative risk of duodenal than gastric ulcers which is the opposite of what we found with misoprostol. An indirect comparison of high dose misoprostol

versus PPIs based on the data from our meta-analysis showed an RRR of 60% in favor of misoprostol that was not statistically significant ($P = 0.12$).

Symptoms

Four omeprazole trials used the same composite endpoints to define treatment success.[71,85,161,162] In these trials omeprazole significantly reduced "dyspeptic symptoms" as defined by the authors. In the combined analysis, dropouts overall and dropouts due to side effects were not different from placebo.

Summary

Collectively these studies demonstrate that PPIs are effective for healing both gastric and duodenal NSAID-induced ulcers irrespective of continued NSAID use or *H. pylori* status. Ala These agents also appear to be effective for the prevention of endoscopically diagnosed NSAID-induced ulcers. However, their efficacy for the prevention of serious NSAID-related gastrointestinal complications is unknown. It is reasonable to recommend its use in eligible patients who are intolerant or otherwise unable to take misoprostol. Interestingly misoprostol appears to be more effective than omeprazole for both the healing and prevention of gastroduodenal erosions and may be more effective than PPIs at reducing the relative risk of NSAID-induced gastric ulcers – although this last point needs to be confirmed in another study. It should be noted that the required high dose of misoprostol is poorly tolerated by many patients.

The appropriate choice of therapy for secondary prophylaxis against NSAID ulcer recurrence among chronic NSAID users is unclear. Currently misoprostol is the only prophylactic agent that has been proved to be of benefit in the prevention of NSAID-induced clinical events. However, in reality most clinicians prescribe a PPI to heal NSAID-induced ulcers, and continue this agent for secondary prophylaxis. Given the results of the OMNIUM and ASTRONAUT studies, this may be appropriate, but a degree of caution is indicated given the limitations of these studies, and the absence of direct evidence of the effectiveness of PPIs against clinical gastrointestinal events. The cost effectiveness of PPIs for the primary or secondary prophylaxis against NSAID-induced upper gastrointestinal toxicity has not been established.

Cyclo-oxygenase-2 inhibitors

Since the first edition of this book was published, much has changed. Several endoscopic studies have demonstrated the safety of COX-2 inhibitors, and two important clinical outcome studies similar to the misoprostol MUCOSA study have been performed. In this section we will present the latest evidence relating to the gastrointestinal safety of COX-2 inhibitors. We will concentrate on the currently available agents that are marketed as COX-2 inhibitors in Canada (celecoxib, rofecoxib, meloxicam). This section is based on a meta-analysis performed for CCOHTA[163] and an ongoing Cochrane Collaboration review.

As described earlier, it is felt that NSAIDs exert their therapeutic anti-inflammatory and analgesic effects through the inhibition of inducible COX-2, whereas their gastric and renal toxicities, and antiplatelet effects arise from the inhibition of the constitutive COX-1 isoform.[24,25] This COX-2 hypothesis, along with the unfavorable safety profile of standard NSAIDs has prompted the development of newer NSAIDs with selectivity for the COX-2 isoform.

Endoscopic ulcer studies

We identified seven studies with a total of 4678 patients that assessed the proportion of patients with endoscopic ulcers while taking a COX-2 inhibitor compared with a standard NSAID.[164–168] Of the five studies that assessed celecoxib, two remain unpublished, and were obtained from the FDA website (FDA studies 21 and 71).[167,168] Two studies assessed rofecoxib.[169,170] The included endoscopic studies are quite similar in design, and share a similar patient population. Overall the proportion of gastric and duodenal ulcers in patients taking non-selective NSAIDs in these trials were 18·9% and 5·6%, respectively. The proportion of gastroduodenal ulcer overall in the standard NSAID arms was 24·2%. As a comparison, in the NSAID prophylaxis studies presented earlier, gastric ulcers occurred in a range of 12–20% for all interventions, while duodenal ulcers occurred in 6% of those taking non-selective NSAIDs. Therefore there is considerable consistency between the control group ulcer risks in the original NSAID prophylaxis studies and the control group risk in the COX-2 selective NSAID studies.

Gastric ulcers

Five studies with a total of 2613 patients compared the safety of COX-2 inhibitors for endoscopic gastric ulcers versus a comparator NSAID over a 3–6-month interval.[164–166,169,170] The use of a COX-2 inhibitor in this setting was associated with an 82% RRR in gastric ulcers (RR 0·18, 95% CI 0·14 to 0·23). This RRR represents a 21% ARR in gastric ulcers (from 26·0% to 5·0%) with COX-2 inhibitors compared with standard NSAIDs. Ala

Duodenal ulcers

The same five studies also compared the effect of low dose COX-2 inhibitors on duodenal ulcers versus standard NSAIDs.[164–166,169,170] COX-2 inhibitors were associated with a 60% RRR in duodenal ulcers compared with standard

NSAIDs (RR 0·40, 95% CI 0·27 to 0·60). This represents only a 4% absolute risk difference (from 6·4% to 2·4%) between COX-2 inhibitors and standard NSAIDs. Ala

Overall, COX-2 inhibitors were more effective at reducing the relative risk of gastric ulcers than the risk of duodenal ulcers (RR 0·18 *v* 0·40). This difference reached statistical significance (*P* < 0·001). This effect was consistent when celecoxib and rofecoxib were analyzed separately.

The results above did not include the two unpublished celecoxib studies obtained from the FDA website.[167,168] Inclusion of these studies did not alter the overall results significantly.

Comparing the COX-2 inhibitors

We identified five studies with a total of 3590 patients that compared celecoxib to standard NSAIDs.[164–168] These studies showed a 72% RRR in total gastroduodenal ulcers in favor of celecoxib (RR 0·28, 95% CI 0·23 to 0·35, 14% ARR). Ala

Only two studies with a total of 1087 patients compared rofecoxib to standard NSAIDs. In this case a 75% RRR is seen in favor of rofecoxib (RR 0·25, 95% CI 0·20 to 0·32, 35% ARR).[169,170] This result was not statistically different from that seen with celecoxib. However, it should be noted that we could not identify any study that directly compared celecoxib with rofecoxib.

COX-2 inhibitors compared with different NSAIDs

Three studies compared celecoxib to naproxen showing a 75% RRR in favor of celecoxib (RR 0·25, 95% CI 0·20 to 0·31).[164,166,167] Ala Likewise, three studies (two rofecoxib, one celecoxib) showed a 73% RRR with COX-2 inhibitors compared with ibuprofen (RR 0·27, 95% CI 0·22 to 0·33).[168–170] However celecoxib was not statistically different from diclofenac (RR 0·45, 95% CI 0·15 to 1·29). Ala

The FDA study 71 compared celecoxib to ibuprofen and diclofenac. In this study there was no significant relative risk reduction between celecoxib and diclofenac for gastric ulcers but there was a significant 66% RRR when compared with ibuprofen (RR 0·34, 95% CI 0·23 to 0·51).[168] Ala Unfortunately, this was the only endoscopic study to compare a COX-2 inhibitor to different standard NSAIDs in one study.

COX-2 inhibitors versus placebo

Four studies with a total of 2576 patients compared COX-2 inhibitors to placebo.[166,167,169,170] In all the same analyses described above for COX-2 inhibitors versus NSAIDS, there were no statistically significant differences between COX-2 inhibitors and placebo. For example the relative risk for combined gastroduodenal ulcers with COX-2 inhibitors versus placebo was a non-significant 1·09 (95% CI 0·74 to 1·60). Ala

Clinical ulcer complications

Clinical ulcer complications in the COX-2 studies are important endpoints derived from the endpoints used in the MUCOSA study.[9] In these studies two endpoints are commonly used: POBs and PUBs. A POB is a hard clinical endpoint of perforation, obstruction or bleeding related to an NSAID ulcer. A PUB is a composite endpoint of POB + a symptomatic ulcer. A PUB endpoint occurs if one of the POB events occurs or if a subject complains of ulcer-like symptoms which subsequently lead to the identification of an ulcer during endoscopy. The difficulty with this last endpoint is that, as described earlier, most endoscopic ulcers remain clinically silent, and that symptoms are poor predictors of the occurrence of true clinical events like perforation, obstruction or bleeding. Further, as will be described, COX-2 inhibitors appear to be associated with less dyspeptic symptoms. This is an important finding in its own right, but using symptoms as a trigger to look for a common finding such as an endoscopic ulcer may bias the PUB result in favor of an agent that produces fewer symptoms even if the compared agents are comparable in terms of producing POBs.

COX-2 versus NSAIDs

At the time of this writing there were seven studies with a total of 61 282 patients that assessed the safety of COX-2 inhibitors using the clinically important endpoint of ulcer complications (POB and PUB).[171,172] Three of these trials used celecoxib,[48,171,172] two used rofecoxib,[173] and two meloxicam.[174] Two of these studies are combined analyses of the early efficacy and the endoscopic studies,[171,173] and one was available only in abstract form.[172]

The two most important studies in this group are the Celecoxib Long-term Arthritis Safety Study (CLASS)[48] and VIOXX™ Gastrointestinal Outcome Research (VIGOR) Arthritis[47] studies and will be discussed in greater detail.

The CLASS study compared celecoxib to ibuprofen and to diclofenac in 8059 patients with osteo or rheumatoid arthritis.[48] This study did not show a statistically significant benefit of celecoxib over the NSAID groups combined for its primary outcome of ulcer complications (POB), though it showed a benefit if the composite PUB endpoint was used (annual incidence of 2·08% *v* 3·54% for celecoxib and NSAIDs, respectively; *P* = 0·02). Ala In subgroup analyses celecoxib was superior to combined NSAIDs in patients not taking ASA (0·44% *v* 1·27%, *P* = 0·04) but not for those on celecoxib and ASA (2·01% *v* 2·12% *P* = 0·92). In fact, the risk of ulcer complications in patients taking celecoxib and ASA was nearly four times that of those who were not taking ASA. There would be no apparent advantage for a patient needing ASA to take celecoxib rather than diclofenac. These data are in stark contrast to the suggestions made based on the initial

endoscopic studies that it may be safer to take ASA with celecoxib than with standard NSAIDs.[175,176]

The CLASS study also presents further problems, which are beyond the scope of this chapter. In brief, according to the original FDA submission the analysis of the CLASS data was to be a stepwise analysis that depended on showing a statistically significant difference between celecoxib and the NSAID group combined for POBs. If this analysis failed than no further analyses or subgroup analyses would be carried out. In the published CLASS study, the POB endpoint failed to reach statistical significance yet multiple subgroup analyses were performed. Furthermore according to multiple documents on the FDA website, multiple letters to the editors of journals,[177,178] and even an article in the *Washington Post*,[179] the CLASS study actually extended to 12 months rather than the published 6 months. The celecoxib sponsors argued that the statistical technique of data imputation was required because more subjects dropped out of the standard NSAID arms than was the case for celecoxib. Therefore those patients who continued on celecoxib remained at risk for gastrointestinal events, while the disproportionate number of those on standard NSAIDs who had already dropped out could not suffer a significant gastrointestinal event. The FDA reviewers refuted these arguments[175,176] (multiple other FDA documents on the FDA website). However from the perspective of this review sensitivity analyses were performed around the CLASS data including both 6-month and 12-month data with the results not impacting on the overall combined analysis. Overall a statistically significant benefit of COX-2 inhibitors over combined standard NSAIDs remained.

The VIGOR study, was a well conducted RCT of rofecoxib versus the relatively gastrointestinal toxic NSAID naproxen in 8000 rheumatoid arthritis patients not taking ASA. The results showed a statistical superiority of rofecoxib over naproxen for both POBs (RR 0·43, *P* = 0·005) Ala and PUBs (RR 0·46, *P* < 0·001). Unfortunately, as evidenced on the FDA website, subjects in the rofecoxib arm were at higher risk of cardiovascular complications than those taking naproxen. This can be interpreted in various ways: as a positive effect of naproxen, a detrimental effect of rofecoxib, or a combination of the two. Currently two large studies are being conducted to further assess the cardiovascular risk associated with rofecoxib (personal communication, F Bertrand, A Gibson, Merck Cardiovascular Safety studies, 9 September 2002) and preliminary data from the Institute for Clinical Evaluative Sciences suggests no increased cardiovascular risk with rofecoxib (personal communication, M Mamdami, cardiovascular risk of rofecoxib, 13 September 2002). The issue still remains that the safety of the coadministration of ASA and rofecoxib is currently unknown, since ASA users were excluded from the VIGOR trial. If the results are similar to those seen in the CLASS study, then one would expect reduced safety of rofecoxib when used with ASA, particularly if it is compared with a less toxic NSAID such as diclofenac.

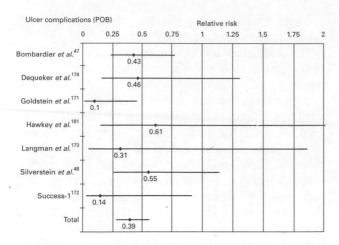

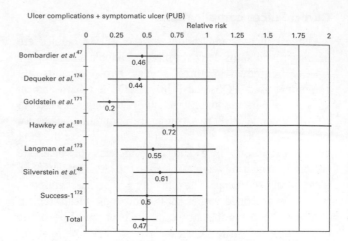

Figures 6.2 and 6.3 The figures show the meta-analysis plots for POB (Figure 6.2) and PUB (Figure 6.3) endpoints. These plots show the relative risk (RR) of developing a POB or PUB on COX-2 inhibitors compared with standard NSAIDs for each study and after combining the studies. The point and line to the right of the studies represent the RR and the 95% confidence interval. If the line representing the 95% confidence interval crosses the vertical line representing a RR of one, then the RR fails to reach statistical significance. As can be seen from the summary RRs, COX-2 inhibitors are associated with statistically significant relative risk of 39% for POBs, and 47% for PUBs. These RRs represent relative risk reductions of 61% for POBs and 53% for PUBs.

In defense of both the CLASS and VIGOR trials, the dosages of the COX-2 inhibitors that were used were two to four times higher than the recommended dosages for rheumatoid and osteoarthritis.

Overall, COX-2 inhibitors are associated with a 61% RRR in the POB outcome compared with standard NSAIDs (RR 0·39, 95% CI 0·27 to 0·56) (Figure 6.2). Ala This however, corresponds to a 0·24% ARR (from 0·36% to 0·12%). The same analysis with the CLASS study[48] 12-month data obtained from the FDA website drops the risk reduction to 55% (RR 0·45, 95% CI 0·32 to 0·63).[180] This difference is not statistically different.

The same seven articles combined the clinically important gastrointestinal outcomes above with a "symptomatic ulcer" endpoint to make a composite endpoint (PUB).[47,48,171–174,181] Using this endpoint, COX-2 inhibitors are associated with a 53% RRR in PUBs compared with standard NSAIDS (RR 0·47, 95% CI 0·38 to 0·57) (Figure 6.3). The same analysis with the CLASS study[48] 12-month data does not significantly alter the results (RR 0·49, 95% CI 0·41 to 0·61).[180]

Analyses stratified by COX-2 inhibitors

Three studies with 30 306 patients compared celecoxib to various NSAIDs.[48,171,172] Significant heterogeneity existed in this analysis most likely due to differing NSAID comparators. Using a random effects model, celecoxib was associated with a 77% RRR over standard NSAIDS (RR 0·23, 95% CI 0·07 to 0·76). Ala

Two studies compared rofecoxib to various NSAIDs.[47,173] In this analysis rofecoxib was associated with a 58% RRR in ulcer complications (RR 0·42, 95% CI 0·24 to 0·73).

Two high quality studies compared meloxicam to a standard NSAID using methodology similar to that of the CLASS and VIGOR trials.[174,181] Individually, the Hawkey *et al.*[181] and Dequeker *et al.* studies[174] failed to show a statistically significant benefit of meloxicam over diclofenac or piroxicam for either POBs or PUBs. Combining these two studies still fails to show a statistical benefit of meloxicam over standard NSAIDs for these endpoints (RR 0·50, 95% CI 0·22 to 1·17 for POBs, RR 0·53, 95% CI 0·26 to 1·05 for PUBs). Ala

We identified an additional eight meloxicam clinical efficacy trials with a total of 3468 patients that also considered gastrointestinal adverse effects as part of their safety analyses.[182–189] Two of these studies compared meloxicam to placebo,[187,189] leaving six studies, with a total of 2300 patients, that compared meloxicam to standard NSAIDs.[182–186,188] Although from an efficacy perspective these trials are of good quality, the reporting of clinical ulcer complications was poor, the criteria by which ulcer complications were adjudicated were not given or poorly described, and all but one of the studies[185] had no ulcer complications in at least one group resulting in empty cell analyses.[190] Therefore we present the combined analysis of the meloxicam studies as a separate analysis. Overall, when these studies are included, there is a RRR of 52% in PUBs with meloxicam (RR 0·48, 95% CI 0·26 to 0·88). Inclusion of these studies in the overall PUB analysis (63 582 patients) did not change the outcome at all (RR 0·47, 95% CI 0·38 to 0·57).

Cost effectiveness of COX-2 inhibitors

The cost-effectiveness of COX-2 inhibitors has recently been assessed by Maetzel *et al.*[191] In this report, a Markov

Table 6.3 Evidence of efficacy

Drug class	NSAID ulcer healing	Clinical events prevention	Gastric ulcers prevention	Duodenal ulcers prevention
Prostaglandin analogs	X	X	X	X
H$_2$ receptor antagonists (standard dose)	X			X
H$_2$ receptor antagonists (double dose)	X		X	X
Proton pump inhibitors	X		X	X
COX-2 inhibitors		X	X	X

NSAID, non-steroidal anti-inflammatory drug; COX, cyclo-oxygenase

model was used to determine the incremental cost effectiveness of celecoxib and rofecoxib compared with the standard NSAIDs naproxen, ibuprofen, and diclofenac with or without PPI prophylaxis in arthritic patients not requiring ASA. The authors used the results of the CLASS and VIGOR trials described previously as the basis of their analysis.

In average risk patients, those without a prior history of a complicated upper gastrointestinal event such as hemorrhage or perforation, the base case results were greater than Can\$ 200 000 per quality-adjusted life years gained for celecoxib versus ibuprofen and rofecoxib versus naproxen and therefore not felt to be cost effective. Diclofenac was found to be more effective and less costly than celecoxib. On the other hand, in older patients (> 76 years) without any other risk factors COX-2 inhibitors were considered to be cost effective. In high risk patients, those with a previous history of a complicated upper gastrointestinal event, the base case results showed COX-2 inhibitors to be more effective and less costly in the cases of celecoxib versus ibuprofen with PPI prophylaxis, and rofecoxib versus naproxen with PPI prophylaxis. Diclofenac was found to be comparable to celecoxib in this setting. Interestingly in the analysis of high risk patients, the cost effectiveness of COX-2 inhibitors was found to drop as the rates of co-prescription of COX-2 inhibitors with PPIs increased, and the cost effective advantage of COX-2 inhibitors was lost altogether if standard NSAIDs were used with a low cost PPI (< 1·90/day).

Summary

The available evidence suggests that the least gastrointestinal toxic NSAID in the lowest effective dose should be used whenever possible to limit the toxicity of these agents. The combination of NSAIDs with other anti-inflammatory agents, including ASA, corticosteroids, and with oral anticoagulants is associated with an increased risk of serious adverse gastrointestinal events, and again should be avoided when possible. Patients with different risk characteristics can have drastically different rates of adverse gastrointestinal events when treated with NSAIDs long term. Therefore, the addition of a second agent for prophylaxis against NSAID-induced adverse gastrointestinal events should likely be reserved for high risk patients, particularly older patients with previous peptic ulcer disease and concomitant coronary artery disease. Misoprostol at 800 micrograms daily is the only prophylactic agent thus far that has been directly shown to reduce the occurrence of significant adverse NSAID-related gastrointestinal events. Lower doses of misoprostol are associated with fewer adverse effects of diarrhea, and cramps, but also appear to be slightly less effective at preventing endoscopic gastric ulcers. The effects of low doses of misoprostol on clinical gastrointestinal events are unknown, so the use of lower doses may be associated with a significant clinical trade-off. Double doses of potent H$_2$-receptor antagonists and standard doses of PPIs appear to be effective at preventing endoscopic duodenal and gastric ulcers, reduce NSAID-related dyspepsia and are significantly better tolerated than misoprostol. However, the effectiveness of these agents at preventing clinical gastrointestinal events is unknown, and their cost effectiveness is dependent on the daily cost of the PPI. Finally, all these agents appear to be effective at healing NSAID ulcers despite continued NSAID use (Table 6.3). However, the more potent acid suppression afforded by PPIs and potent H$_2$-receptor antagonists appears to be most effective.

The accumulating COX-2 literature suggests a fundamental shift in the treatment of arthritic patients. Our meta-analysis demonstrates that celecoxib and rofecoxib appear to be safer than standard NSAIDs overall and are better tolerated. However, one should be cautious in generalizing from comparisons of individual COX-2 inhibitors with individual standard NSAIDs. In fact our data suggest that celecoxib may not offer a clear benefit over diclofenac. Rofecoxib has not been compared with diclofenac in a CLASS or VIGOR style study, and its safety with ASA coadministration is unknown. Meloxicam appears to have similar gastrointestinal toxicity as the standard NSAIDs it was compared with. The VIGOR study has raised concerns regarding the cardiovascular safety of COX-2 inhibitors, while the CLASS study demonstrated no benefit of celecoxib over standard NSAIDs in patients taking ASA. The cardiovascular safety of COX-2 inhibitors is currently being evaluated in several large outcome trials. Lastly, there are currently no studies that support a strategy of combining a gastroprotective such as a PPI with a COX-2 inhibitor.

References

1 Fries JF, Miller SR, Spitz PW, Williams CA, Hubert HB, Bloch DA. Identification of patients at risk for gastropathy associated with NSAID use. *J Rheumatol Suppl* 1990;**20**:12–19.

2 Patr O. Aspirin as an anti-platelet drug. *N Eng J Med* 1994;**330**:1287–94.

3 Stroke prevention in atrial fibrillation investigators. Stroke prevention in atrial fibrillation study: final results. *Circulation* 1991;**84**:527–39.

4 Steering Committee of the physicians' health study research group: final report on the aspirin component of the ongoing physician's health study. *N Eng J Med* 1989;**321**:129–35.

5 The SALT collaborative study group. Swedish aspirin low-dose trial of 75 mg aspirin as secondary prophylaxis after cerebrovascular ischemic events. *Lancet* 1991;**338**: 1345–49.

6 Wallace JL. Nonsteroidal anti-inflammatory drugs and gastroenteropathy: the second hundred years. *Gastroenterology* 1997;**112**:1000–16.

7 Smalley WE, Griffin MR, Fought RL, Ray WA. Excess costs from gastrointestinal disease associated with nonsteroidal anti-inflammatory drugs. *J Gen Intern Med* 1996;**11**: 461–9.

8 Larkai E, Smith J, Lidsky M. Gastroduodenal mucosa and dyspeptic symptoms in arthritic patients during chronic nonsteroidal anti-inflammatory drug use. *Am J Gastroenterol* 1987;**82**:1153–8.

9 Silverstein FE, Graham DY, Senior JR *et al.* Misoprostol reduces serious gastrointestinal complications in patients with rheumatoid arthritis receiving nonsteroidal anti-inflammatory drugs. A randomized, double-blind, placebo-controlled trial. *Ann Intern Med* 1995;**123**:241–9.

10 Stalnikowicz R, Rachmilewitz D. NSAID-induced gastroduodenal damage: is prevention needed? A review and metaanalysis. *J Clin Gastroenterol* 1993;**17**:238–43.

11 Fries JF. NSAID gastropathy: the second most deadly rheumatic disease? Epidemiology and risk appraisal. *J Rheumatol Suppl* 1991;**28**:6–10.

12 Griffin MR, Ray WA, Schaffner W. Nonsteroidal anti-inflammatory drug use and death from peptic ulcer in elderly persons. *Ann Intern Med* 1988;**109**:359–63.

13 Bollini P, Rodriguez G, Gutthann S. The impact of research quality and study design on epidemiologic estimates of the effect of nonsteroidal anti-inflammatory drugs on upper gastrointestinal tract disease. *Arch Intern Med* 1992;**152**: 1289–95.

14 McMahon AD, Evans JM, White G *et al.* A cohort study (with re-sampled comparator groups) to measure the association between new NSAID prescribing and upper gastrointestinal hemorrhage and perforation. *J Clin Epidemiol* 1997;**50**:351–6.

15 Gabriel S, Jaakkimainen L, Bombardier C. Risk for serious gastrointestinal complications related to use of non-steroidal anti-inflammatory drugs: a meta-analysis. *Ann Intern Med* 1991;**115**:787–96.

16 Langman MJ, Weil J, Wainwright P *et al.* Risks of bleeding peptic ulcer associated with individual non-steroidal anti-inflammatory drugs. *Lancet* 1994;**343**:1075–8.

17 MacDonald T, Morant S, Robinson G. Association of upper gastrointestinal toxicity of non-steroidal anti-inflammatory drugs with continued exposure: cohort study. *BMJ* 1997;**315**:1333–7.

18 Armstrong C, Blower A. Nonsteroidal antiinflammatory drugs and life threatening complications of peptic ulceration. *Gut* 1987;**28**:527–32.

19 Kaufmann HJ, Taubin HL. Nonsteroidal anti-inflammatory drugs activate quiescent inflammatory bowel disease. *Ann Intern Med* 1987;**107**:513–16.

20 Wallace JL. NSAID gastroenteropathy: past, present and future. *Can J Gastroenterol* 1996;**10**:451–9.

21 Matsuhashi N, Yamada A, Hiraishi M *et al.* Multiple strictures of the small intestine after long-term nonsteroidal anti-inflammatory drug therapy. *Am J Gastroenterol* 1992; **87**:1183–6.

22 Tannenbaum H, Davis P, Russell AS *et al.* An evidence-based approach to prescribing NSAIDs in musculoskeletal disease: a Canadian consensus. Canadian NSAID Consensus Participants (see comments). *Can Med Assoc J* 1996;**155**:77–88.

23 Lichtenstein DR, Syngal S, Wolfe MM. Nonsteroidal antiinflammatory drugs and the gastrointestinal tract. The double-edged sword. *Arthritis Rheum* 1995;**38**:5–18.

24 Dvornik DM. Tissue selective inhibition of prostaglandin biosynthesis by etodolac. *J Rheumatol Suppl* 1997;**47**:40–7.

25 Robinson DR. Regulation of prostoglandin synthesis by anti-inflammatory drugs. *J Rheumatol* 1997;**24**(Suppl 47): 32–9.

26 Rostom A, Wells G, Tugwell P, Welch V, Dube C, McGowan J. Prevention of NSAID-induced gastroduodenal ulcers. (Update of Cochrane Database Syst Rev. 2000;**(3)**: CD002296;10908548.) (Review) (90 refs). In: Cochrane Collaboration. *Cochrane Library.* Issue 4. Oxford:Update Software, 2002.

27 Rostom A, Wells G, Tugwell P, Welch V, Dube C, McGowan J. The prevention of chronic NSAID induced upper gastrointestinal toxicity: a Cochrane collaboration metaanalysis of randomized controlled trials. *J Rheumatol* 2000;**27**:2203–14.

28 Rostom A, Dube C, Jolicoeur E, Boucher M, Joyce J. Evaluation of pharmacological interventions for the prevention of gastroduodenal ulcers associated with the use of non steroidal antiinflammatory drugs: a systematic review. Canadian Coordinating Office for Health Technology Assessment (CCOHTA) 168. 2003. Ottawa: CCOHTA.

29 Hallas J, Lauritsen J, Villadsen HD, Gram LF. Nonsteroidal anti-inflammatory drugs and upper gastrointestinal bleeding, identifying high-risk groups by excess risk estimates. *Scand J Gastroenterol* 1995;**30**:438–44.

30 Hansen JM, Hallas J, Lauritsen JM, Bytzer P. Non-steroidal anti-inflammatory drugs and ulcer complications: a risk factor analysis for clinical decision-making. *Scand J Gastroenterol* 1996;**31**:126–30.

31 Laporte JR, Carne X, Vidal X, Moreno V. Upper gastrointestinal bleeding in relation to previous use of analgesics and non-steroidal anti-inflammatory drugs. *Lancet* 1991;**337**:85–9.

32 Rodriguez LA. Nonsteroidal anti-inflammatory drugs, ulcers and risks: A collaborative meta-analysis. *Semin Arthritis Rheum* 1997;**26**:16–20.

33 Hochain P, Berkelmans I, Czernichow P *et al.* Which patients taking non-aspirin non-steroidal anti-inflammatory drugs bleed? A case–control study. *Eur J Gastroenterol Hepatol* 1995;**7**:419–26.

34 Scheiman JM. Nsaids, gastrointestinal injury, and cytoprotection. *Gastroenterol Clin North Am* 1998;**25**: 270–98.

35 Gutthann SP, Garcia RL, Raiford DS. Individual nonsteroidal antiinflammatory drugs and other risk factors for upper gastrointestinal bleeding and perforation. *Epidemiology* 1997;**8**:18–24.

36 Henry D, Dobson A, Turner C. Variability in the risk of major gastrointestinal complications from nonaspirin nonsteroidal anti-inflammatory drugs. *Gastroenterology* 1993;**105**:1078–88.

37 Henry D, Lim LL, Garcia RL *et al.* Variability in risk of gastrointestinal complications with individual non-steroidal anti-inflammatory drugs: results of a collaborative meta-analysis. *BMJ* 1996;**312**:1563–6.

38 Smalley WE, Griffin MR. The risks and costs of upper gastrointestinal disease attributable to NSAIDs. *Gastroenterol Clin North Am* 1996;**25**:373–96.

39 Carson JL, Strom BL, Morse ML, West SL. The relative gastrointestinal toxicity of the non-steroidal anti-inflammatory drugs. *Arch Intern Med* 1987;**147**:1054–9.

40 Griffin M, Piper J, Daughterty J, Snowden M. Non-steroidal anti-inflammatory drug use and increased risk for peptic ulcer disease in elderly persons. *Ann Intern Med* 1991;**114**:257–63.

41 Wynne HA, Long A. Patient awareness of the adverse effects of non-steroidal anti-inflammatory drugs (NSAIDs). *Br J Clin Pharmacol* 1996;**42**:253–6.

42 Jorde R, Burhol PG. Asymptomatic peptic ulcer disease. *Scand J Gastroenterol* 1987;**22**:129–34.

43 Graham DY. High-dose famotidine for prevention of NSAID ulcers? *Gastroenterology* 1997;**112**:2143–5.

44 Robbins SL, Cotran RS, Kumar V. *Pathologic Basis of Disease, (3rd edn).* Philadelphia: WB Saunders Co, 1984.

45 Maetzel A, Ferraz MB, Bombardier C. The cost-effectiveness of misoprostol in preventing serious gastrointestinal events associated with the use of nonsteroidal antiinflammatory drugs. *Arthritis Rheum* 1998;**41**:16–25.

46 Wittes J, Lakatos E, Prosbsfeild J. Surrogate endpoints in clinical trial: cardiovascular diseases. *Stat Med* 1989;**8**: 415–25.

47 Bombardier C, Laine L, Reicin A *et al.* Comparison of upper gastrointestinal toxicity of rofecoxib and naproxen in patients with rheumatoid arthritis. *N Engl J Med* 2000; **343**:1520–8.

48 Silverstein FE, Faich G, Goldstein JL *et al.* Gastrointestinal toxicity with celecoxib vs nonsteroidal anti-inflammatory drugs for osteoarthritis and rheumatoid arthritis: the CLASS study: a randomized controlled trial. *JAMA* 2000;**284**: 1247–55.

49 Van Der Hulst R, Rauws E, Koycu B. Recurrence after eradication of *Helicobacter pylori*: a prospective long-term follow-up study. *Gastroenterology* 1997;**113**:1082–6.

50 Rauws EJ, Tytgat GN. *Helicobacter pylori* in duodenal and gastric ulcer disease. (Review) (119 refs). *Baillieres Clin Gastroenterol* 1995;**9**:529–47.

51 Veldhuyzen van Zanten SJ, Sherman PM. *Helicobacter pylori* infection as a cause of gastritis, duodenal ulcer, gastric cancer and nonulcer dyspepsia: a systematic overview. *Can Med Assoc J* 1994;**150**:177–185.

52 Kurata JH, Nogawa AN. Meta-analysis of risk factors for peptic ulcer. Nonsteroidal antiinflammatory drugs, *Helicobacter pylori*, and smoking. *J Clin Gastroenterol* 1997;**24**:2–17.

53 Veldhuyzen Van Zanten S. Ulcers, *H. pylori*, NSAIDs, and dyspepsia. *Gastroenterology* 1997;**113**(Suppl):S90-S92.

54 Borody TJ, George LL, Brandl S. *Helicobacter pylori*-negative duodenal ulcer. *Am J Gastroenterol* 1991;**86**:1154–7.

55 Laine L, Martin-Sorensen M, Weinstein W. NSAID-associated gastric ulcers do not require *H.pylori* for their development. *Am J Gastroenterol* 1992;**87**:1398–402.

56 McColl K, El-Nujumi A, Chittajullu R. A study of the pathogenesis of *Helicobacter pylori*-negative duodenal ulceration. *Gut* 1993;**34**:762–8.

57 Dooley CP, Cohen H, Fitzgibbon Pl. Prevalence of *Helicobacter pylori* infection and histologic gastritis in asymptomatic persons. *N Engl J Med* 1989;**321**:1562–6.

58 Graham DY, Lidsky MD, Cox AM *et al.* Long-term nonsteroidal antiinflammatory drug use and *Helicobacter pylori* infection. *Gastroenterology* 1991;**100**:1653–7.

59 Sontag SJ. Guilty as charged: bugs and drugs in gastric ulcer. *Am J Gastroenterol* 1997;**92**:1255–61.

60 Graham DY. Nonsteroidal anti-inflammatory drugs, *Helicobacter pylori*, and ulcers: where we stand. *Am J Gastroenterol* 1996;**91**:2080–6.

61 Hudson N, Balsitis M, Filipowicz. Effect of *Helicobacter pylori* colonization on gastric mucosal eicosanoid synthesis in patients taking Nsaids. *Gut* 1993;**34**:748–51.

62 Laine L, Cominelli F, Sloane R, Casini-Raggi V, Marin-Sorensen M, Weinstein WM. Interaction of NSAIDs and *Helicobacter pylori* on gastrointestinal injury and prostaglandin production: a controlled double-blind trial. *Aliment Pharmacol Ther* 1995;**9**:127–35.

63 Konturek J, Dembinski A, Konturek SJ. Infection of *Helicobacter pylori* and gastric adaptation to continued administration of aspirin in humans. *Gastroenterology* 1998;**114**:245–55.

64 Loeb DS, Talley NJ, Ahlquist DA, Carpenter HA, Zinsmeister AR. Long-term nonsteroidal anti-inflammatory drug use and gastroduodenal injury: the role of *Helicobacter pylori*. *Gastroenterology* 1992;**102**:1899–905.

65 Lipscomb GR, Wallis N, Armstrong G, Goodman MJ, Rees WD. Influence of *Helicobacter pylori* on gastric mucosal adaptation to naproxen in man. *Dig Dis Sci* 1996;**41**:1583–8.

66 Huang JQ, Sridhar S, Hunt RH. Role of *Helicobacter pylori* infection and non-steroidal anti-inflammatory drugs in peptic-ulcer disease: a meta-analysis. *Lancet* 2002;**359**:14–22.

67 Soll AH. Pathogenesis of peptic ulcer and implications for therapy. *N Engl J Med* 1990;**322**:909–16.

68 Soll AH. Consensus conference. Medical treatment of peptic ulcer disease. Practice guidelines. Practice Parameters Committee of the American College of Gastroenterology (published erratum appears in *JAMA* 1996;**275**:1314) [see comments]. (Review) (99 refs). *JAMA* 1996;**275**:622–9.

69 Somerville K, Faulkner G, Langman M. Non-steroidal anti-inflammatory drugs and bleeding peptic ulcer. *Lancet* 1986;**1**:462–4.

70 Hawkey CJ, Swannell AJ, Yeomans ND. Increased effectiveness of omeprazole compared to ranitidine in non steroidal anti inflammatory drug (NSAID) users with reference to *H. pylori* status. *Gut* 1996;**39**(Suppl 1):A33.

71 Yeomans ND, Tulassay Z, Juhasz L, Racz I, Howard J. A comparison of omeprazole with ranitidine for ulcers associated with nonsteroidal antiinflammatory drugs. *N Eng J Med* 1998;**338**:719–26.

72 Labenz J, Tillenburg B, Peitz U, Idstrom JP. *Helicobacter pylori* augments the pH-increasing effect of omeprazole in patients with duodenal ulcer. *Gastroenterology* 1996;**110**:725–32.

73 Porro GB, Parente F, Imbesi V. Role of *Helicobacter pylori* in ulcer healing and recurrence of gastric and duodenal ulcers in long term Nsaid users: responce to omeprazole dual therapy. *Gut* 1996;**39**:22–6.

74 Hawkey CJ, Tulassay Z, Szczepanski L, van Rensburg CJ, Filipowicz-Sosnowska A, Lanas A *et al.* Randomised controlled trial of *Helicobacter pylori* eradication in patients on non-steroidal anti-inflammatory drugs: HELP NSAIDs study. Helicobacter Eradication for Lesion Prevention. (comment)(erratum appears in *Lancet* 1998 Nov 14;**352**:1634). *Lancet* 1998;**352**:1016–21.

75 Chan FK, Sung JJ, Chung SC *et al.* Randomised trial of eradication of *Helicobacter pylori* before non-steroidal anti-inflammatory drug therapy to prevent peptic ulcers. *Lancet* 1997;**350**:975–9.

76 Chan FKL, To KF, Wu JCY *et al.* Eradication of *Helicobacter pylori* and risk of peptic ulcers in patients starting long-term treatment with non-steroidal anti-inflammatory drugs: a randomised trial. *Lancet* 2002;**359**:9–13.

77 Chan FKL, Chung SC, Suen BY *et al.* Preventing recurrent upper gastrointestinal bleeding in patients with *Helicobacter pylori* infection who are taking low-dose aspirin or naproxen. *N Engl J Med* 2001;**344**:967–73.

78 Fletcher RH, Fletcher SW, Wagner EH. *Clinical Epidemiology: The essentials, (2nd edn).* Baltimore: Williams & Wilkins, 1988.

79 Sackett DL, Haynes RB, Guyatt GH, Tugwell P. *Clinical Epidemiology: A basic science for clinical medicine, (2nd edn).* London: Little, Brown and Company, 1998.

80 Levi S, Goodlad RA, Lee CY *et al.* Inhibitory effect of non-steroidal anti-inflammatory drugs on mucosal cell proliferation associated with gastric ulcer healing. *Lancet* 1990;**336**:840–3.

81 Smedfors B, Johansson C. Stimulation of duodenal bicarbonate secretion by misoprostol. *Dig Dis Sci* 1998; **31**(Suppl):96–100.

82 Walt RP. Misoprostol for the treatment of peptic ulcer and antiinflammatory drug induced gastroduodenal ulceration. *N Eng J Med* 1992;**327**:1575–80.

83 Wilson DE, Quadros E, Rajapaksa T, Adams A. Effects of misoprostol on gastric acid and mucus secretion in man. *Dig Dis Sci* 1986;**31**(Suppl):126–129.

84 Collins PW. Misoprostol: discovery, development, and clinical applications. *Med Res Rev* 1990;**10**:149–72.

85 Hawkey CJ, Karrasch JA, Szczepanski L *et al.* Omeprazole compared to misoprostol for ulcers associated with nonsteroidal antiinflammatory drugs. *N Eng J Med* 1998; **338**:727–34.

86 Graham DY, Agrawal NM, Campbell DR *et al.* Ulcer prevention in long-term users of nonsteroidal anti-inflammatory drugs: results of a double-blind, randomized, multicenter, active- and placebo-controlled study of misoprostol vs lansoprazole. *Arch Intern Med* 2002;**162(2)**: 169–175.

87 Cohen MM, Clark L, Armstrong L, D'Souza J. Reduction of aspirin-induced fecal blood loss with low-dose misoprostol tablets in man. *Dig Dis Sci* 1985;**30**:605–11.

88 Lanza FL, Fakouhi D, Rubin A *et al.* A double-blind placebo-controlled comparison of the efficacy and safety of 50, 100, and 200 micrograms of misoprostol QID in the prevention of ibuprofen-induced gastric and duodenal mucosal lesions and symptoms. *Am J Gastroenterol* 1989;**84**:633–6.

89 Ryan JR, Vargas R, Clay GA, McMahon FG. Role of misoprostol in reducing aspirin-induced gastrointestinal blood loss in arthritic patients. *Am J Med* 1987;**83(1A)**:41–46.

90 Silverstein FE, Kimmey MB, Saunders DR, Levine DS. Gastric protection by misoprostol against 1300 mg of aspirin. An endoscopic study. *Dig Dis Sci* 1986;**31**(Suppl 2): 137S–141S.

91 Hunt JN, Smith Jl, Jiang CL, Kessler L. Effect of synthetic protoglandin E1 anologue on aspirin induced gastric bleeding and secretion. *Dig Dis Sci* 1983;**28**:897–902.

92 Konturek JW, Dembinski A, Stoll R, Domschke W, Konturek SJ. Mucosal adaptation to aspirin induced gastric damage in humans. Studies on blood flow, gastric mucosal growth, and neutrophil activation. *Gut* 1994;**35**:1197–204.

93 Konturek JW, Dembinski A, Konturek SJ, Domschke W. *Helicobacter pylori* and gastric adaptation to repeated aspirin administration in humans. *J Physiol Pharmacol* 1997;**48**:383–91.

94 de Lara A, Gompel H, Baranes C *et al.* Two comparative studies of dosmalfate vs. misoprostol in the prevention of NSAID-induced gastric ulcers in rheumatic patients. *Drug Today* 2000;**36**(Suppl A):73–78.

95 Chan FK, Sung JJ, Ching JY *et al.* Randomized trial of low-dose misoprostol and naproxen vs. nabumetone to prevent recurrent upper gastrointestinal haemorrhage in users of non-steroidal anti-inflammatory drugs. *Aliment Pharmacol Ther* 2001;**15**:19–24.

96 Raskin JB, White RH, Jaszewski R, Korsten MA, Schubert TT, Fort JG. Misoprostol and ranitidine in the prevention of NSAID-induced ulcers: a prospective, double-blind, multicenter study. *Am J Gastroenterol* 1996; **91**:223–7.

97 Agrawal NM, Van KH, Erhardt LJ, Geis GS. Misoprostol coadministered with diclofenac for prevention of gastroduodenal ulcers. A one-year study. *Dig Dis Sci* 1995; **40**:1125–31.

98 Raskin JB, White RH, Jackson JE *et al.* Misoprostol dosage in the prevention of nonsteroidal anti-inflammatory drug-induced gastric and duodenal ulcers: a comparison of three regimens. *Ann Intern Med* 1995;**123**:344–50.

99 Valentini M, Cannizzaro R, Poletti M *et al.* Nonsteroidal antiinflammatory drugs for cancer pain: comparison between misoprostol and ranitidine in prevention of upper gastrointestinal damage. *J Clin Oncol* 1995;**13**:2637–42.

100 Delmas PD, Lambert R, Capron MH. (Misoprostol in the prevention of gastric erosions caused by nonsteroidal anti-inflammatory agents). *Revue du Rhumatisme* 1994; **edition(2)**:126–31.

101 Elliott SL, Yeomans ND, Buchanan RR, Smallwood RA. Efficacy of 12 months' misoprostol as prophylaxis against NSAID-induced gastric ulcers. A placebo-controlled trial. *Scand J Rheumatol* 1994;**23**:171–6.

102 Graham DY, White RH, Moreland LW *et al.* Duodenal and gastric ulcer prevention with misoprostol in arthritis patients taking NSAIDs. Misoprostol Study Group. *Ann Intern Med* 1993;**119**:257–62.

103 Henriksson K, Uribe A, Sandstedt B, Nord CE. *Helicobacter pylori* infection, ABO blood group, and effect of misoprostol on gastroduodenal mucosa in NSAID-treated patients with rheumatoid arthritis. *Dig Dis Sci* 1993; **38**:1688–96.

104 Melo GA, Roth SH, Zeeh J, Bruyn GA, Woods EM, Geis GS. Double-blind comparison of efficacy and gastroduodenal safety of diclofenac/misoprostol, piroxicam, and naproxen in the treatment of osteoarthritis. *Ann Rheum Dis* 1993;**52**:881–5.

105 Roth SH, Tindall EA, Jain AK *et al.* A controlled study comparing the effects of nabumetone, ibuprofen, and ibuprofen plus misoprostol on the upper gastrointestinal tract mucosa. *Arch Intern Med* 1993;**153**:2565–71.

106 Bolten W, Gomes JA, Stead H, Geis GS. The gastroduodenal safety and efficacy of the fixed combination of diclofenac and misoprostol in the treatment of osteoarthritis. *Br J Rheumatol* 1992;**31**:753–8.

107 Geis G, Stead MWC, Nicholson P. Prevalence of mucosal lesions in the stomach and duodenum due to chronic use of NSAID in patients with rheumatoid arthritis or osteoarthritis, and interim report on prevention by misoprostol of diclofenac associated lesions. *J Rheumatol* 1991;**18**:114.

108 Verdickt W, Moran C, Hantzschel H, Fraga AM, Stead H, Geis GS. A double-blind comparison of the gastroduodenal safety and efficacy of diclofenac and a fixed dose combination of diclofenac and misoprostol in the treatment of rheumatoid arthritis. *Scand J Rheumatol* 1992;**21**:85–91.

109 Agrawal NM, Roth S, Graham DY *et al.* Misoprostol compared with sucralfate in the prevention of nonsteroidal anti-inflammatory drug-induced gastric ulcer. A randomized, controlled trial [see comments]. *Ann Intern Med* 1991; **115**:195–200.

110 Chandrasekaran AN, Sambandam PR, Lal HM *et al.* Double blind, placebo controlled trial on the cytoprotective effect of misoprostol in subjects with rheumatoid arthritis, osteoarthritis and seronegative spondarthropathy on NSAIDs [see comments]. *J Assoc Phys India* 1991;**39**:919–21.

111 Saggioro A, Alvisi V, Blasi A, Dobrilla G, Fioravanti A, Marcolongo R. Misoprostol prevents NSAID-induced gastroduodenal lesions in patients with osteoarthritis and rheumatoid arthritis [published erratum appears in Ital J Gastroenterol 1991 Jun;**23**:273]. *Ital J Gastroenterol* 1991;**23**:119–23.

112 Graham DY, Agrawal NM, Roth SH. Prevention of NSAID-induced gastric ulcer with misoprostol: multicentre, double-blind, placebo-controlled trial. *Lancet* 1988;**2**: 1277–80.

113 Bocanegra TS, Weaver AL, Tindall EA *et al.* Diclofenac/misoprostol compared with diclofenac in the treatment of osteoarthritis of the knee or hip: a randomized, placebo controlled trial. Arthrotec Osteoarthritis Study Group. *J Rheumatol* 1998;**25**:1602–11.

114 Graham DY. Critical effect of *Helicobacter pylori* infection on the effectiveness of omeprazole for prevention of gastric or duodenal ulcers among chronic NSAID users. *Helicobacter* 2002;**7**:1–8.

115 Maiden N, Madhok R. Misoprostol in patients taking non-steroidal anti-inflammatory drugs. *BMJ* 1995;**311**: 1518–19.

116 Jonsson B, Haglund U. Cost-effectiveness of misoprostol in Sweden. *Int J Tech Assess Health Care* 1992;**8**:234–44.

117 Knill-Jones R, Drummond M, Kohli H, Davies L. Economic evaluation of gastric ulcer prophylaxis in patients with arthritis receiving non-steroidal anti-inflammatory drugs. *Postgrad Med J* 1990;**66**:639–46.

118 De PG, Bader JP. [Cost-effectiveness of preventive treatment with misoprostol in non-steroidal anti-inflammatory agents related gastric ulcers]. *Gastroenterol Clin Biol* 1991;**15**:399–404.

119 Gabriel SE, Campion ME, O'Fallon WM. A cost-utility analysis of misoprostol prophylaxis for rheumatoid arthritis patients receiving nonsteroidal antiinflammatory drugs. *Arthritis Rheum* 1994;**37**:333–41.

120 Gabriel SE, Jaakkimainen RL, Bombardier C. The cost-effectiveness of misoprostol for nonsteroidal antiinflammatory drug-associated adverse gastrointestinal events. *Arthritis Rheum* 1993;**36**:447–59.

121 Hillman AL, Bloom BS. Economic effects of prophylactic use of misoprostol to prevent gastric ulcer in patients taking nonsteroidal anti-inflammatory drugs. *Arch Intern Med* 1989;**149**:2061–5.

122 Edelson JT, Tosteson AN, Sax P. Cost-effectiveness of misoprostol for prophylaxis against nonsteroidal anti-inflammatory drug-induced gastrointestinal tract bleeding [see comments]. *JAMA* 1990;**264**:41–7.

123 Carrin GJ, Torfs KE. Economic evaluation of prophylactic treatment with Misoprostol in osteoarthritic patients treated with NSAIDs. The case of Belgium. *Rev Epidemiol Sante Publique* 1990;**38**:187–99.

124 Bijlsma JW. Treatment of NSAID-induced gastrointestinal lesions with cimetidine: an international multicentre collaborative study. *Aliment Pharmacol Ther* 1988; **2** Suppl 1:85–95.

125 Croker JR, Cotton PB, Boyle AC, Kinsella P. Cimetidine for peptic ulcer in patients with arthritis. *Ann Rheum Dis* 1980;**39**:275–8.

126 Farah D, Sturrock RD, Russell RI. Peptic ulcer in rheumatoid arthritis. *Ann Rheum Dis* 1988;**47**:478–80.

127 LoIudice TA, Saleem T, Lang JA. Cimetidine in the treatment of gastric ulcer induced by steroidal and nonsteroidal anti-inflammatory agents. *Am J Gastroenterol* 1981;**75**:104–10.

128 O'Laughlin JC, Silvoso GR, Ivey KJ. Healing of aspirin-associated peptic ulcer disease despite continued salicylate ingestion. *Arch Intern Med* 1981;**141**:781–3.

129 Walan A, Bader JP, Classen M, Lamers CB, Piper DW. Effect of omeprazole and ranitidine on ulcer healing and relapse rates in patients with benign gastric ulcers. *N Eng J Med* 1989;**320**:69–75.

130 Mani V. Ranitidine in NSAID ulcers. *Natl Med J India* 1992;**5**:69.

131 O'Laughlin JC, Silvoso GK, Ivey KJ. Resistance to medical therapy of gastric ulcers in rheumatic disease patients taking aspirin. A double-blind study with cimetidine and follow-up. *Dig Dis Sci* 1982;**27**:976–80.

132 Hudson N, Taha AS, Russell RI *et al.* Famotidine for healing and maintenance in nonsteroidal anti-inflammatory drug-associated gastroduodenal ulceration. *Gastroenterology* 1997;**112**:1817–22.

133 Ehsanullah RS, Page MC, Tildesley G, Wood JR. Prevention of gastroduodenal damage induced by non-steroidal anti-inflammatory drugs: controlled trial of ranitidine. *BMJ* 1988;**297**:1017–21.

134 Robinson MG, Griffin JJ, Bowers J *et al.* Effect of ranitidine on gastroduodenal mucosal damage induced by nonsteroidal antiinflammatory drugs. *Dig Dis Sci* 1989;**34**:424–8.

135 Robinson M, Mills RJ, Euler AR. Ranitidine prevents duodenal ulcers associated with non-steroidal anti-inflammatory drug therapy. *Aliment Pharmacol Ther* 1991;**5**:143–50.

136 Taha AS, Hudson N, Hawkey CJ *et al.* Famotidine for the prevention of gastric and duodenal ulcers caused by nonsteroidal antiinflammatory drugs. *N Engl J Med* 1996; **334**:1435–9.

137 Levine LR, Cloud ML, Enas NH. Nizatidine prevents peptic ulceration in high-risk patients taking nonsteroidal anti-inflammatory drugs. *Arch Intern Med* 1993;**153**: 2449–54.

138 Roth SH, Bennett RE, Mitchell CS, Hartman RJ. Cimetidine therapy in nonsteroidal anti-inflammatory drug gastropathy. Double-blind long-term evaluation. *Arch Intern Med* 1987;**147**:1798–801.

139 Bianchi Porro G, Pace F, Caruso I. Why are non-steroidal anti-inflammatory drugs important in peptic ulceration? *Aliment Pharmacol Ther* 1987;**1**(Suppl):547S.

140 Berkowitz JM, Rogenes PR, Sharp JT, Warner CW. Ranitidine protects against gastroduodenal mucosal damage associated with chronic aspirin therapy. *Arch Intern Med* 1987;**147**:2137–9.

141 Simon B, Bergdolt H, Dammann H, Muller P. (Ranitidine in the therapy and prevention of NSAR-induced (non-steroidal anti-rheumatic agents) gastroduodenal lesions in patients with rheumatism). *Z Gastroenterol* 1991;**29**:217–21.

142 Simon B, Muller P. Nizatidine in therapy and prevention of non-steroidal anti-inflammatory drug-induced gastroduodenal ulcer in rheumatic patients. *Scand J Gastroenterol Suppl* 1994;**206**:25–28.

143 Koch M, Dezi A, Ferrario F, Capurso I. Prevention of nonsteroidal anti-inflammatory drug-induced gastrointestinal mucosal injury. A meta-analysis of randomized controlled clinical trials [see comments]. *Arch Intern Med* 1996;**156**: 2321–32.

144 Van Groenendael JH, Markusse HM, Dijkmans BA, Breedveld FC. The effect of ranitidine on NSAID related dyspeptic symptoms with and without peptic ulcer disease of patients with rheumatoid arthritis and osteoarthritis. *Clin Rheumatol* 1996;**15**:450–6.

145 Swift GL, Heneghan M, Williams GT, Williams BD, O'Sullivan MM, Rhodes J. Effect of ranitidine on gastroduodenal mucosal damage in patients on long-term non-steroidal anti-inflammatory drugs. *Digestion* 1989;**44**:86–94.

146 Janssen M, Dijkmans BA, Vandenbroucke JP, Biemond I, Lamers CB. Achlorhydria does not protect against benign upper gastrointestinal ulcers during NSAID use. *Dig Dis Sci* 1994;**39**:362–5.

147 Daneshmend TK, Stein AG, Bhaskar NK, Hawkey CJ. Abolition by omeprazole of aspirin induced gastric mucosal injury in man. *Gut* 1990;**31**:514–17.

148 Scheiman JM, Behler EM, Loeffler KM, Elta GH. Omeprazole ameliorates aspirin-induced gastroduodenal injury. *Dig Dis Sci* 1994;**39**:97–103.

149 Bergmann JF, Chassany O, Simoneau ML. Protection against aspirin induced gastric lesions by lansoprazole: Simultaneous evaluation of functional and morphologic responces. *Clin Pharmacol Ther* 1992;**52**:413–16.

150 Wolde S, Dijkmans BA, Janssen M, Hermans J, Lamers CB. High-dose ranitidine for the prevention of recurrent peptic ulcer disease in rheumatoid arthritis patients taking NSAIDs. *Aliment Pharmacol Ther* 1996;**10**:347–51.

151 Nwokolo CU, Prewett EJ, Sawyerr AM, Hudson M, Lim S, Pounder RE. Tolerance during 5 months of dosing with ranitidine, 150 mg nightly: a placebo-controlled, double-blind study. *Gastroenterology* 1991;**101**:948–53.

152 Smith JT, Gavey C, Nwokolo CU, Pounder RE. Tolerance during 8 days of high-dose H2-blockade: placebo-controlled studies of 24-hour acidity and gastrin. *Aliment Pharmacol Ther* 1990;**4**(Suppl):63.

153 Nwokolo CU, Smith JT, Gavey C, Sawyerr A, Pounder RE. Tolerance during 29 days of conventional dosing with cimetidine, nizatidine, famotidine or ranitidine. *Aliment Pharmacol Ther* 1990;**4**(Suppl):45.

154 Oddsson E, Gudjonsson H, Thjodleifsson B. Comparison between ranitidine and omeprazole for protection against gastroduodenal damage caused by naproxen. *Scand J Gastroenterol* 1992;**27**:1045–8.

155 Lauritsen K, Rutgersson K, Bolling E. Omeprazole 20 or 40 mg daily for healing of duodenal ulcer? A double blind comparative study. *Eur J Gastroenterol Hepato* 1992;**4**: 995–1000.

156 Hawkey CJ, Swannell AJ, Eriksson S. Benefits of omeprazole over misoprostol in healing Nsaid associated ulcers. *Gastroenterology* 1996;**110**(Suppl 4):A131.

157 Hawkey CJ, Foren I, Langstrom G. Omeprazole vs misoprostol: different effectiveness in healing gastric and duodenal ulcers vs erosions in Nsaid users: The Omnium study. *Gut* 1997;**40**(Suppl):A1.

158 Chan FKL, Hung LCT, Suen BY *et al.* Celecoxib versus diclofenac and omeprazole in reducing the risk of recurrent ulcer bleeding in patients with arthritis. *N Eng J Med* 2002;**347**:104–10.

159 Bianchi Porro G, Lazzaroni M, Imbesi V, Montrone F, Santagada T. Efficacy of pantoprazole in the prevention of peptic ulcers, induced by non-steroidal anti-inflammatory drugs: a prospective, placebo-controlled, double-blind, parallel-group study. *Dig Liver Dis* 2000;**32**:201–8.

160 Jensen DM, Ho S, Hamamah S *et al.* A randomized study of omeprazole compared to misoprostol for prevention of recurrent ulcers and ulcer hemorrhage in high risk patients ingesting aspirin or NSAIDs [Abstract]. *Gastroenterology* 2000;**118**(4 Suppl 2 Pt 1):AGA A892.

161 Ekstrom P, Carling L, Wetterhus S *et al.* Prevention of peptic ulcer and dyspeptic symptoms with omeprazole in patients receiving continuous non-steroidal anti-inflammatory drug therapy. A Nordic multicentre study [see comments]. *Scand J Gastroenterol* 1996;**31**:753–8.

162 Cullen D, Bardhan KD, Eisner M *et al.* Primary gastroduodenal prophylaxis with omeprazole for non-steroidal anti-inflammatory drug users. *Aliment Pharmacol Ther* 1998;**12**:135–40.

163 Rostom A, Dubé C, Jolicoeur E, Boucher M, Joyce J. Gastroduodenal ulcers associated with the use of non-steroidal anti-inflammatory drugs: a systematic review of preventive pharmacological interventions. Technology report no 37. 2003. Ottawa, Canadian Coordinating Office for Health Technology Assessment.

164 Goldstein JL, Correa P, Zhao WW *et al.* Reduced incidence of gastroduodenal ulcers with celecoxib, a novel cyclo-oxygenase-2 inhibitor, compared to naproxen in patients with arthritis. *Am J Gastroenterol* 2001;**96**:1019–27.

165 Emery P, Zeidler H, Kvien TK *et al.* Celecoxib versus diclofenac in long-term management of rheumatoid arthritis: randomised double-blind comparison. *Lancet* 1999; **354**:2106–11.

166 Simon LS, Weaver AL, Graham DY *et al.* Anti-inflammatory and upper gastrointestinal effects of celecoxib in rheumatoid arthritis: a randomized controlled trial. *JAMA* 1999;**282**:1921–8.

167 Center for Drug Evaluation and Research, US Food and Drug Administration. Arthritis Drugs Advisory Committee Meeting 12/1/1998: Celebrex. Rockville, MD, USA: The Center; 8 March 2001. Available at: www.fda.gov/cder/foi/adcomm/98/celebrex.htm

168 Witter J. Medical Officer Review. In: *Application no 20-998/S9Celebrex (Celecoxib) Capsules,Company:GD Searle LLC, Approval Date: 6/7/2002 [Supplemental NDA]*: Center for Drug Evaluation and Research, FDA; 2000. Available at: www.fda.gov/cder/foi/nda/2002/20-998S009_Celebrex_medr_P1.pdf

169 Hawkey C, Laine L, Simon T *et al.* Comparison of the effect of rofecoxib (a cyclooxygenase 2 inhibitor), ibuprofen, and placebo on the gastroduodenal mucosa of patients with osteoarthritis: a randomized, double-blind, placebo-controlled trial. *Arthritis Rheum* 2000;**43**:370–7.

170 Laine L, Harper S, Simon T *et al.* A randomized trial comparing the effect of rofecoxib, a cyclooxygenase 2-specific inhibitor, with that of ibuprofen on the gastroduodenal mucosa of patients with osteoarthritis. *Gastroenterology* 1999;**117**:776–83.

171 Goldstein JL, Silverstein FE, Agrawal NM *et al.* Reduced risk of upper gastrointestinal ulcer complications with celecoxib, a novel COX-2 inhibitor. *Am J Gastroenterol* 2000;**95**:1681–90.

172 Singh G, Goldstein J, Bensen W *et al.* Success–1 in Osteoarthritis (OA) Trial: celecoxib significantly reduces the risk of serious upper gi complications compared to NSAIDs while providing similar efficacy in 13,274 randomized patients [Abstract]. *Abstracts Perspective* **5**(1). 2001.

173 Langman MJ, Jensen DM, Watson DJ *et al.* Adverse upper gastrointestinal effects of rofecoxib compared with NSAIDs. *JAMA* 1999;**282**:1929–33.

174 Dequeker J, Hawkey C, Kahan A *et al.* Improvement in gastrointestinal tolerability of the selective cyclooxygenase (COX)-2 inhibitor, meloxicam, compared with piroxicam: results of the Safety and Efficacy Large-scale Evaluation of COX-inhibiting Therapies (SELECT) trial in osteoarthritis. *Br J Rheumatol* 1998;**37**:946–51.

175 Goldkind L. *Medical Officer's Gastroenterology Advisory Committee Briefing Document*. Division of Anti-Inflammatory, Analgesis and Ophthalmologic Drug Products HFD-500, FDA; 2000. NDA 20-998/S-009.

176 Witter J. FDA-NDA 20–998/S-009 Medical Officer Review. Primary-document N49–00–06–035_102, NDA 20–998/S-009 NDA 20–998/S-009. 2000. FDA.

177 Hrachovec JB, Mora M. Reporting of 6-month vs 12-month data in a clinical trial of celecoxib [Letter]. *JAMA* 2001; **286**:2398.

178 Wright JM, Perry TL, Bassett KL, Chambers GK. Reporting of 6-month vs 12-month data in a clinical trial of celecoxib (letter). *JAMA* 2001;**286**:2398–9.

179 Okie S. Missing data on celebrex full study altered picture of drug. *Washington Post* 2001 May 8;A11.

180 Li Q. NDA 21-042: Statistical review of rofecoxib for the treatment of signs and symptoms of osteoarthritis, relief of pain, treatment of primary dysmenorrhea, and improvement of gastrointestinal safety, December 1998–April 1999. In: *Approval package: Vioxx (Rofecoxib) Tablets, Merck Research Laboratories Application No.: 021042 and 021052, Approval Date 5/20/99*. Rockville, MD, USA: Center for Drugs and Evaluation, US Food and Drug Administration; 1999. Available at: www.fda.gov/cder/foi/nda/99/021042_52_vioxx_statr_P1.pdf

181 Hawkey C, Kahan A, Steinbruck K *et al.* Gastrointestinal tolerability of meloxicam compared to diclofenac in osteoarthritis patients. *Br J Rheumatol* 1998;**37**:937–45.

182 Goei Thè HS, Lund B, Distel MR, Bluhmki E. A double-blind, randomized trial to compare meloxicam 15 mg with

diclofenac 100 mg in the treatment of osteoarthritis of the knee. *Osteoarthritis Cartilage* 1997;**5**:283–8.

183 Hosie J, Distel M, Bluhmki E. Efficacy and tolerability of meloxicam versus piroxicam in patients with osteoarthritis of the hip or knee. A six-month double-blind study. *Clin Drug Invest* 1997;**13**:175–84.

184 Hosie J, Distel M, Bluhmki E. Meloxicam in osteoarthritis: a 6-month, double-blind comparison with diclofenac sodium. *Br J Rheumatol* 1996;**35**(Suppl 1):39–43.

185 Lindén B, Distel M, Bluhmki E. A double-blind study to compare the efficacy and safety of meloxicam 15 mg with piroxicam 20 mg in patients with osteoarthritis of the hip. *Br J Rheumatol* 1996;**35**(Suppl 1):35–38.

186 Wojtulewski JA, Schattenkirchner M, Barceló P *et al.* A six-month double-blind trial to compare the efficacy and safety of meloxicam 7.5 mg daily and naproxen 750 mg daily in patients with rheumatoid arthritis. *Br J Rheumatol* 1996; **35**(Suppl 1):22–28.

187 Lemmel EM, Bolten W, Burgos-Vargas R *et al.* Efficacy and safety of meloxicam in patients with rheumatoid arthritis. *J Rheumatol* 1997;**24**:282–90.

188 Yocum D, Fleischmann R, Dalgin P, Caldwell J, Hall D, Roszko P. Safety and efficacy of meloxicam in the treatment of osteoarthritis: a 12-week, double-blind, multiple-dose, placebo-controlled trial. The Meloxicam Osteoarthritis Investigators. *Arch Intern Med* 2000;**160**: 2947–54.

189 Lund B, Distel M, Bluhmki E. A double-blind, randomized, placebo-controlled study of efficacy and tolerance of meloxicam treatment in patients with osteoarthritis of the knee. *Scand J Rheumatol* 1998;**27**:32–7.

190 Deeks JJ, Altman DG, Bradburn MJ. Statistical methods for examining heterogeneity and combining results from several studies in meta-analysis. In: Egger M, Davey Smith G, Altman D (eds). *Systematic Reviews In Health Care: Meta-Analysis In Context.* London: BMJ Publishing Group, 2001.

191 Maetzel A, Krahn M, Naglie G. The cost-effectiveness of celecoxib and rofecoxib in patients with osteoarthritis or rheumatoid arthritis. Canadian Coordinating Office for Health Technology Assessment 2001;(Technology report no 23).

7 Non-variceal gastrointestinal hemorrhage

Nicholas Church, Kelvin Palmer

Introduction

Peptic ulcer is the commonest cause of acute non-variceal bleeding, accounting for approximately half of the cases.[1] Other major causes such as gastroduodenal erosions, gastritis, esophagitis, Mallory–Weiss tears, and vascular malformations are not usually life threatening and respond to conservative therapy.

Approximately 80% of cases pursue a benign course without re-bleeding in hospital and specific intervention is not required. The remaining 20% have severe bleeding due to erosion of a major artery. Most deaths from bleeding arise from this subgroup. The crude death rate from gastrointestinal bleeding has not significantly improved over five decades. Avery Jones in 1957 reported a hospital mortality of 16%[2] whilst a large audit of acute gastrointestinal bleeding carried out in England in 1997 reported very similar mortality of 11%.[3] This disappointing observation must, however, be tempered by the fact that the case mix of patients now admitted is very different from that of previous decades. For example, less that 2% of patients admitted with acute bleeding in 1947 were aged over 80 years whilst approximately a quarter of patients currently admitted are octogenarians. There is a close relationship between increasing age and hospital mortality: increasing age is inevitably associated with a high prevalence of chronic disease, rendering patients susceptible to complications following major hemorrhage.

The risk of death following admission to hospital for gastrointestinal bleeding has been quantified by Rockall et al.[4] (Table 7.1). Independent factors associated with a poor prognosis were identified from data derived from a large population of patients whose clinical course was observed following hospital admission. Whilst the Rockall risk scoring system did well when tested in a cohort of patients subsequently managed in the same geographical area, it has not been widely validated elsewhere. Recently the Rockall score has been shown to correlate well with observed mortality, but not re-bleeding, in a Dutch population.[5] In order to evaluate the use of the scoring system in patients at highest risk, Church et al. calculated Rockall scores for a series of 211 patients who had been entered into randomized trials of endoscopic therapy for major peptic ulcer bleeding in southeast Scotland.[6] Mean scores were higher in those patients who re-bled and those who died following endoscopic therapy when compared with those who had an uneventful course. Patients with a score greater than 8 were significantly more likely to re-bleed or die, and such patients should be managed in a high dependency unit after endoscopic therapy.

As shown in Table 7.2, Rockall et al. showed a good correlation between the risk score, re-bleeding and hospital mortality. Deaths following admission to hospital because of acute gastrointestinal bleeding are rarely due to exsanguination. They are usually a consequence of postoperative complications when an urgent operation is undertaken, or of deterioration of comorbid conditions.

Over the past 10 years the treatment of choice for appropriate bleeding patients has been endoscopic therapy, and surgical intervention has been reserved for the failure of therapeutic endoscopy. Nevertheless, optimum management still relies very much on a team approach with appropriate use of drug therapy, endoscopic intervention, and surgery. Despite much evidence from randomized trials, the management of an individual patient still depends on clinical judgment concerning the probability that attempts at endoscopic intervention are likely to be fruitless and that surgery is inevitable. Management may be best undertaken in a specialized "bleeding unit" in which the patient is treated using agreed protocols and guidelines with endoscopy undertaken once appropriate resuscitation has been achieved and with management decisions based upon endoscopic and surgical opinions. Relatively weak evidence derived from comparison of results in case series with historical controls suggests that this approach may achieve lower hospital mortality and more efficient use of resources than management by generalists working in conventional medical or surgical units.[7,8]

Table 7.1 Rockall scoring system for risk of re-bleeding and death after admission to hospital for acute gastrointestinal bleeding[4]

Variable	Score			
	0	1	2	3
Age	< 60 years	60–79 years	≥ 80 years	
Shock	*No shock* Systolic BP > 100 mmHg Pulse < 100 per minute	*Tachycardia* Systolic BP > 100 mmHg Pulse > 100 per minute	*Hypotension* Systolic BP < 100 mmHg	
Comorbidity	Nil major		Cardiac failure, ischemic heart disease, any major comorbidity	Renal failure, liver failure, disseminated malignancy
Diagnosis	Mallory–Weiss tear, no lesion and no SRH	All other diagnoses	Malignancy of upper gastrointestinal tract	
Major SRH	None, or dark spot		Blood in upper gastrointestinal tract, adherent clot, visible or spurting vessel	

SRH, stigmata of recent hemorrhage

Table 7.2 Correlation between Rockall score and re-bleeding and mortality

Risk score	No. of patients	Re-bleed (%)	Mortality (%)
0	144	7 (5)	0 (0)
1	281	9 (3)	0 (0)
2	337	18 (5)	1 (0·2)
3	444	50 (11)	13 (3)
4	528	76 (14)	28 (5)
5	455	83 (24)	49 (11)
6	312	102 (33)	54 (17)
7	267	113 (44)	72 (27)
8+	190	101 (42)	78 (41)

Specific therapy

For the 80% of patients who have relatively minor bleeding and who do not have major endoscopic stigmata of bleeding, supportive therapy including use of intravenous fluid and the management of comorbidity (particularly cardiorespiratory disease) is sufficient.

Patients who present with clinical shock and who at endoscopy have an actively bleeding peptic ulcer have an 80% risk of continuing to bleed or re-bleed in hospital.[9] Those who have a non-bleeding visible vessel have a 50% risk of further hemorrhage.[10] The "visible vessel" represents a pseudoaneurysm of the involved artery, or adherent blood clot, plugging the arterial defect.[11] Patients who are found to have an adherent blood clot over the ulcer usually have an underlying high risk lesion and should also be regarded as being at considerable risk of further hemorrhage in hospital. Patients who at endoscopy have a clean ulcer base or who have black or red spots are at very little risk of re-bleeding.

It follows from these observations that patients with major endoscopic stigmata should be considered for specific hemostatic treatment and only such patients should be included in clinical trials of therapy for gastrointestinal bleeding. This review will only consider those studies that exclusively included patients having either a non-bleeding visible vessel, active hemorrhage, or adherent blood clot as entry criteria.

Table 7.3   Omeprazole versus placebo for acute upper gastrointestinal bleeding[15]

Outcome	Omeprazole	Placebo
All patients		
n	578	569
Re-bleed (%)	77 (14)	91 (16)
Operation (%)	56 (11)	57 (11)
Death (%)	35 (7)	29 (6)
Gastric ulcer		
n	97	93
Re-bleed (%)	26 (27)	23 (25)
Operation (%)	18 (19)	16 (17)
Death (%)	7 (7)	5 (5)
Duodenal ulcer		
n	149	164
Re-bleed (%)	32 (21)	47 (29)
Operation (%)	27 (18)	34 (21)
Death (%)	16 (11)	8 (5)

The specific non-surgical approaches to hemostasis are drug therapy and endoscopic therapy.

Drug therapy

There are three principles underlying the use of drugs as agents which might stop active hemorrhage and prevent re-bleeding. The first of these is that the stability of a blood clot is poor in an acid environment.[12] Thus agents that suppress acid secretion, including H_2-receptor antagonists (H_2-RA) and proton pump inhibitor (PPI) drugs might reduce re-bleeding. The second is that blood clot may be stabilized by decreasing fibrinolytic mechanisms using agents such as tranexamic acid. The third approach is that, since major gastrointestinal bleeding is due to arterial erosion, reduction of arterial blood flow by agents such as somatostatin and octreotide could achieve hemostasis and prevent re-bleeding.

Acid suppressing drugs

The efficacy of H_2-RA in the management of acute upper gastrointestinal bleeding has been assessed in randomized trials.[13,14] Unfortunately, no trial has shown benefit in terms of reduction of re-bleeding incidence or mortality. Alc

Experience involving the use of PPIs is inconsistent, but recent evidence is beginning to support their use after endoscopic therapy. The largest trial included 1147 patients who were randomized to receive omeprazole (initially intravenously, then orally) or placebo.[15] No significant difference was demonstrated in hospital mortality, operation rate or re-bleeding (Table 7.3). The study was not restricted to the high risk patients who had endoscopic stigmata of recent hemorrhage. Accordingly, event rates were rather low in the placebo group, and this may have limited the power of the study to show a difference. Ala

Khuroo *et al.* randomized 220 bleeding ulcer patients who had major endoscopic stigmata to receive high dose oral omeprazole or placebo.[16] Although all patients had major stigmata of hemorrhage, an adherent clot in the ulcer base was reported in 57% of patients. Re-bleeding, the need for urgent surgery, blood transfusion, and mortality were all reduced in the actively treated group of patients (Table 7.4). The number of patients needed to treat with omeprazole to prevent one death was 25, and to prevent one operation was 7. Alc This trial has been criticized because it included relatively young patients with relatively little comorbidity and because endoscopic therapy was not administered to any patient. The observation that omeprazole reduced re-bleeding and surgery rates when no endoscopic therapy was done suggested a beneficial effect of the PPI. This effect might, however, have been exaggerated by the fact that the majority of patients in the trial were bleeding from ulcers in which adherent clot was found at endoscopy.

Two trials published back to back in the *Scandinavian Journal of Gastroenterology*[17,18] examined the use of high dose intravenous omeprazole after endoscopic hemostasis. All patients had major peptic ulcer bleeding, but as in the trial by Khuroo half the patients had adherent clot as the reported stigma of hemorrhage. The conclusions were that intravenous omeprazole infusion for three days following endoscopic therapy improved outcome. Ald Both trials used composite endpoints which were complex and ill-defined and both were discontinued early due to an unexplained imbalance in mortality in one of the trials,[18] factors that weaken the impact of these results. Villanueva *et al.* randomized 86 patients

Table 7.4 Omeprazole versus placebo for bleeding peptic ulcer[16]

Outcome	Omeprazole (*n* = 110)	Placebo (*n* = 110)	*P* value
Re-bleed (%)	12 (11)	40 (36)	<0·001
Surgery (%)	8 (8)	26 (23)	<0·001
Transfusion (mean units)	2·3	4·1	<0·001
Death	2	6	NS

NS, not significant

Table 7.5 Omeprazole versus placebo for bleeding peptic ulcer treated with endoscopic therapy[21]

Outcome	Omeprazole (*n* = 120)	Placebo (*n* = 120)	*P* value
Re-bleed (%)	8 (7)	27 (23)	<0·001
Surgery (%)	3 (3)	9 (8)	0·14
Transfusion (mean units ±SD)	2·7 +/− 2·5	3·5 +/− 3·8	0·04
Length of stay < 5 days: number of patients (%)	56 (47)	38 (32)	0·02
Death (%)	5 (4)	12 (10)	0·13

following successful endoscopic hemostasis for peptic ulcer bleeding to either intravenous omeprazole or ranitidine. There were no differences between the groups for the endpoints of re-bleeding, surgery or death.[19] Ald In contrast, a similar small trial by Lin and colleagues[20] concluded that intravenous omeprazole was superior to cimetidine in terms of reduction of re-bleeding rates, but not of surgery or mortality rates.

The most important recent trial was performed by Lau et al.[21] Two hundred and forty patients received an infusion of omeprazole or a placebo. Two hundred and forty patients with high risk ulcers with active bleeding or non-bleeding visible vessels in whom endoscopic therapy for major ulcer bleeding had been successful were treated by epinephrine injection followed by heater probe thermocoagulation. Adherent clots were removed to allow therapy to the underlying vessel. The patients were then randomized to receive either an 80 mg bolus dose of intravenous omeprazole followed by an infusion of 8 mg per hour for 72 hours or placebo. Re-bleeding rates, blood transfusion requirements and length of hospital stay were significantly reduced in the omeprazole group compared with placebo. Ala There was a trend toward fewer operations and deaths in the omeprazole group, but these differences were not statistically significant (Table 7.5).

A subsequent trial by the Hong Kong group included 156 patients with peptic ulcers containing non-bleeding visible vessels or adherent clot in the ulcer base.[22] Patients were randomized to endoscopic therapy using epinephrine (adrenaline) injection and heater probe thermocoagulation plus the previously published high dose intravenous PPI

regimen, or to the PPI regimen alone. The probability of re-bleeding within 30 days of the index episode was significantly reduced in the combination therapy group, suggesting that PPI infusion in combination with endoscopic therapy is superior to PPI infusion alone. Alc Seventeen percent of patients with non-bleeding visible vessels re-bled in the PPI-only group (would it be useful to include the percentage of re-bleeds in the combination group), and although a control group receiving no treatment was not included for ethical reasons, this represents a substantial improvement over the expected re-bleeding rate of 50% based on previous studies.

Following the publication of the trial by Lau[21] the use of high dose intravenous PPI after successful endoscopic therapy for bleeding ulcer has become standard management in many centers in the UK and Europe. The 80 mg bolus and 8 mg per hour infusion regimen consistently raises intragastric pH above 6 for the majority of a 24-hour period.[23] It is not known, however, whether this optimum regimen is actually necessary following endoscopic therapy, and whether bolus intravenous or even oral PPI would suffice. Two small studies have attempted to answer these questions.

Udd et al.[24] randomized 142 patients with ulcer bleeding to the high dose 3-day intravenous omeprazole regimen or a single daily bolus dose of 20 mg for 3 days. Rates of re-bleeding (8% for high dose *v* 12% for standard dose), surgery (4% *v* 7%) and death (6% *v* 3%) were comparable between the groups. Only 102 patients had required endoscopic therapy, and around 30% of patients had an ulcer with a black base only. Thus the number of high risk ulcers in the trial was small, the event rates were low and the study

Table 7.6 Tranexamic acid for gastrointestinal bleeding – a meta-analysis[28]

Outcome	POR	95% CI	*P* value
Re-bleeding	0·80	0·61 to 1·10	0·13
Operation	0·72	0·52 to 1·00	0·047
Death	0·60	0·40 to 0·89	0·01

POR, ; CI, confidence interval

may have lacked power to demonstrate a difference between the effects of the two treatments.

The effect of oral omeprazole following endoscopic therapy for bleeding peptic ulcer was studied by Javid *et al.*[25] One hundred and sixty-six patients with actively bleeding ulcers and non-bleeding visible vessels or adherent clots were treated with a combination of 1:10 000 epinephrine plus 1% polidocanol injection. They were then randomized to receive oral omeprazole 40 mg twice daily or placebo. Six (7%) of the 82 patients in the omeprazole group re-bled compared with 18 (21%) of the 84 patients in the placebo group (*P* = 0·02). Alc Surgery was required in two patients in the omeprazole group and seven patients in the placebo group (*P* = 0·17). One death occurred in the omeprazole group compared with two in the placebo group. The results are comparable with those achieved by Lau with the high dose intravenous regimen.[21] However, it should be noted that 40% of patients in this trial had adherent clot, and the number of patients with high risk was therefore correspondingly lower than that in the Hong Kong study. A further high quality trial comparing the use of intravenous and oral omeprazole in patients with high risk ulcer bleeding is now required.

In our view the evidence now supports the use of PPIs following endoscopic hemostasis in patients with major peptic ulcer bleeding. All the trials show a trend for reduction in re-bleeding in omeprazole-treated patients although rates of surgery and mortality are not convincingly reduced. The trials are rather heterogeneous and few in number, making meaningful meta-analysis difficult. Zed *et al.* carried out an analysis of nine trials comparing PPIs with placebo or H$_2$-RAs given after endoscopic therapy.[26] The conclusion was that PPIs are superior to placebo and H$_2$-RAs in terms of reduction of re-bleeding and surgery. Mortality was not reduced in the PPI groups. Ala A second meta-analysis by Gisbert *et al.* included 11 trials and reached similar conclusions, although the beneficial effect of PPI was found only in reduction of the rate of re-bleeding.[27] Ala The group also noted that PPIs were most likely to be beneficial in patients with active bleeding and non-bleeding visible vessels, and in those patients who did not receive endoscopic therapy.

We cannot say with certainty that use of PPIs saves lives, but the effects on surrogate markers such as re-bleeding, transfusion requirements, surgical operation and endoscopic intervention are convincing. There do not appear to be significant hazards associated with the drugs and their cost in the context of an acutely bleeding patient are relatively minor.

Tranexamic acid

A meta-analysis of six controlled trials, which included 1267 patients, did not show a significant reduction in the rate of re-bleeding, but did show a statistically significant reduction in the need for surgery and in mortality (Table 7.6).[28] This meta-analysis included trials in which many patients did not have major endoscopic stigmata of bleeding. Therefore, the results may not be applicable to patient populations at greatest risk. Ala

The largest study was undertaken by the Nottingham group.[29] Seven hundred and seventy-five patients presenting to hospital because of acute gastrointestinal bleeding were randomized to receive oral cimetidine, tranexamic acid or placebo. No significant difference in bleeding or operation rates was demonstrated, but there was a rather surprising large difference in mortality – 11% in cimetidine-treated patients, 10% in tranexamic acid-treated patients, and 20% in the placebo-treated group. Ala The mortality rate of 20% in the placebo-treated group is approximately twice that expected for conservatively treated patients based on the results of other studies. Furthermore, other studies do not demonstrate benefit from the use of cimetidine. It is possible that more high risk patients were inadvertently randomized to the placebo group in this study.

Somatostatin and octreotide

Somatostatin and its analogs have two actions which are theoretically valuable in the management of ulcer bleeding, namely inhibition of acid secretion and reduction of splanchnic blood flow. Mesenteric blood flow falls dramatically during infusions of somatostatin but it is not clear whether this is principally due to vasoconstriction of major blood vessels or peripheral arterioles.

There have been 14 controlled trials of somatostatin versus other therapy in the management of patients presenting with acute gastrointestinal bleeding.[30–43] Two meta-analyses suggest that somatostatin but not octreotide has a primary hemostatic role and reduces the need for surgical

Table 7.7 Somatostatin versus placebo for acute gastrointestinal bleeding

	Somatostatin	Placebo
	Sommerville et al.[30]	
All patients		
n	315	315
Re-bleed (%)	70 (22)	89 (28)
Operation (%)	35 (11)	34 (11)
Death (%)	31 (10)	25 (8)
Subgroup with gastric ulcer		
n	57	57
Re-bleed (%)	18 (32)	21 (37)
Operation (%)	10 (18)	5 (9)
Death (%)	4 (7)	7 (12)
Subgroup with duodenal ulcer		
n	77	81
Re-bleed (%)	21 (27)	31 (38)
Operation (%)	13 (17)	18 (22) $P<0.02$
Death (%)	15 (19)	5 (6)
	Magnusson et al.[31]	
n	46	49
Peptic ulcer bleeding	36	42
Stigmata of major bleeding	38	41
Continued bleeding (%)	8 (17)	16 (33)
Operation (%)	5 (11)	14 (29)
Re-bleeding (%)	6 (13)	5 (10)
Median transfused units	5·8	7·2
Death (%)	4 (9)	1 (2)

intervention.[44,45] Ala However, scrutiny of the relevant trials reveals many problems. Many of the studies were small and inclusion criteria varied widely from gastritis to major active bleeding.

The largest trial was reported by Sommerville *et al.* in 1985 (Table 7.7).[30] Six hundred and thirty of 779 potentially eligible actively bleeding patients were randomized to receive somatostatin (a bolus of 250 micrograms followed by 250 mg hourly for 72 hours) or placebo. No significant differences in re-bleeding, operation rate and mortality were demonstrated between the treatment (one group was placebo) groups. Ala The authors also reported the subgroup analysis of patients who had bled from gastric or duodenal ulcers. There were similar numbers of these in both active and placebo arms. Unfortunately the presence or absence of major stigmata of bleeding were not reported. The operation rate, mortality, and re-bleeding rates were similar in the two groups. However, a statistically significant difference in mortality in duodenal ulcer patients was demonstrated, with more actively bleeding patients dying. Although this was a large study, and patients were randomized early, it may have lacked the power to demonstrate a benefit of somatostatin. Many

patients whose prognosis was excellent because they had relatively trivial bleeding were included, and at the other end of the spectrum, there were also patients included in whom operation and possibly death was inevitable because bleeding was so severe.

A smaller study with contrasting results was reported by Magnusson *et al.* (Table 7.7).[31] This trial only included patients who were in shock and actively bleeding, from peptic ulcers in almost all cases. Patients were randomized to receive somatostatin or placebo infusion. Uncontrolled hemorrhage and need for surgical operation were more common in placebo than somatostatin-treated patients. However, the mortality rate was not improved. Re-bleeding was equally common in both groups and the apparent difference in transfusion requirements was not statistically Ald significant. This small study lacked the power to demonstrate a significant difference in mortality should a true difference exist.

Currently, the evidence for routine use of somatostatin is weak and further studies are needed before this agent can be recommended as routine therapy for non-variceal acute gastrointestinal bleeding.

Endoscopic therapy

Many therapeutic endoscopic treatments have been used to try to stop active ulcer bleeding and prevent re-bleeding. These can be classified into three basic endoscopic approaches (Box 7.1).

Box 7.1   Classification of endoscopic therapeutic modalities for gastrointestinal bleeding

Thermal
- Argon laser
- Nd:YAG laser
- Heater probe
- Electrocoagulation
- Argon plasma coagulation

Injection
- Epinephrine
- Sclerosants
- Alcohol
- Thrombin
- Fibrin glue

Mechanical
- Hemoclips
- Staples
- Sutures

Thermal approaches involving laser, the heater probe and electrocoagulation by monopolar or bipolar probes attempt to induce thermocoagulation with thrombosis of the bleeding point. In experimental bleeding ulcers these approaches are more effective than injection treatments.[46] However, there is no good model of acute peptic ulcer bleeding. Experiments in animals are based upon observation following superficial mucosal injury, which is different from erosion of arteries by chronic or acute peptic ulcer. Injection therapy may produce tamponade by the injection of a relatively large volume of fluid into a rigid compartment, compressing the bleeding artery. Vasoconstriction induced by dilute epinephrine, endarteritis induced by sclerosants, dehydration following absolute alcohol injection or a direct effect upon blood clot formation following injection of thrombin or fibrin glue are other putative mechanisms. Mechanical clips, staples and sewing attempt to produce hemostasis by clamping the bleeding arterial lesion. Many clinical trials of endoscopic therapy for non-variceal bleeding have been published. The quality of these trials varies greatly. In general, the number of patients randomized in any one study is small and clinicians managing the patients have not been blinded to the type of endoscopic therapy. Only one trial has included a placebo control intervention for endoscopic therapy.[47]

Thermal methods

Laser photocoagulation

Lasers were the first endoscopic therapeutic modality shown to be effective in managing acute non-variceal gastrointestinal bleeding. Initial experience involved the use of argon lasers but it became subsequently clear that the tissue characteristics of thermal injury achieved by Nd:YAG (neodymium:yttrium-aluminum-garnet) were more appropriate. In fact, clinical trials showed little difference in outcome in series involving argon or Nd:YAG laser treatment. There have been three randomized trials comparing argon laser therapy and conservative therapy for bleeding peptic ulcer[48–50] and a further nine trials of Nd:YAG laser treatment[51–59] (Table 7.8). Most of these studies show that laser treatment significantly reduced the rates of re-bleeding, transfusion requirement, and operation rate. One trial showed significant improvement in hospital mortality.[51] Ald However, experience has not been universally positive with laser treatment. It is revealing to compare the best conducted study with the large American multicenter study published in the *New England Journal of Medicine*. Swain *et al.* randomized 138 patients to laser treatment or conservative therapy. Swain personally carried out all endoscopic examinations and treatments and was responsible for the clinical management of the treated subjects.[51] The study revealed significant reductions in re-bleeding, need for emergency surgery and mortality in laser-treated patients. In contrast Krejs *et al.* Alc randomized a similar number of patients to laser therapy or to conservative treatment.[52] Patients treated by laser tended to have a poor outcome compared with control patients. Alc It was apparent in this study that endoscopic therapy was undertaken by a large number of endoscopists who varied in their expertise. Of all therapeutic endoscopic modalities, laser therapy is the most difficult to use. Even in Swain's hands up to 17% of ulcers could not be treated. The method is a "no touch" one and an awkwardly placed duodenal ulcer within a deformed duodenum may be extremely difficult to treat adequately. Thus the results in the hands of relatively inexperienced therapeutic endoscopists, each performing few procedures, were likely to have been variable. Furthermore, the patients included in this trial were managed in many units, rather than by a single "bleeding team".

Endoscopic laser therapy has been found to be relatively safe with few complications; in particular, gastrointestinal perforation has been rare. However, since the technique is difficult, relatively expensive and because other approaches are at least as effective, laser therapy for peptic ulcer bleeding is no longer used.

Heater probe

The heater probe transmits preset amounts of energy to the bleeding point via a Teflon tipped catheter. A powerful water

Table 7.8   Results of trials of Nd:YAG laser treatment for bleeding peptic ulcer

Study	Group	No. of patients	Re-bleed (%)	Surgery (%)	Mortality (%)
Swain *et al.* (1986)[51]	Laser	70	7 (10)	7 (10)	1 (1·4)
	Control	68	27 (40)	24 (35)	8 (12)
Krejs *et al.* (1987)[52]	Laser	85	19 (22)	14 (16)	1 (1·2)
	Control	89	18 (20)	15 (17)	1 (1·1)
Rhode *et al.* (1980)[53]	Laser	62	37 (59)	8 (13)	24 (39)
	Control	43	24 (57)	18 (41)	27 (63)
Rutgeerts *et al.* (1982)[54]	Group 2: L[b]	46	3 (7)	1 (2)	6 (13)
	Group 2: C	40	6 (15)[a]	5 (13)	6 (15)
	Group 3: L[c]	17	3 (18)	2 (12)	2 (12)
	Group 3: C	26	8 (31)	6 (23)	4 (15)
MacLeod *et al.* (1983)[55]	Laser	21	6 (29)	5 (24)	1 (5)
	Control	24	8 (33)	8 (33)	2 (8)
Homer *et al.* (1985)[56]	Laser	17	3 (18)	–	0 (0)
	Control	25	8 (32)	–	2 (8)
Trudeau *et al.* (1985)[57]	Laser	18	2 (11)	1 (5)	2 (11)
	Control	15	6 (40)	4 (26)	5 (33)
Buset *et al.* (1988)[58]	Laser	42	10 (24)	3 (7)	1 (2)
	Control	46	17 (37)	2 (4)	2 (4)
Matthewson *et al.* (1990)[59]	Laser	44	9 (20)	9 (20)	1 (2)
	Heater probe	57	16 (28)	13 (22)	6 (10)
	Control	42	18 (43)	13 (30)	4 (9)

[a]6 of 31 where bleeding stopped.
[b]Rutgeerts group 2: active non-spurting bleeding.
[c]Rutgeerts group 3: inactive bleeding with stigmata of recent hemorrhage.

Table 7.9   Results of trials of treatment with the heater probe for gastrointestinal bleeding

Study	Group	Re-bleed (%)	Surgery (%)	Mortality (%)
Fullarton *et al.* (1989)[60]	HP (*n* = 20)	0	0	0
	Sham (*n* = 23)	22*	13**	0
Jensen *et al.* (1988)[61]	BICAP	44	33	3
	HP	22***	3***	3
	Nil	72	41	9
	n (total) = 94			

*$P = 0·05$.
**$P = 0·23$.
***$P < 0·05$.
HP, heater probe; BICAP, bipolar electrocoagulation.

jet is used to clean the ulcer base, help visualize the bleeding point and also to prevent the probe sticking to the bleeding point. Hemostasis is achieved by coaptive coagulation, using both tamponade and the application of heat. Best results are achieved using large sized probes. There have been two trials in which the heater probe has been compared to conservative therapy.[60,61] Both showed benefit in terms of further bleeding, and surgery, and the one published only in abstract form[61] demonstrated a trend towards reduction in mortality (Table 7.9). Ald

The heater probe is "user friendly". Its capacity to apply thermal energy by tangential application and its powerful water jet are particular advantages. Perforations have occurred following treatment, although these are unusual, and are of the order of 1%.[62] In general, medium power settings (20–30 J) are used, but it is not possible to be prescriptive concerning the total amount of energy that should be applied. Most authorities consider that treatment should be continued until active hemorrhage is stopped and until the treated area is blackened and cavitated.

Table 7.10 Results of trials of electrocoagulation for gastrointestinal bleeding

Study	Group	No. of patients	Re-bleed (%)	Surgery (%)	Mean units transfused
O'Brien *et al.* (1987)[63]	Bipolar probe	101	17 (17)*	7 (7)	4·6**
	Nil	103	34 (33)	10 (10)	7.3
Laine (1987)[64a]	MPEC	21	–	3 (14)***	2·4†
	Sham	23	–	10 (43)	5·4
Brearley *et al.* (1987)[65]	Bipolar probe	20	6 (30)	–	–
	Nil	21	8 (38)	–	–
Laine (1988)[66b]	MPEC	37	7 (19)‡	3 (8)	1·6‡
	Sham	37	15 (41)	11 (30)	3·0

*$P = 0.01$.
**$P = 0.13$.
***$P = 0.049$.
†$P = 0.002$.
‡$P < 0.05$.
MPEC, monopolar electrocoagulation.
aStudy included ulcers, Mallory–Weiss tears and vascular malformations.
bStudy was restricted to ulcers with non-bleeding visible vessels. See also Jensen *et al.*[61] (Table 7.9).

Electrocoagulation

Monopolar electrocoagulation uses a metal ball-tipped probe. An electrical circuit is completed by a plate attached to the patient. Application of energy is rather haphazard and perforations and a death were reported in early series. Consequently this device is no longer used. Bipolar electrocoagulation (BICAP) is based upon transmission of electrical energy between adjacent electrodes. The BICAP has eight separate electrodes over its surface. Early studies from the UK involving small numbers of patients showed no benefit for active treatment compared to conservative therapy. Subsequently, however, trials from the UK and the USA showed improved outcomes including primary hemostasis, re-bleeding, the need for surgery and transfusion requirements with BICAP compared with conventionally treated patients.[63–66] (Table 7.10). The efficacy of the heater probe and BICAP appear to be comparable with similar low complication rates.[62,67] Ald

Argon plasma coagulation

This procedure is based upon coagulation through a jet of argon gas. Relatively superficial thermal damage is achieved. The method is particularly applicable to mucosal and superficial bleeding lesions and its final role may be in dealing with vascular malformations such as gastric antral vascular ectasia. One small trial has shown that argon beam coagulation is comparable in efficacy to heater probe therapy for ulcer hemostasis.[68] A second trial compared the argon plasma coagulator with combination injection of epinephrine and polidocanol.[69] Again the two approaches were equally effective. Ald Nevertheless the tissue damage characteristics of argon plasma coagulation are less than ideal for managing arterial bleeding, and it will probably prove to be less appropriate for managing peptic ulcer bleeding than contact methods.

Conclusion

Thermal methods of hemostasis were shown to be superior to conservative management in two meta-analyses. In the study of Cook *et al.* the odds ratio for prevention of re-bleeding was 0·48 (95% CI 0·32 to 0·76); and for avoidance of surgery was 0·47 (95% CI 0·27 to 0·80).[70] Similarly, in the study of Henry and White the odds ratio for prevention of bleeding was 0·32 (95% CI 0·22 to 0·41) and for the avoidance of surgery was 0·31 (95% CI 0·19 to 0·43).[71] Ald Thermal contact methods (heater probe and bipolar coagulation) are technically easier to undertake than laser techniques. There are insufficient data to determine whether the heater probe is better than the BICAP.

The safety profile of thermal modalities is generally very good. Perforations are unusual and treatment-induced exacerbation of bleeding is not usually clinically important.

Injection therapy

Injection treatment is simple to carry out and is the cheapest available hemostatic modality. A large range of injection materials has been studied and it is difficult to prove that any one is superior to the others.

Dilute epinephrine

In 1988 Chung *et al.* reported a controlled trial in which patients with active ulcer bleeding were randomized to receive endoscopic injection with 1:10 000 epinephrine or

Table 7.11 Controlled trial of epinephrine for gastrointestinal bleeding[72]

Outcome	Epinephrine ($n = 34$)	Conservative ($n = 34$)
Primary hemostasis (%)	34 (100)	_a
Surgery (%)	5 (15)	14 (41)
Mortality (%)	3 (9)	2 (6)

a20 patients stopped bleeding spontaneously.

Table 7.12 Summary of results of trials of epinephrine plus sclerosants for gastrointestinal bleeding

Study	Group	No. of patients	Re-bleed (%)	Surgery (%)	Mortality (%)
Panes et al. (1987)[73]	Epi + Pol + Cim	55	3 (5)	3 (5)	2 (4)
	Cim	58	25 (43)	20 (34)	4 (7)
Rajgopal and Palmer (1991)[74]	Epi + Eth	56	7 (13)	6 (11)	2 (4)
	Nil	53	25 (47)	13 (25)	3 (6)
Balanzo et al. (1988)[75]	Epi + Pol	36	7 (19)	7 (19)	–
	Nil	36	15 (42)	15 (42)	–
Oxner et al. (1992)[76]	Epi + Eth	48	8 (17)	4 (8)	4 (8)
	Nil	45	21 (47)	8 (18)	9 (20)

Epi, epinephrine; Pol, polidocanol; Eth, ethanolamine; Cim, cimetidine

were treated conservatively.[72] Primary hemostasis was achieved in all injected patients and the need for subsequent Ald urgent surgery was significantly reduced (Table 7.11). Re-bleeding occurred in 24% of injected patients, suggesting that although dilute epinephrine did stop active bleeding, its effects were temporary.

It seemed logical to combine an injection of epinephrine with that of an agent which might cause permanent sealing of the bleeding arterial defect. For this reason a series of trials were undertaken in which epinephrine injection was combined with a range of sclerosants.

The results of trials in which a combination of epinephrine plus sclerosants were compared with conservative therapy are summarized in Table 7.12.[73–76] All showed that active bleeding stopped more rapidly in treated patients, that re-bleeding rates were less, and that the need for surgery was reduced. No single trial, however, was powerful enough to determine whether mortality was affected. A subsequent meta-analysis, involving thermal contact devices, laser and injection therapy carried out by Cook *et al.* did show a modest reduction in mortality, although this was statistically significant only for laser therapy.[70] Ala

Sclerosants

The sclerosants that have been studied are polidocanol, 5% ethanolamine oleate, and 3% sodium tetradecyl sulfate. There are no controlled trials in which outcome has been assessed in patients randomized to sclerosants versus conservative (no

injection) therapy. Several trials compared the efficacy of sclerosants with other endoscopic therapies. Benedetti *et al.* showed similar efficacy for polidocanol and thrombin injection in patients presenting with a range of bleeding lesions.[77] Strohm *et al.* randomized patients to one of four treatment arms (fibrin glue, 1% polidocanol, dilute epinephrine or epinephrine plus polidocanol) and showed no advantage for any one approach.[78] Rutgeerts *et al.* showed no difference in outcome for patients treated by polidocanol or Nd:YAG laser therapy.[79] In general these studies suffer from the problem of small sample size, and they probably lacked statistical power.

A series of case reports documented complications of injection by sclerosant,[80,81] particularly perforation and necrosis of the upper gastrointestinal tract. These complications did not occur following epinephrine injection and indeed the latter seems remarkably safe. Fears concerning the possible systemic affects of circulating epinephrine have not translated into cardiovascular mishaps. Since complications are mainly due to sclerosant injection, it was important to confirm the importance of combining the sclerosant with the epinephrine injection. Whilst the logic of attempting to induce endarteritis using sclerosants was reasonable, experiments in animals did not demonstrate that this could be achieved by injection using ethanolamine or absolute alcohol.[82] C Three trials compared the efficacy of injection by epinephrine alone versus a combination of epinephrine plus a sclerosant.[83–85] As shown in Table 7.13, these three studies did not show that combination treatment

Table 7.13 Results of studies of epinephrine versus epinephrine plus sclerosant in gastrointestinal bleeding

Study	Group	No. of patients	Primary hemostasis	Re-bleed (%)	Surgery (%)	Transfusion (units +/−range)	Mortality (%)
Chung *et al.* (1993)[83]	Epi + Alc	79	75	6 (8)	9 (11)	2 (0–23)	7 (9)
	Epi	81	79	9 (11)	12 (15)	3 (0–20)	4 (5)
Choudari and Palmer (1994)[84]	Epi + Eth	52	–	7 (14)	4 (8)	8	0 (0)
	Epi	55	–	8 (15)	4 (7)	9	1 (2)
Villanueva *et al.* (1993)[85]	Epi + Pol	33	32	7 (21)	5 (15)	2	1 (3)
	Epi	30	29	3 (10)	4 (13)	2	2 (7)

Epi, epinephrine; Alc, alcohol; Eth, ethanolamine; Pol, polidocanol

Table 7.14 Results of studies of alcohol versus conservative therapy for gastrointestinal bleeding

Study	Group	No. of patients	Re-bleeding (%)	Surgery (%)	Mortality (%)
Pascu *et al.* (1989)[86]	Alcohol	41	1 (2)*	1 (2)	1 (2)
	Conservative	39	5 (13)	14 (36)	6 (15)
Lazo *et al.* (1992)[87]	Alcohol	25	2 (8)**	1 (4)*	–
	Conservative	14	8 (57)	7 (50)	–

*$P < 0.05$.
**$P < 0.001$.

was superior to injection by epinephrine alone. Alc No study has directly compared outcome in patients randomized to dilute epinephrine or to a sclerosant.

Since the addition of sclerosants to an injection of epinephrine offers no proved advantage over injecting epinephrine alone, and because sclerosants have the potential to cause significant local complications following injection, they should no longer be employed as part of the injection treatment regimen.

Alcohol

The efficacy of injecting absolute alcohol into bleeding ulcers has been examined in several clinical trials. Two of these[86,87] (Table 7.14) randomized patients to alcohol injection or to conservative therapy and showed benefit in terms of reduction in re-bleeding rates and need for surgical intervention. Ald

In a randomized controlled trial, Lin *et al.*[88] reported that alcohol injection stopped active bleeding and prevented re-bleeding in 86% of patients whose ulcers were injected, and this result was similar to the proportion of bleeding ulcers responding to injection with 3% sodium chloride, 50% dextrose, or normal saline. Only one small study[88] has attempted to compare the efficacy of alcohol with dilute epinephrine injection, but this study lacked statistical power

to demonstrate differences in the effects of these interventions, should any exist.

The evidence that alcohol stops active bleeding and prevents re-bleeding is stronger than that for the sclerosants. Unfortunately, the potential for adverse effects is probably higher for alcohol than for epinephrine. Deep ulcers commonly follow alcohol injection and perforations have occurred.[90]

Whilst alcohol injection is an effective hemostatic therapy, current evidence suggests that the magnitude of its effect is probably similar to that achieved by injection with epinephrine alone. Because of its propensity for causing adverse effects, alcohol injection is not recommended as treatment for ulcer bleeding.

Thrombin and fibrin glue

The most attractive endoscopic approach is to directly cause blood clot formation by injecting thrombogenic substances. In the 1980s small trials examined the efficacy of bovine thrombin and showed little benefit compared to other modalities.

In 1996 Kubba *et al.* reported a comparison of endoscopic injection therapy using a combination of epinephrine plus human thrombin with dilute epinephrine injection alone (Table 7.15).[91] A proportion of randomized patients had

Table 7.15 Epinephrine plus thrombin versus epinephrine alone for gastrointestinal bleeding

| Outcome | Kubba et al.[91] | | Balanzo et al.[92] | |
	Epi + Throm	Epi alone	Epi + Throm	Epi alone
n	70	70	32	32
Re-bleed (%)	3 (4)	14 (20)*	2 (6)	4 (13)
Transfusion (units)	7	5	3·14	3·94
Surgery (%)	3 (4)	5 (7)	5 (16)	4 (13)
Mortality (%)	0 (0)	7 (10)**	0 (0)	0 (0)

*$P < 0.005$.
**$P < 0.013$.
Epi, epinephrine; Throm, thrombin

Table 7.16 Heater probe plus thrombin versus heater probe plus placebo for gastrointestinal bleeding[47]

Outcome	Heater probe plus Thrombin	Heater probe plus Placebo
n	127	120
Re-bleed (%)	19 (15)	17 (15)
Surgery (%)	16 (13)	13 (11)
Mortality (%)	8 (6)	14 (12)

active bleeding at the time of randomization, while the remainder had non-bleeding visible vessels. Re-bleeding and mortality were significantly reduced in the group receiving combination therapy compared with patients receiving epinephrine alone. The number of patients needed to be treated with combination therapy rather than epinephrine alone to prevent one death is approximately 14. Alc Paradoxically, no statistically significant differences in the need for surgical operation and the overall rate of hemostasis were demonstrated. Indeed, deaths in this study all occurred, as is usually the case, in patients who had significant comorbidity. Complications in this study were minimal. Although this was not a direct comparison of epinephrine versus thrombin, it did strongly suggest that human thrombin is an effective modality.

Balanzo et al. randomized 64 patients with ulcer bleeding to epinephrine injection or epinephrine plus thrombin in a similar, but smaller trial.[92] There were no differences in the rates of primary hemostasis, re-bleeding, surgery or death (see Table 7.15). Ald

To further investigate the use of thrombin as a potential adjunct to standard endoscopic therapy Church et al. randomized 247 patients to treatment with heater probe plus thrombin injection or to heater probe plus placebo injection.[47] This trial included only patients with bleeding peptic ulcers who were at high risk for re-bleeding and death, and was the first trial to include placebo endoscopic therapy. Initial hemostasis was achieved in 97% of patients in both

groups, and the rates of re-bleeding, surgery and mortality were similar (Table 7.16). The results of this trial do not suggest that thrombin is any more effective than placebo when combined with the heater probe for endoscopic hemostasis. Ala

Fibrin glue is a mixture of fibrinogen and thrombin which is injected through a double-channeled endoscopy needle. Its effect was studied by Song et al. in a trial of 127 patients with bleeding ulcers and major stigmata of hemorrhage.[93] Patients were randomized to injection of fibrin glue or hypertonic saline-epinephrine. There were no significant differences between rates of re-bleeding, surgery and death (Table 7.17). Alc This trial is the only one that compared the efficacy of fibrin glue directly with that of another endoscopic therapeutic modality.

In a large multicenter European study (Table 7.18) 850 patients were randomized to endoscopic injection with dilute epinephrine plus a single injection of fibrin glue, to epinephrine and repeated injection of fibrin glue given at daily intervals according to the discretion of the endoscopists, or to epinephrine plus 1% polidocanol.[94] Re-bleeding rates were lowest in patients treated by repeated injection. The rate of serious re-bleeding requiring major blood transfusion or surgical operation, was significantly reduced in patients receiving repeated injections of glue compared with the polidocanol-treated group. Ala A total of seven perforations occurred in this study and these were distributed equally amongst the treated modalities.

Table 7.17   Fibrin glue versus epinephrine injection for gastrointestinal bleeding[93]

Outcome	Fibrin glue	Hypertonic saline/epinephrine
n	64	63
Re-bleed (%)	7 (11)	14 (22)
Surgery (%)	4 (6)	7 (11)
Mortality (%)	1 (2)	4 (6)

Table 7.18   Epinephrine plus fibrin glue versus epinephrine plus polidocanol for gastrointestinal bleeding[94]

Outcome	Epi + rep FG	Epi + single FG	Epi + Pol
n	284	285	281
Re-bleed (%)	43 (15)	55 (19)	64 (23)*
Transfusion (units)	3·7	3·2	3·3
Surgery (%)	9 (3)	14 (5)	14 (5)
Perforation (%)	2 (1)	2 (1)	3 (1)
Mortality (30-day) (%)	12 (4)	15 (5)	13 (5)

*$P < 0.036$.
Epi, epinephrine; FG, fibrin glue; Pol, polidocanol

The most recent trial involving fibrin glue randomized 135 patients to injection of epinephrine plus fibrin glue or to epinephrine alone.[95] Endoscopy was repeated daily with re-treatment of stigmata until the ulcer base contained flat pigmented spots or was clean. The rate of re-bleeding in the combination group was not significantly different from that in the single agent group (24% v 22%). Rates for surgery were also similar (10% v 6%), and mortality was 3% in both groups. A1c

The evidence regarding the use of thrombogenic substances is conflicting. There is evidence of benefit in some studies, but not in others, and currently there is not enough evidence to recommend thrombin or fibrin glue over other injection agents. Thrombin is derived from pooled plasma, and although viral (or other infective agent) transmission has not been reported, this is a possibility. Acute complications are infrequent and no adverse effects have been apparent in terms of systemic coagulation.

Human thrombin is not currently commercially available. It is relatively inexpensive (£35 per vial), although more costly than epinephrine (£1 per vial).

Conclusion

Injection therapy is effective and safe. The optimum injection regimen should probably include dilute epinephrine, which stops active hemorrhage. Re-bleeding rates are not convincingly reduced by the addition of agents such as thrombin or a thrombin–fibrinogen mixture. Sclerosants and alcohol should not be used, since there is no evidence that they are beneficial and they increase the risk of serious complications.

The mechanism of injection therapy is not completely understood. It is thought to work at least in part by exerting a tamponade effect resulting from the injection of a volume of fluid into the rigid ulcer base. This possibility is supported by the study reported by Lin *et al.* who compared injection of normal saline, 3% sodium chloride solution, 50% glucose/water solution and pure alcohol in 200 patients with actively bleeding ulcers or non-bleeding visible vessels.[88] There were no statistical differences between rates of initial hemostasis, re-bleeding and surgery for any group. A1c Larger injected volumes were required to achieve initial hemostasis in the saline and glucose/water groups, suggesting that tamponade was an important factor. These results are challenged by those of Laine and Estrada.[96] In this study patients with high risk ulcers were randomized to injection of normal saline ($n = 48$), or to BICAP ($n = 52$). Twenty-nine percent of patients in the saline group had recurrent bleeding compared with 12% of those treated with the BICAP. The saline-treated patients required significantly more blood, but there were no differences in length of hospital stay or mortality. A1d It is likely that tamponade does not completely explain the mechanism of injection therapy, and active agents should continue to be used.

The optimum volume of injection is not known. Small volumes of alcohol and sclerosants are required in order to reduce the risk of perforation. Much larger volumes of saline and epinephrine can be used without complication. In the trial by Lin discussed above, the mean injection volume in the

Table 7.19 Trials comparing heater probe treatment with injection therapy for gastrointestinal bleeding

Study	Group	No. of patients	Primary hemostasis (%)	Re-bleed (%)	Surgery (%)	Mortality (%)
Lin et al. (1988)[98]	HP	42	42 (100)	5 (12)	–	–
	PA	36	29 (81)	6 (22)	–	–
Lin et al. (1990)[99]	HP	45	44 (98)*	8 (18)	3 (7)**	1 (2)†
	PA	46	31 (67)	2 (4)	2 (4)	0
	Control	46	–	–	12 (26)	7 (15)
Chung et al. (1991)[100]	HP	64	53 (83)‡	6/53 (11)	14 (22)	4 (6)‡
	Epi	68	65 (96)	11 (17)	14 (21)	2 (3)
Choudari et al. (1992)[101]	HP	60	–	9 (15)	7 (12)	3 (5)
	Epi + Eth	60	–	8 (13)	7 (12)	2 (3)
Saeed et al. (1993)[102]	HP	39	35 (90)	4 (10)	–	–
	Ethanol	41	33 (81)	5 (12)	–	–
Llach, et al. (1996)[103]	HP	53	–	3 (6)	2 (4)	1 (2)
	Epi + Pol	51	–	2 (4)	2 (4)	1 (2)

*$P=0.0004$.
**$P=0.0024$ ($P=0.027$ between control and HP; $P=0.012$ between PA and HP).
†$P=0.002$ ($P=0.031$ between control and HP; $P=0.018$ between control and PA).
‡$P<0.05$.
HP, heater probe; PA, pure alcohol; Epi, epinephrine; Eth, ethanolamine; Pol, polidocanol

saline group was 15 ml. Laine and Estrada injected a mean volume of 30 ml. A further trial by Lin et al. compared large with relatively small volume injection.[97] One hundred and fifty-six patients with ulcer bleeding were randomized to injection of 5–10 ml of epinephrine (the small volume group) or injection of 13–20 ml (the large volume group). Re-bleeding occurred in 31% of the small volume patients compared with 15% in the large volume group. Alc The other usual endpoints were similar. The conclusion of this trial is that larger volume injection of epinephrine is safe and more likely to prevent re-bleeding than injection of a smaller volume.

Comparison of injection and thermal treatments

A number of small trials have compared injection with thermal therapies. In general, the two modalities appear to have similar efficacy.

Six trials have compared heater probe with injection[98–103] (Table 7.19). The two trials reported by Lin et al. showed that heater probe treatment was more effective in achieving primary hemostasis.[98,99] These authors noted the heater probe to be better when ulcers were difficult to approach, since it can be applied tangentially. They also found the water jet to be useful in the presence of spurting bleeding. It may be argued that alcohol is a less appropriate injection therapy than epinephrine, which may account for the apparent superiority of the heater probe in these studies. This view was supported by the findings of Chung et al.[100] They concluded that heater

probe and epinephrine were equally effective, but that initial hemostasis was more easily achieved with epinephrine. Choudari et al.[101] compared the heater probe with epinephrine plus ethanolamine (in the table only epi) and found no differences between the modalities. The remaining two trials by Saeed et al.[102] and Llach et al.[103] support this conclusion. Laine showed that electrocoagulation and injection with ethanol were equivalent, although the size of this trial was suboptimal.[104] Alc

Two trials involved the Nd:YAG laser. Carter and Anderson[105] compared laser with epinephrine and Pulanic et al.,[106] in a much larger trial, compared laser with polidocanol. Neither showed a difference in outcome.

Current evidence does not allow a conclusion to be drawn on whether injection or thermal treatment is superior. We advocate the heater probe as the thermal method of choice. Some situations, particularly those involving awkwardly placed posterior duodenal ulcers, lend themselves better to use of the heater probe than to injection therapy.

Combination of injection and thermal treatments

The mechanisms leading to hemostasis associated with thermal treatment and injection therapy may differ, providing a rationale for combining a thermal modality and injection treatment. Currently, only one small study has shown overall benefit from use of such a combination. This trial by Lin et al. used the gold probe, a bipolar coagulation probe containing an injection needle in the center.[107] Using this device heat

Table 7.20 Epinephrine plus heater probe versus epinephrine alone for gastrointestinal bleeding[108]

Outcome	Epi + HP	Epi alone
Overall	*n* = 136	*n* = 134
Primary hemostasis (%)	135 (99)	131 (98)
Re-bleed (%)	5 (4)	12 (9)
Transfusion (units)	3	2
Surgery (%)	8 (6)	14 (11)
Mortality (%)	8 (6)	7 (5)
Subgroup with spurting hemorrhage	*n* = 32	*n* = 28
Primary hemostasis (%)	31 (97)	25 (89)
Re-bleed (%)	2 (6)	6 (21)
Transfusion (units)	4	5
Surgery (%)	2 (6)	8 (29)*
Mortality (%)	Not stated	Not stated

*P = 0.03.
Epi, epinephrine; HP, heater probe

and injection therapy may be applied without removing the probe from the ulcer. Ninety-six patients were randomized to receive injection alone, coagulation alone or combination therapy Re-bleeding rates were lower in the combination group compared with the injection alone and coagulation alone groups (7% *v* 36%, *P* = 0·01 and 7% *v* 30%, *P* = 0·04, respectively). Alc The volume of blood transfused in the combination group was also significantly lower. Although this small trial demonstrated a beneficial outcome following combination endoscopic therapy, confirmation in a larger trial would be desirable.

A further encouraging trend relates to a finding within a study reported by Chung *et al.*[108] This study involved randomization of appropriate patients with ulcer bleeding to injection therapy using 1:10 000 epinephrine or to a combination of epinephrine plus the heater probe (Table 7.20). Although there was no overall difference in outcome between patients randomized to either arm, a *post hoc* subgroup analysis did reveal positive findings. Sixty patients had active spurting hemorrhage from large ulcers, and within this group the primary hemostatic effect of both treatments was similar. However, the need for operation was significantly reduced in the group treated by heater probe and injection. The number of surgical endpoints was very small, and this observation from subgroup analysis requires confirmation in further trials.

Mechanical clips

The hemoclip was first used for non-variceal bleeding by Japanese investigators in the early 1970s.[109] The device has gained favor, particularly in Japan, and is the endoscopic method most analogous to underrunning an ulcer at operative surgery. Three large case series[110–112] support hemoclips as a safe and effective method for the treatment of bleeding peptic

ulcer and there are four randomized trials of reasonable size.[113–116] B

Chung *et al.* published a randomized trial comparing hemoclips with epinephrine injection in 1999.[113] Of 124 patients with actively bleeding ulcers or ulcers with vessels included in the study 41 were treated with hemoclips, 41 with epinephrine and 42 with a combination of the two. Primary hemostasis was achieved in over 95% of patients. Re-bleeding occurred in 2·4%, 14·6% and 9·5%, respectively, but the differences between the groups were not significant (*P* = 0·138). Similarly, rates of surgery and mortality were no different (4·9% *v* 14·6% *v* 2·3% for surgery and 2·4% *v* 2·4% *v* 2·3% for mortality, respectively). Alc Three patients had complications, all in the epinephrine only group. In one patient severe bleeding requiring surgical operation was precipitated; two patients developed submucosal hematoma.

Cipoletta *et al.*[114] randomized 113 patients with endoscopic stigmata of hemorrhage to heater probe thermocoagulation or to application of hemoclips. A mean of three clips per patient were used with up to six being required in some cases. Re-bleeding was dramatically reduced in the hemoclip group with rates in the clip and heater probe groups of 1·8% and 21%, respectively (*P* < 0·05). Surgery and mortality rates were similar in the two groups and there were no complications.

The two previous trials suggested clips to be effective, with re-bleed rates below 3% in the clip only groups. Two subsequent studies, however, have been less encouraging. Eighty patients were randomized to heater probe thermocoagulation or to placement of hemoclips in the trial by Lin *et al.*[115] Primary hemostasis was achieved in only 85% of patients in the clip group versus 100% of those treated with the heater probe (*P* = 0·01). The rates of re-bleeding, surgery and mortality were not different. Ald Gevers *et al.*[116] carried out a similar trial to Chung[113] in which 101 patients were randomized to injection with epinephrine and polidocanol, hemoclip application or a combination of the two. The overall failure rate was significantly higher in the hemoclip alone group than in the injection and combination groups (34%, 6% and 25%, respectively; $P = 0.01$). Alc

The major difficulty with hemoclip placement occurs when ulcers are difficult to reach and tangential application is required. Initial clip applicators resulted in problems with clip alignment, but a rotary applicator has now been developed. Further problems arise when clips are applied to the fibrous base of a chronic ulcer, as in this situation it may not be possible to adequately compress the bleeding vessel. In the trial by Lin[115] a surveillance endoscopy was carried out 72 hours after therapy. Hemoclips had been successfully placed in 31 patients, but at 72 hours the clip was still attached to the ulcer base in only 10 patients. This could have accounted for the disappointing performance of the clip group, and perhaps clips with a more powerful clamping mechanism would improve the efficacy of the device. Further trials with improved clips are required.

Endoscopic therapy for ulcers with adherent blood clot

There is debate concerning the appropriate intervention when blood clot is tightly adherent to an ulcer base. To remove a clot seems counterintuitive in the situation of acute bleeding, but to leave it *in situ* prevents accurate categorization of stigmata of hemorrhage, and may prevent correct application of endoscopic therapy.

Lin *et al.*[117] showed that when clot is tightly adherent after washing for 10 seconds with Water Pik irrigation, the re-bleed rate is 25%. Factors independently associated with re-bleeding in this situation are the presence of shock, comorbid disease and hemoglobin at presentation of < 10 g/dl. In the trial by Sung *et al.*[22] clot was defined as adherent only after 5 minutes irrigation with the 3·2 mm heater probe. Patients received high dose PPI infusion plus or minus endoscopic therapy. Of 39 patients with adherent clot only one (in the combination group) re-bled, suggesting that when clot is truly adherent to an ulcer base a PPI infusion may be all that is required. Bleau *et al.* published a small trial in which patients with adherent clot were randomized to pre-injection with epinephrine followed by clot removal and thermocoagulation of a visible vessel, or to medical therapy with PPI.[118] The patients in the endoscopic therapy group had a significantly lower re-bleeding rate, although the numbers were small (56 patients). Ald A similar but very small trial (32 patients) has been reported by Jensen *et al.*[119] The results again indicate that clot removal and therapy to the underlying stigmata is a safe and effective strategy. Ald A further trial comparing the outcome of endoscopic therapy without removal of adherent clot with that of therapy after clot removal would be of interest.

Elective repeat endoscopic therapy

It is not yet clear whether electively repeating endoscopy and hemostatic therapy in the absence of clinical or endoscopic signs of re-bleeding is a useful strategy. There are clear positive trends from trials by Rutgeerts *et al.*[94] and Villanueva *et al.*[120] toward a better outcome in groups treated repeatedly, but the only statistically significant result in favor of repeated treatment is from a very small study including only 40 patients.[121] Ald Furthermore, Messmann *et al.* randomized 105 patients who had required endoscopic therapy for bleeding ulcers, to daily repeat endoscopy with re-treatment of persistent stigmata, or to close observation. There was no difference between the groups for any of the usual endpoints.[122] Alc The trial by Pescatore *et al.*[95] also reported no clear benefit from the use of an elective repeat endoscopy approach.

Elective repeat endoscopic therapy may be beneficial in patients at very high risk of re-bleeding or surgery, but there is no definite evidence to support this view. Repeat endoscopy should also be considered in cases where the endoscopist is not convinced that adequate hemostasis has been achieved at the time of the initial endoscopy.

Failure of endoscopic therapy

It may be argued that endoscopists can adversely affect outcome in patients who fail endoscopic therapy. Repeated unsuccessful therapeutic endoscopy, large blood transfusion, and delayed surgical operation in those who ultimately fail attempted endoscopic hemostasis all increase the risk of death. Unfortunately, we cannot predict who will fail and who will respond to endoscopic therapy. Two analyses both showed that the presence of active bleeding, large ulcer size, and an ulcer situated in the posterior duodenum were significantly more common in failures of therapy.[123,124] There is an impression that patients who are in shock at presentation also fare worse. However, even in the highest risk group of patients, who present with active spurting hemorrhage from large posterior duodenal ulcers, Choudari *et al.* showed that endoscopic hemostasis can be achieved in approximately 70% of patients.[124] Currently it is not possible to accurately define the subgroup of patients in whom endoscopic therapy should not be attempted. What is clear, however, is that patients who have actively bleeding, large posterior duodenal ulcers should be considered to be at very high risk of requiring urgent operation.

The management of re-bleeding after failed endoscopic therapy has been recently examined by Lau *et al.*[125] Of 3473 patients admitted with bleeding peptic ulcers, 1169 underwent endoscopic therapy in an attempt to achieve hemostasis. Primary hemostasis was achieved in a remarkable 98·5%. Of these 100 re-bled after endoscopic therapy and 92 were randomized to receive endoscopic re-treatment or to

Table 7.21 Repeat endoscopic therapy versus surgery for patients who re-bleed[125]

Outcome	Endoscopic therapy	Surgery
n	48	44
Transfusion (units)	8	7
Complications (no. of patients) (%)	7 (15)	16 (36)*
Mortality (30-day) (%)	5 (10)	8 (18)

*$P = 0.03$.

emergency surgery. The characteristics of the two groups of patients were similar, including the median transfusion requirements before randomization. Endoscopic re-treatment consisted of a combination of epinephrine injection plus the heater probe. Overall, more complications occurred in the group randomized to surgery and there was no significant difference in 30-day mortality between the two groups (Table 7.21). A1c This paper suggests that endoscopic re-treatment rather than immediate, urgent surgery may be undertaken in patients who re-bleed after endoscopic hemostatic therapy.

Endoscopic therapy: summary

Endoscopic therapy for non-variceal hemorrhage is safe and effective, and should be used in the 20% of patients who have major endoscopic stigmata of recent hemorrhage. Combination therapy may produce the best results, but there is no definitive proof that this is the case. It is likely that combination therapy is the best approach for patients with active, spurting hemorrhage. Thermal hemostasis is effective using either the heater probe or multipolar electrocoagulation. No injection agent has been convincingly shown to be superior to dilute epinephrine solution. Injection of larger volumes may improve outcome. The hemoclip requires further development. Re-bleeding should be treated first by further endoscopic intervention, although clinical judgment should dictate when urgent surgery is required for specific high risk cases.

Intravenous infusion of PPI drugs is recommended following successful endoscopic hemostasis. Currently there is no evidence that other drug therapies are effective.

References

1 Fleischen D. Etiology and prevalence of severe persistent upper gastrointestinal bleeding. *Gastroenterology* 1983;**84**:538–43.
2 Avery Jones F. Haematemesis and melaena with special reference to bleeding peptic ulcer. c 1947;**ii**:441–6.
3 Rockall TA, Logan RFA, Devlin HB *et al.* Incidence of and mortality from acute upper gastrointestinal haemorrhage in the United Kingdom. *BMJ* 1995;**311**:222–6.
4 Rockall TA, Logan RFA, Devlin HB *et al.* Risk assessment after acute upper gastrointestinal haemorrhage. *Gut* 1996;**38**:316–21.
5 Vreeburg EM, Terwee CB, Snel P *et al.* Validation of the Rockall risk scoring system in upper gastrointestinal bleeding. *Gut* 1999;**44**:331–5.
6 Church NI, Palmer KR. Relevance of the Rockall score in patients undergoing endoscopic therapy for peptic ulcer haemorrhage. *Eur J Gastroenterol Hepatol* 2001;**13**:1149–52.
7 Holman RAE, Davis M, Gough KR *et al.* Value of centralised approach in the management of haematemesis and melaena: Experience in a district general hospital. *Gut* 1990;**31**:504–8.
8 Sanderson JD, Taylor RFH, Pugh S *et al.* Specialised gastrointestinal units for the management of upper gastrointestinal bleeding. *Postgrad Med J* 1990;**66**:654–6.
9 Bornman PC, Theodorou N, Shuttleworth RD *et al.* Importance of hypovolaemic shock and endoscopic signs in predicting recurrent haemorrhage from peptic ulceration: a prospective evaluation. *BMJ* 1985;**291**:245–7.
10 Griffiths WJ, Neumann DA, Welsh DA. The visible vessels as an indicator of uncontrolled or recurrent gastrointestinal haemorrhage. *N Engl J Med* 1979;**300**:1411–13.
11 Swain CP, Storey DW, Bown SG. Nature of the bleeding vessel in recurrently bleeding gastric ulcers. *Gastroenterology* 1986;**90**:595–606.
12 Patchett SE, Enright l, Afdhal N *et al.* Clot lysis by gastric juice;an in vitro study. *Gut* 1989;**30**:1704–7.
13 Walt RP, Cottrell J, Mann SG *et al.* Continuous intravenous famotidine for haemorrhage from peptic ulcer. *Lancet* 1992;**340**:1058–62.
14 Collins R, Langman M. Treatment with histamine H_2 antagonists in acute upper gastrointestinal haemorrhage: implications of randomised trials. *N Engl J Med* 1985;**313**:660–6.
15 Daneshmend TK, Hawkey CJ, Langman MJS *et al.* Omeprazole versus placebo for acute upper gastrointestinal bleeding: randomised double blind controlled trial. *BMJ* 1992;**304**:143–7.
16 Khuroo MS, Yattoo GN, Javid G *et al.* A comparison of omeprazole and placebo for bleeding peptic ulcer. *N Engl J Med* 1997;**336**:1054–8.
17 Schaffalitzky de Muckadell OB, Havelund T, Harling H *et al.* Effect of omeprazole on the outcome of endoscopically treated bleeding peptic ulcers: randomized double blind

placebo controlled multicenter study. *Scand J Gastroenterol* 1997;**32**:320–7.

18 Hasslegren G, Lind T, Lundell L *et al.* Continuous intravenous infusion of omeprazole in elderly patients with peptic ulcer bleeding: results of a placebo controlled multicentre study. *Scand J Gastroenterol* 1997;**32**:328–33.

19 Villanueva C, Balanzo J, Torras X *et al.* Omeprazole versus ranitidine as adjunct therapy to endoscopic injection in actively bleeding ulcers: a prospective randomized study. *Endoscopy* 1995;**27**:308–12.

20 Lin HJ, Lo WC, Lee FY *et al.* A prospective randomised comparative trial showing that omeprazole prevents rebleeding in patients with bleeding peptic ulcer after successful endoscopic therapy. *Arch Intern Med* 1998;**158**:54–8.

21 Lau JYW, Sung JY, Lee KKC *et al.* Effect of intravenous omeprazole on recurrent bleeding after endoscopic treatment of bleeding peptic ulcers. *N Engl J Med* 2000; **343**:310–16.

22 Sung JJY, Chan FKL, Lau JYW *et al.* The effect of endoscopic therapy in patients receiving omeprazole for bleeding ulcers with nonbleeding visible vessels or adherent clots. *Ann Intern Med* 2003;**139**:237–43.

23 Hasselgren G, Keelan M, Kirdeikis P *et al.* Optimization of acid suppression for patients with peptic ulcer bleeding: an intragastric pH-metry study with omeprazole. *Eur J Gastroenterol Hepatol* 1998;**10**:601–6.

24 Udd M, Mietinnen P, Palmu A *et al.* Regular-dose versus high-dose omeprazole in peptic ulcer bleeding: a prospective randomized double-blind study. *Scand J Gastroenterol* 2001;**36**:1332–8.

25 Javid G, Masoodi I, Zargar SA *et al.* Omeprazole as adjuvant therapy to endoscopic combination injection sclerotherapy for treating bleeding peptic ulcer. *Am J Med* 2001;**111**: 280–4.

26 Zed PJ, Loewen PS, Slavic RS, Marra CA. Meta-analysis of proton pump inhibitors in treatment of bleeding peptic ulcers. *Ann Pharmacother* 2001;**35**:1528–34.

27 Gisbert JP, Gonzalez L, Calvet X *et al.* Proton pump inhibitors versus H2-antagonists: a meta-analysis of their efficacy in treating bleeding peptic ulcer. *Aliment Pharmacol Ther* 2001;**15**:917–26.

28 Henry DA, O'Connell DL. Effect of fibrinolytic inhibitors on mortality from upper gastrointestinal haemorrhage. *BMJ* 1989;**298**:1142–6.

29 Barer D, Ogilvie A, Henry D *et al.* Cimetidine and tranexamic acid in the treatment of acute upper-gastrointestinal-tract bleeding. *N Engl J Med* 1983;**308**: 1571–5.

30 Sommerville KW, Henry DA, Davies JG *et al.* Somatostatin in treatment of haematemesis and melaena. *Lancet* 1985;**i**:130–2.

31 Magnusson I, Ihre T, Johansson C *et al.* Randomised double blind trial of somatostatin in the treatment of massive upper gastrointestinal haemorrhage. *Gut* 1985;**26**:221–6.

32 Basso N, Bagarani M, Bracci F *et al.* Ranitidine and somatostatin. Their effects on bleeding from the upper gastrointestinal tract. *Arch Surg* 1986;**121**:833–5.

33 Coraggio F, Scarpato P, Spina M *et al.* Somatostatin and ranitidine in the control of iatrogenic haemorrhage of the upper gastrointestinal tract. *BMJ* 1984;**289**:224.

34 Coraggio F, Bertini G, Catalona A *et al.* Clinical controlled trial of somatostatin with ranitidine and placebo in the control of peptic haemorrhage of the upper gastrointestinal tract. *Digestion* 1989;**43**:190–5.

35 Galmiche JP, Cassigneul J, Faivre J *et al.* Somatostatin in peptic ulcer bleeding. Results of a double blind controlled trial. *Int J Clin Pharmacol Res* 1983;**III**:379–87.

36 Saperas E, Pique JM, Perez-Ayuso R *et al.* Somatostatin compared with cimetidine in the treatment of bleeding peptic ulcer without visible vessel. *Aliment Pharmacol Ther* 1988;**2**:153–9.

37 Kayasseh L, Gyr K, Keller U *et al.* Somatostatin and cimetidine in peptic ulcer haemorrhage. A randomised controlled trial. *Lancet* 1980;**i**:844–6.

38 Antonioli A, Gandolfo M, Rigo GP *et al.* Somatostatin and cimetidine in the control of acute upper gastrointestinal bleeding. A controlled multicentre study. *Hepato-gastroenterology* 1986;**33**:71–4.

39 Tulassay Z, Gupta R, Papp J *et al.* Somatostatin versus cimetidine in the treatment of actively bleeding duodenal ulcer: a prospective, randomised, controlled trial. *Am J Gastroenterol* 1989;**84**:6–9.

40 Torres AJ, Landa I, Hernandez F *et al.* Somatostatin in the treatment of severe upper gastrointestinal bleeding: a multicentre controlled trial. *Br J Surg* 1986;**73**:786–9.

41 Wagner PK, Rothmund M, Gronniger J. Secretin and somatostatin in treatment of acute upper gastrointestinal haemorrhage: a randomised trial. *Klin Wochenschr* 1983; **61**:285–9.

42 Goletti O, Sidoti F, Lippolis PV *et al.* Omeprazole versus ranitidine and somatostatin in the treatment of acute severe gastroduodenal haemorrhage. *Br J Surg* 1992;**79**(Suppl): S123.

43 Christiansen J, Ottenjann R, Von Arx F. Placebo-controlled trial with the somatostatin analogue sms 201–995 in peptic ulcer bleeding. *Gastroenterology* 1989;**97**:568–74.

44 Jenkins SA, Poulianos G, Coraggio F *et al.* Somatostatin in the treatment of non-variceal upper gastrointestinal bleeding. *Dig Dis Sci* 1998;**16**:214–24.

45 Imperiale TF, Birgisson S. Somatostatin or octreotide compares with H$_2$ antagonists and placebo in the management of acute non-variceal upper gastrointestinal haemorrhage: a meta-analysis. *Ann Intern Med* 1997;**127**: 1062–71.

46 Rutgeerts P, Geboes K, Vantrappen G. Experimental studies of injection therapy for severe nonvariceal bleeding in dogs. *Gastroenterology* 1989;**97**:601–21.

47 Church NI, Dallal HJ, Masson J *et al.* A randomized trial comparing heater probe plus thrombin with heater probe plus placebo for bleeding peptic ulcer. *Gastroenterology* 2003;**125**:396–404.

48 Vallon AG, Cotton PB, Laurence BH *et al.* Randomised trial of endoscopic argon laser photocoagulation in bleeding peptic ulcers. *Gut* 1981;**22**:228–33.

49 Swain CP, Bown SG, Storey DW *et al.* Controlled trial of argon laser photocoagulation in bleeding peptic ulcer. *Lancet* 1981;**ii**:1313–16.

50 Jensen DM, Machicado GA, Tapia JL *et al.* Controlled trial of endoscopic argon laser for severe ulcer haemorrhage. *Gastroenterology* 1984;**86**:1125.

51 Swain CP, Salmon PR, Kirkham JS. Controlled trial of Nd-YAG laser photocoagulation in bleeding peptic ulcers. *Lancet* 1986;**i**:1113–17.

52 Krejs GJ, Little KH, Westergaard H. Laser photocoagulation for the treatment of acute peptic ulcer bleeding. *N Engl J Med* 1987;**316**:1618–21.

53 Rhode H, Thon K, Fischer M. Results of a defined concept of endoscopic Nd-YAG laser therapy in patients with upper gastrointestinal bleeding. *Br J Surg* 1980;**67**:360.

54 Rutgeerts P, Vantrappen G, Broeckhaert. Controlled trial of YAG laser treatment of upper digestive haemorrhage. *Gastroenterology* 1982;**83**:410–16.

55 Macleod I, Mills PR, Mackenzie JF. Neodymium yttrium aluminium garnet laser photocoagulation for major haemorrhage from peptic ulcers and single vessels. *BMJ* 1983;**286**:345–58.

56 Homer AC, Powell S, Vacary FR. Is Nd-YAG laser treatment for upper gastrointestinal bleeds of benefit in a district general hospital? *Postgrad Med J* 1985;**61**:19–22

57 Trudeau W, Siepler JK, Ross K *et al.* Endoscopic Nd-YAG laser photocoagulation of bleeding ulcers with visible vessels. *Gastrointest Endosc* 1985;**31**:138.

58 Buset M, Des Marez B, Vandermeeran A. Laser therapy for non bleeding visible vessel in peptic ulcer haemorrhage: a prospective randomised study. *Gastrointest Endosc* 1988;**34**:173.

59 Matthewson K, Swain CP, Bland M *et al.* Randomised comparison of Nd-YAG laser, heater probe and no endoscopic therapy for bleeding peptic ulcers. *Gastroenterology* 1990;**98**:1234–44.

60 Fullarton GM, Birnie GG, MacDonald A *et al.* Controlled trial of heater probe treatment in bleeding peptic ulcers. *Br J Surg* 1989;**76**:541–4.

61 Jensen DM, Machicado GA, Kovacs TOG. Controlled randomised study of heater probe and BICAP for haemostasis of severe ulcer bleeding. *Gastroenterology* 1988;**94**:A208.

62 Wong SKH, YU L-M, Lau JYW *et al.* Prediction of therapeutic failure after adrenaline injection plus heater probe treatment in patients with bleeding peptic ulcer. *Gut* 2002;**50**:322–5.

63 O'Brien JD, Day SJ, Burnham WR. Controlled trial of small bipolar probes in bleeding peptic ulcers. *Lancet* 1986;**i**:464–8.

64 Laine L. Multipolar electrocoagulation in the treatment of active upper gastrointestinal tract haemorrhage. A prospective controlled trial. *N Engl J Med* 1987;**316**:1613–17.

65 Brearley S, Hawker PC, Dykes PW *et al.* Peri-endoscopic bipolar diathermy coagulation of visible vessels using a 3·2 mm probe – a randomised clinical trial. *Endoscopy* 1987;**19**:160–3.

66 Laine L. Multipolar electrocoagulation for the treatment of ulcers with non bleeding visible vessels: a prospective, controlled trial. *Gastroenterology* 1988;**94**:A246.

67 Pap JP. Heat probe versus BICAP in the treatment of upper gastrointestinal bleeding. *Am J Gastroenterol* 1987;**82**:619–21.

68 Cipolletta L, Bianco MA, Rotondano G *et al.* Prospective comparison of argon plasma coagulator and heater probe in the endoscopic treatment of major peptic ulcer bleeding. *Gastrointest Endosc* 1998;**48**:191–5.

69 Skok P, Ceranic D, Sinkovic A, Pocajt M. Peptic ulcer hemorrhage: argon plasma coagulation versus injection sclerotherapy: a prospective, randomized, controlled study. *Verdauungskrankheiten* 2001;**19**:107–13.

70 Cook DJ, Gayatt GH, Salena BJ *et al.* Endoscopic therapy for acute non-variceal haemorrhage: a meta-analysis. *Gastroenterology* 1992;**102**:139–48.

71 Henry DA, White I. Endoscopic coagulation for gastrointestinal bleeding. *N Engl J Med* 1988;**318**:186–7.

72 Chung SCS, Leung JWC, Steele RJC. Endoscopic injection of adrenaline for actively bleeding ulcers: a randomised trial. *BMJ* 1988;**296**:1631–3.

73 Panes J, Viver J, Forne M *et al.* Controlled trial of endoscopic sclerosis in bleeding peptic ulcers. *Lancet* 1987;1292–4.

74 Rajgopal C, Palmer KR. Endoscopic injection sclerosis: effective treatment for bleeding peptic ulcer. *Gut* 1991;**32**:727–9.

75 Balanzo J, Sainz S, Such J. Endoscopic haemostasis by local injection of epinephrine in bleeding ulcers. A prospective randomised trial. *Endoscopy* 1988;**20**:289–91.

76 Oxner RBG, Simmonds NJ, Gertner DJ *et al.* Controlled trial of endoscopic injection treatment for bleeding peptic ulcers with visible vessels. *Lancet* 1992;**339**:966–8.

77 Benedetti G, Sablich R, Lacchin T. Endoscopic injection sclerotherapy in non-variceal upper gastrointestinal bleeding. A comparative study of epinephrine and thrombin. *Endoscopy* 1990;**22**:157–9.

78 Strohm WD, Rommele UE, Barton E *et al.* Injection therapy of bleeding ulcers with fibrin or polidocanol. *Dtsch Med Wochenschr* 1994;**119**:249–56.

79 Rutgeerts P, Vantrappen G, Brockaert L *et al.* Comparison of endoscopic polidocanol injection and YAG laser for bleeding peptic ulcers. *Lancet* 1989;**i**:1164–7.

80 Levy J, Khakoo S, Barton R *et al.* Fatal injection sclerotherapy of a bleeding peptic ulcer [Letter]. *Lancet* 1991;**337**:504.

81 Loperfido S, Patelli G, La Torre L. Extensive necrosis of gastric mucosa following injection therapy of a bleeding peptic ulcer [Letter]. *Endoscopy* 1990;**22**:785–6.

82 Rajgopal C, Lessles AM, Palmer KR. Mechanisms of action of injection therapy for bleeding peptic ulcer. *Br J Surg* 1992;**79**:782–4.

83 Chung SCS, Leung JWC, Leoug HT *et al.* Adding a sclerosant to endoscopic epinephrine injection in actively bleeding ulcers: randomised trial. *Gastrointest Endosc* 1993;**39**:611–15.

84 Choudari CP, Palmer KR. Endoscopic injection therapy for bleeding peptic ulcer: a comparison of adrenaline alone with adrenaline plus ethanolamine oleate. *Gut* 1994;**35**:608–10.

85 Villanueva C, Balanzo C, Espinos JC. Endoscopic injection therapy of bleeding ulcer: a prospective and randomised comparison of adrenaline alone or with polidocanol. *J Clin Gastroenterol* 1993;**17**:195–200.

86 Pascu O, Draghici A, Acalovschi I. The effect of endoscopic haemostasis with alcohol on the mortality rate of non-variceal upper gastrointestinal haemorrhage: a randomised prospective study. *Endoscopy* 1989;**21**:53–5.

87 Lazo MD, Andrade R, Medina MC *et al.* Effect of injection sclerosis with alcohol on the rebleeding rate of gastroduodenal peptic ulcers with nonbleeding visible vessels: a prospective, controlled trial. *Am J Gastroenterol* 1992;**87**:843–6.

88 Lin HJ, Perng CL, Lee FY. Endoscopic injection for the arrest of peptic ulcer haemorrhage: final results of a prospective, randomised, comparative trial. *Gastrointest Endosc* 1993;**39**:15–19.

89 Chiozzini G, Bortoluzzi F, Pallini P *et al.* Controlled trial of absolute ethanol vs epinephrine as injection agent in gastroduodenal bleeding. *Gastroenterology* 1989;**96**:A86.

90 Nakagawa K, Asaki S, Sato T. Endoscopic treatment of bleeding peptic ulcers. *World J Surg* 1989;**13**:154–7.

91 Kubba AK, Murphy W, Palmer KR. Endoscopic injection for bleeding peptic ulcer: a comparison of adrenaline with adrenaline plus human thrombin. *Gastroenterology* 1996;**111**:623–8.

92 Balanzo J, Villanueva C, Sainz S *et al.* Injection therapy of bleeding peptic ulcer. A prospective, randomized trial using epinephrine and thrombin. *Endoscopy* 1990;**22**:157–9.

93 Song SY, Chung JB, Moon YM *et al.* Comparison of the hemostatic effect of endoscopic injection with fibrin glue and hypertonic saline-epinephrine for peptic ulcer bleeding: a prospective randomized trial. *Endoscopy* 1997;**29**:827–33.

94 Rutgeerts P, Rauws E, Wara P *et al.* Randomised trial of single and repeated fibrin glue compared with injection of polidocanol in treatment of bleeding peptic ulcer. *Lancet* 1997;**350**:692–6.

95 Pescatore P, Jornod P, Borovicka J *et al.* Epinephrine versus epinephrine plus fibrin glue injection in peptic ulcer bleeding: a prospective randomized trial. *Gastrointest Endosc* 2002;**55**:348–53.

96 Laine L, Estrada R. Randomized trial of normal saline solution injection versus bipolar electrocoagulation for treatment of patients with high-risk bleeding ulcers: is local tamponade enough? *Gastrointest Endosc* 2002;**55**:6–10.

97 Lin HJ, Hsieh YH, Tseng GY *et al.* A prospective, randomized trial of large- versus small-volume endoscopic injection of epinephrine for peptic ulcer bleeding. *Gastrointest Endosc* 2002;**55**:615–19.

98 Lin HJ, Tsai YT, Lee SD *et al.* A prospectively randomised trial of heat probe thermocoagulation versus pure alcohol injection in nonvariceal peptic ulcer haemorrhage. *Am J Gastroenterol* 1988;**83**:283–6.

99 Lin HJ, Lee FY, Kang WM *et al.* Heat probe thermocoagulation and pure alcohol injection in massive peptic ulcer haemorrhage: a prospective, randomised controlled trial. *Gut* 1990;**31**:753–7.

100 Chung SCS, Leung JWC, Sung JY *et al.* Injection or heat probe for bleeding ulcer? *Gastroenterology* 1991;**100**:33–7.

101 Choudari CP, Rajgopal C, Palmer KR. Comparison of endoscopic injection therapy versus the heater probe in major peptic ulcer haemorrhage. *Gut* 1992;**33**:1159–61.

102 Saeed ZA, Winchester CB, Michaletz PA *et al.* A scoring system to predict rebleeding after endoscopic therapy of nonvariceal upper gastrointestinal haemorrhage, with a comparison of heat probe and ethanol injection. *Am J Gastroenterol* 1993;**88**:1842–9.

103 Llach J, Bordas JM, Salmeron JM *et al.* A prospective randomised trial of heater probe thermocoagulation versus injection therapy in peptic ulcer haemorrhage. *Gastrointest Endosc* 1996;**43**(2 Pt 1):117–20.

104 Laine L. Multipolar electrocoagulation versus injection therapy in the treatment of bleeding peptic ulcers. *Gastroenterology* 1990;**99**:1303–6.

105 Carter R, Anderson JR. Randomised trial of adrenaline injection and laser photocoagulation in the control of haemorrhage from peptic ulcer. *Br J Surg* 1994;**81**:869–71.

106 Pulanic R, Vucelic B, Rosandic M *et al.* Comparison of injection sclerotherapy and laser photocoagulation for bleeding peptic ulcers. *Endoscopy* 1995;**27**:291–7.

107 Lin HJ, Tseng GY, Perng CL *et al.* Comparison of adrenaline injection and bipolar electrocoagulation for the arrest of peptic ulcer bleeding. *Gut* 1999;**44**:715–19.

108 Chung SCS, Lau JY, Sung JJ. Randomised comparison between adrenaline injection alone and adrenaline injection plus heat probe treatment for actively bleeding peptic ulcers. *BMJ* 1997;**314**:1307–11.

109 Hayashi T, Yonezawa M, Kawabara T. The study on staunch clip for the treatment by endoscopy. *Gastroenterol Endosc* 1975;**17**:92–101.

110 Binmoeller KF, Thonke F, Soehendra N. Endoscopic hemoclip treatment for gastrointestinal bleeding. *Endoscopy* 1993;**25**:167–70.

111 Yokohata T, Takeshima H, Fukushima R *et al.* Limitations of endoscopy injection therapy and efficacy of endoscopic hemoclipping in the treatment of bleeding gastric ulcer. *Japanese Abdominal Emergency Medical Society Magazine* 1996;**16**:1113–19.

112 Nagayama K, Tazawa J, Sakai Y *et al.* Efficacy of endoscopic clipping for bleeding gastroduodenal ulcer: comparison with topical ethanol injection. *Am J Gastroenterol* 1999;**94**:2897–901.

113 Chung IK, Ham JS, Kim HS *et al.* Comparison of the hemostatic efficacy of the endoscopic hemoclip method with hypertonic saline-epinephrine injection and a combination of the two for the management of bleeding peptic ulcers. *Gastrointest Endosc* 1999;**49**:13–18.

114 Cipoletta L, Bianco MA, Marmo R *et al.* Endoclips versus heater probe in preventing early recurrent bleeding from

peptic ulcer: a prospective and randomized trial. *Gastrointest Endosc* 2001;**53**:147–51.

115 Lin HJ, Hsieh YH, Tseng GY *et al.* A prospective, randomized trial of endoscopic hemoclip versus heater probe thermocoagulation for peptic ulcer bleeding. *Am J Gastroenterol* 2002;**97**:2250–4.

116 Gevers AM, De Goede E, Simoens M *et al.* A randomized trial comparing injection therapy with hemoclip and with injection combined with hemoclip for bleeding ulcers. *Gastrointest Endosc* 2002;**55**:466–9.

117 Lin HJ, Wang K, Perng CL *et al.* Natural history of bleeding peptic ulcers with a tightly adherent blood clot: a prospective observation. *Gastrointest Endosc* 1996;**43**: 470–3.

118 Bleau BL, Gostout CJ, Sherman KE *et al.* Recurrent bleeding from peptic ulcer associated with adherent clot: a randomized study comparing endoscopic treatment with medical therapy. *Gastrointest Endosc* 2002;**56**:1–6.

119 Jensen DM, Kovacs TOG, Jutabha R *et al.* Randomized trial of medical or endoscopic therapy to prevent recurrent ulcer hemorrhage in patients with adherent clots. *Gastroenterology* 2002;**123**:407–13.

120 Villanueva C, Balanzo J, Torras X *et al.* Value of second-look endoscopy after injection therapy for bleeding peptic ulcer: a prospective and randomized trial. *Gastrointest Endosc* 1994;**40**:34–9.

121 Saeed ZA, Cole RA, Ramirez FC *et al.* Endoscopic retreatment after successful initial hemostasis prevents ulcer rebleeding: a prospective randomized trial. *Endoscopy* 1996;**28**:288–94.

122 Messmann H, Schaller P, Andus T *et al.* Effect of programmed endoscopic follow-up examinations on the rebleeding rate of gastric or duodenal peptic ulcers treated by injection therapy: a prospective, randomised controlled trial. *Endoscopy* 1998;**30**:583–9.

123 Villanueva C, Balanzo J, Espinos JC. Prediction of therapeutic failure in patients with bleeding peptic ulcer treated with endoscopic injection. *Dig Dis Sci* 1993;**38**: 2062–70.

124 Choudari CP, Rajgopal C, Elton RA *et al.* Failures of endoscopic therapy for bleeding peptic ulcers;an analysis of risk factors. *Am J Gastroenterol* 1994;**89**:1968–72.

125 Lau JYW, Sung JJY, Lam Y *et al.* Endoscopic retreatment compared with surgery in patients with recurrent bleeding after initial endoscopic control of bleeding ulcers. *N Engl J Med* 1999;**340**:751–6.

8 Functional dyspepsia

Sander JO Veldhuyzen van Zanten

Introduction

In this chapter the diagnosis of functional dyspepsia and efficacy of therapeutic interventions will be evaluated. Functional dyspepsia, often referred to as non-ulcer dyspepsia, is an important health problem with a very high prevalence in the general population. Data from Sweden and Canada show that 5–7% of all consultations in primary care are for the symptom of dyspepsia.[1,2] In Sweden, up to 98% of patients receive a prescription if they consult a physician for dyspepsia.[1] Consequently, for the healthcare system the cost of medications, which are often prescribed for long periods of time, adds significantly to the already substantial expenditures for consultations and diagnostic investigations. The following topics will be reviewed: definition of functional dyspepsia, evaluation and diagnostic tests, methodology of trials, and pharmacological treatments including antacids, H_2-receptor antagonists, proton pump inhibitors (PPIs), prokinetic agents and anti-*Helicobacter* therapy. The treatment of functional dyspepsia has been previously reviewed by the author with conclusions similar to those presented in this chapter.[3]

Definition of functional dyspepsia

There is agreement that the cardinal feature of functional dyspepsia is *unexplained pain or discomfort centered in the upper part of the abdomen.* Epigastric pain or discomfort may be accompanied by other symptoms such as excessive burping or belching, nausea, bloating, postprandial fullness, early satiety, or burning sensations. Increasingly, investigators have accepted the definition of the Rome Working Party.[4,5] In 1999 the Rome criteria for functional dyspepsia were updated.[5] The definitions of both dyspepsia in general and functional dyspepsia have remained unchanged. For a diagnosis of functional dyspepsia to be made, it is required that investigations, usually upper gastrointestinal endoscopy, have not revealed abnormalities such as ulcers that could explain the symptoms of the dyspepsia. The Rome II criteria have continued to exclude the symptoms of heartburn and acid regurgitation as these are considered to be diagnostic of

gastroesophageal reflux disease (GERD). Although there is consensus that "dominant" symptoms of heartburn and acid regurgitation make a diagnosis of GERD likely, it is less clear how heartburn should be handled if it is of severity equal to or less than epigastric pain. Furthermore, heartburn and acid regurgitation are often present as associated symptoms in patients who otherwise fit the dyspepsia diagnostic criteria. There is evidence, especially in primary care, that excluding heartburn from the dyspepsia syndrome does not fit with the conceptual framework that primary care physicians have of dyspepsia.[6] This is especially true for uninvestigated dyspepsia patients who are commonly seen in primary care. The Canadian Dyspepsia Working Group (CanDys) has developed a definition for dyspepsia that includes heartburn and acid regurgitation.[6] There is some empiric support for the latter definition as a few studies in *Helicobacter pylori* infected patients have demonstrated that cure of the infection not only led to a decrease in epigastric pain but also in symptoms of heartburn in a small but definite proportion of patients.[7-9]

Diagnosis of functional dyspepsia

There is consensus that there is so much overlap in symptoms among duodenal and gastric ulcers, GERD, and functional dyspepsia that it is impossible to make a definitive diagnosis-based on symptoms alone. This is supported by the results from the Canadian Prompt Endoscopy (CADET-PE) Study.[10] In this study, 1014 patients underwent endoscopy within 10 days without having received acid suppressive therapy. There was a marked overlap in symptoms and it was impossible to distinguish between individuals with ulcers, esophagitis, or functional dyspepsia based on symptoms. In essence, functional dyspepsia is a diagnosis of exclusion, and in the setting of clinical trials generally requires an upper gastrointestinal endoscopy to exclude other diseases. In practice, physicians often decide on a trial of empiric therapy for patients presenting with dyspepsia without worrying about a definitive diagnosis of a particular disease. This strategy is often attractive given that the treatment for duodenal and gastric ulcers, GERD, and functional dyspepsia is similar. The current standard of practice is a trial of acid suppressive therapy. Therefore, subclassification into separate diseases is not always necessary and in primary care may not be feasible. The decision whether or not to refer a patient for further investigation, usually either an upper gastrointestinal endoscopy or a barium study, is based on the severity of the presenting symptoms, age of the patient and on the presence or absence of "alarm symptoms" such as weight loss, evidence of bleeding or anemia, dysphagia and vomiting.

Subgroups of dyspepsia and overlap with GERD

The description of subgroups of dyspepsia has become popular despite evidence of the existence of considerable overlap among them. The four recognized subgroups are: ulcer-like dyspepsia, reflux-like dyspepsia, dysmotility-like dyspepsia, and unclassified dyspepsia.[11,12] These subgroups are attractive because they coincide with current concepts about pathophysiological disturbances which explain specific symptoms. However, a study by Talley *et al.*[12] demonstrated considerable overlap among the different subgroups as did the CADET-PE Study.[10] Although the reflux-like dyspepsia subgroup is easy to define, the Rome Consensus Working Party has not recommended its use. It believed that such patients should be diagnosed as having GERD. In general subclassification into dyspepsia subgroups is not recommended.[5]

Increasingly, endoscopy negative GERD is now recognized as a distinct entity. This is a difficult issue for the methodology of trials of functional dyspepsia. Solely relying on an endoscopy, which does not reveal macroscopic esophagitis, is probably insufficient if one wants to exclude all GERD patients. An example is the study by Klauser *et al.*, in which 17% of patients referred for dyspepsia were diagnosed with esophagitis after an initial work up.[13] However, a further 10% of patients did prove to have endoscopy negative GERD after an extended work up, which included 24-hour pH monitoring and scintigraphy. In practice it seems impossible to exclude all GERD patients in trials of functional dyspepsia. A practical solution is to exclude patients who have heartburn as their dominant symptom, but allow patients who have both epigastric pain and heartburn to enroll as long as the epigastric pain is the predominant symptom.

What constitutes a normal endoscopy has been poorly defined in the literature. Especially important is to determine whether or not patients are still or were recently taking acid suppressive therapy that can mask the presence of esophagitis or ulcers. It would be ideal for trials of functional dyspepsia treatment to require that patients are not allowed to have consumed acid suppressive therapy for at least 4 weeks before the endoscopy. After withdrawal from acid suppressive therapy, it may take longer than 4 weeks for endoscopic abnormalities to become visible; however, a 4-week period of avoidance of acid suppressive therapy seems a reasonable compromise.

Diagnostic investigation: endoscopy or radiographs?

Referral for endoscopy is indicated for older patients presenting with new-onset dyspepsia. Formerly, the recommendation was to use age > 45 years as an indication for investigations,[14] but it seems likely that this can be increased to 50 years or perhaps even higher.[15,16] This cut-off age is largely driven by the incidence of gastric cancer in the population where one practices.[15,16] Interestingly, the recent Scottish guidelines have removed all age criteria as data are insufficient to support them.[17] In family practice, upper gastrointestinal barium studies are still commonly used to rule out peptic ulcer disease and esophageal or gastric cancer in patients with dyspepsia. The technical review of the American Gastroenterology Association (AGA) on Dyspepsia summarizes the consistent evidence of the superiority of upper gastrointestinal endoscopy for detection of structural abnormalities.[14] Radiographs are still frequently used because of their lower cost, wider availability in the community and the speed with which the test can be done. Often there is a significant waiting time before patients can be seen after they are referred to a gastroenterologist. "Open access endoscopy" is one method by which delay in diagnostic endoscopy can be reduced.

The AGA technical review assessed whether patients with new onset of symptoms should be investigated or treated empirically and came to the conclusion that the evidence is equivocal.[14] For example, in the study by Bytzer *et al.*, empiric treatment was compared with direct endoscopy in patients presenting with dyspepsia.[18] Patients in the endoscopy arm were more satisfied, and subsequent healthcare costs were significantly lower in this group. There is further evidence that a patient's quality of life is improved following a normal endoscopy.[14] This is largely due to alleviation of fear of a serious underlying disease since the dyspepsia symptoms persisted. However, a recommendation that endoscopy should be done in all or most patients presenting with dyspepsia would probably be too costly for most healthcare systems. A more rational approach therefore seems to be to stratify patients according to their risk of having serious underlying disease. Factors that can be considered are age of the patient, background prevalence of serious disease, especially of esophageal and gastric cancer, and the presence or absence of alarm symptoms.

Methodological problems in trials of functional dyspepsia

In order to determine whether a treatment does more good than harm, valid and reliable outcome measures must be used in clinical trials. In the case of functional dyspepsia the lack of definite structural or pathophysiological abnormalities which explain the origin of the symptoms of functional dyspepsia has hampered the development of such measures. Clinical trials must use outcome measures that rely on the recording of symptoms and their severity, as is the case in other functional gastrointestinal disorders. A systematic review of drug treatment of functional dyspepsia evaluated the quality of clinical trials in this field.[19] Few studies used validated outcome measures and methodological weaknesses were apparent in several trials. Problems included a lack of definition of functional dyspepsia, unclear inclusion and exclusion criteria, suboptimal study design and short duration of treatment.

The most important problem in randomized controlled trials of interventions for functional dyspepsia is the lack of consensus on outcome measures. Only a small number of outcome measures have been validated. In the systematic review of studies on functional dyspepsia, only five of 52 studies used a validated outcome measure.[19] Subjective endpoints, such as recording of symptoms and their severity, used to measure a clinical outcome in a trial should fulfill four requirements.[20]

1 The range of symptoms included should be important to, and representative of, the disease process.
2 The measurements should be reproducible (producing consistent results when repeated in subjects who have not changed).
3 The measurements should be responsive (able to detect change).
4 Changes in the measurement should reflect a real change in general health status.

Ideally, a separate study is required to demonstrate that an instrument meets these requirements, prior to its use in a randomized controlled trial. Over the past few years, several disease-specific quality of life questionnaires for (functional) dyspepsia have been published.[21–25] As part of the 1999 Rome initiative, a special working party reported on the design of trials of clinical treatment of functional gastrointestinal disorders.[26] This working party also strongly recommended the use of validated outcome measures. In addition, the group strongly endorsed the use of a primary outcome measure that integrates the global overall severity of symptoms, although it did not specify how this should be done. Several recently completed trials of functional dyspepsia used 4- or 7-point Likert scales to measure overall severity of symptoms of dyspepsia or epigastric pain. However, to date, none of these scales has been sufficiently validated to be unequivocally recommended for general use in functional dyspepsia trials.

Another important weakness of many trials has been the relatively short duration of treatment. The duration of treatment was 4 weeks or less in 44 trials evaluated in the systematic review of 52 studies.[19] It was 8 weeks or longer in only four studies. Only seven studies had a follow up period (varying from 3 to 52 weeks) after treatment was discontinued. The short duration of treatment is surprising given the known chronicity of the symptoms of functional dyspepsia.

The placebo response rate is high in clinical trials in patients with functional dyspepsia and other functional gastrointestinal disorders, such as the irritable bowel syndrome.[26,27] In the systematic review of trials of functional dyspepsia it varied from 13% to 73%.[19] An explanation for the high placebo response rate may be the reassurance effect of a "normal" endoscopy. Fear of cancer is a frequent reason for concern among patients with functional dyspepsia undergoing gastroscopy.[14,16] Wiklund *et al.* measured quality of life and gastrointestinal symptoms just prior to endoscopy and 7 days later.[28] In patients in whom no significant endoscopic abnormalities were found overall quality of life improved, although there was little change in the severity of individual gastrointestinal symptoms. This observation supports the concept that endoscopy has a powerful placebo effect through reassurance of patients. The higher satisfaction with care in the study by Bytzer *et al.*[18] may also be explained by a reassurance effect.

Functional versus uninvestigated dyspepsia

It is important to distinguish between uninvestigated dyspepsia and functional dyspepsia. The diagnosis of functional dyspepsia is generally considered to require an endoscopy. Most studies to date have dealt with investigated dyspepsia. Studies of uninvestigated dyspepsia will include a proportion of patients with duodenal or gastric ulcer, esophagitis and, rarely, gastric cancer. The frequency with which structural abnormalities are found has changed over the past decade.[14] With the declining prevalence of duodenal and gastric ulcers, reflux esophagitis now by far is the most common abnormality. Its prevalence ranges from 20% to 40% among patients and is far more common than duodenal and gastric ulcers which, for example, were 3% and 4% in the previously mentioned Canadian CADET-PE Study.[10] However, these rates clearly depend on the prevalence of these disorders in the population being studied. Gastric cancer is rare below the age of 50 years.[14,29] In most endoscopic dyspepsia studies the rate of functional dyspepsia is high and varies between 30% and 60%.[14] Several studies of patients with uninvestigated dyspepsia are currently being carried out in general practice. Such studies are contaminated with patients with undiagnosed duodenal or gastric ulcer and GERD. However, this situation will better mimic the real life situation in general practice, where treatment for most patients is instituted without endoscopic investigations. In this chapter we will focus on patients with investigated dyspepsia, that is functional dyspepsia.

Given the problems in study design, especially the large variation in the way outcome measures have been used, it is difficult to do quantitative meta-analysis. Over the past few years, several meta-analyses have been reported including Cochrane reviews. Although several of these systematic reviews have statistically combined results of individual trials, it is important to stress that this is usually done by transforming the various outcome measures. For example, in one of the Cochrane meta-analyses, all outcomes of included studies were dichotomized into improved versus not improved.[30] No evidence has been provided that such an approach is valid although some kind of transformation is required if one wants to combine studies which have used substantially different outcome measures. In this chapter the results are mainly presented in a qualitative fashion. As several meta-analyses have been published for the different treatments the question whether treatments are efficacious is largely based on the results of the five systematic reviews presented here.

Drug treatment

Antacids

Over-the-counter medications, especially antacids, are commonly prescribed as first-line treatment. Many patients will probably have tried these medications before consulting a physician. As several reviews have been written on the use of antacids, the details of individual studies will not be discussed here. Clinical trials have generally not shown significant benefit from antacids.[14,30,31] The frequently cited and methodologically strong randomized controlled trial reported by Nyren *et al.* did not show benefit of antacids over placebo over a 3-week treatment period.[32] Ald

H$_2$-receptor antagonists

These agents continue to be used extensively especially in primary care.[33] Over the past few years, four systematic reviews have evaluated the use of H$_2$-blockers in functional dyspepsia.[30,34–36] The number of studies that met the inclusion criteria varied in these reviews. All four came to the same conclusion: that there is some evidence that these agents provide benefit in functional dyspepsia patients (Box 8.1). However, it is important to point out several methodological issues. The reason why the results for H$_2$-blockers have varied is that several of the included studies which showed benefit probably included GERD patients. This factor may explain why the meta-analysis by Dobrilla *et al.* showed a therapeutic gain of 18% of active treatment over placebo.[34] Ala Two methodologically strong studies did not show a benefit of either cimetidine or nizatidine over placebo.[32,37] Alc It is also worth pointing out that most studies have used low doses

---

Box 8.1 Results of meta-analyses of clinical trials of treatment of functional dyspepsia with H$_2$-blockers

1 Dobrilla *et al.*[34]: Therapeutic gain H$_2$-blockers compared with placebo 18%
2 Bytzer[36]: Therapeutic gain H$_2$-blockers compared with placebo 22%
3 Soo *et al.*[30]: Relative risk reduction of ongoing dyspepsia of H$_2$-blockers compared with placebo 22%
4 Redstone *et al.*[35]: Odds ratio studies of H$_2$-blockers compared with placebo reporting complete relief from epigastric pain 1·8 (95% CI 1·2 to 2·8)
   Odds ratio studies of H$_2$-blockers compared with placebo reporting global improvement dyspepsia symptoms 1·48 (95% CI 0·9 to 2·3)

---

of H$_2$-receptor antagonists (H$_2$-RA), for example ranitidine 150 mg twice a day. It is possible that higher doses of H$_2$-RA might yield larger and more consistent treatment effects, but this needs to be assessed in future studies.

Proton pump inhibitors

Until recently, PPIs were mainly restricted to patients with peptic ulcer disease or GERD. This increased efficacy compared with H$_2$-RA in these patient populations is explained by the more profound acid suppression induced by proton pump inhibition. The BOND-OPERA report consisted of two large randomized controlled trials evaluating the role of PPI therapy in functional dyspepsia.[38] Over a 4-week period, 1262 functional dyspepsia patients received either omeprazole (20 mg or 10 mg) or placebo. Complete relief of symptoms was achieved in 38% of patients on omeprazole 20 mg, 36% on omeprazole 10 mg, and 28% on placebo ($P < 0.001$). The absolute risk reduction (ARR) of 10% and 8% correspond to an NNT (the number of patients needed to treat with omeprazole to yield one additional patient with a complete response) of 10 for 20 mg omeprazole and 12 for 10 mg omeprazole. Ald Subgroup analysis suggested that patients with ulcer-like and reflux-like dyspepsia benefited from omeprazole therapy, while patients fulfilling the criteria for dysmotility-like dyspepsia did not. Although it is generally not useful to make a diagnosis of specific dyspepsia subgroups, the results of this study suggest that use of the two subgroups – ulcer-like and reflux-like dyspepsia – may be useful to predict a response to PPI therapy. Interestingly, reflux patients were excluded but despite this a proportion of patients reported heartburn as their most bothersome symptom. Further randomized trials are needed to confirm the results of this subgroup analysis. It remains to be determined whether the dyspepsia responders to omeprazole are in fact patients with unrecognized endoscopy negative GERD. Alternatively, associated but not dominant heartburn may be the driver of response to PPI therapy. In other studies, omeprazole was superior to antacids in combination with ranitidine[39] or alone[40] and in patients with ulcer-like or reflux-like dyspepsia.[41]

In contrast to the BOND-OPERA[38] study the recent study of 453 patients in Hong Kong by Wong *et al.*[42] using lansoprazole had negative results. Patients were randomized to receive either lansoprazole 30 mg or 15 mg a day or placebo. The severity of the symptoms of dyspepsia was assessed by a 5-point Likert scale. In this study there was no difference in the proportion of patients with complete relief of symptoms: lansoprazole 30 mg 23%, lansoprazole 50 mg 23% and placebo 30%. Ala It is possible that one of the reasons this study had these results is that in Hong Kong the prevalence of GERD is low.[43] Such patients were excluded from the study. The discrepancy between the two studies once again highlights the methodological difficulties that exist especially with regard to possible overlap between GERD and dyspepsia and whether associated heartburn may be an important predictor of response to acid suppression.

Domperidone and cisapride

Prokinetics have been evaluated in functional dyspepsia because of the hypothesis that disturbed gastrointestinal motility may in part be responsible for the symptoms of dyspepsia. Domperidone is a dopamine receptor antagonist, which has shown a benefit in several randomized placebo-controlled trials of functional dyspepsia. However, as a systematic review pointed out many of these trials enrolled only small numbers of patients and had other weaknesses.[44] Cisapride, a prokinetic agent with $5-HT_4$-agonist activity specifically targeted patients with dysmotility-like dyspepsia. The drug had also been proved to be effective in patients with mild GERD and in patients with delayed gastric emptying. Due to rare but serious cardiac side effects this drug has now been removed from most markets. The three systematic reviews that have looked at the efficacy of cisapride in functional dyspepsia all came to the same conclusion that there was some evidence that the drug improved the symptoms of dyspepsia (Box 8.2).[30,36,44] Alc However, several of the cisapride studies suffered from serious methodological weaknesses, which made the conclusions about efficacy tentative. Furthermore, on funnel plots there was also evidence of a publication bias,[30] almost certainly due to the fact that there was an overrepresentation of small studies with positive results. In addition, it is worth pointing out that two recent methodologically strong studies with adequate sample size did not show a benefit of cisapride over placebo.[37,45] Ala In the study of 330 patients by Hansen *et al.*[37] there were no statistically significant differences in response to 2 weeks' treatment with cisapride 10 mg three times daily (62%), nizatidine 300 mg once daily (54%) or placebo (62%). In the study of 123 patients by Champion *et al.* there were no statistically significant differences in good or

excellent response to treatment among patients treated with cisapride 10 mg three times daily (47%), cisapride 20 mg three times daily (38%) and placebo (33%).[45] As cisapride no longer is available and evidence for domperidone is weak it can not be recommended.

Anti-Helicobacter therapy

The prevalence of *H. pylori* in functional dyspepsia varies from 30% to 70%, but this is in large part dependent on known risk factors for *H. pylori* infection: age, socioeconomic status and race.[46,47] Due to differences in study design and problems with selection bias, it is still unclear whether the prevalence of *H. pylori* infection is increased in patients with functional dyspepsia compared with normal controls, although a meta-analysis suggested that it is.[48]

A hotly debated issue over the past 10 years has been the question of whether cure of *H. pylori* infection leads to a sustained improvement in symptoms of functional dyspepsia. Fortunately, several studies with large sample sizes have been published. Not surprisingly, many authors have attempted to combine the results of the different studies into a formal meta-analysis. The two systematic reviews which have received the most attention are the ones by Moayyedi *et al.*[49] and by Laine *et al.*[50] (Box 8.3). The first review combined the results from approximately 2500 patients and concluded that after 6–12 months patients were 9% less likely to have ongoing symptoms of dyspepsia, a small but statistically significant benefit (95% CI 4 to 14%).[49] Ala In contrast the second review found no evidence of a treatment benefit as a result of anti-*Helicobacter* therapy.[50] Ala The discrepancy between the two reviews can best be explained by differences in the studies that met the inclusion criteria and the timing of the final searches. It is worth mentioning that most of the studies conducted in North America have shown negative results.

The study that most clearly showed a positive result was the UK Medical Research Council trial of *H. pylori* eradication therapy for functional dyspepsia. This was a single center randomized controlled trial conducted in Scotland.[51] Three hundred and eighteen patients were randomized to 14 days of treatment with anti-*Helicobacter* therapy (omeprazole,

---

> **Box 8.2 Results of meta-analyses of clinical trials of treatment of functional dyspepsia with cisapride**
>
> 1 Soo *et al.*[30]: Relative risk reduction of ongoing dyspepsia of prokinetic compared with placebo 50% *(funnel plot indicates publication bias)*
> 2 Bytzer[36]: Therapeutic gain cisapride compared with placebo >20%, exact gain difficult to estimate
> 3 Veldhuyzen van Zanten *et al.*[44]: Odds ratio of benefit of cisapride compared with placebo − global assessment of improvement by the investigator or patient odds ratio 2·9 (95% CI 1·5 to 5·8); epigastric pain odds ratio 0·19 (95% CI 0·05 to 0·7)

Box 8.3   Results of meta-analyses of clinical trials of treatment of functional dyspepsia with anti-*Helicobacter* therapy versus placebo

1   Moayyedi *et al.*[49]: Relative risk reduction of ongoing dyspepsia of anti-*Helicobacter* therapy relative to placebo 9% (95% CI 4% to 14%)
2   Laine *et al.*[50]: Odds ratio for treatment success of anti-*Helicobacter* therapy relative to placebo 1·29 (95% CI 0·89 to 1·89, *P* = 0·18)

metronidazole and amoxicillin) or omeprazole alone and followed for 12 months. The primary outcome measure was the validated Glasgow Dyspepsia Severity Scale (GDSS).[24] This score assesses the frequency of dyspepsia symptoms and the impact they have on daily activities, the number of doctor visits and diagnostic tests for dyspepsia, and the need for either over-the-counter medication or prescription drugs to treat the symptoms. The proportion of patients who became *H. pylori* negative was 87% for patients randomized to anti-*Helicobacter* therapy compared with 4% for the omeprazole group. Improvement, defined as a score of 0 or 1 on the dyspepsia score, was achieved in 21% of anti-*Helicobacter* treated patients and 7% of the control group (*P* < 0·001, ARR 14%, NNT = 7).[51] A1a

The methodically strong OCAY, ORCHID and the USA Dyspepsia Trials, all with adequate sample sizes, had negative results.[52–54] A1a One of the explanations for the markedly positive results in the McColl *et al.* study was that patients were recruited at a single center and may have been more homogeneous than those in the other trials. The disadvantage that accompanies this greater homogeneity is that results may be less generalizable. The population in which such a study is carried out may influence outcome. Endoscopic studies of asymptomatic *H. pylori* positive individuals or *H. pylori* positive blood donors have revealed marked differences in the prevalence of peptic ulcers. For example, in an Italian study 42% of 1010 predominantly asymptomatic blood donors were *H. pylori* positive. Of the *H. pylori* positive patients, 15% had a duodenal ulcer and 5% a gastric ulcer.[55] In contrast, in a study of asymptomatic *H. pylori* positive volunteers in Texas the point prevalence of duodenal ulcer was only 1%.[56] McColl *et al.* found the prevalence of duodenal ulcer to be 40% in patients presenting with dyspepsia in Scotland.[57] The incidence and prevalence of duodenal and gastric ulcers have been in decline now for quite some time in Western countries, and individual countries may be at different stages on this slope of change. The consequence for interpretation of *H. pylori* eradication trials is that in countries with a continuing high background of duodenal ulcers there will also be a higher proportion of patients among the functional dyspepsia patients who ultimately will develop duodenal ulcers. It is possible that trials of functional dyspepsia carried out in these countries are more likely to demonstrate a beneficial effect on symptoms after eradication of *H. pylori*. It is worth pointing out that studies in *H. pylori* positive uninvestigated dyspepsia patients have shown positive results. It is possible that the benefit seen in these studies is explained by the presence of underlying ulcer disease in a proportion of patients.[7,58] C5

Summarizing all the data on *H. pylori* eradication in functional dyspepsia, the conclusion is that this either has no or a small positive effect on symptoms. If one believes the data from the Moayyedi analysis the NNT is 11. However, given that *H. pylori* is a true pathogen that leads to peptic ulcer disease in 5–15% of infected individuals and is associated with gastric cancer in up to 1% of patients, it seems reasonable that patients with chronic dyspepsia symptoms who come to endoscopy are tested for the infection and treated if positive. However, one should be aware that the large majority of such patients will continue to have ongoing symptoms of dyspepsia requiring further treatment.

Conclusion

There are methodological shortcomings in many of the trials of treatment of functional dyspepsia which make it difficult to provide firm guidelines. There are no trials comparing the main treatment options. These options include H$_2$-receptor antagonists, PPIs and anti-*Helicobacter* therapy for patients who are *H. pylori* positive. With cisapride no longer available the evidence is insufficient to recommend other prokinetic agents. Endoscopy may give a patient reassurance that there is no serious underlying disease and this may have a powerful beneficial therapeutic effect. It is reasonable to prescribe a period of acid suppression with either an H$_2$-RA or a PPI in patients with functional dyspepsia. The evidence for effectiveness of PPIs is stronger. For all these treatments it is possible that patients with unrecognized GERD represent the main responders to acid suppression and or that associated heartburn is a driver of response. Whether eradication therapy for *H. pylori* will lead to a sustained improvement of the symptoms of functional dyspepsia is currently unresolved. At best this will occur in a small proportion of patients. However, given that *H. pylori* is a true pathogen, capable of producing peptic ulcers and sometimes gastric cancer, the author recommends that patients coming for endoscopy are tested and treated if positive.

References

1   Nyrén O, Lindberg G, Lindstrom E *et al. Economic costs of functional dyspepsia.* PharmacoEconomics, Adis International Ltd, 1992.
2   Chiba N, Bernard L, O'Brien BJ *et al.* A Canadian physician survey of dyspepsia management. *Can J Gastroenterol* 1998; **12**:183–90.

3   Veldhuyzen van Zanten SJO. Treatment of functional dyspepsia. *Balliere's Clin Gastroenterol* 1998;**12**:573–86.

4   Talley NJ, Colin-Jones D, Koch KL *et al.* Functional dyspepsia: a classification with guidelines for diagnosis and management. *Gastroenterol Int* 1991;**4**:145–60.

5   Talley NJ, Stanghellinin V, Heading RC, Koch KL, Malageleda JR, Tytgat GNJ. Functional gastroduodenal disorders. *Gut* 1999;**45(Suppl II)**:37–42.

6   Veldhuyzen van Zanten SJ, Flook N, Chiba N *et al.* An evidence-based approach to the management of uninvestigated dyspepsia in the era of *Helicobacter pylori.* Canadian Dyspepsia Working Group. *Can Med Assoc J* 2000:**162(12 Suppl):**S3–23.

7   Chiba N, Van Zanten SJ, Sinclair P, Ferguson RA, Escobedo S, Grace E. Treating *Helicobacter pylori* infection in primary care patients with uninvestigated dyspepsia: the Canadian adult dyspepsia empiric treatment – *Helicobacter pylori* positive (CADET-Hp) randomised controlled trial. *BMJ* 2002;**324**:1012–16.

8   Moayyedi P, Feltbower R, Brown J *et al.* Effect of population screening and treatment for *Helicobacter pylori* on dyspepsia and quality of life in the community: a randomised controlled trial. Leeds HELP Study Group. *Lancet* 2000;**355**:1665–9.

9   Wildner-Christensen M, Moller Hansen J, Schaffalitzky De Muckadell OB. Rates of dyspepsia one year after *Helicobacter pylori* screening and eradication in a Danish population. *Gastroenterology* 2003;**125**:372–9.

10 Thomson AB, Barkun AN, Armstrong D *et al.* The prevalence of clinically significant endoscopic findings in primary care patients with uninvestigated dyspepsia: the Canadian Adult Dyspepsia Empiric Treatment – Prompt Endoscopy (CADET-PE) study. *Aliment Pharmacol Ther* 2003;**17**:1481–91.

11 Talley NJ, Zinsmeister AR, Schleck CD *et al.* Dyspepsia and dyspepsia subgroups: a population-based study. *Gastroenterology* 1992;**102**:1259–68.

12 Talley NJ, Weaver AL, Tesmer DL *et al.* Lack of discriminant value of dyspepsia subgroups in patients referred for upper endoscopy. *Gastroenterology* 1993;**105**:1378–86.

13 Klauser AG, Schindlbeck NE, Muller-Lissner SA. Symptoms in gastrooesophageal reflux disease. *Lancet* 1990;**335**:205–8.

14 Talley NJ, Silverstein MC, Agreus L *et al.* AGA Technical Review: evaluation of dyspepsia. *Gastroenterology* 1998;**114**:582–95.

15 Veldhuyzen van Zanten SJO. Can the age limit for endoscopy be increased in dyspepsia patients who do not have alarm symptoms? *Am J Gastroenterol* 1999;**94**:9–11.

16 Axon ATR. Chronic dyspepsia: who needs endoscopy? *Gastroenterology* 1997;**112**:1376–80.

17 Scottish Intercollegiate Guideline Network (SIGN) Clinical Guidelines No. 68, Dyspepsia. A national clinical guideline. March 2003. www.sign.ac.uk (accessed September 2003).

18 Bytzer P, Hansen JM, Schaffalitzky de Muckadell OB. Empirical H2-blocker therapy or prompt endoscopy in management of dyspepsia. *Lancet* 1994;**343**;811–16.

19 Veldhuyzen van Zanten SJO, Cleary C, Talley NJ *et al.* Drug treatment of functional dyspepsia: a systematic analysis of trial methodology with recommendations for design of future trials. *Am J Gastroenterol* 1996;**91**:660–71.

20 Guyatt GH, Veldhuyzen van Zanten SJO, Feeney DH *et al.* Measuring quality of life in clinical trials. A taxonomy and review. *Can Med J Assoc* 1989;**140**:1441–8.

21 Nyrén O, Adami HO, Bates S *et al.* Self-rating of pain in non-ulcer dyspepsia. *J Clin Gastroenterol* 1987;**9**:408–14.

22 Dimenas E, Glise H, Ballerback B *et al.* Well-being and gastrointestinal symptoms among patients referred to endoscopy due to suspected duodenal ulcer. *Scand J Gastroenterol* 1995;**30**:1046–52.

23 Veldhuyzen van Zanten SJO, Tytgat KMAJ, Pollak PT *et al.* Can severity of symptoms be used as outcome measures in trials of non-ulcer dyspepsia and *Helicobacter pylori. J Clin Epidemiol* 1993;**46**:273–9.

24 El-Omar EM, Banerjee S, Wirz A *et al.* The Glasgow Dyspepsia Severity Score – a tool for the global measurement of dyspepsia. *Eur J Gastroenterol Hepatol* 1996;**8**:967–71.

25 Buckley MJ, Seatko C, McGuigan J *et al.* A validated dyspepsia symptom score. *Int J Gastroenterol* 1998;**18**: 495–500.

26 Veldhuyzen van Zanten SJO, Talley NJ, Bytzer P, Klein KB, Whorwell PJ, Zinsmeister AR. Design of treatment trials for functional gastrointestinal disorders. *Gut* 1999; **45(Suppl II)**:1169–77.

27 Klein KB. Controlled treatment trials in the irritable bowel syndrome: a critique. *Gastroenterology* 1988;**95**:232–41.

28 Wiklund I, Glise H, Jerndal PI *et al.* Does endoscopy have a positive impact on quality of life in dyspepsia? *Gastrointest Endosc* 1998;**47**:449–54.

29 Christie J, Shepherd NA, Codling BW *et al.* Gastric cancer below the age of 55: implications for screening patients with uncomplicated dyspepsia. *Gut* 1997;**41**:513–17.

30 Soo S, Moayyedi P, Deeks J, Delaney B, Innes M, Forman D. Pharmacological interventions for non-ulcer dyspepsia. *Cochrane Database Syst Rev* 2000;**2**:CD01960.

31 Talley NJ. Drug treatment of functional dyspepsia. *Scand J Gastroenterol* 1991;**26(S182)**:47–60.

32 Nyren O, Adami HO, Bates S *et al.* Absence of therapeutic benefit from antacids or cimetidine in non-ulcer dyspepsia. *N Engl J Med* 1986;**314**:339–43.

33 Bodger K, Daly MJ, Heatley RV. Prescribing patterns for dyspepsia in primary care: a prospective study of selected general practitioners. *Aliment Pharmacol Ther* 1996;**10**: 889–95.

34 Dobrilla G, Comberlato L, Steele A *et al.* Drug treatment of functional dyspepsia. A meta-analysis of randomized controlled clinical trials. *J Clin Gastroenterol* 1989;**11**: 169–77.

35 Redstone HA, Barrowman N, Veldhuyzen van Zanten SJO. H2-receptor antagonists in the treatment of functional (non-ulcer) dyspepsia: a meta-analysis of randomized controlled clinical trials. *Aliment Pharmacol Ther* 2001;**15**:1291–9.

36 Bytzer P. H2-receptor antagonists and prokinetics in dyspepsia: a critical review. *Gut* 2002;**50(Suppl 4):iv**: 58–62.

37 Hansen JM, Bytzer P, Schaffalitzky de Muckadell OB. Placebo-controlled trial of cisapride and nizatidine in

unselected patients with functional dyspepsia. *Am J Gastroenterol* 1998;**93**:368–74.

38 Talley NJ, Meineche-Schmidt V, Pare P *et al.* Efficacy of omeprazole in functional dyspepsia: double-blind, randomized placebo-controlled trials (the Bond and Opera studies). *Aliment Pharmacol Ther* 1998;**12**:1055–65.

39 Mason I, LJ Millar, RR Sheikh *et al.* The management of acid-related dyspepsia in general practice: a comparison of an omeprazole versus an antacid-alginate/ranitidine management strategy. *Aliment Pharmacol Ther* 1998;**12**: 263–71.

40 Goves H, Oldring JK, Kerr D *et al.* First line treatment with omeprazole provides an effective and superior alternative strategy in the management of dyspepsia compared to antacid/alginate liquid: a multicentre study in general practice. *Aliment Pharmacol Ther* 1998;**2**:147–57.

41 Meineche-Schmidt V, Krag E. Anti-secretory therapy in 1017 patients with ulcerlike or reflux-like dyspepsia in general practice. *Eur J Gen Prac* 1997;**3**:125–30.

42 Wong WM, Wong BCY, Hung WK *et al.* Double blind, randomized, placebo controlled study of four weeks of lansoprazole for the treatment of functional dyspepsia in Chinese patients. *Gut* 2002;**51**:502–6.

43 Wong WM, Lam SK, Hui WM *et al.* Long-term prospective follow-up of endoscopic oesophagitis in southern Chinese – prevalence and spectrum of the disease. *Aliment Pharmacol Ther* 2002;**16**:2037–42.

44 Veldhuyzen van Zanten SJ, Jones MJ, Verlinden M, Talley NJ. Efficacy of cisapride and domperidone in functional (nonulcer) dyspepsia: a meta-analysis. *Am J Gastroenterol* 2001;**96**:689–96.

45 Champion MC, MacCannell K, Thomson A *et al.* A double-blind randomized study of cisapride in the treatment of non-ulcer dyspepsia. The Canadian Cisapride NUD study group. *Can J Gastroenterol* 1997;**11**:127–34.

46 Graham DY, Malaty HM, Evans DG *et al.* Epidemiology of *H. pylori* in an asymptomatic population in the United States: effect of age, race and socioeconomic status. *Gastroenterology* 1991;**100**:1495–501.

47 Veldhuyzen van Zanten SJO. *H. pylori*, socioeconomic status, marital status and occupation. *Aliment Pharmacol Ther* 1995;**9(S2)**:41–4.

48 Armstrong D. *H. pylori* and dyspepsia. *Scand J Gastroenterol* 1996;**31(Suppl 215)**:38–47.

49 Moayyedi P, Soo S, Deeks J *et al.* Eradication of helicobacter pylori for non-ulcer dyspepsia. *BMJ* 2000;**321**:659–64.

50 Laine L, Schoenfeld P, Fennerty MB. Therapy for *Helicobacter pylori* in patients with nonulcer dyspepsia. A meta-analysis of randomized, controlled trials. *Ann Intern Med* 2001;**134**:361–9.

51 McColl KEL, Murray LS, El-Omar E *et al.* Symptomatic benefit from eradicating *H. pylori* in patients with non-ulcer dyspepsia. *N Engl J Med* 1998;**339**:1869–74.

52 Talley NJ, Vakil N, Ballard ED II, Fennerty MB. Absence of benefit of eradicating *Helicobacter pylori* in patients with non-ulcer dyspepsia. *N Engl J Med.*1999;**34**:1106–11.

53 Blum AL, Talley NJ, O'Morain C *et al.* Lack of effect of treating *H. pylori* infection in patients with non-ulcer dyspepsia. *N Engl J Med* 1998;**339**:1875–81.

54 Talley NJ, Janssens J, Lauritsen K *et al.* Cure of *H. pylori* and symptoms in functional dyspepsia. A randomized double-blind placebo-controlled trial. *BMJ* 1999;**318**:823–7.

55 Vaira D, Miglioli M, Mule P *et al.* Prevalence of peptic ulcer in *H. pylori* positive blood donors. *Gut* 1994;**35**:309–12.

56 Anand BS, Raed AK, Malaty HM *et al.* Low point prevalence of peptic ulcer in normal individuals with *H. pylori* infection. *Am J Gastroenterol* 1996;**91**:1112–15.

57 McColl KEL, El-Nujumi A, Murray L *et al.* The *H. pylori* breath test: a surrogate marker for peptic ulcer disease in dyspeptic patients. *Gut* 1997;**40**:302–6.

58 McColl KE, Murray LS, Gillen D *et al.* Randomised trial of endoscopy with testing for *Helicobacter pylori* compared with non-invasive *H. pylori* testing alone in the management of dyspepsia. *BMJ* 2002;**324**:999–1002.

9 Celiac disease

James Gregor, Diamond Sherin Alidina

Introduction

Since its first description in children by Gee[1] over a century ago, the term celiac disease has been used interchangeably with such designations as primary malabsorption, gluten-sensitive enteropathy, and non-tropical or celiac sprue. Due to the protean nature of its clinical manifestations and their consistent improvement with appropriate therapy, few medical conditions can rival celiac disease for both the frustration and gratification experienced by clinicians and patients.

The first clinical description of celiac disease in adults was provided by Thaysen[2] in 1932. In the early 1950s, Dicke first reported a putative link between the disease and the ingestion of certain grains.[3] Over the next decade the characteristic intestinal lesion was described in both surgical specimens[4] and those obtained using the newly developed peroral suction biopsy technique.[5]

Epidemiology

Celiac disease is most common in Western Europeans and in immigrants from this area to North America and Australia; it is less common in non-Caucasoids, and although reported in Indians, Arabs, Hispanics, Israeli Jews, Sudanese and people of Cantonese extraction, it is very rare in those of Afro-Caribbean extraction. The true prevalence of celiac disease remains difficult to ascertain, and the prevalence varies with the intensity of screening.[6]

Until the advent of new, accurate serologic tests, celiac disease was presumed to be a rare entity, with a prevalence of 1:1500 in Europe and 1:3000 in the USA.[7] The recognition of atypical presentations of disease has led to intensified serologic screening followed by intestinal biopsy, and this protocol has revealed a true prevalence ranging from 1:300 in the UK[8] to 1:150 in Ireland.[9,10] In the USA screening of blood from 2000 blood donors has revealed a prevalence of raised anti-endomysial antibodies of 1:250,[11] while a retrospective cohort of 3654 school-aged subjects in Finland estimated a prevalence approaching one in 99.[12] The suggestion has been made that celiac disease detected by screening is not silent, but rather undetected, given the range of pathology and symptomatology that may be present in this disease.[13,14]

Clinical manifestations

The clinical manifestations of celiac disease are largely due to nutrient malabsorption, with iron-deficiency anemia being the most common presenting finding in an adult celiac patient.[15] Other symptoms such as severe abdominal pain, nausea and vomiting are much less common. Although some patients may even complain of constipation, most describe increased stool volume. The diarrhea of celiac disease is classically described as high volume, pale, loose to semi-formed, and foul-smelling. However, in many cases it is watery, probably due to the effects of malabsorbed fat and its bacterial degradation products on the secretory mechanisms of intestinal mucosal cells. A high fat content may produce an oily or frothy appearance, and a high gas content can make the stools difficult to flush from the toilet bowl.

Constitutional symptoms of fatigue, weakness and weight loss, often despite a history of hyperphagia, are common. Many of these symptoms can be attributed to the presence of nutritional deficiencies. In some patients insufficient calories and protein are absorbed to meet nutritional requirements, and weight loss and muscle wasting ensue. Specific deficiencies resulting in anemia, bleeding diathesis, tetany, neuropathy and dermatitis can also occur.

Given the genetic and immunological factors felt to be important in the pathogenesis of the disease, it is not surprising that investigators have sought and reported an association between celiac disease and over 100 medical conditions.[16] By far the most common of these is dermatitis herpetiformis. This pruritic rash is typically papulovesicular and characterized by IgA deposits at the dermal–epidermal junction. If adequate biopsies are performed, villous atrophy has been identified in up to 95% of these patients. In support of the validity of this association is the observation that the characteristic blistering skin lesions tend to improve in response to a gluten-free diet, although at a slower rate (up to 2 years) than the intestinal lesions.[17]

Lymphocytic infiltration of the epithelium of the colon and even stomach has been widely reported in celiac disease. Recent data suggest, however, that the majority of patients with microscopic or collagenous colitis do not have serological evidence of disease.[18]

Type I diabetes mellitus has been described in up to 5% of patients with celiac disease[16] and a similar proportion of patients with insulin dependent diabetes have been reported to have occult villous atrophy.[19,20] Autoimmune thyroid disease and selective IgA deficiency[21] also appear to be more prevalent in patients with celiac disease. Studies linking celiac disease to other autoimmune diseases such as ulcerative colitis,[22] primary biliary cirrhosis[23] and sclerosing cholangitis[24] are primarily family studies or small case series.

Screening studies suggest an increased prevalence (up to 7%) of celiac disease in patients with Down's syndrome.[25,26] In one study this generated an odds ratio as high as 100, compared to the general population.[27] However, due to the small number of celiac patients diagnosed in the groups with Down's syndrome, a statistically significantly increased prevalence has not been demonstrated uniformly.

Pathology

Celiac disease primarily affects the mucosal layer of the small intestine, often involving only duodenum and jejunum, with damage decreasing in severity more distally. In severe disease, the entire length of the small bowel may be involved, and there have even been occasional reports of abnormalities of the gastric and rectal mucosa.[14] The characteristic lesion includes lymphocytic infiltration of the lamina propria and, in particular, the surface epithelium, resulting in villous atrophy and crypt hyperplasia. The degree of villous damage ranges from mere blunting to total atrophy. The degree and extent of disease involvement grossly correlates with the severity of gastrointestinal symptoms.[28] In some studies the prevalence of asymptomatic celiac disease is four-fold greater than the prevalence of symptomatic disease.[29]

Historically, the gold standard for the diagnosis of celiac disease has required not only the identification of the typical histological lesion, but also clinical and histological improvement with appropriate dietary therapy. It has been clearly demonstrated in human subjects that the instillation into the small bowel of wheat, rye, or barley flour or their alcohol-soluble protein components, "prolamins", produces both clinical symptoms and histological lesions.[30]

Wheat gluten must be processed into alcohol soluble prolamins in order to develop antigenicity. Although the exact epitope(s) within gluten remain unknown, the generation of this epitope from the antigenic wheat protein is accomplished by a brush border enzyme known as tissue transglutaminase (tTG). Once the epitope has been generated by the tTG enzyme, the enzyme itself becomes one of the targets of the autoimmune response.[14]

Although the environmental trigger of wheat gluten is implicated in the development of this disease, it is apparent that genetic factors also play a prominent role. Concordance between identical twins approaches 100%, and first-degree relatives of celiac disease have a 10% prevalence of celiac disease, which is higher than that cited in the general population.[15] Current theories of disease pathogenesis therefore focus on the interaction between the antigen (wheat gluten) and the human leukocyte antigen (HLA) predisposition of affected individuals. Over 95% of patients with celiac disease express the HLA DQ(a1*501,β1*02) heterodimer (HLA-DQ2). This class II major histocompatibility complex (MHC) molecule exists on antigen-presenting cells, including the gluten-sensitive T helper cells, which preferentially present gluten-derived gliadin peptide epitopes to intestinal mucosal T cells. A Th1/Th0 type inflammatory response is mounted, thus producing the observed mucosal damage. One of the targets of this autoimmune response is the tTG brush border enzyme which generates the gluten-derived epitope. An anti-tTG assay may therefore be used to screen populations for celiac disease.[14,15]

Much of the fundamental research relating to celiac disease in recent years has focused on the immunologic and genetic factors associated with sensitivity to gliadin and the other prolamins. In clinical practice the diagnosis and treatment of the disease are well defined. Thus most of the recently published clinical research has addressed a few specific questions, namely:

1 **Diagnosis:** the role of the anti-endomysial antibody and the anti-tissue transglutaminase antibody for screening populations at risk, diagnosing symptomatic individuals, and following the response to a gluten-free diet.
2 **Treatment:** whether oats (or specifically the oat prolamin avenin) can safely be consumed by patients with celiac disease or dermatitis herpetiformis.
3 **Prognosis:** whether patients are at an increased risk of malignancy and other autoimmune diseases, and whether adherence to a gluten-free diet reduces that risk.

Serological testing

In patients with typical signs, symptoms and laboratory parameters the diagnosis of celiac disease is usually made by performing a mucosal biopsy of the small bowel. Though the differential diagnosis of villous injury is long (including tropical sprue, lymphoma, cows' milk-induced enteritis, Zollinger–Ellison syndrome, Whipple's disease, eosinophilic gastroenteritis, bacterial overgrowth, and even viral gastroenteritis), in most patients the diagnosis is not in doubt. From the 1950s until the introduction of flexible endoscopic equipment, specimens were usually obtained using peroral suction instruments, a cumbersome procedure which was uncomfortable for the patient. With the recognition of the immunologic nature of the disease it was predictable that serological testing would be developed and evaluated to simplify diagnosis and to facilitate the institution of screening programs in areas of high prevalence.

A number of serological tests have been developed employing antireticulin antibodies (ARA), antigliadin antibodies (AGA), and more recently antibodies to smooth muscle endomysium (EMA). Given that the pathogenesis of celiac disease appears to involve the interaction between cereal grain gluten, or more specifically the alcohol-soluble gliadins, it is not surprising that many of the early reports have focused on AGA as the primary serological test. As is often the case following the introduction of a new diagnostic test, the initial promise has to some degree yielded to acknowledgement of the test's limitations. Most studies have examined both the IgG and IgA subsets of AGA.[31,32] The data demonstrate reasonable sensitivity (69–91%) but poor specificity (2–79%) for the IgG antibody, suggesting that it may be a general marker for increased gut permeability of any cause rather than an important factor in disease pathogenesis. The IgA AGA has improved specificity (9–94%) at the expense of sensitivity (66–87%).

The development of the EMA test has produced a renewed interest in serological diagnosis. Initial reports suggested almost perfect test accuracy in subjects not restricted to a gluten-free diet. Because it employs an IgA antibody, it is acknowledged that the test may be falsely negative in a celiac patient with associated IgA deficiency. The test is generally performed on serum diluted at 1:10 and 1:20 concentrations, using an immunofluorescence technique. The substrate used is derived from monkey esophagus which has the disadvantages of being expensive (US$20–40) and morally controversial. Recently studies have shown that using human umbilical cord as a substrate produces similar test results.[33–36]

One of the largest studies evaluating the EMA assay involved 22 pediatric gastroenterology centers throughout Italy.[37] Almost 4000 children underwent testing with both AGA (IgA and IgG) and IgA EMA. "Gold standard" biopsies had been obtained from all patients with a diagnosis of celiac disease who had not yet been placed on dietary therapy ($n = 688$) and from those with compatible gastrointestinal symptoms who subsequently were given a different diagnosis ($n = 797$). Limiting the analysis to these two groups, the EMA assay was more sensitive than the IgG AGA assay (94% *v* 90%) and more specific than the IgA AGA assay (97% *v* 90%), both differences being statistically significant. Healthy first-degree relatives ($n = 599$) were also studied. Of the 46 positive EMA results (7·6%), 32 underwent biopsy. Ninety

percent of these patients were found to have pathological changes consistent with a diagnosis of celiac disease. In patients on a strict gluten-free diet ($n = 96$) it was found that 81% were negative for EMA, suggesting that the test may have a role in monitoring intestinal response after diagnosis.

There have been many studies from several countries[29,33–49] which have evaluated the diagnostic accuracy of EMA (Table 9·1). One useful way of summarizing the utility of a test is to consider both its positive and negative likelihood ratios (LR). In bayesian analysis the appropriate LR (depending on the positivity or negativity of the test) is multiplied by the estimated pretest odds to determine the likelihood that a particular condition is present or absent. Positive LRs greater than 10 and negative LRs less than 0·1 are generally agreed to be quite useful. Consider an example of a patient with non-specific symptoms and a family history of celiac disease in whom the pretest likelihood of celiac disease was estimated to be 8% (odds of 2:23). Using the LRs from the large Italian study[37] of 31 and 0·06, respectively, the post-test likelihood of celiac disease after a positive test would be 65% and after a negative test 0·5%. In a patient with more specific symptoms and therefore a higher pretest probability estimated at 50%, a positive test would produce a post-test likelihood of 97% while a negative test would reduce this likelihood to 6%. Similarly if one screened the general population (with a prevalence of 0·25%) the post-test probabilities would be much different at 8% and 0·02%, respectively, significantly lower than a high risk or symptomatic population.

Though obviously highly dependent on pretest probabilities, the utility of a particular LR also has to be interpreted in light of the implications of misdiagnosis, which in the case of celiac disease would include weighing the tribulations of a gluten-free diet against the potential for future symptoms and complications in an untreated patient. In one recent economic model,[48] it was estimated that using EMA alone for the diagnosis of celiac disease was potentially more costly than small bowel biopsy if the test specificity was under 95%. The authors concluded that the most cost-effective strategy for most patients presenting to a gastroenterologist was to use EMA as the initial diagnostic test and to confirm all positive results with a small bowel biopsy.

Although most studies suggest good diagnostic accuracy, due to differences in test interpretation and the populations studied there are considerable differences of opinion as to whether EMA is more useful in ruling out celiac disease (high sensitivity/negative LR) or confirming the diagnosis (high specificity/positive LR). Of the 17 studies listed in Table 9.1, 13 produced positive LRs above 10, and 11 produced negative LRs below 0·1. EMA appears to be a useful diagnostic test that should replace other serological tests, but it probably should not replace small bowel biopsy for the diagnosis of celiac disease.

Table 9.1 Recent studies examining the operating properties of the anti-endomysial antibody in patients who have undergone small bowel biopsy[a]

Study	Subjects	% Celiac	Sensitivity (%)	Specificity (%)	Positive LR[a]	Negative LR[b]
Cataldo et al. 1995[37]	1485 children with GI disease	46	94	97	**31**	**0·06**
Grodzinsky et al. 1995[39]	97 children with GI symptoms	28	78	99	**78**	0·22
Vogelsang et al. 1995[40]	102 patients with suspected celiac disease	48	100	100	**100**	**0·01**
Volta et al. 1995[33]	160 patients with GI disease	38	95	100	**95**	**0·05**
Pacht et al. 1995[41]	35 children with GI symptoms	63	100	100	**100**	**0·01**
Stern et al. 1996[42]	66 patients with GI disease	71	98	89	**8·9**	0·02
Grodzinsky 1996[29]	49 AGA-positive blood donors	14	71	100	**71**	0·29
Valdimarsson et al.1996[43]	144 patients with suspected celiac disease	17	74	100	**74**	0·26
Ascher et al. 1996[44]	120 patients with GI symptoms	46	98	100	**98**	**0·02**
Sacchetti et al. 1996[45]	74 children with GI symptoms	43	297	100	**97**	**0·03**
de Lecea et al. 1996[46]	65 children of short stature	34	88	91	**9·7**	0·13
Yiannakou et al. 1996[38]	154 patients – celiac, IBD or normal	30	89	100	**89**	0·11
Carroccio et al. 1996[35]	108 children – celiac or milk allergy	33	97	100	**97**	**0·03**
Bottaro et al. 1997[47]	50 children – celiac or normal	67	96	96	**24**	**0·04**
Atkinson et al. 1997[48]	66 patients with GI symptoms	33	95	64	2·6	**0·08**
Corazza et al. 1997[49]	78 patients with GI symptoms	45	91	80	4·6	0·11
Kolho and Savilahti 1997[34]	167 children with GI symptoms	32	94	100	**94**	**0·06**

Positive LR greater than 10 and negative LR less than 0·1 are shown in bold type because they are generally considered to be quite useful.

[a] Calculated using sensitivity/1 – specificity and assuming specificity = 99% when reported as 100%.

[b] Calculated using 1 – sensitivity/specificity and assuming specificiity = 99% when reported as 100%.

LR, likelihood ratio; GI, gastrointestinal; AGA, antigliadin antibody; IBD, inflammatory bowel disease

The discovery that the protein cross-linking enzyme tTG is the autoantigen for EMA has resulted in the development of an ELISA assay for the antibody to tTG (anti-tTG). The anti-tTG may be carried out using either guinea pig liver or human erythrocyte substrate. Large studies comparing anti-tTG to EMA have generally shown comparable sensitivities (93–98%) and specificities (94–99%)[15] with the human tTG antigen producing slightly superior results. Recent reports have suggested that even human anti-tTG may miss some cases of EMA positive celiac disease.[50,51] Despite this, given the ease and cost advantages of the anti-tTG, it is likely that the trend toward the use of this test will continue.

Therapy

The mainstay of therapy for celiac disease is a lifelong gluten-free diet. Because biopsy findings suggesting celiac disease may also be compatible with other conditions, some clinicians advocate a follow up biopsy to confirm remission after implementation of a gluten-free diet. However, most are satisfied with a symptomatic response. In addition to a gluten-free diet, supplemental vitamins such as iron, folic acid or vitamin K should be given where deficiencies are documented. Calcium and vitamin D may be deficient, and consideration may be given to measuring bone mineral density, particularly in women. Although it is suggested that the institution of a gluten-free diet protects against increasing bone loss, some patients may be candidates for hormone replacement or bisphosphonate therapy.[52]

Poor dietary compliance is the most common reason for failure of a gluten-free diet. However, the complications of intestinal lymphoma and adenocarcinoma must be considered. Patients with persistent symptoms in whom other diagnoses are excluded are described as having refractory sprue.[53] There are considerable uncontrolled data to support the use of corticosteroids for this indication. Anecdotal evidence suggests that azathioprine[54] and cyclosporin[55] may also be effective in patients who do not respond to corticosteroids. In one known case of steroid-refractory celiac disease, infliximab followed by azathioprine was successfully used to induce and maintain remission.[56] C5

Currently, the greatest controversy pertaining to therapy is the safety of including modest amounts of oats in the diet. Historically, wheat and rye were the first grains with demonstrated toxicity in celiac patients, followed subsequently by reports of toxicity with oats and barley. Similar injurious effects were not found with corn, rice, and potatoes.[57] Although it appears that grain prolamins contain the antigen responsible for the toxic immune response, the exact amino acid sequence of the responsible peptide has yet to be fully elucidated. Certain prolamins appear to be more antigenic than others, and the proline content of certain amino acid sequences in the prolamins are determinants of antigenicity. The specificity of tTG for proline-rich sequences may render the proline-rich proteins of the Triticeae tribe grasses (wheat gluten, rye secalin and barley hordein) more antigenic than the proline-poor oat avenin, giving biological plausibility to the hypothesis that oats may be less toxic.[14] Contrary immunological evidence exists to suggest immune reactivity with avenin proteins[58]; however, the relevance of this finding is questionable, since this study also demonstrated immune reactivity with corn extract, and subsequent *in vitro* immunofluorescence tests have demonstrated induction of EMA production with partially-digested gliadin fractions, but not with avenin.[59]

Mounting clinical and biological evidence is now accumulating to demonstrate a lack of toxicity of oats in newly diagnosed patients with celiac disease, and in celiac disease patients in remission. However, the clinical trials which address the issue of long-term safety of oat consumption are still limited in number. A small cohort study

followed 10 patients with celiac disease for 3 months during which time they consumed porridge containing 50 g of oats daily.[60] The patients remained symptom-free without showing an elevation in EMA or AGA or any histological deterioration. B4 Based only on this result, and the estimation that the upper limit of the 95% confidence interval for a harmful effect in a study failing to show harm is approximately $3/n$, where n is the number of subjects,[61] the true incidence of toxic effects could be as high as 30%.

A study using a similar design was undertaken to determine the effects of oats on patients with dermatitis herpetiformis. This manifestation often requires even longer periods of gluten withdrawal (2 years on average) to achieve clinical remission, while recurrence usually occurs within 12 weeks of gluten reintroduction.[8] All 10 patients in the study continued with the diet, consuming on average 62·5 g of oats daily. No symptomatic, antibody or histological relapse was noted. B4

More recent data on the use of oats in newly diagnosed celiac disease are limited. One small scale cohort study in a pediatric population was carried out in 2000, and followed 10 patients for 6 months following diagnosis, during which time they consumed a gluten-free diet with 24 g of oat cereal per day ($1·2 \pm 0·9$ g/kg per day). At study completion, the patients demonstrated a significant decrease in the primary outcome variables of intestinal biopsy score, intraepithelial lymphocyte (IEL) count, tTG titer and number of symptoms. However, this study was limited by its size and by a lack of long-term follow up.[62] B4

A larger Finnish study randomized 92 patients with newly diagnosed celiac disease to a strict gluten-free diet or one containing 50 g of oats daily for 6 months.[63] The authors excluded patients who had severe disease or were not well controlled on their present diet and those with comorbid illnesses. The patients were well matched with regards to clinical, histologic and nutritional parameters. The investigators but not the patients were blinded to treatment. Seventy-six percent of the oat group consumed more than 30 g daily. Six patients in the oat consuming group withdrew because of cutaneous or abdominal symptoms or for unspecified reasons, but a similar withdrawal rate was observed in the control group. No significant change was found in nutritional laboratory parameters or in small bowel histology. The authors concluded that moderate amounts of oats were safe in most patients. A1d However, skeptics could point out that even under these controlled circumstances, 24% of patients may have been intolerant, since the 95% confidence interval was calculated as 12–36%. The issue of oat contamination with other grains secondary to crop rotation and processing was not addressed in this study.

A 5-year follow up study of a subset of 63 of the above patients was carried out by the same authors. The patients selected for this study were those who consented to reassessment by laboratory nutritional and immunologic

Table 9.2 A subjective assessment of current evidence attempting to establish a causal or non-causal relationship (see text for details)

	Hypothesis	
Criteria	Untreated celiac causes gastrointestinal malignancy/lymphoma	Oats may be consumed as part of a gluten-free diet
Biological plausibility	Yes	Yes
Study design	Case–control/cohort	Randomized controlled
Study consistency	**Moderate**	Good
Control groups used	Yes	Yes
Group similarity	**Questionable**	Yes
Adequate follow up	Yes	**Questionable**
Temporal relationship	Probable	Yes
Exposure gradient	**Not shown**	**Not shown**
Strength of association	Strong	Strong
Precision of estimate	**Poor**	Good

parameters and duodenal biopsy.[64] Twelve of the 35 oat consuming patients discontinued the oat consuming diet, citing lack of data on long-term safety as the primary reason for discontinuation of the diet. The results of the follow up study demonstrated no significant differences or changes in body mass index, nutritional status, or routine laboratory data between the two groups at the 5-year examination. Given the limitations of the study, and the small number of study patients, these data might be interpreted as preliminary support of the long-term safety of oats in celiac disease in remission. B4

Prognosis

Celiac disease, if left unrecognized and untreated, has the potential to result in severe complications which are for the most part secondary to malnutrition. When appropriate dietary therapy is instituted, the prognosis for celiac disease is usually good; however, untreated, the morbidity and mortality, and the risk of certain malignancies has been postulated to be increased in a celiac population. Past studies have suggested an increase in age-adjusted mortality attributable to the disease itself.[28] However, these studies may have been biased because of the inclusion of substantial numbers of untreated patients. More recent studies have suggested that at least short-term survival is not different from that of the general population.[16] Despite this finding there is evidence, both from retrospective and cohort studies, which suggests an increased risk of certain malignancies.[6]

Immunologic stimulation and increased permeability are among the characteristics of the gut in celiac disease which lend biological credence to the possibility that celiac patients are at increased risk for malignancies such as lymphoma and adenocarcinoma of the small bowel. Although the epidemiological studies are heterogeneous in their design and findings, most of the epidemiologic evidence to date confirms a general increase in morbidity. The left-hand column of Table 9.2 summarizes some of the data from these studies.

Most of the reports are based on case–control studies. This design is particularly subject to problems with *bias* and *confounding*. A *selection bias* toward the inclusion of particularly ill or refractory patients is one of the most frequently cited criticisms of the studies which show a mortality rate increased as much as 3·4-fold over that of the general population[66–69] and complicating malignancy rates as high as 14%.[67] *Measurement bias* is another potential problem. Patients presenting with abdominal symptoms secondary to a malignancy may be more likely to undergo investigations like small bowel biopsy, which could lead to a diagnosis of celiac disease. Finally, some of the risk factors for celiac disease such as ethnic/geographic origin or immune markers (for example the class II HLA antigens HLA-DR3 and HLA-DQw2) could potentially be independent risk factors for certain diseases.

Despite these concerns, it is unlikely that the excess risk of small bowel lymphoma and adenocarcinoma seen in most studies can be explained by methodological flaws. In the early 1980s, a British registry collected data on approximately 400 cases of celiac disease and various cancers. The data were analyzed and compared to individual cancer rates in the local population.[70] Of the 259 histologically confirmed tumors, slightly more than half were lymphomas, the majority of which had arisen in the small bowel. Two-thirds were discovered after the diagnosis of celiac disease was established at a mean interval of 7·3 years. A number of other studies have shown similarly high rates of lymphoma with death rates due to this complication varying from 2·6% to 8·9%, translating into relative risks of 25–122 with respect to the general population.[71]

Of non-lymphomatous malignancies only those of the gastrointestinal tract were seen in excess, compared to the general population. A statistically significant increased risk of adenocarcinomas of the pharynx, esophagus and small bowel was observed. The relative risk of pharyngeal or esophageal cancer was relatively small (5–6) and could possibly be explained by confounding risk factors. However, the relative risk of small bowel carcinoma, a rare malignancy in the general population, was markedly increased at 83 (95% CI 46 to 117).

Another British series of 210 patients reported in 1976[72] produced similar results. It was followed by a prospective cohort study published in 1989[73] which also demonstrated increased cancer risk. The patients were *a priori* divided into three groups – patients following a strict gluten-free diet ($n = 108$), patients intermittently adherent or adherent less than 5 years ($n = 56$), and patients not adhering to any dietary restrictions ($n = 46$). Increased risk was seen overall for cancers of the mouth, pharynx and esophagus (ratio of observed to expected (O/E) approached 10). The increase in risk was particularly strong for non-Hodgkin's lymphoma ($n = 9$, O/E = 42·7). For these cancers there was a statistically significant reduced risk for the strict gluten-free diet group. In a follow up article by the same author[74] on the same cohort of patients, *excess morbidity* for those not observing a gluten-free diet was confirmed. B2

Retrospective cohort and genetic studies on celiac patients who develop malignancy has yielded information on possible prognostic indicators of malignant disease. Refractory sprue, or celiac disease which does not respond to dietary treatment, is a negative prognostic indicator, possibly because of the ongoing immune stimulation which may predispose to malignant transformation. Non-response to therapy may be present from diagnosis or after a period of response to dietary therapy, but is always a negative prognostic indicator.[74] A confounding factor may exist in that other disease types which produce villous atrophy and inflammatory infiltrates may be present, such as ulcerative jejunitis or jejunoileitis or mesenteric lymph node cavitation syndrome, and thus the diagnosis of underlying celiac disease may be questionable. Genetic prognostic indicators are less well studied still. A small case study of six refractory sprue patients demonstrated the replacement of the normal IEL population with morphologically normal and phenotypically abnormal cells with intracytoplasmic CD3, no surface CD3, CD4, CD8 or TCR, and restricted TCR γ gene rearrangements. On this basis, the authors postulated a spectrum of disease ranging from celiac disease to refractory sprue to enteropathy-associated T cell lymphoma (EATL), with refractory sprue being the transitional disease state between celiac disease and malignancy.[75] The same study showed a poorer prognosis for the three patients with the aberrant phenotype TCR γ gene rearrangement, intracytoplasmic CD3 + , surface CD8 –, and a better prognosis (in terms of treatment response to diet and

steroid therapy) for the three patients without this phenotype. This finding could be of practical importance, as non-response to treatment, coupled with the above phenotype implying a poor prognosis, would warrant closer follow up for the implicated patient. Non-response to treatment in the absence of this phenotype would suggest non-compliance with dietary therapy.

The risk of malignancy in patients with dermatitis herpetiformis has also been studied. One study used a retrospective cohort design[76] to evaluate 109 patients who were followed for 13 years at one clinic, with almost complete follow up. Seven patients (6·4%) developed a malignancy, three of which were lymphomas, one without small intestinal involvement. This translated into a relative risk of lymphoma of 100· The overall relative risk of malignancy was 2·38 (95% CI 1·22 to 3·56). However, in those patients adhering to a gluten-free diet, no increased risk was seen. B2 A subsequent Finnish study[77] of 305 patients in whom 81% were compliant with a gluten-free diet also showed no excess risk of malignancy with the exception of non-Hodgkin's lymphoma ($n = 4$) (RR = 10, 95% CI 2·8 to 26·3). B2 A cohort study of 487 patients with dermatitis herpetiformis reported a 2% incidence of lymphoma while on a normal diet or a gluten-free diet for less than 5 years.[78] B2

In contrast to these results, another retrospective cohort study originating in Finland[16] compared 335 celiac patients to age and sex-matched controls with other gastrointestinal disease and normal villous architecture. A statistically significant increased incidence of endocrine disease (12%) and connective tissue disease (7%) was observed, but no increased incidence of malignancy was detected. B2 Notably, no cases of small bowel adenocarcinoma or non-Hodgkin's lymphoma were identified. This negative finding may be accounted for by either the relatively short mean follow up (3·1 years) or the high rate of dietary compliance with a strict gluten-free diet (83%).

Though debate persists on the magnitude and type of cancer for which untreated celiac patients are at risk, there is general acceptance among clinicians that the risk is significant enough to warrant lifelong strict dietary compliance even in asymptomatic patients. This concern is foremost among those advocating that oats should not be included in a gluten-free diet.[79] Table 9.2 suggests that the evidence supporting the view that the inclusion of modest amounts of oats in a celiac diet is safe may actually be stronger than the data demonstrating an increased cancer risk in celiac patients.

Strict dietary therapy is warranted in adolescent and pediatric populations alone on the sole basis of prevention of morbidity, even if the questions of malignancy and mortality are set aside. A large retrospective cohort analysis of 909 pediatric and adolescent celiac patients, 1268 control subjects and 163 patients with Crohn's disease was undertaken to determine the effect of duration of gluten exposure on the development of autoimmune disease in patients with celiac disease.[80] The prevalence of autoimmune disorders was noted to be significantly increased in the celiac population (14%) with respect to the control population (2·8%) but not with respect to the Crohn's disease population (12·9%). When the celiac population was subdivided into groups according to age at diagnosis, a surrogate for duration of gluten exposure, it was noted that the first group (< 2 years at diagnosis; 5.1% prevalence) did not have a significantly different prevalence of autoimmune disease compared to the control group, but that the second group (2–10 years; 17·0% prevalence) and the third group (> 10 years; 23·8% prevalence) did have a significantly increased comparative prevalence of autoimmune disease. Furthermore, a logistic regression model predicted increased odds of developing autoimmunity of 1·1% per year of diagnosis delay, with the expected numbers derived from this model correlating well with the observed study numbers. A second analysis of a subset of the 374 celiac disease patients who were diagnosed before the age of 2 years was subdivided on the basis of exposure to a gluten challenge following diagnosis, and those exposed to gluten for an additional "challenge" period following diagnosis were susceptible to an increased prevalence of autoimmune disorders. The implications of this study support early clinical diagnosis with serologic and histologic confirmation, and avoidance of prolonged exposure to gluten, even in the form of a gluten challenge. B2

This study has been challenged by a subsequent similar study in an adult population.[81] This retrospective cohort analysis analyzed 605 controls and 422 celiac disease patients. Although the prevalence of autoimmunity was three-fold higher in the celiac population than in controls, the duration of gluten exposure did not correlate with the development of autoimmunity in an adult population. B2 The two studies may be reconciled by the pathogenesis of the disease; it is possible that immune modulation and gluten exposure play a role in the development of disease early in life, and that once exposure has occurred in youth, circulating autoantibodies to various organs arise and the risk of later development of autoimmune disorders is subsequently increased in the adult celiac population. [82]

Other complications of celiac disease exist in addition to those listed above, but are more rarely seen than autoimmune disease and malignancy. These include refractory sprue which often requires immunosuppressive therapy. Ulcerative jejunoileitis manifesting as chronic ulcers of the small and occasionally large bowel can rarely occur and can lead to the diagnosis of celiac disease.[65] This condition can be difficult to distinguish from intestinal lymphoma and may actually progress to this disease. Collagenous sprue, an even more rare complication of celiac disease, is histologically distinguished by a thick subepithelial band of collagen. No effective therapy has been described and patients generally go on to parenteral alimentation.[6,83]

Conclusion

The gold standard for the diagnosis of celiac disease remains the small bowel biopsy. Serological testing, particularly the EMA and tTG, can be very useful in the appropriate clinical situation to diagnose the disease and to monitor the response to a gluten-free diet. The threshold for initial and follow up biopsy if necessary should be low given the limitations of the test and the general ease of upper gastrointestinal endoscopy and biopsy. A gluten-free diet remains the cornerstone of management. The available evidence suggests that a substantial proportion of patients will tolerate a moderate amount of oats in their diet with the appropriate clinical follow up. To prevent symptomatic recurrences, nutritional deficiencies (particularly bone disease), and malignant and autoimmune complications, a strict gluten-free diet should be encouraged in all patients.

References

1 Gee S. On the coeliac affection. *St Barth Hosp Rep* 1888;**24**:17–20.
2 Thaysen TEH. *Non-tropical sprue.* Copenhagen: Levin & Munksgaard, 1932.
3 Dicke WK, Weijers HA, van de Kamer JH. Coeliac disease. II: The presence in wheat of a factor having a deleterious effect in cases of coeliac disease. *Acta Paediatr Scand* 1953;**42**:34–42.
4 Paulley LW. Observations on the aetiology of idiopathic steatorrhea. *BMJ* 1954;**2**:1318–21.
5 Rubin CE, Brandborg LL, Phelps PC *et al.* Studies of coeliac disease I. The apparent identical and specific nature of the duodenal and proximal jejunal lesion in coeliac disease and idiopathic sprue. *Gastroenterology* 1960;**38**:28–49.
6 Trier JS. Coeliac sprue. *N Engl J Med* 1991;**325**:1709–19.
7 Fasano A. Where have all the American celiacs gone? *Acta Paediatrica Suppl* 196;**412**:20–4.
8 Hin H, Bird G, Fisher P, Mahy N, Jewell D. Coeliac disease in primary care: a case finding study. *BMJ* 1999;**318**:164–7.
9 Mylotte M, Egan-Mitchell B, McCarthy CE, McNicholl B. Coeliac disease in the west of Ireland. *BMJ* 1973;**3**:498–9.
10 Catassi C, Fabiani E, Ratsch IM *et al.* The coeliac iceberg in Italy: a multicentre antigliadin antibodies screening for coeliac disease in school-age subjects. *Acta Paediatr Suppl* 1996;**412**:29–35.
11 Not T, Horvath K, Hill ID *et al.* Celiac disease risk in the USA: high prevalence of antiendomysium antibodies in healthy blood donors. *Scand J Gastroenterol* 1998;**33**:494–8.
12 Maki M, Mustalahti K *et al.* Prevalence of celiac disease among children in Finland. *N Engl J Med* 2003;**348**:2517–24.
13 Johnston SD, Watson RG, McMillan SA, Slaon J, Love AH. Coeliac disease detected by screening is not silent – simply unrecognized. *Q J Med* 1998;**91**:853–60.
14 Ciclitira, PJ. AGA Technical review on celiac sprue. AGA Practice Guidelines. *Gastroenterology* 2001;**120**:1–26.

15 Farrell RJ, Kelly, CP. Celiac sprue. *N Engl J Med* 2002;**346**:180–8.

16 Collin R, Reunala T, Pukkala E *et al.* Coeliac disease – associated disorders and survival. *Gut* 1994;**35**:1215–18.

17 Hardman C, Garioch JJ, Leonard JN *et al.* Absence of toxicity of oats in patients with dermatitis herpetiformis. *N Engl J Med* 1997;**337**:1884–7.

18 Bohr J, Tysk C, Yang P *et al.* Autoantibodies and immunoglobulins in collagenous colitis. *Gut* 1996;**39**:73–6.

19 Mäki M, Huupponen T, Holm K *et al.* Seroconversion of reticulin autoantibodies predicts coeliac disease in insulin dependent diabetes mellitus. *Gut* 1995;**36**:239–42.

20 Rensch MJ, Merenich JA, Lieberman M *et al.* Gluten-sensitive enteropathy in patients with insulin-dependent diabetes mellitus. *Ann Intern Med* 1996;**124**:564–7.

21 Rittmeyer C, Rhoads JM. IgA deficiency causes false-negative endomysial antibody results in coeliac disease. *J Pediatr Gastroenterol Nutr* 1996;**23**:504–6.

22 Shah A, Mayberry JF, Williams G *et al.* Epidemiological survey of coeliac disease and inflammatory bowel disease in first-degree relatives of coeliac patients. *Q J Med* 1990; **74**:283–8.

23 Logan RF, Finlayson NDC, Weir DG. Primary biliary cirrhosis and coeliac disease: an association? *Lancet* 1978;**i**:230–3.

24 Hay JE, Wiesner RH, Shorter R *et al.* Primary sclerosing cholangitis and coeliac disease. *Ann Intern Med* 1988;**109**: 713–17.

25 George EK, Mearin ML, Bouquet J *et al.* High frequency of coeliac disease in Down's syndrome. *J Pediatr* 1996;**128**: 555–7.

26 Bonamico M, Rasore-Quartino A, Mariani P *et al.* Down syndrome and coeliac disease: usefulness of antigliadin and antiendomysium antibodies. *Acta Paediatr* 1996;**85**:1503–5.

27 Gale L, Wimalaratna H, Brotodihargo A *et al.* Down's syndrome is strongly associated with coeliac disease. *Gut* 1997;**40**:492–6.

28 Trier JS. *Coeliac sprue and refractory sprue.* Toronto: WB Saunders, 1998.

29 Grodzinsky E. Screening for coeliac disease in apparently healthy blood donors. *Acta Paediatr* 1996;**412**(Suppl): 36–8.

30 van de Kamer JH, Weijers HA, Dicke WK. Coeliac disease. IV. An investigation into the injurious constituents of wheat in connection with their action on patients with coeliac disease. *Acta Paediatr Scand* 1953;**42**:223–31.

31 Berger R, Schmidt G. Evaluation of six anti-gliadin antibody assays. *J Immunol Methods* 1996;**91**:77–86.

32 Chartrand LJ, Agulnik J, Vanounou T *et al.* Effectiveness of antigliadin antibodies as a screening test for coeliac disease in children. *Can Med Assoc J* 1997;**157**:527–33.

33 Volta U, Molinaro N, De Franceshi L *et al.* IgA anti-endomysial antibodies on human umbilical cord tissue for coeliac disease screening save both money and monkeys. *Dig Dis Sci* 1995;**40**:1902–5.

34 Kolho KL, Savilahti E. IgA endomysium antibodies on human umbilical cord: an excellent diagnostic tool for coeliac disease in childhood. *J Pediatr Gastroenterol Nutr* 1997;**24**:563–7.

35 Carroccio A, Cavataio F, Iacono G *et al.* IgA antiendomysial antibodies on the umbilical cord in diagnosing coeliac disease. Sensitivity, specificity, and comparative evaluation with the traditional kit. *Scand J Gastroenterol* 1996;**31**: 759–63.

36 Sulkanen S, Halttunen T, Laurila K *et al.* Tissue transglutaminase autoantibody enzyme-linked immuno-sorbent assay in detecting celiac disease. *Gastroenterology* 1998;**115**:1322–8.

37 Cataldo F, Ventura A, Lazzari R *et al.* Antiendomysium antibodies and coeliac disease: solved and unsolved questions. An Italian multicentre study. *Acta Paediatr* 1995;**84**:1125–31.

38 Yiannakou JY, Dell'Olio D, Saaka M *et al.* Detection and characterization of anti-endomysial antibody in celiac disease using human umbilical cord. *Int Arch Allergy Immunol* 1997;**112**:140–4.

39 Grodzinsky E, Jansson G, Skogh T *et al.* Anti-endomysium and anti-gliadin antibodies as serological markers for coeliac disease in childhood: a clinical study to develop a practical routine. *Acta Paediatr* 1995;**84**:294–8.

40 Vogelsang H, Genser D, Wyatt J *et al.* Screening for coeliac disease: a prospective study on the value of noninvasive tests. *Am J Gastroenterol* 1995;**90**:394–8.

41 Pacht A, Sinai N, Hornstein L. The diagnostic reliability of anti-endomysial antibody in coeliac disease: the north Israel experience. *Isr J Med Sci* 1995;**31**:218–20.

42 Stern M, Teuscher M, Wechmann T. Serological screening for coeliac disease: methodological standards and quality control. *Acta Paediatr Suppl* 1996;**412**:49–51.

43 Valdimarsson T, Franzen L, Grodzinsky E. Is small bowel biopsy necessary in adults with suspected coeliac disease and IgA anti-endomysium antibodies? 100% positive predictive value for coeliac disease in adults. *Dig Dis Sci* 1996;**41**:83–7.

44 Ascher H, Hahn-Zoric M, Hanson LÅ *et al.* Value of serologic markers for clinical diagnosis and population studies of coeliac disease. *Scand J Gastroenterol* 1996;**31**:61–7.

45 Sacchetti L, Ferrajolo A, Salerno G *et al.* Diagnostic value of various serum antibodies detected by diverse methods in childhood coeliac disease. *Clin Chem* 1996;**42**:1838–42.

46 de Lecea A, Ribes-Koninckx C, Polanco I, Calvete JF. Serological screening (antigliadin and antiendomysium antibodies) for non-overt coeliac disease in children of short stature. *Acta Paediatr* 1996;**412**(Suppl):54–5.

47 Bottaro G, Volta U, Spina M *et al.* Antibody pattern in childhood coeliac disease. *J Pediatr Gastroenterol Nutr* 1997;**24**:559–62.

48 Atkinson K, Tokmakajian S, Watson W. Evaluation of the endomysial antibody for coeliac disease: operating properties and associated cost implications in clinical practice. *Can J Gastroenterol* 1997;**11**:673–7.

49 Corazza GR, Biagi F, Andreani ML *et al.* Screening test for coeliac disease. *Lancet* 1997;**349**:325–6.

50 Green P, Barry M and Matsutani M. Serologic tests for celiac disease. *Gastroenterology* 2003;**124**:585–6.

51 Dickey W, McMillan SA, Hughes DF. Sensitivity of serum tissue transglutaminase antibodies for endomysial antibody

positive and negative celiac disease. *Scand J Gastroenterol* 2001;**36**:511–14.

52 Valdimarsson T, Löfman O, Toss G *et al.* Reversal of osteopenia with diet in adult coeliac disease. *Gut* 1996;**38**:322–7.

53 Trier JS. Coeliac sprue and refractory sprue. *Gastroenterology* 1978;**75**:307–8.

54 Sinclair TS, Kumar PJ, Dawson AM. Azathioprine responsive villous atrophy [Abstract]. *Gut* 1983;**24**:A494.

55 Longstreth GF. Successful treatment of refractory sprue with cyclosporine. *Ann Intern Med* 1993;**119**:1014–16.

56 Gillett HR, Arnott IDR, McIntyre M *et al.* Successful infliximab treatment for steroid-refractory celiac disease: a case report. *Gastroenterology* 2002;**122**:800–5.

57 Schmitz J. Lack of oats toxicity in coeliac disease (editorial). *BMJ* 1997;**314**:159–60.

58 Vainio E, Varjonen E. Antibody response against wheat, rye, barley, oats and corn: comparison between gluten-sensitive patients and monoclonal antigliadin antibodies. *Int Arch Allerg Immunol* 1995;**106**:134–8.

59 Picarelli A, Di Tola M, Sabbatella L *et al.* Immunologic evidence of no harmful effect of oats in celiac disease. *Am J Clin Nutr* 2001;**74**:137–40.

60 Srinivasan U, Leonard N, Jones E *et al.* Absence of oats toxicity in adult coeliac disease. *BMJ* 1996;**313**:1300–1.

61 Hanley J, Lippman-Hand A. If nothing goes wrong is everything all right? Interpreting zero numerators. *JAMA* 1983;**249**:1743–5.

62 Hoffenberg EJ, Haas J, Drescher A *et al.* A trial of oats in children with newly diagnosed celiac disease. *J Pediatr* 2000;**137**:361–6.

63 Janatuinen EK, Pikkarainen PH, Kemppainen TA *et al.* A comparison of diets with and without oats in adults with coeliac disease. *N Engl J Med* 1995;**333**:1033–7.

64 Janatuinen EK, Kemppainen TA, Julkunen RJK *et al.* No harm from five-year ingestion of oats in celiac disease. *Gut* 2002;**50**:332–5.

65 Holmes GKT. Coeliac disease and malignancy. *J Pediatr Gastroenterol Nutr* 1997;**24**:S20–4.

66 Nielsen OH, Jacobsen O, Pedersen EF *et al.* Non-tropical sprue: malignant diseases and mortality rate. *Scand J Gastroenterol* 1985;**20**:13–18.

67 Logan RF, Rifkind EA, Turner ID *et al.* Mortality in coeliac disease. *Gastroenterology* 1989;**97**:265–71.

68 Ferguson A, Kingstone K. Coeliac disease and malignancies. *Acta Paediatr* 1996;**412**(Suppl):78–81.

69 Harris OD, Cooke WT, Thompson H *et al.* Malignancy in adult coeliac disease and idiopathic steatorrhoea. *Am J Med* 1967;**42**:899–912.

70 Swinson CM, Coles EC, Slavin G *et al.* Coeliac disease and malignancy. *Lancet* 1983;**i**:111–15.

71 Mathus-Vliegen EMH. Coeliac disease and lymphoma: current status. *Neth J Med* 1996;**49**:212–20.

72 Holmes GKT, Stokes PL, Sorahan TM *et al.* Coeliac disease, gluten-free diet, and malignancy. *Gut* 1976;**17**:612–19.

73 Holmes GKT, Prior P, Lane MR *et al.* Malignancy in coeliac disease – effect of a gluten free diet. *Gut* 1989;**30**:333–8.

74 Holmes GKT. Coeliac disease and malignancy. *Dig Liver Dis* 2002;**34**:229–37.

75 Cellier C, Delabesse E, Helmer C *et al.* Refractory sprue, coeliac disease and enteropathy-associated T-cell lymphoma. *Lancet* 2000;**356**:202–8.

76 Leonard JN, Tucker WFG, Fry JS *et al.* Increased incidence of malignancy in dermatitis herpetiformis. *BMJ* 1983;**286**:16–18.

77 Collin P, Pukkala E, Reunala T. Malignancy and survival in dermatitis herpetiformis: a comparison with coeliac disease. *Gut* 1996;**38**:528–30.

78 Lewis HM, Renaula RL, Garioch JN *et al.* Protective effect of gluten-free diet against development of lymphoma in dermatitis herpetiformis. *Br J Dermatol* 1996;**135**:363–7.

79 Branski D, Shine M. Oats in coeliac disease [Letter]. *N Engl J Med* 1996;**334**:865–6.

80 Ventura A, Magazzu G, Greco L. Duration of exposure to gluten and risk for autoimmune disorders in patients with celiac disease. *Gastroenterology* 1999;**117**:297–303.

81 Guidetti CS, Solerio E, Scaglione N, Aimo G, Mengozzi G. Duration of gluten exposure in adult coeliac disease does not correlate with the risk for autoimmune disorders. *Gut* 2001;**49**:502–5.

82 Ventura A, Magazu G, Gerarduzzi T, Greco L. Coeliac disease and the risk of autoimmune disorders [Author reply]. *Gut* 2002;**51**(**6**):897–8.

83 Trier JS. Complications of coeliac sprue and potentially related diseases with similar intestinal histopathology. *Gastroenterology* 1978;**75**:314–15.

10 Crohn's disease

Brian G Feagan, John WD McDonald

Introduction

The use of non-specific anti-inflammatory drugs such as the 5-aminosalicylates, glucocorticoids, and antimetabolites is the foundation of the current treatment for Crohn's disease (CD). However, recent advances in molecular biology have yielded novel approaches for therapy which may be more relevant to the pathophysiology of the disease. This review offers an evidence-based approach to the management of active CD. An overview of maintenance therapy is also provided.

Induction of remission

An ideal treatment for active CD should rapidly and reliably induce remission of symptoms. In clinical trials the most frequently used metric is a decrease in the Crohn's Disease Activity Index (CDAI) of from 50 to 100 points with a final score below 150.[1,2] A substantial placebo response (20–30%) is observed in short-term (8–16 week) studies. Four classes of drugs have been most frequently evaluated for treatment of active disease: 5-aminosalicylates (5-ASA), glucocorticoids, antibiotics, and monoclonal antibodies.

5-aminosalicylates

The prototypic 5-ASA compound sulfasalazine has been used to treat CD for more than 40 years.[3] Although highly effective for ulcerative colitis, randomized trials showed that sulfasalazine was only marginally superior to a placebo for the induction of remission in active CD (Figure 10.1).[4,5] Alc Since the sulfa-related adverse effects of sulfasalazine often limit the maximum drug dose that can be administered, the development of 5-ASA formulations which lack a sulfa moiety and which target specific regions of the gastrointestinal tract raised the possibility that greater efficacy was possible. Multiple randomized controlled trials (RCTs) have compared the newer 5-ASA compounds with either a placebo (Table 10.1) or an active treatment (sulfasalazine, glucocorticoids). Although many of these trials were at a high risk of a type II statistical error due to a small sample size, some definite conclusions can be derived.

Initial experience with 5-ASA doses of 1·5 g/day showed no clear benefit over a placebo.[6,7] These negative studies led

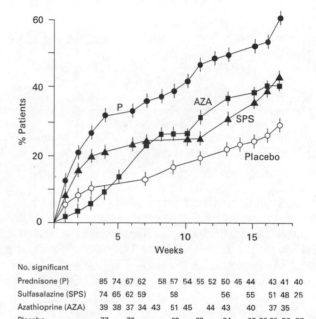

Figure 10.1 Cumulative percentage of patients in remission week by week: comparison of prednisone, sulfasalazine, azathioprine, and placebo. Remission is defined as Crohn's Disease Activity Index (CDAI) less than 150 and continuing below 150 through week 17 (life-table using Kaplan–Meier method). (Adapted with permission from Summers RW *et al. Gastroenterology* 1979;**77**:847–69[4])

to the evaluation of higher dose regimens. Singleton and colleagues[8] allocated over 300 patients with moderate disease activity to receive either 1 g, 2 g or 4 g of Pentasa daily or a placebo for a period of 16 weeks. Although 5-ASA was well tolerated, only a modest benefit of treatment was observed; 43% of the patients who received 4 g/day of Pentasa entered remission as compared with 18% of those who were assigned to the placebo (absolute risk reduction (ARR) 25%, number needed to treat (NNT) 4; *P* = 0·017). Alc No improvement over placebo was observed for those individuals who received the lower doses of 5-ASA. Subgroup analyses failed to identify any specific predictors of response. Pentasa was well tolerated; more patients who received the placebo were withdrawn from treatment due to adverse events than those who received the highest dose of the active drug.

Table 10.1 Response rates of remission in studies comparing 5-ASA to placebo or glucocorticoid therapy

Study	Drug dose	No. of patients	Duration (weeks)	Placebo	% remission 5-ASA	GL
NCCDS (1979)[4]	SPS 4–6 g/day	236	17	30	43	–
ECCDS (1984)[5]	SPS 3 g/day	159	18	38	50	82
Rasmussen *et al.* (1987)[6]	Pentasa 1·5 g/day	67	16	30	40	–
Mahida and Jewell *et al.* (1990)[7]	Pentasa 1·5 g/day	40	6	–	–	–
Singleton *et al.* (1993)[8]	Pentasa 1,2,4 g	310	16	18 placebo vs 4 g 18	43	–
Schölmerich *et al.* (1990)[11]	Pentasa 2 g	62	24	–	27	66
Martin *et al.* (1990)[12]	Salofalk 3 g/day	55	12	–	47	46
Maier *et al.* (1990)[14]	Salofalk 3 g/day	52	12	–	83	88
Thomsen *et al.* (1996)[13]	Pentasa 4 g	182	16	–	36	62
Prantera *et al.* (1993)[15]	Asacol 4 g, 5-ASA microgranules	94	12	–	60	61
Gross (1995)[16]	Salofalk 4·5 g	34	8	–	40	56·3

Source: Feagan B. *Eur J Surg* 1998;**164**:903–9:
SFS sulfasalazine; GL, glucocorticoids; 5-ASA, 5-aminosalicylate; NCCDS, National Cooperative Crohn's Disease Study;
ECCDS, European Cooperative Crohn's Disease Study

Although this trial suggested a benefit of high dose 5-ASA therapy, a cautionary note was raised subsequently by the principal investigator,[9] who described a second evaluation of Pentasa in 232 patients. Recently data from this trial and a third unpublished study have been combined in a meta-analysis[10] which suggested that patients assigned to 4 g/day Pentasa (*n* = 304) improved on average only 18 points more on the CDAI score than those who received a placebo (*n* = 311). Ala No difference in remission rates were observed. Readers should be aware that a minimum clinically important difference in CDAI score is approximately 50 points.

No trials of adequate power have compared the efficacy of the newer 5-ASA drugs and sulfasalazine. However, several studies have compared 5-ASA to glucocorticoid therapy for induction of remission (see Table 10.1). Schölmerich[11] randomized 62 patients to receive either 5-ASA at a dose of 2 g/day or a standard tapering regimen of methyl prednisolone. In this 24-week trial 73% of the 5-ASA-treated patients failed therapy compared with 34% of those who received methyl prednisolone (ARR 39%, NNT = 3; *P* = 0·0019). Alc The authors concluded that treatment with 5-ASA, although well tolerated, was inferior· to steroid therapy. Martin *et al.*[12] compared a 3 g/day dose of Salofalk to a standard oral prednisone regimen. Although a similar proportion of individuals in the two treatment groups entered remission (47% 5-ASA *v* 46% prednisone; *P* = 0·59), an analysis of the change in mean CDAI and quality of life scores demonstrated a more rapid improvement in patients treated with prednisone. A study by Thomsen and colleagues provides important information on the relative efficacy of glucocorticoids and 5-ASA.[13] In this methodologically rigorous trial 182 patients

with active disease were assigned to receive either 9 mg/day of a controlled ileal release preparation of budesonide (a locally active steroid) or 4 g/day of Pentasa. Following 16 weeks of treatment, 62% of budesonide treated patients were in remission compared with only 36% of the patients who received 5-ASA (ARR 26%, NNT = 4, *P* < 0·01). Ald

What conclusions can be drawn from these trials? The existing data show that the newer 5-ASA compounds are not more effective than sulfasalazine and are, at best, only marginally superior to a placebo for the induction of remission. A single clinical trial has demonstrated the superiority of budesonide over high dose 5-ASA with no increased frequency of adverse events. Although many clinicians prescribe 5-ASA compounds as first-line therapy for mild disease activity and treat those patients who fail to achieve a remission with glucocorticoids, the wisdom of this approach is questionable. Although the reluctance of physicians to expose individuals to glucocorticoid therapy is understandable, the likelihood of a response to the newer 5-ASA formulations is so low that the strategy is inefficient. Most patients will ultimately require glucocorticoid treatment to induce remission. In any event, if a 5-ASA drug is used for induction remission in patients with mild disease the best evidence supports the use of sulfasalazine. Alc

Glucocorticoids

Conventional steroids

The conventional glucocorticoid compounds, prednisone and 6-methyl prednisolone, are highly effective drugs for the treatment of active CD. The National Cooperative Crohn's Disease Study (NCCDS) and the European Cooperative Crohn's Disease Study (ECCDS) both showed that approximately 70% of patients who are treated with 40–60 mg/day of prednisone for 3–4 months enter remission,[4,5] compared with 30% of patients treated with placebo (see Figure 10.1). Ala

Budesonide

Glucocorticoids have pluripotent actions on the immune system, including effects on the synthesis of inflammatory mediators, cellular immunity and neutrophil function.[17] Since the glucocorticoid receptor is widely expressed in tissues, the biological actions of these drugs are not restricted to the immune system. Unpleasant cosmetic effects (acne, moon faces, bruising) and more serious metabolic disturbances (hypertension, metabolic bone disease, and diabetes) are common[18] and limit the usefulness of these agents. An ideal glucocorticoid should retain the efficacy of conventional glucocorticoid drugs while minimizing systemic effects. One possible means of achieving this objective is to specifically target the bowel wall as the therapeutic compartment of interest.[19] The development of budesonide as a treatment for active CD is an example of this approach.

Budesonide is a novel glucocorticoid with a potency approximately five times that of prednisone. The systemic effects of budesonide are reduced in comparison to conventional steroid drugs as a result of extensive first pass metabolism to inactive compounds. Thus a high local anti-inflammatory effect on mucosal surfaces is possible with low systemic activity.[20] Proof of this concept was first demonstrated in asthma therapy, where topical budesonide was shown to be highly effective with few or no systemic adverse effects.[21] An oral controlled ileal release formulation of budesonide was developed for the treatment of active CD of the ileum and right colon. A Canadian multicenter dose finding study[22] found that, first, 9 mg/day of budesonide was more effective than a placebo for the induction of remission in patients with moderately active CD (51% v 20%, P < 0·001) and, second, the proportion of patients experiencing glucocorticoid-related adverse effects with this drug was not greater than with placebo treatment (26% 9 mg budesonide v 26% placebo, P > 0·05). Alc In a second study, Rutgeerts and colleagues[23] compared 9 mg/day of budesonide with a standard prednisolone regimen. Although a favorable trend in response rate was observed in favor of prednisolone therapy, the difference in efficacy between the treatment groups was not large (65% v 52%, P = 0·12). There were fewer glucocorticoid-related adverse events in patients who received budesonide (budesonide 29%, prednisolone 55%, ARR 26%, NNT = 4, P = 0·003). Alc Finally, as described earlier, Thomsen and colleagues[13] have shown that 9 mg/day of budesonide is more effective than 4 g/day of 5-ASA and is

equally well tolerated. Data from the studies have been summarized in a meta-analysis by Kane and colleagues[24] who estimated that budesonide was approximately 13% less effective than conventional glucocorticoid therapy but was 35% less likely to cause glucocorticoid-related adverse events. Ala Thus, budesonide is an attractive alternative to 5-ASA or prednisone for induction of remission in patients whose disease is restricted to the appropriate anatomical sites.

Antibiotics

A substantial body of experimental evidence supports the notion that bacteria play an important role in initiating and/or sustaining the pathological inflammatory reaction in the bowel wall.[25,26] Antibiotics have been used empirically for the treatment of active CD for many years, and review articles and textbooks of medicine commonly advocate their use. However, few good data exist to support this endorsement. The Cooperative Crohn's Disease Study in Sweden[27] compared 800 mg/day of metronidazole to 1·5 g/day of sulfasalazine in 78 patients with active disease. A 25% response rate for both treatments was shown. Accordingly, it is debatable whether these results are more consistent with an equivalent benefit of metronidazole or the lack of any therapeutic effect for either treatment. The largest trial of metronidazole, carried out by Sutherland and colleagues,[28] randomized patients to receive metronidazole (10 or 20 mg/kg per day) or a placebo for 16 weeks (n = 105). Metronidazole therapy produced a dose-dependent decrease of disease activity (decrease in CDAI: metronidazole 20 mg/kg 97, 10 mg/kg 60, placebo 1; P = 0·001). However, no difference in remission rate was observed (proportion in remission: placebo 25%, metronidazole 10 mg/kg 36%, 20 mg/kg 27%). Thus, the controlled data that support the efficacy of metronidazole are not impressive. Ald

More recently the quinolone antibiotic ciprofloxacin has been used in combination with metronidazole. Prantera and colleagues[29] randomized 41 patients to receive combined antibiotics (ciprofloxacin 500 mg twice daily *and* 250 mg of metronidazole four times daily) or methyl prednisolone 0·7–1·0 mg/kg for 12 weeks. A statistically significant difference in patients entering remission was not demonstrated (combined antibiotic therapy 10/22 (46%), steroid therapy 12/19 (63%), P > 0·05). The small number of patients in this trial does not permit any definitive conclusion regarding the value of combined antibiotic therapy; however, the 17% difference in remission rates in favor of methyl prednisolone is most consistent with a clinically meaningful treatment advantage in favor of glucocorticoid therapy. Ald

Steinhart *et al.*[30] conducted a double blind study of oral ciprofloxacin and metronidazole, (both 500 mg twice daily), or placebo for 8 weeks in 134 patients with active CD of the ileum, right colon or both. All patients received oral budesonide 9 mg once daily. At week 8, 21 patients (33%) assigned to antibiotics were in remission, compared with 25 patients (38%) in the placebo group ($P = 0.55$; 95% confidence interval (CI) −21% to 11%). Ala An interaction ($P = 0.025$) between treatment allocation and disease location on treatment response was identified. Among patients with disease of the colon, 9 of 17 (53%) were in remission after treatment with antibiotics, compared with 4 of 16 (25%) of those who received placebo ($P = 0.10$). Discontinuation of therapy because of adverse events occurred in 13 of 66 (20%) patients treated with antibiotics, compared with 0 of 68 in the group who received placebo ($P < 0.001$). In patients with active CD of the ileum, the addition of ciprofloxacin and metronidazole to budesonide was an ineffective intervention. Although this antibiotic combination may improve outcome when there is involvement of the colon, the evidence supporting this possibility comes only from a *post hoc* analysis of a small number of patients and was not statistically significant.

In summary, glucocorticoids are the most effective treatment for active CD. For those patients whose disease is confined to the terminal ileum and/or right colon, budesonide is an attractive alternative to the conventional glucocorticoids because of the lower incidence of adverse events. Sulfasalazine is modestly effective in patients with mild disease activity. Although the newer 5-ASA compounds and antibiotics are used by many clinicians to treat patients with milder forms of the disease, current data do not support the efficacy of these drugs.

Treatment of therapy-resistant or steroid-dependent patients

Munkholm and colleagues[31] have documented the natural history of an acute exacerbation of CD in a cohort of patients from Copenhagen county. One year after an initial course of treatment a high proportion (56%) of their patients were either therapy resistant (20%) or steroid dependent (36%). This observation has led many clinicians to conclude that earlier and more aggressive treatment with immunosuppressives may be warranted in selected patients.

Conventional immunosuppressive drugs

Three classes of drugs have been most frequently used: the purine antimetabolites (azathioprine (AZA)/6-mercaptopurine), cyclosporin, and methotrexate.

Purine antimetabolites

Until recently the use of the purine antimetabolites for the treatment of refractory patients was not widely accepted,

perhaps because of the inconsistent results obtained from the early randomized trials of these drugs. However, recent studies have for the most part confirmed their efficacy. One of the more important trials was conducted by Candy *et al.*,[32] who randomized 63 patients with active CD to receive a standard tapering induction regimen of prednisone over 3 months and either AZA 2.5 mg/kg daily or a placebo for 15 months. Although no early (3 months) benefit of AZA was identified with respect to remission rates (CDAI < 150 and no prednisone), the proportion of patients who remained in remission over the entire follow up time was greater in the AZA group (42% v 7%, ARR 35%, NNT = 3; $P = 0.001$). Alc This result is consistent with observational data that suggest that the purine antimetabolites require a minimum of 3 months to show a treatment effect. In an attempt to overcome this theoretical limitation Sandborn *et al.*[33] did a small, uncontrolled study in which patients with active CD received an intravenous 1800 mg loading dose of AZA. This strategy rapidly achieved stable erythrocyte concentrations of the thiol metabolites, which are believed to be responsible for the immunosuppressive effects of AZA. Despite this promising finding, a subsequent RCT which evaluated 96 patients showed equally low (8-week) remission rates in patients who received either loading or conventional AZA regimens (25% v 24%)[34] in spite of achieving steady state nucleotide levels by week 2. Ald Furthermore, the proportion of patients entering remission did not increase after 8 weeks of treatment. It should be noted that all patients in this study received oral AZA in a dose of 2 mg/kg and that the proportion of these patients who entered remission and withdrew completely from steroids was only 24%, a figure roughly comparable with the expected response to a placebo in many induction of remission studies. The data are consistent with a slow onset of effect for the purine antimetabolites.

The data from the RCTs which have evaluated the purine antimetabolites for the treatment of active CD in adults have been summarized in a meta-analysis[35] in which the pooled ARR for AZA treatment for induction of remission is approximately 20% (NNT = 5) (Figure 10.2). Ald In the majority of these studies patients were receiving concomitant corticosteroid therapy. A steroid-sparing effect was also demonstrated in this analysis: the NNT for steroid sparing (the NNT with AZA for one additional patient to reduce steroids to < 10 mg/day) was estimated to be 3. These results should be interpreted with a degree of caution, since important clinical heterogeneity exists among the studies in their definitions of treatment response, duration, and the use of cointerventions. No single large, well-designed trial that resulted in a clinically and statistically significant benefit compared with placebo exists. Nevertheless, the meta-analysis suggests that some beneficial effect is present on disease activity, and the use of these drugs can be recommended for treatment of patients who fail to respond to steroid therapy or develop steroid dependence.

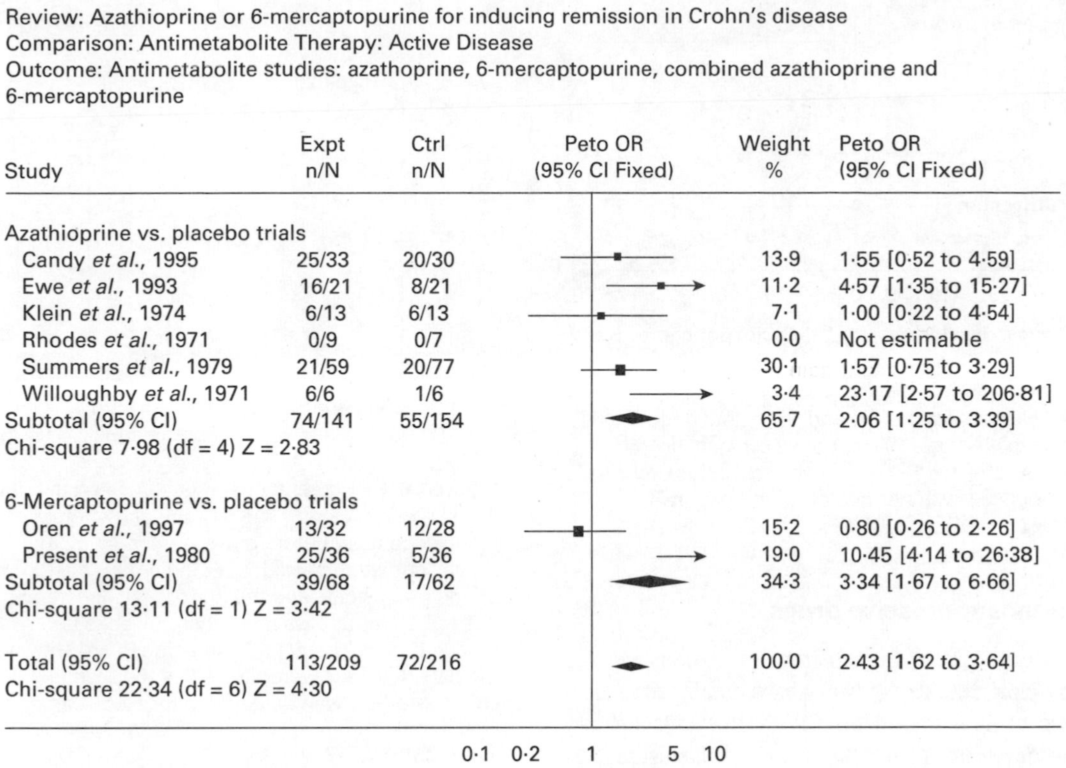

Review: Azathioprine or 6-mercaptopurine for inducing remission in Crohn's disease
Comparison: Antimetabolite Therapy: Active Disease
Outcome: Antimetabolite studies: azathioprine, 6-mercaptopurine, combined azathioprine and
6-mercaptopurine

Study	Expt n/N	Ctrl n/N	Peto OR (95% CI Fixed)	Weight %	Peto OR (95% CI Fixed)
Azathioprine vs. placebo trials					
Candy *et al.*, 1995	25/33	20/30		13·9	1·55 [0·52 to 4·59]
Ewe *et al.*, 1993	16/21	8/21		11·2	4·57 [1·35 to 15·27]
Klein *et al.*, 1974	6/13	6/13		7·1	1·00 [0·22 to 4·54]
Rhodes *et al.*, 1971	0/9	0/7		0·0	Not estimable
Summers *et al.*, 1979	21/59	20/77		30·1	1·57 [0·75 to 3·29]
Willoughby *et al.*, 1971	6/6	1/6		3·4	23·17 [2·57 to 206·81]
Subtotal (95% CI)	74/141	55/154		65·7	2·06 [1·25 to 3·39]
Chi-square 7·98 (df = 4) Z = 2·83					
6-Mercaptopurine vs. placebo trials					
Oren *et al.*, 1997	13/32	12/28		15·2	0·80 [0·26 to 2·26]
Present *et al.*, 1980	25/36	5/36		19·0	10·45 [4·14 to 26·38]
Subtotal (95% CI)	39/68	17/62		34·3	3·34 [1·67 to 6·66]
Chi-square 13·11 (df = 1) Z = 3·42					
Total (95% CI)	113/209	72/216		100·0	2·43 [1·62 to 3·64]
Chi-square 22·34 (df = 6) Z = 4·30					

0·1   0·2   1   5   10

Figure 10.2 Azathioprine or 6-mercaptopurine for inducing remission in Crohn's disease. (*Source*: Sandborn WJ *et al.* In: *Cochrane Library*, issue 2. Oxford: Update Software, 1999[35])

Cyclosporine

The emergence of this drug as a standard therapy for organ transplantation led to large scale evaluations for the treatment of chronically active CD. The results of four RCTs (Figure 10.3)[36] have shown that the therapeutic index of cyclosporin is low,[37–40] if there is any efficacy. Alc The study of Brynskov *et al.*,[38] which demonstrated only a modest benefit, used a high cyclosporin dose (7·6 mg/kg per day), which cannot be recommended for chronic treatment, since the risk of nephrotoxicity is unacceptably high.[41] The three trials[37–39] which assessed a dose of cyclosporin that is tolerable for long-term treatment (5 mg/kg per day) showed no benefit with this drug. Thus cyclosporin is not a practical therapy for long-term management. Although uncontrolled studies[42,43] have suggested that short duration, high dose intravenous therapy may be beneficial in patients with refractory CD, data from controlled trials are required before this intervention can be advocated for widespread use.

Methotrexate

The success of low dose (5–25 mg/weekly) methotrexate as a treatment for rheumatoid arthritis led to its evaluation in patients with chronically active CD. In 1989 Kozarek *et al.*[44]

reported the results of an open study in which two-thirds of patients with steroid refractory disease showed an improvement in symptoms and a concomitant reduction in prednisone requirements. B4 Some patients demonstrated an endoscopic remission. A controlled trial[45] was subsequently conducted in which 141 patients who had failed previous attempts to discontinue prednisone were randomized to receive either methotrexate 25 mg/weekly intramuscularly or a placebo for 16 weeks. All of the patients received 20 mg of prednisone per day at the initiation of the trial; a standardized prednisone withdrawal regimen was then used. Patients who responded to therapy discontinued prednisone entirely 12 weeks following randomization. A significant benefit of methotrexate therapy was observed for the primary outcome measure, the proportion of patients who were completely withdrawn from prednisone *and* in clinical remission as defined by a CDAI score of < 150 points (methotrexate 39%, placebo 19%, ARR 20%, NNT = 5; *P* = 0·025) (Figure 10.4). Ala Improvements in the median prednisone dose, Health Related Quality of Life and mean CDAI scores, and concentration of serum acute phase reactants were also associated with methotrexate therapy. In this short-term trial, no serious toxicity was observed, although withdrawals from treatment due to nausea were more common with methotrexate.

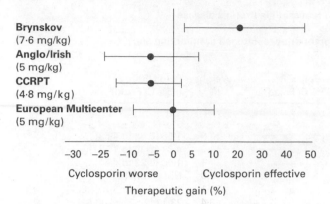

Figure 10.3 Point estimates (•) and 95% confidence limits (|–|) of the therapeutic gain (% response cyclosporin–% response placebo) for four RCTs of cyclosporin for Crohn's disease. (Reproduced with permission from Feagan B. *Inflamm Bowel Dis* 1995;**1**:335–9[36])

Novel immunosuppressive drugs

New knowledge of the human immune system and the growth of the biotechnology industry have combined to yield an abundance of new treatments for chronic inflammatory diseases. The development of infliximab and natalizumab as therapies for CD are examples of the promise of this new technology.

Infliximab

Tumor necrosis factor (TNF)-α is a proinflammatory cytokine which plays an important part in the pathophysiology of CD.[46] Following the successful treatment of a young woman with a chimeric anti-TNF-α antibody by investigators in Amsterdam,[47] a series of controlled studies were initiated. Targan and colleagues[48] carried out a multicenter dose finding study that evaluated 108 patients whose disease was refractory to other forms of treatment. Patients with moderately severe disease received one of three doses of infliximab (5, 10, 20 mg/kg) or a placebo administered as a single intravenous infusion. Patients continued to receive other treatments at a fixed dose. The primary endpoint of the study was the occurrence of a clinical response as defined by a decrement of 70 points in the CDAI score from the baseline value. No dose–response relationship was identified; 81·5% of infliximab-treated patients responded compared with 16·7% of those who received the placebo (ARR 65%, NNT = 2; $P < 0.001$). Ala Minor allergic reactions to the antibody occurred infrequently but clinically significant adverse effects were not encountered in this short-term study.

In a second pivotal trial colleagues evaluated the efficacy of infliximab for the treatment of patients with fistulizing CD[49] (no previous controlled trials had evaluated this population of patients). The patients studied had active, fistulizing

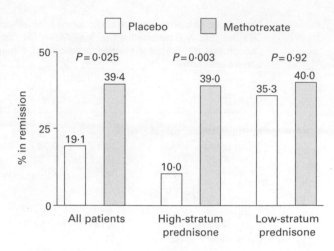

Figure 10.4 Percentages of patients in remission at week 16 according to study group and stratum of daily prednisone dose before entry into the study. The high prednisone stratum was receiving a daily dose of more than 20 mg prednisone, and the low prednisone stratum a daily dose of 20 mg or less more than 2 weeks before randomization. The actual percentages are shown above the bars. *P* values were derived by the Mantel–Haenszel chi-square test, with adjustment for study center. (Reproduced with permission from Feagan BG *et al. N Engl J Med* 1995;**332**:292–7[45])

disease for a minimum of 3 months prior to randomization. Concomitant treatment with steroids, 6-mercaptopurine or AZA, and antibiotics was permitted although the dose of these cointerventions was maintained at a stable level throughout the trial. The primary measure of response was a 50% reduction in the number of open fistulae. Ninety-four patients received three intravenous infusions of either a placebo or one of two dose regimens of antibody (5 or 10 mg/kg) during a total of 18 weeks of follow up. Patients treated with infliximab were significantly more likely to respond (61·9% *v* 25·8%, ARR 36·1%, NNT = 3; $P = 0.002$). Ala The response to treatment was rapid and in many cases dramatic. Again, no dose–response relationship was identifiable.

It is clear that infliximab is effective for induction of remission of CD in a patient population refractory to other treatments and that serious short-term toxicity is uncommon. However, potential safety concerns include the formation of autoantibodies, the risk of infusion reactions with re-treatment, and a possible increased risk of lymphoproliferative disease. Currently it is most appropriate to reserve infliximab as an induction treatment for individuals who have failed to respond to or are intolerant of conventional drug treatments.

Natalizumab

Natalizumab, a recombinant, humanized monoclonal antibody against the $\alpha 4$ integrin, was evaluated in a randomized trial in 248 patients with moderate to severe CD (CDAI > 220, < 450).[50] Approximately half the patients were receiving steroids (< 25 mg daily) and about one-third were receiving AZA or mercaptopurine. Patients received two infusions four weeks apart: two placebo infusions, or one infusion of natalizumab 3 mg/kg and one placebo infusion, or two infusions of natalizumab, either 3 or 6 mg/kg. The primary endpoint for this study was remission (CDAI < 150) at 6 weeks. The remission rates for patients receiving placebo and two infusions of natalizumab 3 mg/kg were 27% and 44% (ARR = 17%, NNT = 6; *P* = 0·027). Ala Significant differences in rates of remission were observed as early as 2 weeks and were maintained for 12 weeks. Statistically significant differences in the primary were not observed between the other treatment groups. However, patients receiving two infusions of the higher dose were more likely to be in remission than placebo-treated patients at both 4 and 8 weeks following infusions. Furthermore, response rates (decrease in CDAI of ≥ 70) and disease-specific quality of life scores Inflammatory Bowel Disease Questionnaire (IBDQ) were found to be greater with all three regimens of natalizumab infusion than with placebo at most time intervals. No serious adverse events were attributable to treatment with this antibody preparation. However, antibodies to natalizumab were detected in 7% of treated patients. Mild infusion reactions occurred in two patients. Despite these promising initial results, preliminary data from a follow up study of similar design failed to confirm a benefit of natalizumab for induction of remission.[51] A large scale RCT evaluating the role of natalizumab maintenance therapy will be reported later this year.

Maintenance of remission

The objectives of maintenance therapy are to prevent the recurrence of symptoms, to reduce the risk of complications, and to avoid the need for surgery and hospitalization. One year after a medically induced remission of CD approximately 30–40% of patients will experience a relapse of disease[52]; and following surgery symptoms recur at a rate of approximately 15% per year.[53] The failure of the maintenance therapy components of the NCCD[4] and ECCDS[5] trials to demonstrate a long-term benefit of sulfasalazine or conventional, low dose glucocorticoid therapy Alc led to the extensive evaluation of the newer 5-ASA and budesonide for this indication.

5-Aminosalicylates

Over 20 clinical trials have compared a 5-ASA drug with a placebo for the prevention of a symptomatic recurrence following either surgery or a medically induced remission. A number of the studies that have evaluated 5-ASA for the latter indication showed a 1-year reduction in the rate of relapse of about 10–20%. In the "typical" trial the size of the treatment

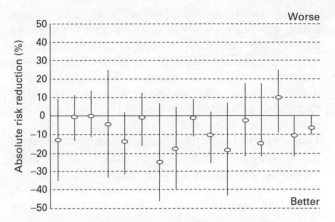

Figure 10.5 Meta-analysis of 5-aminosalicylate drugs for maintenance therapy in Crohn's disease. (Adapted with permission from Camma C *et al.* Mesalamine in the maintenance treatment of Crohn's disease: a meta-analysis adjusted for confounding variables. *Gastroenterology* 1997;**13**:1465–73[57])

effect observed is less than that which the investigators considered to be clinically important when the sample size for the trial was determined. Thus statistical significance has not often been demonstrated. To illustrate this point, consider the results of the trial of Sutherland *et al.*,[54] who randomized 293 patients with quiescent disease to receive either 3 g/day of 5-ASA or placebo for 1 year. A total of 25% of the patients who received the active treatment experienced a relapse compared with 36% of those who received the placebo (ARR 11%, *P* = 0·056). Ala

In an attempt to provide a more precise estimate of the magnitude of the treatment effect of 5-ASA several meta-analyses[55–57] have been done. Some caution is warranted when considering the data from these overview analyses. First, meta-analysis is an observational procedure (unlike the RCT) which is susceptible to bias.[58] As noted previously, Singleton has documented the occurrence of publication bias with respect to the trials which evaluated 5-ASA for the therapy of active disease.[9] Another issue is the considerable heterogeneity which exists in the published literature. The variability of study design, patient populations, and the drug formulations/doses which have been evaluated is a concern. Notwithstanding these considerations, meta-analysis does provide important information.

A meta-analysis performed by Camma *et al.*[57] (Figure 10.5) evaluated 15 maintenance trials, which included a total of 2097 patients and suggested an overall ARR of 6·3% per year for 5-ASA therapy in comparison with a placebo (95% CI − 2·1% to − 10·4%). Ala The results of a subgroup analysis demonstrated that the benefit of 5-ASA was most apparent in the post-surgical trials where an ARR of 13·1% was calculated (95% CI − 4·5% to − 21·8%). No statistically significant result was observed for those trials that evaluated 5-ASA after a medically induced remission (ARR 4·7%; 95% CI − 9·6% to 2·8%). Ala Patients with ileal disease and prolonged disease duration were most likely to benefit from therapy. Thus it seemed that a relatively clear picture of the efficacy of 5-ASA maintenance therapy had emerged. The majority of RCTs showed a modest effect of treatment. If the ARR of 13% identified by the Camma meta-analysis is accepted as the best estimate of the true value of 5-ASA therapy, the NNT for 1 year to prevent one symptomatic recurrence of the disease is 8. Whether a benefit of this magnitude is meaningful given the cost[58] and inconvenience of the drug depends on patients' wishes, previous disease severity, the anatomical location of disease and whether or not maintenance treatment follows surgery.

Subsequent to this meta-analysis, two additional large randomized trials have been done. Lochs et al.[59] randomized 318 patients within 10 days of resection of all severe visible disease (approximately 30% of patients had some residual disease judged to be not severe) to receive 4 g of mesalamine (Pentasa) or a placebo for 18 months. Clinical relapse was defined as an increase in CDAI above 250, or a CDAI score above 200 but with a minimum 60-point increase from the lowest postoperative value for 2 consecutive weeks. The observed proportions of clinical relapse (± 1 SE) were not significantly different (placebo 31·4 ± 3·7%, mesalamine 24·5 ± 3·6%; $P = 0·1$, 1-sided test). Ala Although study medication was discontinued by 32% of mesalamine and 26% of placebo-treated patients, two separate per protocol analyses failed to reveal significant differences between the treatment groups. Subgroup analysis revealed a difference in recurrence between mesalamine and placebo-treated patients with disease confined to the small intestine: (placebo 39·7 ± 6·1%, mesalamine 21·8 ± 5·6%, $P = 0·002$, 1-sided log-rank test).

The second study[60] which randomized 328 patients to 2 g of olsalazine or placebo for 82 weeks following a medically induced remission, again, failed to show a benefit for 5-ASA maintenance therapy. (relapse rate 48·5% olsalazine v 45% placebo). Ala

Sutherland[61] repeated the meta-analysis of Camma *et al.*[57] incorporating the data from Lochs' study, and calculated an ARR of only 4% for this treatment in postsurgical patients, compared to 13% reported by Camma *et al.* Ala On the basis of these data it is increasingly difficult to support the chronic use of mesalamine therapy in CD.

Budesonide

The efficacy of budesonide for induction of remission in CD suggested that chronic therapy might be an effective and safe maintenance strategy. Four randomized placebo controlled trials[62–64] have evaluated the use of either 6 mg/day or 3 mg/day of budesonide for 1 year of treatment. The first three studies were of similar design, following treatment of

active CD with either budesonide, prednisolone or a placebo. Patients who responded to treatment were randomized to receive either one of the two doses of budesonide or a placebo. No other treatments for CD were permitted. The primary outcome measure of these studies was the proportion of symptomatic relapses of CD as defined by a 60 point increase in the CDAI and a minimum CDAI score of 200 at the time of the disease exacerbation.

Greenberg *et al.*[62] ($n = 105$) found that the median time to relapse or withdrawal from treatment differed significantly between the three treatment groups: budesonide-treated patients remained in remission longer than those who received the placebo (178 days 6 mg v 124 days 3 mg v 39 days placebo; $P = 0·027$); however, the treatment effect was not durable. The greatest difference in remission rates was observed 3 months after randomization whereas at 1 year no significant differences were present (39% 6 mg v 30% 3 mg v 33% placebo). Ala Budesonide therapy was well tolerated. No differences were observed among the treatment groups in the proportion of patients who experienced adverse events (78% 6 mg v 70% 3 mg v 89% placebo). Although glucocorticoid-related adverse events occurred more frequently in patients who were treated with budesonide, the proportion of patients who reported these events decreased throughout the follow up period and the most common steroid-related adverse event identified was easy bruising. A dose-dependent depression of the plasma cortisol concentration was noted in the budesonide-treated groups.

Similar results were obtained by Löfberg and colleagues[63] ($n = 90$) who observed that the median time to relapse or discontinuation of therapy was 258 days for the 6 mg/day group, 139 days for the 3 mg/day group, and 92 days for the patients who received a placebo ($P = 0·021$). Again, the time in remission was significantly prolonged for those patients who received budesonide, but the therapeutic effect was not sustained. At 12 months following randomization, 41%, 26% and 37% of the 6 mg/day, 3 mg/day, and placebo group, respectively remained in remission ($P = 0·44$). Ala Thirty-eight percent of those patients who had received 6 mg/day reported glucocorticoid-related adverse events compared with 20% of those who received 3 mg/day and 12% of those who received the placebo.

The third trial, by Ferguson *et al.*,[64] which evaluated the smallest number of patients ($n = 75$), failed to demonstrate any benefit of budesonide treatment. The median time to relapse or discontinuation of therapy was 272 days in the 6 mg/day group, 321 days in the 3 mg/day group, and 290 days in the placebo group ($P = 0·80$). Alc A similar proportion of patients in the three treatment groups experienced glucocorticoid-related adverse events (18% 6 mg/day v 36% 3 mg/day and 15% placebo; $P = 0·79$).

An analysis of the pooled data from these studies[65] and a fourth, as yet unpublished trial (Hanauer S and Sandborn WJ, personal communication), show that on average an additional 114 days of remission is attributable to the continued use of 6 mg/day of budesonide over 1 year compared with placebo ($P = 0.002$). Ala Examination of the pooled toxicity data from these studies confirms the absence of serious glucocorticoid-related adverse effects, although moon face and acne were more common in patients who received active treatment.

Two additional randomized trials that used endoscopic relapse following surgery as endpoints have not demonstrated significant prolongation of remission with this therapy. Hellers et al.[66] randomized 129 patients following ileal or ileocecal resection to receive budesonide 6 mg daily or a placebo.[5] Ileocolonoscopy including biopsy was carried out 3 and 12 months after surgery. The frequency of endoscopic recurrence did not differ between the groups. Ala The investigators reported a subgroup analysis which suggested that recurrence at 12 months was lower in patients who had undergone surgery for control of disease activity rather than for stricture (budesonide 32%, placebo 65%; $P = 0.047$). However, this *post hoc* analysis should be viewed with caution.

Ewe et al.[67] randomized 88 patients to receive budesonide 3 mg (pH-modified release formulation) or a placebo for 1 year. Endoscopic recurrence at 3 and 12 months was the primary measure of efficacy. The recurrence rate was not reduced by active treatment (budesonide 57%, placebo 70%; $P < 0.05$). Survival analysis also failed to show prolongation of remission with active therapy. Alc

Given the lack of sustained benefit observed in any of these trials we do not recommend continued budesonide therapy for patients who have entered remission during treatment with this intervention.

Antituberculous therapy

A systematic review[68] of antituberculous therapy for maintenance of remission in CD demonstrated a possible small benefit in patients in whom remission was induced by steroid. However, this observation was derived from a meta-analysis of subgroups from only two trials involving 90 patients, and the authors of the review do not recommend this form of therapy in the absence of further trials.

Nitroimadazole antibiotics

Only one RCT[69] has assessed metronidazole for postoperative maintenance therapy. In this study 66 patients were randomized to 2 weeks of therapy with 20 mg/kg per day of metronidazole or placebo within 1 week of surgical resection of all visible disease. Following 12 weeks of therapy endoscopic recurrence occurred in 52% of patients assigned to metronidazole compared with 75% of those who received placebo ($P = 0.09$). Alc Furthermore, significant effect was

shown for clinical recurrence at 1 year (4% for metronidazole v 25% for placebo ($P = 0.046$). However, peripheral neuropathy was common making continuous therapy impracticable. A second trial[70] of a potentially less neurotoxic nitroimadazole, ornidazole, also suggested a maintenance benefit of antibiotic therapy; unfortunately clinically relevant neuropathy was also observed. These two trials indicate that manipulation of the endogenous bacterial flora with antibiotics may ultimately prove to be effective strategy for the prevention of postoperative recurrence. Unfortunately the problems of antibiotic resistance and neuropathy mitigate against the use of nitroimadazole antibiotics as long-term treatments.

Azathioprine

A systematic review published by Pearson et al.[71] analyzed the results of five randomized trials of AZA, of which two[72,73] studied only patients with quiescent disease and three[4,8,25] enrolled patients in a separate phase of a trial which also included patients with active disease. These trials were all relatively small, with a total of 319 patients included. The overall rate of maintenance of remission was 91/136 (67%; CI 59 to 75%) for treatment compared with 96/183 (52%; CI 45 to 60%) for placebo (Figure 10.6). The analysis suggested that higher doses of AZA were more effective than a dose of 1 mg/kg. The Peto odds ratio for response to azathioprine was 2·16 (CI 1·35 to 3·47). The NNT to prevent one recurrence was 7. Ala There was some evidence of a steroid-sparing effect, although this was based on the analysis of only 30 patients in two trials. Patients who received AZA were at greater risk of withdrawal from studies due to adverse events compared with those on placebo (Peto odds ratio 4·36, CI 1·63 to 11·67). The number needed to harm (NNH) was estimated to be 19. Ala Withdrawals due to adverse effects were noted in 5·8% of those patients receiving therapy, and 1·3% of the patients who were not. Common events for withdrawal included pancreatitis, leukopenia, nausea, "allergy", and infection.

Markowitz et al.[74] conducted a study that included 55 children (age 13 +/− 2 years) who were randomized within 8 weeks of initial diagnosis to receive treatment with 6-mercaptopurine (1·5 mg/kg per day) or a placebo for 18 months in addition to prednisone (40 mg/day), with prednisone dosage withdrawal based on a defined schedule. Although remission was induced in 89% of both groups, only 9% of the remitters in the 6-mercaptopurine group relapsed compared with 47% of controls ($P = 0.007$) (Figure 10.7). Alc In the 6-mercaptopurine group, the duration of steroid use was shorter ($P < 0.001$) and the cumulative steroid dose lower at 6, 12, and 18 months ($P < 0.01$).

Growth was comparable in both groups. No clinically significant adverse events occurred, although mild leukopenia and increases in aminotransferase activity were noted in the 6-mercaptopurine group. 6-Mercaptopurine decreased the

Review: Azathioprine for maintaining remission of Crohn's disease
Comparison: Antimetabolite vs. placebo: quiescent disease
Outcome: Maintenance of remission

Study	Expt n/N	Ctrl n/N	Peto OR (95% CI Fixed)	Weight %	Peto OR (95% CI Fixed)
Azathioprine dose 2·5 mg/kg/day					
Candy *et al.*, 1995	14/25	2/20		15·1	7·12 [2·11 to 23·99]
Summers *et al.*, 1979	16/19	15/20		9·4	1·73 [0·37 to 8·05]
Subtotal (95% CI)	30/44	17/40		24·5	4·13 [1·59 to 10·71]
Chi-square 2·00 (df = 1) Z = 2·92					
Azathioprine dose 2·0 mg/kg/day					
O'Donoghue *et al.*, 197	13/23	8/27		17·9	2·95 [0·97 to 9·00]
Rosenberg *et al.*, 1975	7/10	4/10		7·5	3·16 [0·57 to 17·62]
Willoughby *et al.*, 1971	4/5	2/5		3·9	4·48 [0·41 to 49·43]
Subtotal (95% CI)	24/38	14/42		29·3	3·17 [1·33 to 7·59]
Chi-square 0·10 (df = 2) Z = 2·60					
Azathioprine dose 1·0 mg/kg/day					
Summers *et al.*, 1979	37/34	65/101		46·2	1·20 [0·60 to 2·41]
Subtotal (95% CI)	37/54	65/101		46·2	1·20 [0·60 to 2·41]
Chi-square 0·00 (df = 0) Z = 0·52					
Total (95% CI)	91/136	96/183		100·0	2·16 [1·35 to 3·47]
Chi-square 7·37 (df = 5) Z = 3·20					

0·1 0·2   1   5   10

Favors Placebo   Favors Azathioprine

Figure 10.6 Azathioprine for maintaining remission of Crohn's disease. (*Source*: Pearson DC *et al.* In: *Cochrane Library*, issue 2. Oxford: Update Software, 1999[68])

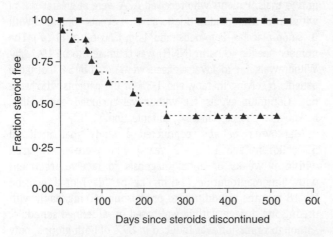

Figure 10.7 Time (days) off of corticosteroid treatment after initial discontinuation, depicted as a Kaplan–Meier survival curve.[74] ■ 6-mercaptopurine; ▲ controls; *P* < 0·0001

need for corticosteroids and decreased the frequency of relapses.

Minor toxicity, such as nausea, fatigue, skin rash, fever and arthralgias, is relatively common with the purine antimetabolites. Asymptomatic elevation of liver and pancreatic enzymes also occur frequently. Clinically important pancreatitis occurs in 3% of patients. Although leukopenia, defined by a white blood cell count of < 3·8, develops in approximately 20% of patients per year, infection associated with severe neutropenia is uncommon.[75] Whether therapeutic drug monitoring can improve efficacy and/or reduce toxicity remains controversial[76] and is being investigated by a National Institute for Health sponsored RCT. In the USA the Food and Drug Administration has recommended genotype testing prior to the initiation of treatment so that patients with low thiopurine methyltransferase activity can be identified. These individuals develop profound leukopenia following treatment with either agent. No studies have compared this strategy to the usual clinical practice of initiating treatment with a relatively low drug dose and following the white blood cell count each week.

In summary, AZA or 6-mercaptopurine are moderately effective for maintenance of remission in adults and children and are relatively well tolerated.

Methotrexate

The efficacy of methotrexate in a dose of 15 mg per week for maintaining remission was evaluated in 76 patients with quiescent CD. Patients who entered remission and were

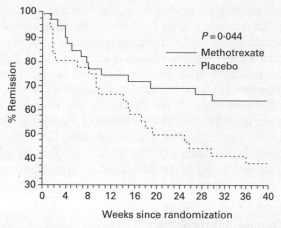

% Remission vs Weeks since randomization

$P = 0.044$

— Methotrexate
---- Placebo

Methotrexate	40	36	30	29	28	27	27	26	25	24	19
Placebo		36	29	28	24	21	18	18	16	15	15	12

Figure 10.8 6-MP for maintenance of remission of Crohn's disease in children. Adapted from Markowitz *et al.*[74]

totally withdrawn from steroids during the induction phase of the trial methotrexate for induction of remission described above[8] and additional patients who entered remission on a similar regimen outside the trial were randomized to receive methotrexate 15 mg weekly (40 patients) or a placebo (36 patients) for 40 weeks.[77] Methotrexate was effective for maintaining remission (proportion in remission at 40 weeks: methotrexate 65%, placebo 38·9%, ARR 0·26, NNT 4; $P = 0.01$). Alc The survival data for maintenance of remission are shown in Figure 10.8, Methotrexate also reduced the requirement for prednisone use (methotrexate 27·5%, placebo 58·3%, $P = 0.01$) and mean disease activity (CDAI) score at week 40 (methotrexate 135 ± 16, placebo 196 ± 18; $P = 0.005$). Only one methotrexate-treated patient withdrew because of nausea and no serious adverse events occurred. A low dose of methotrexate is safe and effective for maintaining remission in patients who have responded to methotrexate for inducing remission of active disease. The available data regarding the short-term efficacy of methotrexate have been summarized in a recently published systematic review.[78]

The adverse event profile of low dose methotrexate is well established.[79] The most common minor adverse effect is nausea, which tends to develop for a period of 24–48 hours after the weekly injection. This problem, which occurs in at most 15% of patients, can usually be managed by coadministration of oral folate (1 mg every day), use of antinauseants around the time of dosing (metoclopramide, odansetron), or, uncommonly, dose reduction. As with the purine antimetabolites, leukopenia and associated opportunistic infections occur uncommonly. Methotrexate is teratogenic and must not be given to women of childbearing potential. This issue is the most important limitation to the use of the drug. Hepatotoxicity was first documented in psoriatic patients. Subsequent understanding of pharmacokinetics and the conversion to weekly, from daily,

dosing has virtually eliminated this problem. Patients should be monitored according to the American Rheumatological Association guidelines,[80] paraphrased as follows: (i) avoid treating patients with risk factors for hepatotoxicity (obesity, diabetes, excessive alcohol use), and (ii) measure transaminases every 4–6 weeks. If, over the course of 1 year, more than half of the transaminase values are abnormal, take a liver biopsy before continuing treatment. Finally, no good data indicate that methotrexate is associated with malignancy.

Monoclonal antibodies

Infliximab

The first RCT to evaluate the efficacy of infliximab as a maintenance therapy was carried out by Rutgeerts *et al.*[81] Seventy-six patients with moderate to severe disease who had responded to induction therapy with the antibody were re-randomized to receive infliximab 10 mg/kg or a placebo at weeks 12, 20, 28, and 36. Cointerventions permitted in the induction phase (6-mercaptopurine, AZA or mesalamine) were continued at the same dose in the maintenance phase.

The proportions of patients in clinical remission 8 weeks after the last infusion in the infliximab and placebo groups were 52·9% and 20%, respectively (ARR 0·329, NNT 3, $P = 0.013$). Alc The time to loss of response in these patients was also significantly prolonged by active treatment (infliximab > 47 weeks, placebo 37 weeks, $P = 0.057$).

Data from the recently published ACCENT I[82] ($n = 573$) trial confirm the efficacy of infliximab as a maintenance therapy. In this study, patients who responded to infliximab induction therapy were randomly assigned to receive continued treatment with the drug at one of two doses (5 mg/kg *v* 10 mg/kg) or placebo, administered every 8 weeks. The design of this trial is complex and since patients were permitted to receive other forms of treatment, such as corticosteroids and antimetabolites, interpretation of the results is somewhat problematic. The most clinically relevant information can be obtained by examining a subgroup of approximately one-half of the patients who were receiving corticosteroid therapy at the baseline visit. Patients who received infusions of infliximab every 8 weeks were more likely to discontinue corticosteroid therapy and remain in remission compared with those who received placebo (Figure 10.9). Twenty-four percent of patients who received continuous infliximab therapy, 5 mg/kg every 8 weeks, were in remission and off corticosteroid therapy, at the end of the trial compared with 9% of those who received a placebo ($P = 0.03$). Alc Thus ACCENT 1 provides strong evidence for a maintenance benefit of infliximab in a group of high-risk patients.

Similar results regarding the long-term efficacy of infliximab in patients with fistulizing disease have also been obtained from the ACCENT II trial.[83] This RCT randomized 306 patients with draining abdominal or perianal fistulas to receive a three-dose induction regimen of infliximab 5 mg/kg

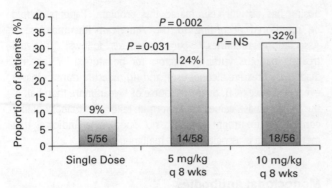

Figure 10.9 Clinical remission with complete steroid withdrawal at week 54 in ACCENT 1 (Adapted from Hanauer SB *et al. Lancet* 2002;**359**:1541–9[82]

at weeks 0, 2 and 6. Patients who achieved a response, defined by closure of 50% or more of the fistula orifices, were randomized to receive either continued treatment with infliximab 5 mg/kg every 8 weeks or placebo. Patients who received active treatment were significantly less likely to relapse during the course of the trial. The median time to loss of response was 14 weeks for placebo-treated patients compared with more than 40 weeks for those who received active drug. At week 54, 36% of patients treated with infliximab had complete closure or all draining fistulas compared with 19% of those who received only the three-dose induction regimen followed by placebo (*P* = 0·009). Ala

Although multiple concerns have been raised regarding the safety of infliximab therapy the initial experience with this agent has been for the most part favorable. Approximately 420 000 patients had been treated for rheumatoid arthritis and CD since the introduction of infliximab in the late 1990s. The most serious adverse events associated with TNF inhibition are tuberculosis, opportunistic infections and the risk of lymphoma. Tuberculosis following administration of anti-TNF inhibitors is usually the result of disease reactivation.[84,85] Since the introduction of appropriate screening methods[86] (identification of high-risk patients, tuberculin testing, chest radiography) the incidence of tuberculosis has declined. With respect to opportunistic infection, aspergillosis,[87–89] listeriosis and *Pneumocystis carinii* infections have been reported. The estimated rate of opportunistic infection is estimated at 0·43 cases per 1000 patient exposures. Many of the reported lymphomas have occurred in patients with rheumatoid arthritis. This disease has a greatly increased risk of lymphoma, that is correlated with disease activity. A recent FDA advisory meeting concluded that the rate of lymphoma associated with TNF-inhibitors may be no higher than that in the general rheumatoid arthritis population. The association between anti-TNF inhibitors and the development of congestive heart failure is also a concern.[90] Most cases have developed in patients with pre-existing congestive heart failure and thus a causal relationship is not clear. Finally, the immunogenicity of infliximab has been increasingly recognized as an important clinical issue. The development of antibodies to the drug may be associated with a wide array of allergic reactions. Moreover formation of neutralizing antibodies may result in diminished efficacy.[91] For this reason, interventions that are effective in reducing the incidence of antibody formation, such as coadministration of antimetabolites (AZA, 6-mercaptopurine, methotrexate) or infusion of hydrocortisone prior to treatment,[92] should be considered as part of a standard treatment regimen.

Omega-3 fatty acids

ω-3 fatty acids are polyunsaturated long-chain fatty acids derived from fish. Diets high in marine fish oils increase the concentrations of the ω-3 fatty acids, eicosapentaenoic acid and docosahexaenoic acid, in cell membranes. As a consequence, the concentration of the pro-inflammatory eicosanoid precursor, arachidonic acid is reduced which theoretically should attenuate inflammatory responses.[93,94]

A preliminary randomized controlled trial by Belluzzi and colleagues[95] evaluated the efficacy of an ω-3 fatty acid formulation in 78 patients with CD who were at a high risk for the development of a relapse. Patients were randomly assigned to receive either 4·5 g/day of ω-3 fatty acids or placebo for 1 year. At the end of treatment, 59% of the patients assigned to active treatment remained in remission as compared with 26% of those who received placebo (*P* < 0·001). Alc The only adverse event attributable to treatment was diarrhea which occurred in 10% of patients. No serious adverse events were observed. Two large-scale trials are currently underway that will further evaluate this approach to maintenance therapy.

Summary

An algorithm for the treatment of Crohn's disease is given in Figure 10.10. Several concepts are inherent to this treatment plan. First, only a minority of patients with active disease are considered to be suitable candidates for treatment with sulfasalazine, primarily those with mild disease involving the colon. Patients with moderately severe disease and involvement of the terminal ileum and or right colon may be treated with budesonide at a dose of 9 mg/day. Patients with more extensive colonic involvement, those who fail to respond to budesonide or sulfasalazine or those with severe disease activity should receive either prednisone or parenteral steroids. Failure to achieve control of disease activity with these drugs (therapy-resistant disease) is an indication for addition of azathioprine (or 6-mercaptopurine), methotrexate, infliximab or surgery. Individuals who respond to glucocorticoid

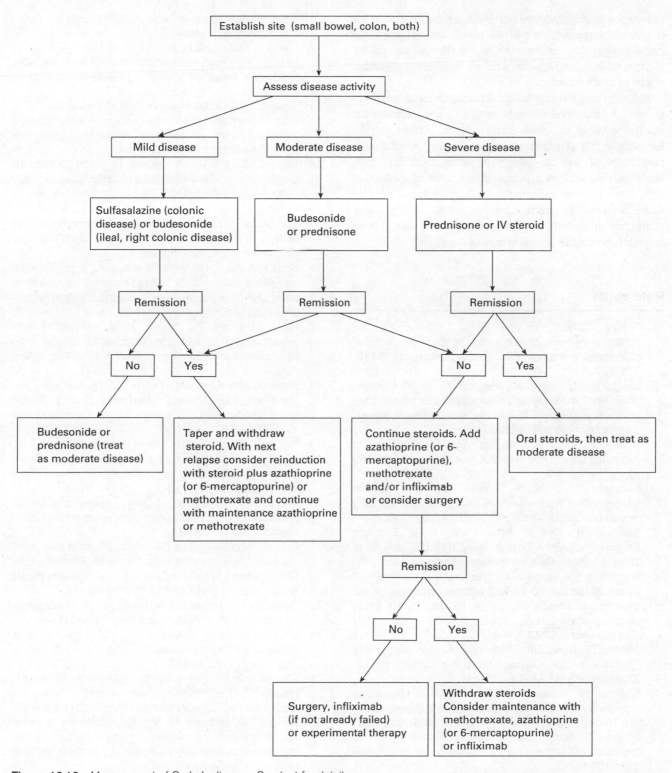

Figure 10.10 Management of Crohn's disease. See text for details

therapy should be withdrawn from steroid therapy over a 12–16 week period. In those patients who fail to successfully discontinue prednisone without a reactivation of disease activity (steroid-dependent disease), the introduction of either azathioprine, (or 6-mercaptopurine) or methotrexate treatment is warranted. Furthermore, individuals who experience frequent relapses of the disease are candidates for long-erm therapy with one of the purine antimetabolites or methotrexate. Surgery remains a highly effective therapy for patients with limited disease who are experiencing adverse effects of medical therapy.

Although our existing medical management is relatively effective for induction of remission of CD, and improves the quality of life of the majority of patients, current therapy for maintenance of remission is less effective. A substantial proportion of patients still experience morbidity from chronically active disease, complications, or adverse effects of drug therapy. Many patients require surgery and a majority undergo more than one resection. In the future it is highly likely that drugs will become available which are able to favorably modify the natural history of the disease.

References

1 Feagan BG, McDonald JWD, Koval JJ. Therapeutics and inflammatory bowel disease: a guide to the interpretation of randomized controlled trials. *Gastroenterology* 1996;**110**: 275–83.

2 Sandborn WJ, Feagan BG, Hanauer SB *et al.* A review of activity indices and efficacy endpoints for clinical trials of medical therapy in adults with Crohn's disease. *Gastroenterology* 2002;**122**:512–30.

3 Azad Khan AK, Piris J, Truelove SC. An experiment to determine the active therapeutic moeity of sulphasalazine. *Lancet* 1977;**ii**:892–5.

4 Summers RW, Switz DM, Sessions JT Jr *et al.* National Cooperative Crohn's Disease Study: results of drug treatment. *Gastroenterology* 1979;**77**:847–69.

5 Malchow H, Ewe K, Brandes JW *et al.* European Cooperative Crohn's Disease Study (ECCDS): Results of Drug Treatment. *Gastroenterology* 1984;**86**:249–266.

6 Rasmussen SN, Lauritsen K, Tage-Jensen U, Nielsen OH, Bytzer P, Jacobsen O *et al.* 5-aminosalicylic acid in the treatment of Crohn's Disease. A 16-week double blind, placebo-controlled, multicentre study with Pentasa. *Scand J Gastroenterol* 1987;**22**:877–83.

7 Mahida YR, Jewell DP. Slow-release 5-amino-salicylic acid (Pentasa) for the treatment of active Crohn's disease. *Digestion* 1990;**45**:88–92.

8 Singleton JW, Hanauer SB, Gitnick GL *et al.* Mesalamine capsules for the treatment of active Crohn's disease: results of a 16-week trial. *Gastroenterology* 1993;**104**:1293–301.

9 Singleton J. Second trial of mesalamine therapy in the treatment of Active Crohn's Disease. *Gastroenterology* 1994;**107**:632–3.

10 Hanauer SB, Stromberg U. Efficacy of oral Pentasa 4/g day in the treatment of active Crohn's disease: a meta-analysis of double blind, placebo-controlled trials. *J Gastroenterol Hepatol* 2004;(in press).

11 Schölmerich J, Jenss H, Hartmann F. The German 5-ASA Study Group. Oral 5-aminosalicyclic acid versus 6-methylprednisolone in active Crohn's disease. *Can J Gastroenterol* 1990;**4**:446–51.

12 Martin F, Sutherland L, Beck IT *et al.* Oral 5-ASA versus prednisone in short term treatment of Crohn's disease: a multicentre controlled trial. *Can J Gastroenterol* 1990;**4**: 452–7.

13 Thomsen OO, Cortot A, Jewell D *et al.* Budesonide CIR is more effective than mesalazine in active Crohn's disease. a 16-week, international randomized, double-blind multicentre trial. *AGA Abstracts* 1996;**112**:A1104.

14 Maier K, Frick H-J, von Gaisberg U, Teufel T, Klotz U. Clinical efficacy of oral mesalazine in Crohn's disease. *Can J Gastroenterol* 1990;**4(1)**:13–18.

15 Prantera C, Pallone F, Brunetti G, Cottone M, Miglioli M, The Italian IBD Study Group. Oral 5-aminosalicylic acid (Asacol) in the maintenance treatment of Crohn's disease. *Gastroenterology* 1992;**103**:363–8.

16 Gross V, Andus T, Fischbach W *et al.* Comparison between high dose 5-aminosalicylic acid and 6-methylprednisolone in active Crohn's ileocolitis. A multicenter randomized double-blind study. *Z Gastroenterol* 1995;**33(10)**:581–4.

17 Fahey JV, Guyer PM, Munck A. Mechanisms of anti-inflammatory actions of glucocorticoids. In: Weissman G, ed. *Advances in inflammation research.* New York: Raven Press, 1981.

18 Singleton JW, Law DH, Kelley ML Jr, Mekhjian HS, Sturdevant RAL. National Cooperative Crohn's Disease Study: adverse reactions to study drugs. *Gastroenterology* 1979;**77**:870–82.

19 Hamedani R, Feldman RD, Feagan BG. Review article: drug development in inflammatory bowel disease: budesonide – a model of targeted therapy. *Aliment Pharmacol Ther* 1997;**11(Suppl 3)**:98–108.

20 Brattsand R. Overview of newer gluco-corticosteroid preparations for inflammatory bowel disease. *Can J Gastroenterol* 1990;**4**:414.

21 Pauwels RALCG, Postma DS. Effect of inhaled formoterol and budesonide on exacerbations of asthma. Formoterol and Corticosteriods Establishing Therapy (FACET) International Study Group. *N Engl J Med* 1997;**337**:1405–11.

22 Greenberg GR, Feagan BG, Martin F *et al.* Oral budesonide for active Crohn's disease. *N Engl J Med* 1994;**331**:836–41.

23 Rutgeerts P, Lofberg R, Malchow H *et al.* A comparison of budesonide with prednisolone for active Crohn's disease. *N Engl J Med* 1994;**331**:842–5.

24 Kane SV, Schoenfeld SP, Sandborn WJ, Tremaine W, Hofer T, Feagan BG. The effectiveness of budesonide therapy for Crohn's disease. *Aliment Pharmacol Ther* 2002;**16**:1509–17.

25 Herfarth HH, Mohanty SP, Rath HC, Tonkonogy S, Sartor RB. Interleukin 10 suppresses experimental chronic, granulomatous inflammation induced by bacterial cell wall polymers. *Gut* 1996;**39**:836–45.

26 Duchmann R, Schmitt E, Knolle P *et al.* Tolerance towards resident intestinal flora in mice is abrogated in experimental colitis and restored by treatment with interleukin-10 or antibodies to interleukin-12. *Eur J Immunol* 1996;**26**:934–8.

27 Ursing B, Alm T, Báràny F *et al.* A comparative study of metronidazole and sulfasalazine for active Crohn's disease:

the Cooperative Crohn's Disease Study in Sweden. *Gastroenterology* 1982;**83**:550–62.

28 Sutherland L, Singleton J, Sessions J *et al.* Double blind, placebo controlled trial of metronidazole in Crohn's disease. *Gut* 1991;**32**:1071–5.

29 Prantera C, Zannoni F, Scribano ML *et al.* An antibiotic regimen for the treatment of active Crohn's disease: a randomized, controlled clinical trial of metronidazole plus ciprofloxacin. *Am J Gastroenterol* 1996;**91**:328–32.

30 Steinhart AH, Feagan BG, Wong CJ *et al.* Combined budesonide and antibiotic therapy for active Crohn's disease: a randomized controlled trial. *Gastroenterology* 2002;**123**:33–40.

31 Munkholm P, Langholz E, Davidsen M, Binder V. Disease activity courses in a regional cohort of Crohn's disease patients. *Scand J Gastroenterol* 1995;**30**:699–706.

32 Candy S, Wright J, Gerber M, Adams G, Gerig M, Goodman R. A controlled double blind study of azathioprine in the management of Crohn's disease. *Gut* 1995;**37**:674–8.

33 Sandborn WJ, Van O EC, Zins BJ *et al.* An intravenous loading dose of azathioprine decreases the time to response in patients with Crohn's disease. *Gastroenterology* 1995;**109**:1808–17.

34 Sandborn WJ, Tremaine WJ, Wolf DC *et al.* Lack of effect of intravenous administration on time to respond to azathioprine for steroid-treated Crohn's disease. North American Azathioprine Study Group. *Gastroenterology* 1999;**117**:527–35.

35 Sandborn WJ, Sutherland L, Pearson D *et al.* Azathioprine or 6-mercaptopurine for induction of remission of Crohn's disease (Cochrane Review). In: Cochrane Collaboration. *Cochrane Library.* Issue 3. Oxford: Update Software, 2003

36 Feagan B. Cyclosporin has no proven role as a therapy for Crohn's disease. *Inflammatory Bowel Diseases* 1995;**1**:335–9.

37 Feagan BG, McDonald JWD, Rochon J *et al.* Low-dose cyclosporine for the treatment of Crohn's disease. *N Engl J Med* 1994;**330**:1846–51.

38 Brynskov J, Freund L, Rasmussen SN *et al.* A placebo-controlled, double blind, randomized trial of cyclosporine therapy in active chronic Crohn's disease. *N Engl J Med* 1989;**321**:845–50.

39 Jewell DP, Lennard-Jones JE, Cyclosporin Study Group of Great Britain and Ireland. Oral cyclosporin for chronic active Crohn's disease: a multicentre controlled trial. *Eur J Gastroenterol Hepatol* 1994;**6**:499–505.

40 Stange EF, Modigliani R, Peña AS *et al.* European trial of cyclosporine in chronic active Crohn's disease: a 12-month study. *Gastroenterology* 1995;**109**:774–82.

41 Feutren G, Mihatsch MJ. Risk factors for cyclosporine-induced nephropathy in patients with autoimmune diseases. international kidney biopsy registry of cyclosporine in autoimmune diseases. *N Engl J Med* 1992;**326**:1654–60.

42 Hanauer SB, Smith MB. Rapid closure of Crohn's disease fistulas with continuous intravenous cyclosporin A. *Am J Gastroenterol* 1993;**88**:646–9.

43 Present DH, Lichtiger S. Efficacy of cyclosporine in treatment of fistula of Crohn's disease. *Dig Dis Sci* 1994;**39**:374–80.

44 Kozarek RA, Patterson DJ, Geland MD, Botoman VA, Ball TJ, Wilske KR. Methotrexate induces clinical and histologic remission in patients with refractory inflammatory bowel disease. *Ann Intern Med* 1989;**110**:353–6.

45 Feagan BG, Rochon J, Fedorak RN *et al.* Methotrexate for the treatment of Crohn's disease. *N Engl J Med* 1995;**332**:292–7.

46 van Deventer SJH. Tumour necrosis factor and Crohn's disease. *Gut* 1997;**40**:443–8.

47 Derkx HH, Taminiau J, Radema SA. Tumour necrosis factor antibody treatment in Crohn's disease. *Lancet* 1993;**342**:173–4.

48 Targan SR, Hanauer SB, van Deventer SJ *et al.* A short-term study of chimeric monoclonal antibody ca2 to tumor necrosis factor for Crohn's disease. *N Engl J Med* 1997;**337**:1029–35.

49 Present DH, Rutgeerts P, Targan S *et al.* Infliximab for the treatment of fistulas in patients with Crohn's disease. *N Engl J Med* 1999;**340**:1398–405.

50 Ghosh S, Goldin E, Gordon FH *et al.* Natalizumab for Crohn's disease. *N Engl J Med* 2003;**348**:24–32.

51 Elan: Website News Release: Analysis of Antegren Phase III Induction Clinical Trial in Crohn's Disease. www.elan.com 2003.

52 Feagan BG. Aminosalicylates for active disease and in the maintenance of remission in Crohn's disease. *Eur J Surg* 1998;**164**:903–9.

53 Lapidus A, Bernell O, Hellers G, Lofberg R. Clinical course of colorectal Crohn's disease: a 35-year follow-up study of 507 patients. *Gastroenterology* 1998;**114**:1151–60.

54 Sutherland LR, Martin F, Bailey RJ *et al.* A randomized, placebo-controlled, double-blind trial of mesalamine in the maintenance of remission of Crohn's disease. *Gastroenterology* 1997;**112**:1069–77.

55 Messori A, Brignola C, Trallori G *et al.* Effectiveness of 5-aminosalicylic acid for maintaining remission in patients with Crohn's disease: a meta-analysis. *Am J Gastroenterol* 1994;**89**:692–8.

56 Steinhart AH, Hemphill D, Greenberg GR. Sulfasalazine and mesalazine for the maintenance therapy of Crohn's disease: a meta-analysis. *Am J Gastroenterol* 1994;**89**:2116–24.

57 Camma C, Giunta M, Rosselli M, Cottone M. Mesalamine in the maintenance treatment of Crohn's disease: a meta-analysis adjusted for confounding variables. *Gastroenterology* 1997;**113**:1465–73.

58 Trallori G, Messori A. Drug treatments for maintaining remission in Crohn's disease. a lifetime cost-utility analysis. *PharmacoEconomics* 1997;**11**:444–53.

59 Lochs H, Mayer M, Fleig WE *et al.* Prophylaxis of postoperative relapse in Crohn's disease with mesalazine (Pentasa) in comparison to placebo. *Gastroenterology* 2000;**119**:264–73.

60 Mahmud N, Kamm MA, Dupas JL *et al.* Olsalazine is not superior to placebo in maintaining remission of inactive Crohn's colitis and ileocolitis: a double blind, parallel, randomised, multicentre study. *Gut* 2001;**49**:552–526.

61 Sutherland LR. Mesalamine for the prevention of postoperative recurrence: is nearly there the same as being there? *Gastroenterology* 2000;**118**:264–73.

62 Greenberg GR, Feagan BG, Martin F *et al.* Oral budesonide as maintenance treatment for Crohn's disease: a placebo-controlled, dose-ranging study. *Gastroenterology* 1996;**110**: 45–51.

63 Löfberg R, Rutgeerts P, Malchow H *et al.* Budesonide prolongs time to relapse in ileal and ileocaecal Crohn's disease. a placebo controlled one year study. *Gut* 1996;**39**: 82–6.

64 Ferguson A, Campieri M, Doe W, Persson T, Nygard G. Oral budesonide as maintenance therapy in Crohn's disease – results of a 12-month study. Global Budesonide Study Group. *Aliment Pharmacol Ther* 1998;**12**:175–83.

65 Sandborn W, Feagan B, Lofberg R, Campieri M, Greenberg AG, Hanauer S. Budesonide Capsules Prolong Time to Relapse in Crohn's Disease Patients with Medically induced Remission. *Dig Dis Week* 2003;Abstract No. M1600.

66 Hellers G, Cortot A, Jewell D *et al.* Oral budesonide for prevention of postsurgical recurrence in Crohn's disease: The IOIBD Budesonide Study Group. *Gastroenterology* 1999;**116**:294–300.

67 Ewe K, Bottger T, Buhr HJ, Ecker KW, Otto HF. Low-dose budesonide treatment for prevention of postoperative recurrence of Crohn's disease: a multicentre randomized placebo-controlled trial. German Budesonide Study Group. *Eur J Gastroenterol Hepatol* 1999;**11**:277–82.

68 Borgaonkar MR, MacIntosh D, Fardy J. Anti-tuberculous therapy for maintaining remission of Crohn's disease. In: Cochrane Collaboration. *Cochrane Library* (database on disk and CD-ROM) Issue 3. Oxford: Update Software, 2003.

69 Rutgeerts P, Hiele M, Geboes K *et al.* Controlled trial of metronidazole treatment for prevention of Crohn's recurrence after ileal resection. *Gastroenterology* 1995;**108**:1617–21.

70 Rutgeerts P. Strategies in the prevention of post-operative recurrence in Crohn's disease. *Best Pract Res Clin Gastroenterol* 2003;**17**:63–73.

71 Pearson C, May GR, Fick G, Sutherland LR. Azathioprine for maintaining remission in Crohn's disease. In: Cochrane Collaboration. *Cochrane Library*. Issue 3. Oxford: Update Software, 2003

72 Rosenberg JL, Levin B, Wall AJ *et al.* A controlled trial of azathioprine in Crohn's disease. *Am J Dig Dis* 1975;**20**: 721–6.

73 O'Donoghue DP, Dawson AM, Powell-Tuck J, Bown RL, Lennard-Jones JE. Double-blind withdrawal trial of azathioprine as maintenance treatment for Crohn's disease. *Lancet* 1978;**ii**:955–7.

74 Markowitz J, Grancher K, Kohn N, Lesser M, Daum F, The Pediatric 6MP Collaborative Group. A multicenter trial of 6-mercaptopurine and prednisone in children with newly diagnosed Crohn's disease. *Gastroenterology* 2000;**119**: 895–902.

75 Present DH, Meltzer SJ, Krumholz MP, Wolke A, Korelitz BI. 6-Mercaptopurine in the Management of Inflammatory Bowel Disease: Short- and Long-Term Toxicity. *Ann Intern Med* 1989;**111**:641–9.

76 Reuther LO, Sonne J, Larsen NE *et al.* Pharmacological monitoring of azathioprine therapy. *Scan J Gastroenterol* 2003;**38**:972–7.

77 Feagan BG, Fedorak RN, Irvine EJ *et al.* A comparison of methotrexate with placebo for the maintenance of remission in Crohn's disease. North American Crohn's Study Group Investigators. *N Engl J Med* 2000;**342**:1627–32.

78 Alfadhli AAF, McDonald JWD, Feagan BG. Methotrexate for induction of remission in refractory Crohn's disease (Cochrane Review). In: Cochrane Collaboration. *Cochrane Library*. Issue 1. Chichester: John Wiley & Sons Ltd, 2004.

79 McKendry RJ. The remarkable spectrum of methotrexate toxicities. *Rheum Dis Clin North Am* 1997;**23**:939–54.

80 Kremer JM, Alarcon GS, Lightfoot RW Jr *et al.* Methotrexate for rheumatoid arthritis. Suggested guidelines for monitoring liver toxicity. American College of Rheumatology. *Arthritis Rheum* 1994;**37**:1829–30.

81 Rutgeerts P, D'Haens G, Targan S *et al.* Efficacy and safety of retreatment with antitumor necrosis factor antibody (infliximab) to maintain remission in Crohn's disease. *Gastroenterology* 1999;**117**:761–9.

82 Hanauer SB, Feagan BG, Lichtenstein GR, Mayer LF, Schreiber S, Colombel JF *et al.* Maintenance infliximab for Crohn's disease: The ACCENT 1 randomised trial. *Lancet* 2002;**359**:1541–9.

83 Sands BE, Anderson F, Bernstein C *et al.* A randomized controlled trial of infliximab maintenance therapy for fistulizing Crohn's disease (ACCENT II). *N Engl J Med* 2004; (in press).

84 Long R, Gardam M. Tumour necrosis factor-alpha inhibitors and the reactivation of latent tuberculosis infection. *Can Med Assoc J* 2003;**168**:1153–6.

85 Keane J, Gershon S, Wise RP *et al.* Tuberculosis associated with infliximab, a tumor necrosis factor alpha-neutralizing agent. *N Engl J Med* 2001;**345**:1098–104.

86 Gardam MA, Keystone EC, Menzies R *et al.* Anti-tumour necrosis factor agents and tuberculosis risk: mechanisms of action and clinical management. *Lancet Infect Dis* 2003;**3**: 148–55.

87 Warris A, Bjorneklett A, Gaustad P. Invasive pulmonary aspergillosis associated with infliximab therapy. *N Engl J Med* 2001;**344**:1099–100.

88 Gluck T, Linde HJ, Scholmerich J, Muller-Ladner U, Fiehn C, Bohland P. Anti-tumor necrosis factor therapy and listeria monocytogenes infection: report of two cases. *Arthritis Rheum* 2002;**46**:2255–7.

89 Tai TL, O'Rourke KP, McWeeney M, Burke CM, Sheehan K, Barry M. *Pneumocystis carinii* pneumonia following a second infusion of infliximab. *Rheumatology (Oxford)* 2002;**41**:951–2.

90 Kwon HJ, Cote TR, Cuffe MS, Kramer JM, Braun MM. Case reports of heart failure after therapy with a tumor necrosis factor antagonist. *Ann Intern Med* 2003;**138**:807–11.

91 Baert F, Norman MR, Vermeire S *et al.* Influence of immunogenicity on the long-term efficacy of infliximab in Crohn's disease. *N Engl J Med* 2003;**348**:601–8.

92 Farrell RJ, Alsahli M, Jeen YT, Falchuk KR, Peppercorn MA, Michetti P. Intravenous hydrocortisone premedication reduces antibodies to infliximab in Crohn's disease: a randomized controlled trial. *Gastroenterology* 2003;**124**:917–24.

93 Endres S, Ghorbani R, Kelley VE *et al.* The effect of dietary supplementation with n-3 polyunsaturated fatty acids on the synthesis of interleukin-1 and tumour necrosis factor by mononuclear cells. *N Engl J Med* 1989;**320**:265–71.

94 Teitelbaum JE, Allan Walker W. Review: the role of omega 3 fatty acids in intestinal inflammation. *J Nutr Biochem* 2001; **12**:21–32.

95 Belluzzi A, Brignola C, Campieri M, Pera A, Boschi S, Miglioli M. Effect of an enteric-coated fish-oil preparation on relapses in Crohn's disease. *N Engl J Med* 1996;**334**: 1557–60.

11 Ulcerative colitis

Derek P Jewell, Lloyd R Sutherland

Introduction

Patients with ulcerative colitis have a variety of questions for those practitioners who treat their disease. This chapter focuses on the evidence on which decisions relating to patient advice (prognosis for the first attack, extension of disease, risk of cancer) and treatment options should be made. Our recommendations are based wherever possible on evidence from published population-based studies and randomized controlled clinical trials. Where several clinical trials have addressed the same question we have frequently used meta-analyses to summarize the results.

Histological diagnosis

The diagnosis of ulcerative colitis and Crohn's disease together with accurate differentiation between them and other inflammatory diseases of the colon relies on a combination of clinical, radiological, endoscopic and histological features. Accurate histological interpretation is crucial but is confounded by at least four major problems.

- Variability in assessing normal colorectal histology and assessing minimal degrees of inflammation.
- Considerable overlap in the histological changes of most colonic inflammatory conditions.
- Accuracy and reproducibility of many of the histological features commonly used for diagnosis have not been determined.
- Absence of standard nomenclature.

Recently, a working party of the British Society of Gastroenterology has published guidelines for the biopsy diagnosis of suspected chronic inflammatory bowel disease.[1] Databases were searched for papers relating to reproducibility, sensitivity, and specificity of histological features used for the differential diagnosis of inflammatory bowel disease (IBD). Only those achieving moderate reproducibility (a minimum κ statistic of 0·4 or a percentage agreement of 80% or more) were included. Precise definitions of mucosal architectural changes, lamina propria cellularity, neutrophil infiltration and epithelial cell abnormalities were derived from the systematic review of the literature. Then the quality of the evidence for these features with respect to differential diagnosis was rated according to the criteria recommended by the Evidence Based Working Party. Features for which the literature review provided high quality evidence for their use in differential diagnosis are shown in Figure 11.1. These histopathological criteria formed the basis of guidelines for clinical practice, thereby helping to ensure uniformity and consistency of reporting. Subsequently, a workshop was set up to examine the value of these guidelines.[2] A group of histopathologists were asked to report on a series of colonoscopic biopsies from 60 patients. The group consisted of 13 pathologists with a special interest in IBD and 12 general pathologists. Following this, there was a discussion with regard to the evidence-based guidelines and the biopsy specimens were then renumbered and then re-reported. For ulcerative colitis, the accuracy of reporting was similar in both the first and second rounds and there was little difference between the expert pathologists and the generalists. However, there was improved accuracy in reporting Crohn's disease following discussion of the guidelines: for the experts accuracy improved from 56% to 64% and for the general pathologists from 50% to 60%. The same workshop was also able to show that multiple, as opposed to single, biopsies led to better and more reproducible diagnoses, especially for Crohn's disease. Thus, the introduction of evidence-based guidelines and training in their use is helpful, predominantly for Crohn's disease, but results in a more accurate histopathological diagnosis only in one in 10 colonoscopic series reported.

Prognosis

Population-based studies

The importance of recognizing that the prognosis for referred patients differs from that of a regional population was recognized by Truelove and Pena nearly three decades ago.[3] They found that the survival of patients who were referred to

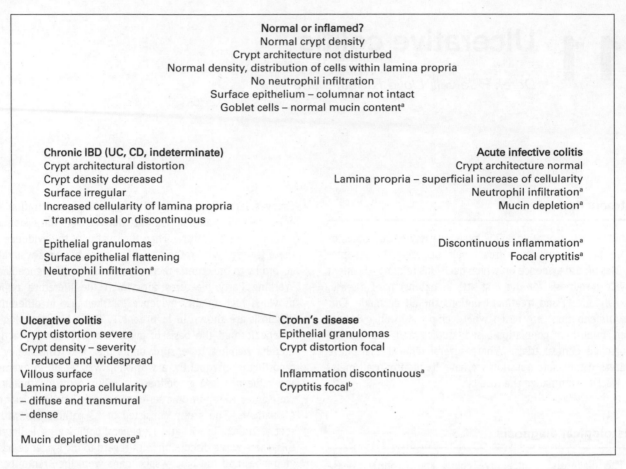

Normal or inflamed?
Normal crypt density
Crypt architecture not disturbed
Normal density, distribution of cells within lamina propria
No neutrophil infiltration
Surface epithelium – columnar not intact
Goblet cells – normal mucin content[a]

Chronic IBD (UC, CD, indeterminate)
Crypt architectural distortion
Crypt density decreased
Surface irregular
Increased cellularity of lamina propria
– transmucosal or discontinuous

Epithelial granulomas
Surface epithelial flattening
Neutrophil infiltration[a]

Acute infective colitis
Crypt architecture normal
Lamina propria – superficial increase of cellularity
Neutrophil infiltration[a]
Mucin depletion[a]

Discontinuous inflammation[a]
Focal cryptitis[a]

Ulcerative colitis
Crypt distortion severe
Crypt density – severity
  reduced and widespread
Villous surface
Lamina propria cellularity
– diffuse and transmural
– dense

Mucin depletion severe[a]

Crohn's disease
Epithelial granulomas
Crypt distortion focal

Inflammation discontinuous[a]
Cryptitis focal[b]

Figure 11.1 Evidence-based features for histological diagnosis of colonic biopsy specimens. Note: All features have the highest quality of evidence except for: [a]evidence of diagnostic value from single studies only and [b]no published evidence of accuracy or reproducibility. IBD, inflammatory bowel disease; UC, ulcerative colitis; CD, Crohn's disease

Oxford (UK) from other regions was significantly reduced compared with that of patients who actually resided in the Oxford catchment area.

There are several population-based studies on the prognosis for patients with ulcerative colitis. Sinclair and associates described the prognosis of 537 patients with ulcerative colitis, seen between 1967 and 1976 in northeastern Scotland.[4] They found a high proportion of cases with distal disease (70%). The overall mortality and surgical resection rates in the first attack were both 3%. During this period of time, the mortality for severe, first-time attacks was 23%. However, there were only modest differences in the observed and expected mortality for the ulcerative colitis population. The colectomy rate after 5 years was 8%.

The prognosis and mortality associated with ulcerative colitis in Stockholm county was reported by Persson *et al.*[5] In their review of 1547 patients followed from 1955 to 1984, they found that the mortality in the patient population was higher than that expected in the general population. After 15 years of follow up, the survival rate was 94% of that expected based on the study population's age and sex. The

relative survival rates differed more for patients with pancolitis than for patients with proctitis, but the confidence intervals overlapped. While ulcerative colitis was the most important influence on the increased mortality, deaths from colorectal cancer, asthma, and non-alcoholic liver disease were also increased.

Danish investigators have also reported the results of their population-based assessment of the prognosis of ulcerative colitis. Their population included 1161 patients with ulcerative colitis followed for up to 25 years (median 11 years).[6] Of the 1161 patients, 235 underwent colectomy. Interestingly, 60 of these patients presented with proctosigmoiditis initially. The cumulative colectomy rate was 9%, 24%, 30% and 32% at 1, 10, 15, and 25 years, respectively, after diagnosis. At any one time, nearly half of the clinic population was in remission. Prognostic factors associated with frequent relapses included: the number of relapses in the first 3 years after diagnosis and the year of diagnosis (1960s *v* 1970s *v* 1980s). Surprisingly, signs and symptoms of weight loss or fever were associated with fewer relapses on follow up. A recent report on the same inception cohort of patients,[7] published nearly 10 years after these initial observations, has shown that overall life expectancy is normal for patients with ulcerative colitis, but patients over 50 years of age with extensive colitis at diagnosis have an increased mortality within the first 2 years, due to colitis-associated postoperative complications and comorbidity.

Another report by the same investigators focused on the prognosis in children with ulcerative colitis.[8] Eighty of the 1161 patients in the cohort were children who presented with more extensive disease compared with adults. The cumulative colectomy rate did not differ from that of adults (29% at 20 years). At any interval from diagnosis, the majority of children were thought to be in remission.

Two prospective population studies are in progress in Europe (the European Collaborative Study on Inflammatory Bowel Diseases and Inflammatory Bowel South Eastern Norway (IBSEN) cohort) but only 1-year follow up data have so far been reported[9,10]

Extension of disease

Ayres and associates reported their experience with extension of disease in 145 patients presenting with proctitis or proctosigmoiditis, followed prospectively for a median of 11 years. By life-table analysis, extension occurred in 16% and 31% of patients at 5 and 10 years follow up, respectively. Extension was associated with a clinical exacerbation of disease in most cases but no specific clinical factors were associated with disease extension.[11]

Much higher rates of progression have been reported, largely in retrospective non-population-based series. However, in the IBSEN cohort, 22% of 130 patients with a new diagnosis of ulcerative colitis had progressed to more extensive disease during the first year of follow up.[12] The most recent study from Italy included 273 patients with proctitis.[13] It is retrospective and not population-based (patients were identified in 13 hospitals) but it is the largest cohort yet reported. Overall, proximal extension occurred in 27·1% during clinical and endoscopic follow up: 20% at 5 years and 54% at 10 years. However, the disease only extended into the sigmoid in the majority and into the splenic flexure in only 10% of the patients. An interesting observation was that smoking protected against disease progression on univariate analysis.

While research for the most part has focused on *extension* of disease, Langholz and colleagues report a much more dynamic pattern. After 25 years of follow up, 53% of patients with limited disease had extension of disease, but in 75% of patients with extensive disease, the disease boundary had *regressed*.[14] This dynamic process, if confirmed by others, could have implications in terms of cancer surveillance programs. One potential explanation for these findings is that in the early years of the study, disease extent was assessed by radiological techniques.

Cancer surveillance (see also Chapter 15)

Although ulcerative colitis is a premalignant condition, the proportion of patients who develop cancer is small. In a population study using a retrospectively assembled cohort of patients the cumulative risk at 20 years of disease was about 7% and rose to 12% at 30 years.[15] This study is likely to have included all or nearly all patients with ulcerative colitis in two regions of England and one of Sweden and referral bias is probably minimal. Follow up was both of long duration (17–38 years) and thorough (97%). On the other hand, in centers with an aggressive policy of colectomy, no increased cancer risk has been seen.[16] In all studies, length of history and extent of disease are important factors. Thus, left-sided colitis carries only a slightly increased risk while extensive colitis increases the risk about 20 times over that of an age and sex-matched population. Whether early age of onset of ulcerative colitis is an independent risk factor is controversial. Children tend to have extensive disease and have greater life expectancy than adults; they are, therefore, more likely to be at risk.

There is some controversy concerning the role of colonoscopic surveillance in detection of cancer. Most centers carry out colonoscopy in patients with extensive disease 8–10 years after diagnosis. Even at that stage, a few patients with dysplasia or a frank carcinoma will be identified. However, the subsequent pickup rate during the surveillance program is small – about 11% – and in one center only two cancers were detected in 200 patients over a 20-year period.[17] Furthermore, cancers can develop outside the screening program. Thus, the need for colonoscopic surveillance has been questioned and no controlled study has shown that surveillance reduces mortality. However, in the published studies, the 5-year survival rates for cancers detected in asymptomatic patients have been considerably higher than was observed in those presenting with symptoms. B4, C5

A second controversial area is the management of patients with endoscopically visible lesions. Where such lesions are associated with dysplasia in the adjacent mucosa (dysplasia-associated lesions or masses (DALMs)) the incidence of cancer appears to be very high and prophylactic colectomy is recommended [18,19] However, polyps for which there is no associated dysplasia in adjacent mucosa do not appear to carry this high risk of cancer, and in such cases conservative management rather than colectomy is recommended.[20,21] B4, C5

Reviewing the evidence for dysplasia surveillance, Riddell recommended obtaining three to four biopsies every 10 cm.[22] Annual colonoscopy is probably ideal, but 2-yearly colonoscopy with intervening flexible sigmoidoscopy in alternate years is a compromise. Dysplasia detected at the initial screening colonoscopy should lead to colectomy, as there is a high chance of concomitant cancer. Indeed, most clinicians advocate colectomy whenever dysplasia is found, even when it is low grade. There is no doubt that such a policy abolishes the cancer risk but justification for it for patients with low grade dysplasia remains controversial[23,24] The development of molecular markers may help to resolve the issue.

Treatment

The treatment of ulcerative colitis can be conveniently discussed for each category or class of medications, and in terms of either induction or maintenance of remission.

Aminosalicylates

With the discovery of sulfasalazine by Svartz,[25] the first effective agent for the treatment of ulcerative colitis became available. The first trial that established the efficacy of sulfasalazine for the *induction of remission* was reported in 1962.[26] Alc Misiewicz and colleagues were the first to study its efficacy as *maintenance therapy*.[27] An early randomized trial in the UK established the importance of continuous therapy.[28] Alc Azad Khan and the Oxford group established that 2 g/day of sulfasalazine provided the optimal trade-off between efficacy and adverse effects.[29]

The finding that mesalamine (5-ASA) is the active moiety of sulfasalazine[30,31] stimulated a decade of trials of induction and maintenance of remission. Numerous aminosalicylate delivery systems have been developed. These include drugs that release 5-ASA upon bacterial splitting of the azo bond (for example sulfasalazine, olsalazine and balsalazide), pH-dependent release formulations (for example Asacol (pH 7) and Claversal/Mesasal/Salofalk (pH 6)), and a microsphere preparation (Pentasa).[32]

The efficacy of oral mesalamine has been evaluated by meta-analyses of randomized controlled trials.[33–35] As shown in Figure 11.2a, mesalamine is more effective than placebo for the induction of remission (pooled odds ratio 0·51, CI 0·35 to 0·76).[34] Ala The newer 5-ASA preparations were not significantly more effective than sulfasalazine, however, for active disease (pooled odds ratio 0·75, CI 0·50 to 1·13) (Figure 11.2b). On the other hand, adverse events were less frequently noted with mesalamine than with sulfasalazine: the number of patients needed to treat (NNT) with mesalamine rather than sulfasalazine to avoid an adverse event in one patient is approximately 7. Ala

Figure 11.3a illustrates the results of a meta-analysis that demonstrates the superiority of aminosalicylates over placebo for maintenance of remission (pooled odds ratio 0·47, CI 0·36 to 0·62).[35] Ala Conflicting results were obtained in studies comparing sulfasalazine with mesalamine for maintenance therapy. The overall results are shown in Figure 11.3b; sulfasalazine appeared to be more effective than mesalamine (pooled odds ratio 1·29, CI 1·05 to 1·57). Ala When only

studies with a minimum of 12 months' follow up were included in the analysis, however, there was no statistically significant advantage for sulfasalazine (pooled odds ratio 1·15, CI 0·89 to 1·50). There are a number of possible explanations for this discrepancy. First, the observation in the overall analysis may be correct: sulfasalazine may be a more effective delivery system than mesalamine. Second, the analysis that was restricted to studies with 12 months' follow up might have lacked sufficient statistical power to detect a small difference in efficacy. Third, the high dropout rate with olsalazine therapy might have biased the overall results against mesalamine. Finally, it is possible that the comparison studies suffered from selection bias. With the exception of one trial,[36] the inclusion criteria included tolerance to sulfasalazine. This factor would tend to minimize the occurrence of adverse events with sulfasalazine therapy.

Several oral 5-ASA preparations are available, but two warrant special mention. Olsalazine and balsalazide appear to be approximately as effective as sulfasalazine and mesalamine in the treatment of active ulcerative colitis and in the maintenance of remission. There have been concerns about the development of secretory diarrhea with olsalazine,[37,38] due to interference with Na^+/K^+-ATPase, but the frequency of this adverse effect can be minimized by taking the medication in divided doses with meals[39,40] Moreover, systemic absorption of 5-ASA and its metabolites is less with olsalazine than with mesalamine, which might translate into a smaller risk of nephropathy[41,42] Several randomized controlled trials have demonstrated a slight (and statistically insignificant) advantage of balsalazide (in a dosage of 6·75 g/day) to sulfasalazine 3 g/day or mesalamine 2·4 g/day in the treatment of active ulcerative colitis. Ald The newer agent may provide relief of symptoms and sigmoidoscopic healing more quickly than mesalamine,[43–45] and may be better tolerated.[46] Balsalazide 3 g/day appears to be as effective as mesalamine 1·2 g/day at maintaining remission, and may provide better relief of nocturnal symptoms in the first 3 months of maintenance therapy.[47] It should be noted that these observations suggesting small advantages of balsalazide over mesalamine depend on *post hoc* subgroup analyses of relatively small groups of patients and should be interpreted with some caution.

Topical therapy is a logical option for patients with disease limited to the distal colon. In theory, it presents a high concentration of mesalamine to the affected area, while minimizing systemic absorption. Marshall and Irvine have published two meta-analyses of topical therapy[48,49] The first analysis established that topical mesalamine was effective for both induction and maintenance therapy in patients with distal disease.[48] Alc The second analysis found that mesalamine was more effective than topical corticosteroids for the induction of remission.[49] Alc Foam enemas can reliably deliver mesalamine to the rectum and sigmoid colon, and sometimes

Review: Ulc. colitis: induction of remission, 5-ASA
Comparison: 5-ASA vs. placebo
Outcome: Failure to induce global/clinical remission

Study	Expt n/N	Ctrl n/N	Peto OR (95% CI Fixed)	Weight (%)	Peto OR (95% CI Fixed)
Dose of 5-ASA: < 2 g					
Hanauer *et al.*, 1993	73/92	26/30		13·8	0·62 (0·22 to 1·78)
Schroeder *et al.*, 1986	10/11	36/38		2·0	0·52 (0·03 to 8·31)
Sninsky *et al.*, 1991	47/53	25/28		5·6	0·40 (0·08 to 2·07)
Subtotal (95% CI)	130/156	87/94		21·4	0·55 (0·23 to 1·27)
Chi-square 0·20 (df = 2) Z = 1·41					
Dose of 5-ASA: 2–2·9 g					
Hanauer *et al.*, 1993	69/97	26/30		17·2	0·44 (0·17 to 1·13)
Hanauer *et al.*, 1996	81/92	39/45		13·1	1·13 (0·39 to 3·33)
Sninsky *et al.*, 1991	47/53	25/26		5·6	0·40 (0·08 to 2·07)
Subtotal (95% CI)	197/242	90/101		35·9	0·61 (0·32 to 1·17)
Chi-square 1·98 (df = 2) Z = 1·48					
Dose of 5-ASA: ≥3 g					
Hanauer *et al.*, 1993	67/95	27/30		17·0	0·35 (0·14 to 0·91)
Hanauer *et al.*, 1996	75/91	39/45		16·3	0·73 (0·28 to 1·93)
Schroeder *et al.*, 1996	29/38	36/38		9·4	0·23 (0·06 to 0·82)
Subtotal (95% CI)	171/224	102/113		42·6	0·43 (0·23 to 0·77)
Chi-square 2·25 (df = 2) Z = 2·81					
Total (95% CI)	498/622	279/306		100·0	0·51 (0·35 to 0·76)
Chi-square 5·12 (df = 8) Z = 3·37					

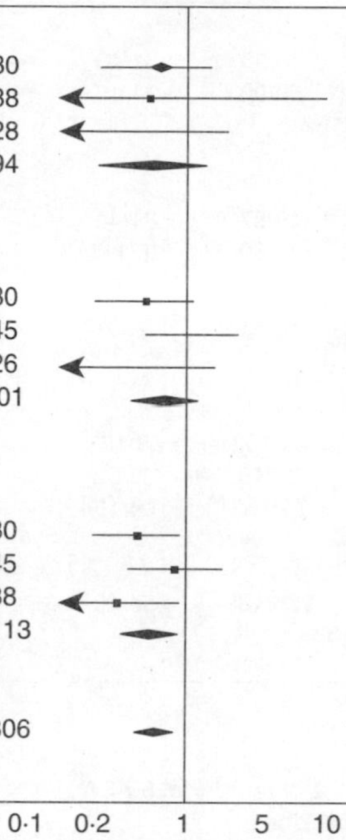

0·1   0·2   1   5   10

(a)

Review: Ulc. colitis: induction of remission, 5-ASA
Comparison: 5-ASA vs. sulfasalazine
Outcome: Failure to induce global/clinical remission

Study	Expt n/N	Ctrl n/N	Peto OR (95% CI Fixed)	Weight (%)	Peto OR (95% CI Fixed)
5-ASA/SASP < 1/2	14/20	7/9		5·7	0·69 (0·12 to 3·87)
Riley *et al.*, 1988	14/20	7/9		5·7	0·69 (0·12 to 3·87)
Subtotal (95% CI)					
Chi-square 0·00 (df = 0) Z = 0·43					
1/1 > 5-ASA/SASP ≥ 1/2					
Andreoli *et al.*, 1987	2/6	3/6		3·5	0·53 (0·06 to 4·80)
Rachmilewitz *et al.*, 1989	78/115	70/105		54·1	1·05 (0·60 to 1·85)
Rijk *et al.*, 1991	13/27	17/28		15·5	0·61 (0·21 to 1·74)
Subtotal (95% CI)	93/148	90/139		73·2	0·91 (0·56 to 1·47)
Chi-square 1·05 (df = 2) Z = 0·39					
5-ASA/SASP ≥ 1/1					
Green *et al.*, 1993	6/28	12/29		14·0	0·40 (0·13 to 1·22)
Riley *et al.*, 1988	12/21	8/10		7·1	0·38 (0·08 to 1·79)
Subtotal (95% CI)	18/49	20/39		21·1	0·40 (0·16 to 0·97)
Chi-square 0·00 (df = 1) Z = 2·02					
Total (95% CI)	125/217	117/187		100·0	0·75 (0·50 to 1·13)
Chi-square 3·60 (df = 5) Z = 1·37					

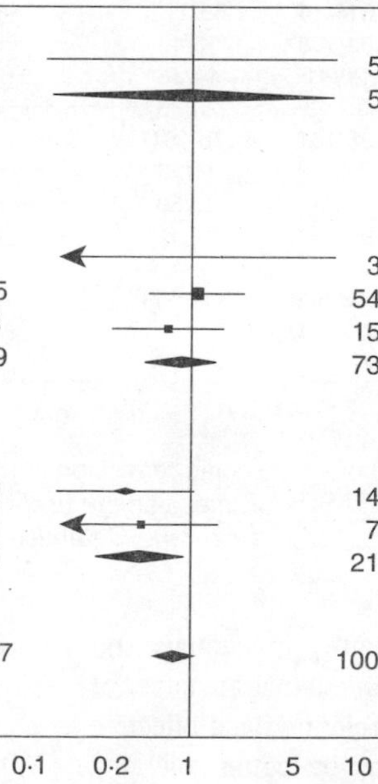

(b)   0·1   0·2   1   5   10

Figure 11.2   Failure to induce clinical or endoscopic remission in ulcerative colitis. Randomized controlled clinical trials of mesalamine (5-ASA) and sulfasalazine (SASP): (a) mesalamine (Expt) versus placebo (Ctrl), (b) mesalamine (Expt) versus sulfasalazine (Ctrl). (Source: Sutherland LR *et al. Cochrane Database Syst Rev* 2000;**2**:CD000543[34])

Review: Ulc. colitis: maintenance of remission, 5-ASA
Comparison: 5-ASA vs. placebo
Outcome: Failure to maintain clinical or endoscopic remission

Study	Expt n/N	Ctrl n/N	Peto OR (95% CI Fixed)	Weight (%)	Peto OR (95% CI Fixed)
Dose of 5-ASA: <1 g					
Hanauer *et al.,* 1996	50/90	31/43		13·6	0·50 (0·24 to 1·05)
Subtotal (95% CI)	50/90	31/43		13·6	0·50 (0·24 to 1·05)
Chi-square 0·00 (df = 0) Z = 0·182					
Dose of 5-ASA: 1–1·9 g					
Hanauer *et al.,* 1996	49/87	31/44		13·7	0·56 (0·28 to 1·16)
Hawkey *et al.,* 1997	40/99	66/111		25·6	0·47 (0·27 to 0·80)
Sandberg *et al.,* 1986	12/52	22/49		1·1	0·38 (0·17 to 0·86)
Subtotal (95% CI)	101/238	119/204		50·4	0·47 (0·32 to 0·69)
Chi-square 0·45 (df = 2) Z = 3·86					
Dose of 5-ASA: ≥ 2 g					
Miner *et al.,* 1995	44/103	68/102		24·9	0·38 (0·22 to 0·66)
Wright *et al.,* 1993	31/49	36/52		11·1	0·77 (0·34 to 1·75)
Subtotal (95% CI)	75/152	104/154		36·0	0·47 (0·30 to 0·75)
Chi-square 1·91 (df = 1) Z = 3·21					
Total (95% CI)	226/480	254/401		100·0	0·47 (0·36 to 0·62)
Chi-square 2·39 (df = 5) Z = 5·33					

(a)

0·1 0·2 0 5 10

Review: Ulc. colitis: maintenance of remission, 5-ASA
Comparison: 5-ASA vs. sulfasalazine
Outcome: Failure to maintain clinical or endoscopic remission

Study	Expt n/N	Ctrl n/N	Peto OR (95% CI Fixed)	Weight (%)	Peto OR (95% CI Fixed)
Anderoli *et al.,* 1987	3/7	1/6		0·8	3·11 (0·32 to 30·11)
Ardizzone *et al.,* 1989	20/44	27/44		5·7	0·53 (0·23 to 1·22)
Ireland *et al.,* 1988	35/82	21/82		9·6	2·13 (1·12 to 4·05)
Killerich *et al.,* 1992	61/114	55/112		14·7	1·19 (0·71 to 2·01)
Kruis *et al.,* 1995	39/108	13/40		6·9	1·17 (0·55 to 2·50)
McIntyre *et al.,* 1988	20/41	14/38		5·1	1·62 (0·67 to 3·92)
Mulder *et al.,* 1988	19/42	20/36		5·1	0·67 (0·27 to 1·61)
Nilsson *et al.,* 1995	88/161	76/161		20·9	1·35 (0·87 to 2·08)
Rijk *et al.,* 1992	14/23	11/23		3·0	1·67 (0·53 to 5·27)
Riley *et al.,* 1988	20/50	23/60		6·4	0·78 (0·36 to 1·73)
Rutgeerts *et al.,* 1989	90/167	70/167		21·7	1·61 (1·05 to 2·48)
Total (95% CI)	409/839	331/759		100·0	1·29 (1·05 to 1·57)
Chi-square 12·61 (df = 10) Z = 2·47					

(b)

0·1 0·2 0 5 10

Figure 11.3 Failure to maintain clinical or endoscopic remission in ulcerative colitis. Randomized controlled clinical trials of mesalamine (5-ASA) and sulfasalazine (SASP): (a) mesalamine (Expt) versus placebo (Ctrl), (b) mesalamine (Expt) versus sulfasalazine (Ctrl). (Source: Sutherland LR *et al. Cochrane Database Syst Rev* 2002;**4**:CD000544[35])

even to the descending colon, in healthy individuals and patients with ulcerative colitis.[50–53] Foam enemas are superior to placebo,[53] and are at least as easily tolerated and effective as liquid enemas.[54–56] Gel enemas may be better tolerated than foam preparations.[57] Mesalamine suppositories have been shown to be effective for the maintenance of remission of ulcerative proctitis.[58] Ald

Corticosteroids

Corticosteroids remain the standard therapy for moderate to severe ulcerative colitis. Truelove and Witts were the first to undertake a randomized controlled trial of cortisone in patients with active colitis, and showed that 100 mg/day, followed by tapering over 6 weeks, was an effective

Table 11.1   Clinical course during trial in two treatment groups of patients according to whether patients entered trial in first attack of ulcerative colitis or in relapse

	Admitted in first attack		Admitted in relapses	
No. of relapses	Azathioprine group	Control group	Azathioprine group	Control group
0	7	6	9	3
1–2	5	6	8	7
3 or failed	4	3	7	15
Total	16	15	24	25
Significance of differences[a]	NS		$P = 0.055$	

[a]Fisher's exact test.

Reproduced from Jewell DP *et al. BMJ* 1974;**iv**:627–30.[69]

treatment.[59] Alc Lennard-Jones and associates reported similar efficacy for prednisone.[60] It appears that once daily dosage yields similar effectiveness as divided doses of the medication.[61]

The assumption that there is no additional benefit from the use of more than 40 mg/day of prednisone is based on a small comparative trial conducted by Baron and colleagues.[62] This trial compared the outcomes of 58 outpatients who were randomized to 20, 40, or 60 mg of prednisone per day. Although either 40 or 60 mg/day yielded better results than 20 mg/day, no difference in results were observed in patients given 40 *versus* 60 mg/day. The study included too few patients, however, to have sufficient statistical power to rule out a relative benefit from the 60 mg dose. Ald

Budesonide is a potent second-generation corticosteroid with 90% first pass metabolism, resulting in decreased systemic toxicity.[63] A randomized controlled trial demonstrated that a targeted colonic release formulation of budesonide appeared to be as effective as prednisolone and exhibited a more favorable adverse event profile.[64] Ald

Budesonide enemas have also been used for active distal disease. A meta-analysis published by Marshall and Irvine documented that they are as effective as conventional steroid enemas.[49] Alc The only published trial comparing budesonide enemas with 5-ASA enemas revealed no differences in endoscopic or histopathologic scores between the treatment groups, but the clinical remission rate was greater with 5-ASA (60% *v* 38%, $P = 0.03$).[65]

Most reported trials have demonstrated no benefit for corticosteroids in the maintenance of remission of ulcerative colitis.[66–68]

Azathioprine and 6-Mercaptopurine

Most trials of anti-metabolite drugs in ulcerative colitis have been small. There is no evidence that azathioprine (2·5 mg/kg/day) combined with prednisolone induces remission more effectively than steroids alone.[69] Alc

Nevertheless, azathioprine has been shown to have a steroid-sparing effect at doses between 1·5 and 2·5 mg/kg/day, and the major indication for this drug in ulcerative colitis is for patients who require continuing steroid therapy.[70,71]

In the double blind randomized controlled trial conducted by Jewell and Truelove, patients who had gone into remission during the acute stage were weaned off steroids and given either placebo or maintenance therapy with azathioprine for 1 year.[69] Overall, azathioprine offered no statistically significant advantage over placebo for reducing the relapse rate. There may have been some benefit to azathioprine, however, in the subgroup of patients who were treated for relapsing disease, as opposed to those who presented with their first episode of colitis, as illustrated in Table 11.1. Specifically, nine of 24 azathioprine-treated patients in the former group had no relapse during follow up, compared with three of 25 patients given placebo. More detailed *post hoc* analysis revealed that only seven patients in the azathioprine group experienced at least three relapses or failed therapy, compared with 15 patients in the placebo group ($P = 0.055$). These analyses should be interpreted with caution because they represent *post hoc* subgroup analyses of small numbers of patients.

Hawthorne and colleagues conducted an azathioprine withdrawal trial that suggested a benefit for this drug in the maintenance of remission.[72] In this study, patients who were in long-term remission while taking azathioprine were randomized to continue with the medication or take placebo. During the subsequent year of follow up, patients receiving placebo relapsed significantly more often than did those who remained on azathioprine. Ald It should be pointed out, however, that this type of trial design cannot be used to estimate the size of the treatment effect from an intervention. It is possible that only a small proportion of patients can be maintained in remission with azathioprine, and that most of these patients would relapse if the drug were withdrawn. More recently, Sood *et al.*[73] randomized 35 patients with newly diagnosed ulcerative colitis, all of whom received corticosteroids to induce remission, to receive either sulfasalazine and azathioprine, or sulfasalazine and a placebo for one year. Four patients (23·5%) who received azathioprine suffered relapse of disease, compared to 10 (55·6%) who received sulfasalazine alone (*P* < 0·05). Ald This is somewhat stronger evidence that azathioprine is beneficial for maintenance of remission in ulcerative colitis, but the results should be confirmed with a larger study.

A single small randomized trial reported by Maté-Jimenez et al.[74] using 6-mercaptopurine rather than azathioprine showed 6-mercaptopurine to be more effective than methotrexate or 5-ASA for induction and maintenance of remission in ulcerative colitis (see below). Ald

Methotrexate

There have been anecdotal reports of the steroid-sparing effects of methotrexate in patients with chronic active ulcerative colitis. In a double blind randomized controlled trial 67 patients with steroid-dependent disease were randomized to either oral methotrexate 12·5 mg per week (30 patients) or placebo (37 patients) for 9 months.[75] No benefit was demonstrated for methotrexate in terms of disease activity, remission rate or steroid dosage. Alc The dosage of methotrexate employed in this study, however, was smaller than those used in case reports (up to 25 mg intramuscularly per week). A subsequent small study using oral methotrexate at a dose of 15 mg/week in steroid-dependent ulcerative colitis found that the dosage of corticosteroids could be reduced acutely but that the benefit was not maintained over the subsequent 76 weeks.[74] In this study Maté-Jimenez et al. compared 6-mercaptopurine (1·5 mg/kg), methotrexate (15 mg orally weekly), and 5-ASA (3 g daily) for induction and maintenance of remission in 34 steroid-dependent patients with ulcerative colitis.[74] They reported that 6-mercaptopurine was more effective than either methotrexate or 5-ASA for both induction and maintenance of remission in these patients. Ald Larger studies using higher doses of methotrexate would be of interest.

Cyclosporin

There have been no randomized controlled trials of oral cyclosporin in patients with ulcerative colitis, and case reports have not suggested impressive efficacy. Anecdotal reports of benefit from intravenous cyclosporin led to a randomized controlled trial by Lichtiger and associates, involving 20 patients with severe ulcerative colitis unresponsive to 7–10 days of intravenous hydrocortisone therapy.[76] Patients received either cyclosporin (4 mg/kg) or placebo by continuous intravenous infusion. Nine of the 11 cyclosporin-treated patients went into remission without surgery, compared with none of the patients in the placebo group.

Moreover, five of the placebo-treated patients achieved remission after receiving intravenous cyclosporin. Ald

Since publication of Lichtiger's trial, intravenous cyclosporin has been extensively used for severe disease. Response rates between 60% and 85% have been reported outside of controlled trials, but many patients subsequently relapse and require colectomy[77,78] B4 Nevertheless, intravenous cyclosporin may be useful especially for patients with their first episode of severe colitis and for those who need time before deciding to undergo surgery. Although most clinical investigators have continued to use 4 mg/kg intravenously, 2 mg/kg was as effective as the higher dose in a randomized trial of 73 patients with severe colitis.[79] Alc Further trials are necessary to determine the optimal length of treatment and especially to decide what to do with the responders. Many clinicians discontinue cyclosporin and add azathioprine on the basis that this approach may provide sufficient time for azathioprine to become effective while the corticosteroids are being tapered. For patients who either refuse intravenous corticosteroids or who have previously had major adverse effects (for example psychoses), no difference in effectiveness was demonstrated in a small randomized trial between intravenous cyclosporin as monotherapy and intravenous hydrocortison.[80] Ald

Several clinical trials have shown that oral cyclosporin is not an effective maintenance therapy in patients with steroid-resistant ulcerative colitis who achieved remission with either intravenous or oral cyclosporin.[81–83] Most patients either relapsed (and underwent colectomy) or required corticosteroid therapy. Uncontrolled trials suggest that azathioprine may be effective in maintaining remission in patients whose disease remitted with intravenous cyclosporin.[84–86] B4

Topical cyclosporine has been used for patients with resistant proctitis or distal colitis. Enemas containing 250 mg of the drug have yielded minimal plasma concentrations and no systemic adverse effects. Small clinical series have been reported from Copenhagen, the Mayo Clinic and Oxford. These patients had failed to respond to oral or topical mesalamine, corticosteroids or antimetabolites. Approximately 70% of the patients seemed to improve with topical cyclosporin, although many relapsed when treatment was discontinued. B4 No formal clinical trial has been conducted in patients with resistant proctitis, largely because of the negative results found by Sandborn and colleagues in a small randomized controlled trial.[87] Ald Because this study enrolled only 40 patients, it may not have had sufficient power to exclude a small therapeutic benefit. Furthermore, Sandborn's trial differed from the open series in that it involved patients with active distal colitis instead of resistant proctitis.

Nicotine

Cigarette smoking seems to protect against the development of ulcerative colitis; ex-smokers and non-smokers are at increased risk.[88] Three randomized controlled trials have examined the efficacy of transdermal nicotine, given concurrently with mesalamine and/or corticosteroids, in the treatment of ulcerative colitis.[89–91] Pullan and associates found that the nicotine patch was more effective than placebo (49% v 24%) for the induction of remission.[89] Sandborn and colleagues showed that nicotine was superior to placebo (39% v 9%) at producing clinical improvement.[90] The NNT to induce remission or result in clinical improvement in these two trials was 4 and 3, respectively. Alc

A 6-week trial failed to demonstrate any benefit of transdermal nicotine over prednisolone 15 mg/day.[91] A more recent randomized controlled trial involving patients with left-sided ulcerative colitis that relapsed despite taking mesalamine 1 g twice daily, compared nicotine patches with prednisone, each given for 5 weeks.[92] The study found that the rate of relapse after nicotine was less than with prednisone (20% v 60%), and that patients in the latter group relapsed earlier. Ald

Two pilot studies found that nicotine enemas were effective for distal colitis,[93,94] and randomized controlled trials are warranted.

Thomas and associates reported the only randomized controlled trial of transdermal nicotine as maintenance therapy for ulcerative colitis.[95] The study demonstrated no benefit of nicotine 15 mg/day over placebo over a 6-month period, but this may be explained by poor compliance with the patch. Ald

New agents

Many new approaches are being developed for the treatment of moderate–severe ulcerative colitis. Apheretic techniques in which leukocytes are removed by passing venous blood through absorption columns have been widely reported to be effective but virtually all the data are anecdotal, mainly from Japan. A single small randomized controlled trial has been carried out[96] in which 19 ulcerative colitis patients were randomized to receive apheresis or a sham procedure in addition to continuing their conventional therapy. Apheresis appeared to be significantly more "effective" than the sham procedure (remission rates: apheresis 8/10, sham procedure 3/9, $P < 0.05$) and was well tolerated. A European trial is in progress.

Monoclonal anti-bodies to adhesion molecules, ($\alpha4\beta7$ integrin) are also being investigated in clinical trials, based on the hypothesis that inhibiting the recruitment of lymphocytes into the lamina propria might lead to a downregulation of the inflammation. Feagan et al. carried out a randomized placebo-controlled trial of two doses (0.5 and 2.0 mg/kg) of the humanized $\alpha_4\beta_7$ anti-body MLN02 in 181 patients with mildly to moderately active ulcerative colitis (median Ulcerative Colitis Clinical Score 7, median Modified Baron

Score 3, minimum disease extent 25 cm).[97] Remission rates 2 weeks after the two infusions were significantly greater in the MLN02-treated patients (MLN02 0.5 mg/kg 33%, 2.0 mg/kg 34%, placebo 15%; $P = 0.03$). Ald A single patient experienced mild angioedema following MLN02 infusion. Further studies of this agent are required.

Based on the favorable experience with intravenous cyclosporine, it is plausible that inhibition of interleukin-2 by other, better tolerated, agents might be an effective therapeutic strategy. Preliminary studies have evaluated two different humanized monoclonal anti-bodies to the interleukin-2 receptor.[98,99] Although these trials were uncontrolled preliminary results seemed promising. B4

The anti-tumor necrosis factor (TNF) strategies have primarily been directed towards Crohn's disease. Nevertheless, there are many anecdotal reports of the use of infliximab for severe ulcerative colitis not responding to intravenous corticosteroids.[100] Randomized trials are in progress but the only one published so far has been negative.[101] This trial included 43 patients with steroid-resistant ulcerative colitis. Some patients were receiving azathioprine, and about 70% had extensive disease. They were all symptomatic, but rectal inflammation on sigmoidoscopy was mostly mild and C-reactive protein (CRP) in both groups was low at entry into the study. Patients were randomized in a blinded fashion to receive an infusion of infliximab 5 mg/kg or placebo at week 0 and week 2. Final assessment was at week 6. Outcome measures included a fall in the clinical activity and sigmoidoscopic scores. There was a trend in favor of infliximab but no statistically significant differences were found at 6-weeks. Ald However, the reduction in steroid use was significantly greater in the infliximab group compared with the placebo group. The authors conclude that infliximab should not be used in the routine treatment of steroid-resistant colitis. However, larger studies in better defined groups of patients are needed before that conclusion can stand with confidence. In a small randomized trial in patients with severe pancolitis,[102] no difference in remission between infliximab and steroid-treated patients was demonstrated (infliximab 5/6, steroid 6/7), although this study clearly lacked power to demonstrate significant differences in response and larger trials are needed.

Pegylated interferon alpha in one of two doses (0.5 micrograms/kg or 1.0 micrograms/kg) infused weekly for 12 weeks was compared with placebo in a randomized trial in 60 patients who continued to receive conventional therapies (5-ASA, steroids, azathioprine) in stable doses.[103] A trend toward benefit with the lower dose of interferon was reported, but further studies are required. Ald

Sinha et al.[104] randomized 12 patients with active left-sided colitis or proctitis to receive daily enemas of the potent mitogenic epidermal growth factor (EGF), and 12 to receive placebo enemas for 14 days. All patients received oral mesalamine. At two weeks 10 of the 12 patients given EGF enemas were in clinical remission, as compared with 1 of 12 in the control group ($P < 0.001$). Ald At the 2-week assessment, disease-activity scores, sigmoidoscopic scores, and histologic scores were all significantly better in the EGF group than in the placebo group ($P < 0.01$ for all comparisons), and this benefit was maintained at 4 weeks and at 12 weeks. Sandborn et al.[105] conducted a randomized placebo-controlled trial of the fibroblast growth factor repifermin at doses of 1–50 micrograms/kg infused daily for 5 days in patients with active ulcerative colitis who were receiving 5-ASA, steroids or azathioprine. They found this agent to be safe but not effective at these doses. Ald

Probiotics

A popular theory regarding the pathogenesis of IBD contends that chronic inflammation is the result of an abnormal host response to the endogenous microflora. Thus, a sound rationale exists for attempts to modify host bacteria in the hope that this would downregulate the pathological immune response.[106] Experiments in rodents have demonstrated the potential of this approach[107,108] and preliminary studies in humans have been reported. Kruis[109] randomly assigned 120 patients with ulcerative colitis in remission to receive either 1.5 g/day of 5-ASA or identically appearing tablets that contained *Escherichia coli* strain Nissle 1917. At the end of this 1-year study 11.3% of patients who received 5-ASA relapsed as compared with 16.0% of those who received the probiotic ($P > 0.05$). Alc No serious adverse events were associated with active treatment. This study can be criticized because of the very low relapse rate observed in the control group despite the rather modest dose of 5-ASA that was used. Moreover, the trial was not designed as a formal non-superiority study and therefore lacked sufficient statistical power to assess whether the treatments were clinically equivalent. In another study of this agent, Rembacken et al.[110] randomized 116 patients with active disease to receive 5-ASA or the *E. coli* strain. Treatment was continued for 1 year. At the end of the trial 73% of the patients who had entered remission with conventional therapy relapsed as compared with 67% of those assigned to the probiotic ($P > 0.05$). The authors concluded that the two strategies were of equivalent efficacy. Alc Finally, a third randomized controlled trial of *E. coli* Nissle 1917 has been reported in abstract form. This trial, which was designed as a formal non-superiority study,[109] randomized 327 patients with quiescent disease to 200 mg once daily of the probiotic or 500 mg three times daily of 5-ASA for 12 months of treatment. The rate of relapse was 45% in patients who received *E. coli* Nissle 1917 compared with 36% (absolute difference 9%) in favor of 5-ASA and met the investigators prespecified criterion for therapeutic equivalence. Ala

In summary these preliminary results from relatively large studies suggest that the concept of using probiotics to maintain remission deserves further investigation.

Surgery

Colectomy with construction of an ileal pouch–anal anastomosis has become the operation of choice for ulcerative colitis in major centers. Precise details of pouch construction may affect the eventual functional outcome, although a "J" pouch with 20-cm limbs and a stapled anastomosis 1.0–1.5 cm above the dentate line is the best for most patients.[111–113] Pouch dysfunction remains a frequent problem, and is often due to "pouchitis". The management of this disorder is addressed in Chapter 12.

References

1 Jenkins D, Balsitis M, Gallivan S *et al.* Guidelines for the initial biospy diagnosis of suspected chronic inflammatory bowel disease. The British Society of Gastroenterology Initiative. *J Clin Pathol* 1997;**50**:93–105.

2 Bentley E, Jenkins D, Campbell F and Warren B. How could pathologists improve the initial diagnosis of colitis? Evidence from an international workshop. *J Clin Pathol* 2003;**55**:955–60.

3 Truelove SC, Pena AS. Course and prognosis of Crohn's disease. *Gut* 1976;**17**:192–201.

4 Sinclair TS, Brunt PW, Mowat NAG. Non-specific protocolitis in northeastern Scotland: a community study. *Gastroenterology* 1983;**85**:1–11.

5 Persson PG, Bernell O, Leijonmarck CE *et al.* Survival and cause-specific mortality in inflammatory bowel disease: a population-based cohort study. *Gastroenterology* 1996;**110**: 1339–45.

6 Langholz E, Munkholm P, Davidsen M *et al.* Course of ulcerative colitis: analysis of changes in disease activity over years. *Gastroenterology* 1994;**107**:3–11.

7 Winther KV, Jess T, Langholz E, Munkholm P, Binder V. Survival and cause-specific mortality in ulcerative colitis: follow up of a population-based cohort in Copenhagen county. *Gastroenterology* 2003;**125**:1576–82.

8 Langholz E, Munkholm P, Krasilnikoff PA *et al.* Inflammatory bowel diseases with onset in childhood-clinical features, morbidity, and mortality in a regional cohort. *Scand J Gastroenterol* 1997;**32**:139–47.

9 Lennard-Jones JE, Shivananda S. Clinical uniformity of inflammatory bowel disease a presentation and during the first year of disease in the north and south of Europe. EC-IBD Study Group. *Eur J Gastroenterol Hepatol* 1997;**9**:353–9.

10 Moum B, Ekbom A, Vatn MH *et al.* Clinical course during the 1st year after diagnosis in ulcerative colitis and Crohn's disease. Results of a large, prospective population-based study in southeastern Norway, 1990–93. *Scand J Gastroenterol* 1997;**32**:1005–12.

11 Ayres RC, Gillen CD, Walmsley RS, Allan RN. Progression of ulcerative proctosigmoiditis: incidence and factors influencing progression. *Eur J Gastroenterol Hepatol* 1996; **8**:555–8.

12 Moum B, Ekbom A, Vatn MH, Elgjo K. Change in the extent of colonoscopic and histological involvement in ulcerative colitis over time. *Am J Gastroenterol* 1999;**94**:1564–9.

13 Meucci G, Vecchi M, Astegiano M *et al*. The natural history of ulcerative proctitis: a multicenter, retrospective study. Gruppo di Studio per le Malattie Infiammatorie Intestinali (GSMII). *Am J Gastroenterol* 2000;**95**:469–73.

14 Langholz E, Munkholm P, Davidsen M *et al*. Changes in extent of ulcerative colitis – a study on the course and prognostic factors. *Scand J Gastroenterol* 1996;31:260–6.

15 Gyde SN, Prior P, Allan RN *et al*. Colorectal cancer in ulcerative colitis: a cohort study of primary referrals from three centres. *Gut* 1988;**29**:206–17.

16 Langholz E, Munkholm P, Davidsen M *et al*. Colorectal cancer risk and mortality in patients with ulcerative colitis. *Gastroenterology* 1992;**103**:1444–51.

17 Lynch DAF, Lobo AJ, Sobala GM *et al*. Failure of colonoscopic surveillance in ulcerative colitis. *Gut* 1993;**34**:1075–80.

18 Blackstone M, Riddell R, Rogers B, Levin B. Dysplasia-associated lesion or mass (DALM) detected by colonoscopy in longstanding ulcerative colitis: an indication for colectomy. *Gastroenterology* 1981;**80**:366.

19 Butt J, Konishi F, Morson BC *et al*. Macroscopic lesions in dysplasia and carcinoma complicating ulcerative colitis. *Dig Dis Sci* 1983;**28**:18.

20 Engelsgjerd M, Farraye FA, Odze RD. Polypectomy may be adequate treatment for adenoma-like dysplastic lesions in chronic ulcerative colitis. *Gastroenterology* 1999;**117**:1288.

21 Rubin PH, Friedman S, Harpaz N *et al*. Colonoscopic polypectomy in chronic colitis: conservative management after endoscopic resection of dysplastic polyps. *Gastroenterology* 1999;**117**:1295.

22 Riddell RH. Cancer surveillance in IBD does not work: the argument against. In: Tytgat GNJ, Bartelsman JFWM, Deventer SJH (eds). *Inflammatory bowel diseases*. New York: Kluwer Academic, 1995.

23 Lim CH. Low grade dysplasia: non-surgical treatment. *Inflamm Bowel Dis* 2003;**9**:270–2.

24 Ullman TA. Patients with low-grade dysplasia should be advised to undergo colectomy. *Inflamm Bowel Dis* 2003;**9**:267–9.

25 Svartz N. Salazopyrin, a new sulfanilamide preparation. A. Therapeutic results in rheumatic polyarthritis. B. Therapeutic results in ulcerative colitis. C. Toxic manifestations in treatment with sulfanilamide preparation. *Acta Med Scand* 1942;**110**:557–90.

26 Baron JH, Connell AM, Lennard-Jones JE *et al*. Sulphasalazine and salicylazosulphadimidine in ulcerative colitis. *Lancet* 1962;**i**:1094–6.

27 Misiewicz JJ, Lennard-Jones JE, Connell AM *et al*. Controlled trial of sulphasalazine in maintenance therapy for ulcerative colitis. *Lancet* 1965;**i**:185–8.

28 Dissanayake AS, Truelove SC. A controlled therapeutic trial of long-term maintenance treatment of ulcerative colitis with sulphasalazine (Salazopyrin). *Gut* 1973;**14**:923–6.

29 Azad Khan AK, Piris J, Truelove SC. An experiment to determine the active therapeutic moiety of sulphasalazine. *Lancet* 1977;**ii**:892–5.

30 Azad Khan AK, Howes DT, Piris J, Truelove SC. Optimum dose of sulphasalazine for maintenance treatment in ulcerative colitis. *Gut* 1980;**21**:232–40.

31 Van Hees PAM, Bakker JH, Van Tongeren JHM. Effect of sulphapyridine, 5-aminosaliylic acid, and placebo in patients with idiopathic proctitis: a study to determine the active therapeutic moiety of sulphasalazine. *Gut* 1980;**21**:632–5.

32 Williams CN. Overview of 5-ASA in the therapy of IBD. In: Sutherland LR, Collins SM, Martin F *et al* (eds). *Bowel Disease: Basic Research, Clinical Implications and Trends in Therapy*. Dordecht: Kluwer Academic, 1994.

33 Sutherland LR, Roth DE, Beck PL. Alternatives to sulfasalazine: a meta-analysis of 5-ASA in the treatment of ulcerative colitis. *Inflamm Bowel Dis* 1997;**3**:65–78.

34 Sutherland LR, Roth DE, Beck PL, May GR, Makiyama K. Oral 5-aminosalicylic acid for inducing remission in ulcerative colitis. Cochrane Database of Systematic Reviews 2000;**2**:CD000543.

35 Sutherland LR, Roth DE, Beck PL, May GR, Makiyama K. Oral 5-aminosalicylic acid for maintenance of remission in ulcerative colitis. Cochrane Database of Systematic Reviews 2002;**4**:CD000544.

36 Rao SSC, Dundas SAC, Holdsworth CD, Cann PA, Palmer KR, Corbett CL. Olsalazine or sulphasalazine in the first attacks of ulcerative colitis? A double blind study. *Gut* 1989;**30**:675–9.

37 Nilsson A, Danielsson A, Löfberg R, *et al*. Olsalazine versus sulphasalazine for relapse prevention in ulcerative colitis: a multicenter study. *Am J Gastroenterol* 1995;**90**:381–7.

38 Travis SP, Tysk C, de Silva HJ, Sandberg-Gertzen H, Jewell DP, Järnerot G. Optimum dose of olsalazine for maintaining remission in ulcerative colitis. *Gut* 1994;**35**:1282–6.

39 Wadworth AN, Fitton A. Olsalazine. A review of its pharmacodynamic and pharmacokinetic properties, and therapeutic potential in inflammatory bowel disease. *Drugs* 1991;**41**:647–64.

40 Järnerot G. Withdrawal rates because of diarrhoea in Dipentum-treated patients with ulcerative colitis are low when Dipentum is taken with food and dose titrated [Abstract]. *Gastroenterology* 1996;**110**:A932.

41 Gionchetti P, Campieri M, Venturi A *et al*. Systemic availability of 5-aminosalicylic acid: comparison of delayed release and an azo-bond preparation. *Aliment Pharmacol Ther* 1996;**10**:601–5.

42 Stoa-Birketvedt G, Florholmen J. The systemic load and efficient delivery of active 5-aminosalicylic acid in patients with ulcerative colitis on treatment with olsalazine or mesalazine. *Aliment Pharmacol Ther* 1999;**13**:357–61.

43 Green JRB, Lobo AJ, Holdsworth CD *et al*. and the Abacus Investigator Group. Balsalazide is more effective and better tolerated than mesalamine in the treatment of acute ulcerative colitis. *Gastroenterology* 1998;**114**:15–22.

44 Levine DS, Riff DS, Pruitt R *et al.* A randomized, double blind, dose-response comparison of balsalazide (6.75 g), balsalazide (2.25 g), and mesalamine (2.4 g) in the treatment of active, mild-to-moderate ulcerative colitis. *Am J Gastroenterol* 2002;**97**:1398–407.

45 Pruitt R, Hanson J, Safdi M *et al.* Balsalazide is superior to mesalamine in the time to improvement of signs and symptoms of acute mild-to-moderate ulcerative colitis. *Am J Gastroenterol* 2002;**97**:3078–86.

46 Green JRB, Mansfield JC, Gibson JA, Kerr GD, Thornton PC. A double blind comparison of balsalazide, 6.75 g daily, and sulfasalazine, 3 g daily, in patients with newly diagnosed or relapsed active ulcerative colitis. *Aliment Pharmacol Ther* 2002;**16**:61–8.

47 Green JRB, Gibson JA, Kerr GD *et al.* Maintenance of remission of ulcerative colitis: a comparison between balsalazide 3 g daily and mesalazine 1.2 g daily over 12 months. ABACUS Investigator group. *Aliment Pharmacol Ther* 1998;**12**:1207–16.

48 Marshall JK, Irvine EJ. Rectal aminosalicylate therapy for distal ulcerative colitis: a meta-analysis. *Aliment Pharmacol Ther* 1995;**9**:293–300.

49 Marshall JK, Irvine EJ. Rectal corticosteroids versus alternative treatments in ulcerative colitis: a meta-analysis. *Gut* 1997;**40**:775–81.

50 Brown J, Haines S, Wilding IR. Colonic spread of three rectally administered mesalazine (Pentasa) dosage forms in healthy volunteers as assessed by gamma scintigraphy. *Aliment Pharmacol Ther* 1997;**11**:685–91.

51 Wilding IR, Kenyon CJ, Chauhan S *et al.* Colonic spreading of a non-chlorofluorocarbon mesalazine rectal foam enema in patients with quiescent ulcerative colitis. *Aliment Pharmacol Ther* 1995;**9**:161–6.

52 Campieri M, Corbelli C, Gionchetti P *et al.* Spread and distribution of 5-ASA colonic foam and 5-ASA enema in patients with ulcerative colitis. *Dig Dis Sci* 1992;**37**:1890–7.

53 Pokrotnieks J, Marlicz K, Paradowski L, Margus B, Zaborowski P, Greinwald R. Efficacy and tolerability of mesalazine foam enema (Salofalk foam) for distal ulcerative colitis: a double-blind, randomized, placebo-controlled study. *Aliment Pharmacol Ther* 2000;**14**:1191–8.

54 Campieri M, Paoluzi P, D'Albasio G, Brunetti G, Pera A, Barbara L. Better quality of therapy with 5-ASA colonic foam in active ulcerative colitis. A multicenter comparative trial with 5-ASA enema. *Dig Dis Sci* 1993;**38**:1843–50.

55 Ardizzone S, Doldo P, Ranzi T *et al.* Mesalazine foam (Salofalk foam) in the treatment of active distal ulcerative colitis. A comparative trial vs Salofalk enema. The SAF-3 study group. *Ital J Gastroenterol Hepatol* 1999;**31**:677–84.

56 Malchow H, Gertz B, CLAFOAM Study group. A new mesalazine foam enema (Claversal Foam) compared with a standard liquid enema in patients with active distal ulcerative colitis. *Aliment Pharmacol Ther* 2002;**16**:415–23.

57 Gionchetti P, Ardizzone S, Benvenuti ME *et al.* A new mesalazine gel enema in the treatment of left-sided ulcerative colitis: a randomized controlled multicentre trial. *Aliment Pharmacol Ther* 1999;**13**:381–8.

58 D'Albasio G, Paoluzi P, Campieri M *et al.* Maintenance treatment of ulcerative proctitis with mesalazine suppositories: a double-blind placebo-controlled trial. The Italian IBD Study Group. *Am J Gastroenterol* 1998;**93**: 799–803.

59 Truelove SC, Witts LJ. Cortisone in ulcerative colitis. Final report on a therapeutic trial. *BMJ* 1955;**4947**:1041–8.

60 Lennard-Jones JE, Longmore AJ, Newell AC *et al.* An assessment of prednisone, salazopyrin, and topical hydrocortisone hemisuccinate used as out-patient treatment for ulcerative colitis. *Gut* 1960;**1**:217–22.

61 Powell-Tuck J, Bown RL, Lennard-Jones JE. A comparison of oral prednisolone given as single or multiple daily doses for active proctocolitis. *Scand J Gastroenterol* 1978;**13**:833–7.

62 Baron JH, Connell AM, Kanaghinis TG *et al.* Out-patient treatment of ulcerative colitis. Comparison between three doses of oral prednisone. *BMJ* 1962;**2**:441–3.

63 Brattsand R. Overview of newer glucocorticosteroid preparations for inflammatory bowel disease. *Can J Gastroenterol* 1990;**4**:407–14.

64 Löfberg R, Danielsson A, Suhr O *et al.* Oral budesonide versus prednisolone in patients with active extensive and left-sided colitis. *Gastroenterology* 1996;**110**:1713–18.

65 Lemann M, Galian A, Rutgeerts P. Comparison of budesonide and 5-aminosalicylic acid enemas in active distal ulcerative colitis. *Aliment Pharmacol Ther* 1995;**9**:557–62.

66 Truelove SC, Witts LJ. Cortisone and corticotrophin in ulcerative colitis. *BMJ* 1959;**i**:387–94.

67 Truelove SC. Treatment of ulcerative colitis with local hydrocortisone hemisuccinate sodium: a report on a controlled therapeutic trial. *BMJ* 1958;**ii**:1072–7.

68 Lennard-Jones JE, Misiewicz JJ, Connell AM. Prednisone as maintenance treatment for ulcerative colitis in remission. *Lancet* 1965;**i**:188–9.

69 Jewell DP, Truelove SC. Azathioprine in ulcerative colitis: final report on controlled therapeutic trial. *BMJ* 1974;**iv**: 627–30.

70 Rosenberg JL, Wall AJ, Levin B, Binder HJ, Kirsner JB. A controlled trial of azathioprine in the management of chronic ulcerative colitis. *Gastroenterology* 1975;**69**: 96–9.

71 Kirk AP, Lennard-Jones JE. Controlled trial of azathioprine in chronic ulcerative colitis. *BMJ* 1982;**284**:1291–2.

72 Hawthorne AB, Logan RFA, Hawkey CJ *et al.* Randomised controlled trial of azathioprine withdrawal in ulcerative colitis. *BMJ* 1992;**305**:20–2.

73 Sood A, Kaushal V, Midha V, Bhatia KL, Sood N, Malhotra V. The beneficial effect of azathioprine on maintenance of remission in severe ulcerative colitis. *J Gastroenterol* 2002; **37**:270–4.

74 Maté-Jimenez J, Hermida C, Cantero-Perona J, Moreno-Otero R. 6-mercaptopurine or methotrexate added to prednisone induces and maintains remission in steroid-dependent inflammatory bowel disease. *Eur J Gastroenterol Hepatol* 2000;**12**:1227–33.

75 Oren R, Arber N, Odes S *et al.* Methotrexate in chronic active ulcerative colitis: a double blind, randomized, Israeli multicenter trial. *Gastroenterology* 1996;**110**:1416–21.

76 Lichtiger S, Present DH, Kornbluth A *et al.* Cyclosporine in severe ulcerative colitis refractory to steroid therapy. *N Engl J Med* 1994;**330**:1841–5.

77 Hyde GM, Thillainayagam AV, Jewell DP. Intravenous cyclosporin as rescue therapy in severe ulcerative colitis: time for a reappraisal? *Eur J Gastroenterol Hepatol* 1998; **10**:411–13.

78 Jewell DP, Hyde GM. Severe ulcerative colitis: cyclosporin or colectomy? A European view. In: Modigliani R, ed. *IBD and Salicylates 3*. Tunbridge Wells: Wells Medical, 1998.

79 Van Assche G, D'Haens G, Noman M *et al.* Randomized, double blind comparison of 4 mg/kg versus 2 mg/kg intravenous cyclosporine in severe ulcerative colitis. *Gastroenterology* 2003;**125**:1025–31.

80 D'Haens G, Leumens L, Geboes K *et al.* Intravenous cyclosporin versus intravenous corticosteroids as single therapy for severe attacks of ulcerative colitis. *Gastroenterology* 2001;**120**:1323–9.

81 Treem WR, Cohen J, Davis PM, Justinich CJ, Hyams JS. Cyclosporine for the treatment of fulminant ulcerative colitis in children. Immediate response, long-term results, and impact on surgery. *Dis Colon Rectum* 1995;**38**:474–9.

82 Gurudu SR, Griffel LH, Gialanella RJ, Das KM. Cyclosporine therapy in inflammatory bowel disease: short-term and long-term results. *J Clin Gastroenterol* 1999;**29**:151–4.

83 Rowe FA, Walker JH, Karp LC, Vasiliauskas EA, Plevy SE, Targan SR. Factors predictive of response to cyclosporin treatment for severe, steroid-resistant ulcerative colitis. *Am J Gastroenterol* 2000;**95**:2000–8.

84 Fernández-Bañares F, Bertran X *et al.* Azathioprine is useful in maintaining long-term remission induced by intravenous cyclosporine in steroid-refractory severe ulcerative colitis. *Am J Gastroenterol* 1996;**91**:2498–9.

85 Actis GC, Bresso F, Astegiano M *et al.* Safety and efficacy of azathioprine in the maintenance of ciclosporin-induced remission of ulcerative colitis. *Aliment Pharmacol Ther* 2001;**15**:1307–11.

86 Domenech E, Garcia-Planella E, Bernal I *et al.* Azathioprine without oral cyclosporine is enough to maintain long-term remission induced by intravenous cyclosporine in steroid-refractory severe ulcerative colitis. Digestive Diseases Week (DDW) 2002; Abstract T1661.

87 Sandborn WJ, Tremaine WJ, Schroeder KW *et al.* A placebo-controlled trial of cyclosporine enemas for mildly to moderately active left-sided ulcerative colitis. *Gastroenterology* 1994;**106**:1429–35.

88 Calkins BM. A meta-analysis of the role of smoking in inflammatory bowel disease. *Dig Dis Sci* 1989;**34**:1841–54.

89 Pullan RD, Rhodes J, Ganesh S *et al.* Transdermal nicotine for active ulcerative colitis. *N Engl J Med* 1994;**330**: 811–15.

90 Sandborn WJ, Tremaine WJ, Offord KP *et al.* Transdermal nicotine for mildly to moderately active ulcerative colitis. A randomized, double blind, placebo-controlled trial. *Ann Intern Med* 1997;**126**:364–71.

91 Thomas GAO, Rhodes J, Ragunath K *et al.* Transdermal nicotine compared with oral prednisolone therapy for active ulcerative colitis. *Eur J Gastroenterol Hepatol* 1996;**8**:769–76.

92 Guslandi M, Tittobello A. Outcome of ulcerative colitis after treatment with transdermal nicotine. *Eur J Gastroenterol Hepatol* 1998;**10**:513–15.

93 Sandborn WJ, Tremaine WJ, Leighton JA *et al.* Nicotine tartrate liquid enemas for mildly to moderately active left-sided ulcerative colitis unresponsive to first-line therapy: a pilot study. *Aliment Pharmacol Ther* 1997;**11**: 663–71.

94 Green JT, Thomas GAO, Rhodes J *et al.* Nicotine enemas for active ulcerative colitis – a pilot study. *Aliment Pharmacol Ther* 1997;**11**:859–63.

95 Thomas GAO, Rhodes J, Mani V *et al.* Transdermal nicotine as maintenance therapy for ulcerative colitis. *N Engl J Med* 1995;**332**:988–92.

96 Sawada K, Kusugam K, Suzuki Y *et al.* Multicenter randomized double blind controlled trial for ulcerative colitis therapy with leukocytapheresis. *Gastroenterology* 2003;**124(4 Suppl 1)**:A67–A68.

97 Feagan B, Greenberg G, Wild G *et al.* A randomized controlled trial of a humanized α4β7 anti-body in ulcerative colitis (UC). Presented at Digestive Diseases Week annual meeting of the American Gastroenterology Association, Orlando, May 2003.

98 Van Assche G, Dalle I, Noman M *et al.* A pilot study on the use of the humanized anti-interleukin-2 receptor anti-body dacluzimab in active ulcerative colitis. *Am J Gastroenterology.* 2003;**98**:369–76.

99 Creed TJ, Norman MR, Probert CS *et al.* Basiliximab (anti-CD25) in combination with steroids may be an effective new treatment for steroid-resistant ulcerative colitis. *Aliment Pharmacol Ther* 2003;**18**:65–75.

100 Gornet JM, Couve S, Hassani Z *et al.* Infliximab for refractory ulcerative colitis or indeterminate colitis: an open label study. *Aliment Pharmacol Ther* 2003;**18**: 175–81.

101 Probert CS, Hearing SD, Schreiber S *et al.* Infliximab in moderately severe glucocorticoid-resistant ulcerative colitis: a randomised controlled trial. *Gut* 2003;**52**: 998–1002.

102 Ochsenkuhn T, Sackmann M, Goeke B. Infliximab for acute severe ulcerative colitis: A randomized pilot study in non-steroid refractory patients. *Gastroenterology* 2003; **124(4 Suppl 1)**:A62.

103 Tilg H, Vogelsang H, Ludwiczek O *et al.* A randomised placebo-controlled trial of pegylated interferon alpha in active ulcerative colitis. *Gut* 2003;**52**:1728–33.

104 Sinha A, Nightingale J, West KP, Berlanga-Acosta J, Playford RJ. Epidermal growth factor enemas with oral mesalamine for mild-to-moderate left-sided ulcerative colitis or proctitis. *N Engl J Med* 2003;**349**:350–7.

105 Sandborn WJ, Sands BE, Wolf DC *et al.* Repifermin (keratinocyte growth factor 2) for the treatment of active ulcerative colitis: a randomized, double blind, placebo-controlled, dose-escalation trial. *Gastroenterology* 2002; **122(Suppl 1)**:A61.

106 Shanahan F. Probiotics and inflammatory bowel disease: from fads and fantasy to facts and future. *Br J Nutr* 2002; **88**:S5–S9.

107 McCarthy J, O'Mahony L, O'Callaghan L *et al*. Double blind, placebo-controlled trial of two probiotic strains in interleukin 10 knockout mice and mechanistic link with cytokine balance. *Gut* 2003;**52**:975–80.

108 Madsen KL. Inflammatory bowel disease: lessons from the IL-10 gene-deficient mouse. *Clin Invest Med* 2001;**24**:250–7.

109 Kruis W. Maintenance of remission in ulcerative colitis is equally effective with *Escherichia coli* Nissle 1917 and with standard mesalamine. Digestive Disease Week 2001;Abstract 680.

110 Rembacken BJ, Snelling AM, Hawkey PM, Chalmers DM, Axon ATR. Non-pathogenic *Escherichia coli* versus mesalazine for the treatment of ulcerative colitis: a randomised trial. *Lancet* 1999;**354**:635.

111 Romanos J, Samarasekera DN, Stebbing J, Jewell DP, Kettlewell MG, Mortensen NJ. Outcome of 200 restorative proctocolectomy operations: the John Radcliffe Hospital experience. *Br J Surg* 1997;**84**:814–18.

112 Setti-Carraro P, Ritchie JK, Wilkinson KH, Nicholls RJ, Hawley PR. The first 10 years' experience of restorative proctocolectomy for ulcerative colitis. *Gut* 1994;**35**:1070–5.

113 McIntyre PB, Pemberton JH, Wolff BG, Beart RW, Dozois RR. Comparing functional results one year and ten years after ileal pouch-anal anastomosis for chronic ulcerative colitis. *Dis Colon Rectum* 1994;**37**:303–7.

12 Pouchitis after restorative proctocolectomy

William J Sandborn

Introduction

Pouchitis is an idiopathic chronic inflammatory disease which may occur in the ileal pouch after restorative proctocolectomy with ileal pouch–anal anastomosis (IPAA) for ulcerative colitis (UC).[1] It is expected that the total number of patients with pouchitis in the USA will eventually stabilize at 30 000–45 000 persons (prevalence of 12–18/100 000).[2] Thus, pouchitis is emerging as an important third form of inflammatory bowel disease (IBD).

Because pouchitis is a relatively new disease, criteria for diagnosis, classification and measurement of disease activity are still evolving. The previous lack of consensus on these issues has hampered the design and conduct of randomized, double blind, placebo-controlled treatment trials, and medical therapy for pouchitis was largely empirical. In 1994 an instrument to measure efficacy of therapy, the pouchitis disease activity index (PDAI) was developed.[3] This facilitated clinical research in this area, and there are now 11 controlled trials of various agents for pouchitis, evaluating treatment with metronidazole, ciprofloxacin, budesonide enemas, dietary fiber, probiotic bacteria, allopurinol, and bismuth carbomer foam enemas.[4-14] The medical therapies reported to be of benefit for pouchitis are shown in Box 12.1. This chapter will assist physicians and surgeons in becoming familiar with the diagnosis and classification of pouchitis, and will review the clinical results from empirical medical therapies and controlled trials, and the rationale for using them.

Diagnosis and disease activity measurement

The diagnosis of pouchitis is suggested by variable clinical symptoms of increased stool frequency, rectal bleeding, abdominal cramping, rectal urgency and tenesmus, incontinence, and fever. A clinical diagnosis of pouchitis should be confirmed by endoscopy and mucosal biopsy of the pouch.[1] Endoscopic examination shows inflammatory changes, which may include mucosal edema, granularity,

---

Box 12.1 Treatments reported to be beneficial for pouchitis

Class example

Antibiotics
- Metronidazole
- Ciprofloxacin
- Amoxicillin/clavulanic acid
- Erythromycin
- Tetracycline
- Rifaximin + ciprofloxacin
- Metronidazole + ciprofloxacin

Probiotic bacteria
- Lactobacilli, Bifidobacteria, *Streptococcus salivarius* sp. *thermophilus*
- *Escherichia coli* strain Nissle 1917

5-Aminosalicylates
- Mesalamine enemas
- Sulfasalazine
- Oral mesalamine

Corticosteroids
- Conventional corticosteroid enemas
- Budesonide suppositories
- Budesonide enemas
- Oral corticosteroids

Immune modifier agents
- Cyclosporin enemas
- Azathioprine, 6-mercaptopurine
- Infliximab

Nutritional agents
- Short chain fatty acids enemas or suppositories
- Glutamine suppositories
- Dietary fiber (pectin, methylcellulose, inulin)

Oxygen radical inhibitors
- Allopurinol

Antidiarrheal/antimicrobial
- Bismuth carbomer enemas
- Bismuth subsalicylate

Modified with permission from Mahadevan and Sandborn. *Gastroenterology* 2003;**124**:1636–50.

Table 12.1   Pouchitis disease activity index (PDAI)

Clinical criteria	Score
Stool frequency	
Usual postop stool frequency	0
1–2 stools/day > postop usual	1
3 or more stools/day > postop usual	2
Rectal bleeding	
None or rare	0
Present daily	1
Fecal urgency/abdominal cramps	
None	0
Occasional	1
Usual	2
Fever (temperature > 100·5° F)	
Absent	0
Present	1
Endoscopic criteria	
Edema	1
Granularity	1
Friability	1
Loss of vascular pattern	1
Mucus exudate	1
Ulceration	1
Acute histological criteria	
Polymorph infiltration:	
Mild	1
Moderate + crypt abscess	2
Severe + crypt abscess	3
Ulceration per low power field:	
(average) < 25%	1
≥ 25% ≥ 50%	2
≥ 50%	3

*Pouchitis is defined as a total PDAI
score ≥ 7 points*

Adapted with permission from Sandborn WJ *et al. Mayo Clin Proc* 1994;**69**:409–15.[3]

contact bleeding, loss of vascular pattern, hemorrhage, and ulceration.[15,16] Histologic examination shows acute inflammation including neutrophil infiltration and mucosal ulceration, superimposed on a background of chronic inflammation including villous atrophy, crypt hyperplasia and chronic inflammatory cell infiltration.[16,17] Endoscopic examination of the neo-terminal ileum above the ileal pouch should be normal. The PDAI is a quantitative 19-point index of pouchitis activity based on both clinical symptoms and endoscopic and histologic findings (Table 12.1).[3] Active pouchitis is defined as a PDAI score ≥ 7 points and remission is defined as a PDAI score < 7 points in a patient with a history of pouchitis. The PDAI has now been used as the endpoint in a number of clinical trials.[6,7,10–12,14] The Heidelberg pouchitis activity score has been proposed as an alternative to the PDAI, but has not been used to assess efficacy in clinical trials.[18]

Classification

Patients with pouchitis can be classified according to disease activity, symptom duration and disease pattern.[2] Disease activity can be classified as: remission (no active pouchitis), mildly to moderately active (increased stool frequency, urgency, infrequent incontinence), or severely active (hospitalization for dehydration, frequent incontinence). Symptom duration can be classified as: acute (< 4 weeks) or chronic (≥ 4 weeks). Finally, the disease pattern can be classified as: infrequent (one to two acute episodes), relapsing (three or more acute episodes), or continuous.

These classifications allow the physician to predict, based on the natural history of pouchitis, the need for suppressive medical therapy.

Treatment with antibiotics and probiotic bacteria

Rationale

After IPAA, the primary function of the terminal ileum changes from absorption to storage, and bacterial overgrowth occurs with bacterial concentrations increasing to levels that are intermediate between end ileostomy and colon.[19,20] There is no correlation between fecal bacterial concentrations and histologic changes of acute inflammation,[19,20] demonstrating that pouchitis and bacterial overgrowth are not directly related. However, anaerobic bacterial overgrowth of the pouch is associated with transformation of the ileal mucosa to a "colon-like" morphology (villous atrophy, chronic inflammatory cell infiltration).[19,21] Thus, pouch bacterial overgrowth may indirectly set the stage for pouchitis to the extent that "colon-like" ileal mucosa may be more susceptible to a recurrence of UC. Strategies directed towards reducing fecal concentrations of anaerobic bacteria through the use of antibiotics, or altering the relative balance of anaerobes and other bacteria using probiotic bacteria therapy, may be useful in treating pouchitis.

Clinical results

Antibiotic therapy

Clinicians have observed that most patients with pouchitis who are empirically treated with antibiotics experience clinical improvement. Although there are few controlled

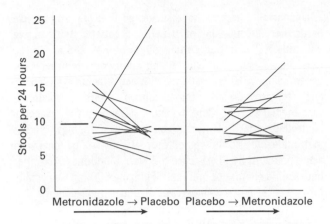

Figure 12.1 Stool frequency before and after metronidazole and placebo. Bars represent mean values. (Reproduced with permission from Madden MV *et al. Dig Dis Sci* 1994;**39**:1193–6[5])

trials, antibiotics have become the *de facto* "standard medical therapy" for pouchitis. The most commonly used antibiotic for pouchitis is metronidazole.[1,4–7,16,20,22–34] The primary alternative to metronidazole is ciprofloxacin.[6,29] Amoxicillin/clavulanic acid, erythromycin and tetracycline have also been reported to be of benefit.[31] Most patients with pouchitis initially appear to respond to metronidazole at doses of 750–1500 mg/day. Symptomatic improvement usually occurs within 1–2 days. Patients with relapsing or continuous pouchitis may require chronic maintenance metronidazole therapy, with doses ranging from 250 mg every third day up to 750 mg/day. In the first controlled trial of this form of therapy reported Madden *et al.* treated 13 patients with active chronic pouchitis in a crossover trial of oral metronidazole 400 mg three times daily or placebo for 14 days.[5] Each patient had a 7-day washout period before crossing over from the first to the second therapy. Eleven of 13 patients completed the study. Metronidazole reduced the daily stool frequency from $10·0 ± 2·8$ to $9·0 ± 5·2$ (mean ± SD) in 12 patients whereas the 11 placebo-treated patients had an increase in daily stool frequency from $8·9 ± 2·5$ up to $10·7 ± 4·1$ (mean ± SD, $P < 0·05$) (Figure 12.1). Ald The clinical significance of such a small change in mean stool frequency may be questioned, and the confidence limits around the difference in means would be very wide in this small study. A second randomized controlled trial by Shen *et al.* compared 2 weeks of treatment with metronidazole 20 mg/kg per day with ciprofloxacin 1000 mg/day in patients with acute pouchitis.[6] Both drugs significantly reduced the PDAI score, but ciprofloxacin had a greater reduction in overall PDAI score ($6·9 ± 1·2$ *v* $3·8 ± 1·7$, $P = 0·002$), symptom score ($2·4 ± 0·9$ *v* $1·3 ± 0·9$, $P = 0·03$) and endoscopic score ($3·6 ± 1·3$ *v* $1·9 ± 1·5$, $P = 0·03$) compared with metronidazole. Ald A third randomized controlled trial

comparing metronidazole 1000 mg/day and budesonide enemas 2 mg/day is described below.[7] Adverse effects occurred in 33–55% of patients during metronidazole treatment, including nausea, vomiting, abdominal discomfort, headache and skin rash.[5–7]

In an attempt to reduce adverse effects from metronidazole, Nygaard *et al.* used a topical metronidazole suspension to treat pouchitis in patients with an IPAA ($n = 4$) or a Kock continent ileostomy ($n = 7$).[35] Seven of the 11 patients had active chronic pouchitis, and three metronidazole-intolerant patients had active acute pouchitis. In this uncontrolled study therapy a liquid metronidazole suspension (40 mg) was instilled into the IPAA or continent ileostomy one to four times per day. All 11 patients improved within 2–3 days of beginning treatment with topical metronidazole. Nine of the 11 patients had continued improvement on either maintenance ($n = 3$) or intermittent ($n = 8$) treatment. Four of eight patients had undetectable serum metronidazole concentrations and four had low serum concentrations following instillation of metronidazole into the pouch. In another uncontrolled study a vaginal formulation of metronidazole (37·5 mg) was administered transanally two to four times per day with an applicator into the ileal pouch of six patients with active pouchitis (four of whom were metronidazole-intolerant).[36] All patients improved, and only one of six patients experienced metronidazole-induced adverse effects. Gionchetti *et al.* also used this "topical" antibiotic approach, reporting that oral ciprofloxacin 1 g/day in combination with an orally administered non-absorbable antibiotic, rifaximin, was beneficial in patients with active chronic pouchitis resistant to standard antibiotic therapy.[37]

Probiotic bacteria

Another therapeutic approach to altering pouch bacterial contents is to administer probiotic bacteria. Three controlled trials have been performed.[10–12] Gionchetti *et al.* randomized 40 patients with chronic pouchitis in remission (PDAI score = 0 after induction therapy with antibiotics) to treatment with either a new oral probiotic preparation (VSL-3) 6 g/day or placebo for 9 months.[10] The VSL-3 preparation contained 10^{11}/g of viable lyophilized bacteria: four strains of lactobacilli (*Lactobacillus acidophilus*, *L. delbrueckii* sp. *bulgaricus*, *L. plantarum* and *L. casei*), three strains of bifidobacteria (*Bifidobacterium infantis*, *B. longum*, *B. breve*), and one strain of *Streptococcus salivarius* sp. *thermophilus*. Relapse was defined as an increase in the clinical component of the PDAI of > 2 points (6 points is the maximum possible). At 9 months, the relapse rate in the VSL-3 group was 15% compared with 100% in the placebo group ($P < 0·01$). Ald The NNT, the number of patients needed to treat with this therapy to prevent one relapse, is 2, indicating that this is a very effective form of therapy. Fecal concentrations of lactobacilli, bifidobacteria, and *S. thermophilus* increased significantly from baseline in the VSL-3 group but not in the placebo group. There was no change from baseline in the fecal concentrations of anaerobic bacteria in either group. In a second controlled trial, 36 patients with recurrent or refractory pouchitis were treated with antibiotics and then randomized to maintenance therapy with VSL-3 or placebo for 1 year. The relapse rates were 10% in the VSL-3 group and 94% in the placebo group ($P < 0.0001$).[11] Ald In a third study, patients undergoing colectomy and IPAA were randomized to prophylactic therapy with VSL-3 or placebo for 1 year.[12] The rate of developing pouchitis during the first year was 10% in the VSL-3 group and 40% in the placebo group ($P < 0.05$). Ald A case report of two patients suggested that another probiotic, *Escherichia coli* strain Nissle 1917, may be of benefit for the treatment of active pouchitis and for maintenance therapy.[38]

Treatment with anti-inflammatory and immune modifier agents

Rationale

Pouchitis may be a recurrence of IBD in the ileoanal pouch.[1] Data to support this view include: an increased frequency of pouchitis in patients with UC as compared with familial polyposis; an increased frequency of pouchitis in patients with extra-intestinal manifestations of UC; an increased frequency of pouchitis in patients with primary sclerosing cholangitis; an increased frequency of pouchitis in patients with anti-neutrophil cytoplasmic antibodies with a perinuclear staining pattern (pANCA); and a protective effect against developing pouchitis in current smokers. Strategies directed towards empirical medical therapy with agents known to be efficacious in UC may be useful in treating pouchitis. Unfortunately few controlled trials have been reported to provide evidence for the efficacy of these approaches.

Clinical results

Uncontrolled studies suggest that topical mesalamine (enemas or suppositories) may be beneficial for active pouchitis.[15,20,30,39,40] B4 Anecdotal experience suggests that sulfasalazine and oral mesalamine may also be of benefit. An *in vitro* study measuring the azoreductase enzyme activity of fecal bacteria from patients with ileoanal pouches demonstrated adequate enzyme activity to cleave the azo bond necessary to activate sulfasalazine.[41] An *in vivo* study demonstrated that the azo bond of sulfasalazine was cleaved in patients with ileal pouches.[42] It is reasonable to assume that at least a portion of the Pentasa formulation of mesalamine will release into the ileoanal pouch. Whether the Asacol formulation of mesalamine will release into the pouch is unknown.

Uncontrolled reports have suggested that oral and topical corticosteroids may be of benefit in patients with active pouchitis.[20,30,31,33] Budesonide suppositories 0·5 mg three times daily resulted in clinical and endoscopic improvement or remission in 10/10 patients with active acute pouchitis,[43] and decreased pouch luminal concentrations of inflammatory mediators.[40,43] More recently, a randomized, placebo-controlled trial of 2 mg budesonide enemas versus metronidazole also showed efficacy.[7] Twenty-six patients with acute pouchitis by PDAI score ≥ 7 were randomized to either budesonide enemas or oral metronidazole 500 mg twice daily for 6 weeks. Fifty-eight percent of budesonide patients and 50% of metronidazole patients improved. Fifty-seven percent of metronidazole patients had adverse events versus only 25% Ald of budesonide patients. Oral controlled release budesonide has not been reported for the treatment of pouchitis, but anecdotal experience suggests that it may be effective (WJ Sandborn, unpublished data).

Cyclosporin enemas (250 mg/day) were reported to be beneficial in one patient with active chronic pouchitis[44] although a small placebo-controlled trial of cyclosporin enemas in patients with left-sided UC was negative. Ald Two studies involving 11 patients with both IPAA for UC and liver transplantation for primary sclerosing cholangitis have reported on the clinical disease course of pouchitis following liver transplantation.[45,46] Five of 11 patients had chronic pouchitis following liver transplantation, despite immunosuppression with ciclosporin or tacrolimus, prednisone, and azathioprine, suggesting that immuno-suppression may not be efficacious for pouchitis. B4 Two small reports have suggested a beneficial effect of azathioprine in patients with Crohn's disease and an IPAA.[47,48] Recently, infliximab has been reported to be of benefit in patients with pouchitis[49,50] and patients with Crohn's disease of the ileoanal pouch.[51,52]

Treatment with nutritional agents

Rationale

In the well-functioning ileal pouch, the bacterial flora produce short chain fatty acids (SCFA) including acetate, propionate and butyrate at concentrations similar to those in the colon of healthy controls, and increased compared with stomal SCFA concentrations in ileostomy patients.[19,53] Some[54,55] but not all[19] studies have reported that patients with pouchitis have significantly lower fecal concentrations of SCFAs than patients with well functioning IPAAs, perhaps from dilution.[54] Strategies directed at replacing fecal SCFA deficiencies by administering SCFA enemas or suppositories, or by increasing intake of fermentable dietary fiber may theoretically be useful in treating pouchitis. C5 Another nutritional therapeutic approach to improving pouch function is through use of non-fermentable dietary fiber, with the goal of improving stool consistency.

Clinical results

SFCA 60 ml enemas containing 60 mmol sodium acetate, 30 mmol sodium propionate, 40 mmol sodium n-butyrate, and sodium chloride titrated to a concentration of 280–290 mosmol, were not of benefit in two patients with active pouchitis.[56] Similarly, another study using an identical SCFA enema formulation reported improvement in only 3/8 patients with active pouchitis.[57] In contrast, a third study in patients with active chronic pouchitis reported improvement in 3/9 patients treated with 40 mmol sodium butyrate suppositories compared with 6/10 patients treated with 1 g L-glutamine suppositories.[55] Finally, a case report using the SCFA enema formulation described above reported success in a single patient with active chronic pouchitis.[58] Inulin is a dietary fiber that is fermented to SCFAs. Twenty patients with ileoanal pouches (included both patients with and without pouchitis) were randomized to treatment with inulin 24 g/day or placebo for 3 weeks.[9] Patients treated with inulin had higher fecal butyrate concentrations, lower fecal pH, lower fecal concentrations of *Bacteroides fragilis* and lower concentrations of some secondary bile acids in the feces compared with patients treated with placebo. The mean PDAI scores were lower in patients treated with inulin compared with placebo-treated patients (4·1 v 5·4, P = 0·01). Ald Because not all of these patients had pouchitis, the effectiveness of inulin for the treatment of pouchitis is unclear. Thirlby and Kelly randomized 13 patients with ileoanal pouches (included both patients with and without pouchitis) in a crossover trial to treatment for 3 weeks with pectin (a soluble fermentable fiber supplement) or Citrucel (a methyl cellulose-based non-fermentable fiber) and found that neither fiber compound resulted in improved stool frequency, pouch function, bloating or stool consistency after IPAA.[8] Thus, the low overall clinical response rates in these small studies suggest that neither SCFA enemas or suppositories, nor inulin, are highly effective therapies for active pouchitis. B4, Ald

Treatment with allopurinol

Rationale

During surgical construction of the IPAA, the mesenteric vessels may be divided to avoid tension on the pouch–anal anastomosis.[59] This ligation of the arterial blood supply has the potential to cause ischemic injury to the ileal pouch, and oxygen free radical formation is known to be one the mechanisms by which ischemic injury occurs. However, there have been no studies that measured either ileal blood flow or

oxygen free radical formation in patients with and without pouchitis. Thus, there are no objective data demonstrating that pouch ischemia occurs, much less data demonstrating a relationship between pouch ischemia and pouchitis. If intestinal ischemia contributed to the pathogenesis of pouchitis, then medical therapy directed toward reducing oxygen free radical formation might be a useful strategy. For this reason, the xanthine oxidase inhibitor allopurinol has been proposed as a treatment for pouchitis.

Clinical results

An uncontrolled study reported that allopurinol 300 twice daily induced clinical improvement in 4/8 patients with active acute pouchitis and maintained remission despite the withdrawal of suppressive antibiotic therapy in 7/14 patients with chronic pouchitis.[60] However, a randomized, double blind, placebo-controlled trial of allopurinol 200 mg/day for the prophylaxis of pouchitis in 184 patients undergoing colectomy with ileoanal pouch was negative.[13] Ald The cumulative frequency of pouchitis was 31% in the allopurinol group and 28% in the placebo group. Additionally, there was no difference in overall pouch function between these two groups. These findings do not support the idea that ischemic damage and free radical injury contribute to the pathogenesis of pouchitis.

Treatment with bismuth

Rationale

Bismuth has both antimicrobial and antidiarrheal properties, and has been useful in the treatment of traveler's diarrhea. A randomized, double blind controlled trial suggested that bismuth citrate may have efficacy comparable with mesalamine for the treatment of active left-sided UC.[61] Given the proved benefit of bismuth for traveler's diarrhea, and its potential benefit in UC, therapeutic trials of bismuth in patients with pouchitis seemed reasonable. C5

Clinical results

An uncontrolled study of bismuth complexed to carbomer (an acrylic acid polymer) suggested beneficial effects for both inducing improvement and maintaining remission in patients with chronic pouchitis.[62] A randomized, double blind placebo controlled trial of bismuth carbomer foam enemas in 40 patients with active chronic pouchitis showed no benefit of bismuth carbomer compared with a placebo containing xanthan gum (45% response in both groups).[14] Ald However, the fact that the placebo response rate is rather high and that a recent uncontrolled study suggests that *Boswella serrata* gum resin may be beneficial in patients with active UC,[63]

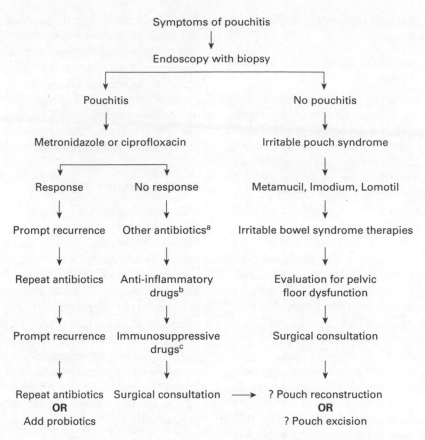

Figure 12.2 Treatment algorithm for pouchitis. [a]Rifaximin; amoxicillin/clavulanate; erythromycin; tetracycline; and cycling of multiple antibiotics. [b]Bismuth subsalicylate, mesalamine enemas; sulfasalazine; and oral mesalamine. [c]Budesonide, steroid enemas; oral steroids; azathioprine. (Reproduced with permission from Mahadevan U and Sandborn WJ. *Gastroenterology* 2003;**124**:1636–50[1])

there is the possibility that both the bismuth carbomer and the xanthan gum were effective therapies, and that the controlled trial simply demonstrated therapeutic equivalence of the two agents. A long-term uncontrolled maintenance/ toxicity study of bismuth carbomer foam enemas in patients with pouchitis demonstrated minimal systemic absorption of bismuth, no toxicity and possible continued clinical benefit in patients with chronic pouchitis after treatment for 9–128 weeks.[64] B4 Further support for a potential therapeutic effect of bismuth in pouchitis comes from an uncontrolled study of oral bismuth subsalicylate, administered as two 262 mg tablets four times per day for 4 weeks, which suggested a beneficial effect in 11/13 patients with active chronic pouchitis.[65] Controlled trials, using an inactive placebo control, are needed to determine whether bismuth has a role in the treatment of pouchitis.

Treatment algorithm for pouchitis

An algorithm of the approach to treatment of pouchitis is shown in Figure 12.2. A presumptive diagnosis of pouchitis in patients with compatible symptoms should be confirmed by pouch endoscopy and biopsy. After the diagnosis is confirmed, treatment with metronidazole or ciprofloxacin is initiated. A1d Responding patients who experience recurrent episodes and are able to tolerate the medication should be re-treated with the same regimen. Some patients with chronic pouchitis will require long-term suppressive or maintenance antibiotic therapy. When patients who require suppressive antibiotic therapy develop bacterial resistance after prolonged treatment, cycling of three or four antibiotics in 1-week intervals may be beneficial. Probiotic therapy can also be considered in patients with chronic pouchitis. A1d Those patients who do not respond to metronidazole or other antibiotics should receive topical pouch therapy with mesalamine enemas or suppositories, or with steroid enemas. In more refractory cases, sulfasalazine, oral mesalamine in the form of Pentasa, oral steroids, and possibly azathioprine or 6-mercaptopurine may be useful. B4 Some patients may require combination therapy with multiple agents as is the case for some patients with IBD, although there are no data to support this approach. There are few data and limited rationale to support empirical therapy with SCFA enemas, glutamine suppositories, inulin or allopurinol. A small number of

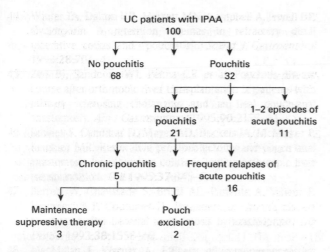

Figure 12.3 Clinical outcome with regard to pouchitis in 100 patients with ulcerative colitis (UC) undergoing abdominal colectomy with ileal pouch–anal anastomosis (IPAA). (Reproduced with permission from Sandborn WJ. In: *Trends in inflammatory bowel disease.* Lancaster, UK: Kluwer Academic, 1997[2])

patients will be refractory to all forms of medical therapy, and these patients should be referred to a surgeon for consideration of permanent ileostomy with pouch exclusion or excision.

Response to treatment of pouchitis (natural history)

In patients with IPAA for UC, the cumulative risk of developing at least one episode of pouchitis is 32%.[66] Of those patients who develop pouchitis, 36% have one or two acute pouchitis episodes which respond to treatment with antibiotics, 49% relapse more frequently (at least three acute episodes) but respond to antibiotics, and 15% require maintenance suppressive therapy and have been classified as having chronic pouchitis.[2,66] Of patients with chronic pouchitis, almost 50% require surgical exclusion or excision of the pouch. An algorithm showing the clinical course of pouchitis in IPAA patients is shown in Figure 12.3.

Conclusion

Medical treatment of acute and chronic pouchitis is often required. Small controlled trials have suggested superior efficacy of metronidazole compared with placebo and similar efficacy for metronidazole compared with both ciprofloxacin and budesonide enemas for active chronic pouchitis. Three somewhat larger placebo-controlled trials suggested that treatment with probiotic bacteria may be useful in maintaining remission of chronic pouchitis and as prophylaxis against pouchitis. A small placebo-controlled trial of bismuth

carbomer foam enemas did not demonstrate efficacy in active chronic pouchitis. A large controlled trial with allopurinol did not demonstrate efficacy for prophylaxis against pouchitis. Uncontrolled studies suggest possible benefit from empirical therapy with antibiotics, sulfasalazine, mesalamine, corticosteroids and bismuth. There are few data that immune modifiers, SCFA enemas or inulin are of benefit. Natural history studies suggest that most patients with pouchitis respond to a short course of antibiotic therapy. Some patients with chronic pouchitis require suppressive medical therapy with antibiotics or probiotics, and some will require permanent ileostomy with pouch exclusion or excision. Additional randomized, double blind placebo-controlled trials are needed to determine the efficacy of empirical medical therapies currently being used in patients with pouchitis.

References

1 Mahadevan U, Sandborn WJ. Diagnosis and management of pouchitis. *Gastroenterology* 2003;**124**:1636–50.

2 Sandborn WJ. Pouchitis: definition, risk factors, frequency, natural history, classification, and public health perspective. In: McLeod RS, Martin F, Sutherland LR *et al* (eds). *Trends in inflammatory bowel disease.* Lancaster, UK: Kluwer Academic, 1997.

3 Sandborn WJ, Tremaine WJ, Batts KP, Pemberton JH, Phillips SF. Pouchitis after ileal pouch-anal anastomosis: a Pouchitis Disease Activity Index. *Mayo Clin Proc* 1994;**69**:409–15.

4 McLeod RS, Taylor DW, Cohen Z, Cullen JB. Single-patient randomised clinical trial. Use in determining optimum treatment for patient with inflammation of Kock continent ileostomy reservoir. *Lancet* 1986;**1**:726–8.

5 Madden MV, McIntyre AS, Nicholls RJ. Double-blind crossover trial of metronidazole versus placebo in chronic unremitting pouchitis. *Dig Dis Sci* 1994;**39**:1193–6.

6 Shen B, Achkar JP, Lashner BA *et al.* A randomized clinical trial of ciprofloxacin and metronidazole to treat acute pouchitis. *Inflamm Bowel Dis* 2001;**7**:301–5.

7 Sambuelli A, Boerr L, Negreira S *et al.* Budesonide enema in pouchitis – a double-blind, double-dummy, controlled trial. *Aliment Pharmacol Ther* 2002;**16**:27–34.

8 Thirlby RC, Kelly R. Pectin and methyl cellulose do not affect intestinal function in patients after ileal pouch-anal anastomosis. *Am J Gastroenterol* 1997;**92**:99–102.

9 Welters CF, Heineman E, Thunnissen FB, van den Bogaard AE, Soeters PB, Baeten CG. Effect of dietary inulin supplementation on inflammation of pouch mucosa in patients with an ileal pouch-anal anastomosis. *Dis Colon Rectum* 2002;**45**:621–7.

10 Gionchetti P, Rizzello F, Venturi A *et al.* Oral bacteriotherapy as maintenance treatment in patients with chronic pouchitis: a double-blind, placebo-controlled trial. *Gastroenterology* 2000;**119**:305–9.

11 Mimura T, Rizzello F, Schreiber S *et al.* Once daily high dose probiotic therapy maintains remission and improved quality of life in patients with recurrent or refractory pouchitis: a

randomised, placebo-controlled, double-blind trial. *Gastroenterology* 2002;**122**:A-81.

12 Gionchetti P, Rizzello F, Helwig U *et al.* Prophylaxis of pouchitis onset with probiotic therapy: a double-blind, placebo-controlled trial. *Gastroenterology* 2003;**124**:1202–9.

13 Joelsson M, Andersson M, Bark T *et al.* Allopurinol as prophylaxis against pouchitis following ileal pouch-anal anastomosis for ulcerative colitis. A randomized placebo-controlled double-blind study. *Scand J Gastroenterol* 2001;**36**:1179–84.

14 Tremaine WJ, Sandborn WJ, Wolff BG, Carpenter HA, Zinsmeister AR, Metzger PP. Bismuth carbomer foam enemas for active chronic pouchitis: a randomized, double-blind, placebo-controlled trial. *Aliment Pharmacol Ther* 1997;**11**:1041–6.

15 Di Febo G, Miglioli M, Lauri A *et al.* Endoscopic assessment of acute inflammation of the ileal reservoir after restorative ileo-anal anastomosis. *Gastrointest Endosc* 1990;**36**:6–9.

16 Moskowitz RL, Shepherd NA, Nicholls RJ. An assessment of inflammation in the reservoir after restorative proctocolectomy with ileoanal ileal reservoir. *Int J Colorectal Dis* 1986;**1**:167–74.

17 Shepherd NA, Jass JR, Duval I, Moskowitz RL, Nicholls RJ, Morson BC. Restorative proctocolectomy with ileal reservoir: pathological and histochemical study of mucosal biopsy specimens. *J Clin Pathol* 1987;**40**:601–7.

18 Heuschen UA, Autschbach F, Allemeyer EH *et al.* Long-term follow-up after ileoanal pouch procedure: algorithm for diagnosis, classification, and management of pouchitis. *Dis Colon Rectum* 2001;**44**:487–99.

19 Sandborn WJ, Tremaine WJ, Batts KP *et al.* Fecal bile acids, short-chain fatty acids, and bacteria after ileal pouch-anal anastomosis do not differ in patients with pouchitis. *Dig Dis Sci* 1995;**40**:1474–83.

20 Shepherd NA, Hulten L, Tytgat GN *et al.* Pouchitis. *Int J Colorectal Dis* 1989;**4**:205–29.

21 Natori H, Utsunomiya J, Yamamura T, Benno Y, Uchida K. Fecal and stomal bile acid composition after ileostomy or ileoanal anastomosis in patients with chronic ulcerative colitis and adenomatosis coli. *Gastroenterology* 1992;**102**:1278–88.

22 Zuccaro G Jr, Fazio VW, Church JM, Lavery IC, Ruderman WB, Farmer RG. Pouch ileitis. *Dig Dis Sci* 1989;**34**:1505–10.

23 Lohmuller JL, Pemberton JH, Dozois RR, Ilstrup D, van Heerden J. Pouchitis and extraintestinal manifestations of inflammatory bowel disease after ileal pouch-anal anastomosis. *Ann Surg* 1990;**211**:622–7; discussion 627–9.

24 Svaninger G, Nordgren S, Oresland T, Hulten L. Incidence and characteristics of pouchitis in the Kock continent ileostomy and the pelvic pouch. *Scand J Gastroenterology* 1993;**28**:695–700.

25 Kelly DG, Phillips SF, Kelly KA, Weinstein WM, Gilchrist MJ. Dysfunction of the continent ileostomy: clinical features and bacteriology. *Gut* 1983;**24**:193–201.

26 Boerr LA, Sambuelli AM, Sugai E, Graziano A, Valero J, Kogan Z, Bai J. Faecal alpha 1-antitrypsin concentration in the diagnosis and management of patients with pouchitis. *Eur J Gastroenterol Hepatol* 1995;**7**:129–33.

27 Boerr LA, Sambuelli AM, Filinger E *et al.* Increased mucosal levels of leukotriene B4 in pouchitis: evidence for a persistent inflammatory state. *Eur J Gastroenterol Hepatol* 1996;**8**:57–61.

28 Kmiot WA, Hesslewood SR, Smith N, Thompson H, Harding LK, Keighley MR. Evaluation of the inflammatory infiltrate in pouchitis with 111In-labeled granulocytes. *Gastroenterology* 1993;**104**:981–8.

29 Hurst RD, Molinari M, Chung TP, Rubin M, Michelassi F. Prospective study of the incidence, timing and treatment of pouchitis in 104 consecutive patients after restorative proctocolectomy. *Arch Surg* 1996;**131**:497–500; discussion 501–2.

30 Tytgat GN, van Deventer SJ. Pouchitis. *Int J Colorectal Dis* 1988;**3**:226–8.

31 Scott AD, Phillips RK. Ileitis and pouchitis after colectomy for ulcerative colitis. *Br J Surg* 1989;**76**:668–9.

32 Bonello JC, Thow GB, Manson RR. Mucosal enteritis: a complication of the continent ileostomy. *Dis Colon Rectum* 1981;**24**:37–41.

33 Klein K, Stenzel P, Katon RM. Pouch ileitis: report of a case with severe systemic manifestations. *J Clin Gastroenterol* 1983;**5**:149–53.

34 Knobler H, Ligumsky M, Okon E, Ayalon A, Nesher R, Rachmilewitz D. Pouch ileitis – recurrence of the inflammatory bowel disease in the ileal reservoir. *Am J Gastroenterol* 1986;**81**:199–201.

35 Nygaard K, Bergan T, Bjorneklett A, Hoverstad T, Lassen J, Aase S. Topical metronidazole treatment in pouchitis. *Scand J Gastroenterol* 1994;**29**:462–7.

36 Isaacs K, Klenzak J, Koruda M. Topical metronidazole for the treatment of pouchitis. *Gastrointest Endosc* 1997;**45**:AB108.

37 Gionchetti P, Rizzello F, Venturi A *et al.* Antibiotic combination therapy in patients with chronic, treatment-resistant pouchitis. *Aliment Pharmacol Ther* 1999;**13**:713–18.

38 Kuzela L, Kascak M, Vavrecka A. Induction and maintenance of remission with nonpathogenic *Escherichia coli* in patients with pouchitis. *Am J Gastroenterol* 2001;**96**:3218–19.

39 Miglioli M, Barbara L, Di Febo G *et al.* Topical administration of 5-aminosalicylic acid: a therapeutic proposal for the treatment of pouchitis. *N Engl J Med* 1989;**320**:257.

40 Belluzzi A, Campieri M, Gionchetti P *et al.* Acute pouchitis:5-aminosalicylic acid and budesonide suppositories effectiveness on inflammatory mediator production. *Gastroenterology* 1993;**104**:A665.

41 Rafii F, Ruseler-Van Embden JG, Asad YF. Azoreductase and nitroreductase activity of bacteria in feces from patients with an ileal reservoir. *Dig Dis Sci* 1997;**42**:133–6.

42 Ciribilli JM, Chaussade S, Perrin S *et al.* Metabolism of sulfasalazine (SLZ) in patients with ileo-anal anastomosis (IAA) and reservoir. *Gastroenterology* 1991;**100**:A203.

43 Belluzzi A, Campieri M, Miglioli M *et al.* Evaluation of flogistic pattern in "pouchitis" before and after the treatment with budesonide. *Gastroenterology* 1992;**102**:A593.

44 Winter TA, Dalton HR, Merrett MN, Campbell A, Jewell DP. Cyclosporin A retention enemas in refractory distal ulcerative colitis and "pouchitis". *Scand J Gastroenterol* 1993;**28**:701–4.

45 Zins BJ, Sandborn WJ, Penna CR *et al*. Pouchitis disease course after orthotopic liver transplantation in patients with primary sclerosing cholangitis and an ileal pouch-anal anastomosis. *Am J Gastroenterol* 1995;**90**:2177–81.

46 Rowley S, Candinas D, Mayer AD, Buckels JA, McMaster P, Keighley MR. Restorative proctocolectomy and pouch anal anastomosis for ulcerative colitis following orthotopic liver transplantation. *Gut* 1995;**37**:845–7.

47 Berrebi W, Chaussade S, Bruhl AL, Pariente A, Valleur P, Hautefeuille P, Couturier D. Treatment of Crohn's disease recurrence after ileoanal anastomosis by azathioprine. *Dig Dis Sci* 1993;**38**:1558–60.

48 MacMillan F, Warner A. Efficacy of immunosuppressive therapy for the treatment of chronic pouchitis following ileal pouch-anal anastomosis. *Am J Gastroenterol* 1999;**94**: 2677.

49 Arnott ID, McDonald D, Williams A, Ghosh S. Clinical use of infliximab in Crohn's disease: the Edinburgh experience. *Aliment Pharmacol Ther* 2001;**15**:1639–46.

50 Viscido A, Habib FI, Kohn A *et al*. Infliximab in refractory pouchitis complicated by fistulae following ileo-anal pouch for ulcerative colitis. *Aliment Pharmacol Ther* 2003;**17**: 1263–71.

51 Ricart E, Panaccione R, Loftus EV, Tremaine WJ, Sandborn WJ. Successful management of Crohn's disease of the ileoanal pouch with infliximab. *Gastroenterology* 1999; **117**:429–32.

52 Colombel JF, Ricart E, Loftus EV *et al*. Management of Crohn's disease of the ileoanl pouch with infliximab. *Am J Gastroenterol* 2003 (in press).

53 Nasmyth DG, Godwin PG, Dixon MF, Williams NS, Johnston D. Ileal ecology after pouch-anal anastomosis or ileostomy. A study of mucosal morphology, fecal bacteriology, fecal volatile fatty acids, and their interrelationship. *Gastroenterology* 1989;**96**:817–24.

54 Clausen MR, Tvede M, Mortensen PB. Short-chain fatty acids in pouch contents from patients with and without pouchitis after ileal pouch-anal anastomosis. *Gastroenterology* 1992;**103**:1144–53.

55 Wischmeyer P, Pemberton JH, Phillips SF. Chronic pouchitis after ileal pouch-anal anastomosis: responses to butyrate and glutamine suppositories in a pilot study. *Mayo Clin Proc* 1993;**68**:978–81.

56 de Silva HJ, Ireland A, Kettlewell M, Mortensen N, Jewell DP. Short-chain fatty acid irrigation in severe pouchitis. *N Engl J Med* 1989;**321**:1416–17.

57 Tremaine WJ, Sandborn WJ, Phillips SF, Pemberton JH, Carpenter HA. Short chain fatty acid (SCFA) enema therapy for treatment-resistant pouchitis following ileal pouchanal anastomosis (IPAA) for ulcerative colitis (UC). *Gastroenterology* 1994;**106**:784.

58 den Hoed PT, van Goch JJ, Veen HF, Ouwendijk RJ. Severe pouchitis successfully treated with short-chain fatty acids. *Can J Surg* 1996;**39**:168–9.

59 Smith L, Friend WG, Medwell SJ. The superior mesenteric artery. The critical factor in the pouch pull-through procedure. *Dis Colon Rectum* 1984;**27**:741–4.

60 Levin KE, Pemberton JH, Phillips SF, Zinsmeister AR, Pezim ME. Role of oxygen free radicals in the etiology of pouchitis. *Dis Colon Rectum* 1992;**35**:452–6.

61 Pullan RD, Ganesh S, Mani V, Morris J, Evans BK, Williams GT, Rhodes J. Comparison of bismuth citrate and 5-aminosalicylic acid enemas in distal ulcerative colitis: a controlled trial. *Gut* 1993;**34**:676–9.

62 Gionchetti P, Rizzello F, Venturi A *et al*. Long-term efficacy of bismuth carbomer enemas in patients with treatment-resistant chronic pouchitis. *Aliment Pharmacol Ther* 1997; **11**:673–8.

63 Gupta I, Parihar A, Malhotra P, Singh GB, Ludtke R, Safayhi H, Ammon HP. Effects of *Boswellia serrata* gum resin in patients with ulcerative colitis. *Eur J Med Res* 1997;**2**: 37–43.

64 Tremaine WJ, Sandborn WJ. Safety of long term open treatment with bismuth carbomer foam enemas for chronic pouchitis. *Gastroenterology* 1997;**112**:A1105.

65 Tremaine WJ, Sandborn WJ, Kenan ML. Bismuth subsalicylate tablets for chronic antibiotic-resistant pouchitis. *Gastroenterology* 1998;**114**:A1101.

66 Penna C, Dozois R, Tremaine W, Sandborn W, LaRusso N, Schleck C, Ilstrup D. Pouchitis after ileal pouch-anal anastomosis for ulcerative colitis occurs with increased frequency in patients with associated primary sclerosing cholangitis. *Gut* 1996;**38**:234–9.

randomised, placebo-controlled, double-blind trial. *Gastroenterology* 2002;122:A-81.

12 Gionchetti P, Rizzello F, Helwig U *et al.* Prophylaxis of pouchitis onset with probiotic therapy: a double-blind, placebo-controlled trial. *Gastroenterology* 2003;124:1202–9.

13 Joelsson M, Andersson M, Bark T *et al.* Allopurinol as prophylaxis against pouchitis following ileal pouch anal anastomosis for ulcerative colitis. A randomized placebo-controlled double-blind study. *Scand J Gastroenterol* 2001;36:1179–84.

14 Tremaine WJ, Sandborn WJ, Wolff BG, Carpenter HA, Zinsmeister AR, Metzger PP. Bismuth carbomer foam enemas for active chronic pouchitis: a randomized, double-blind, placebo-controlled trial. *Aliment Pharmacol Ther* 1997;11:1041–6.

15 Di Febo G, Miglioli M, Lauri A *et al.* Endoscopic assessment of acute inflammation of the ileal reservoir after restorative ileo-anal anastomosis. *Gastrointest Endosc* 1990;36:6–9.

16 Moskowitz RL, Shepherd NA, Nicholls RJ. An assessment of inflammation in the reservoir after restorative proctocolectomy with ileoanal ileal reservoir. *Int J Colorectal Dis* 1986;1:167–74.

17 Shepherd NA, Jass JR, Duval I, Moskowitz RL, Nicholls RJ, Morson BC. Restorative proctocolectomy with ileal reservoir: pathological and histochemical study of mucosal biopsy specimens. *J Clin Pathol* 1987;40:601–7.

18 Heuschen UA, Autschbach F, Allemeyer EH *et al.* Long-term follow-up after ileoanal pouch procedure: algorithm for diagnosis, classification, and management of pouchitis. *Dis Colon Rectum* 2001;44:487–99.

19 Sandborn WJ, Tremaine WJ, Batts KP *et al.* Fecal bile acids, short-chain fatty acids, and bacteria after ileal pouchanal anastomosis do not differ in patients with pouchitis. *Dig Dis Sci* 1995;40:1474–83.

20 Shepherd NA, Hultén L, Tytgat GN *et al.* Pouchitis. *Int J Colorectal Dis* 1989;4:205–29.

21 Natori H, Utsunomiya J, Yamamura T, Benno Y, Uchida K. Fecal and stomal bile acid composition after ileostomy or ileoanal anastomosis in patients with chronic ulcerative colitis and adenomatosis coli. *Gastroenterology* 1992;102:1278–88.

22 Zuccaro G Jr, Fazio VW, Church JM, Lavery IC, Ruderman WB, Farmer RG. Pouch ileitis. *Dig Dis Sci* 1989;34:1505–10.

23 Lohmuller JL, Pemberton JH, Dozois RR, Ilstrup D, van Heerden J. Pouchitis and extraintestinal manifestations of inflammatory bowel disease after ileal pouch-anal anastomosis. *Ann Surg* 1990;211:622–7; discussion 627–9.

24 Svaninger G, Nordgren S, Oresland T, Hultén L. Incidence and characteristics of pouchitis in the Kock continent ileostomy and the pelvic pouch. *Scand J Gastroenterol* 1993;28:695–700.

25 Kelly DG, Phillips SF, Kelly KA, Weinstein WM, Gilchrist MJ. Dysfunction of the continent ileostomy: clinical features and bacteriology. *Gut* 1983;24:193–201.

26 Boerr LA, Sambuelli AM, Sugai E, Graziano A, Valero J, Kogan Z, Bai J. Faecal alpha 1-antitrypsin concentration in the diagnosis and management of patients with pouchitis. *Eur J Gastroenterol Hepatol* 1995;7:129–33.

27 Boerr LA, Sambuelli AM, Filinger E *et al.* Increased mucosal levels of leukotriene B4 in pouchitis: evidence for a persistent inflammatory state. *Eur J Gastroenterol Hepatol* 1996;8:57–61.

28 Kmiot WA, Hesslewood SR, Smith N, Thompson H, Harding LK, Keighley MR. Evaluation of the inflammatory infiltrate in pouchitis with 111In-labeled granulocytes. *Gastroenterology* 1993;104:981–8.

29 Hurst RD, Molinari M, Chung TP, Rubin M, Michelassi F. Prospective study of the incidence, timing and treatment of pouchitis in 104 consecutive patients after restorative proctocolectomy. *Arch Surg* 1996;131:497–500; discussion 501–2.

30 Tytgat GN, van Deventer SJ. Pouchitis. *Int J Colorectal Dis* 1988;3:226–8.

31 Scott AD, Phillips RK. Ileitis and pouchitis after colectomy for ulcerative colitis. *Br J Surg* 1989;76:668–9.

32 Bonello JC, Thow GB, Manson RR. Mucosal enteritis: a complication of the continent ileostomy. *Dis Colon Rectum* 1981;24:37–41.

33 Klein K, Stenzel P, Katon RM. Pouch ileitis: report of a case with severe systemic manifestations. *J Clin Gastroenterol* 1983;5:149–53.

34 Knobler H, Ligumsky M, Okon E, Ayalon A, Nesher G, Rachmilewitz D. Pouch ileitis — recurrence of the inflammatory bowel disease in the ileal reservoir. *Am J Gastroenterol* 1986;81:199–201.

35 Nygaard K, Bergan T, Bjorneklett A, Hoverstad T, Lassen J. Topical metronidazole treatment in pouchitis. *Scand J Gastroenterol* 1994;29:462–7.

36 Isaacs K, Klenzak J, Koruda M. Topical metronidazole for the treatment of pouchitis. *Gastrointest Endosc* 1997;45:AB108.

37 Gionchetti P, Rizzello F, Venturi A *et al.* Antibiotic combination therapy in patients with chronic, treatment-resistant pouchitis. *Aliment Pharmacol Ther* 1999;13:713–18.

38 Kuisma J, Jarvinen H, Mayranpaa M. Induction and maintenance of remission with nonpathogenic *Escherichia coli* in patients with pouchitis. *Aliment Pharmacol Ther* 2001;96:3218–99.

39 Miglioli M, Barbara L, Di Febo G *et al.* Topical administration of 5-aminosalicylic acid: a therapeutic proposal for the treatment of pouchitis. *N Engl J Med* 1989;320:257.

40 Belluzzi A, Campieri M, Gionchetti P *et al.* Acute pouchitis: 5 aminosalicylic acid and budesonide suppositories effect on inflammatory mediator production. *Gastroenterology* 1993;104:A665.

41 Ruseler-van Embden JG, Schouten WR, van Lieshout LM. Pouchitis: result of microbial imbalance? *Dig Dis Sci* 1997;42:133–6.

42 Cramai IM, Ghanssic S, Pettit S *et al.* Metabolism of sulfasalazine (SZ) in patients with ileo-anal anastomosis (IAA) and reservoirs. *Gastroenterology* 1991;100:A203.

43 Belluzzi A, Campieri M, Miglioli M *et al.* Evaluation of lipidic pattern in pouchitis before and after treatment with budesonide. *Gastroenterology* 1992;102:A591.

13 Microscopic and collagenous colitis

Robert Löfberg

Introduction

Microscopic colitis is characterized clinically by chronic, non-bloody diarrhea and a macroscopically normal or near-normal colonic mucosa, in the presence of specific histopathologic features on microscopic examination of mucosal biopsies. Collagenous colitis and lymphocytic colitis constitute the two main forms of microscopic colitis. Collagenous colitis was first described by Lindström in 1976.[1] The term lymphocytic colitis was introduced by Lazenby *et al.* in 1989, to reflect the fact that the major feature of lymphocytic colitis was an increased number of intraepithelial lymphocytes.[2]

Epidemiology

Collagenous colitis was initially regarded as being rare, until the first epidemiologic studies showed the incidence to be 0·8/100 000 and 2·7/100 000 and the prevalence 15·7/100 000.[3,4] Recent epidemiologic studies, however, show that collagenous colitis is more common and incidence figures of 5·2/100 000 and 6·1/100 000 have been reported (Table 13.1).[5,6] If these figures are representative, the incidence of collagenous colitis is equal to the incidence of Crohn's disease in Sweden. Patients with collagenous colitis are typically middle-aged women, the age at diagnosis being around 65 years, and the female:male ratio around 7:1 (Figure 13.1).[3–6] However, 25% of 163 patients were diagnosed before the age of 45 years so this diagnosis must be considered even in younger subjects with chronic watery diarrhea.[7] Only four children below the age of 12 years have been reported.[8]

Epidemiologic data for lymphocytic colitis have been reported from three different regions in Europe during the 1990s (see Table 13.1).[4–6] The data are fairly consistent and an annual incidence of 3·1–5·7/100 000 inhabitants has been reported. The incidence of lymphocytic colitis is also similar to the incidence of Crohn's disease and the combined rates for collagenous colitis and lymphocytic colitis approach the incidence of ulcerative colitis. The data illustrate that these conditions are more common than was considered earlier. Microscopic colitis may be diagnosed in 10% of

patients investigated for chronic non-bloody diarrhea, and in 20% of patients older than 70 years with these symptoms.[6] The age at onset of symptoms in lymphocytic colitis is around 60–65 years but the female predominance is less pronounced than is the case for collagenous colitis (Figure 13.2).

Histopathology

The following histopathologic features are the hallmarks of collagenous colitis: diffuse non-continuous thickening of a subepithelial collagen layer is seen beneath the basement membrane (Figure 13.3); the thickness of the subepithelial layer must be 10 μm or more on a well-orientated section of the mucosa in comparison to 0–3 μm in normal individuals; chronic inflammation in the lamina propria dominated by lymphocytes and plasma cells; flattening and vacuolization of the epithelial cells and detachment of the surface epithelium; intraepithelial lymphocyte infiltration may be present, although this feature is not as prominent as in lymphocytic colitis.[2,11] Cryptitis does not exclude the diagnosis of collagenous colitis.[12] In the matrix containing the thickened collagen layer collagen type I, III and VI and fibronectin have been identified.[13,14]

Table 13.1 Annual incidence per 100 000 in population-based epidemiological studies of collagenous and lymphocytic colitis

Region and study period	Collagenous colitis	Lymphocytic colitis
Örebro, Sweden, 1984–88[3]	0·8	
Örebro, Sweden, 1989–93[3]	2·7	
Örebro, Sweden, 1993–95[6]	3·7	3·1
Örebro, Sweden, 1996–98[6]	6·1	5·7
Franche-Comté, France, 1987–92[9]	0·6	
Uppsala, Sweden, 1992–94[10]	1·9	
Terrassa, Spain, 1993–97[4]	2·3	3·7
Iceland, 1995–99[5]	5·2	4·0

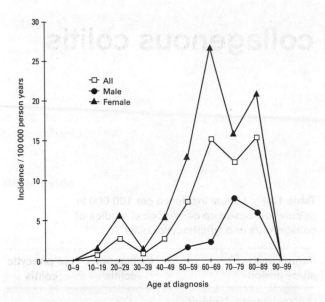

Figure 13.1 Age- and sex-specific incidence of collagenous colitis. (Reprinted with permission from Olesen M *et al. Gut* 2004;**53**:346–50.[6])

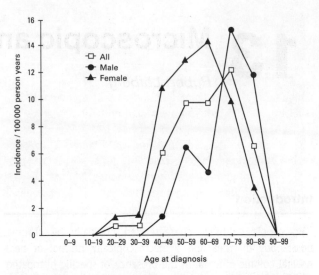

Figure 13.2 Age- and sex-specific incidence of lymphocytic colitis. (Reprinted with permission from Olesen M *et al. Gut* 2004;**53**:346–50.[6])

The histopathologic findings are mainly located in the colon and the rectum. The collagen layer is most prominent in the proximal colon, and may be absent in the rectal mucosa in between 18% and 73% of biopsy specimens.[4,5,15,16] However, an increased subepithelial collagen layer in the stomach and duodenum as well as in the terminal ileum, so called collagenous gastritis and collagenous enterocolitis, has been reported occasionally.[17–26]

The histopathologic diagnostic criteria of lymphocytic colitis are epithelial lesions, an increase in intraepithelial lymphocytes (> 20 lymphocytes per 100 epithelial cells), and infiltration of the lamina propria with lymphocytes and plasma cells, in the absence of an increase in the collagen layer (Figure 13.4).[2,27] An increased number of intraepithelial T-lymphocytes may be seen in the terminal ileum.[26]

Etiology and pathophysiology

The etiology of microscopic colitis is largely unknown. At present, both collagenous and lymphocytic colitis are considered to be caused by an abnormal immunologic reaction to various mucosal insults in predisposed individuals.

Genetics

Data on genetics are sparse. A small number of familial cases with collagenous and lymphocytic colitis, and with mixed collagenous and lymphocytic colitis have been reported.[28–32] Twelve per cent of patients with lymphocytic colitis reported a family history of other bowel disorders such as inflammatory bowel disease, celiac disease or collagenous

colitis.[33] Whether these associations are due to genetics, environmental factors or chance cannot be assessed.

Reaction to a luminal agent

The increased number of T lymphocytes in the epithelium has supported the theory that collagenous colitis may be caused by an abnormal immunologic reaction to a luminal agent.[34–36] The observation that diversion of the fecal stream by an ileostomy normalizes or reduces the characteristic histopathologic changes in collagenous colitis, further supports this theory.[37] B4 Recurrence of symptoms and histopathologic changes was seen after closure of ileostomy. Furthermore, abnormalities of colonic histology resembling lymphocytic colitis have been reported in untreated celiac disease.[38]

Infectious agent

The sudden onset of the disease in some patients, and the effect of various antibiotics support a possible infectious cause.[7] An association with microscopic colitis and infection with *Campylobacter jejuni*[39] and *Clostridium difficile*[40–42] has been reported. In another study, *Yersinia enterocolitica* was detected in three of six patients prior to the collagenous colitis diagnosis, and a serologic study showed that antibodies to *Yersinia* spp. were more common in collagenous colitis patients than in healthy controls.[43,44] Of interest is "Brainerd diarrhea", which refers to outbreak of chronic watery diarrhea characterized by acute onset and prolonged duration.[45] An infectious cause is likely, but no agent has been identified. Colonic biopsies in these patients show

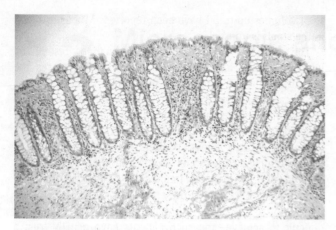

Figure 13.3 A biopsy from the colon showing typical findings of collagenous colitis: increased subepithelial collagen layer, inflammation of lamina propria and epithelial lesions with intraepithelial lymphocytes

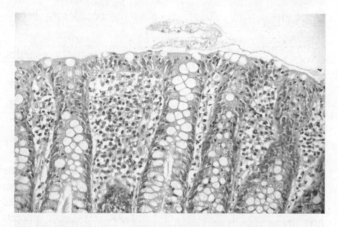

Figure 13.4 A biopsy from the colon showing typical findings of lymphocytic colitis: epithelial lesions with intraepithelial lymphocytes and inflammation in the lamina propria

epithelial lymphocytosis similar to lymphocytic colitis but the surface epithelial lesions are absent.

Drugs

There are several reports of drug-induced microscopic colitis, especially lymphocytic colitis (Box 13.1). Most reports concern ticlopidine and Cyclo 3 Fort. In a case–control study the use of non-steroidal anti-inflammatory drugs (NSAIDs) was significantly more common among collagenous colitis patients than in controls and discontinuation of NSAIDs was followed by improvement of the diarrhea in some patients.[46] Others found that use of NSAIDs at presentation was associated with a greater need for 5-aminosalicylic acid (5-ASA) and steroid therapy, possibly reflecting a more

Box 13.1   Drugs reported to be associated with microscopic colitis

Lymphocytic colitis

- Ticlopidine[48–50]
- Cyclo 3 Fort[53–55]
- Ranitidine[56]
- Vinburnine[58]
- Tardyferon[59]
- Flutamide[50]
- Acarbose[60]
- Piroxicam[61]
- Levodopa-benserazide[62]
- Carbamazepine[33,63,64]
- Sertraline[33]
- Paroxetine[33]
- Oxetorone[65]
- Lanzoprazole[52,66]

Collagenous colitis

- Lanzoprazole[51,52]
- Non-steroidal anti-inflammatory drugs[46]
- Cimetidine[57]

resistant form of disease, but that withdrawal of NSAIDs did not improve clinical symptoms.[47] The increased use of NSAIDs in patients with collagenous colitis is probably due to the occurrence of concomitant arthritis. The number of reported cases of drug-induced microscopic colitis is small and a chance association is possible. It is, however, important to assess concomitant drug use in patients and consider withdrawal of drugs that might worsen the condition.

Autoimmunity

Both collagenous and lymphocytic colitis are associated with autoimmune diseases. An autoimmune pathogenesis has therefore been proposed, possibly initiated by a foreign luminal agent, which causes an immunologic cross-reaction with an endogenous antigen. A study of autoantibodies and immunoglobulins in collagenous colitis showed that the mean level of IgM in collagenous colitis patients was significantly increased,[67] similar to observations in primary biliary cirrhosis. A specific autoantibody in collagenous colitis has not been reported.

Bile acids

Data on bile acid malabsorption in microscopic colitis are conflicting. In one study no association was found,[68] whereas others found bile acid malabsorption in 27–44% of patients with collagenous colitis and in 9–60% of patients with lymphocytic colitis.[69–71] The coexistence of bile acid malabsorption seems to worsen the diarrhea in patients with collagenous colitis.[69] These observations are the rationale for recommendations of bile acid binding treatment, which was reported effective in a majority of patients with microscopic colitis and concomitant bile acid malabsorption.[69,71] B4 Even patients without bile acid malabsorption may respond to this treatment. This emphasizes the importance of the fecal stream, and the therapeutic effect may possibly be related to binding of luminal toxins.[72]

Nitric oxide

Colonic nitric oxide (NO) production is greatly increased in active microscopic colitis caused by an upregulation of inducible nitric oxide synthase (iNOS) in the colonic epithelium.[73–75] The levels of NO correlated with clinical activity and histopathologic status of the colonic mucosa, i.e. patients in histopathologic remission had normal levels of colonic NO in contrast to increased levels in patients with histologically active disease.[75] The role of NO in microscopic colitis is uncertain. NO is an inflammatory mediator but whether its role is proinflammatory or protective remains unclear. NO may furthermore be involved in the diarrheal pathophysiology as infusion into the colon of N^G-monomethyl-L-arginine, an inhibitor of NOS, reduced colonic net secretion by 70% and the addition of L-arginine increased colonic net secretion by 50%.[76]

Secretory or osmotic diarrhea

Diarrheal pathophysiology in collagenous colitis has been regarded as secretory caused by the epithelial lesions, the inflammatory infiltrate in the lamina propria and the collagenous band that might be a barrier for reabsorption of electrolytes and water.[77,78] Furthermore, an impaired epithelial barrier function due to downregulation of tight junction molecules was found to contribute to diarrheal pathophysiology.[78] Studies on the influence of fasting on diarrhea in collagenous colitis indicated, however, that osmotic diarrhea was predominant.[79] Many patients report that fasting reduces their diarrhea in accordance with this observation.

Clinical features and diagnosis

The main symptom in collagenous colitis is non-bloody diarrhea that may be accompanied by nocturnal diarrhea, fecal incontinence, crampy abdominal pain and distension.[7] Weight loss of up to 5 kg is common initially and occasionally is even more pronounced. Serious dehydration is rare, although 25% of the patients had 10 daily stools or more and stool volumes up to 5 l have been reported. Mucus or blood in the stools is unusual.

The onset of the disease may be sudden, resembling infectious diarrhea, in some patients.[7] In most cases the clinical course is chronic relapsing and benign. Serious complications are rare, although a small number of patients with colonic perforation have been reported.[80–82] The risk of developing colorectal cancer in collagenous colitis is not increased.[83,84] In a follow up study, 63% of the patients had lasting remission after 3·5 years.[85] Another cohort study showed that all patients improved 47 months after the diagnosis and only 29% of these required medications.[86] In a number of collagenous colitis patients, however, remission is difficult to achieve, and such patients have usually tried a large variety of medications in vain.[7,87]

Patients with collagenous colitis often have concomitant diseases. Up to 40% have one or more associated autoimmune diseases. The most common are rheumatoid arthritis, thyroid disorders, celiac disease, asthma/allergy and diabetes mellitus. Crohn's disease or ulcerative colitis concomitant with collagenous colitis has occasionally been reported.[7,88]

Lymphocytic colitis is clinically indistinguishable from collagenous colitis and the predominant symptom is chronic watery diarrhea. In a recent report, however, it was found that symptoms in lymphocytic colitis were milder and more likely to disappear than in collagenous colitis.[50] Similar to collagenous colitis, lymphocytic colitis has also been reported in association with autoimmune diseases.[50] The prognosis of lymphocytic colitis is good. There is no increased mortality and no increased risk of subsequent bowel malignancy reported. A benign course was reported in 27 cases with resolution of diarrhea and normalization of histology in over 80% of the patients within 38 months.[89] Others reported that the clinical course was a single attack in 63% of the patients with a median duration of 6 months from onset of symptoms to remission.[33]

Only microscopic assessment of colonic mucosal biopsies can verify the diagnosis of collagenous or lymphocytic colitis. Merely non-specific, minor laboratory abnormalities are found, and there are at present no blood tests available for screening purposes. Analyses of pANCA (anti-neutrophil cytoplasmic antibody)[90] or serum procollagen III propeptide are of no diagnostic value in collagenous colitis.[91] Stool examinations reveal no pathologic organisms, though increased excretion of fecal leukocytes in more than half of the collagenous colitis patients has been reported.[24] Barium enema and endoscopy are usually normal, though subtle endoscopic changes such as mucosal edema, granularity or erythema may be seen in up to 30% of cases.[7,33] Pancolonoscopy is preferred to sigmoidoscopy as a thickened collagenous layer in collagenous colitis may be absent in between 18% and 73% of rectal biopsy specimens.

Table 13.2   Data from three randomized placebo-controlled studies of oral budesonide in collagenous colitis

Author year	No. of patients	Dosage of budesonide; formulation; trial duration	Clinical response: budesonide v placebo	Histologic response; budesonide v placebo	Adverse events
Baert et al. 2002[99]	28	9 mg/day Budenofalk; 8 weeks	Improvement: 8/14 v 3/14 (P = 0·05)	Reduction of lamina propria inflammation in 9/13 v 4/12 (P < 0·001). No difference in collagen layer	Mild; no difference between treatment groups
Miehlke et al. 2002[100]	45[a]	9 mg/day Entocort; 6 weeks	Remission: 15/23 v 0/22 (P < 0·0001).	Improvement in 17/23 v 5/22 (P < 0·01). No difference in collagen layer	Mild; 38% v 12% P = 0·052
Bonderup et al. 2003[101]	20	9 mg/day Entocort; 8 weeks	10/10 v 2/10 (P < 0·001)	Reduction of overall inflammation (P < 0·01) and of collagen layer in sigmoid colon (P < 0·02)	None

[a]Per protocol analysis, 51 patients were randomized but six were withdrawn early due to lack of efficacy or adverse events

One or two diseases?

It has been questioned whether lymphocytic colitis and collagenous colitis are the same disease in different stages of development or rather two different but related conditions. They have a similar clinical expression and similar histopathologic features except for the subepithelial collagenous layer in collagenous colitis. Conversion of lymphocytic colitis to collagenous colitis or the opposite has been reported,[92,93] but the fact that conversion happens fairly seldom, and the observed differences in sex ratio and human leukocyte antigen (HLA) pattern[94] makes it more likely that collagenous colitis and lymphocytic colitis are two separate but related entities.

Treatment of microscopic colitis

The enigmatic etiology of microscopic colitis has led to a wide range of antidiarrheal and anti-inflammatory drugs being evaluated for medical treatment. Few controlled studies have been conducted, and recommendations on therapy have largely been based on retrospective reports and uncontrolled data.[7,95] The benign course of microscopic colitis in general has led to suggestions of an algorithm with a "step-up" type of approach to medical treatment, depending on clinical response and outcome in the individual patient. Milder symptoms may be well controlled using drugs such as loperamide or cholestyramine.[69,96] B4 However, in patients with moderate to intense symptoms potent anti-inflammatory treatment is required. In a retrospective study, the degree of

lamina propria inflammation in colonic biopsies was found to predict the response to therapy, and greater inflammation may indicate the need of corticosteroid therapy.[47] A finding of a substantial degree of inflammation at time of diagnosis may thus aid in the clinical decision-making.

Randomized controlled trials

Only the medical treatment of collagenous colitis has been properly evaluated in randomized controlled trials (RCTs) – level of evidence 1b. A Cochrane review carried out in 2003 identified all published reports between 1970 and 2002, and four studies that fulfilled the criteria for a meta-analysis (evidence level 1a) were found.[97] In one study bismuth subsalicylate was evaluated[98] and three trials[99–101] studied oral formulations of budesonide (Table 13.2).

Bismuth subsalicylate

In the small pilot trial with oral bismuth subsalicylate (n = 14 of which nine had collagenous colitis) the efficacy of 2·4 g daily versus placebo for 8 weeks was studied. The patients randomized to active treatment were more likely to improve clinically (P = 0·003) as well as histologically (P = 0·003). A1d All patients on bismuth therapy demonstrated clinical improvement, and six out of seven also displayed histological regression. In contrast, no patient in the placebo group improved. When placebo patients were crossed over to bismuth therapy in a blinded manner, five out of six improved (one dropped out due to nausea).

Budesonide

The use of oral preparations of budesonide has been well proved for induction of remission in active ileocolonic Crohn's disease. This glucocorticosteroid has a high potency and a rapid first pass metabolism rendering it a topical mode of action and less systemic impact than conventional steroids. A total of 94 patients were enrolled in three placebo-controlled trials of budesonide (9 mg daily for 6–8 weeks) in collagenous colitis. Fifty patients received active budesonide therapy. The pooled odds ratio for clinical response with budesonide was 12·32 (95% CI 5·53 to 27·46), with number needed to treat of 2. A1a Most responders had a decrease in the number of loose stools after 2–4 weeks of therapy. After cessation of active therapy most patients were reported to experience a flare-up of symptoms. Histological improvement was significant in all three trials with oral budesonide. A decrease in the grade of infiltration of lamina propria mononuclear cells was observed in most patients, whereas a reduction in the thickness of the collagen layer was found less consistently. One of the trials demonstrated a significant decrease of the collagen band in the sigmoid colon with almost a normalization of the mean thickness to 10·2 μm.[101]

Other anti-inflammatory compounds

Sulfasalazine and mesalamine have been extensively tried in microscopic colitis but never evaluated in RCTs. Observational studies of sulfasalazine and mesalamine have reported benefit in 34–50% of patients.[7,95] B4 Antibiotics such as metronidazole and erythromycin have also been used but no controlled studies have been done.

Oral prednisolone may be effective with a reported response rate in uncontrolled studies of 70–80%. The effect, however, is generally not sustained after withdrawal, and the dose required to maintain remission is often unacceptably high; more than 20 mg per day.[7]

Recommended therapy

Based on a meta-analysis and RCTs, oral budesonide is the drug of choice (short or medium duration therapy) for the treatment of collagenous colitis in patients with significant symptoms that cannot be controlled with loperamide, cholestyramine or aminosalicylates. A1a Of interest is the observation indicating that oral budesonide may even be more efficacious than conventional systemic corticosteroids (for example prednisolone).[102] Corticosteroids may, in addition to their anti-inflammatory effects, also ameliorate ileal bile acid malabsorption.[103] There are as yet no RCTs evaluating the long-term role of budesonide for maintenance of remission. Budesonide has a benign safety profile, as proved in other inflammatory bowel disease-conditions, but it would be prudent to taper the dose to the minimum necessary for controlling symptoms in patients with microscopic colitis if more than 8 weeks of therapy is indicated. C5 Most candidates for longer-term budesonide treatment would be women aged 50–70 years, a group at increased risk for osteoporosis. In this respect, budesonide has been demonstrated to have less impact than prednisolone on bone mineral density in patients with Crohn's disease during treatment for up to 2 years. Budesonide therapy given on-demand may be an attractive option for long-term control of symptoms. Although we have positive experience from this approach in our own clinical practice, controlled data are lacking.

Bismuth subsalicylate therapy may be an alternative to budesonide, but it is not available in all countries due to concerns regarding toxicity.

Severe attacks of microscopic colitis are rare, but a small number of patients may require hospitalization, intravenous steroid therapy, bowel rest and total parenteral nutrition.

For steroid-refractory or steroid-dependent patients immunomodulators may be of value. An open trial with azathioprine gave partial or complete remission in eight of nine patients with microscopic colitis.[104] Low dose methotrexate (median dose 7·5 mg/week) was effective in 10 of 11 patients with prednisolone-refractory collagenous colitis.[105] C5 There are no controlled trials of these agents in patients with microscopic colitis.

Surgical treatment

If medical therapy fails and alternative diagnoses are ruled out surgery may be considered in a patient with intractable microscopic colitis. Split ileostomy was conducted successfully in nine women with collagenous colitis[37] and successful outcomes both in collagenous colitis and lymphocytic colitis have been reported after total or subtotal colectomy.[106–110] B4

References

1 Lindström CG. "Collagenous colitis" with watery diarrhoea – a new entity? *Pathol Eur* 1976;**11**:87–9.

2 Lazenby AJ, Yardley JH, Giardiello FM *et al.* Lymphocytic ("microscopic") colitis: a comparative histopathologic study with particular reference to collagenous colitis. *Hum Pathol* 1989;**20**:18–28.

3 Bohr J, Tysk C, Eriksson S *et al.* Collagenous colitis in Örebro, Sweden, an epidemiological study 1984–1993. *Gut* 1995;**37**:394–7.

4 Fernandez-Banares F, Salas A, Forne M *et al.* Incidence of collagenous and lymphocytic colitis: a 5-year population-based study. *Am J Gastroenterol* 1999;**94**:418–23.

5 Agnarsdottir M, Gunnlaugsson O, Orvar KB *et al.* Collagenous and lymphocytic colitis in Iceland. *Dig Dis Sci* 2002;**47**:1122–8.

6 Olesen M, Eriksson S, Bohr J *et al.* Microscopic colitis – a common diarrhoeal disease. An epidemiologic study in Örebro, Sweden 1993–1998. *Gut* 2004;**53**:346–50.

7 Bohr J, Tysk C, Eriksson S *et al.* Collagenous colitis:a retrospective study of clinical presentation and treatment in 163 patients. *Gut* 1996;**39**:846–51.

8 Gremse DA, Boudreaux CW, Manci EA. Collagenous colitis in children. *Gastroenterology* 1993;**104**:906–9.

9 Raclot G, Queneau P, Ottignon Y *et al.* Incidence of collagenous colitis. A retrospective study in the east of France. *Gastroenterology* 1994;**106**:A23.

10 Taha Y, Kraaz W, Lööf L. Förekomst av kollagen kolit i biopsier vid kolonoskopi med makroskopiskt normal slemhinna [Swedish]. *Sv Läkarsällskapets handl Hygiea* 1995;**104**:167.

11 Levy AM, Yamazaki K, Van Keulen VP *et al.* Increased eosinophil infiltration and degranulation in colonic tissue from patients with collagenous colitis. *Am J Gastroenterol* 2001;**96**:1522–8.

12 Jessurun J, Yardley JH, Giardiello FM *et al.* Chronic colitis with thickening of the subepithelial collagen layer (collagenous colitis): histopathologic findings in 15 patients. *Hum Pathol* 1987;**18**:839–48.

13 Flejou JF, Grimaud JA, Molas G *et al.* Collagenous colitis. Ultrastructural study and collagen immunotyping of four cases. *Arch Pathol Lab Med* 1984;**108**:977–82.

14 Aigner T, Neureiter D, Muller S *et al.* Extracellular matrix composition and gene expression in collagenous colitis. *Gastroenterology* 1997;**113**:136–43.

15 Tanaka M, Mazzoleni G, Riddell RH. Distribution of collagenous colitis: utility of flexible sigmoidoscopy. *Gut* 1992;**33**:65–70.

16 Offner FA, Jao RV, Lewin KJ *et al.* Collagenous colitis: a study of the distribution of morphological abnormalities and their histological detection. *Hum Pathol* 1999;**30**:451–7.

17 Eckstein RP, Dowsett JF, Riley JW. Collagenous enterocolitis: a case of collagenous colitis with involvement of the small intestine. *Am J Gastroenterol* 1988;**83**:767–71.

18 Stolte M, Ritter M, Borchard F *et al.* Collagenous gastroduodenitis on collagenous colitis. *Endoscopy* 1990;**22**:186–7.

19 Lewis FW, Warren GH, Goff JS. Collagenous colitis with involvement of terminal ileum. *Dig Dis Sci* 1991;**36**:1161–3.

20 Meier PN, Otto P, Ritter M *et al.* Collagenous duodenitis and ileitis in a patient with collagenous colitis. *Leber Magen Darm* 1991;**21**:231–2.

21 McCashland TM, Donovan JP, Strobach RS *et al.* Collagenous enterocolitis: a manifestation of gluten-sensitive enteropathy. *J Clin Gastroenterol* 1992;**15**:45–51.

22 Chatti S, Haouet S, Ourghi H *et al.* Collagenous enterocolitis. Apropos of a case and review of the literature. *Arch Anat Cytol Pathol* 1994;**42**:149–53.

23 Veress B, Lofberg R, Bergman L. Microscopic colitis syndrome. *Gut* 1995;**36**:880–6.

24 Zins BJ, Tremaine WJ, Carpenter HA. Collagenous colitis: mucosal biopsies and association with fecal leukocytes. *Mayo Clin Proc* 1995;**70**:430–3.

25 Pulimood AB, Ramakrishna BS, Mathan MM. Collagenous gastritis and collagenous colitis: a report with sequential histological and ultrastructural findings. *Gut* 1999;**44**:881–5.

26 Padmanabhan V, Callas PW, Li SC *et al.* Histopathological features of the terminal ileum in lymphocytic and collagenous colitis: a study of 32 cases and review of literature. *Mod Pathol* 2003;**16**:115–19.

27 Bogomoletz WV. Collagenous, microscopic and lymphocytic colitis. An evolving concept. *Virchows Arch* 1994;**424**:573–9.

28 van Tilburg AJ, Lam HG, Seldenrijk CA *et al.* Familial occurrence of collagenous colitis. A report of two families. *J Clin Gastroenterol* 1990;**12**:279–85.

29 Järnerot G, Hertervig E, Grännö C *et al.* Familial occurrence of microscopic colitis: a report on five families. *Scand J Gastroenterol* 2001;**36**:959–62.

30 Abdo AA, Zetler PJ, Halparin LS. Familial microscopic colitis. *Can J Gastroenterol* 2001;**15**:341–3.

31 Freeman HJ. Familial occurrence of lymphocytic colitis. *Can J Gastroenterol* 2001;**15**:757–60.

32 Thomson A, Kaye G. Further report of familial occurrence of collagenous colitis. *Scand J Gastroenterol* 2002;**37**:1116.

33 Olesen M, Eriksson S, Bohr J *et al.* Lymphocytic colitis in Sweden – a retrospective clinical study of 199 patients. *Scand J Gastroenterol* 2003;**38**(Suppl 238):20.

34 Giardiello FM, Lazenby AJ. The atypical colitides. *Gastroenterol Clin North Am* 1999;**28**:479–90.

35 Stampfl DA, Friedman LS. Collagenous colitis: pathophysiologic considerations. *Dig Dis Sci* 1991;**36**:705–11.

36 Armes J, Gee DC, Macrae FA *et al.* Collagenous colitis: jejunal and colorectal pathology. *J Clin Pathol* 1992;**45**:784–7.

37 Järnerot G, Bohr J, Tysk C *et al.* Faecal stream diversion in patients with collagenous colitis. *Gut* 1996;**38**:154–5.

38 Fine KD, Lee EL, Meyer RL. Colonic histopathology in untreated celiac sprue or refractory sprue: is it lymphocytic colitis or colonic lymphocytosis? *Hum Pathol* 1998;**29**:1433–40.

39 Perk G, Ackerman Z, Cohen P *et al.* Lymphocytic colitis: a clue to an infectious trigger. *Scand J Gastroenterol* 1999;**34**:110–12.

40 Vesoulis Z, Lozanski G, Loiudice T. Synchronous occurrence of collagenous colitis and pseudomembranous colitis. *Can J Gastroenterol* 2000;**14**:353–8.

41 Khan MA, Brunt EM, Longo WE *et al.* Persistent *Clostridium difficile* colitis: a possible etiology for the development of collagenous colitis. *Dig Dis Sci* 2000;**45**:998–1001.

42 Byrne MF, McVey G, Royston D *et al.* Association of *Clostridium difficile* infection with collagenous colitis. *J Clin Gastroenterol* 2003;**36**:285.

43 Makinen M, Niemela S, Lehtola J *et al.* Collagenous colitis and *Yersinia enterocolitica* infection. *Dig Dis Sci* 1998;**43**:1341–6.

44 Bohr J, Nordfelth R, Jarnerot G *et al. Yersinia* species in collagenous colitis: a serologic study. *Scand J Gastroenterol* 2002;**37**:711–14.

45 Bryant DA, Mintz ED, Puhr ND *et al.* Colonic epithelial lymphocytosis associated with an epidemic of chronic diarrhea. *Am J Surg Pathol* 1996;**20**:1102–9.

46 Riddell RH, Tanaka M, Mazzoleni G. Non-steroidal anti-inflammatory drugs as a possible cause of collagenous colitis: a case–control study. *Gut* 1992;**33**:683–6.

47 Abdo A, Raboud J, Freeman HJ *et al.* Clinical and histological predictors of response to medical therapy in collagenous colitis. *Am J Gastroenterol* 2002;**97**:1164–8.

48 Brigot C, Courillon-Mallet A, Roucayrol AM *et al.* Lymphocytic colitis and ticlopidine. *Gastroenterol Clin Biol* 1998;**22**:361–2.

49 Berrebi D, Sautet A, Flejou JF *et al.* Ticlopidine induced colitis: a histopathological study including apoptosis. *J Clin Pathol* 1998;**51**:280–3.

50 Baert F, Wouters K, D'Haens G *et al.* Lymphocytic colitis: a distinct clinical entity? A clinicopathological confrontation of lymphocytic and collagenous colitis. *Gut* 1999;**45**:375–81.

51 Wilcox GM, Mattia A. Collagenous colitis associated with lansoprazole. *J Clin Gastroenterol* 2002;**34**:164–6.

52 Thomson RD, Lestina LS, Bensen SP *et al.* Lansoprazole-associated microscopic colitis: a case series. *Am J Gastroenterol* 2002;**97**:2908–13.

53 Pierrugues R, Saingra B. Lymphocytic colitis and Cyclo 3 fort: 4 new cases. *Gastroenterol Clin Biol* 1996;**20**:916–17.

54 Beaugerie L, Luboinski J, Brousse N *et al.* Drug induced lymphocytic colitis. *Gut* 1994;**35**:426–8.

55 Bouaniche M, Chassagne P, Landrin I *et al.* Lymphocytic colitis caused by Cyclo 3 Fort. *Rev Med Interne* 1996;**17**:776–8.

56 Beaugerie L, Patey N, Brousse N. Ranitidine, diarrhoea, and lymphocytic colitis. *Gut* 1995;**37**:708–11.

57 Duncan HD, Talbot IC, Silk DB. Collagenous colitis and cimetidine. *Eur J Gastroenterol Hepatol* 1997;**9**:819–20.

58 Chauveau E, Prignet JM, Carloz E *et al.* Lymphocytic colitis likely attributable to use of vinburnine (Cervoxan). *Gastroenterol Clin Biol* 1998;**22**:362.

59 Bouchet-Laneuw F, Deplaix P, Dumollard JM *et al.* Chronic diarrhea following ingestion of tardyferon associated with lymphocytic colitis. *Gastroenterol Clin Biol* 1997;**21**:83–4.

60 Piche T, Raimondi V, Schneider S *et al.* Acarbose and lymphocytic colitis. *Lancet* 2000;**356**:1246.

61 Mennecier D, Gros P, Bronstein JA *et al.* Chronic diarrhea due to lymphocytic colitis treated with piroxicam beta cyclodextrin. *Presse Med* 1999;**28**:735–7.

62 Rassiat E, Michiels C, Sgro C *et al.* Lymphocytic colitis due to Modopar. *Gastroenterol Clin Biol* 2000;**24**:852–3.

63 Mahajan L, Wyllie R, Goldblum J. Lymphocytic colitis in a pediatric patient: a possible adverse reaction to carbamazepine. *Am J Gastroenterol* 1997;**92**:2126–7.

64 Linares Torres P, Fidalgo Lopez I, Castanon Lopez A *et al.* Lymphocytic colitis as a cause of chronic diarrhea: possible association with carbamazepine. *Aten Primaria* 2000;**25**:366–7.

65 Macaigne G, Boivin JF, Chayette C *et al.* Oxetorone-associated lymphocytic colitis. *Gastroenterol Clin Biol* 2002;**26**:537.

66 Ghilain JM, Schapira M, Maisin JM *et al.* Lymphocytic colitis associated with lansoprazole treatment. *Gastroenterol Clin Biol* 2000;**24**:960–2.

67 Bohr J, Tysk C, Yang P *et al.* Autoantibodies and immunoglobulins in collagenous colitis. *Gut* 1996;**39**:73–6.

68 Eusufzai S, Lofberg R, Veress B. Studies on bile acid metabolism in collagenous colitis: no evidence of bile acid malabsorption as determined by the SeHCAT test. *Eur J Gastroentol Hepatol* 1992;**4**:317–21.

69 Ung KA, Gillberg R, Kilander A *et al.* Role of bile acids and bile acid binding agents in patients with collagenous colitis. *Gut* 2000;**46**:170–5.

70 Ung KA, Kilander A, Willen R *et al.* Role of bile acids in lymphocytic colitis. *Hepatogastroenterology* 2002;**49**:432–7.

71 Fernandez-Banares F, Esteve M, Salas A *et al.* Bile acid malabsorption in microscopic colitis and in previously unexplained functional chronic diarrhea. *Dig Dis Sci* 2001;**46**:2231–8.

72 Andersen T, Andersen JR, Tvede M *et al.* Collagenous colitis: are bacterial cytotoxins responsible? *Am J Gastroenterol* 1993;**88**:375–7.

73 Lundberg JO, Herulf M, Olesen M *et al.* Increased nitric oxide production in collagenous and lymphocytic colitis. *Eur J Clin Invest* 1997;**27**:869–71.

74 Perner A, Nordgaard I, Matzen P *et al.* Colonic production of nitric oxide gas in ulcerative colitis, collagenous colitis and uninflamed bowel. *Scand J Gastroenterol* 2002;**37**:183–8.

75 Olesen M, Middelveld R, Bohr J *et al.* Luminal nitric oxide and epithelial expression of inducible and endothelial nitric oxide synthase in collagenous and lymphocytic colitis. *Scand J Gastroenterol* 2003;**38**:66–72.

76 Perner A, Andresen L, Normark M *et al.* Expression of nitric oxide synthases and effects of L-arginine and L-NMMA on nitric oxide production and fluid transport in collagenous colitis. *Gut* 2001;**49**:387–94.

77 Rask-Madsen J, Grove O, Hansen MG *et al.* Colonic transport of water and electrolytes in a patient with secretory diarrhea due to collagenous colitis. *Dig Dis Sci* 1983;**28**:1141–6.

78 Burgel N, Bojarski C, Mankertz J *et al.* Mechanisms of diarrhea in collagenous colitis. *Gastroenterology* 2002;**123**:433–43.

79 Bohr J, Järnerot G, Tysk C *et al.* Effect of fasting on diarrhoea in collagenous colitis. *Digestion* 2002;**65**:30–4.

80 Taylor S, Haggitt R, Bronner M. Colonic perforation complicating colonoscopy in collagenous colitis. *Gastroenterology* 1999;**116**:A938.

81 Freeman HJ, James D, Mahoney CJ. Spontaneous peritonitis from perforation of the colon in collagenous colitis. *Can J Gastroenterol* 2001;**15**:265–7.

82 Bohr J, Larsson L, Tysk C *et al.* Spontaneous colonic perforation in collagenous colitis. (Swedish). *Sv Läkarsällkapets Handl Hygiea* 2003;**112**:170.

83 Bonderup OK, Folkersen BH, Gjersoe P *et al.* Collagenous colitis: a long-term follow-up study. *Eur J Gastroenterol Hepatol* 1999;**11**:493–5.

84 Chan JL, Tersmette AC, Offerhaus GJ *et al.* Cancer risk in collagenous colitis. *Inflamm Bowel Dis* 1999;**5**:40–3.

85 Goff JS, Barnett JL, Pelke T *et al.* Collagenous colitis: histopathology and clinical course. *Am J Gastroenterol* 1997;**92**:57–60.

86 Bonner GF, Petras RE, Cheong DM *et al.* Short- and long-term follow-up of treatment for lymphocytic and collagenous colitis. *Inflamm Bowel Dis* 2000;**6**:85–91.

87 Järnerot G, Tysk C, Bohr J *et al.* Collagenous colitis and fecal stream diversion. *Gastroenterology* 1995;**109**:449–55.

88 Pokorny CS, Kneale KL, Henderson CJ. Progression of collagenous colitis to ulcerative colitis. *J Clin Gastroenterol* 2001;**32**:435–8.

89 Mullhaupt B, Guller U, Anabitarte M *et al.* Lymphocytic colitis: clinical presentation and long term course. *Gut* 1998;**43**:629–33.

90 Yang P, Bohr J, Tysk C *et al.* Antineutrophil cytoplasmic antibodies in inflammatory bowel disease and collagenous colitis. No association with lactoferrin, b-glucuronidase, myeloperoxidase, or proteinase 3. *Inflamm Bowel Dis* 1996;**2**:173–7.

91 Bohr J, Jones I, Tysk C *et al.* Serum procollagen III propeptide is not of diagnostic predictive value in collagenous colitis. *Inflamm Bowel Dis* 1995;**1**:276–9.

92 Bowling TE, Price AB, al-Adnani M *et al.* Interchange between collagenous and lymphocytic colitis in severe disease with autoimmune associations requiring colectomy: a case report. *Gut* 1996;**38**:788–91.

93 Tremaine WJ. Collagenous colitis and lymphocytic colitis. *J Clin Gastroenterol* 2000;**30**:245–9.

94 Giardiello FM, Lazenby AJ, Yardley JH *et al.* Increased HLA A1 and diminished HLA A3 in lymphocytic colitis compared to controls and patients with collagenous colitis. *Dig Dis Sci* 1992;**37**:496–9.

95 Pardi DS, Ramnath VR, Loftus EV Jr *et al.* Lymphocytic colitis: clinical features, treatment, and outcomes. *Am J Gastroenterol* 2002;**97**:2829–33.

96 Pardi DS, Smyrk TC, Tremaine WJ *et al.* Microscopic colitis: a review. *Am J Gastroenterol* 2002;**97**:794–802.

97 Chande N, McDonald JW, MacDonald JK. Interventions for treating collagenous colitis. *Cochrane Database Syst Rev* 2003;**1**:CD003575.

98 Fine KD, Ogunji L, Lee E *et al.* Randomized, double-blind, placebo-controlled trial of bismuth subsalicylate for microscopic colitis. *Gastroenterology* 1999;**116**:A880.

99 Baert F, Schmit A, D'Haens G *et al.* Budesonide in collagenous colitis: a double-blind placebo-controlled trial with histologic follow-up. *Gastroenterology* 2002;**122**:20–5.

100 Miehlke S, Heymer P, Bethke B *et al.* Budesonide treatment for collagenous colitis: a randomized, double-blind, placebo-controlled, multicenter trial. *Gastroenterology* 2002;**123**:978–84.

101 Bonderup OK, Hansen JB, Birket-Smith L *et al.* Budesonide treatment of collagenous colitis: a randomised, double blind, placebo controlled trial with morphometric analysis. *Gut* 2003;**52**:248–51.

102 Lanyi B, Dries V, Dienes HP *et al.* Therapy of prednisone-refractory collagenous colitis with budesonide. *Int J Colorectal Dis* 1999;**14**:58–61.

103 Jung D, Fantin AC, Scheurer U *et al.* Human ileal bile acid transporter gene ASBT (SLCIOAZ) is transactivated by the glucocorticoid receptor. *Gut* 2004;**53**:78–84.

104 Pardi DS, Loftus EV, Jr., Tremaine WJ *et al.* Treatment of refractory microscopic colitis with azathioprine and 6-mercaptopurine. *Gastroenterology* 2001;**120**:1483–4.

105 Hillman L, Ashton C, Chirigakis L *et al.* Collagenous colitis remission with methotrexate. *Gastroenterology* 2001;**120**:A278.

106 Alikhan M, Cummings OW, Rex D. Subtotal colectomy in a patient with collagenous colitis associated with colonic carcinoma and systemic lupus erythematosus. *Am J Gastroenterol* 1997;**92**:1213–15.

107 Yusuf TE, Soemijarsih M, Arpaia A *et al.* Chronic microscopic enterocolitis with severe hypokalemia responding to subtotal colectomy. *J Clin Gastroenterol* 1999;**29**:284–8.

108 Williams RA, Gelfand DV. Total proctocolectomy and ileal pouch anal anastomosis to successfully treat a patient with collagenous colitis. *Am J Gastroenterol* 2000;**95**:2147.

109 Varghese L, Galandiuk S, Tremaine WJ *et al.* Lymphocytic colitis treated with proctocolectomy and ileal J-pouch-anal anastomosis: report of a case. *Dis Colon Rectum* 2002;**45**:123–6.

110 Riaz AA, Pitt J, Stirling RW *et al.* Restorative procto-colectomy for collagenous colitis. *J R Soc Med* 2000;**93**:261.

14 Metabolic bone disease in gastrointestinal disorders

Ann Cranney, Catherine Dube, Alaa Rostom, Peter Tugwell, George Wells

Introduction

Metabolic bone disease is seen in patients suffering from a variety of gastrointestinal disorders, including chronic liver disease, inflammatory bowel disease (IBD), and malabsorption syndromes such as celiac disease. In the setting of gastrointestinal disorders, bone disease can be broadly divided into osteoporosis and osteomalacia. Osteoporosis is the systemic skeletal disorder of reduced bone mass per unit volume (i.e. bone density) and disrupted micro-architecture, resulting in decreased bone strength and an increased risk of fragility fractures mainly of the hip, wrist, and vertebrae.[1] Bone mass is the major determinant of bone strength. Osteomalacia, however, is characterized by defective mineralization of bone matrix, usually due to a disturbance of vitamin D and calcium homeostasis. It is clinically associated with pain, bone fractures, occasionally muscle weakness and radiologically with pseudofractures (radiolucent bands perpendicular to surface of bone) and loss of trabeculae.

There are two types of bone: cortical, which primarily makes up the long bones, and trabecular bone, which makes up most of the axial skeleton. Bone formation and resorption is a continuous process in which osteoblasts are responsible for the formation of new bone including the mineralization of bone, and osteoclasts are responsible for bone resorption. Metabolic bone disease results from abnormalities in the normal remodeling cycle. Osteoporosis is associated with disability, impaired quality of life and fractures can be associated with increased mortality.[2]

This chapter will focus on metabolic bone disease associated with chronic liver disease and IBD and will review corticosteroid-induced osteoporosis.

Assessment of bone mass

Age-related bone loss begins during the fourth decade, and in women there is an accelerated bone loss at the time of the menopause (5–15% in the initial 5 years after menopause).

Women experience greater rates of bone loss than men and their lifetime risk of an osteoporotic fracture is about 15% compared with 5% in men.[3] Osteoporosis can be detected by measurement of bone mineral density. Bone density is the most accurate predictor of fracture risk and it is a useful guide for monitoring therapy.[4] Prospective trials have established the ability of bone density to predict site-specific fractures.[5] For each reduction in bone density of the hip by 1 SD from the mean for young normal individuals, the risk of hip fracture increases by a factor of 1·5–2·6.[6] In men, low bone mineral density (BMD) has been demonstrated to be predictive of vertebral fractures.[7] In a prospective study which included 1690 men, it was estimated that a 1 SD decrease in femoral neck bone density was associated with a two-fold increase in risk of atraumatic fracture.[8] Increasing age and a history of a previous vertebral fracture are very important predictors of fracture.

Bone mass can be evaluated at a number of sites, such as the proximal femur, spine and distal radius. The most commonly used technique to evaluate BMD is dual energy x ray absorptiometry (DXA). The reproducibility, accuracy and precision of DXA are excellent, with a coefficient of variation of 2%. Another technique, quantitative computed tomography (QCT), provides a three-dimensional image which makes it possible to separate trabecular and cortical bone. The accuracy of QCT is not as good (5–15%) as DXA, and is associated with a higher radiation dose.

Bone mineral content (BMC) is the total amount of mineralized tissue (g) in the bone scan, usually normalized to the length of the scan path (grams per mineral per centimeter of bone or g/cm). BMD, on the other hand, is the amount of mineralized tissue in the scanned area (g/cm^2). BMD can be expressed as a T score (comparison of the patient's bone density with the peak bone mass in young normal individuals) or Z score (comparison of patient's BMD to other age-matched controls). Individuals with a T score or BMD less than 1 SD below the mean in young adults are considered to be osteopenic, while those with a BMD less than 2·5 SDs below the young normal value are osteoporotic.[1] A study group on densitometry hosted by the World Health Organization (WHO) in 1993 defined these four diagnostic thresholds based on reference populations of healthy young women. Since these thresholds are based on young women, this definition does not account for biological variation and age-related bone loss and many have argued against the use of T scores. The increased use of DXA has resulted in more gastroenterology patients being diagnosed with osteoporosis. However, it is not clear what a diagnosis of osteopenia in gastrointestinal patients means in terms of increased fracture risk. On the basis of BMD osteomalacia cannot be distinguished from osteoporosis.

Hepatic osteodystrophy

Hepatic osteodystrophy, or chronic liver disease-associated metabolic bone disease, was previously thought to arise mainly in cholestatic liver diseases, as a result of calcium and vitamin D malabsorption. However, hepatic osteodystrophy has now been described in association with most types of chronic liver diseases, whether cholestatic or non-cholestatic.[9] Increased bone loss and/or increased incidence of fractures have been described in primary biliary cirrhosis (PBC),[10] primary sclerosing cholangitis (PSC),[11] alcoholic liver disease (ALD),[12,13] autoimmune hepatitis (AIH),[14] hemochromatosis, as well as viral cirrhosis.[15,16] Additionally, hepatic osteodystrophy has important clinical repercussions in the early period after liver transplant, where immobilization, comorbidity, corticosteroids and immunosuppressive drugs further reduce an already compromised bone mass,[10] resulting in spontaneous vertebral fractures.[17,18]

Prevalence

The prevalence of hepatic osteodystrophy varies from 13% to 56%,[11,15,19] while the incidence of fractures in ambulant and non-alcoholic patients with chronic liver disease ranges from 6% to 18%. The prevalence of vertebral fractures ranges from 7% to 44% and is approximately twice that of age and sex-matched controls with the highest rates in those individuals with AIH.[15,19] The degree of bone loss correlates with the severity of the cirrhosis and increasing age, making patients with endstage liver disease the group most at risk of fractures.[5,19,20]

The fracture risk in chronic liver disease was best studied by Diamond *et al.*, in a case–control study of 115 patients with chronic liver disease (72 men and 43 women), who were matched for age, sex and menopausal status with healthy controls.[19] The etiology of the chronic liver disease was ALD ($n = 40$), chronic active hepatitis ($n = 27$), hemochromatosis ($n = 25$), PBC ($n = 10$), and PSC ($n = 13$).

Fifty-two per cent of the patients were cirrhotic, while 30% had clinical and biochemical evidence of hypogonadism. It is important to note that, in men, hypogonadism correlates with the degree of liver dysfunction. All patients were ambulatory and none were on cholestyramine, vitamin D, estrogen, or calcium. From the data in this study, the relative risk (RR) of either spinal or peripheral fractures can be calculated, based on the absolute number of fractures (as opposed to the number of patients with fractures). In men this RR is 3·03 (95% CI 1·35 to 11·09), while in women the RR is 2·13 (95% CI 1·38 to 7·46). These authors did a stepwise regression analysis to define the main predictors of fracture and osteoporosis. Variables used were: age, sex, gonadal status, presence of cirrhosis, type of liver disease, liver function, 25(OH) vitamin D_3 level and parathyroid hormone (PTH) level. Spinal bone density, liver dysfunction and hypogonadism were the main predictors of spinal fracture while hypogonadism and the presence of cirrhosis were the main predictors of peripheral fractures. There was no association with serum PTH or 25-hydroxy-vitamin D_3.

Because of the potential for impaired absorption of calcium and vitamin D,[21,22] as well as impaired hepatic uptake and metabolism of vitamin D,[23] osteomalacia was initially thought to be the major cause of hepatic osteodystrophy in cholestatic liver diseases.[23,24] However, it then became evident that bone disease was still prevalent despite treatment with calcium and vitamin D, and that most patients with cholestatic liver disease and osteopenia did not have low 25-hydroxy-vitamin D_3 levels[11] or histomorphometric characteristics of osteomalacia.[20,25,26] Osteoporosis appears to be the major metabolic bone disease found with chronic liver disease.

The mechanisms responsible for the osteoporosis in this setting are uncertain, and evidence exists for both decreased bone formation[20,27–29] and increased bone resorption.[11,25,30] The presence of cirrhosis seems to play an important role through several mechanisms. Testosterone, 25-hydroxy-vitamin D, and insulin-like growth factor 1 (IGF-1) levels are all reduced in advanced liver disease and correlate inversely with the degree of osteopenia.[15,19] As well, bone mass starts to increase within 6 months to a year after liver transplantation.[10] Other factors may also affect bone metabolism independently of cirrhosis: bone formation is directly suppressed by alcohol,[13,31] and possibly by iron in hemochromatosis. The majority of patients with advanced PBC are also postmenopausal females, which adds to the list of pathogenic factors of hepatic osteodystrophy.[19] Malnutrition, treatment with corticosteroids[14,32] or immunosuppressives plays a role in some cases.

Treatment

Osteomalacia

Osteomalacia secondary to vitamin D deficiency is characterized by low serum v25-hydroxy-vitamin D, low or

Table 14.1   Case series of interventions for hepatic osteodystrophy

Study	Disease (no. of patients)	Therapy (duration)	Measurement (site)	Comments
Wagonfeld *et al.* (1976)[23]	PBC (8)	PO or SC D *v* 25-OH-D$_3$ 100–200 micrograms/day (3 months)	X-ray and PBA (hand)	Failure of oral or parenteral vitamin D to normalize 25-OH-D or to prevent accelerated bone loss
Matloff *et al.* (1982)[35]	PBC (10)	25-OH-D$_3$ 40–120 micrograms/day (1 year)	PBA (radius)	Normalization of 25-OH-D levels but ongoing bone loss and fractures
Herlong *et al.* (1982)[30]	PBC (15)	25-OH-D$_3$ 50–100 micrograms/day (1 year)	PBA (radius)	Normalization of 25-OH-D levels but ongoing bone loss
Floreani *et al.* (1997)[36]	PBC (34)	1,25(OH)$_2$-D$_3$ 1 micrograms/day × 5d, calcitonin 40 U IM 3/week and; 4 week, CaCO$_3$ 1·5 g/day × 4 week (3 years)	DPA (LS)	?Reduced bone loss in treated (uncontrolled)
Neuhaus *et al.* (1995)[37]	OLT (150)	25-OHD$_3$ 0·25–0·5 micrograms/day ± Ca 1 g/day ± NaF 25 mg/day (2 year)	DXA (LS/FN)	Reduced bone loss in any of the treatment groups compared with untreated controls
Riemens *et al.* (1996)[38]	OLT (53)	1-OHD 1 microgram/day; Ca 1 g/day; etidronate 400 mg/day 2/15 week (1 year)	DPA (LS)	No reduction in bone loss compared with historical controls
Crippin *et al.* (1994)[39]	PBC (107)	Estrogen (low dose oral or patch) (1 year)	DPA (LS)	Reduction in bone loss in estrogen group

PBC, primary biliary cirrhosis; OLT, orthotopic liver transplantation; CAH, chronic active hepatitis; ALD, alcoholic liver disease; HA, hydroxyapatite; NaF, sodium fluoride; UDCA, ursodeoxycholic acid; DPA, dual photon absorptiometry; DXA, dual x ray absorptiometry; PBA, photon beam absorptiometry; SPA, single photon absorptiometry; LS, lumbar spine; FN, femoral neck, 25-OH-D$_3$, 25-hydroxy-vitamin D$_3$, PO, per os; SC, subcutaneous; IM, intramuscular

normal calcium, low phosphate and elevated alkaline phosphatase levels. Based on measurement of 25-hydroxy-vitamin D level and bone histomorphometry, osteomalacia can be successfully treated and prevented with combined calcium and vitamin D supplementation (oral or parenteral).[33,34] B4 Vitamin D does not need to be given as its 25-hydroxy metabolite, since the capacity of the liver to hydroxylate vitamin D is maintained, even in advanced liver disease. However, since its absorption and/or hepatic uptake may be decreased, sufficient doses should be administered.[22] Successful treatment of osteomalacia has been achieved with calcium and either oral vitamin D$_2$ 2000–4000 IU daily, intramuscular vitamin D$_2$ 150 000 IU weekly,[33] or oral 25-hydroxy-D$_3$ 1000–4000 IU daily,[34] for a duration of 3–6 months. B4

Osteoporosis

The evidence for interventions for the treatment of osteoporosis in chronic liver disease is summarized in Tables 14.1 and 14.2. There are a number of observational trials and more recently randomized controlled trials (RCTs), most of which have relatively small numbers of patients.

Vitamin D and calcium   Therapy with vitamin D has been studied in osteoporotic patients with either cholestatic[30,35] or non-cholestatic liver disease[12] and low 25-hydroxy-vitamin D levels. Uncontrolled studies in PBC (Table 14.1) suggest that normalization of 25-hydroxy-vitamin D levels failed to arrest bone loss[30] or to prevent spontaneous fractures.[35] B4 In one of these two reports, improvements in bone mass occurred only in patients whose calcium absorption increased as a result of the therapy.[35] However, in an RCT of 18 abstinent patients with alcoholic liver disease, Mobarhan *et al.* showed that normalization of 25-hydroxy-vitamin D levels was associated with a significant increase in BMD after a mean duration of 10 months (Table 14.2).[12] A1d Unfortunately, bone biopsy to rule out osteomalacia was done in only nine out of the 18 patients.

Table 14.2 Randomized trials of interventions for hepatic osteodystrophy

Study	Disease (no. of patients)	Intervention (duration)	Measurement (site)	Comments
Guanabens *et al.* (2003)[40]	PBC (36)	2 year cyclical etidronate *v* alendronate	DXA, LS, FN	Both treatments increased BMD, but increases with alendronate were significantly larger
Shiomi *et al.* (2002)[41]	Viral hepatitis (50)	2 years cyclical etidronate	DXA LS	Significant reduction in bone loss in etidronate treated group
Lindor *et al.* (2000)[42]	PBC (67)	1 year cyclical etidronate	DXA LS, FN	No significant difference from placebo
Shiomi *et al.* (1999)[43]	Cirrhosis, PBC and secondary to hepatitis B and C (76)	0·5 micrograms calcitriol twice daily 15 months	DXA (LS)	Significant reduction in bone loss in calcitriol group
Guanabens *et al.* (1997)[44]	PBC (32)	Etidronate 400 mg/day 2/15 week *v* NaF 50 mg/day (2 years)	DPA (LS)	Significant reduction in bone loss in etidronate group
Camisasca *et al.* (1994)[45a]	PBC (25)	Carbicalcitonin 40 U SC every day *v* porcine calcitonin IU SC 2/week (15 months)	DPA (LS)	No difference between groups
Wolfhagen *et al.* (1997)[46]	PBC (12)	Etidronate 400 mg/day × 2 week + Ca 500 mg/day, 11/13 week *v* Ca 500 mg/day. (1 year)	DXA (LS/FN)	Significant reduction in LS bone loss in etidronate group
Guanabens *et al.* (1992)[47]	PBC (22)	NaF 50 mg/day *v* placebo (2 years)	DPA (LS)	Significant reduction in bone loss in NaF group
Lindor *et al.* (1995)[48]	PBC (88)	UDCA 13–15 mg/kg/day (3 years)	DPA (LS)	No difference between groups
Stellon *et al.* (1985)[49]	CAH (36)	HA 8 g/day (2 years)	*x* ray/SPA	Reduced bone loss in HA group
Mobarhan *et al.* (1984)[12]	ALD (18)	D_2 50 000 U 2–3x/wk *v* 25-OH-D 20–50 micrograms/day *v* control (1 year)	DPA (LS)	Significant increase in BMD compared to baseline in all groups

[a]Crossover design.
For abbreviations see Table 14.1.

Shiomi *et al.* studied the efficacy of 1,25-dihydroxy-vitamin D_3 (0·5 micrograms) on lumbar spine BMD in 76 individuals with cirrhosis secondary to hepatitis B or C infection. The results suggest that calcitriol may be effective in increasing bone mass at the lumbar spine over a 12 month period.[43] B4

Calcium supplementation appeared to prevent or diminish bone loss compared with untreated controls.[50]

Antiresorptive and anabolic agents A retrospective study of 107 females with PBC suggested that hormone replacement therapy (HRT) is associated with a significant reduction of annual bone loss[39] (Table 14.1). B4

Table 14.2 summarizes the results of randomized trials of a variety of other interventions. Guanabens *et al.* in a 2-year RCT of 32 women with PBC, compared cyclical etidronate at a dose of 400 mg for 2 weeks every 78 days, to sodium fluoride (NaF) 50 mg per day.[44] In the fluoride-treated group, the bone density of the lumbar spine decreased by 1·94% and the femoral neck decreased by 1·4%. By contrast, etidronate increased bone mass in the lumbar spine by 0·53% and femoral neck BMD was stable and was better tolerated. Ald

Wolfhagen *et al.* compared etidronate plus calcium with calcium alone in a randomized trial in 12 women with PBC on corticosteroids.[46] There was a statistically significant difference in the percentage change in mean lumbar BMD between the etidronate and calcium-treated groups (etidronate +0·4%, calcium −3·0%, $P = 0.01$).[46] Ald In a randomized trial that was not blinded, Shiomi *et al.* evaluated etidronate in 45 women with cirrhosis due to underlying viral hepatitis and also found a statistically significant difference in the percentage change in lumbar spine BMD.[41] Guanabens *et al.* compared alendronate with etidronate in an RCT of 36 women with PBC.[40] After 2 years, both treatments increased bone density but the increase was significantly greater in women on alendronate. Ald

Camisasca *et al.*[45] evaluated the effect of a 6-month course of calcitonin 40 IU every other day, given subcutaneously in a trial with a crossover design. The control group received 1 IU of porcine calcitonin (no metabolic effect). Both groups received calcium and 100 000 IU of parenteral vitamin D_2 ($n = 25$). Treatments were administered for 6 months with a 3-month washout. There was no difference in bone density between the two treatment groups in either of the crossover periods. It is possible that this study was inadequately powered to detect a significant difference. Ald

In another trial of 22 women with PBC followed for 2 years, Guanabens *et al.*[47] compared NaF to calcium in a 2-year RCT In the NaF group, the bone density of the lumbar spine increased by 2·9% compared with the control group in which it decreased by 6·6%. However, there was a high frequency of adverse effects, mainly gastrointestinal. Since NaF therapy was also less effective than etidronate in another study, this intervention is not recommended.

In summary, both cholestatic and non-cholestatic types of liver disease may be complicated by metabolic bone disease, predominately osteoporosis. The prevalence of bone disease increases with the degree of cirrhosis. Accelerated bone loss is most severe after liver transplantation. Patients with advanced liver disease, awaiting transplantation, on prolonged corticosteroid therapy or with a history of low trauma fractures, C5 should be investigated with BMD testing. Low 25-hydroxy-vitamin D_3 levels should be corrected and calcium supplementation given. Bisphosphonates should be considered in patients with known osteoporosis or vertebral fractures, based on the evidence from a number of small randomized trials. Ala Testosterone therapy should be considered in males with hypogonadism. C5

There is a need for population-based studies of fracture risk in patients with chronic liver disease.

Inflammatory bowel disease

Prevalence

The importance of metabolic bone disease in patients with IBD has been recognized for some time. However, the point prevalence of bone disease in this population varies greatly

Table 14.3 Factors influencing interpretation of studies of bone disease in gastrointestinal patients

Definition of osteopenia	Z scores of ≤ 1
Diagnostic method	*x* ray, SPA, DPA, QCT, DXA, US
Results expressed	BMD, BMC, radiological or clinical fracture
Bone site studied	Spine, forearm, femoral neck or total hip
High risk patients	Included or excluded
Control of confounders	Smoking, steroid use

SPA, single photon absorptiometry; QCT, quantitative computed tomography; DPA, dual photon absorptiometry; DXA, dual energy *x* ray absorptiometry; BMD, bone mineral density; BMC, bone mineral content

from one study to another, with estimates as low as 5% to as high as 78%. This variation reflects a number of factors, including the definition of osteoporosis used, the site of bone density measurement, and the heterogeneous nature of the IBD population. A list of potential factors that need to be considered when evaluating studies in this area is provided in Table 14.3.

In a well conducted study, Abitbol *et al.*[51] evaluated the BMD of 84 consecutive patients with IBD (34 Crohn's disease, 50 ulcerative colitis, excluding proctitis). Overall, 43% had osteopenia in the lumbar spine. Steroid users were at significantly greater risk of osteopenia (58% *v* 28% in non-users, $P = 0.03$). Six patients with a mean age of 50 had vertebral crush fractures (mean Z score was −1·63). Five patients were found to have low 25-hydroxy-vitamin D_3 levels; however, the cause of this deficiency was felt to be extraintestinal in all but one case. Multiple regression analysis of the lumbar Z score revealed a significant correlation between osteopenia and age, cumulative corticosteroid dose, inflammatory status as assessed by the erythrocyte sedimentation rate (ESR), and low osteocalcin levels ($r^2 = 0.76$, $P < 0.05$).

The rate of bone loss in IBD has been studied in several longitudinal studies.[52–57] In the majority of the studies the annual rate of bone loss appears to be greater in the spine than at the radius, and varies from 2% to 6%. Schulte *et al.* studied the rate of BMD change in 80 IBD patients and found that the annual rate of bone loss was small (0·8 %/year for spine).[56] Corticosteroid use[52] and low body mass index[53] were found, in some studies, to negatively affect bone mass. Overall, metabolic bone disease is an important problem among patients with IBD, with an estimated prevalence in the range of 45%.

Malabsorption of calcium and vitamin D because of small bowel disease appears to play a minor role in the pathogenesis of the metabolic bone disease of IBD. Both low and normal vitamin D levels have been documented in patients with

Crohn's disease and there is no clear correlation between vitamin D levels and bone mass.[58,59] Osteomalacia appears to be much less common than osteoporosis in IBD. Hessov *et al.*[60] did bone biopsy and serum vitamin D determinations on 36 randomly selected Crohn's disease patients with previous surgical resections (mean length 105 cm). Only two patients were found to have below normal 25-hydroxy-vitamin D_3 levels and/or histomorphometric evidence of osteomalacia. However, the mean trabecular bone volume was reduced in this group compared with controls, suggestive of osteoporosis. This finding did not correlate with any of the measured clinical characteristics, including length of resection and serum vitamin D level. Another bone histomorphometry study in IBD revealed decreased bone formation without evidence of osteomalacia.[61]

Comparisons between Crohn's disease and ulcerative colitis patients suggest that osteoporosis may be more prevalent in the former.[62–64] However, careful review of these publications suggests that the analysis may not have been fully controlled for the effects of disease activity and/or steroid use. Jahnsen *et al.* in an age and sex-matched cross-sectional study of 60 Crohn's disease patients, 60 ulcerative colitis patients and 60 controls, found no differences in BMD between the patients with ulcerative colitis and the controls.[63] However, Crohn's disease patients had significantly lower BMD. Overall 16% of ulcerative colitis patients and controls had Z scores ≤ 1 compared with 23% of Crohn's disease patients.[63] However, significantly more Crohn's disease than ulcerative colitis patients used corticosteroids (72% *v* 47%), and smoked (57% *v* 28%). Although the disease activity was not specifically addressed in this study, 53% of the ulcerative colitis group had left-sided disease, with 40% having proctosigmoiditis or less. As well, the BMD of Crohn's disease patients who were not using steroids was not significantly different from that of the other two groups. Ghosh *et al.*[62] evaluated 30 IBD patients at the time of diagnosis and found that those with Crohn's disease had significantly lower bone density than those with ulcerative colitis. The mean lumbar spine Z score for Crohn's disease patients was −1·06 versus −0·03 for those with ulcerative colitis. However, seven of 15 ulcerative colitis patients had proctitis alone, and one had a "distal colitis". As well, the mean duration of disease before diagnosis (18·6 *v* 12 weeks), and of steroid use (1·2 *v* 0·5 weeks) before BMD, measurements are slightly longer in the Crohn's group, again suggesting that disease severity rather than diagnosis may be the important factor. Bernstein *et al.* in a study of 26 Crohn's disease and 23 ulcerative colitis patients, also found a greater prevalence of osteopenia among the former.[64] However, using stepwise discriminant analysis, the authors found that steroid use rather than disease type was the most important predictive factor.

A cross sectional study of 51 Crohn's disease, 40 ulcerative colitis patients and 30 age and sex-matched controls by Ardizzone *et al.* found no significant difference in mean T score values between patients with Crohn's or ulcerative colitis but did find that 37% of Crohn's and 18% of ulcerative colitis patients were osteoporotic based on WHO criteria.[65] Stepwise regression showed that in Crohn's disease, the femoral neck T score was inversely related to disease duration and lumbar spine T score was inversely related to age. There were baseline differences in disease duration between the two groups. Schulte studied the rate of BMD change in 80 patients with IBD. The results indicated that the average annual rate of bone loss was small. There was a large range reported bone density in these patients, suggesting that certain subgroups may lose bone more quickly than others.

The study of metabolic bone disease in ulcerative colitis before and after restorative proctocolectomy also suggests that disease activity plays an important role, since BMD increases significantly with time after colectomy, with a mean annual increase of around 2%.[66]

Fracture prevalence estimates in IBD from cross-sectional and prospective studies have been variable with larger series reporting vertebral fractures in 7–22%[67] and non-vertebral fractures in 27% of patients, although these data may have been affected by referral bias. There have been three recent population-based studies of fracture risk in IBD. Bernstein *et al.* identified 6027 IBD patients through an administrative database in a Canadian population and matched them to 60 270 controls by age, sex and geographic residence.[68] The overall fracture rate was higher than for controls with a 41% overall increased incidence of hip, spine, wrist and rib fractures among IBD patients (RR 1·41, 95% CI 1·27 to 1·56). The incidence rate ratio was 1·59 (95% CI 1·27 to 2·00) for hip fractures. There were no difference in fracture rates between males and females or between Crohn's and ulcerative colitis patients, except that males with ulcerative colitis had a higher fracture rate than females with ulcerative colitis. Although the fracture risk of IBD patients was higher than controls, the increase was one patient per 100 patient years. Another North American study in Olmsted County, Minnesota assessed fracture risk in 238 Crohn's disease patients through reviews of radiology reports and found that compared with age and sex-matched controls the overall risk ratio for any fracture was 0·9 (95% CI, 0·6 to 1·4) but this was statistically non-significant. The risk ratio for vertebral fracture was 2·2 (95% CI 0·9 to 5·5), and the relative risk for an osteoporotic fracture was 1·4 (95% CI 0·7–2·7), all statistically non-significant.[69] Age was the only significant predictor of fracture risk in a multivariate analysis and fracture risk was not increased in comparison with the general population except in the elderly patients. The findings were similar for the ulcerative colitis patients. Vestergaard and Mosekilde in a population-based study from hospital discharge data did not find an increase in fracture risk except for a small increase risk of fracture that required hospitalization in Crohn's disease patients.[70] The difference from fracture rates seen in ulcerative colitis patients was not significant. A potential weakness of this study was the use of administrative databases which could result in the under-reporting of fractures that do not require hospitalization. In addition, the diagnosis of Crohn's disease and ulcerative colitis was only validated in a small sample of patients.

A recent nested case–control study of 231 778 fracture cases from the UK General Practice Research Database demonstrated an increased risk of vertebral (OR 1.72 (95% CI 1·13–2·61) and hip fracture (OR 1·59 (95% CI 1·14–2·23) in patients with IBD. There was a greater risk of hip fracture seen in Crohn's patients compared with ulcerative colitis patients. This study also noted that only 13% of IBD patients who had already sustained a fracture were on osteoporosis treatment.[71] Corticosteroid use was associated with an increased risk of fracture and this persisted after adjustment for disease severity (OR 1·10 (95% CI 1·00–1·20). Limitations of this study include method of ascertainment of fractures and the fact that only clinically diagnosed fractures were included.

The literature suggests that there is a discrepancy between BMD findings and fracture risk in the IBD population and that the greatest risk is in elderly patients with IBD.

Treatment

Clements *et al.* in an uncontrolled 2-year prospective study of HRT in 47 postmenopausal women with IBD (25 ulcerative colitis, 22 Crohn's disease), found that radial and spine BMD rose significantly over baseline with HRT.[72] B4 The authors found no differences in the responses between patients with ulcerative colitis and Crohn's disease. Patients using cortico-steroids also seemed to respond.

Vogelsang *et al.* randomized 75 Crohn's disease patients, without short bowel syndrome, to 1000 IU vitamin D_3 + calcium or placebo. The BMD of the forearm decreased in 80% of the control group versus 50% of the treatment group at 1 year. BMD decreased less in calcium/vitamin D-treated patients (median decrease in BMD: treated 0·2%, interquartile range 3·8–(+14)%; control 7%, range 12·6–(+14)%; $P < 0·005$). Ald The correlation between the change in vitamin D and change in BMC was low (r = 0·19).[73] Bernstein *et al.*[74] in a pilot study of 17 IBD patients with a history of steroid use (14 men, 10 Crohn's disease), assessed the efficacy of calcium supplementation (1000 mg/day) and vitamin D 250 IU on BMD by DXA. The authors found that the dose of prednisone in the year prior to the study inversely correlated with bone density at the hip and Ward's triangle, but not at the spine. There was no effect on bone density demonstrated after 1 year. Ald However, there is a significant risk of a type 2 error in this small study.

Robinson *et al.*[75] assessed the effect of low impact exercise in a randomized controlled trial. Although no statistically significant increase in BMD was observed in the exercise group, secondary analysis revealed that the number of exercise sessions correlated significantly with increased BMD at the hip and spine. Ald

Haderslev *et al.* assessed the impact of alendronate in Crohn's disease patients with osteopenia in a 12-month RCT. Alendronate increased the BMD of the lumbar spine by 5·5 % compared with control over a 1-year period. Fractures were not evaluated.[76] Ald

von Tirpitz *et al.* studied the effectiveness of NaF (75 mg SR) on 33 subjects with Crohn's disease in a 12-month RCT. The results indicated that NaF is effective at increasing mean spine Z score ($P = 0·02$). The control arm of calcium 1000 mg/day and vitamin D 1000 IU/day did not result in increases in spine BMD.[77] Ald

In summary, osteopenia is an important problem among patients with IBD, even at initial diagnosis. The risk appears to be greatest among those with the greatest disease activity and duration, and those treated with corticosteroids. It is difficult to distinguish the impact on bone density of corticosteroid use from that of disease activity, since these factors are linked. The risk of osteoporosis and facture in ulcerative colitis is similar to that seen in Crohn's disease and after proctocolectomy the bone density of ulcerative colitis patients increases. The risk for osteoporosis and fractures appears to be similar in males and females. Crohn's and ulcerative colitis patients seem to have comparable risks for fracture; although the overall rate for fracture is increased, the rate is affected by age.

There is evidence that IBD patients with low BMD benefit from a combination of vitamin D and calcium. HRT may be a less attractive option based on recent results from the Women's Health Initiative study and concerns about unfavorable risk profile. Existing studies have used surrogate outcome measures, particularly measures of BMD, and management has been based on results from treatment trials of postmenopausal osteoporosis. Further studies are needed to assess the impact of bisphosphonates on the clinically important outcome of fracture. Current recommendations are that for individuals with T scores < −2·5 or vertebral compression fractures, therapy should include calcium and vitamin D in addition to bisphosphonates. Ald For those with T scores between −2·5 and −1·0, therapy should include calcium and vitamin D and bisphosphonate therapy for patients on prolonged corticosteroid therapy. In patients with active Crohn's disease parenteral administration of a bisphosphonate may be indicated. C

Celiac disease

Prevalence

Osteoporosis

Prevalence rates of osteoporosis in celiac disease vary depending on the population studied (adults *v* children) and whether the disease has been treated. Lower BMD values have been noted in untreated populations, including those individuals who are asymptomatic at presentation. A number of cross-sectional studies have evaluated the prevalence of osteoporosis in (i) newly diagnosed celiac patients and (ii) individuals treated with a gluten-free diet.[78–85] In general, studies in untreated celiac disease demonstrate diminished bone density. When compared with age-matched controls (Z score of < −2 at the spine), the prevalence of osteopenia in untreated patients varied among studies from 15% to 40%.[80,83] Serum PTH levels have been shown to correlate inversely with BMD[80,86] and levels of 25-hydroxy-vitamin D correlate positively with BMD in untreated celiac disease patients.[86]

Fractures

Vasquez *et al.* estimated the incidence of fractures from a case–control study and found that 25% of patients had a history of previous fractures, compared with 8% of age and sex-matched controls (odds ratio (OR) 3·5, 95% CI 1·8 to 7·2), with the majority of fractures occurring prior to diagnosis or in those individuals who were non-compliant.[85] The most common fracture was a wrist fracture and there was a trend to increased vertebral fractures. Vasquez studied patients from a malabsorption clinic and therefore this rate may not be representative of the general celiac population. BMD or body mass index did not correlate with the presence of fractures, suggesting that there are other factors beside BMD, such as disease duration that account for increased fracture risk.

Vestergaard and Mosekilde in Denmark in a retrospective case–control study examined hospital discharge abstracts for patients previously hospitalized with celiac disease and did not detect a difference in fracture rates compared with controls.[70] Age was the only significant risk factor for fracture. There are potential sources of bias in using hospital-based discharge data including the fact that outpatient fracture diagnoses are not included. Thomason *et al.* in a case–control study did not find an increased fracture risk in Crohn's disease patients compared with controls, and other small longitudinal studies have yielded similar findings.[81,87,88] Further clarification of the risk of fracture in celiac disease with a large prospective study would be helpful.

Pathogenesis

Reduced calcium absorption can result in hypersecretion of PTH, enhanced 1,25-dihydroxy vitamin D and decreased 25-hydroxy-vitamin D.[89] In addition, systemic inflammatory effects may result in bone loss via action of interleukin (IL)-1 and IL-6, the levels of which have been shown to correlate with BMD.[90] It is also thought that zinc deficiency may lead to reduced IGF-1 levels which in turn results in impaired

bone metabolism.[91] It is not clear what proportion of individuals with celiac disease have osteomalacia, due to the lack of bone biopsy data, but many individuals are vitamin D deficient.

Treatment

Longitudinal studies of patients with celiac disease have demonstrated increases in BMD after starting on a gluten-free diet and the majority of the change occurs within the first year, particularly at the lumbar spine.[92] B4 The average increase in lumbar spine BMD is approximately 5% within the initial year. A number of observational studies have shown that children will often normalize their BMD after a gluten-free diet.[92,93] B4 Adults, however, may continue to have BMDs below average (Z score of −1 at the spine).[81,95] Premenopausal females have shown a greater increase in BMD than postmenopausal females.[95]

Valdimarsson *et al.* found that patients with secondary hyperparathyroidism at baseline did not increase their BMD to normal by 3 years in comparison to those who had a normal baseline PTH, and did achieve a normal BMD.[80]

The goal of treatment should be to maintain normal serum vitamin D levels, with vitamin D supplements if necessary. Bone density scans should be recommended in newly diagnosed adult celiac patients after 1 year on a gluten-free diet. Initial evaluation should also include serum calcium, 25-hydroxy-vitamin D and PTH levels. Additional therapies may be considered depending on the severity of bone loss.

Glucocorticoid-induced bone loss

Glucocorticoids are widely used in the treatment of inflammatory bowel disease, and were discussed earlier are a risk factor for bone loss. Cross-sectional studies have demonstrated a relationship between cumulative corticosteroid dose and bone loss, in multiple populations, but some prospective studies have failed to support this relationship, perhaps because of a beneficial effect of corticosteroids on disease activity.[96]

Data from cross-sectional studies of patients on corticosteroids estimate that the incidence of fractures varies from 30% to 50%.[67,97] In a study by Adinoff and Hollister, 11% of asthma patients on oral steroids for 1 year developed vertebral fractures.[98] In a case–control study, Cooper *et al.* (Van Staa *et al.*[99]) found that use of oral steroids resulted in an RR of 1·16 (CI 1·47 to 1·76) for hip fracture and 2·6 (CI 2·31 to 2·92) for vertebral fracture. A nested case–control study from the Study for Osteoporotic Fractures Cohort confirmed an increase incidence of hip fractures in patients on corticosteriods with an adjusted relative risk of hip fracture of 2·1 (95% CI 1·0 to 4·4).[100] There is evidence

Table 14.4 Randomized trials of calcium/vitamin D for prevention and treatment of steroid-induced osteoporosis and fractures[a]

Study	Disease (no. of patients)	Placebo (M:F)	Treatment (M:F)	Intervention (duration)	Control	Lumbar BMD (% change)	Vertebral fractures RR (95% CI)
Sambrook et al. (1993)[109]	PMR/RA (103)	29 (7:22)	34 (7:27)	Calcitriol 0·5–1·0 micrograms (2 years)	Calcium 1000 mg	−1·3	Efficacy: 0·43 (0·04 to 4·47)
Adachi et al. (1996)[110]	PMR/TA (62)	31	31	50 000 U vit D (3 years)	Placebo	−0·7	ITT: 0·56 (0·24 to 1·32)
Dyckman et al. (1984)[111]	Rheumatic disease (23)	10 (1:9)	13 (3:10)	Calcium + 1,25 vit D (18 months)	Placebo + 500 mg calcium		Efficacy: 0·58 (0·17 to 2·01)

[a]Only studies in which vertebral fractures were included as an outcome measure have been listed.
ITT, intention to treat analysis; PMR, polymyalgia rheumatica; RA, rheumatoid arthritis; TA, temporal arteritis; RR, relative risk

that the relationship between bone density and fracture may underestimate the risk of fracture in patients on corticosteroids.[101]

Glucocorticoid-induced bone loss is greatest in the initial 6–12 months of treatment,[102] and involves areas of the skeleton which have the greatest turnover, in particular, the lumbar spine, cortical rim of the vertebral body and Ward's triangle of the femoral neck. Hahn et al. demonstrated that trabecular bone loss is greater than cortical bone loss in rheumatoid arthritis patients on prednisone (preferential loss at the distal metaphysis of the forearm).[103]

Pathogenesis

The mechanism of corticosteroid-induced osteoporosis (CSOP) is multifactorial.[104] CSOP differs from other forms of osteoporosis in that bone formation is greatly decreased at a time of increased bone resorption. This results in an imbalance between formation and resorption – "remodeling imbalance" and a pattern of low bone turnover. Corticosteroids cause a reduction in bone formation by increasing the apoptosis of osteoblasts.[105] Steroids stimulate osteoclastic activity through various growth factors such as IGF, IL-1 and transforming growth factor-β (TGF-β). Steroids may also cause an inhibition of intestinal calcium absorption and an increase in urinary excretion of calcium, which in turn leads to an elevation of PTH.[106] Secondary hyperparathyroidism causes increased osteoclast resorption and an increase in urinary phosphate excretion. Glucocorticoids also suppress the hypothalamic–pituitary–gonadal axis that leads to a functional hypogonadism and increased bone loss.[107] Women who are receiving steroids have adrenal suppression that results in decreased adrenal androgen secretion. Finally, steroids cause loss of muscle mass, and muscle strength is correlated with bone density.

The understanding of the coupling of bone resorption and formation has been enhanced by the discovery of a receptor ligand expressed by osteoblasts – RANKL (osteoprotegerin ligand) which binds to osteoclast precursors, RANK and results in the maturation of osteoclasts and bone resorption. Osteoprotegerin is an osteoblast-derived soluble decoy receptor that blocks the interaction between RANK and RANKL (receptor activator of nuclear factor κB ligand) and inhibits osteoclast formation.[108] Corticosteroids stimulate RANKL expression and inhibit osteoprotegerin production resulting in an increase in osteoclastic activity.

Prevention and treatment

A baseline bone density measurement is recommended for patients who are to remain on steroids for a prolonged period and in patients who are at risk of other types of osteoporosis, such as postmenopausal osteoporosis. The first principle of prevention is to minimize the dose of steroids. C5 Maintenance of muscle mass through exercise is also beneficial. Supplemental calcium 1000–1500 mg/day and vitamin D 800 IU/day should be recommended.

A number of medications have been used for the prevention and treatment of CSOP. Tables 14·4–14·6 summarize the results of those controlled trials of prevention and treatment of CSOP, which had vertebral fractures as an endpoint. These tables show results according to intention to treat analysis. Efficacy results are indicated. Unfortunately, patients with IBD have been underrepresented in these trials. WMD is the weighted mean average of the trials and the weight given to each study is the inverse of the variance. To calculate the WMD, the mean percentage change from baseline in the treatment and control groups was multiplied by the inverse of the associated variance.

Table 14.5 Randomized trials of calcitonin for prevention and treatment of steroid-induced osteoporosis and fractures[a]

Study	Disease (no. of patients)	Placebo (M:F)	Treatment (M:F)	Dose (duration)	Control	Lumbar BMD (% change)	Vertebral fractures RR (95% CI)
Healey *et al.* (1996)[112]	PMR/TA (48)	23 (3:20)	25 (9:16)	100 IU 3/week SC (1 year)	Calcium/vit D	−1·5	Efficacy: 0·74 (0·14 to 3·95)
Kotaniemi *et al.* (1996)[113]	RA/all women (78)	31	32	100 IU intranasal (1 year)	Placebo + calcium	10·9	ITT: 0·32 (0·01 to 7·65)
Luengo *et al.* (1994)[114]	Asthma (44)	22 (3:19)	22 (3:19)	200 IU every 2 days intranasal (1 year)	Placebo + calcium	0·6	ITT: 1·00 (0·15 to 0·48)
Sambrook *et al.* (1993)[109]	RA, PMR (103)	29 (7:22)	29 (6:23)	400 IU intranasal (2 years)	Calcium	1·1	Efficacy: 1·00 (0·15 to 6·63)
Ringe *et al.* (1987)[115]	Lung disease (36)	18 (4:14)	18 (3:15)	100 IU every 2 days SC (6 months)	Placebo + calcium		Efficacy: 0·14 (0·01 to 2·58)

[a]Only studies in which vertebral fractures were included as an outcome measure have been listed.
For abbreviations see in Tables 14.1 and 14.4.

Table 14.6 Randomized trials of bisphosphonates for prevention or treatment of steroid-induced osteoporosis and fractures[a]

Study	Disease (no. of patients)	Placebo (M:F)	Treatment (M:F)	Intervention (duration)	Control	LS BMD (% change)	Vertebral fractures RR (95% CI)
Worth *et al.* (1994)[114]	Asthma (40)	20 (3:11)	20 (9:10)	Etidronate 400 mg (6 months)	Calcium	9·3	0·11 (0·01 to 1·94)
Adachi *et al.* (1997)[117]	PMR/TA (116)	74 (28:46)	67 (26:41)	Etidronate 400 mg (1 year)	Placebo + calcium	3·8	0·58 (0·20 to 1·60) Men: 1·44 (0·35 to 5·81) Women: 0·15 (0·02 to 1·13)
Saag *et al.* (1998)[118]	RA/PMR/ IBD/ asthma (288)	159 (52:107)	318 (89:229)	Alendronate 5 or 10 mg 48 week	Placebo + calcium/ vitamin D	2·5	0·60 (0·19 to 1·94) Men: 1·18 (0·35 to 4·01) Women: 0·51 (0·14 to 1·83)
Boutsen *et al.* (1997)[119]	PMR/TA (15)	17	15	Pamidronate IV (1 year)	Placebo	–	0·38 (0·02 to 8·57)
Roux *et al.* (1998)[120]	PMR/RA	58	59	Etidronate 400 mg (1 year)	Placebo + calcium	3·1	0·79 (0·22 to 2·78)
Reid *et al.* (2000)[121]	(290)	(36:60)	194	Risedronate 2·5; 5·0 mg	Calcium, vitamin D	2·7	0·33 (0·12 to 0·89)
Cohen *et al.* (1999)[122]	(224)	(25:52)	25:50 (2·5)	Risedronate 2·5 mg/5·0 mg	Calcium/ vitamin D	4·4	0·34 (0·13 to 0·93)

[a]Only studies in which vertebral fractures were included as an outcome measure have been listed.
PM, postmenopausal; IV, intravenous; for other abbreviations see Tables 14.1 and 14.4

Recent guidelines have been developed by consensus groups for the primary and secondary prevention of glucocorticoid osteoporosis, based on evidence from recent clinical trials.[101] This group recommends that patients be considered for therapeutic intervention if the BMD T score is below −1·5. Follow up bone densitometry is recommended after 1 year and then every 1–3 years depending on the result.

Calcium and vitamin D

Calcium and vitamin D have been used to prevent losses that occur from decreased calcium absorption, increased renal excretion of calcium and secondary hyperparathyroidism.

Buckley conducted a 2-year RCT with calcium (1000 mg/day) and vitamin D_3 (500 IU/day) in rheumatoid arthritis patients on steroids and found that the loss of BMD in the lumbar spine and trochanter was prevented.[123] B4 Adachi *et al.* evaluated the efficacy of vitamin D (50 000 U per week) and 1000 mg calcium in patients on moderate to high dose corticosteroids and found that vitamin D and calcium prevented the early loss of bone but did not seem to be beneficial in the long term. A Cochrane meta-analysis found that calcium and vitamin D prevented bone loss at the lumbar spine with a pooled weighted mean difference of 2·6% (95% CI 0·76 to 4·53).[124] Ala Another meta-analysis by Amin *et al.* that examined all therapies concluded that vitamin D and calcium is more effective that placebo or calcium alone.[125] Ala Three trials using vitamin D and calcium have assessed vertebral fractures as an outcome (Table 14.4). Neither the individual trials nor a meta-analysis of the three trials demonstrated a statistically significant reduction in vertebral fractures (pooled relative risk 0·56, 95% CI 0·24 to 1·32). Alc However, the number of patients included in these trials was small.

Antiresorptive agents

Since steroids increase bone resorption, antiresorptive agents such as bisphosphonates, calcitonin and hormone replacement have been used for the treatment and prevention of osteoporosis.

There have been six published RCTs of calcitonin (intranasal or subcutaneous) for prevention of osteoporosis in patients on corticosteroids with fracture data. These trials show a positive effect of calcitonin on lumbar spine bone density at 1 year. However, no statistically significant reduction in fractures was demonstrated in the five trials in which this was analyzed (Table 14.5). Meta-analysis of these five trials did not demonstrate a significant reduction in fractures (pooled relative risk was 0·60, 95% CI 0·24 to 1·46).[126] Alc

HRT was compared to calcium supplementation in a 2-year RCT in 200 patients with rheumatoid arthritis, of whom 41 were receiving corticosteroids.[127] BMD in the spine fell by 1·19% (95% CI 2·29 to 0·09) in the control group, but increased in HRT-treated patients (2·22%, 95% CI 0·72 to 3·72; $P < 0.001$). Ala Subgroup analysis of the steroid treated group also showed benefit of HRT treatment on spine BMD (3·75%, 95% CI 0·72 to 6·78). There are no published data on fracture reduction with HRT in CSOP. Similarly, there is little evidence to support the use of testosterone in men on corticosteroids. A small RCT of 15 men with asthma on oral glucocorticoids demonstrated that monthly testosterone injections were effective in preventing bone loss.[128] Ald

We were unable to locate any trials of selective estrogen receptor modulators such as raloxifene in the setting of corticosteroid-induced osteoporosis.

Bisphosphonates have been used for the treatment and prevention of CSOP (Table 14.6). A Cochrane meta-analysis of 13 trials ($n = 842$) published in 2000 found that the weighted mean difference of percent change in lumbar spine BMD between bisphosphonates and placebo groups was 4·3% (95% CI 2·7–5·9) at one year, using a random effects model.[129] There was significant heterogeneity between trials. In the Cochrane review, the pooled RR from four studies that reported outcomes on vertebral fractures was 0·76 (95% CI 0·4–1·5) a result that was not statistically significant.

Since the Cochrane review was published there have been additional randomized trials with vertebral fractures as an endpoint and the results of these are summarized in Table 14.6[118,121,122,130] The baseline characteristics (BMD, prevalent fractures) were different among these trials. The relative risk reduction for vertebral fractures in these trials ranged from 40% to 70%, although the upper limit of the 95% CI overlaps 1·0. Ala The individual trials did not reveal statistically significant effects of bisphosphonates. However, if all seven prevention and treatment trials with bisphosphonates are pooled, the RR of vertebral fractures is 0·50 (95% CI 0·30–0·80), consistent with an absolute risk reduction of 6·3%. A one year extension study of the original alendronate trial demonstrated a significant reduction in morphometric vertebral fractures (ARR of 6·1%).[130]

Amin *et al.* conducted a meta regression of all therapies for CSOP, using lumber spine as the outcome and found that bisphosphonates were more effective than calcitonin, vitamin D or fluoride,[131] with an effect size of 1·03, 95%, CI 0·85–1·17). The authors also found that the efficacy of bisphosphonates was enhanced with the concomitant use of vitamin D.

Bone formation (anabolic) agents

Monosodium fluoride has been shown to increase BMD at the lumbar spine.[132,133] Ald However, efficacy of fluoride for vertebral fracture reduction has not been demonstrated for CSOP.[132,133] Other agents that hold promise for the future include injections of human PTH 1-34 (hPTH 1-34) fragment. Lane *et al.* compared daily injections of hPTH 1-34 along with estrogens with estrogen therapy alone in 51 osteoporotic postmenopausal women receiving glucocorticoids for rheumatic diseases. These women had been taking HRT for more than 1 year and were randomized to receive either HRT and parathyroid hormone PTH 25 micrograms daily or HRT alone. All subjects received calcium and vitamin D. None of the patients had liver disease or IBD. The mean steroid dose was 8·0+3·8 for PTH with estrogen group and 9·5+4·5 for the estrogen alone group. At 12 months the mean difference in the lumbar spine was 9·8% favoring PTH and estrogen over estrogen alone. Ald There were no significant differences seen between treatment and control at the distal radius, femoral neck, trochanter and hip.[135]

A second publication presented 24-month follow up after patients had discontinued medication at 12 months. The lumbar spine BMD was maintained at 24 months with a mean difference of 11·9%. The study was not powered to assess a difference in fractures.[136]

Other anabolic agents such as strontium ranelate have proved antifracture efficacy in postmenopausal osteoporosis and may be useful for CSOP.

Conclusion

Metabolic bone disease is an important problem in patients with liver disease and inflammatory bowel disease and the pathogenesis is multifactorial. Osteomalacia does not appear to be common in IBD and osteoporosis appears to be the major metabolic bone disorder in IBD, Crohn's disease and chronic liver disease. The use of corticosteroids in IBD and chronic liver disease is an important, but not precisely defined contributing factor since it is difficult to distinguish corticosteroid use from disease activity. Few controlled trials have evaluated the efficacy of treatments in the absence of steroid therapy and the inflammatory cytokines that are involved in the immune response have been linked to increased bone resorption. In patients on corticosteroids, however, there is information from a number of RCTs about the efficacy of therapeutic agents in other patient populations.

Patients at particular risk for osteoporosis and fracture include: patients on glucocorticoids for IBD, those with endstage liver disease and liver transplant patients, postmenopausal women who may already be osteopenic, patients with Crohn's disease and patients with low trauma fractures. In these individuals bone density measurement early in their treatment is recommended, although bone density does not exactly correlate with fracture risk in these populations. Minimization of steroid use and use of preventive agents such as calcium and vitamin D are indicated. In those individuals who are on corticosteroids (> 3 months) or have osteoporosis (T score below −2·5) or a fragility fracture, then bisphosphonates should be recommended.

While the evidence for prevention and treatment of steroid-induced osteoporosis is convincing, additional trials of interventions specifically for the bone disease associated with IBD and liver disease are needed. RCTs with fracture as the primary outcome may be difficult to conduct given the sample sizes required. Clarification of the risk of the fracture in patients with liver disease, IBD, and celiac disease is required, with identification of high risk subgroups. Evidence-based guidelines of strategies to prevent osteoporosis in these populations are needed[137,138] in addition to the development of better tools to predict the risk of fracture in individuals with IBD and celiac disease.

References

1 Assessment of fracture risk and its application to screening for postmenopausal osteoporosis. *World Health Organization Report No 843,* 1994.

2 Center JR, Nguyen TV, Schneider D, Sambrook PN, Eisman JA. Mortality after all major types of osteoporotic fracture in men and women: an observational study. *Lancet* 1999;**353**:878–82.

3 Eastell R, Boyle IT. Management of male osteoporosis: report of the UK Consensus Group. *QJM* 1998;**91**:71–92.

4 Melton LJ, Atkinson EJ, O'Fallon WM *et al.* Long term fracture prediction by bone mineral assessed at different skeletal sites. *J Bone Miner Res* 1993;**8**:1227–33.

5 Hui SL, Slemenda CW, Johnston CC. Age and bone mass as predictors of fractures in a prospective study. *J Bone Miner Res* 1988;**81**:1804–9.

6 Marshall D, Johnell O, Wedel H. Meta-analysis of how well measures of bone mineral density predict occurence of osteoporotic fractures. *BMJ* 1996;**312**:1254–9.

7 Lunt M, Felsenberg D, Adams J *et al.* Population based geographic variations in DXA bone density in Europe: the EVOS study. *Osteoporos Int* 1997;**7**:175–89.

8 Nguyen T, Ambrook P, Elly P *et al.* Prediction of osteoporotic fractures by postural instability and bone density. *BMJ* 1993;**307**:1111–15.

9 Compston JE. Hepatic osteodystrophy: vitamin D metabolism in patients with liver disease [Review]. *Gut* 1986;**27**:1073–90.

10 Eastell R, Dickson ER, Hodgson SF *et al.* Rates of vertebral bone loss before and after liver transplantation in women with primary biliary cirrhosis. *Hepatology* 1991;**14**:296–300.

11 Hay JE, Lindor KD, Wiesner RH, Dickson ER, Krom RAF, LaRusso NF. The metabolic bone disease of primary sclerosing cholangitis. *Hepatology* 1991;**14**:257–61.

12 Mobarhan SA, Russell RM, Recker RR, Posner DB, Iber FL, Miller P. Metabolic bone disease in alcoholic cirrhosis: a comparison of the effect of vitamin D2, 25-hydroxyvitamin D, or supportive treatment. *Hepatology* 1984;**4**:266–73.

13 Chappard D, Plantard B, Fraisse H, Palle S, Alexandre C, Riffat G. Bone changes in alcoholic liver cirrhosis, a histomorphometrical analysis of 52 cases. *Pathol Res Pract* 1989;**184**:480–5.

14 Stellon AJ, Webb A, Compston JE. Bone histomorphometry and structure in corticosteroid treated chronic active hepatitis. *Gut* 1988;**29**:378–84.

15 Chen CC, Wang SS, Jeng FS, Lee SD. Metabolic bone disease of liver cirrhosis: is it parallel to the clinical severity of cirrhosis? *J.Gastroenterol Hepatol* 1996;**11**:417–21.

16 Gallego-rojo FJ. Bone mineral density, serum insulin-like growth factor I and bone turnover markers in viral cirrhosis. *Hepatology* 1998;**28**:695–9.

17 Porayko MK, Wiesner RH, Hay JE *et al.* Bone disease in liver transplant recipients: incidence, timing, and risk factors. *Transplant Proc* 1991;**23**:1462–5.

18 Park KM, Hay JE, Lee SG *et al.* Bone loss after orthotopic liver transplantation: FK 506 versus cyclosporine. *Transplant Proc* 1996;**28**:1738–40.

19 Diamond T, Stiel D, Lunzer M, Wilkinson M, Roche J, Posen S. Osteoporosis and skeletal fractures in chronic liver disease. *Gut* 1990;**31**:82–7.

20 Diamond TH, Stiel D, Lunzer M, McDowall D, Eckstein RP, Posen S. Hepatic osteodystrophy. Static and dynamic bone histomorphometry and serum bone Gla-protein in 80 patients with chronic liver disease. *Gastroenterology* 1989;**96**:213–21.

21 Krawitt EL, Grundman MJ, Mawer EB. Absorption, hydroxylation, and excretion of vitamin D3 in primary biliary cirrhosis. *Lancet* 1977;**2**(8051):1246–9.

22 Davies M, Mawer EB, Klass HJ *et al.* Vitamin D deficiency, osteomalacia, and primary biliary cirrhosis. Response to orally administered vitamin D3. *Dig Dis Sci* 1983;**28**:145–53.

23 Wagonfeld JB, Nemchausky BA, Bolt M *et al.* Comparison of vitamin D and 25-hydroxy-vitamin D in the therapy of primary biliary cirrhosis. *Lancet* 1976;**ii**:391–4.

24 Dibble JB, Sheridan P, Hampshire R, Hardy GJ, Losowsky MS. Osteomalacia, vitamin D deficiency and cholestasis in chronic liver disease. *QJM* 1982;**51**:89–103.

25 Cuthbert JA, Pak CY, Zerwekh JE, Glass KD, Combes B. Bone disease in primary biliary cirrhosis: increased bone resorption and turnover in the absence of osteoporosis or osteomalacia. *Hepatology* 1984;**4**:1–8.

26 Jung RT, Davie M, Siklos P, Chalmers TM, Hunter JO, Lawson DE. Vitamin D metabolism in acute and chronic cholestasis. *Gut* 1979;**20**:840–47.

27 Hodgson SF, Dickson ER, Wahner HW, Johnson KA, Mann KG, Riggs BL. Bone loss and reduced osteoblast function in primary biliary cirrhosis. *Ann Intern Med* 1985;**103**:855–60.

28 Maddrey WC. Bone disease in primary biliary cirrhosis. *Prog Liv Dis* 1990;**9**:537–54.

29 Stellon AJ, Webb A, Compston J *et al.* Low bone turnover state in primary biliary cirrhosis. *Hepatology* 1987;**7**:137–42.

30 Herlong HF, Recker RR, Maddrey WC. Bone disease in primary biliary cirrhosis: histologic features and response to 25-hydroxyvitamin D. *Gastroenterology* 1982;**83**:103–8.

31 Peris P, Pares A, Guanabens N *et al.* Bone mass improves in alcoholics after 2 years of abstinence. *J Bone Miner Res* 1994;**9**:1607–12.

32 Mitchison HC, Bassedine MF, Malcolm AJ *et al.* A pilot, double-blind, controlled 1-year trial of prednisolone treatment in primary biliary cirrhosis: increased bone resorption and turnover in the absence of osteoporosis or osteomalacia. *Hepatology* 1989;**10**:420–9.

33 Compston JE, Horton LW, Thompson RP. Treatment of osteomalacia associated with primary biliary cirrhosis with parenteral vitamin D2 or oral 25-hydroxyvitamin D3. *Gut* 1979;**20**:133–6.

34 Reed JS, Meredith SC, Nemchausky BA *et al.* Bone disease in primary biliary cirrhosis: reversal of osteomalacia with oral 25-hydroxyvitamin D. *Gastenterology* 1980;**78**:512.

35 Matloff DS, Kaplan MM, Neer RM *et al.* Osteoporosis in primary biliary cirrhosis: effects of 25-hydroxyvitamin D3 treatment. *Gastroenterology* 1982;**83**:97–102.

36 Floreani A, Zappala F, Fries W *et al.* A 3-year pilot study with 1,25-dihydroxyvitamin D, calcium, and calcitonin for severe osteodystrophy in primary biliary cirrhosis. *J Clin Gastroenterol* 1997;**24**:239–44.

37 Neuhaus R, Lohmann R, Platz KP *et al.* Treatment of osteoporosis after liver transplantation. *Transplan Proc* 1995;**27**:1226.

38 Riemens SC, Oostdijk A, van DJ *et al.* Bone loss after liver transplantation is not prevented by cyclical etidronate, calcium and alphacalcidol. The liver transplant group. *Osteoporos Int* 1996;**6**:213–18.

39 Crippin JS, Jorgensen RA, Dickson ER, Lindor KD. Hepatic osteodystrophy in primary biliary cirrhosis: effects of medical treatment. *Am J Gastroenterol* 1994;**89**:47–50.

40 Guanabens N, Pares A, Ros I, Alvarez L, Pons F, Caballeria L *et al.* Alendronate is more effective than etidronate for increasing bone mass in osteopenic patients with primary biliary cirrhosis. *Am J Gastroenterol* 2003;**98**:2268–74.

41 Shiomi S, Nishiguchi S, Kurooka H *et al.* Cyclical etidronate for treatment of osteopenia in patients with cirrhosis of the liver. *Hepatol Res* 2002;**22**:102–6.

42 Lindor KD, Jorgensen RA, Tiegs RD, Khosla S, Dickson ER. Etidronate for osteoporosis in primary biliary cirrhosis: a randomized trial. *J Hepatol* 2000;**33**:878–82.

43 Shiomi S, Masaki K, Habu D, Takeda T, Nishiguchi S, Kuroki T. Calcitriol for bone disease in patients with cirrhosis of the liver. *J Gastroenterol Hepatol* 1999;**14**:547–52.

44 Guanabens N, Pares A, Monegal A *et al.* Etidronate versus fluoride for treatment of osteopenia in primary biliary cirrhosis: preliminary results after 2 years. *Gastroenterology* 1997;**113**:219–24.

45 Camisasca M, Crosignani A, Battezzati PM *et al.* Parenteral calcitonin for metabolic bone disease associated with primary biliary cirrhosis. *Hepatology* 1994;**20**:633–7.

46 Wolfhagen FHJ, van Buuren HR, den Ouden JW, Hop WCJ, van Leeuwen JPTM. Cyclical etidronate in the prevention of bone loss in corticosteroid treated primary biliary cirrhosis. *J Hepatol* 1997;**26**:325–30.

47 Guanabens N, Pares A, Del R *et al.* Sodium fluoride prevents bone loss in primary cirrhosis. *J Hepatol* 1992;**15**:345–9.

48 Lindor KD, Janes CH, Crippin JS *et al.* Bone disease in primary biliary cirrhosis: does ursodeoxycholic acid make a difference? *Hepatology* 1995;**21**:389–92.

49 Stellon A, Davies A, Webb A *et al.* Microcrystalline hydroxyapatite compound in prevention of bone loss in corticosteroid-treated patients with chronic active hepatitis. *Postgrad Med J* 1985;**61**:791–6.

50 Epstein O, Kato Y, Dick R *et al*. Vitamin D, hydroxyapatite, and calcium gluconate in treatment of cortical bone thinning in postmenopausal women with primary biliary cirrhosis. *Am J Clin Nutr* 1982;**36**:426–30.

51 Abitbol V, Roux C, Chaussade S *et al*. Metabolic bone assessment in patients with inflammatory bowel disease. *Gastroenterology* 1995;**108**:417–22.

52 Motley RJ, Clements D, Evans WD *et al*. A four-year longitudinal study of bone loss in patients with inflammatory bowel disease. *Bone Miner* 1993;**23**:95–104.

53 Motley RJ, Crawley EO, Evans C, Rhodes J, Compston JE. Increased rate of spinal trabecular bone loss in patients with inflammatory bowel disease. *Gut* 1988;**29**:1332–6.

54 Ryde SJ, Clements D, Evans WD *et al*. Total body calcium in patients with inflammatory bowel disease: a longitudinal study. *Clin Sci (Lond)* 1991;**80**:319–24.

55 Dinca M, Fries W, Luisetto G *et al*. Evolution of osteopenia in inflammatory bowel disease. *Am J Gastroenterol* 2003;**94**:1292–7.

56 Schulte C, Dignass AU, Mann K, Goebell H. Bone loss in patients with inflammatory bowel disease is less than expected: a follow-up study. *Scand J Gastroenterol* 1999;**34**:696–702.

57 Roux C, Abitbol V, Chaussade S *et al*. Bone loss in patients with inflammatory bowel disease: a prospective study. *Osteoporos Int* 1995;**5**:156–60.

58 Bernstein CN, Leslie WD. The pathophysiology of bone disease in gastrointestinal disease. *Eur J Gastroentrol Hepatol* 2003;**15**:857–64.

59 Andreassen H, Rungby J, Dahlerup JF, Mosekilde L. Inflammatory bowel disease and osteoporosis. *Scand J Gastroenterol* 1997;**32**:1247–55.

60 Hessov I, Mosekilde L, Melsen F *et al*. Osteopenia with normal vitamin D metabolites after small-bowel resection for Crohn's disease. *Scand J Gastroenterol* 1984;**19**:691–6.

61 Croucher PI, Vedi S, Motley RJ, Garrahan NJ, Stanton MR, Compston JE. Reduced bone formation in patients with osteoporosis associated with inflammatory bowel disease. *Osteoporos Int* 1993;**3**:236–41.

62 Ghosh S, Cowen S, Hannan WJ, Ferguson A. Low bone mineral density in Crohn's disease, but not in ulcerative colitis, at diagnosis. *Gastroenterology* 1994;**107**:1031–9.

63 Jahnsen J, Falch JA, Aadland E *et al*. Bone mineral density is reduced in patients with Crohn's disease but not in patients with ulcerative colitis: a population based study. *Gut* 1997;**40**:313–19.

64 Bernstein CN, Seeger LL, Sayre JW, Anton PA, Artinian L, Shanahan F. Decreased bone density in inflammatory bowel disease is related to corticosteroid use and not disease diagnosis. *J Bone Miner Res* 1995;**10**:250–6.

65 Ardizzone S, Bollani S, Bettica P, Bevilacqua M, Molteni P, Bianchi PG. Altered bone metabolism in inflammatory bowel disease: there is a difference between Crohn's disease and ulcerative colitis. *J Intern Med* 2000;**247**:63–70.

66 Clements D, Motley RJ, Evans WD *et al*. Longitudinal study of cortical bone loss in patients with inflammatory bowel disease. *Scand J Gastroenterol* 1992;**27**:1055–60.

67 Klaus J, Armbrecht G, Steinkamp M *et al*. High prevalence of osteoporotic vertebral fractures in patients with Crohn's disease. *Gut* 2002;**51**:654–58.

68 Bernstein CN, Blanchard JF, Leslie W, Wajda A, Yu N. The incidence of fracture among patients with inflammatory bowel disease. *Ann Intern Med* 2000;**133**:795–9.

69 Loftus EV, Crowson CS, Sandborn WJ *et al*. Long-term fracture risk in patients with Crohn's disease: a population-based study in Olmssted county, Minnesota. *Gastroenterology* 2002;**123**:468–75.

70 Vestergaard P, Mosekilde L. Fracture risk in patients with Celiac disease, Crohn's disease and ulcerative colitis: a nationwide follow-up study of 16 416 in Denmark. *Am J Epidemiol* 2002;**156**:1–10.

71 Van Staa TP, Cooper C, Samuels Brusse L *et al*. Inflammatory bowel disease and the risk of fracture. *Gastroenterology* 2003;**125**:1591–7.

72 Clements D, Compston JE, Evans WD, Rhodes J. Hormone replacement therapy prevents bone loss in patients with inflammatory bowel disease. *Gut* 1993;**34**:1543–6.

73 Vogelsang H, Ferenci P, Resch H *et al*. Prevention of bone mineral loss in patients with Crohn's disease by long-term oral vitamin D supplementation. *Eur J Gastroenterol Hepatol* 1995;**7**:609–14.

74 Bernstein CN, Seeger LL, Anton PA *et al*. A randomized, placebo-controlled trial of calcium supplementation for decreased bone density in corticosteroid-using patients with inflammatory bowel disease: a pilot study. *Aliment Pharmacol Ther* 1996;**10**:777–86.

75 Robinson RJ, Iqbal SJ, Wolfe R, Patel K, Abrams K, Mayberry JF. The effect of rectally administered steroids on bone turnover: a comparative study. *Aliment Pharmacol Ther* 1998;**12**:213–17.

76 Haderslev KL, Tjellesen L, Sorensen HA, Staun M. Alendronate increases lumbar spine bone mineral density in patients with Crohn's disease. *Gastroenterology* 2000;**119**:639–46.

77 von Tirpitz C, Klaus J, Bruckel J *et al*. Increase of bone mineral density with sodium fluoride in patients with Crohn's disease. *Eur J Gastroenterol Hepatol* 2000;**12**:19–24.

78 DiStefano M, Jorizzo RA, Veneto G *et al*. Bone mass and metabolism in dermatitis herpetiformis. *Dig Dis Sci* 1999;**44**:2139–43.

79 Valdimarsson T, Lofman O, Toss G, Strom M. Reversal of osteopenia with diet in adult coeliac disease. *Gut* 1996;**38**:322–7.

80 Valdimarsson T, Toss G, Lofman O, Strom M. Three years' follow-up of bone density in adult coeliac disease: significance of secondary hyperparathyroidism. *Scand J Gastroenterol* 2000;**35**:274–80.

81 Bai JC, Gonzalez D, Mautalen C *et al*. Long-term effect of gluten restriction on bone mineral density of patients with coeliac disease. *Aliment Pharmacol Ther* 1997;**11**:157–64.

82 Meyer D, Stavropolous S, Diamond B, Shane E, Green PH. Osteoporosis in a North American adult population with celiac disease. *Am J Gastroenterol* 2001;**96**:112–19.

83 McFarlane XA, Bhalla AD, Robertson DA. Effect of a gluten-free diet on osteopenia in adults with newly diagnosed celiac disease. *Gut* 1996;**39**:180–4.

84 Kemppainen T, Kroger H, Janatuinen E *et al.* Osteoporosis in adult patients with celiac disease. *Bone* 1999;**24**: 249–55.

85 Vasquez H, Mazure R, Gonzalez D *et al.* Risk of fractures in celiac disease patients: a cross-sectional, case–control study. *Am J Gastroenterol* 2000;**95**:183–9.

86 Kemppainen T, Kroger H, Janatuinen E *et al.* Osteoporosis in adult patients with celiac disease. *Bone* 1999;**24**:249–55.

87 Thomason K, West J, Logan RFA, Coupland C, Holmes GKT. Fracture experience of patients with celiac disease: a population based survey. *Gut* 2003;**52**:518–22.

88 Valdimarsson T, Toss G, Lofman O, Strom M. Bone mineral density in coeliac disease. *Scand J Gastroenterol* 1994;**29**: 457–61.

89 Selby PL, Davies M, Adams JE, Mawer EB. Bone loss in celiac disease is related to secondary hyperparathyroidism. *J Bone Miner Res* 1999;**14**:652–7.

90 Fornari MC, Pedreira S, Niveloni S *et al.* Pre- and post-treatment serum levels of cytokines IL-1 beta, IL-6 and Il-1 receptor anatagonist in celiac disease: are they related to the associated osteopenia? *Am J Gastroenterol* 1998;**93**: 413–18.

91 Jameson S. Coeliac disease, insulin-like growth factor, bone mineral density and zinc. *Scand J Gastroenterol* 2000;**35**: 894–96.

92 Kemppainen T, Kroger H, Janatuinen E *et al.* Bone recovery after a gluten-free diet: A 5-year follow-up study. *Bone* 1999;**25**:355–60.

93 Mora S, Barera G, Ricotti A, Weber G, Bianchi C, Chiumello G. Reversal of low bone density with a gluten-free diet in children and adolescents with celiac disease. *Am J Clin Nutr* 1998;**67**:477–81.

94 Mora S, Weber G, Barera G *et al.* Effect of gluten-free diet on bone mineral content in growing patients with celiac disease. *Am J Clin Nutr* 1993;**57**:224–8.

95 Ciaccia C, Maurelli L, Klain M, Savino G, Salvatore M, Mazzaacca G CM. Effect of dietary treatment on bone mineral density in adults with celiac disease: factors predicting response. *Am J Gastroenterol* 1997;**92**: 992–6.

96 Lane NE. An update on glucocorticoid-induced osteoporosis. *Rheum Dis Clin North Am* 2001;**27**:235–53.

97 Lukert BP, Raisz LG. Glucocorticoid-induced osteoporosis: pathogenesis and management. *Ann Intern Med* 1990; **112**:352–64.

98 Adinoff AD, Hollister JR. Steroid-induced fractures and bone loss in patients with asthma. *N Engl J Med* 1983; **309**:265–8.

99 Van Staa TP, Leufkens HGM, Abenhaim L, Zhang B, Cooper C. Use of oral corticosteroids and risk of fractures. *J Bone Miner Res* 2000;**15**:993–1000.

100 Baltzan MA, Suissa S, Bauer DC, Cummings SR. Hip fractures attributable to corticosteroid use. *Lancet* 1999; **353**:1327.

101 Eastell R, Reid DM, Compston J *et al.* A UK Consensus Group on management of glucocorticoid-induced osteoporosis: an update. *J Intern Med* 1998;**244**:271–92.

102 Hahn BH, Mazzaferri EL. Glucocorticoid-induced osteoporosis. *Hosp Pract (Off Ed)* 1995;**30**:45–3.

103 Hahn TJ, Boisveau VC, Avioli LV. Effect of chronic corticosteroid administration on diaphyseal and metaphyseal bone mass. *J Clin Endocrinol Metab* 1974; **39**:274–82.

104 Manolagas SC, Weinstein RS, Jilka RL, Parfitt AM. Parathyroid hormone and corticosteroid-induced osteoporosis. *Lancet* 1998;**352**:1940.

105 Manolagas SC, Weinstein RS. New developments in the pathogenesis and treatment of steroid-induced osteoporosis. *J Bone Miner Res* 1999;**14**:1061–6.

106 Suzuki Y, Ichikawa Y, Saito E *et al.* Importance of increased urinary calcium excretion in the development of secondary hyperparathyroidism of patients under glucocorticoid therapy. *Metabolism* 1983;**32**:151–6.

107 Sambrook PN. Corticosteroid induced osteoporosis. *J Rheumatol* 1996;**45**:19–22.

108 Aubin JE, Bonnelye E. Osteoprotegerin and its ligand: a new paradigm for regulation of osteoclastogenesis and bone resorption. *Osteoporos Int* 2000;**11**:905–13.

109 Sambrook P, Birmingham J, Kelly P *et al.* Prevention of corticosteroid osteoporosis. A comparison of calcium, calcitriol, and calcitonin. *N Engl J Med* 1993;**328**:1747–52.

110 Adachi JD, Bensen WG, Bianchi F *et al.* Vitamin D and calcium in the prevention of corticosteroid induced osteoporosis: a 3 year follow-up. *J Rheumatol* 1996;**23**: 995–1000.

111 Dykman TR, Haralson KM, Gluck OS *et al.* Effect of oral 1,25 dihydroxyvitamin D and calcium on glucocorticoid-induced osteopenia in patients with rheumatic diseases. *Arthritis Rheum* 1984;**27**:1336–43.

112 Healey JH, Paget SA, Williams-Russo P *et al.* A randomized controlled trial of salmon calcitonin to prevent bone loss in corticosteroid-treated temporal arteritis and polymyalgia rheumatica. *Calcif Tissue Int* 1996;**58**:73–80.

113 Kotaniemi A, Piirainen H, Paimela L *et al.* Is continuous intranasal salmon calcitonin effective in treating axial bone loss in patients with active rheumatoid arthritis receiving low dose glucocorticoid therapy? *J Rheumatol* 1996; **23**:1875–9.

114 Luengo M, Pons F, Martinez de Osaba MJ, Picado C. Prevention of further bone mass loss by nasal calcitonin in patients on long term glucocorticoid therapy for asthma: a two year follow up study. *Thorax* 1994;**49**:1099–102.

115 Ringe JD, Welzel D. Salmon calcitonin in the therapy of corticosteroid-induced osteoporosis. *Eur J Clin Pharmacol* 1987;**33**:35–9.

116 Worth H, Stammen D, Keck E. Therapy of steroid induced bone loss in adult asthmatics with calcium, vitamin D and a diphosphonate. *Am J Respir Crit Care Med* 1994;**150**: 394–7.

117 Adachi JD, Bensen WG, Brown J *et al.* Intermittent etidronate therapy to prevent corticosteroid-induced osteoporosis. *N Engl J Med* 1997;**337**:382–7.

118 Saag KG, Emkey R, Schnitzer TJ *et al.* Alendronate for the prevention and treatment of glucocorticoid-induced osteoporosis. Glucocorticoid-Induced Osteoporosis Intervention Study Group. *N Engl J Med* 1998;**339**:292–9.

119 Boutsen Y, Jamart J, Esselinckx W, Stoffel M, Devogelaer JP. Primary prevention of glucocorticoid-induced osteoporosis with intermittent intravenous pamidronate: a randomized trial. *Calcif Tissue Int* 1997;**61**:266–71.

120 Roux C, Oriente P, Laan R *et al.* Randomized trial of effect of cyclical etidronate in the prevention of corticosteroid-induced bone loss. Ciblos Study Group. *J Clin Endocrinol Metab* 1998;**83**:1128–33.

121 Reid DM, Hughes RA, Laan RFJM *et al.* Efficacy and safety of daily risedronate in the treatment of corticosteroid-induced osteoporosis in men and women: a randomized trial. *J Bone Miner Res* 2000;**15**:1006–13.

122 Cohen S, Levy RM, Keller M *et al.* Risedronate therapy prevents corticosteroid-induced bone loss. *Arthritis Rheum* 1999;**42**:2309–18.

123 Buckley LM. Calcium and Vitamin D3 supplementation prevents bone loss in the spine secondary to low-dose corticosteroids in patients with rheumatoid arthritis. *Ann Intern Med* 1996;961–8.

124 Homik J, Suarez-Almazor ME, Shea B, Cranney A, Wells G, Tugwell P. Calcium and vitamin D for corticosteroid-induced osteoporosis. *Cochrane Database Syst Rev* 2000; CD000952.

125 Amin S, LaValley MP, Simms RW, Felson DT. The role of vitamin D in corticosteroid-induced osteoporosis: a meta-analytic approach. *Arthritis Rheum* 1999;**42**: 1740–51.

126 Cranney A, Welch V, Adachi JD *et al.* Calcitonin for the treatment and prevention of corticosteroid-induced osteoporosis. *Cochrane Database Syst Rev* 2000; CD001983.

127 Hall GM, Daniels M, Doyle D, Spector TD. Effect of hormone replacement therapy on bone mass in rheumatoid arthritis patients treated with and without steroids. *Arthritis Rheum* 1994;**37**:1499–505.

128 Reid IR, Wattie DJ, Evans MC, Stapleton JP. Testosterone therapy in glucocorticoid-treated men. *Arch Intern Med* 1996;**156**:1173–7.

129 Homik J, Cranney A, Shea B *et al.* Bisphosphonates for steroid induced osteoporosis. *Cochrane Database Syst Rev* 2000;CD001347.

130 Adachi JD, Saag KG, Delmas P *et al.* Two-year effects of alendronate on bone mineral density and vertebral fracture in patients receiving glucocorticoids: a randomized, double-blind placebo-controlled extension trial. *Arthritis Rheum* 2001;**44**:202–11.

131 Amin S, Lavalley MP, Simms RW *et al.* The comparative efficacy of drug therapies used for the management of corticosteroid-induced osteoporosis: a meta-regression. *J Bone Miner Res* 2002;**17**:1512–26.

132 Lems WF, Jacobs WG, Bijlsma JW *et al.* Effect of sodium fluoride on the prevention of corticosteroid-induced osteoporosis. *Osteoporos Int* 1997;**7**:575–82.

133 Lippuner K, Hallerr B, Casez JP *et al.* Effect of disodium monofluorophosphate, calcium and vitamin D supplementation on bone mineral density in patients chronically treated with glucocorticoids: a prospective, randomized, double-blind study. *Miner Electrolyte Metabol* 1996;**22**: 207–13.

134 Guaydier-Souquieres G, Kotzki P, Sabatier J *et al.* In corticosteroid-treated respiratory diseases, monoflurophosphate increases lumbar bone density: a double-masked randomized study. *Osteoporos Int* 1996;**6**:171–7.

135 Lane NE, Sanchez S, Modin GW, Genant HK, Pierini E, Arnaud CD. Parathyroid hormone treatment can reverse corticosteroid-induced osteoporosis. Results of a randomized controlled clinical trial. *J Clin Invest* 1998;**102**:1627–33.

136 Lane NE, Sanchez S, Modin G, Genant HK, Pierini E, Arnaud CD. Bone mass continues to increase at the hip after parathyroid hormone treatment is discontinued in glucocorticoid-induced osteoporosis: results of a randomized controlled clinical trial. *J Bone Miner Res* 2000;**14**:944–51.

137 Brown JP, Josse RG, for the Scientific Advisory Council of the Osteoporosis Society of Canada. 2002 clinical practice guidelines for the diagnosis and management of osteoporosis in Canada. *Can Med Assoc J* 2002;**167**:S1–S34.

138 Bernstein CN, Leslie WD, LeBoff MS. AGA technical review on osteoporosis in gastrointestinal diseases. *Gastroenterology* 2003;**124**:795–841.

15 Colorectal cancer in ulcerative colitis: surveillance

Bret A Lashner, Alastair JM Watson

Epidemiological investigation

Many questions are posed by patients, clinicians and investigators regarding the recommended methods of cancer surveillance in ulcerative colitis. In the absence of scientific rigor conferred by randomized clinical trials, answers to these questions only can be inferred from observational studies. The evidence from cohort studies, case–control studies, and studies of diagnostic testing coupled with surveillance theory and perceived patient preferences can be used to answer some of the more pressing questions and provide recommendations.

Cohort studies are epidemiological investigations that address specific "natural history" questions.[1] Groups of ulcerative colitis patients and controls are followed from the inception of disease until the development of specific outcomes, such as dysplasia or cancer, and incidence rates are compared between groups. Cohort studies are particularly useful for quantifying cancer risk as well as for identifying risk factors for disease outcome.[2–12] For example, recent cohort studies mostly have found primary sclerosing cholangitis to be a risk factor for dysplasia or colorectal cancer in patients with ulcerative colitis (Table 15.1).[13–20] However, incorrect conclusions related to prognosis can be made if cohort studies are carried out without careful attention to issues of bias and confounding variables. Standards have been published delineating the scientific requirements for the performance of valid cohort studies on cancer risk in ulcerative colitis. These include assembly of an inception cohort, blind assessment of objective outcomes, complete follow up, and a description of the referral pattern.[21]

Case–control studies also can be used to examine etiological associations.[1] Patients with ulcerative colitis with cancer or dysplasia are compared with controls without neoplasia to test for differences in the odds of exposure to possible causative agents. Case–control studies are highly susceptible to bias and confounding variables. For a putative etiological factor to be considered valid it must be strong, consistent from study to study, occur before the effect, be biologically plausible, and exhibit a dose–response relationship to the event of interest. As an example, case–control studies are best for identifying agents such as folic acid that may prevent the development of cancer or dysplasia.[22–24]

Two case–control studies have shown that colonoscopic surveillance may be effective by identifying patients at high risk of developing cancer for colectomy. Karlen and colleagues from Stockholm compared 40 ulcerative colitis patients who died from colorectal cancer with 102 ulcerative colitis controls.[25] Patients who had undergone a surveillance colonoscopy had a 71% decrease in risk of cancer mortality (odds ratio (OR) 0·29, 95% CI 0·06 to 1·31). B3 Having two or more examinations had an even greater beneficial effect (OR 0·22, 95% CI 0·03 to 1·74). Similarly, Eaden *et al.* compared 102 patients with ulcerative colitis and colorectal cancer with an equal number of ulcerative colitis controls matched for age, sex, and extent and duration of disease.[26] Surveillance colonoscopy was associated with a decreased risk of developing colorectal cancer (one to two examinations OR 0·22, 95% CI 0·09 to 1·10; more than two examinations OR 0·42, 95% CI 0·16 to 1·10). B3

Studies of diagnostic testing provide important insights into the optimization of parameters related to cancer surveillance.[1,27] Studies comparing the sensitivity and specificity of different diagnostic tests can help choose the best test. Studies examining the sensitivity–specificity trade-off between different cut-points of the same test can help choose the optimal criterion for a positive test. Among surveillance tests examined in ulcerative colitis (such as DNA aneuploidy, salicyl-Tn expression, *p53* suppressor gene overexpression and dysplasia), dysplasia is the best studied and the test with the best surveillance program performance.[28] When evaluating biopsy specimens for dysplasia, the optimal criterion for a positive test is low grade dysplasia (a criterion with high sensitivity), rather than high grade dysplasia (a criterion with high specificity).

Table 15.1 Cohort studies of primary sclerosing cholangitis (PSC) as a risk factor for dysplasia or cancer in ulcerative colitis

Study	Center	No. of patients	Dysplasia or cancer (%)	Relative risk (95% CI)
Broome et al. (1992)[13]	Huddinge	5 PSC	4 (80)	6·7 (2·6 to 17·4)
		67 controls	8 (12)	
Gurbuz et al. (1995)[14]	Baltimore	35 PSC	13 (37)	Increased
Broome et al. (1995)[15]	Huddinge	40 PSC	16 (40)	3·2 (1·6 to 6·2)
		80 controls	10 (12)	
Brentnall et al. (1996)[16]	Seattle	20 PSC	9 (45)	4·9 (1·4 to 17·7)
		25 controls	4 (16)	
Loftus et al. (1996)[17]	Rochester	143 PSC	8 (6)	4·9 (0·1 to 27)
Marchesa et al. (1997)[18]	Cleveland	27 PSC	18 (67)	10·4 (4·1 to 26·1)
		1185 controls	145 (12)	
Shetty et al. (1999)[19]	Cleveland	132 PSC	33 (25)	3·2 (1·4 to 7·3)
		196 controls	11 (16)	
Lindberg et al. (2001)[20]	Huddinge	19 PSC	12 (63)	3·1 (1·1 to 8·9)
		124 controls	31 (30)	

Axioms

Many accepted practices related to cancer surveillance in ulcerative colitis have not been studied, but are assumed to be valid. Indeed, there are certain axiomatic statements that must be true for surveillance to be at all accepted by patients and physicians.

1. The cancer risk is elevated in ulcerative colitis patients and is too high to ignore There have been many epidemiological studies investigating the cancer risk in ulcerative colitis[3–12] mostly from northern Europe or North America where the incidence of ulcerative colitis is high and accurate and complete databases exist. From these studies, it is reasonable to assume that the lifetime incidence of colorectal cancer in a patient with pan-ulcerative colitis is approximately 6%, since a risk of this magnitude has been established for the background risk in the American population,[29] and the risk of cancer-related mortality is approximately 3%. These figures are too high to ignore, assuming there is either effective surveillance available or acceptable prophylactic treatment. Furthermore, in some countries like the USA, either prophylactic colectomy or cancer surveillance colonoscopy have become the standard of care for ulcerative colitis patients, especially those diagnosed at a young age. In older patients, especially those with severe comorbidity or disability, the case for surveillance is much less clear since they may be more likely to die from other diseases and not be fit for proctocolectomy.

2. Most patients would rather not have prophylactic colectomy Colectomy prior to the development of dysplasia or cancer is sure to dramatically reduce, if not eliminate, the mortality from colorectal cancer.[30] The existence of cancer surveillance programs, whether or not they are effective, has convinced some patients that the excess cancer mortality risk with ulcerative colitis can be minimized, and that the minimized risk is preferred to the morbidity following proctocolectomy.

3. Patients would agree to proctocolectomy if the cancer risk is very high, as it is with a positive test from surveillance There is no point to performing surveillance colonoscopy if a patient will refuse to have a proctocolectomy for a positive test. Clinicians need to counsel patients carefully so they understand that surveillance is meant to identify the patients at very high cancer risk for proctocolectomy and allow the remaining patients to continue in the cancer surveillance program. From that approach, a majority of patients, those without dysplasia, will not have a colectomy recommended.

In an optimally performing program, all cancer deaths will be averted through colectomy on high risk patients, and no cancer deaths will occur among patients not having colectomy. There has been no perfectly performing surveillance program reported. Program performance is likely to improve following the development of a diagnostic test with better sensitivity and specificity than the presence or absence of dysplasia and/or with more frequent testing than is currently done.

Questions

Existing evidence can only partially answer some of the questions related to cancer surveillance in ulcerative colitis.

Understanding the limits of this evidence and identifying priorities for future investigation could improve technical aspects of surveillance and, ultimately, decrease cancer-related mortality. Questions regarding expected outcomes, the method of surveillance, testing intervals and the criterion for a positive test will be addressed.

1. How effective will a surveillance program be for reducing cancer-related mortality? The number of patients needed to be enrolled in a surveillance program who comply with all of its parameters (i.e. repeated testing with colectomy for a positive test) in order to avert one cancer death can be calculated using expected risk reductions. The number needed to treat (NNT) is the inverse of the absolute risk reduction.[1] Assuming the cancer-related mortality in high risk patients is 3%, the NNT in a perfectly performing program in which colectomy for dysplasia is highly effective for prevention of death from cancer and results in the complete elimination of cancer-related mortality is 1/0·03 or 33. For an absolute risk reduction from surveillance of 1% (i.e. 3% to 2%), the NNT is 100, and for an absolute risk reduction of 2% (i.e. 3% to 1%), the NNT is 50. It is reasonable to assume that surveillance will have some benefit and the NNT most likely will fall between 33 and 100. Therefore, for every 100 patients with pan-ulcerative colitis who are entered into and faithfully comply with the parameters of a surveillance program, between one and three cancer deaths will be averted.

2. What is the best testing method for cancer surveillance? Using colonoscopy with multiple biopsies of the colon as a testing method is problematical, but is still the best and most accepted method of testing for cancer surveillance in ulcerative colitis. Since dysplasia can be present focally, and not necessarily diffusely, biopsies must be taken throughout the colon. The more biopsies taken, the better will be the sensitivity for detecting dysplasia. However, the more biopsies taken, the higher will be the pathology costs, the longer will be the time (and the associated costs) of the procedure, and the greater will be the morbidity of the colonoscopy. Even the most intensive sampling protocols sample less than 0·05% of the colon. While it has not been studied, it seems to be a reasonable trade-off between sensitivity and cost/morbidity to sample the colon with two biopsies taken from each 10-cm colonic segment and of any lesion suspicious of a dysplasia-associated lesion or mass (DALM). DALMs can be suspected by an irregular, furry appearance that resembles a sessile adenoma, but can only be confirmed by detecting dysplasia histologically.[31]

Problematical issues involve pseudopolyps and strictures. A patient with multiple pseudopolyps that cannot be adequately biopsied could easily harbor dysplastic tissue that would not be biopsied. These patients need to be informed of the poor sensitivity of surveillance, and the benefits of prophylactic colectomy. Likewise, colonic strictures that do not allow passage of the colonoscope and adequate sampling could, and very often do, harbor dysplasia.[32] Once again, these patients should be considered for prophylactic colectomy since surveillance of these patients is insensitive.

While it does not appear that other tests will have adequate sensitivity or specificity to be used in the near future for cancer surveillance, research is progressing in the area of testing alternatives. Acquired genetic abnormalities such as DNA aneuploidy, *p53* suppressor gene mutations, and salicyl-Tn expression could be used with dysplasia to improve sensitivity.[22] Patients would be considered to have a positive test if either dysplasia or a genetic abnormality is present. Of course, improved sensitivity will be at the cost of specificity and result in increased numbers of false positives. The penalty for lowering specificity is high – a proctocolectomy in a patient who might not have developed cancer. These alternative tests would be acceptable for use in a surveillance program if the cost were relatively low, the availability high, the gain in sensitivity great and the loss of specificity minimal.

3. What is the best testing interval? The more tests that are carried out in a lifetime, the higher the likelihood that dysplasia will be detected and treated prior to the development of cancer and the lower the cancer-related mortality. Of course, the more tests that are done, the higher will be the cost, morbidity and patient intolerance to colonoscopy. A balance between benefits and costs needs to be struck.[33, 34]

While patients could progress at a slower or faster rate, the mean value for the time between the development of low grade dysplasia and cancer (lead time) is believed to be 3 years.[35,36] Therefore, testing at intervals longer than 3 years should be discouraged, as the majority of patients who develop cancer would not have had an opportunity for dysplasia to be detected at surveillance examinations.

The risk of developing cancer or dysplasia increases with increasing duration of disease. The benefits of frequent testing (short interval) also increase with increasing duration of disease. It can be concluded that uniform testing intervals over a lifetime of disease is not an efficient way to allocate the performance of costly and invasive test procedures. A decision analysis suggests that efficient testing is characterized by decreasing the testing interval with increasing duration of disease.[35] One reasonable method, which certainly can be adjusted according to patient and physician preferences, specifies testing every 3 years for the first 20 years of disease, every 2 years for the next 10 years of disease, and yearly thereafter. C5 Such an approach would require at least 20 tests over a 40-year lifetime of disease, with most allocated in the later years when the risk is the highest.

4. What is the best criterion for a positive test? The type of dysplastic lesion to be used as a criterion for a positive

Table 15.2 Contingency table for calculating sensitivity and specificity of dysplasia for the diagnosis of cancer

	Cancer	No Cancer
Dysplasia	a	b
No Dysplasia	c	d

test is best determined by weighing the trade-off between sensitivity and specificity. Sensitivity is defined as the proportion of patients with disease who are positive for the test in question. Likewise, specificity is defined as the proportion of patients without disease who are negative for the test in question. A standard 2×2 contingency table for n patients ($n = a + b + c + d$) is shown in Table 15.2.

In normally distributed populations, sensitivity ($a/[a + c]$) and specificity ($d/[b + d]$) are stable values that do not vary with prevalence of disease. Sensitivity and specificity will vary though, when the "cut-point" or the criterion for a positive test changes. For example, if the criterion for a positive test changes from high grade dysplasia to low grade dysplasia, the sensitivity will increase (more "a"s and less "c"s) and the specificity will decrease (more "b"s and less "d"s). As the criterion for a positive test changes, there is a trade-off between sensitivity and specificity – as one increases the other decreases.

The sensitivity and specificity of screening for dysplasia to identify patients with asymptomatic cancer has been studied with remarkably consistent results. A blinded review from the University of Chicago of all regions in colectomy specimens in 22 ulcerative colitis patients with cancer identified dysplasia distant from the malignancy in 16 (73% sensitivity for any dysplasia).[37] Eleven patients had high grade dysplasia (50% sensitivity for high grade dysplasia). In a comparable group of 22 ulcerative colitis patients without cancer, six had dysplasia (73% specificity for any dysplasia) and two had high grade dysplasia (91% specificity for high-grade dysplasia). Nearly identical results were found in a study from the Mayo Clinic, where 100 colectomy specimens from patients with ulcerative colitis, 50 of whom had cancer, were studied.[38] The sensitivity for any dysplasia was 74% (37/50) and the sensitivity for high grade dysplasia was 32% (16/50). The specificity of any dysplasia was 74% (37/50) and the specificity of high grade dysplasia was 98% (49/50). Both studies acknowledged that only a small minority of patients were followed in cancer surveillance programs. In a study from St Mark's Hospital, London, principally of ulcerative colitis patients participating in surveillance programs, 37 of 50 colectomy specimens with cancer had dysplasia distant from the malignancy (74% sensitivity for any dysplasia).[39] Sixteen of those patients had high grade dysplasia (32% sensitivity for high grade dysplasia). A large review from Mount Sinai Hospital in New York of 590 colectomy specimens from ulcerative colitis patients, 38 (6%) of whom

had colorectal cancer, found that multifocal dysplasia was highly associated with cancer (OR 6·0, 95% CI 2·5 to 14·4).[40] Another large review from Heidelberg, Germany of 595 colectomy specimens in ulcerative colitis patients, found that high grade dysplasia, low grade dysplasia and backwash ileitis were highly associated with colorectal cancer.[41] Collectively from these studies, both the sensitivity and specificity of testing for any dysplasia is at least 74% (Table 15.3). If high grade dysplasia were to be used as a criterion for a positive test, the sensitivity would fall to about 50% and the specificity would rise to greater than 90%.

Definitions for sensitivity and specificity for surveillance are somewhat different from these definitions for screening. The endpoint of interest in the former situation is death from colon cancer in distinction to its detection alone. Over the course of the disease, patients in a surveillance program will have several colonoscopic examinations with biopsies for dysplasia or cancer. The sensitivity of a surveillance program may be regarded as the proportion of patients with cancer who are successfully treated with colectomy. Those who die from colorectal cancer are false negative patients (group "c" in Table 15.2) in whom surveillance has failed to prevent a cancer-related death. This definition of sensitivity represents a conservative value, since there are patients who had a colectomy for dysplasia in whom cancer would have developed if the colectomy had not been done. Since it is impossible to know which patients with dysplasia would have developed cancer, these patients are not included in the calculations of sensitivity. The specificity of a surveillance program is the proportion of patients who do not develop cancer and who do not have dysplasia detected. Since cancer is rare in a surveillance program, specificity is very well estimated by the proportion of patients in the surveillance program who do not develop dysplasia ($[c + d]/n$). For the purposes of this review, sensitivity of surveillance is defined as the proportion of patients with cancer who survive following colectomy and specificity is defined as the proportion of patients without cancer who do not develop dysplasia. Using these definitions, estimates of sensitivity and specificity from 11 large surveillance programs are shown in Table 15.4.[42–52] Specificity from surveillance is approximately 85%. The estimate of sensitivity is much less stable from study to study due to the low number of cancers in each program, but is for the most part over 50%.

If high grade dysplasia is used as the criterion for a positive test, specificity will increase. The trade-off between specificity and sensitivity is impossible to determine, since patients with low grade dysplasia often are not observed for the development of cancer; rather colectomy or more intensive surveillance is recommended. The increase in specificity with high grade dysplasia rather than low grade dysplasia as the criterion for a positive test is shown in Table 15.5. Specificity using high grade dysplasia as a criterion for a positive test is approximately 95%.

Table 15.3   The sensitivity and specificity of dysplasia to diagnose colorectal cancer in ulcerative colitis patients stratified by degree of dysplasia

Study center	Sensitivity (%)	Specificity (%)
University of Chicago (1985)[37]		
Any dysplasia	73	73
High grade dysplasia	50	91
Mayo Clinic (1992)[38]		
Any dysplasia	74	74
High grade dysplasia	32	98
St Mark's Hospital (1994)[39]		
Any dysplasia	74	–
High grade dysplasia	32	–
Mount Sinai (2000)[40]		
Any dysplasia	84	93
High grade dysplasia	61	95
Heidelberg (2001)[41]		
Any dysplasia	71	83
High-grade dysplasia	55	90

Table 15.4   The sensitivity and specificity of 11 large colorectal cancer surveillance programs for patients with ulcerative colitis

Study center	No. of patients	Sensitivity	Specificity
University of Leeds (1980)[42]	43	2/2 (100%)	34/41 (83%)
Cleveland Clinic (1985)[43]	248	6/7 (86%)	194/241 (80%)
University of Chicago (1989)[44]	99	4/8 (50%)	73/91 (80%)
Karolinska Institute (1990)[45]	72	2/2 (100%)	54/70 (77%)
Lahey Clinic (1991)[46]	213	4/10 (40%)	171/203 (84%)
Helsinki University (1991)[47]	66	0/0	57/66 (86%)
Lennox Hill Hospital (1992)[48]	121	4/7 (57%)	91/114 (80%)
St Mark's Hospital (1994)[49]	284	13/17 (76%)	205/267 (77%)
Ornskoldsvik Hospital (1994)[50]	131	2/4 (50%)	103/127 (81%)
Tel Aviv Medical Center (1995)[51]	154	3/4 (75%)	141/150 (94%)
University of Bologna (1995)[52]	65	4/4 (100%)	58/61 (95%)

The optimal criterion for a positive test also depends on the consequences of false positive (group "b", Table 15.2) and false negative (group "c", Table 15.2) testing. Patients who have a false positive test have dysplasia but are not destined to develop malignancy. These are the patients who have a proctocolectomy without truly needing one. Unfortunately, there is currently no way to predict which patients will fall into this false positive category. In the future, alternative markers of malignancy, such as the presence of *p53* suppressor gene mutations, may help in determining which patient with dysplasia is a true positive patient (group "a") and which is a false positive patient (group "b"). Likewise, patients with false negative examinations die of cancer without having proctocolectomy recommended from the detection of dysplasia. In these patients, either the testing interval was too long or the imperfect specificity of testing (mostly due to the focality of dysplasia) led to a false negative test. While both false positive and false negative errors are difficult to accept, false negative errors are the more grievous and the category that should be minimized with the most vigor. Therefore, the criterion for a positive test should be the detection of any dysplasia, low grade or high grade, on any biopsy of any examination. Also, since the mortality rate of proctocolectomy is very low, less than 1%, the risk/benefit ratio of opting for surgery in patients with dysplasia against no surgery favors surgical management.[53]

Improving cancer surveillance programs in ulcerative colitis

Evidence-based recommendations can be made to improve and optimize cancer surveillance strategies using currently available techniques. Factors related to the disease, the test

Table 15.5 Comparisons of specificity with low grade dysplasia or high grade dysplasia used as the criterion for a positive test in colorectal cancer surveillance from 11 large surveillance programs

Study center	Specificity using low grade dysplasia as a cut-point	Specificity using high grade dysplasia as a cut-point
University of Leeds (1980)[42]	34/41 (83%)	40/41 (98%)
Cleveland Clinic (1985)[43]	194/241 (80%)	231/241 (96%)
University of Chicago (1989)[44]	73/91 (80%)	87/91 (96%)
Karolinska Institute (1990)[45]	54/70 (77%)	64/70 (91%)
Lahey Clinic (1991)[46]	171/203 (84%)	182/203 (90%)
Helsinki University (1991)[47]	57/66 (86%)	58/66 (88%)
Lennox Hill Hospital (1992)[48]	91/114 (80%)	114/114 (100%)
St Mark's Hospital (1994)[49]	205/267 (77%)	255/267 (96%)
Ornskoldsvik Hospital (1994)[50]	103/127 (81%)	123/127 (97%)
Tel Aviv Medical Center (1995)[51]	141/150 (94%)	144/150 (96%)
University of Bologna (1995)[52]	58/61 (95%)	61/61 (100%)

and the treatment can be optimized based on the above discussion.

Preferentially test high risk patients, such as patients with pan-ulcerative colitis of at least 8 years or patients with primary sclerosing cholangitis, with colonoscopy and extensive biopsy. Patients with lower cancer risk, such as ulcerative colitis patients with left-sided ulcerative colitis or Crohn's colitis, should receive cancer surveillance if resources exist.

The testing interval should shorten with increasing duration of disease to maximize the efficiency of a surveillance program.

The criterion for a positive test should optimize sensitivity. A positive test is defined as the presence of any dysplasia on any biopsy on any examination. "Confirmatory" testing is unnecessary. A positive test places the patient at extremely high risk of dying from colorectal cancer and thus necessitates a strong recommendation for proctocolectomy. C5

References

1 Sackett DL, Hayes RB, Guyatt GH *et al. Clinical epidemiology: a basic science for clinical medicine,* 2nd edn. Boston: Little, Brown, 1991.

2 Greenstein AJ, Sachar DB, Smith H *et al.* Cancer in universal and left-sided ulcerative colitis: factors determining risk. *Gastroenterology* 1979;**77**:290–4.

3 Brostrom O, Lofberg R, Nordenvall B *et al.* The risk of colorectal cancer in ulcerative colitis: an epidemiologic study. *Scand J Gastroenterol* 1987;**22**:1193–9.

4 Gyde SN, Prior P, Allen RN *et al.* Colorectal cancer in ulcerative colitis: a cohort study of primary referrals from three centers. *Gut* 1988;**29**:206–17.

5 Gilat T, Fireman Z, Grossman A *et al.* Colorectal cancer in patients with ulcerative colitis: a population study in central Israel. *Gastroenterology* 1988;**94**:870–7.

6 Lashner BA, Kane SV, Hanauer SB. Colon cancer surveillance in chronic ulcerative colitis: an historical cohort study. *Am J Gastroenterol* 1990;**85**:1083–7.

7 Lennard-Jones JE, Melville DM, Morson BC *et al.* Precancer and cancer in ulcerative colitis: findings among 401 patients over 22 years. *Gut* 1990;**31**:800–6.

8 Ekbom A, Helmick C, Zack M *et al.* Ulcerative colitis and colorectal cancer: a population-based study. *N Engl J Med* 1990;**323**:1228–33.

9 Farmer RG, Easley KA, Rankin GB. Clinical patterns, natural history, and progression of ulcerative colitis: a long-term follow-up of 1 116 patients. *Dig Dis Sci* 1993;**38**:1137–46.

10 Lashner BA, Provencher K, Bozdech JM *et al.* Worsening risk for the development of cancer or dysplasia in patients with ulcerative colitis. *Am J Gastroenterol* 1995;**90**: 377–80.

11 Wandell EP, Damlier P, Moller Pederson F *et al.* Survival and incidence of colorectal cancer in patients with ulcerative colitis in Funen County diagnosed between 1973 and 1993. *Scand J Gastroenterol* 2000;**35**:312–17.

12 Ishibashi N, Hirota Y, Ikeda M, Hirohata T. Ulcerative colitis and colorectal cancer: a follow-up study in Fukuoka, Japan. *Int J Epidemiol* 1999;**28**:609–13.

13 Broome U, Lindberg G, Lofberg R. Primary sclerosing cholangitis in ulcerative colitis – a risk factor for the development of dysplasia and DNA aneuploidy? *Gastroenterology* 1992;**102**:1877–80.

14 Gurbuz AK, Giardiello FM, Bayless .TM. Colorectal neoplasia in patients with ulcerative colitis and sclerosing cholangitis. *Dis Colon Rectum* 1995;**38**:37–41.

15 Broome U, Lofberg R, Veress B *et al.* Primary sclerosing cholangitis and ulcerative colitis: evidence for increased neoplastic potential. *Hepatology* 1995;**22**:1404–8.

16 Brentnall TA, Haggitt RC, Rabinovitch PS *et al.* Risk and natural history of colonic neoplasia in patients with primary sclerosing cholangitis and ulcerative colitis. *Gastroenterology* 1996;**110**:331–8.

17 Loftus EV Jr, Sandborn WJ, Tremaine WJ III *et al.* Risk of colorectal neoplasia in patients with primary sclerosing cholangitis. *Gastroenterology* 1996;**110**:432–40.

18 Marchesa P, Fazio VW, Lavery IC *et al.* The risk of cancer and dysplasia among ulcerative colitis patients with

primary sclerosing cholangitis. *Am J Gastroenterol* 1997; **92**:1285–8.

19   Shetty K, Rybicki L, Brezinski A, Carey WD, Lashner BA. The risk of cancer or dysplasia in ulcerative colitis patients with primary sclerosing cholangitis. *Am J Gastroenterol* 1999;**94**:1643–9.

20   Lindberg BU, Broome U, Persson B. Proximal colorectal dysplasia or cancer in ulcerative colitis: the impact of primary sclerosing cholangitis and sulfasalazine. *Dis Colon Rectum* 2001;**44**:77–85.

21   Sackett DL, Whelan G. Cancer risk in ulcerative colitis: scientific requirements for the study of prognosis. *Gastroenterology* 1980;**78**:1632–5.

22   Lashner BA, Heidenreich PA, Su GL *et al.* Effect of folate supplementation on the risk of dysplasia and cancer in ulcerative colitis. *Gastroenterology* 1989;**97**:255–9.

23   Lashner BA. Red blood cell folate is associated with cancer and dysplasia in ulcerative colitis. *J Cancer Res Clin Oncol* 1993;**119**:549–54.

24   Lashner BA, Provencher KS, Seidner DL *et al.* The effect of folic acid supplementation on the risk for cancer or dysplasia in ulcerative colitis. *Gastroenterology* 1997;**112**: 29–32.

25   Karlen P, Kornfeld D, Brostrom O *et al.* Is cancer surveillance reducing colorectal cancer mortality in ulcerative colitis? A population based case–control study. *Gut* 1998;**42**:711–14.

26   Eaden J, Abrams K, Ekbom A, Jackson E, Mayberry J. Colorectal cancer prevention in ulcerative colitis: a case–control study. *Aliment Pharmacol Ther* 2000;**14**:145–53.

27   Cole P, Morrison AS. Basic issues in population screening for cancer. *J Natl Cancer Inst* 1980;**64**:1263–72.

28   Shapiro BD, Lashner BA. Cancer biology in ulcerative colitis and potential use in endoscopic surveillance. *Gastrointest Clin North Am* 1997;**7**:453–68.

29   Byers T, Levin B, Rothenberger D *et al.* American Cancer Society guidelines for screening and surveillance for early detection of colorectal polyps and cancer: Update 1997. *CA Cancer J Clin* 1997;**47**:154–60.

30   Provenzale D, Kowdley KV, Arora S, Wong JB. Prophylactic colectomy or surveillance for chronic ulcerative colitis? A decision analysis. *Gastroenterology* 1995;**109**:1188–96.

31   Blackstone MO, Riddell RH, Rogers BHG *et al.* Dysplasia-associated lesion or mass (DALM) detected by colonoscopy in long-standing ulcerative colitis: an indication for colectomy. *Gastroenterology* 1981;**80**:366–74.

32   Lashner BA, Turner BC, Bostwick DG *et al.* Dysplasia and cancer complicating strictures in ulcerative colitis. *Dig Dis Sci* 1990;**35**:349–52.

33   Provenzale D, Wong JB, Onken JE *et al.* Performing a cost-effectiveness analysis: surveillance of patients with ulcerative colitis. *Am J Gastroenterol* 1998;**93**:872–80.

34   Provenzale D, Onken J. Surveillance issues in inflammatory bowel disease. *J Clin Gastroenterol* 2001;**32**:99–105.

35   Lashner BA, Hanauer SB, Silverstein MD. Optimal timing of colonoscopy to screen for cancer in ulcerative colitis. *Ann Intern Med* 1988;**108**:274–8.

36   Lashner BA, Shapiro BD, Husain A, Goldblum JR. Evaluation of the usefulness of testing for *p53* mutations in colorectal cancer for ulcerative colitis. *Am J Gastroenterol* 1999;**94**:456–62.

37   Ransohoff DF, Riddell RH, Levin B. Ulcerative colitis and colonic cancer: problems in assessing the diagnostic usefulness of mucosal dysplasia. *Dis Colon Rectum* 1985;**28**:383–8.

38   Taylor BA, Pemberton JH, Carpenter HA *et al.* Dysplasia in chronic ulcerative colitis: Implications for colonoscopic surveillance. *Dis Colon Rectum* 1992;**35**:950–6.

39   Connell WR, Talbot IC, Harpaz N *et al.* Clinicopathological characteristics of colorectal carcinoma complicating ulcerative colitis. *Gut* 1994;**35**:1419–23.

40   Gorfine SR, Bauer JJ, Harris MT, Kreel I. Dysplasia complicating chronic ulcerative colitis: is immediate colectomy warranted? *Dis Colon Rectum* 2000;**43**:1575–81.

41   Heuschen UA, Hinz U, Allemeyer EH *et al.* Backwash ileitis is strongly associated with colorectal carcinoma in ulcerative colitis. *Gastroenterology* 2001;**120**:841–7.

42   Dickenson RJ, Dixon MF, Axon ATR. Colonoscopy and the detection of dysplasia in patients with longstanding ulcerative colitis. *Lancet* 1980;**2**:620–2.

43   Rosenstock E, Farmer RG, Petras R *et al.* Surveillance for colonic carcinoma in ulcerative colitis. *Gastroenterology* 1985;**89**:1342–6.

44   Lashner BA, Silverstein MD, Hanauer SB. Hazard rates for dysplasia and cancer in ulcerative colitis: results from a surveillance program. *Dig Dis Sci* 1989;**34**:1536–41.

45   Lofberg R, Brostrom O, Karlen O *et al.* Colonoscopic surveillance in longstanding ulcerative colitis: a 15-year follow-up study. *Gastroenterology* 1990;**99**:1021–31.

46   Nugent FW, Haggitt RC, Gilpin PA. Cancer surveillance in ulcerative colitis. *Gastroenterology* 1991;**100**:1241–8.

47   Leidenius M, Kellokumpu I, Husa A *et al.* Dysplasia and carcinoma in longstanding ulcerative colitis: an endoscopic and histologic surveillance program. *Gut* 1991;**32**:1521–5.

48   Woolrich AJ, DaSilva MD, Korelitz BI. Surveillance in the routine management of ulcerative colitis: the predictive value of low-grade dysplasia. *Gastroenterology* 1992;**103**: 431–8.

49   Connell WR, Lennard-Jones JE, Williams CD *et al.* Factors affecting the outcomes of endoscopic surveillance for cancer in ulcerative colitis. *Gastroenterology* 1994;**107**:934–44.

50   Jonsson B, Ahsgren L, Andersson LO *et al.* Colorectal cancer survival in patients with ulcerative colitis. *Br J Surg* 1994; **81**:689–91.

51   Rozen P, Baratz M, Fefer F *et al.* Low incidence of significant dysplasia in a successful endoscopic surveillance program of patients with ulcerative colitis. *Gastroenterology* 1995;**108**:1361–70.

52   Biasco G, Brandi G, Paganelli GM *et al.* Colorectal cancer in patients with ulcerative colitis: a prospective cohort study in Italy. *Cancer* 1995;**75**:2045–50.

53   Fazio VW, Ziv Y, Church JM, Oakley JR, Lavery IC, Milsom JW, Schroeder TK. Ileal pouch–anal anastomoses complications and function in 1005 patients. *Ann Surg* 1995;**222**:120–7.

16 Colorectal cancer: population screening and surveillance

Bernard Levin

Epidemiology

Worldwide, colorectal cancer is the third most frequently occurring cancer in both sexes; however, it ranks second in developed countries. Although the developed world includes only about a quarter of the world's population, approximately two-thirds of the estimated world total of 875 000 new cases a year in 1996 occurred in this group.[1] In the USA, the cumulative lifetime risk of developing colorectal cancer is about 6%.[2] In spite of the advances in the treatment of this disease, the 5-year survival is only about 55%.[3] Studies have shown that survival improves with diagnosis at an earlier stage, thus providing a rationale for screening.[4]

Biology of colorectal cancer

The adenoma–carcinoma sequence

An understanding of the biology of colorectal cancer is essential to guide the application of available screening tests. It is generally accepted that most colorectal cancers evolve from adenomatous polyps. Direct evidence supporting this belief is limited, since ethical concerns preclude observing the natural history of polyps. However, indirect studies have demonstrated that cancers rarely arise in the absence of adenomatous polyps, individuals with a history of adenomatous polyps are at increased risk of developing cancer[5] and removal of these premalignant lesions reduces the incidence of colorectal cancer.[6,7]

A series of genetic alterations appears to be the impetus from which normal colonic mucosa develops into an adenomatous polyp and ultimately transforms into a cancer.[8] The time required for the transformation of a small adenomatous polyp to localized cancer and ultimately to invasive cancer, the so-called "polyp dwell time", is of great interest in colorectal cancer screening. Knowledge of the polyp dwell time can be used to determine the window of opportunity during which screening is effective in the prevention and early detection of colorectal cancer.

The average polyp dwell time is not precisely known. An interdisciplinary expert panel originally convened by the Agency of Health Care Policy and Research (USA) to establish colorectal cancer screening guidelines estimated that it takes an average of about 10 years for an adenomatous polyp to transform into invasive cancer.[4] Knowledge of this transformation time has been the basis on which the frequency of accepted screening tests is determined. However, it has recently been suggested that up to one-third of colorectal cancers arise through alternative mechanisms that include origin in serrated adenomas and hyperplastic polyps and involve micro-satellite instability rather than loss of heterozygosity as the fundamental defect responsible for neoplastic transformation.[9] This remains an area of controversy.

Screening for colorectal cancer

Five different tests for the screening of colorectal cancer are presented. Of all the modalities mentioned, the strongest evidence exists for fecal occult blood testing. Intermediate level evidence is available for flexible sigmoidoscopy and only indirect evidence supports the use of colonoscopy and double contrast barium enema.

Fecal occult blood test

Screening for the presence of blood in the stool is based on the fact that most cancers and some polyps bleed.[10] The bleeding is intermittent and blood is unevenly distributed throughout the stool. Additionally, the amount of bleeding is dependent on the size of the polyp or cancer. Screening for the presence of blood in the stool is far less sensitive for polyps than for cancers. Polyps, especially small ones, do not bleed or do so only infrequently.[11] However, screening by fecal occult blood testing may detect the presence of polyps because large polyps, those most likely to be precancerous, do bleed. Furthermore, false positive results lead to diagnostic testing that discovers polyps whether or not they have bled.

Guaiac-based tests for peroxidase activity are the most commonly used means of testing for blood in the stool. Dietary restrictions are important to eliminate the possibility of false positive results. False negative tests may result if the cancer or premalignant lesion did not bleed when the test was carried out. A positive test for occult blood does not confirm the presence of a cancer or polyp but only suggests its presence. Further diagnostic testing, preferably by colonoscopy, must be undertaken to ascertain the source of the occult blood.

Current recommendations are that testing be conducted on two samples from three different stool specimens on consecutive days as multiple, consecutive samplings increase the likelihood of detecting blood. The sensitivity of the test is improved if the test is performed as a part of a program of testing over a period of several years instead of a one-time test, as this offers several opportunities to detect intermittent bleeding.[4] The sensitivity of this test is also dependent on the hydration status of the developed sample cards. Rehydration of the samples with a few drops of distilled water prior to the addition of the developing reagent increases the sensitivity at the expense of the specificity and is not recommended.

To date, four randomized controlled studies have investigated fecal occult blood testing for colorectal cancer screening. Three of the trials have been completed and the fourth is still in progress.[12–14] These trials incorporate a program of screening with multiple, consecutive tests on an annual or biennial basis rather than a single test in time. In studies using non-rehydrated samples, sensitivities ranged from 72% to 78% with a specificity of 98% and a positive predictive value of 10–17%. The sensitivity increased to 88–92% when rehydrated samples were used; however, the specificity dropped to 90–92% and the positive predictive value fell to 2–6%.[4]

The Minnesota trial[12] was initiated using non-rehydrated samples but slide processing was modified early in the trial to incorporate rehydration; ultimately, 83% of the slides were developed after rehydration. Participants were randomly assigned to annual or biennial screening or to a control group. After 13 years, the group receiving annual screening showed a 33% reduction in colorectal cancer mortality while the group receiving biennial screening showed a non-significant 5% reduction.[12] Ala Combination of the annual and the biennial groups resulted in an overall reduction of 19% in the risk of colorectal cancer death with screening. Adverse events related to diagnostic colonoscopy, perforation or hemorrhage, were reported to occur at the rate of 12 complications per 10 000 colonoscopies. There is some question as to how much of the mortality reduction demonstrated in this trial is due to the high rate of colonoscopy carried out as a result of the increased positivity of the rehydrated sample. In an analysis of the study by other authors, it was estimated that one-third to one-half of the mortality reduction was due to the increased number of colonoscopies done and not attributable to fecal occult blood testing alone.[15,16] The assumptions in that

analysis have been disputed by the authors of the Minnesota study. Using actual data in a model, they concluded that 16–25% of the reduction in colorectal cancer deaths effected by fecal occult blood testing was due to chance detection.[17]

The question has been raised as to the effect that biennial screening, as opposed to the annual screening employed in this study, would have on colorectal cancer mortality. Two other randomized controlled trials offered biennial screening and did not perform rehydration of the fecal occult blood slides. Diagnostic evaluation of positive tests in both studies was performed by colonoscopic evaluation. Both studies had a low colonoscopy rate as compared to the Minnesota study. The Nottingham trial had a mean follow up of 7·8 years and showed a 15% reduction in colorectal cancer mortality.[13] The Funen study showed an 18% reduction in mortality after 10 years.[14] Ald

Unpublished results from the Goteborg trial, published in the Cochrane Review with information supplied by the principal investigator of that study, indicates that there is a 12% reduction in colorectal cancer mortality with biennial screening after 8 years of follow up. Ala The investigators reported a 0·3% complication rate (30 complications per 10 000 endoscopies), as evidenced by perforation and hemorrhage, out of 2298 endoscopies (colonoscopies and sigmoidoscopies).

Using data from these four randomized controlled studies, a systematic review including a meta-analysis was performed and published in the Cochrane Library[18] (Figure 16.1). This analysis showed an overall significant reduction in colorectal cancer mortality with screening by fecal occult blood testing of 16% (RR 0·84, CI 0·77 to 0·93). Ala When the relative risk is adjusted for attendance for screening in individual studies, the mortality reduction is 23%. Overall, if 10 000 persons were offered screening and approximately two-thirds attended for at least one fecal occult blood test, there would be 8·5 deaths (CI 3·6 to 13·5) from colorectal cancer prevented over 10 years. Stating this another way, in order to prevent one death from colorectal cancer over 10 years, 1173 persons would need to be screened. However, the screening program would also result in 2800 participants having at least one colonoscopy. If harmful effects of screening from the Minnesota trial are considered, there would be 3·4 colonoscopy complications. If harmful effects of screening from the Goteborg trial are considered, approximately 600 participants would need at least one sigmoidoscopy and double contrast enema, resulting in 1·8 perforations or hemorrhage.

The estimate of mortality reduction from the randomized controlled trials of fecal occult blood tests is now well quantified and the confidence intervals are narrow enough to allow the conclusion that colorectal cancer screening is likely to be beneficial in a program of colorectal cancer screening. However, the wide range of mortality reduction seen in these studies and the overall modest mortality reduction indicates a

Review: Screening for colorectal cancer using Hemoccult
comparison: All Hemoccult screening programs *v* control
outcome: colorectal cancer mortality

Study	Expt n/N	Ctrl n/N	Peto OR (95% CI fixed)	Weight %	Peto OR (95% CI fixed)
Randomized controlled trials					
Funen	205/30 967	249/30 966		24·7	0·82 (0·66 to 0·99)
Goteborg	121/34 144	138/34 164		14·1	0·88 (0·69 to 1·12)
Minnesota	199/31 157	121/15 394		15·4	0·81 (0·64 to 1·02)
Nottingham	360/76 466	420/76 384		42·5	0·86 (0·74 to 0·99)
Subtotal (95% CI)	885/172 734	928/156 908		96·6	0·84 (0·77 to 0·92)
Chi-square 0·35 (df = 3) Z = 3·6					

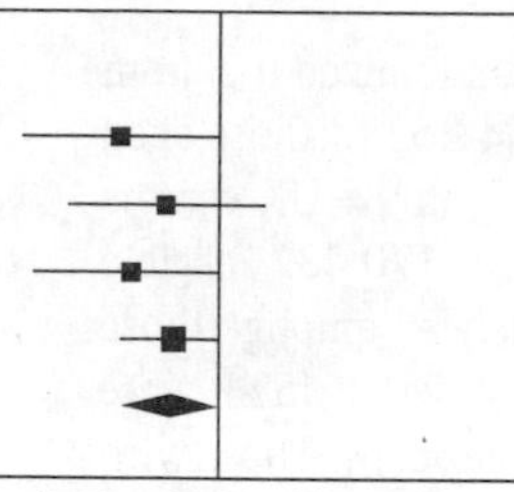

0·5   0·7   1   1·5   2

Figure 16.1 Meta-analysis of randomized controlled trials of Hemoccult screening programs as an intervention for reducing mortality from colorectal cancer. (Source: Towler BP *et al.* Cochrane Review. In: *Cochrane Library*, Issue 3. Oxford: Update Software, 2002[18])

need for continued improvement in fecal occult blood test technology. Detection of gene mutations or loss of heterozygosity in DNA from stool samples may facilitate early diagnosis in the future.

Other benefits of fecal occult blood testing are emerging. Most notably, a reduction in the incidence of colorectal cancer of 20% in subjects screened annually, has been observed in the Minnesota trial.[19] AId Additionally, treatment of early stage colorectal cancers may involve less invasive surgery.

In all three randomized studies evaluating the effectiveness of fecal occult blood testing, a favorable stage shift to earlier stage disease, which has better outcomes, was seen. In the Nottingham study, 90% of the screened group had Dukes' A or B compared with 40% of the control group.[13] A similar stage shift was seen in the other two randomized controlled trials described.

Immunochemical tests use monoclonal and/or polyclonal antibodies that detect the intact globin portion of human hemoglobin. If hemoglobin is present in the stool, the labeled antibody will attach to its antigens, creating a positive test result. Diet does not affect the immunochemical tests thus obviating a potential source of false positive tests and also likely enhancing patient acceptance. While only a limited number of individuals have been screened using the immunochemical tests, it appears as if these tests are at least as sensitive and specific as the guaiac-based tests.[20]

Flexible sigmoidoscopy

The rationale for screening with sigmoidoscopy is that it provides direct visualization of the colon, and suspicious lesions can be biopsied. The most obvious disadvantage is that it examines only that portion of the distal colon within reach of the endoscope. Approximately 65–75% of adenomatous polyps and 40–65% of colorectal cancers are within the reach of a 60-cm flexible sigmoidoscope.[21–24] As with the fecal occult blood test, patients with a positive examination require further evaluation by colonoscopy. It has been well established that patients with an adenomatous polyp found on sigmoidoscopy have an increased probability of additional lesions located more proximally.[25–27]

The sensitivity of flexible sigmoidoscopy is 96·7% for cancer and large polyps and 73·3% for small polyps. The specificity is 94% for cancer and large polyps with a 92% specificity for small polyps.[4]

Only indirect evidence derived from several case–control studies using either rigid sigmoidoscopy or a combination of rigid with flexible sigmoidoscopy currently exists to support the effectiveness of flexible sigmoidoscopy.[28,29] B3 The best designed trial, by Selby *et al.*, avoided many of the biases inherent in case–control studies.[28] The screening histories of persons who died of colorectal cancer were compared against controls and a 59% reduction in mortality from cancers of the rectum and distal colon was found in individuals who had undergone sigmoidoscopic evaluation.[25] Newcomb *et al.* reported an 80% reduction in mortality from cancer of the rectum and distal colon in persons who had ever undergone sigmoidoscopic examination compared with individuals who had never done so.[29] B3 Several potential biases limit the applicability of this study; however, it does provide independent collaboration of the effectiveness of sigmoidoscopy in a colorectal cancer screening program.

Of great interest is the optimal interval for screening sigmoidoscopy. In the study by Selby *et al.* described above, the effectiveness of screening sigmoidoscopy was found to be just as great for patients who had undergone the procedure 9–10 years before as compared to those who had just undergone the examination.[30] A modeling study evaluating the optimal interval for sigmoidoscopic screening found that 90% of the effectiveness of annual screening was preserved with an interval of 10 years.[24] This model assumes that adenomatous polyps take 10–14 years to evolve into invasive cancers.

The baseline findings of a multicenter randomized trial from the UK have been reported.[31] Out of 354 262 of those aged 55–64 years invited to undergo screening in 14 UK centers 194 726 (55%) accepted. Out of these 170 432 eligible individuals were randomized. Attendance among those assigned screening was 71%. A total of 2131 (5%) were classified as high risk and referred for colonoscopy. Those with no polyps or detected with only low risk polyps ($n = 38\,525$) were discharged. Distal adenomas were detected in 493 (12%) and distal cancer in 131 (0·3%). Proximal adenomas were detected in 386 (18·8% of those undergoing colonoscopy) and proximal cancer in nine cases (10·4%). Sixty-two percent of cancers were Dukes' A. There was one perforation after flexible sigmoidoscopy and four after colonoscopy.

The baseline findings of a multicenter randomized trial in Italy in individuals aged 55–64 years have also been reported.[32] Distal adenomas were detected in 1070 subjects (10·8%). Proximal adenomas were detected in 116 of 747 (15·5%) subjects without cancer at sigmoidoscopy who then underwent colonoscopy. A total of 54 subjects were found to have colorectal cancer, a rate of 5·4 per 1000 (54% of which were Dukes' A). Two perforations occurred (one in 991 sigmoidoscopies and one in 77 colonoscopies) and one hemorrhage requiring hospitalization. The long-term results of these randomized trials are awaited with interest.

Double contrast barium enema

Evidence for the use of double contrast barium enema in screening is limited. The fact that detecting polyps and early cancers in other screening studies has resulted in a reduction in the incidence and mortality of colorectal cancer provides indirect evidence that double contrast barium enema, which detects many of these lesions, would be beneficial. The sensitivity of double contrast barium enema is 84% for cancer, 82% for large polyps and 67% for small polyps. The specificity is 97·5% for cancer, 83·3% for large polyps and 75% for small polyps.[4]

One randomized controlled trial investigated the addition of double contrast barium enema to sigmoidoscopy compared to colonoscopy. Colonoscopy was found to be more sensitive in detecting small polyps but no difference was found between the groups for large polyps and cancers.[33] A1c

The frequency at which double contrast barium enema should be carried out has not been well studied. An interval of 5–10 years has been suggested based on the estimated polyp dwell time of 10 years and the performance characteristics of the double contrast barium enema, which is known to be less sensitive in detecting small polyps. C5 For this reason, a shorter time interval of 5 years is a part of the recommended screening procedure.[4]

Colonoscopy

Colonoscopy is the only technique that offers screening, diagnostic and, at times, therapeutic management all in one procedure. Most data available on the effects of colonoscopy are derived either from studies of colonoscopy in a diagnostic and surveillance setting or from indirect evidence as outlined above for double contrast barium enema. There are no studies currently available that evaluate colonoscopy as a screening test in terms of reduction of colorectal cancer mortality. However, to the extent that colonoscopy is a significant part of the fecal occult blood test program, these trials of occult blood testing also provide evidence of the effectiveness of colonoscopy.[12] Additional support is provided from one case–control study which showed that persons who had undergone colonoscopy had a 70–80% reduction in colorectal cancers.[7] B3 A feasibility trial of screening colonoscopy has been launched in the USA (Winawer S, personal communication, 2002).

Colonoscopy can detect both polyps and cancers, although it is less accurate when the lesions are small. In studies evaluating the performance of colonoscopy, it has been demonstrated that 15% of small polyps but few large polyps are missed.[34] False positive results are rare but about one-third of polyps removed are not adenomatous.[35] Colonoscopic sensitivity is 96·7% for cancers, 85% for large polyps, and 78·5% for small polyps; specificity is 98% for all lesions.[4]

No studies address the optimal frequency with which screening with colonoscopy should be carried out. Based on the natural history of the disease and the high accuracy of colonoscopy in the detection of polyps, it has been suggested that a screening interval of 10 years would be protective.[4] C5 This is supported by the case–control study of Selby *et al.* evaluating sigmoidoscopy, which suggests a protective effect for up to 10 years.[28] B3

Although no randomized trials of colonoscopy have been performed, two large-scale demonstration projects have been recently reported.[36,37] The first was from a group of Veterans Affairs centers (USA) involving 3212 individuals (97% men) and the other one included 2000 men and women, who were employed by Eli Lilly, Inc. (Indianapolis, Indiana, USA) The adenomatous polyp rate was 38% in the Veterans cohort and 20% in the Lilly cohort. The rate of advanced proximal lesions varied from 2% to 4% and about half of these would have been missed by sigmoidoscopy. The complication rate was low; 97% of examinations reached the cecum with a perforation rate of 0·02% without any deaths.

It remains to be seen whether colonoscopy will become a primary screening test in view of its expense and invasiveness.

The emerging technology of virtual colonoscopy (three-dimensional colography) is anticipated with enthusiasm in the hope that a non-invasive method of imaging the entire colon will increase compliance with colorectal cancer screening. Results from major specialized centers in the USA show accuracy of CT colonography to be comparable with conventional colonoscopy for the detection of polyps greater than 10 mm with few false positives.[37] In expert centers, polypoid lesions larger than 10 mm can be detected with sensitivity and specificity approaching 90% with sensitivity falling to 50% for polyps 5 mm in size. CT colonography, in some studies, has been shown to be accurate in detecting colon cancer with a sensitivity of 100%.[38]

Further study is required to evaluate the performance characteristics of virtual colonoscopy in a typical screening setting. In the future, avoidance of the need to undergo bowel preparation and advances in software design may enhance the public appeal of this method of colonic examination.

Digital rectal examination

Less than 10% of colorectal cancers are within the 7–8-cm reach of the examining finger.[39] Additionally, stool obtained during the course of a digital rectal examination is an inadequate sample upon which to screen for the presence or absence of blood and this type of fecal occult blood testing is not recommended. Finally, there is no evidence that digital rectal examination reduces morbidity or mortality from colorectal cancer, and it is not currently indicated as a screening test for the prevention or early detection of colorectal cancer.[4]

Screening recommendations

Using the above evidence, the interdisciplinary Task Force, initially convened by the Agency for Health Care Policy and Research and completed with funding from seven professional societies, developed recommendations for the screening of colorectal cancer.[4] In 1997, the American Cancer Society published its recommendations for screening, which were based largely on, and nearly identical to those developed by the Agency for Health Care Policy and Research Task Force and the Society updated these recommendations in 2001.[2]

The appropriate age at which to stop screening has not been well established; however, logic and indirect evidence suggest that screening would appropriately cease when significant comorbid conditions exist. In addition, consideration must be given to an individual's ability to tolerate the screening procedures as well as any further diagnostic evaluation that may be necessary.

Risk stratification

A key component of the American Cancer Society's Guidelines for Screening and Surveillance for Early Detection of Colorectal Polyps and Cancer (Table 16.1) is the stratification of individuals based on their risk profile. To better understand average risk, a definition of moderate and high risk must first be outlined.

Moderate risk individuals are those with a personal history of adenomatous polyps. In addition, a history of adenomatous polyps or colorectal cancer in a first-degree relative younger than 60 years or in two first-degree relatives of any age increases the risk of developing colorectal cancer. Approximately 15–20% of colorectal cancers occur in persons of moderate risk.

Persons at high risk of developing colorectal cancer fall into two categories. Those with one of two hereditary syndromes, familial adenomatous polyposis (FAP) and hereditary non-polyposis colorectal cancer (HNPCC) syndrome, and those with inflammatory bowel disease including both ulcerative colitis and Crohn's disease. Persons in the high risk category who develop colorectal cancer comprise approximately 5–10% of the colorectal cancers diagnosed.

Individuals in the average risk category are by definition those persons who do not meet the criteria for either the moderate or high risk categories. Approximately 70–80% of colorectal cancers diagnosed occur in this risk category. The proportions of hereditary and sporadic colorectal cancer in the population are depicted in Figure 16.2.

Average risk screening recommendations

Persons at average risk should begin colorectal cancer screening at age 50 years with either an annual fecal occult blood test or a flexible sigmoidoscopy every 5 years although the combination is preferred (see Table 16.1), or total colonic examination either by colonoscopy every 10 years or double contrast barium enema every 5–10 years. The decision as to which screening modality to use should be made between the patient and clinician. Factors to consider are the availability of trained and competent clinicians to perform the examination as well as cost and patient acceptability. Any positive fecal occult blood test, abnormal flexible sigmoidoscopy or double contrast barium enema should usually be followed up by colonoscopy for diagnostic evaluation. Consideration should be given to performing a supplemental double contrast barium enema or virtual colonoscopy for those in whom colonoscopy is not complete, i.e. to the cecum.

Moderate risk screening recommendations

Persons diagnosed with one or more adenomatous polyps on flexible sigmoidoscopy should undergo further evaluation

Table 16.1 ACS guidelines for screening and surveillance for early detection of colorectal polyps and cancers

Risk category	Recommendation[b]	Age to begin	Interval
Average risk			
All people 50 years or older who are not in the categories below	One of the following:		
	FOBT plus flexible sigmoidoscopy[c] or	50 years	FOBT every year and flexible sigmoidoscopy every 5 years
	TCE[d]	50 years	Colonoscopy every 10 years or DCBE every 5–10 years
Moderate risk			
People with single, small (<1 cm) adenomatous polyps	Colonoscopy	At time of initial polyp diagnosis	TCE within 3 years after initial polyp removal; if normal, as per average risk recommendations (above)
People with large (≥1 cm) or multiple adenomatous polyps of any size	Colonoscopy	At time of initial polyp diagnosis	TCE within 3 years after initial polyp removal; if normal, TCE every 5 years
Personal history of curative-intent resection of colorectal cancer	TCE[e]	Within 1 year after resection	If normal, TCE in 3 years; If normal, TCE every 5 years
Colorectal cancer or adenomatous polyps in first-degree relative younger than 60 years or in two or more first-degree relatives of any ages	TCE	Age 40 or 10 years before the youngest case in the family, whichever is earlier	Every 5 years
Colorectal cancer in other relatives (not included above)	As per average risk recommendations (above); may consider beginning screening before age 50 years		
High risk			
Family history of familial adenomatous polyposis	Early surveillance with endoscopy, counseling to consider genetic testing, and referral to a specialty center	Puberty	If genetic test positive or polyposis confirmed, consider colectomy; otherwise, endoscopy every 1–2 years
Family history of hereditary non-polyposis colon cancer	Colonoscopy and counseling to consider genetic testing	21 years	If genetic test positive or if patient has not had genetic testing, colonoscopy every 2 years until age 40 years, then every year
Inflammatory bowel disease	Colonoscopies with biopsies for dysplasia	8 years after the start of pancolitis; 12–15 years after the start of left-sided colitis	Every 1–2 years

[a]Approximately 70–80% of cases are from average risk individuals, approximately 15–20% are from moderate risk individuals and 5–10% are from high risk individuals.
[b]Digital rectal examination should be done at the time of each sigmoidoscopy, colonoscopy or DCBE.
[c]Annual FOBT has been shown to reduce mortality from colorectal cancer, so it is preferable to no screening; however, the ACS recommends that annual FOBT be accompanied by flexible sigmoidoscopy to further reduce the risk of colorectal cancer mortality.
[d]TCE includes either colonoscopy or DCBE. The choice of procedure should depend on the medical status of the patient and the relative quality of the medical examinations available in a specific community. Flexible sigmoidoscopy should be performed in those instances in which the rectosigmoid colon is not well visualized by DCBE. DCBE would be performed when the entire colon has not been adequately evaluated by colonoscopy.
[e]This assumes that a perioperative TCE was done.
DCBE, double contrast barium enema; FOBT, fecal occult blood testing; TCE, total colon examination; ACS, American Cancer Society
Modified from Smith RA et al. *CA Cancer J Clin* 2002;**52**:8–22.

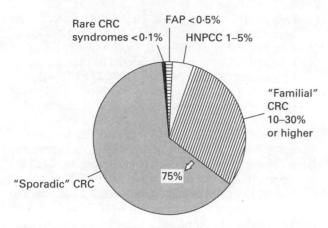

Figure 16.2 Familial causes of colorectal cancer. The rare CRC syndromes include the hamartomatous polyposis conditions and other extremely rare diseases. FAP accounts for about 0·5% of cases and HNPCC for 1–5%. Epidemiological studies suggest that familial CRC outside the well-defined syndromes involves adenomatous polyps and suggest that this proportion is much higher and that familial factors, probably inherited, may be present in the majority of colonic neoplasms. CRC, colorectal cancer; FAP, familial adenomatous polyposis; HNPCC, hereditary non-polyposis colorectal cancer. (Reproduced with permission from Burt RW and Petersen GM. In: *Familial colorectal cancer; diagnosis and management.* London: WB Saunders, 1996[40])

of the entire colon by colonoscopy to complete the diagnostic evaluation for additional polyps. Interval screening, or surveillance, for individuals with a history of adenomatous polyps should be carried out by total colonic examination within 3 years of initial polyp removal. If this evaluation is normal, subsequent examinations can be carried out every 5 years unless the polyp was single and small (less than 1 cm), in which case screening can return to the average risk guidelines.

For persons with a family history of either colorectal cancer or adenomatous polyps in a first-degree relative younger than 60 years of age or in more than one first-degree relative of any age, screening should be carried out by total colonic examination every 5 years beginning at age 40 years or 10 years prior to the index case, whichever is earlier.

High risk screening recommendations

Familial adenomatous polyposis is a hereditary syndrome in which persons expressing the gene develop hundreds of polyps early in life and have nearly 100% probability of developing colorectal cancer. Recommendations for individuals thought to be at risk for this condition include genetic counseling and testing in addition to endoscopic evaluation every 1–2 years beginning at puberty. Because the polyps are distributed throughout the colon, flexible sigmoidoscopy is considered to be as effective as colonoscopy

to monitor for the initial development of polyps. Due to the vast number of polyps that develop in these individuals, it would be impossible to manage these patients by colonoscopic polypectomy. The only feasible preventive strategy at present in this group is colectomy, and the main decision to be made is the timing of this preventive measure. However, chemopreventive strategies are being developed aimed at preventing the development of adenomas or their malignant transformation.[41]

The other major hereditary condition which places an individual in the high risk category is the HNPCC syndrome. Risk for colorectal cancer is increased by 21 years and is very high by 40 years. Individuals suspected of having this syndrome should undergo genetic counseling and testing. Additionally, screening with colonoscopy, necessary because of the proximal distribution of the lesions, should be carried out every 2 years beginning at age 21 and yearly beginning at age 40. Because of the increased risk of endometrial cancer, consideration should be given to screening for this malignancy.

Persons with inflammatory bowel disease, comprising both ulcerative colitis and Crohn's disease of the colon, are at increased risk of developing colorectal cancer and this risk is related to the duration and extent of the disease. Recommendations are to begin screening with colonoscopy and perform random biopsies for dysplasia beginning 8 years after the onset of pancolitis and 15 years after the start of left-sided colitis. While there is no direct evidence demonstrating a reduction in mortality for these individuals with this screening regimen, the rationale is that early detection of dysplasia would result in management, i.e. colectomy, that would lower the risk of developing an invasive cancer.

Cost effectiveness of colorectal cancer screening

Increasingly, decisions about preventive services are being made after due consideration of the cost effectiveness of the screening regimen. Cost analyses of colorectal cancer screening programs have been carried out to provide a basis from which legislation can be influenced and benefit plans can be constructed. While these analyses are limited by the assumptions that were made, they provide a means by which healthcare decisions can be made with the benefit of some economic input.

The cost effectiveness of colorectal cancer screening is estimated to be approximately US$30 000–US$40 000 per year of life gained.[43] This compares favorably with the costs of other preventive services; for example, annual breast screening with mammography would cost approximately US$34 500 per year of life gained. In the analysis by the Congressional Office of Technology Assessment and the National Cancer Institute (USA), it was demonstrated that the cost of missing an early curable cancer, or of failing to prevent cancers, is greater than the cost of screening.[42] As a result of this and other analyses, colorectal cancer screening services are now provided by law in the USA as a Medicare benefit.

In conclusion, there is sufficient evidence supporting the colorectal cancer screening recommendations discussed in this chapter. This evidence arises from both observed mortality reduction and from a calculated economic benefit. It is more cost effective to treat early stage disease and even more cost effective to prevent colorectal cancer than it is to treat it at an advanced stage.

References

1 World Health Organization. *The World Health Report*. Geneva: WHO, 1997.

2 Smith RA, Cokkinides V, von Eschenbach AC *et al.* American Cancer Society guidelines for the early detection of cancer. *CA Cancer J Clin* 2002;**52**:8–22.

3 Bond JH, Levin B. Screening and surveillance for colorectal cancer. *Am J Managed Care* 1998;**4**:H431–7.

4 Winawer SJ, Fletcher RH, Miller L *et al.* Colorectal cancer screening: clinical guidelines and rationale. *Gastroenterology* 1997;**112**:594–642.

5 Atkin WS, Morson BC, Cuzick J. Long-term risk of colorectal cancer after excision of rectosigmoid adenomas. *N Engl J Med* 1992;**326**:658–62.

6 Winawer SJ, Zauber AG, Ho MN *et al.* Prevention of colorectal cancer by colonoscopic polypectomy. The National Polyp Study Workgroup. *N Engl J Med* 1993; **329**:1977–81.

7 Muller AD, Sonnenberg A. Prevention of colorectal cancer by flexible endoscopy and polypectomy. A case–control study of 32 702 veterans. *Ann Intern Med* 1995;**123**: 904–10.

8 Vogelstein B, Fearon ER, Hamilton SR *et al.* Genetic alterations during colorectal tumor development. *N Engl J Med* 1988;**319**:525–32.

9 Jass JR. Pathogenesis of colorectal cancer. *Surg Clin North Am* 2002;**82**:891–904.

10 Simon JB. Occult blood screening for colorectal carcinoma: a critical review. *Gastroenterology* 1985;**88**:820–37.

11 Macrae FA, St.John DJ. Relationship between patterns of bleeding and Hemoccult sensitivity in patients with colorectal cancers and adenomas. *Gastroenterology* 1982; **82**:891–8.

12 Mandel JS, Bond JH, Church TR *et al.* Reducing mortality from colorectal cancer by screening for fecal occult blood. Minnesota Colon Cancer Control Study. *N Engl J Med* 1993;**328**:1365–71.

13 Hardcastle JD, Chamberlain JO, Robinson MHE *et al.* Randomised controlled trial of faecal-occult-blood screening for colorectal cancer. *Lancet* 1996;**348**:1472–7.

14 Kronberg O, Fenger C, Olsen J *et al.* Randomised study of screening for colorectal cancer with faecal-occult-blood test. *Lancet* 1996;**348**:1467–71.

15 Ahlquist DA, Moertel CG, McGill DB. Screening for colorectal cancer [Letter]. *N Engl J Med* 1993;**329**:1351.

16 Lang CA, Ransohoff DF. Fecal occult blood screening for colorectal cancer. Is mortality reduced by chance selection for screening colonoscopy? *JAMA* 1994;**271**:1011–13.

17 Ederer F, Church TR, Mandel JS. Fecal occult blood screening in the Minnesota study: role of chance detection of lesions. *J Natl Cancer Inst* 1997;**89**:1423–8.

18 Towler BP, Irwig L, Glasziou P *et al.* Screening for colorectal cancer using the faecal occult blood test, Hemoccult (Cochrane Review). In: Cochrane Collaboration. *Cochrane Library*, Issue 3. Oxford: Update Software, 2002.

19 Mandel JS, et al. The effect of fecal occult blood screening on the incidence of colorectal cancer. *N Engl J Med* 2000; **343**:1603–07.

20 Levin B, Brooks S, Smith RA, Stone A. Emerging technologies in screening for colorectal cancer: CT colonography, immunochemical fecal occult tests and stool screening using molecular markers. *CA Cancer J Clin* 2003;**53**:44–55.

21 Tedesco JF, Wave JD, Avella JR *et al.* Diagnostic implications of the spatial distribution of colonic mass lesions (polyps and cancers): a prospective colonoscopic study. *Gastrointest Endosc* 1980;**26**:95–7.

22 Shinya H, Wolff WI. Morphology, anatomic distribution and cancer potential of colonic polyps: an analysis of 7000 polyps endoscopically removed. *Ann Surg* 1979;**190**: 679–83.

23 Winawer SJ, Gottlieb LS, Stewart ET *et al.* First progress report of the National Polyp Study. *Gastroenterology* 1983;**84**:1352.

24 Report of the US Preventive Services Task Force. *Guide to clinical preventive services*, *2nd edn.* Baltimore, MD: Williams & Wilkins, 1996.

25 Winawer SJ, Zauber AG, O'Brien MJ *et al.* The National Polyp Study. 1. Design, methods and characteristics of patients with newly diagnosed polyps. The National Polyp Study Workgroup. *Cancer* 1992;**70**(Suppl 5):1236–45.

26 Grossman S, Milos ML, Tekawa IS *et al.* Colonoscopic screening of persons with suspected risk factors for colon cancer. II. Past history of colorectal neoplasms. *Gastroenterology* 1989;**96**:299–306.

27 Tripp MR, Morgan TR, Sampliner RE *et al.* Synchronous neoplasms in patients with diminutive colorectal adenomas. *Cancer* 1987;**60**:1599–603.

28 Selby JV, Friedman GD, Quesenberry CP Jr *et al.* A case–control study of screening sigmoidoscopy and mortality from colorectal cancer. *N Engl J Med* 1992;**326**: 653–7.

29 Newcomb PA, Norfleet RG, Storer BE. Screening sigmoidoscopy and colorectal cancer mortality. *J Natl Cancer Inst* 1992;**84**:1572–5.

30 Selby JV, Friedman GD, Quesenberry CP Jr *et al.* Effect of fecal occult blood testing on mortality from colorectal cancer. A case–control study. *Ann Intern Med* 1993;**118**: 1–6.

31 Flexible Sigmoidoscopy Screening Trial Investigators. Single flexible sigmoidoscopy screening to prevent colorectal

cancer: baseline findings of a UK multicentre randomised trial. *Lancet* 2002;**359**:1291–300.

32 Segnan N, Semone C, Andreoni B *et al.* Baseline findings of the Italian Multi-center randomized control trial of "once-only sigmoidoscopy"-SCORE *J Natl Cancer Inst* 2002;**94**: 1763–72.

33 Rex DK, Weddle RA, Lehman GA *et al.* Flexible sigmoidoscopy plus air contrast barium enema versus colonoscopy for suspected lower gastrointestinal bleeding. *Gastroenterology* 1990;**98**:855–61.

34 Hixson LJ, Femerty MB, Sampliner RE *et al.* Prospective study of the frequency and size distribution of polyps missed by colonoscopy. *J Natl Cancer Inst* 1990;**82**:1769–72.

35 Bernstein MA, Feczko PJ, Halpert RD *et al.* Distribution of colonic polyps: increased incidence of proximal lesions in older patients. *Radiology* 1985;**155**:35–8.

36 Lieberman DA, Weiss DG, Bond JH, Ahnen DJ. Use of colonoscopy to screen asymptomatic adults for colorectal cancer. Veterans Affairs Cooperative Study Group 380. *N Engl J Med* 2000;**343**:162–8.

37 Imperiale TF, Wagner DR, Lin CY, Larkin GN. Risk of advanced proximal neoplasms in asymptomatic adults according to the distal colorectal findings. *N Engl J Med* 2000;**343**:169–74

38 Ferrucci JT. Colon cancer screening with virtual colonoscopy: Promise, polyps, politis. *Am J Roentgenl* 2001;**177**:974–88.

39 Yee J, Akerkar GA, Hung RK *et al.* Colorectal neoplasia: Performance characteristics of CT colonography for detection in 300 patients. *Radiology* 2001;**219**:685–92.

40 Burt RW, Petersen GM. Prevention and early detection of colorectal cancer. In: Young G, Rozen P, Levin B (eds). *Familial colorectal cancer: diagnosis and management.* London: WB Saunders, 1996.

41 Winawer SJ. Surveillance overview. In: Cohen AM, Winawer SJ (eds). *Cancer of the colon, rectum and anus.* New York: McGraw-Hill, 1995.

42 Giardiello FM, Hamilton SR, Krush AJ *et al.* Treatment of colonic and rectal adenomas with sulindac in familial adenomatous polyposis. *N Engl J Med* 1993;**328**:1313–16.

43 Wagner JL, Tunis S, Brown M *et al.* The cost-effectiveness of colorectal cancer screening in average-risk adults. In: Young G, Levin B, Rozen A (eds), *Prevention and early detection of colorectal cancer.* London: WB Saunders, 1996.

17 Irritable bowel syndrome

Albena Halpert, Douglas A Drossman

Introduction

Patients with functional gastrointestinal disorders are commonly seen in medicine. They comprise 12% of patient encounters in primary care practice[1] and 41% of those in a general gastrointestinal practice.[2–4] These patients account for an estimated 2·4–3·5 million physician visits per year in the USA.[5,6] Irritable bowel syndrome (IBS), the most common functional bowel disorder, is characterized by abdominal pain, bloating, and disturbed defecation. Functional gastrointestinal disorders result in significant use of healthcare resources. A recent community-based study showed that subjects with IBS incurred on average annual healthcare costs of US$742 (1992 dollars) compared to US$429 for patients without IBS.[7]

Rationale for symptom-based diagnostic criteria

The first reported account of IBS was published by Powell in 1818.[8] The syndrome remained poorly understood, but recently there has been a substantial increase in research and publications related to this illness.[9] The reasons for the increased interest in IBS include several historical factors. The primary reason is the development of newer investigative techniques. Previously altered motility was considered the underlying pathophysiologic basis for IBS. Early studies, however, did not fully explain pain symptoms. More recent studies have demonstrated the role of visceral hypersensitivity, the involvement of inflammatory mediators and brain–gut interaction.[1,10] Also, the clinical observation that stress exacerbates the symptoms of IBS has led to the hypothesis that there may be a psychophysiological component to the illness. This hypothesis was elaborated and supported by newer technologies such as positron emission tomography (PET) and functional magnetic resonance imaging (MRI) of the brain.[11–13]

Another reason for the increase in research is based on the biopsychosocial model as a framework to elaborate upon biomedical reductionism proposed by George Engel in late 1970s. This framework also provided a model to reconcile the emerging data that were beginning to suggest that the social environment could contribute to the clinical expression of a disease.[14] Engel advocated that illness is the product of biological, psychological, and social subsystems interacting at multiple levels. This framework provided the conceptual basis for understanding gastrointestinal symptoms not easily attributed to specific diseases. Using biopsychosocial research, we recognize that IBS is not caused solely by intestinal dysmotility, but may reflect dysregulation of CNS–enteric nervous system linkages. The phenomenon of enhanced visceral sensitivity may amplify even subthreshold gastrointestinal regulatory input to the brain, and cortical processes may regulate symptom perception either intrinsically or through descending influences on the spinal cord.[1,15]

Finally, diagnostic criteria came to be used to define and classify functional gastrointestinal disorders. The first IBS criteria, described by Manning *et al.*,[16] were identified using discriminate function analysis. Subsequently, efforts emerged to develop diagnostic criteria by international consensus. The first international consensus conference on IBS took place at the 13th International Congress of Gastroenterology in 1988 in Rome.[17] Soon after that, consensus committees developed a classification system referred to as the "Rome Criteria"[18] for 21 functional gastrointestinal disorders. These criteria categorize patients by symptom clusters into five anatomical regions: esophageal, gastroduodenal, bowel, biliary and anorectal. The symptom clusters are based on disturbances in sensory or motor function by target organ. The approach to treatment varies depending on the target organ involved. The Rome Criteria have become the standard for diagnosis of functional gastrointestinal disorders. The latest revised version of the criteria (Rome II) was published in 2000.[19] These criteria are shown in Box 17.1.

Box 17.1 Diagnostic criteria (Rome II Criteria) for irritable bowel syndrome

At least 12 weeks, which need not be consecutive, in the preceding 12 months of abdominal discomfort or pain that has two out of three features:

- Relieved with defecation; and/or
- Onset associated with a change in frequency of stool; and/or
- Onset associated with a change in form (appearance) of stool

Symptoms that cumulatively support the diagnosis of irritable bowel syndrome:

- Abnormal stool frequency (for research purposes "abnormal" may be defined as greater than three bowel movements per day and less than three bowel movements per week)
- Abnormal stool form (lumpy/hard or loose/watery stool)
- Abnormal stool passage (straining, urgency, or feeling of incomplete evacuation)
- Passage of mucus
- Bloating or feeling of abdominal distension

Within the bowel grouping of functional gastrointestinal disorders, IBS is a prototype. In addition, functional abdominal bloating, functional constipation, and functional diarrhea are distinct functional bowel disorders with their own criteria. Chronic or recurrent functional abdominal pain is not considered to be at least entirely a bowel disorder since it occurs independently of known physiological activity in the gut. Diagnosis of each of these syndromes depends on the clinical features, and each syndrome has a unique differential diagnosis. The adoption of multinational symptom-based criteria, particularly for clinical research studies, has increased diagnostic precision, and may lead to a reduction in unnecessary diagnostic studies.

The Rome Criteria for IBS were derived from discriminate function analyses that differentiated patients with the symptoms of IBS from normal subjects or patients with other gastrointestinal disorders.[20] Two factor analysis studies validated Rome II criteria for IBS.[21,22] Palsson *et al.* administered a questionnaire containing 85 questions that corresponded to 17 of the 21 functional gastrointestinal disorders to 895 patients seen at the University of North Carolina gastroenterology clinic.[23] Using principal components factor analysis 13 symptom clusters corresponded to the Rome Criteria functional gastrointestinal diagnoses. Recently, further validation of the Rome Criteria was reported by Vanner *et al.*[24] In this study, 98 patients fulfilling at least one of the Rome Criteria were studied with respect to diagnosis made by application of the criteria versus the gastroenterologist's diagnosis. The latter was considered to be the gold standard. Using the Rome Criteria for diagnosis, there were no false positives and 16 false negatives, giving a sensitivity of 63% and a specificity of 100%. Furthermore, of the 30 true positives, follow up over 2 years showed no errors in diagnosis. The most recent revision of symptom-based diagnosis uses the Rome II criteria.

Epidemiology

Prevalence data

IBS is a common condition in population surveys of adults. The prevalence rate varies depending on the population being surveyed and the nature of the questions used to elicit the information. Many prevalence estimates were drawn from study samples that are not representative of the general population; however, in large population-based studies, such as in those carried out by the National Center for Health Statistics (USA), the functional gastrointestinal disorders are not given a specific diagnostic code, but are categorized into more general codes such as "gastritis" or "unspecified enteritis". The true prevalence of IBS in the population cannot be determined from population-based studies that do not include the symptom criteria for IBS. Five population-based surveys have used Manning and Rome II criteria specific for IBS and these surveys provide the prevalence rates of 14–24% for women and 5–19% for men.[25–29] More recent estimates using the more specific Rome II Criteria yielded rates under 10%.[1]

The first presentation of IBS to the physician usually occurs between the ages of 30 and 50 years, although children also have the illness.[30] The prevalence decreases after 60 years.[25] There is a strong gender difference; the female-to-male prevalence is 2–3:1; in referral centers it is 4–5:1[1]. The data on racial differences are scarce. In the five randomly sampled surveys of American and European adults,[25–29] blacks were underrepresented. One study of culturally diverse American college students,[31] however, showed a prevalence rate in blacks that was similar to whites. The prevalence of IBS may be lower in Hispanics.[32] There are few data that address the prevalence of IBS in non-Western countries. A study of 4178 residents in south China found point prevalence of IBS to be 10·0% if modified Manning criteria were used and 4·9% according to the Rome Criteria, with male-to-female ratio of 1:1·34.[33] Differences may be determined by cultural influences. Available data suggest that IBS is as common in Japan, South America and the Indian subcontinent as it is in Western countries.[9] The symptoms of IBS tend to wax and wane. When the prevalence is examined in the same population at two different time points, the incidence of new cases at the second time point is approximately half of the prevalence noted at the first time point.[25,29] Once the diagnosis of IBS has been made, it is considered to be a chronic disease, and approximately 75% of patients will continue to be symptomatic. In a study of 25 patients with

IBS, symptoms were evaluated over 8 weeks using time series analysis. In these patients, IBS severity was predictable over more than 1 day, and symptoms tended to occur in clusters rather than randomly.[31]

Healthcare utilization

One of the most notable features of patients with IBS is their increased rate of health care utilization. This increase is for both gastrointestinal and non-gastrointestinal illnesses. Patients with IBS have an increased incidence of other chronic diseases, including fibromyalgia, chronic fatigue syndrome, endometriosis, migraine headaches and depression. In one study, patients with fibromyalgia and IBS had poorer health status than those with either disease alone. In the US householder survey,[28] people with IBS had visited physicians for non-gastrointestinal complaints 3·88 times in the previous year. These same people visited a physician for gastro-intestinal complaints 1·64 times. The risk of abdominal surgery is increased in patients with IBS,[34] and women with IBS are three times more likely to undergo a hysterectomy.[35]

A study in England evaluated the healthcare utilization and outcome of 20 female patients with chronic functional abdominal pain, a subgroup of the functional gastrointestinal disorders that is distinct from IBS because of the absence of motility disturbances. In this study, the patients were seen by an average of 5·7 consultants, underwent 6·4 endoscopic or radiological procedures, and had 2·7 major operations.[36] Similarly, patients with IBS have increased pain reporting with anxiety or acute stress. Although it may be assumed that more frequent visits are associated with greater disease activity or physiological dysfunction, several studies have shown that psychological distress and psychosocial disturbance independently influence who will seek health care.[37-41]

IBS is second only to esophageal reflux in its prevalence (15·4 million people) in the USA. It is associated with US$1·6 billion in direct costs, and US$19·2 billion in indirect costs.[42] The prevalence for lower functional bowel disorders approximates that of gastroesophageal reflux if patients suffering from chronic diarrhea (3·5 million) are included.[42]

Prevalence of psychological disturbances

Psychological stress or emotional reactions to stress can affect gastrointestinal function in both normal and IBS patients.[43] Even though the effects of stress on gut function are universal, patients with IBS seem to report more symptoms in response to stress.[44] The role of psychosocial factors in patients with functional gastrointestinal disorders can be summarized as follows: (i) psychological stress exacerbates gastrointestinal symptoms; (ii) psychological distress and other psychological factors affect health status

and clinical outcome; (iii) psychological factors influence which patients consult physicians; and (iv) IBS has psychosocial impact in terms of impaired quality of life.[9]

Most studies suggest that IBS patients report more lifetime and daily stressful events than both medical comparison groups and healthy controls.[37,44,45] In addition, for IBS patients stress is strongly associated with symptom onset.[45-47] Psychological factors that adversely affect health status and clinical outcome include: (i) a history of emotional, sexual or physical abuse[41,48-51]; (ii) stressful life events[47,52]; (iii) chronic social stress[53,53] or anxiety disorder[54,55]; and (iv) maladaptive coping style.[49] Three psychiatric diagnoses are more frequently seen in patients with IBS: anxiety disorders (panic and generalized anxiety disorder), mood disorders (major depression and dysthymic disorder) and somatoform disorders (hypochondriasis and somatization disorder).[56]

The coexistence of a psychiatric disorder with IBS is seen more frequently in referral centers than in the community setting. In a review of the prevalence of psychiatric diagnoses, psychiatric disorder and IBS coexisted in 42–61% of patients seen in gastroenterology clinics.[56] The presence of a psychiatric disorder is even higher in studies from tertiary care centers, when lifetime psychiatric diagnosis is considered.[57] One study examined the difference in the prevalence of psychological disturbances between patients with IBS who had seen a doctor and those who had never seen a doctor and compared them to a control group of subjects without bowel symptoms. They found that people with IBS who do not consult physicians were not psychologically different from normal subjects without the disorder. People with IBS who chose to see doctors had greater psychological disturbances than both "non-consulters" with IBS and controls without bowel symptoms.[37] Thus, the psychological difficulties in IBS relate primarily to patients who see physicians.

Although psychological disturbance is not part of IBS *per se*, it influences health seeking behavior. The increased use of health care by patients with IBS may be influenced by cultural factors, family role modeling, illness behavior, coping mechanisms and the tendency towards somatization. A series of studies[37-40] has shown that individuals who seek care for functional gastrointestinal disorders have more psychological distress, a higher proportion of abnormal personality patterns and greater illness behaviors than those who do not.

Patients with unexplained, severe or refractory symptoms and a high rate of use of health care often have contributing psychosocial factors. Psychosocial stresses, such as a history of physical or sexual abuse, major loss (for example death or divorce) and other major trauma, influence the development of the clinical expression of IBS.[51] The loss of an intimate relationship is closely associated with the onset of symptoms of IBS.[58] In one study, severely stressful life events or chronic social difficulties were associated with the onset of symptoms.[47] Stressful life events also had a significant impact on healthcare visits and disability days.[52]

Additionally, sexual and physical abuse history is more common in IBS patients with severe symptoms, and patients with IBS have more severe history of abuse than patients with structural diagnoses. Drossman *et al.*[41,59–61] reported a prevalence of history of abuse in 44% of patients seen at a gastrointestinal referral center. In another study comparing IBS patients to healthy controls, the prevalence of sexual abuse was 31·6% in the IBS group compared with 7·6% in the controls.[62] A history of abuse does not determine that IBS will necessarily occur, since it is also associated with other chronic syndromes (pelvic pain, headaches, fibromyalgia, bulimia, substance abuse).[63] The significance of a history of abuse relates to the tendency of persons with such a history to communicate psychological distress through physical symptoms. In gastrointestinal patients with history of abuse, there is more severe pain and poorer daily function, three times as many days spent in bed, and 30% more physician visits and surgeries.[41,64]

Over time, the changes in gastrointestinal function that result from stress modify the person's appraisal of bodily symptoms and may lead to unwarranted feelings of lack of control, helplessness or guilt. These factors can produce a chronic state of symptom amplification originating at the CNS (hypervigilance to body sensations) or the gut level (visceral hypersensitivity and conditioned hypermotility). Eventually a vicious cycle of seeking health care, refractoriness and repeated referral may develop.[65]

Finally, maladaptive cognitive strategies such as "catastrophizing" or perceived inability to decrease symptoms can amplify subjective experiences and behaviors leading to poorer clinical outcome[49]; therefore, it is critically important that psychosocial factors be considered and properly addressed by the physician in order to achieve an effective clinical response.

Diagnosis of irritable bowel syndrome

Diagnostic approaches

There is no single diagnostic test that confirms the presence of IBS. Assessment of the pattern of the abdominal pain and abnormal defecation is the cornerstone of diagnosing IBS. Although the exacerbation of gastrointestinal symptoms by stress factors is an important observation in persons with IBS, it is not a diagnostic criterion; however, this observation can be helpful in planning treatment. The Rome Criteria specify that the abdominal pain is associated with change of bowel habits and is relieved by a bowel movement. In addition to obtaining diagnostic criteria the interview process determines the patient's concerns, responds to the patient's expectations, involves the patient in the treatment plan and establishes a long-term relationship with the primary care provider.

Two algorithms for the evaluation of patients with IBS seen in primary care settings have been recently presented.[66] The algorithms are shown in Figures 17.1 and 17.2 and summarized below.[1] In general, if Rome Criteria are fulfilled, "alarm signs" or "red flags" are not present, and screening studies are negative, further testing is not necessary.[67] Rome II Criteria have a sensitivity of 65%, a specificity of 100%, and a positive predictive value of 100% (98% in prospective studies).[24] In addition, patients generally do not require revisions of their diagnosis at 2 years.[24] For screening purposes, a complete blood count and stool hemoccult are recommended. A sedimentation rate (particularly in a young person), serum chemistry, testing of stool for ova and parasites and thyroid stimulating hormone may be added based on symptom pattern and the geographic area. Studies generally do not support a role for these tests without supportive clinical features.[8]

In a research setting, visceral hypersensitivity has been proposed as a biological marker of IBS. Pain thresholds elicited with a rectal barostat appear lower in IBS patients when compared with controls or even functional dyspepsia patients (at 40 mmHg rectal barostat sensitivity to identify IBS patients is 95·5%, specificity is 71·8%, positive and negative predictive values are 85·4% and 90·2% respectively).[69]

Use of diagnostic tests

Patients presenting with typical symptoms and no alarm signs are rarely found to have another diagnosis.[68,70] This observation supports the approach of ongoing care and symptomatic management instead of continued diagnostic evaluation. If initial treatment fails, or certain clinical features requiring further evaluation are present as discussed above, the algorithm outlined in Figure 17.1 may be followed. Many IBS studies are carried out by gastroenterologists in specialty centers. The studies should be targeted toward the predominant symptoms.

Predominant symptom: diarrhea

If diarrhea is present in large amounts, stool volume should be determined. Patients with IBS typically have frequent, but small volume, stools (< 300 ml/day) which does not usually require this type of assessment or additional studies. If large stool volume is present, however, the diarrhea is more physiologically based and stool osmolality and electrolytes can differentiate between osmotic and secretory causes of diarrhea. A laxative screen is often helpful to identify surreptitious laxative abuse. Other tests to consider in patients with diarrhea are a small bowel biopsy for *Giardia lamblia* or sprue, anti-endomysial and antigliadin antibodies (EMA and AGA) for celiac sprue and random colonic biopsy for microscopic colitis. A jejunal biopsy and aspirate may be

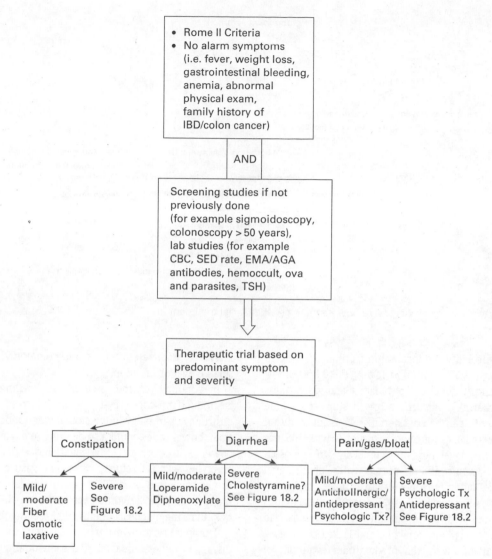

Figure 17.1 Initial evaluation by the gastroenterologist for patients with irritable bowel syndrome.[1] IBD, inflammatory bowel disease; CBC, complete blood count; SED, sedimentation; EMA, anti-endomysial antibody; AGA; anti-gliadin antibody; TSH, thyroid stimulating hormone

done to obtain samples to assess malabsorption or to obtain samples to rule out *Giardia* infection and bacterial overgrowth.

There has been growing evidence and interest in the use of EMA and AGA to diagnose celiac sprue.[67,71–73] The sensitivity and positive predictive values range from 90% to 100%,[74] making the above tests potentially useful for screening; however, in populations in which the prevalence of this disorder is low, there will be many false positive results. Such testing thus must be put into clinical perspective as determined by presence of symptom pattern, ethnicity and other clinical features suggestive of the disease. Upper endoscopy with duodenal biopsy is almost always needed to confirm this diagnosis.[67] There does, however, seem to be a subgroup of patients with latent or potential celiac sprue

among people thought to have IBS. These patients do not have the histopathological findings characteristic of sprue (i.e. villous atrophy or mucosal inflammation) when exposed to a gluten but may respond clinically to a gluten-free diet.[72] Two surrogate markers (HLA-DQ2 alleles DQA1*050/DQB1*0201 and intestinal IgA titer against tissue transglutaminase and/or gliadin), have been proposed in research settings for the diagnosis of sprue in these patients.[72]

Another area of interest in IBS diagnosis has been surrogate laboratory markers such as fecal calprotectin, a calcium-binding protein that can be measured in feces. This protein has been shown to be abnormally elevated in patients with IBD, colorectal carcinoma and non-steroidal enteropathy, but not in those without inflammation (for example IBS). In patients with positive Rome II Criteria and a combination of

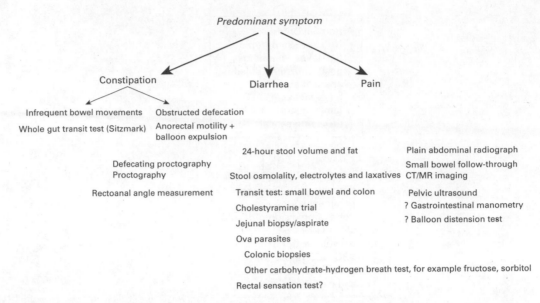

Figure 17.2 Further evaluation of irritable bowel syndrome when initial treatment fails

both normal permeability and fecal calprotectin level, the odd ratio for IBS is 46·1 (95% CI 20·0 to 106·4, $P = 0.0001$).[75]

When postprandial symptoms of bloating and gaseousness accompany the diarrhea, a hydrogen breath study to exclude bacterial overgrowth can be considered.[76] A recent study on prevalence of bacterial overgrowth in patients with IBS has resulted in increased awareness of bacterial overgrowth as an entity that can mimic IBS (reported rates of bacterial overgrowth in IBS and improvement with antibiotic treatment are 73% and 50%, respectively).[76] B4 However, these figures should be regarded with some caution since the study had some limitations, primarily referral bias and lacked controls.

Finally, in patients with the predominant symptom of diarrhea, a therapeutic trial of cholestyramine may also be considered, particularly if the symptoms began and/or worsened following a cholecystectomy.

Predominant symptom: constipation

If constipation is the predominant symptom, a radio-opaque Sitzmark study[77] will determine whole gut transit time for the diagnosis of colonic inertia. Symptoms of dyschezia or incomplete evacuation are evaluated by anorectal manometry or pelvic floor electromyography. A balloon expulsion test or defecography is indicated in cases of possible obstructive defecation. Patients with hypothyroidism or medication-induced constipation should be identified before the diagnosis of IBS is made.

Predominant symptom: pain and bloating

When pain and bloating symptoms predominate, a plain abdominal radiograph can be helpful to exclude aerophagia,

increased stool retention, or less commonly, an overlooked small bowel obstruction.

If vomiting is the predominant symptom, esophago-gastroduodenoscopy (EGD) is useful to diagnose organic obstructive pathology in the stomach or duodenum. A barium small bowel series could also be done to exclude partial small bowel obstruction or other small bowel disease. A gastric emptying scan is useful to determine gastric emptying time. In extreme cases, a small bowel motility study will measure the migrating motor complexes in the small intestine and be helpful in the diagnosis of intestinal pseudo-obstruction.

The impulse to investigate in an effort to rule out organic disease is understandable. The individual symptoms of IBS have a long list of rare causes that can be responsible for that individual symptom. When the symptom is longstanding and previous evaluations have been negative, follow up studies of adults yield specific etiologies in less than 10% of patients.[9] It is important to remember that the individual symptoms of IBS need to be evaluated in the context of the Rome Criteria, with a focus on the psychosocial factors that contribute to the perception and reporting of symptoms. If the diagnosis is in doubt, it is best to re-evaluate the clinical features over one or more visits.

Treatment

Validity of clinical trials

Clinical trials for various therapeutic agents have had several methodological limitations.[1] The validity of clinical trials of interventions for IBS must be evaluated within a framework that recognizes the considerations discussed below.

- *Long-term efficacy of various treatments is unknown.* A wide variety of interventions have been developed to treat patients with IBS, yet most of the relevant clinical trials have been seriously flawed.[78] Since 1966, there have been 58 randomized, double blind, placebo-controlled studies. The trials were generally of short duration, ranging from 3 days to 24 weeks. Only 16 trials evaluated an intervention for 12 weeks or longer. Careful analysis of the duration of response to treatment is important to determine the efficacy of various treatments in IBS.[79]

- *The therapeutic relationship affects prognosis in IBS patients.* The value of the therapeutic relationship is supported by the observation that 30–88% of patients with IBS respond to a placebo in clinical trials.[9] In one retrospective study, the establishment of a long-term relationship with a primary care provider was associated with a reduction in healthcare visits.[80] Reassurance has therapeutic value, since IBS tends to be chronic and characterized by exacerbation and remissions.

- *Recruitment for clinical trials of patients who satisfy the Rome Criteria results in more homogeneous groups of patient.* Patients with IBS tend to fluctuate from one symptom subtype to another, yet patients with diarrhea-predominant IBS are clinically distinct from those with constipation-predominant IBS. Trials that separate IBS patients into symptom subgroups by application of the Rome Criteria are more clinically useful than trials where the patients are lumped into one group. Trials that exclude patients with mild, irregular or intermittent IBS symptoms have a similar advantage.

- *The severity of the IBS also affects prognosis and treatment.* Patients with mild IBS require a different treatment approach than patients with severe symptoms.[1,81] A Functional Bowel Disorder Severity Index has been developed by Drossman *et al.*[82] and has been used by clinicians to rate and stratify patients into mild, moderate or severe categories. One validation study confirmed that patient self-administered rating was highly correlated with a physician severity rating.[82] Another severity index developed by Francis *et al.* incorporated pain, distension, bowel dysfunction and quality of life/global well-being into a severity index.[83] Very few published studies of treatment trials include an analysis of the severity of the disorder in the study population, making the ability to generalize the treatment results uncertain.

- *Treatment trials without a placebo group are not recommended.* This statement is based on the fact that the placebo response rate in patients with IBS may be higher than 70%.[9] Since there is no accepted standard treatment for IBS, all treatment trials of IBS should be placebo controlled.

Outcome measures

Subjective global assessment

A variety of measures have been used to assess efficacy of interventions for IBS.[9] Historically, abdominal pain has been the most commonly employed outcome measure (83% of trials), followed by alternating diarrhea and constipation (50% of trials). This approach seems too simplistic, considering that patients' illness experience, perception and functional status do not always correlate with the amount of pain or number of bowel movements. This discrepancy has lead to the development and use of more global measures of outcome, for the purposes of clinical trials, which reflect patients' overall global well-being, satisfaction with care, and quality of life related to illness.

Currently for the purpose of drug development and outcome measures, the consensus is to use global measures of relief (e.g. "adequate relief" and patient satisfaction) as primary outcomes, as opposed to changes in specific symptoms, such as pain, number of bowel movements, or severity of symptoms.[84]

Symptom-based outcome measures such as abdominal distension and urgency/frequency of bowel movements continue to be used in clinical practice and as secondary outcome measures in clinical trials.

Pain Pain is the most important symptom that predicts physician visits and patient distress[37] in IBS patients. No specific disease measures for IBS exist, and most trials have used standard pain indices to evaluate the response to pain. The Rome Committee has recommended 7–10-step adjectival ordinal scales or a 10-cm visual analog scale to increase sensitivity of the measurement of pain in IBS trials.[9]

Bowel habits A change in bowel habits is a prominent feature of IBS, and patients should be questioned about the form and appearance of their stools. The Bristol Stool Form Scale is the most commonly used instrument in clinical trials, and describes the stool in seven categories ranging from separate, hard lumps (1) to watery (7). This scale has been shown to correlate with transit time in patients with IBS.[85] Stool form alone does not evaluate the other features of disturbed defecation seen in IBS patients. Symptoms often reported by IBS patients include: urgency, unproductive calls to stool, anal pain during defecation, excessive straining at stool, feeling of incomplete evacuation, altered stool frequency and passage of mucus. Measuring defecation symptoms is important, yet no valid objective assessment exists that is reproducible.

Health-related quality of life

The lack of clearly defined structural and biochemical indices for persons with IBS has led to the development of health-related quality of life (QOL) outcome measures. The most commonly used instrument, the IBS-QOL, was developed to evaluate the patient's perceptions, illness experience and functional status. This instrument has 34 questions and assesses dysphoria, interference with activity, body image, health worry, food avoidance, social reaction, sexual function and relationships.[86,87] The internal consistency reliability of the summed score was 0·95, and the intraclass correlation coefficient 0·86.[86] The convergent and discriminate validity of the IBS-QOL was compared with the short form 3b questionnaire and symptom checklist 90 (revised). Correlations were strongest with bodily pain, social functioning, somatization, and obsessive-compulsiveness.[88] Persons with diarrhea-predominant symptoms reported the lowest overall quality of life. Patients with IBS have significantly poorer health-related quality of life (SF-36) than the general population or patients with gastroesophageal reflux disease, and have selected impairments in health-related quality of life relative to patients with diabetes and endstage renal disease.[89] However, the degree of impairment also relates to the population being studied. Quality of life improves in relation to changes in pain severity and daily function after psychological or antidepressant treatment.[87] The IBS-QOL instrument[86] was independently rated the best currently available health-related quality of life instrument for IBS in clinical trials based on a recent panel evaluation of symptom scales and health-related quality of life instruments[90]; furthermore, the adequate relief question appears to be the first choice when assessing global symptom as an outcome in IBS studies. For a more detailed assessment of outcome and quality of life measures in IBS see Bijkerk *et al.*[91]

Approaches to treatment

General approach

Diagnostic and treatment strategies for IBS depend on a biopsychosocial approach that incorporates both physiological and psychosocial information.[15] The first step is determination of the type and severity of the symptoms, followed by adopting individualized treatment plans. Patients with IBS can be classified as diarrhea or constipation predominant, or with mixed or alternating bowel habits. They can also be classified as mild, moderate or severe. These distinctions are based on the nature, frequency and constancy of symptoms, concurrent psychosocial difficulties, recognition of stress and the frequency of use of health care. Table 17.1 provides a practical guide, supported by recent empiric evidence[81] for differentiating patients into subgroups of severity based primarily on patients' pain reports and behaviors.[1,82,92,93] In general, milder symptoms relate primarily to visceral hyperactivity and/or hypersensitivity and are commonly treated symptomatically with pharmacological agents directed at the gut, whereas more severe symptoms are associated with

greater levels of psychosocial difficulties and illness behavior and often require psychological treatments and antidepressant medications. Several factors that predict disease severity among patients with functional bowel disease have been identified.[81] Patients with severe functional bowel disease are characterized by greater depression and psychological functioning, negative health-related quality of life, more maladaptive coping styles and greater health care utilization.[81]

The therapeutic relationship plays an important role in the approach to treatment. Empathy has been shown to be correlated with the patient's evaluation of physician competence, compliance with medical visits, and an overall positive effect on patient's coping. A therapeutic relationship implies a non-judgmental approach, the ability to offer warmth and genuineness, addressing fears, providing explanations and involving the patient in management decisions.[94] When IBS is severe, the therapeutic relationship has been shown to affect outcome by promoting a sense of control or mastery over the symptoms.[95,96] B4

The approach to therapy for the three symptom groups – abdominal pain and bloating, diarrhea and constipation – is very different. Each symptom will be considered individually. In cases where the predominant symptom is not determined, a symptom diary is helpful. The patient is asked to record the time and severity of the symptoms and the presence of associated factors that aggravate or alleviate the symptoms. After 2–3 weeks, the physician can review the diary and consider diet, lifestyle or behavioral modifications with the patient. This approach has the additional benefit of encouraging active patient engagement in the approach to treatment. Many patients take a passive attitude toward their illness and feel that the illness is controlling them. A symptom diary allows patients to feel they are collaborators in their care.

Dietary approach

Lactose restriction

Dietary modification has not been well studied, except for the role of lactose and fiber in patients with IBS. The symptoms of lactose malabsorption are nearly identical to those of IBS. In one study, almost 25% of patients with a diagnosis of IBS had evidence of lactose malabsorption by hydrogen breath tests.[97] In a population-based study, subjective intolerance to lactose and the prevalence of symptoms determined by questionnaire were studied and formal lactose tolerance testing was performed in 580 subjects. In this population, 24% were lactose maldigesters with no known organic gastrointestinal disease. In the population of both lactose maldigesters and lactose digesters, 15% of the subjects met the Rome Criteria for IBS. Using logistic regression analysis, subjective lactose intolerance was strongly associated with IBS with an odds ratio of 4·6 (CI 2·1 to 10·1). The symptoms of IBS tend to improve after a lactose

Table 17.1 Double blind placebo-controlled trials of fiber supplementation in patients with irritable bowel syndrome

Authors	Study type	Grams of fiber daily	Duration (months)	Difference between treatment groups	Symptom response
Soltoft, 1976[98]	Crossover	14·4	1·5	NS	None
Manning, 1977[99]	Parallel group	7·0	1·5	NS	Pain improved
Ornstein, 1981[100]	Crossover	7·0	4	NS	Constipation improved
Longstreth, 1981[101]	Crossover	9·8	2	NS	None
Cann, 1984[102]	Crossover	9·6	1	NS	Constipation improved
Arrfman, 1985[103]	Crossover	9·6	1·5	NS	Constipation improved
Lucey, 1987[104]	Crossover	12·8	3	NS	None
Cook, 1990[105]	Crossover	20	7	NS	Improvement with time, not fiber
Badiali, 1995[106]	Crossover	24	1	NS	Increased transit time with fiber

NS = $P > 0.05$

restricted diet is introduced, but the co-mingling of subjective lactose intolerance and IBS tends to confound the clinical response. Only patients with a positive lactose intolerance test should eliminate lactose from the diet. For patients with subjective lactose intolerance, who fulfill the Rome Criteria for IBS, symptom-based and psychological treatment may be more effective.

One systematic review of the literature[107] identified seven double blind, placebo-controlled clinical trials of dietary exclusion in IBS. Problem foods were identified in 6–58% of cases. Milk, wheat and eggs were most frequently identified to cause symptom exacerbation; of the foods identified, the most common feature was a high salicylate and amines content. Overall, the positive response to an elimination diet ranged from 15% to 67%; however, all the studies had major limitations in their trial designs, including inadequate patient selection, appropriateness of and duration of exclusion diets, and methods of food challenge. There may be a role in using food elimination based on IgG food antibodies in some patients with IBS.[108]

Fiber supplementation

An increase in dietary fiber is recommended for constipation and possibly for constipation-predominant IBS symptoms, but not for those with predominant pain or severe or refractory symptoms. Randomized trials of fiber supplementation in patients with IBS are evaluated in Table 17.2.[109–112] The response rate to added fiber was 31–75% in these trials, while the response rate to placebo was 38–71%. These trials were flawed by inadequate sample size, short duration of treatment (median 8 weeks), ill-defined inclusion criteria, other design flaws, and a high withdrawal rate. Despite these pitfalls, addition of bran to the diet is a very common recommendation of physicians because it is cheap and unlikely to cause harm. Quantitative analysis of the trials

is not possible; however, perusal of the data suggests that the symptoms more likely to benefit from fiber supplementation are the passage of hard stools, constipation and urgency. AId

Approach to abdominal pain

Anticholinergic agents

The most frequently prescribed class of medications for abdominal pain in the USA are anticholinergic agents. The rationale for their use lies in their ability to reduce postprandial colonic motor activity through inhibition of cholinergic receptors. Older anticholinergics inhibit both nicotinic and muscarinic receptors and have been associated with more adverse effects than the newer antimuscarinic agents (hyoscyamine). A recent meta-analysis of smooth muscle relaxants/antispasmodics included 26 randomized controlled trials that studied these preparations in IBS.[113] The analysis showed that these medications were significantly better than placebo for treatment of abdominal pain. In one meta-analysis of smooth muscle relaxants in IBS,[113] five drugs showed efficacy over the placebo: cimetropium bromide, pinaverium bromide, octilium bromide, trimebutine and mebeverine. Other meta-analyses have been published with similar conclusions.[114–116] AIc As noted in these reviews, however, most of all studies had limitations and none of these agents is available in the USA.

Drugs acting on neurotransmitters

Newer agents take advantage of growing knowledge about neuropeptides that act on receptors in the enteric and central nervous systems, the brain–gut axis.

These agents include: 5-hydroxytryptamine (5-HT$_3$), the neurokinins (bradykinin, tachykinins), calcitonin gene-related peptide, and the enkephalins, to name a few. 5-HT$_3$-receptors

Table 17.2 Randomized trials of psychological interventions for irritable bowel syndrome

Authors	Psychological intervention	Treatment effect	Follow up period (months)	Comments
Svedlund, 1983[143]	Psychodynamic	Psychodynamic better	12	Improvement sustained
Whorwell et al., 1984[144]	Hypnotherapy or psychotherapy v placebo	Psychodynamic better	18	Improvement sustained
Bennett and Wilkinson, 1985[138]	CBT v usual care for IBS	Not significant		CBT better for anxiety
Guthrie et al., 1993[140]	Psychodynamic v supportive listening for 12 weeks	Psychodynamic better	12	Reduced number of physician visits
Shaw et al., 1991[142]	CBT v usual IBS care	CBT better than conventional therapy for IBS	12	CBT superior in improvement of psychological and physical symptoms. Improvement sustained
Rumsey, 1991[141]	CBT	Medical better	6	CBT better for depression and anxiety
Corney et al., 1991[139]	CBT or relaxation v standard medical therapy[a] for IBS	CBT better	9	Improvement in GI symptoms correlated with improvement in psychological scores
Boyce et al., 2001[146]	CBT Relaxation	All groups equivalent	10	No difference between groups: CBT v relaxation v standard medical therapy
Heymann-Mönnikes et al., 2000[148]	Multicomponent behavior therapy and conventional medical therapy for IBS v conventional medical therapy	Reduced bowel and psychological symptoms at 6 months follow up	6	Improvement sustained at 6 months follow up. Improved "well being" and improved "control over the illness"
Creed et al., 2001[149]	Interpersonal therapy v SSRI v standard medical therapy	No difference in psychological status or bowel habits at 12 months follow up	6	No difference between treatment groups
Drossman et al., 2003[150]	12-week trial of CBT v education in patients with moderate and severe IBS	CBT was more effective than education (70% v 37%)	12	CBT better than education in patients with moderate to severe IBS

[a]Medical therapy: antispasmodics, general medical therapy.
IBS, irritable bowel syndrome; CBT, cognitive behavioral therapy

are distributed on enteric motor neurons, on peripheral terminals of visceral afferent nerves, and on central locations (vomiting center). Antagonism of these receptors reduces visceral pain, colonic transit and small bowel intestinal secretion.[117] Alosetron hydrochloride, a selective 5-HT_3 antagonist was shown to be effective in relieving pain and normalizing bowel frequency, and reducing urgency in female patients with diarrhea-predominant IBS (absolute risk

reduction 12–15%).[118] Ala It was more effective than placebo for inducing adequate relief of pain and discomfort and improved bowel frequency, consistency and urgency.[118–120] The most common adverse effect is constipation (28%). A serious adverse effect is acute ischemic colitis, estimated to occur in 0·1–1% of patients. The drug was withdrawn from the US market in November 2000 because of this adverse effect, but after further evaluation was re-approved by the

Food and Drug Administration (FDA) in the spring of 2002 under restrictive guidelines. Another 5-HT$_3$ antagonist, cilansetron, has demonstrated similar efficacy in phase II trials[121] and was shown to be effective in male patients, possibly because of the larger number of males studied. Alc

For constipation-predominant IBS, a new partial 5-HT$_4$ agonist is being used. Tegaserod was shown to result in global improvement of IBS symptoms and constipation in females with constipation-predominant IBS.[123] A dosage of 12 mg a day (6 mg PO twice daily) has produced an absolute risk reduction of 10% compared with placebo in females with constipation. Ala Tegaserod appears safe, with no serious adverse effects reported in clinical trials in contrast to other 5-HT$_4$ agonists such as the substituted benzamide (cisapride). Tegaserod was approved by the FDA in July 2002 for females with constipation-predominant IBS symptoms.

Other new treatments being explored include: newer type 3 antimuscarinic agents; NK1- and NK3-receptor antagonists; cholecystokinin antagonists; the α2 adrenergic agonists; clonidine[124]; a 5-HT$_1$ agonist (buspirone)[125]; a selective serotonin reuptake inhibitor (SSRI; citalopram)[126,127]; probiotics; neostigmine; and κ opiates (fedotozine and asimadoline). Narcotic analgesics in the control of abdominal pain are contraindicated as they may lead to narcotic bowel syndrome.[128]

Approach to diarrhea

When the predominant symptom is diarrhea, the opioid derivatives (loperamide and diphenoxylate) may be useful. Loperamide exerts an opioid effect on colonic muscle tone. Diphenoxylate exerts an antisecretory effect at the mucosal level and delays intestinal transit by inhibiting the opiate receptor in the myenteric plexus. Loperamide has been shown to be effective in reducing the number of stools in IBS patients in placebo-controlled clinical trials, Alc but no controlled trials have been performed for diphenoxylate. One recent study suggested that bile acid malabsorption is responsible for 30% of diarrhea-like symptoms in IBS. For patients who have suspected bile acid malabsorption, cholestryamine was an effective treatment in one study reported in abstract form.[129]

As indicated above, alosetron hydrochloride (Lotronex), a selective 5-HT$_3$ antagonist, may be used in diarrhea-predominant IBS under restricted conditions to reduce the risk of ischemic colitis and severe constipation.

Tricyclic antidepressants may also be used for diarrhea (see below).

Approach to constipation

Severe constipation that is unresponsive to fiber supplementation requires more aggressive therapy. Surfactants (ducosate sodium) have been associated with impairment of small intestinal water absorption and disruption of intestinal epithelium. Stimulant laxatives, such as phenolphthalein, cascara, senna and bisacodyl, are not recommended for chronic use. Long-term use of these laxatives have been associated with a "cathartic colon".[130,131] B4 The most effective therapies for severe constipation are osmotic laxatives, colonic lavage with polyethylene glycol (PEG), and bowel retraining. Lactulose and sorbitol have been shown to increase intraluminal bulk and stimulate peristalsis in placebo-controlled trials.[132,133] Ald The use of an oral isotonic solution containing PEG is safe and not associated with net ion absorption or loss. In one randomized placebo-controlled trial, PEG ingestion was associated with an improvement in stool frequency and consistency.[134] Alc Bowel retraining involves sitting on the commode for a distraction free period of 15 or 20 minutes each day without the obligation to perform, in addition to using a high fiber diet and an osmotic laxative. If no bowel movement occurs, an enema every 2–3 days is added to the bowel retraining. An uncontrolled study showed an improvement in bowel regularity using this method in 50–75% of affected children.[135] B4 No controlled clinical trials of bowel retraining have been published for adults with IBS, yet clinical experience has shown an improvement in bowel regularity by this behavioral technique. Tegaserod, a partial 5-HT$_4$ agonist 6 mg twice daily has been shown as indicated above to result in global improvement in symptoms of constipation-predominant IBS in females in a 12-week study and is now approved for the treatment of constipation-predominant IBS patients.[122] Ala The most frequent adverse effect is diarrhea, which seems to subside after the first week of treatment. Subtotal colectomy should be performed only in selected patients with severe colonic inertia, who have failed medical therapy.[136,137] B4

Psychological interventions

Five types of psychological interventions have been studied in the treatment of IBS: relaxation therapy, hypnosis, biofeedback, cognitive behavior therapy (CBT) and psychodynamic therapy. Relaxation methods reduce sympathetic nervous system activity and produce skeletal muscle relaxation. Hypnosis may be effective for IBS by reducing pain perception in the gut.[138] Biofeedback uses audio or visual instruments to reduce skeletal muscle activity. CBT involves identifying stressors recognizing thoughts that increase distress, and learning new ways to cope with stress by restructuring personal reactions to the cause. Interpersonal or brief psychodynamic therapy helps patients to modify interpersonal conflicts that contribute to symptoms. The choice of psychological intervention depends on the ability of the patient to perceive it as part of a treatment plan.

Randomized controlled trials of psychological interventions have typically used conventional pharmacotherapy as the control intervention[138-144] (Table 17.3). There appears to be no difference in outcome based on the specific psychological

Table 17.3 Placebo-controlled trials of tricyclic antidepressants in irritable bowel syndrome

Authors	Treatment	Clinical outcome	Comments
Heefner et al., 1978[152]	Desipramine v placebo	No difference between groups	Combined constipation and diarrhea patients
Greenbaum et al., 1987[153]	Desipramine v placebo	Diarrhea and pain improved with drug	Constipation patients did not improve
Myren et al., 1984[154]	Trimipramine v placebo	Vomiting and mucous content of stool improved on drug	Depression improved on drug
Ritchie and Truelove, 1980[156]	Nortriptyline and fluphenazine	Improved pain and diarrhea on drug	Constipation patients did not improve. No placebo group
Lancaster-Smith et al., 1982[158]	Nortriptyline and fluphenazine v placebo	Improved pain and diarrhea on drug	
Tripathi et al., 1989[157]	Trimipramine v placebo	Improved pain on drug	
Drossman et al., 2003[159]	Desipramine v placebo	Patients on desipramine more satisfied with care in per protocol analysis	Patients who take desipramine are likely to benefit

technique. *Post hoc* subgroup analysis of these studies has identified the patients who are more likely to respond to psychological interventions: (i) Patients who have insight about the role of stressors; (ii) patients who are under 50 years of age; (iii) patients with lower levels of trait anxiety; (iv) patients with a predominant symptom of abdominal pain or diarrhea and not constipation; (v) symptoms that wax and wane (rather than being constant) in response to eating, defecation or stress; (vi) symptoms that are of relatively short duration. Also, it has been postulated that patients who exhibit maladaptive coping styles or cognition (for example "catastrophizing") relating to their symptoms, or perceive an inability to decrease them, may be particularly responsive to CBT.[49] C5

A randomized multicenter trial of 431 IBS patients on desipramine versus placebo and CBT versus education[135] demonstrated that 12 weeks of CBT was more effective than education ($P = 0.0001$). The response rate was 70% versus 37%, and the number of patients needed to be treated (NNT) with CBT to produce one additional response was 3.1. A1a CBT appeared to be less effective in patients with severe depression. Psychological treatment is initially expensive because it requires multiple, long sessions; however its benefits persist or even increase over time.[146] In the long run, there may be a net reduction in clinic visits and healthcare costs[147] which offsets the cost of psychological treatments.

Antidepressant medications

It is now recognized that antidepressants have neuromodulatory and analgesic properties, independent of their psychotropic effect. Antidepressants have been used successfully in other chronic pain syndromes, such as neuropathic pain (60% response rate) and chronic headaches (75% response rate).[151] The analgesic effects are similar in depressed and non-depressed patients.[151] Both tricyclic antidepressants (amitriptyline, imipramine, desipramine) and SSRIs (fluoxetine, sertraline, paroxetine, fluvoxamine) are frequently used to treat patients with IBS. The decision to use the SSRIs versus the tricyclics is based on the specific subgroup of IBS symptoms, and the profile of adverse effects of the particular drug. The patient with diarrhea, nausea, and abdominal pain is a candidate for tricyclic antidepressant therapy, while the SSRIs are more appropriate for the patient with constipation-predominant IBS. A patient with considerable anxiety might do better on an antidepressant that tends to be more sedating, for example, trazadone or doxepin.

Of seven randomized trials of tricyclic antidepressants, six[152-158] showed a significant improvement in symptoms (Table 17.4).[160] The adverse effects profile of the various antidepressants is shown in Table 17.5. In a meta-analysis of randomized controlled trials of tricyclic antidepressants[161] improvement in global gastrointestinal symptoms against placebo was highly significant (OR 4.2, 95% CI 2.3 to 7.9). There was also improvement in standardized pain scores by 0.9 SD (95% CI 0.6 to 1.2). The NNT, the number of patients needed to treat with an antidepressant to yield one improved patient was 3. A1a

A recent large, randomized multicenter trial comparing the clinical outcome of IBS patients treated with desipramine (DES) versus placebo (PLA), and CBT versus education[145] demonstrated that for patients with moderate to severe IBS, desipramine was significantly effective in the per protocol analysis (response of 69% DES v 49% PLA; $P = 0.02$, NNT = 5), but not in the intention to treat analysis.[145] A1c This finding suggests that patients who take the medication as prescribed are likely to benefit.[145] In general, the tricyclic antidepressant doses used were lower than those used to treat major depression, suggesting that the therapeutic effect is largely unrelated to the antidepressant effect.[162] C5

Table 17.4 Antidepressant drugs: effects on CNS receptor sites and adverse effects

	Anticholinergic effect	5-HT receptor uptake	Histaminic effects	Daily dosage range	Adverse effects
Tricyclic antidepressants					
Amitriptyline	++++	+++	++++	50–300 mg	Sedation, orthostasis, dry mouth, constipation
Desipramine	+	+++	+	50–300 mg	Diaphoresis, dry mouth, orthostasis
Doxepin	++	+++	++++	50–300 mg	Sedation, dry mouth
Maprotiline	+	Nil	++++	100–150 mg	Orthostasis, dry mouth, seizure, sedation
Nortriptyline	++	+	++	75–150 mg	Dry mouth
SSRIs					
Fluoxetine	Nil	++++	Nil	10–60 mg	N+V, bruxism, HA, diarrhea
Fluvoxamine	Nil	+++	Nil	50–300 mg	N+V, bruxism, HA, diarrhea
Paroxetine	Nil	++++	Nil	20–60 mg	N+V, bruxism, HA, diarrhea
Sertraline	Nil	++++	Nil	50–200 mg	N+V, bruxism, HA, diarrhea
Comipramine	++++	+++	+	25–250 mg	Sedation
Atypical antidepressants					
Bupropion		Nil	Nil	200–450 mg	Seizures (>450 mg/day), parkinsonian symptoms
Trazodone	Nil	+++	+++	50–600 mg 100–150 mg	Sedation, priapism
Nefazodone	Nil	++	+++	200–600 mg 20–60 mg 50–200 mg	Sedation
Venlafaxine	Nil	+++	Nil	50–200 mg	N+V, diarrhea

N+V, nausea and vomiting; HA, headache; SSRI, selective serotonin reuptake inhibitors; Atypical antidepressants, mixed adrenergic/serotonergic activator (NE/5HT)
Source: Psych Working Team Report for the Rome II Committee (1999)

The use of SSRIs in the therapy of IBS has increased, since up to 30% of patients experience adverse reactions to tricyclic antidepressants. The lower incidence of adverse effects and rapid onset of efficacy with the use of SSRIs provide rationale for their use in IBS; however, there are no randomized controlled trials demonstrating the efficacy of SSRIs in IBS. One case series showed efficacy of fluoxetine in controlling abdominal pain in IBS,[163] but this study was not a randomized controlled trial. B4 A large trial comparing paroxetine to psychotherapy and usual care showed no benefit to the other groups at 12 weeks, but there was reduced cost at 1 year for the group receiving CBT.[164] The prokinetic effects of the SSRIs make them particularly useful in patients with constipation and/or abdominal bloating. Specific agents may be considered. Fluoxetine is an SSRI with a long half-life. If compliance is an issue, citalopram has a low side effect profile and may prove beneficial because of peripheral effects on colonic tone and sensitivity in IBS.[127] Paroxetine, because of its greater anticholinergic effect, may be selected for patients with diarrhea. C5 In addition, there are novel antidepressants such as mirtazapine, which has the potentially beneficial 5-HT_3-receptor blocking effect and is particularly indicated in

patients with insomnia and inability to gain weight. Venlafaxine produces combined serotonin and norepinephrine uptake inhibition and has shown to increase simulated pain thresholds.[165] It has been suggested for treatment of certain naturopathic disorders.[166]

Anxiolytic medications (benzodiazepines or azapirones) have been prescribed for patients with IBS because of the frequent comorbidity of anxiety disorders with IBS.[167] Recently, there is preliminary evidence suggesting that 5-HT_1 agonists like buspirone may have a role in decreasing gastrointestinal symptoms due to their effect on relaxing visceral organs.[125,168] C5 There is also preliminary growing evidence to suggest an augmenting effect of combining psychological treatment with an antidepressant for depression and certain other medical conditions like headache.[169,170] A1a

Prognosis

Functional gastrointestinal disorders differ from other gastrointestinal diseases in that the organic pathology is not well defined. Because there are no biological markers to define IBS, symptom-based criteria have been validated for the diagnosis.[9] Clinical expertise is needed to individualize therapy for these patients. The nature of symptoms, predisposing factors, altered physiology, psychosocial modifiers, and illness behavior all interact to influence clinical decision making and the ultimate prognosis.

IBS is a chronic disease, with over 75% of patients continuing to have fluctuating symptoms. The goal should be judicious use of medical testing, within the atmosphere of an empathetic patient–doctor relationship. Recurrences should be treated by a symptom-based approach, with careful attention to the psychosocial triggers that contribute to exacerbation. In a cohort study reported by Harvey *et al.*,[30] 104 patients with IBS were studied prospectively to determine their prognosis over a 5-year period. The response to treatment was better in men than in women, in patients with predominant constipation rather than with diarrhea, in patients whose symptoms had initially been triggered by an episode of acute diarrhea, and in patients with a relatively short history. With a few simple investigations, sympathetic explanation and appropriate treatment most patients with IBS have a good prognosis.

Conclusion

IBS is one of the most common medical conditions seen in clinical practice. Patients with IBS and other functional gastrointestinal disorders comprise 40% of gastroenterology practice. This illness is responsible for a considerable economic burden because of the high frequency of physician visits and work absenteeism. After consideration of demographic features, the nature of the symptoms and the severity index, only limited investigations to rule out organic disease are indicated. The variety of symptoms, the lack of understanding of the pathophysiology, the complex interaction of the enteric and central nervous systems and their receptors, suggest that no single drug will cure IBS. A strong physician–patient relationship is essential in treating patients with IBS and helps control the use of health care by these patients.

References

1 Drossman DA, Camilleri M, Mayer EA, Whitehead WE. AGA Technical review on irritable bowel syndrome. *Gastroenterology* 2002;**123**:2108–31.

2 Switz DM. What the gastroenterologist does all day. A survey of a state society's practice. *Gastroenterology* 1976;**70**:1048–50.

3 Ferguson A, Sircus W, Eastwood MA. Frequency of "functional" gastrointestinal disorders. *Lancet* 1977;**2**: 613–14.

4 Mitchell CM, Drossman DA. Survey of the AGA membership relating to patients with functional gastrointestinal disorders. *Gastroenterology* 1987;**92**: 1282–4.

5 Sandler R. Epidemiology of irritable bowel syndrome in the United States. *Gastroenterology* 1990;**99**:409–15.

6 Everhart JE, Renault PF. Irritable bowel syndrome in office-based practice in the United States. *Gastroenterology* 1991;**100**:998–1005.

7 Talley NJ, Gabriel SE, Harmsen WS, Zinsmeister AR, Evans RW. Medical costs in community subjects with irritable bowel syndrome. *Gastroenterology* 1995;**109**:1736–41.

8 Powell R. On certain painful afflictions of the intestinal canal. *Med Trans Royal Coll Phys* 1818;**6**:106–17.

9 Drossman DA, Corazziari E, Talley NJ, Thompson WG, Whitehead WE. *Rome II. The Functional Gastrointestinal Disorders. Diagnosis, Pathophysiology and Treatment: A Multinational Consensus.* McLean, Virginia: Degnon Associates, 2000.

10 Mayer EA, Gebhart GF. Basic and clinical aspects of visceral hyperalgesia. *Gastroenterology* 1994;**107**:271–93.

11 Mertz H, Morgan V, Tanner G *et al.* Regional cerebral activation in irritable bowel syndrome and control subjects with painful and nonpainful rectal distension. *Gastroenterology* 2000;**118**:842–8.

12 Drossman DA, Ringel Y, Vogt B *et al.* Alterations of brain activity associated with resolution of emotional distress and pain in a case of severe IBS. *Gastroenterology* 2003;**124**: 754–61.

13 Silverman DHS, Munakata JA, Ennes H, Mandelkern MA, Hoh CK, Mayer EA. Regional cerebral activity in normal and pathologic perception of visceral pain. *Gastroenterology* 1997;**112**:64–72.

14 Engel GL. The need for a new medical model: a challenge for biomedicine. *Science* 1977;**196**:129–36.

15 Drossman DA. Presidential address: gastrointestinal illness and biopsychosocial model. *Psychosom Med* 1998;**60**: 258–67.

16 Manning AP, Thompson WG, Heaton KW, Morris AF. Towards positive diagnosis of the irritable bowel. *BMJ* 1978;**2**:653–4.

17 Thompson WG, Dotevall G, Drossman DA, Heaton KW, Kruis W. Irritable bowel syndrome: Guidelines for the diagnosis. *Gastroenterol Int* 1989;**2**:92–5.

18 Drossman DA, Thompson WG, Talley NJ, Funch-Jensen P, Janssens J, Whitehead WE. Identification of subgroups of functional bowel disorders. *Gastroenterol Int* 1990;**3**: 159–72.

19 Drossman DA, Corazziari E, Talley NJ, Thompson WG, Whitehead WE. Diagnostic criteria for functional gastrointestinal disorders. In: Drossman DA, Corazziari E, Talley NJ, Thompson WG, Whitehead WE, eds. *Rome II. The Functional Gastrointestinal Disorders. Diagnosis, Pathophysiology and Treatment: A Multinational Consensus.* McLean, Virginia: Degnon Associates, 2000.

20 Drossman DA. The functional gastrointestinal disorders and their diagnosis: a coming of age. In: Drossman DA, Richter JE, Talley NJ, Thompson WG, Corazziari E, Whitehead WE,

eds. *The Functional Gastrointestinal Disorders: Diagnosis, Pathophysiology and Treatment.* McLean, Virginia: Degnon Associates, 1994.

21 Whitehead WE, Crowell MD, Bosmajian L *et al.* Existence of irritable bowel syndrome supported by factor analysis of symptoms in two community samples. *Gastroenterology* 1990;**98**:336–40.

22 Talley NJ, Phillips SF, Melton LJ, Wiltgen C, Zinsmeister AR. A patient questionnaire to identify bowel disease. *Ann Intern Med* 1989;**111**:671–4.

23 Palsson OS, Taub E, Cook E III, Burnett CK, McCommons JJ, Whitehead WE. Validation of Rome Criteria for functional gastrointestinal disorders by factor analysis. *Am J Gastroenterol* 91, 2000. 1996. Type: Abstract

24 Vanner SJ, Depew WT, Paterson W *et al.* Predictive value of the Rome Criteria for diagnosing the irritable bowel syndrome. *Am J Gastroenterol* 1999;**94**:2912–7.

25 Kay L, Jorgensen T, Jensen KH. The epidemiology of irritable bowel syndrome in a random population: prevalence, incidence, natural history and risk factors. *J Intern Med* 1994;**236**:23–30.

26 Jones R. Irritable bowel syndrome. *Practitioner* 1991;**235**:811–14.

27 Heaton KW. Epidemiology of irritable bowel syndrome. *Eur J Gastroenterol Hepatol* 1994;**6**:465–9.

28 Drossman DA, Li Z, Andruzzi E *et al.* US Householder Survey of functional gastrointestinal disorders: prevalence, sociodemography and health impact. *Dig Dis Sci* 1993;**38**:1569–80.

29 Talley NJ, O'Keefe EA, Zinsmeister AR, Melton I. Prevalence of gastrointestinal symptoms in the elderly: a population-based study. *Gastroenterology* 1992;**102**:895–901.

30 Harvey RF, Mauad EC, Brown AM. Prognosis in the irritable bowel syndrome: a five-year prospective study. *Lancet* 1987;**I**:963–5.

31 Taub E, Cuevas JL, Cook EW, Crowell M, Whitehead WE. Irritable bowel syndrome defined by factor analysis: Gender and race comparisons. *Dig Dis Sci* 1995;**40**:2647–55.

32 Zuckerman MJ, Guerra LG, Drossman DA, Foland JA, Gregory GG. Comparison of bowel patterns in Hispanics and non-Hispanic whites. *Dig Dis Sci* 1995;**40**:1761–9.

33 Xiong L, Minhu C, Chen H, Xu A, Wang W, Hu P. A population based epidemiologic study of irritable bowel syndrome in South China: stratified randomized study by cluster sampling [Abstract]. *Gastroenterology* 2003;**124**

34 Burns DG. The risk of abdominal surgery in irritable bowel syndrome. *South Afr Med J* 1986;**70**:91.

35 Whitehead WE, Cheskin LJ, Heller BR *et al.* Evidence for exacerbation of irritable bowel syndrome during menses. *Gastroenterology* 1990;**98**:1485–9.

36 Maxton DG, Whorwell PJ. Use of medical resources and attitudes to health care of patients with "chronic abdominal pain". *Br J Med Econ* 1992;**2**:75–9.

37 Drossman DA, McKee DC, Sandler RS *et al.* Psychosocial factors in the irritable bowel syndrome. A multivariate study of patients and nonpatients with irritable bowel syndrome. *Gastroenterology* 1988;**95**:701–8.

38 Smith RC, Greenbaum DS, Vancouver JB *et al.* Psychosocial factors are associated with health care seeking rather than diagnosis in irritable bowel syndrome. *Gastroenterology* 1990;**98**:293–301.

39 Whitehead WE, Bosmajian L, Zonderman AB, Costa PTJr, Schuster MM. Symptoms of psychologic distress associated with irritable bowel syndrome. Comparison of community and medical clinic samples. *Gastroenterology* 1988;**95**:709–14.

40 Drossman DA. Illness behaviour in the irritable bowel syndrome. *Gastroenterol Int* 1991;**4**:77–81.

41 Drossman DA, Li Z, Leserman J, Toomey TC, Hu Y. Health status by gastrointestinal diagnosis and abuse history. *Gastroenterology* 1996;**110**:999–1007.

42 Sandler RS, Everhart JE, Donowitz M *et al.* The burden of selected digestive diseases in the United States. *Gastroenterology* 2002;**122**:1500–11.

43 Holtmann G, Enck P. Stress and gastrointestinal motility in humans: a review of the literature. *J Gastrointest Mot* 1991;**3**:245–54.

44 Drossman DA, Sandler RS, McKee DC, Lovitz AJ. Bowel patterns among subjects not seeking health care. Use of a questionnaire to identify a population with bowel dysfunction. *Gastroenterology* 1982;**83**:529–34.

45 Levy RL, Cain KC, Jarrett M, Heitkemper MM. The relationship between daily life stress and gastrointestinal symptoms in women with irritable bowel syndrome. *J Behav Med* 1997;**20**:177–93.

46 Walker LS, Garber J, Smith CA, Van Slyke DA, Claar RL. The relation of daily stressors to somatic and emotional symptoms in children with and without recurrent abdominal pain. *J Consult Clin Psychol* 2001;**69**:85–91.

47 Creed FH, Craig T, Farmer RG. Functional abdominal pain, psychiatric illness and life events. *Gut* 1988;**29**:235–42.

48 Ali A, Toner BB, Stuckless N *et al.* Emotional abuse, self-blame and self-silencing in women with irritable bowel syndrome. *Psychosom Med* 2000;**62**:76–82.

49 Drossman DA, Li Z, Leserman J, Keefe FJ, Hu YJ, Toomey TC. Effects of coping on health outcome among female patients with gastrointestinal disorders. *Psychosom Med* 2000;**62**:309–17.

50 Talley NJ, Fett SL, Zinsmeister AR, Melton LJ. Gastrointestinal tract symptoms and self-reported abuse: A population-based study. *Gastroenterology* 1994;**107**:1040–9.

51 Drossman DA, Talley NJ, Olden KW, Leserman J, Barreiro MA. Sexual and physical abuse and gastrointestinal illness: review and recommendations. *Ann Intern Med* 1995;**123**:782–94.

52 Whitehead WE, Crowell MD, Robinson JC, Heller BR, Schuster MM. Effects of stressful life events on bowel symptoms: subjects with irritable bowel syndrome compared to subjects without bowel dysfunction. *Gut* 1992;**33**:825–30.

53 Bennett EJ, Tennant CC, Piesse C, Badcock CA, Kellow JE. Level of chronic life stress predicts clinical outcome in irritable bowel syndrome. *Gut* 1998;**43**:256–61.

54 Fowlie S, Eastwood MA, Ford MJ. Irritable bowel syndrome: the influence of psychological factors on the symptom complex. *J Psychosom Res* 1992;**36**:169–73.

55 Blanchard EB, Schwartz SP, Neff DF, Gerardi MA. Prediction of outcome from the self-regulatory treatment of irritable bowel syndrome. *Behav Res Ther* 1988;**26**:187–90.

56 Drossman DA, Creed FH, Olden KW, Svedlund J, Toner BB, Whitehead WE. Psychosocial aspects of the functional gastrointestinal disorders. In: Drossman DA, Corazziari E, Talley NJ, Thompson WG, Whitehead WE, eds. *Rome II. The Functional Gastrointestinal Disorders: Diagnosis, Pathophysiology and Treatment; A Multinational Consensus. Rome II. The Functional Gastrointestinal Disorders. Diagnosis, Pathophysiology and Treatment: A Multinational Consensus.* McLean, Virginia: Degnon Associates, 2000.

57 Walker EA, Gelfand AN, Gelfand MD, Katon WJ. Psychiatric diagnoses, sexual and physical victimization, and disability in patients with irritable bowel syndrome or inflammatory bowel disease. *Psychol Med* 1995;**25**:1259–67.

58 Craig TKJ, Brown GW. Goal frustration and life events in the aetiology of painful gastrointestinal disorder. *J Psychosom Res* 1984;**28**:411–21.

59 Drossman DA, Leserman J, Hu YJB. Gastrointestinal diagnosis, abuse history and effects on health status. *Gastroenterology* 1996;**111**:1159–61.

60 Li Z, Drossman DA, Leserman J, Toomey T, Hu Y. Relationship of a new severity of abuse scale and gastrointestinal diagnosis with daily functional status [Abstract]. *Gastroenterology* 1996;**110**:706.

61 DA, Leserman J, Nachman G *et al.* Sexual and physical abuse in women with functional or organic gastrointestinal disorders. *Ann Intern Med* 1990;**113**:828–33.

62 Delvaux M, Denis P, Allemand H, French Club of Digestive Motility. Sexual and physical abuses are more frequently reported by IBS patients than by patients with organic digestive diseases or controls. Results of a multicenter inquiry. *Euro J Gastroenterol Hepatol* 1997;**9**:345–52.

63 Laws A. Does a history of sexual abuse in childhood play a role in women's medical problems? A review. *J Women's Health* 1993;**2**:165–72.

64 Longstreth GF, Wolde-Tsadik G. Irritable bowel-type symptoms in HMO examinees. Prevalence, demographics, and clinical correlates. *Dig Dis Sci* 1993;**38**:1581–9.

65 Drossman DA. Irritable bowel syndrome and sexual/physical abuse history. *Eur J Gastroenterol Hepatol* 1997;**9**:327–30.

66 Fass R, Longstreth G, Pimentel M *et al.* Evidence- and consensus-based practice guidelines for the diagnosis of irritable bowel syndrome. *Arch Intern Med* 2001;**161**:2081–8.

67 Drossman DA. Irritable bowel syndrome: How far do you go in the workup? *Gastroenterology* 2001;**121**:1512–15.

68 Hamm LR, Sorrells SC, Harding JP *et al.* Additional investigations fail to alter the diagnosis of irritable bowel syndrome in subjects fulfilling the Rome criteria. *Am J Gastroenterol* 1999;**94**:1279–82.

69 Bouin M, Plourde V, Boivin M *et al.* Rectal distention testing in patients with irritable bowel syndrome: sensitivity, specificity, and predictive values of pain sensory thresholds *Gastroenterology* 2002;**122**:1771–7.

70 Tolliver BA, Herrera JL, DiPalma JA. Evaluation of patients who meet clinical criteria for irritable bowel syndrome. *Am J Gastroenterol* 1994;**89**:176–8.

71 Ciclitira PJ. American Gastroenterological Association medical position statement: Celiac sprue. *Gastroenterology* 2001;**120**:1522–5.

72 Wahnschaffe U, Ullrich R, Riecken EO, Schulzke JD. Celiac disease-like abnormalities in a subgroup of patients with irritable bowel syndrome. *Gastroenterology* 2001;**121**: 1329–38.

73 Sanders DS, Carter MJ, Hurlstone DP *et al.* Association of adult coeliac disease with irritable bowel syndrome: a case–control study in patients fulfilling ROME II criteria referred to secondary care. *Lancet* 2001;**358**:1504–8.

74 Ciclitira PJ. AGA technical review on celiac sprue. *Gastroenterology* 2001;**120**:1526–40.

75 Tibble JA, Sigthorsson G, Foster R, Forgacs I, Bjarnason I. The use of surrogate markers of intestinal inflammation and symptom based criteria to distinguish organic from non-organic intestinal disease. *Gastroenterology* 2002;**123**: 450–60.

76 Pimentel M, Chow EJ, Lin HC. Eradication of small intestinal bacterial overgrowth reduces symptoms of irritable bowel syndrome. *Am J Gastroenterol* 2000;**95**:3503–6.

77 Metcalf AM, Phillips SF, Zinsmeister AR, MacCarty RL, Beart RW, Wolff BG. Simplified assessment of segmental colonic transit. *Gastroenterology* 1987;**92**:40–7.

78 Talley NJ, Nyren O, Drossman DA *et al.* The irritable bowel syndrome: toward optimal design of controlled treatment trials. *Gastroenterol Int* 1993;**4**:189–211.

79 Veldhuyzen van Zanten SJO, Talley NJ, Bytzer P, Klein K, Whorwell PJ, Zinsmeister AR. Design of treatment trials for the functional gastrointestinal disorders. In: Drossman DA, Corazziari E, Talley NJ, Thompson WG, Whitehead WE, eds. *Rome II. Functional Gastrointestinal Disorders: Diagnosis, Pathophysiology, and Treatment. A Multinational consensus.* McLean, Virginia: Degnon Associates, 2000.

80 Owens DM, Nelson DK, Talley NJ. Irritable bowel: it helps to have a friendly physician – or so it would seem. *Gastroenterology* 1995;**109**:1711–13.

81 Drossman DA, Whitehead WE, Toner BB *et al.* What determines severity among patients with painful functional bowel disorders? *Am J Gastroenterol* 2000;**95**:974–80.

82 Drossman DA, Li Z, Toner BB *et al.* Functional bowel disorders: a multicenter comparison of health status, and development of illness severity index. *Dig Dis Sci* 1995;**40**:986–95.

83 Francis CY, Morris J, Whorwell PJ. The irritable bowel severity scoring system: a simple method of monitoring irritable bowel syndrome and its progress. *Aliment Pharmacol Ther* 1997;**11**:395–402.

84 Mangel A, Hahn B, Heath A *et al.* Adequate relief as an endpoint in clinical trials in irritable bowel syndrome [Abstract]. *Gastroenterology* 1998;**14**.

85 Heaton KW, Ghosh S, Braddon FEM. How bad are the symptoms and bowel dysfunction of patients with the irritable bowel syndrome? A prospective, controlled study with emphasis on stool form. *Gut* 1991;**32**:73–9.

86 Patrick DL, Drossman DA, Frederick IO, DiCesare J, Puder KL. Quality of life in persons with irritable bowel syndrome: development of a new measure. *Dig Dis Sci* 1998;**43**: 400–11.

87 Drossman DA, Patrick DL, Whitehead WE, Toner BB, Diamant NE, Hu YJB *et al.* Further validation of the IBS-QOL: A disease specific quality of life questionnaire. *Am J Gastoenterology* 2000;**95**:999–1007.

88 Patrick DL, Drossman DA, Frederick IO. A quality of life measure for persons with irritable bowel syndrome (IBS-QOL). User's manual and scoring diskette. Seattle: University of Washington, 1997.

89 Gralnek IM, Hays RD, Kilbourne A, Naliboff B, Mayer E. The impact of irritable bowel syndrome on health-related quality of life. *Gastroenterology* 2000;**119**:655–60.

90 Bijkerk CJ, de Wit NJ, Muris JW, Jones RH, Knottnerus JA, Hoes AW. Outcome measures in irritable bowel syndrome: comparison of psychometric and methodological characteristics. *Am J Gastroenterol* 2003;**98**:122–7.

91 Bijkerk CJ, de Wit NJ, Muris JW, Jones RH, Knottnerus JA, Hoes AW. Outcome measures in irritable bowel syndrome: comparison of psychometric and methodological characteristics. *Am J Gastroenterol* 2003;**98**:122–7.

92 Sperber AD, Carmel S, Atzmon Y *et al.* Use of the Functional Bowel Disorder Severity Index (FBDSI) in a study of patients with the irritable bowel syndrome and fibromyalgia. *Am J Gastroenterol* 2000;**95**:995–8.

93 Shapiro MS, Olden KW. Symptom expression in pain-predominant functional bowel syndrome: is visceral hyperalgesia the whole truth? *Am J Gastroenterol* 2000; **95**:862–3.

94 Lipkin M Jr. The medical interview and related skills. In: Branch WT, ed. *Office Practice of Medicine*. Philadelphia: WB Saunders, 1994.

95 Drossman DA. Diagnosing and treating patients with refractory functional gastrointestinal disorders. *Ann Intern Med* 1995;**123**:688–97.

96 Drossman DA, Creed FH, Fava GA *et al.* Psychosocial aspects of the functional gastrointestinal disorders. *Gastroenterol Int* 1995;**8**:47–90.

97 Bohmer CJ, Tuynman HA. The clinical relevance of lactose malabsorption in irritable bowel syndrome. *Eur J Gastroenterol Hepatol* 1996;**8**:1013–16.

98 Soltoft J, Gudmund-Hoyer AG, Krag B *et al.* A double-blind trial of the effects of wheat bran on symptoms of irritable bowel syndrome. *Lancet* 1976;**i**:270–2.

99 Manning AP, Heaton KW, Harvey RF *et al.* Wheat bran and irritable bowel syndrome. *Lancet* 1977;**ii**:417–18.

100 Ornstein MH, Littlewood ER, Baird IM *et al.* Are fibre supplements really necessary in diverticular disease of the colon? Controlled clinical trial. *Br Med J* 1981;**282**: 1353–6.

101 Longstreth GF, Fox DD, Youkeles L *et al.* Psyllium therapy in the irritable bowel syndrome. A double-blind trial. *Ann Intern Med* 1981;**95**:53–6.

102 Cann PA, Read NWH, Holdsworth CD. What is the benefit of coarse bran in patients with irritable bowel syndrome? *Gut* 1984;**25**:168–71.

103 Arrfman S, Andersen JR, Hegnoj J *et al.* The effect of coarse wheat bran in the irritable bowel syndrome. A double-blind cross-over study. *Scand J Gastroenterol* 1985;**20**:295–8.

104 Lucey MR, Clark ML, Lowndes JO *et al.* Is bran efficacious in irritable bowel syndrome? A double-blind placebo-controlled study. *Gut* 1987;**21**:221–5.

105 Cook IJ, Irvine EJ, Campbell D *et al.* Effect of dietary fiber on symptoms and rectosigmoid motility in patients with irritable bowel syndrome. A controlled crossover study. *Gastroenterology* 1990;**98**(1):66–72.

106 Badiali D, Corazziari E, Habib FI *et al.* Effect of wheat bran in treatment of chronic nonorganic constipation. A double-blind controlled trial. *Dig Dis Sci* 1995;**40**(2):349–56.

107 Niec AM, Frankum B, Talley NJ. Are adverse food reactions linked to irritable bowel syndrome? *Am J Gastroenterol* 1998;**93**:2184–90.

108 Atkinson W, Gurney R, Sheldon TA, Whorwell PJ. Do food elimination diets improve irritable bowel syndrome? A double blind trial based on IgG antibodies to food [Abstract]. *Gastroenterology* 2003;**124**.

109 Longstreth GF, Fox DD, Youkeles L, Forsythe AB, Wolochow DA. Psyllium therapy in the irritable bowel syndrome. *Ann Intern Med* 1981;**95**:53–6.

110 Cann PA, Read NW, Holdsworth CO. What is the benefit of coarse wheat bran in patients with irritable bowel syndrome? *Gut* 1984;**25**:168–73.

111 Lucey MR, Clark ML, Lowndes J, Dawson AM. Is bran efficacious in irritable bowel syndrome? A double-blind placebo-controlled crossover study. *Gut* 1987;**28**:221–5.

112 Cook IJ, Irvine EJ, Campbell D, Shannon S, Reddy SN, Collins SM. Effect of dietary fiber on symptoms and rectosigmoid motility in patients with irritable bowel syndrome. *Gastroenterology* 1990;**98**:66–72.

113 Poynard T, Naveau S, Mory B, Chaput JC. Meta-analysis of smooth muscle relaxants in the treatment of irritable bowel syndrome. *Aliment Pharmacol Ther* 1994;**8**:499–510.

114 Poynard T, Regimbeau C, Benhamou Y. Meta-analysis of smooth muscle relaxants in the treatment of irritable bowel syndrome. *Aliment Pharmacol Ther* 2001;**15**: 355–61.

115 Jailwala J, Imperiale TF, Kroenke K. Pharmacologic treatment of the irritable bowel syndrome: A systematic review of randomized, controlled trials. *Ann Intern Med* 2000;**133**:136–47.

116 Akehurst R, Kaltenthaler E. Treatment of irritable bowel syndrome: a review of randomised controlled trials. *Gut* 2001;**48**:272–82.

117 Kozlowski CM, Green A, Grundy D, Boissonade FM, Bountra C. The 5-HT$_3$ receptor antagonist alosetron inhibits the colorectal distention induced depressor response and spinal *c-fos* expression in the anaesthetized rat. *Gut* 2000;**46**:474–80.

118 Camilleri M, Northcutt AR, Kong S, Dukes GE, McSorley D, Mangel AW. Efficacy and safety of alosetron in women with irritable bowel syndrome: a randomised, placebo-controlled trial. *Lancet* 2000;**355**:1035–40.

119 Bardhan KD, Bodemar G, Geldof H *et al.* A double-blind, randomized, placebo-contolled dose-ranging study to

evaluate the efficacy of alosetron in the treatment of irritable bowel syndrome. *Aliment Pharmacol Ther* 2000; **14**:23–34.

120 Mangel AW, Camilleri M, Chey WY *et al.* Alosetron, a 5-HT$_3$ receptor antagonist, in the treatment of non-constipated female IBS patients [Abstract]. *Am J Gastroenterol* 1999;**94**:2677.

121 Caras S, Krause G, Biesheuvel E, Steinborn C. Cilansetron shows efficacy in male and female non-constipated patients with irritable bowel syndrome in a United States study [Abstract]. *Gastroenterology* 2001;**120**:A217.

122 Mueller-Lissner S, Fumagalli I, Bardhan KD *et al.* Tegaserod, a 5-HT4 receptor partial agonist, relieves key symptoms of irritable bowel syndrome. *Gastroenterology* [Abstract] 2000;**118**:A175.

123 Muller-Lissner SA, Fumagalli I, Bardhan KD *et al.* Tegaserod, a 5-HT$_4$ receptor partial agonist, relieves symptoms in irritable bowel syndrome patients with abdominal pain, bloating and constipation. *Aliment Pharmacol Ther* 2001;**15**:1655–66.

124 Camilleri M, Kim DY, McKinzie S *et al.* A randomized, controlled exploratory study of clonidine in diarrhea-predominant irritable bowel syndrome. *Clinical Gastroenterol Hepatol* 2003;**1**:111–21.

125 Tack J, Piessevaux H, Coulie B, Fischler B, De Gucht V, Janssens J. A placebo-controlled trial of buspirone, a fundus-relaxing drug, in functional dyspepsia: effect on symptoms and gastric sensory and motor function [Abstract]. *Gastroenterology* 1999;**116**:A325.

126 Tack JF, Vos R, Broekaert D, Fischler B, Janssens J. Influence of citalopram, a selective serotonin reuptake inhibitor, on colonic tone and sensitivity in man [Abstract]. *Gastroenterology* 2000;**118**:A175.

127 Broekaert D, Vos R, Gevers AM *et al.* A double-blind randomised placebo-controlled crossover trial of citalopram, a selective 5-hydroxytryptamine reuptake inhibitor, in irritable bowel syndrome [Abstract]. *Gastroenterology* 2001;**120**:A641.

128 Sandgren JE, McPhee MS, Greenberger NJ. Narcotic bowel syndrome treated with clonidine. *Ann Intern Med* 1984;**101**:331–4.

129 Smith M, Cherian P, Raju GS, Mahon S, Bardhan K. Bile acid malabsorption (BAM)-related diarrhea: common, easily diagnosed and treatable. [Abstract]. *Gastroenterology* 1998;(Suppl.):90170.

130 Smith B. Effect of irritant purgatives on the myenteric plexus in man and the mouse. *Gut* 1968;**9**:139.

131 Cummings JH, Sladen GE, James OFW, Sarner M, Misiewicz JJ. Laxative-induced diarrhoea: a continuing clinical problem. *BMJ* 1974;537–41.

132 Lederle FA, Busch DL, Mattox KM, West MJ, Aske DM. Cost-effective treatment of constipation in the elderly: a randomized double-blind comparison of sorbitol and lactulose. *Am J Med* 1990;**89**:597–601.

133 Lederle FA, Busch DL, Mattox KM, West MJ, Aske DM. Cost-effective treatment of constipation in the elderly: a randomized double-blind comparison of sorbitol and lactulose. *Am J Med* 1990;**89**:597–601.

134 Andorsky RI, Goldner F. Colonic lavage solution (polyethylene glycol electrolyte lavage solution) as a treatment for chronic constipation: A double-blind, placebo-controlled study. *Am J Gastroenterol* 1990;**85**: 261–5.

135 Sarahan T, Weintraub WH, Coran AG, Wesley JR. The successful management of chronic constipation in infants and children. *J Pediatr Surg* 1982;**17**:171–4.

136 Leon SH, Krishnamurthy S, Schuffler MD. Subtotal colectomy for severe idiopathic constipation: a follow up study of 13 patients. *Dig Dis Sci* 1987;**32**:1249–54.

137 Gasslander T, Larsson J, Wetterfors J. Experience of surgical treatment for chronic idiopathic constipation. *Acta Chir Scand* 1987;**153**:553–5.

138 Bennett P, Wilkinson S. A comparison of psychological and medical treatment of the irritable bowel syndrome. *Br J Clin Psychol* 1985;**24**:215–16.

139 Corney RH, Stanton R, Newell R, Clare A, Fairclough P. Behavioural psychotherapy in the treatment of irritable bowel syndrome. *J Psychosom Res* 1991;**35**: 461–9.

140 Guthrie E, Creed F, Dawson D, Tomenson B. A randomised controlled trial of psychotherapy in patients with refractory irritable bowel syndrome. *Br J Psychiatry* 1993;**163**:315–21.

141 Rumsey N. Group stress management programmes v pharmacological treatment in the treatment of the irritable bowel syndrome. In: Heaton KW, Creed F, Goeting NLM, eds. *Current Approaches Towards Confident Management of Irritable Bowel Syndrome*. Lyme Regis: Lyme Regis Printing Company, 1991.

142 Shaw G, Srivastava ED, Sadlier M, Swann P, James JY, Rhodes J. Stress management for irritable bowel syndrome: a controlled trial. *Digestion* 1991;**50**:36–42.

143 Svedlund J. Psychotherapy in irritable bowel syndrome: a controlled outcome study. *Acta Psychiatr Scand* 1983;**67**(Suppl 306):1–86.

144 Whorwell PJ, Prior A, Faragher EB. Controlled trial of hypnotherapy in the treatment of severe refractory irritable bowel syndrome. *Lancet* 1984;**2**:1232–3.

145 Drossman DA, Toner BB, Whitehead WE *et al.* Cognitive-behavioral therapy vs. education and desipramine vs. placebo for moderate to severe functional bowel disorder. *Gastroenterology.* 2003;**125**:19–31.

146 Boyce PM, Talley NJ, Koloski NA, Balaam B, Nandurkar S. A randomized controlled trial of cognitive behavioural therapy, relaxation therapy and routine medical care for irritable bowel syndrome (IBS) [Abstract]. *Gastroenterology* 2001;**120**:A115.

147 Creed F, Ratcliffe J, Fernandez L *et al.* Health-related quality of life and health care costs in severe, refractory irritable bowel syndrome. *Ann Intern Med* 2001;**134**: 860–8.

148 Heymann-Mönnikes I, Arnold R *et al.* The combination of medical treatment plus multicomponent behavioral therapy is superior to medical treatment alone in the therapy of irritable bowel syndrome. *Am J Gasteroenterol* 2000;**95**:981–94.

149 Creed FH, Fernandes L, Guthrie E *et al.* The cost-effectiveness of psychotherapy and SSRI antidepressants for

severe irritable bowel syndrome [Abstract]. *Gastroenterology* 2001;**120**:A115.

150 Drossman DA, Toner BB, Whitehead WE *et al.* A multi-center randomized trial of cognitive-behavioral treatment (cbt) vs. education (edu) in moderate to severe functional bowel disorder (fbd). [Abstract] *Gastroenterology* 2003: **124**:A-530.

151 Egbunike IG, Chaffee BJ. Antidepressants in the management of chronic pain syndromes. *Pharmacotherapy* 1990;**10**:262–70.

152 Heefner JD, Wilder RM, Wilson JD. Irritable colon and depression. *Psychosomatics* 1978;**19**:540–7.

153 Greenbaum DS, Mayle JE, Vanegeren LE *et al.* The effects of desipramine on IBS compared with atropine and placebo. *Dig Dis Sci* 1987;**32**:257–66.

154 Myren J, Lovland B, Larssen S-E, Larsen S. A double-blind study of the effect of trimipramine in patients with the irritable bowel syndrome. *Scand J Gastroenterol* 1984;**19**:835–43.

155 Myren J, Groth H, Larssen SE, Larsen S. The effect of trimipramine in patients with the irritable bowel syndrome. *Scand J Gastroenterol* 1982;**17**:871–5.

156 Ritchie JA, Truelove SC. Comparison of various treatments for irritable bowel syndrome. *BMJ* 1980;**281**:1317–19.

157 Tripathi BM, Misra NP, Gupta AK. Evaluation of tricyclic compound (trimipramine) vis-a-vis placebo in irritable bowel syndrome. (Double-blind randomized study). *J Assoc Phys India* 1989;**31**:201–3.

158 Lancaster-Smith MJ, Prout BJ, Pinto T, Anderson JA, Schiff AA. Influence of drug treatment on the irritable bowel syndrome and its interaction with psychoneurotic morbidity. *Acta Psychiatr Scand* 1982;**66**:33–41.

159 Drossman DA, Toner BB, Whitehead WE *et al.* A multi-center randomized trial of desipramine (des) vs. placebo (pla) in moderate to severe functional bowel disorder (fbd) [Abstract]. *Gastroenterology* 2003;**124**:A-30.

160 Cannon RO, Quyyumi AA, Mincemoyer R *et al.* Imipramine in patients with chest pain despite normal coronary angiograms. *New Engl J Med* 1994;**20**:1411–17.

161 Jackson JL, O'Malley PG, Tomkins G, Balden E, Santoro J, Kroenke K. Treatment of functional gastrointestinal disorders with anti-depressants: a meta-analysis. *Am J Med* 2000;**108**:65–72.

162 Halpert AD, Dalton CB, Diamant N *et al.* Is clinical response to tricyclic antidepressants in functional bowel disorders related to dosage? *Gastroenterology* [Abstract] 2003;**124**:A-223.

163 Eisendrath SJ, Kodama KT. Fluoxetine management of chronic abdominal pain. *Psychosomatics* 1992;**33**:229.

164 Creed F, Fernandes L, Guthrie E *et al.* The cost-effectiveness of psychotherapy and paroxetine for severe irritable bowel syndrome. *Gastroenterology* 2003;**124**:303–17.

165 Enggaard TP, Klitgaard NA, Gram LF, Arendt-Nielsen L, Sindrup SH. Specific effect of venlafaxine on single and repetitive experimental painful stimuli in humans. *Clin Pharmacol Ther* 2001;**69**:245–51.

166 Pernia A, Micó JA, Calderón E, Torres LM. Venlafaxine for the treatment of neuropathic pain. *J Pain Symptom Manage* 2000;**19**:408–10.

167 Lydiard RB, Falsetti SA. Experience with anxiety and depression treatment studies: implications for designing irritable bowel syndrome clinical trials. *Am J Med* 1999;**107**:65S-73S.

168 Tack J, Piessevaux H, Coulie B, Caenepeel P, Janssens J. Role of impaired gastric accommodation to a meal in functional dyspepsia. *Gastroenterology* 1998;**115**:1346–52.

169 Keller MB, McCullough JP, Klein DN *et al.* A comparison of nefazodone, the cognitive behavioral-analysis system of psychotherapy, and their combination for the treatment of chronic depression. *N Engl J Med* 2000;**342**:1462–70.

170 Holroyd KA, O'Donnell FJ, Stensland J, Lipchik GL, Cordingley GE, Carlson BW. Management of chronic tension-type headache with tricyclic antidepressant medication, stress management therapy, and their combination: a randomized controlled trial. *JAMA* 2001;**285**:2208–15.

18 Clostridium difficile disease

Lynne V McFarland, Christina M Surawicz

Introduction

Clostridium difficile-associated disease (CDAD) has been described in the literature since the early 1980s.[1,2] Although important work has been accomplished on the epidemiology, clinical diagnosis and control of hospital outbreaks, CDAD continues to persist as a leading cause of nosocomial gastrointestinal illness.[3–7] In addition, other forms of CDAD have become recognized which include recurrent CDAD, toxic megacolon, *C. difficile*-associated arthritis and septicemia.[8–14] These forms occur sporadically and may cause significant clinical problems for patients and a challenge for healthcare providers. Vancomycin and metronidazole are effective for the treatment of the first episode (initial CDAD). However, from 10% to 24% of patients with primary CDAD have at least one recurrence after the first antibiotic treatment is discontinued. Recurrent CDAD may occur intermittently over several years despite treatment.[15–18] The objectives of this chapter are to describe the epidemiology, diagnosis, evidence-based treatment strategies and guidelines for prevention of initial and recurrent CDAD.

Epidemiology

Incidence/prevalence

The prevalence of CDAD ranges from 0·15% to 10% in hospitalized patients during non-outbreak situations and increases to 16–29% during hospital outbreaks.[4,19–23] The prevalence of community-acquired CDAD is 7·7–12 per 100 000 person years.[24,25]

Nosocomial outbreaks

Documented hospital outbreaks due to *C. difficile* were initially described in the 1980s and have been reported in hospitals and long-term care facilities around the world with increasing frequency.[4,26–32] CDAD continues to be the leading cause of nosocomial gastrointestinal disease in adult patients.[33]

A variety of patient populations has been shown to be susceptible to nosocomial CDAD. Outbreaks or nosocomial acquisition have occurred in patients in general medicine wards,[4,5] in surgical wards,[34,35] and in long-term care facilities,[36,37] in elderly patients,[38–40] pediatric patients,[41–43] in patients immunocompromised by human immunodeficiency virus infection,[30,44] by cancer,[45] or by transplantation,[46] and, less commonly, in new mothers.[47]

Strain typing techniques have been valuable tools to track the routes of transmission during hospital outbreaks and also to document that hospitals may harbor both endemic and epidemic strains of *C. difficile*.[4,27,48] Strain typing of isolates from hospitalized patients has also shown that half of clinical recurrences may be reinfections with different strains of *C. difficile*, adding support to the importance of nosocomial acquisition of new strains.[17,49]

Nosocomial transmission

Transmission within the hospital has been shown to be largely due to horizontal transmission via environmental surface contamination, hand carriage by hospital personnel and infected roommates.[4,27,31,32,50–52] In a cohort of 3500 patients, a multivariate analysis found that physical proximity to a patient with CDAD significantly increased the risk of CDAD (RR 1·86, 95% CI 1·06 to 3·28).[51] New admissions who are *C. difficile* positive have been shown to be a source of infection for susceptible patients.[53] In a prospective study of 428 patients admitted to one general medicine ward, a multivariate analysis documented that the risk of nosocomial acquisition of *C. difficile* was significantly higher (RR 1·73, 95% CI 1·15 to 2·55) after exposure to an infected roommate.[4]

Complications

Complications of recurrent CDAD in one study included repeated hospitalizations for cases of severe recurrences (three hospitalizations of 100 patients), development of toxic megacolon (0·5 of 100), septicemia (0·5 of 100) and

C difficile-associated arthritis (0·5 of 100).[16] In addition to the types of complications above, *C. difficile* septicemia and acute abdomen have been associated with cases of primary CDAD, but the rates of these complications have not been reported.[8–10,13,54–56]

Costs

Studies of patients with CDAD have shown that the cost of medical care associated with CDAD cases ranges from US$2000–6000 per patient.[56–58] Recurrent CDAD has a higher impact on the medical care system due to the high costs of medical care, rehospitalizations for severe cases of recurrent episodes, and complications (toxic megacolon, septicemia, arthritis). In one study of 209 patients with recurrent CDAD, the total lifetime cost for direct medical expenses (including all prior episodes, enrollment episodes and prospective recurrences) totaled US$2 292 856, or an average of US$10 970 per person.[16] The average cost of diagnosis and treatment for episodes other than the enrollment episode was US$3103 per patient. These costs do not include lost time from work, costs of complications, additional clinic visits or any indirect costs.

In one prospective study, the average length of stay for a hospitalization due to a CDAD recurrence was 8·8 ± 8·6 days (ranging from 3 to 26 days).[16] Other studies have documented that CDAD extends hospital stays for hospitalized patients from 4 to 36 days.[40,57–60]

Risk factors

Risk factors for primary CDAD usually involve factors in one of three general areas: (i) factors that disrupt normal colonic flora, such as broad spectrum antibiotics or surgery, (ii) host factors, such as age, sex, diet, immune status, concurrent medical conditions or diseases such as cancer, transplantation, other gastrointestinal conditions, or coinfection with other enteric pathogens, and (iii) exposure to the organism, usually through admission to a hospital with endemic *C. difficile* or admission when an outbreak is occurring.

The normal colonic microflora has been shown to be protective of colonization by *C. difficile* through a multifocal mechanism known as colonization resistance. This complex interaction of the intestinal microflora produces a wide variety of protective effects that may include spatial interference, attachment inhibition, production of bacteriocins, production of toxin degrading proteases and stimulation of immunoglobulins that act as a barrier to the colonization of newly introduced pathogens.[61] Factors that disrupt this colonization resistance, such as exposure to antibiotics, surgery or medications, have been shown in epidemiologic studies to increase the risk of CDAD. Exposure to broad spectrum antibiotics is the strongest risk factor

associated with CDAD, but narrow spectrum antibiotics have also been implicated. Neither the dose nor the total duration of antibiotic therapy seems to be correlated with the risk of acquiring CDAD.[7,30,34,36,39,40,51,57,59,62–67] Gastrointestinal surgery or manipulation and nasogastric tube feeding have also been shown to be significant risk factors for CDAD in epidemiologic studies.[36,59,62–64]

Several host factors have also been shown to be significant risk factors for CDAD including increasing age,[16,18,39,57,62,63] female sex,[34,57] serious underlying illness and the presence of other concurrent disease.[16,36,39,62,63,65,68] Long stay in a hospital has been shown to increase the risk of *C. difficile* acquisition.[46,62,63,65] Brown *et al.* compared 37 hospitalized patients with cytotoxin positive CDAD with 37 hospitalized patients without CDAD and used multivariate analysis to show that age over 65 years (OR 14·1, 95% CI 1·4 to 141), stay in an intensive care unit (OR 39·2, 95% CI 2·2 to 713), gastrointestinal procedures (OR 23·2, 95% CI 2·1 to 255) and over 10 days of antibiotics (OR 16·1, 95% CI 2·2 to 117) were significant risk factors for CDAD.[64] Nelson *et al.* studied 33 hospitalized patients with CDAD and 32 controls (patients without CDAD) and showed that the use of second or third generation cephalosporins was a significant risk factor (OR 8·3, 95%CI 1·4 to 48·9), as was the use of two or more antibiotics (OR 18·7, 95%CI 4·1 to 85·8).[67] McFarland *et al.* followed 428 patients admitted to a general medicine ward and found seven risk factors using multivariate analysis[59]: increasing age, extreme severe underlying disease (RR 5·18, 95%CI 1·2 to 22·2), cephalosporin use for at least one week (RR 2·1, 95%CI 1·1 to 3·8), penicillin use for 2 weeks (RR 3·4, 95% CI 1·5 to 7·9), and use of gastrointestinal stimulants (RR 3·1, 95% CI 1·7 to 5·6), enemas (RR 3·3, 95% CI 1·5 to 7·0) and stool softeners (RR 1·7, 95% CI 1·02 to 3·0).

The two most strongly implicated sources of *C. difficile* infection are hospital personnel (including other infected patients) and environmental surfaces or fomites.[4,69] Longer length of stay in hospitals has been shown to increase the risk of acquiring nosocomial CDAD.[70,71]

Recurrent disease

Prospective studies of risk factors for recurrent CDAD may help to define this subset of highly susceptible patients who have a tendency to develop the recurrent form of CDAD. The risk factors for recurrent CDAD have been found to be slightly different from risk factors found for primary CDAD and from risk factors for nosocomial CDAD.[15,59,64,66,67,69,72,73] In a prospective study of 209 patients with recurrent CDAD, logistic regression revealed two significant independent risk factors for CDAD recurrence: increased age and a lower quality of health scale at enrollment ($\chi^2 = 9·03$, $P = 0·01$).[16] Patients who had recurrent disease were older (mean age 64·8 ± 1·65 years) than patients who did not (mean age 54·6 ± 19·6 years). Recurrent disease was also associated with a lower quality of health index ($\bar{x}$ = 42·9 ± 17·8) compared with no recurrence ($\bar{x}$ = 50·3 ± 18·5). The estimates of risk for CDAD recurrence were as follows: age (OR 1·04, 95% CI 1·01 to 1·08) and a lower mean quality of health index (OR 0·96, 95% CI 0·93 to 0·99). There were no significant interactions in the model. No other risk factor was significant including sex, number of prior episodes, type, dose or duration of antibiotic therapy, duration of follow up, number of medications or prior surgeries, allergies, severity of enrollment episode, study center, or type of patient (inpatient or outpatient).

In another study comparing 34 patients with recurrent CDAD with 33 patients with non-recurrent CDAD, the risk factors for subsequent recurrences included a higher number of prior episodes (RR 3·87, 95% CI 1·12 to 13·34), spring onset of initial episode (RR 7·73, 95% CI 1·07 to 55·89) and the use of more than one antibiotic (RR 2·97, 95% CI 1·11 to 7·93).[15] Do *et al.* analyzed 13 patients with recurrent CDAD and 46 patients with an initial episode of CDAD in a case–control study.[74] Risk factors for recurrent CDAD in these patients included a history of chronic renal insufficiency, and a white blood cell count over 15 000/mm^3.

Tal *et al.* carried out a case–control study of 43 patients with recurrent CDAD and 38 patients with initial CDAD followed at a subacute geriatric department for 18 months.[72] Risk factors for recurrent CDAD included fecal incontinence (OR 2·75, 95% CI 1·05 to 7·54), longer duration of fever from admission until first episode of CDAD (OR 1·11, 95% CI 1·02 to 1·25) and H2 antagonist exposure (OR 1·03, 95% CI 1·14 to 7·29).

Diagnosis

For the diagnosis of CDAD, three criteria must be fulfilled: (i) clinical presentation of diarrheal disease, (ii) presence of the organism or its toxins and (iii) the exclusion of other causes of diarrhea. Errors in diagnosis have occurred if not all of these three criteria are present. Clinical diarrhea must be present, as the asymptomatic carrier state of *C. difficile* is a common finding in hospital patients.[4,33] Due to the numerous causes of diarrhea, the other causes must also be eliminated from the differential diagnosis (other enteric pathogens, chronic gastrointestinal conditions and drugs). Finally, the presence of either the organism (culture positive) or its toxins should be documented.

Clinical presentation

Diarrhea due to CDAD has been defined as a change in bowel habits with at least three loose or watery bowel movements per day for at least two consecutive days or greater than eight loose or watery stools within 48 hours.[69,75]

The symptoms of CDAD can also include fever, nausea and abdominal cramping or pain.[11,57]

The incubation period after acquisition of *C. difficile* is usually 1 week or less, but can be up as long as 8 weeks after exposure to antibiotics.[11,52] Asymptomatic carriers may also become symptomatic after exposure to antibiotics.

Presence of *Clostridium difficile*

Laboratory diagnosis of CDAD rests on culture and toxin detection in the stools. Infection can be suggested by fecal white blood cells or their byproduct lactoferrin, but these are non-specific indications of colonic inflammation and are not specific for *C. difficile* disease. Guidelines developed for testing for *C. difficile* toxin include testing on non-solid stools, recent history (30 days) of antibiotic therapy and recent hospitalization.[11,33,76,77]

Stool culture alone is very sensitive, but is not specific because it does not differentiate asymptomatic carriers from patients with clinical disease.

Tissue culture cytotoxin assays for toxin B have long been the gold standard for diagnosis of CDAD with excellent sensitivity (94–100%) and specificity (99%). The disadvantages of this approach are the time necessary to perform the test (24–48 hours) and the cost.[11]

Enzyme immunoassay (EIA) tests have been developed which are rapid (2 hours), and less expensive and do not require specially trained personnel.[78] These tests vary in specificity and sensitivity. Various EIA kits can detect toxin A, B or both. Tests that detect only toxin A have lower sensitivity than tests that detect both toxin A and B.[79,80]

The Premier cytoclone A + B EIA showed sensitivity of 75–85% and specificity of 95–100% in several studies.[81,82] The Biosite Triage test detects *C. difficile* antigen and toxin A with sensitivity and specificity of 100% and 83%, respectively.[82] A disadvantage of this test is its failure to diagnose toxin A negative, toxin B positive patients, and therefore its inability to distinguish carriers from those with disease when only the common antigen is positive.[82] A prospective study of 400 stools using this test showed the accuracy of the test to be 85%.[83]

A more comprehensive study of six commercial assays showed the highest sensitivity (95%), and highest negative predictive value for the Triage test followed by the Clearview and ColorPac tests.[84] The detection of toxin A and B by the Techlab immunoassay showed high sensitivity and specificity (33% and 100%, respectively).[85] A single negative EIA test does not exclude CDAD. A repeated test can improve the sensitivity by 12%.[86]

Recommendations

An ELISA for toxin A or B is appropriate as a screening test for CDAD. If toxins are not detected and diarrhea persists, empiric therapy should be initiated and one or two repeat stool samples should be tested for toxin B. This approach will identify an additional 5–10% of cases.

Treatment for the initial episode

If possible, the inciting antibiotic should be discontinued. Fluid support (oral or intravenous) may be needed. Antiperistaltic or opiate drugs should be avoided. There is no role for treatment of asymptomatic carriers.[87] If the index of suspicion for CDAD is high, it is best to begin empiric therapy rather than wait for confirmatory stool tests. C5

Antibiotic treatment

Given the number and variety of clinical trials of antibiotics for treatment of CDAD, a meta-analysis was performed.[88] Of nine trials with suitable methodology for systematic review, only two were placebo controlled. Six other trials compared vancomycin with other antibiotics (fusidic acid, bacitracin, teicoplanin, metronidazole) and demonstrated no superiority of any single antibiotic.[88–96]

Vancomycin

Several trials have demonstrated the efficacy of oral vancomycin for therapy of initial CDAD, given orally at doses of 500–1225 mg four times a day for 7–14 days (Table 18.1). Wenisch *et al.* performed a randomized controlled trial of four antibiotics.[89] Patients with *C. difficile* toxin positive diarrhea were randomized to receive 10 days of one of the four antibiotic regimens and followed for initial resolution of symptoms ("cure") and for relapse within 30 days of antibiotic being discontinued ("relapse"). The four groups were comparable in terms of age, sex and previous antibiotic exposure. The recurrence rate was significantly lower in patients receiving teicoplanin (7%) than in patients treated with fusidic acid (28%, $P = 0.04$) and there were no other statistically significant differences between treatment groups. There were no reported adverse reactions to any of the four antibiotic treatments. A1c

Two randomized trials[89,90] did not show differences in efficacy of metronidazole and vancomycin (Table 18.1) for either initial "cure" (94% to 100%) or recurrence rate (5% to 16%). A1c In a 10-year observational surveillance study of 908 patients at the Minneapolis VA Medical Center[97] Olson *et al.* reported that the initial responses to metronidazole and vancomycin (in a variety of dosage regimens) were 98% and 99%, respectively. B4 Figure 18.1 shows the relative risks for treatment failure or subsequent *C. difficile* recurrence observed in comparative trials of antibiotics for the treatment

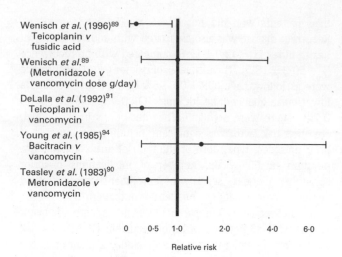

Figure 18.1 Point estimates (black circles) and 95% confidence limits for the risk of recurrence in patients with an initial episode of *Clostridium difficile*-associated disease by antibiotic treatment in randomized controlled trials

of initial episodes of CDAD. Vancomycin and metronidazole appear to be equally effective. A1a

Fekety *et al.*[92] (see Table 18.1) did not show differences in initial cure or recurrence rates in a randomized trial comparing 500 mg and 2 g daily doses of vancomycin. A1d These authors encouraged the use of the lower dose, less expensive regimen.

While intravenous vancomycin has little efficacy, the use of vancomycin enemas is an alternative when the oral route is not feasible, for example for patients with ileus. A small observational study in nine patients and other case reports suggest that this approach may be effective[98] but there are no randomized trials. B4

Metronidazole

Oral metronidazole has been used for treatment of initial CDAD, and several practice guidelines suggest that it should be the first antibiotic to be administered in a dose of 250–500 mg orally four times a day for 7–14 days. Randomized trials showed good "cure" rates >95% (see Table 18.1).[89,90] A1c There is no good explanation for the failure of metronidazole in a small proportion of patients. Analysis of pretreatment isolates in 14 such patients showed no decreased susceptibility to the antibiotic.[99] A more recent study from Spain documented metronidazole resistance in 6·3% of strains over an 8-year period.[100]

The oral route of administration is preferred, but case reports and an observational study in 10 patients suggest that the intravenous route is effective for patients with paralytic ileus or toxic megacolon.[101] B4 There are no controlled trials of the parenteral administration of this antibiotic.

Table 18.1 Randomized controlled trials of treatments for patients with initial *Clostridium difficile*-associated disease

Reference	Antibiotic	Daily dose	Duration (days)	No. of patients	Initial cure (%)	Recurred (%)
Wenisch *et al.*, 1996[89]	Teicoplanin	400 mg two times daily	10	28	96	7*
	Fusidic acid	500 mg three times daily	10	29	93	28
	Vancomycin	500 mg three times daily	10	31	94	16 (NS)
	Metronidazole	500 mg three times daily	10	31	94	16 (NS)
DeLalla *et al.*, 1992[91]	Teicoplanin	100 mg two times daily	10	26	96	8*
	Vancomycin	500 mg four times daily	10	20	100	20
Fekety *et al.*, 1989[92]	Vancomycin	125 mg four times daily	10	24	100	21
	Vancomycin	500 mg four times daily	10	22	100	18 (NS)
Dudley *et al.*, 1986[93]	Bacitracin	25 000 U four times daily	10	15	80	33
	Vancomycin	500 mg four times daily	10	15	93	20 (NS)
Young *et al.*, 1985[94]	Bacitracin	20 000 U four times daily	10	21	76	24
	Vancomycin	125 mg four times daily	10	21	86	29 (NS)
Teasley *et al.*, 1983[90]	Vancomycin	500 mg four times daily	10	52	100	11
	Metronidazole	250 mg four times daily	10	42	95	5 (NS)
Mogg *et al.*, 1982[95]	Colestipol	10 g four times daily	5	12	25	NR
	Placebo		5	14	21	NR
Keighley *et al.*, 1978[96]	Vancomycin	125 mg four times daily	5	12	92	0*
	Placebo	125 mg four times daily	5	9	22	44

*$P < 0.05$
NS, not significant; NR, not reported

Bacitracin

Bacitracin is a non-absorbable antibiotic, for oral administration with the disadvantages of an unpleasant taste and significant expense. Two uncontrolled trials in 1980 showed response to therapy in very small numbers of patients.[102,103] Two randomized controlled trials did not show significantly different initial cure rates for bacitracin and vancomycin (see Table 18.1). Ald However, the bacitracin treated patients were reported to subsequently have higher rates of *C. difficile* carriage in the stools.[93,94] The authors[94] suggest that bacitracin be used as a first line alternative to vancomycin, but the important trial comparing bacitracin and metronidazole has not been done.

Teicoplanin

The oral antibiotic teicoplanin has been studied for treatment of initial CDAD. DeLalla *et al.* compared teicoplanin with oral vancomycin in a randomized controlled trial in 46 patients with CDAD[91] (see Table 18.1) and did not show differences in initial cure rate. [Ald] However, the recurrence rate appeared to be significantly lower following teicoplanin. Teicoplanin was also found to be significantly more effective for prevention of recurrent disease than fusidic acid (Table 18.1 and Figure 18.1).[89] [Ald]

Fusidic acid

A randomized trial did not show significant differences in initial cure rate for fusidic acid, metronidazole, vancomycin and teicoplanin[89] (Table 18.1). [Ald] Fusidic acid is an alternative for patients who are unable to tolerate, or who do not respond to metronidazole.

Ion exchange resins

In vivo studies of two resins, cholestyramine and colestipol, demonstrated binding of cytotoxin (as well as some binding of vancomycin), and cholestyramine delayed death in the hamster model of clindamycin-induced cecitis.[104] [C5] Trials of ion exchange resins to bind toxins have been disappointing. However, a placebo-controlled randomized trial of colestipol in 38 patients with postoperative diarrhea showed no difference in fecal excretion of *C. difficile* toxin, and treatment with ion exchange resins is not recommended.[95] [Ald]

Probiotics

Probiotics are mono or mixed cultures of live micro-organisms which, when administered to animal or man, benefit the host by improving the properties of the indigenous microflora.[105] [C5] Probiotics have no proved role in treatment of initial CDAD. The closest evidence that they may have a role comes from studies for the prevention of antibiotic associated diarrhea (AAD). Both the bacteria *Lactobacillus* spp. and the yeast *Saccharomyces boulardii* have been shown to reduce the occurrence of AAD when given in conjunction with antibiotics. In four placebo-controlled randomized trials (adults given erythromycin, two pediatric studies and adults being treated for *Helicobacter pylori*) there was less diarrhea in the patients receiving *Lactobacillus GG* than in those receiving placebo[106–109] [Ald] However, a more recent placebo-controlled trial failed to show efficacy of *Lactobacillus GG*.[110] [Ald] The commercial preparation Lactinex, a mixture of *L. acidophilus* and *L. bulgaricus*, has not shown significant benefit in reduction of AAD in three trials.[111–113] [Ald] Two controlled trials of *Enterococcus faecium* showed modest efficacy in prevention of AAD.[114,115] Two small trials of bifidobacteria showed less diarrhea associated with antibiotics.[107,116] [Ald] Additional randomized controlled trials with sufficient power to show differences, should they exist, are needed.

The non-pathogenic yeast *S. boulardii* has been shown to decrease AAD in four randomized controlled trials.[117–120]

[Alc] A fifth trial did not show efficacy in elderly patients, but the duration of follow up may have been inadequate.[121]

Evidence for efficacy of probiotics for AAD was provided by a randomized placebo-controlled trial of three different probiotic regimens for the prevention of diarrhea associated with antibiotic therapy for *H. pylori* eradication. *Lactobacillus GG, S. boulardii* and a mixture of *L. acidophilus* and *Bifidobacterium lactus* all resulted in a significant decrease in diarrhea.[122] [Alc]

Treatment of recurrent CDAD

Most patients (76–98%) with an initial episode of CDAD are cured by treatment with either vancomycin or metronidazole.[15,97] A proportion of patients develops recurrent episodes of CDAD that may recur for several years, despite antibiotic treatment.[15,16] Following a second episode of CDAD, 60% of affected patients experience subsequent episodes and are considered to have an especially difficult form of CDAD, designated "recurrent CDAD".[15,16] Treatment of recurrent CDAD has relied on antibiotics (usually vancomycin or metronidazole), toxin binding resins, fecal enemas and the use of probiotics or biotherapeutic agents.[11,69,75,118,123,124]

Vancomycin or metronidazole

There is a limited number of randomized trials comparing antibiotics for patients with recurrent CDAD after exclusion of all patients who are experiencing an initial episode (Table 18.2). Most randomized trials have been carried out in patients with initial disease, or patients in whom the prior history of CDAD has not been clarified. A randomized, double blind, placebo-controlled trial of an investigational probiotic treatment for patients with recurrent CDAD allowed the analysis of the effect of the antibiotic treatments in the 78 patients who received antibiotics and placebo (and excluded patients who received antibiotics and the investigational probiotic).[125] Patients were randomized to 10 days of either high dose vancomycin (2 g/day), low dose vancomycin (500 mg/day) or metronidazole (1 g/day) and followed for recurrence over 2 months. No differences in recurrence rates were found between the groups (Table 18.2). [Ald]

An earlier double-blinded, placebo controlled trial also showed similar recurrence rates in vancomycin and metronidazole treated patients.[75] [Ald] An observational study of 163 patients, of whom 125 received vancomycin and 38 received metronidazole also showed similar recurrence rates.[124] [B4]

Similar rates of recurrence are seen despite the differences in the pharmacokinetics of vancomycin and metronidazole in the intestine as seen in Table 18.3.[75,126,127] In the healthy intestine, fecal levels of metronidazole are rapidly absorbed

Table 18.2   Randomized trial of vancomycin, metronidazole, and prolonged vancomycin and probiotic therapy for recurrent CDAD[125]

Initial antibiotic therapy (10 days)	Probiotic therapy (28 days)	No. of patients	Patients with recurrent CDAD (%)
Vancomycin 500 mg four times daily	–	14	7 (50)
Vancomycin 125 mg four times daily	–	38	17 (45)
Metronidazole 250 mg four times daily	–	26	13 (50)
Vancomycin 500 mg four times daily	*S. boulardii* 500 mg two times daily	18	3 (17)
Vancomycin 500 mg four times daily	Placebo	14	7 (50)

CDAD, *Clostridium difficile*-associated disease

Table 18.3   Randomized trial of vancomycin, metronidazole and probiotic therapy for initial and recurrent CDAD[75]

Initial antibiotic therapy (11 or 12 days)	Prolonged antibiotic therapy (20 days)	Probiotic therapy (28 days)	No. of patients	No. with recurrent CDAD (%)
Vancomycin 200 mg four times daily		–	65	28 (43)
Metronidazole 300 mg four times daily	–	–	37	12 (32)
	Standard antibiotic[a]	*S. boulardii* 500 mg two times daily	26	9 (35)
	Standard antibiotic	Placebo	34	22 (65)

[a]Standard antibiotic was physician's choice of vancomycin or metronidazole (dose not regulated by study protocol).
CDAD, *Clostridium difficile*-associated disease

and so the concentration within the lumen of the gut is low. Once an acute episode of CDAD occurs, high concentrations of metronidazole have been documented in the infected intestine.[128] Vancomycin is bacteriostatic for *C. difficile* organisms, thus allowing the persistence of vegetative cells of *C. difficile* and the rapid increase in *C. difficile* after therapy is discontinued.[127,129] The time required for spore germination, *C. difficile* overgrowth, and acute toxigenic symptoms may be extremely short (usually between 3 and 5 days) once antibiotics have been discontinued. Ninety-seven percent of the recurrences during a prospective follow up of antibiotic-treated patients occurred within four weeks of stopping antibiotic treatment (median of 7 days).[16] The short interval between the end of antibiotic therapy and the recurrence of symptoms was confirmed by two other studies of patients with recurrent CDAD.[15,97] Delayed onsets of new episodes (4–8 weeks later) reported in some studies may be attributed to exposure to exogenous spores or to germination of asymptomatic carriage of *C. difficile* during the time when

the normal colonic flora has not yet recovered. A previous study has shown that antibiotics may disrupt the normal flora for up to 6 weeks after their use is discontinued.[130] Continuing or restarting inciting antibiotics after successful treatments has been shown to increase the risk of recurrence.[131]

The treatment of recurrent CDAD must consider the possible role of residual *C. difficile* spores in the intestinal tract and the time the intestine is susceptible to *C. difficile* overgrowth. Short antibiotic treatment regimens may be effective in initially resolving the symptoms of diarrhea, but do nothing during the "window of susceptibility", i.e. the time required for re-establishment of the intestinal microflora and resistance to the overgrowth of *C. difficile* and recurrence of disease. Several strategies have been tested including the provision of extended protection by tapering the dose or pulsing antibiotics, use of biotherapeutic agents ("beneficial microbes") and the restoration of intestinal microflora using fecal infusions of bacteria or normal stool contents.

Vancomycin taper/pulse

There have been two studies of patients with recurrent CDAD treated with either tapering or pulsed dosing of vancomycin. A prospective case series of 163 patients with recurrent CDAD documented the rate of CDAD recurrences over a 2-month period in patients who were treated with a variety of strategies using either vancomycin or metronidazole.[132] The overall recurrence rates for all patients receiving vancomycin or metronidazole were not significantly different. B2 Two strategies appeared to result in significantly reduced recurrence rates: vancomycin tapering and vancomycin pulsed dosing. The recurrence rates in patients treated with vancomycin (1–1·5 g/day for 10 days), with a tapering dose of vancomycin (over a mean of 21 days), or with pulsed dosing of vancomycin (125–500 mg every 3 days over a mean of 18 days) were 71%, 31%, and 14%, respectively. B2 Tedesco *et al.* reported a case series of 22 patients with recurrent CDAD who appeared to be successfully treated with a regimen of vancomycin tapered over 21 days (500 mg/day for 1 week, 250 mg/day for 1 week, 125 mg/day for 1 week, 125 mg every other day) followed by vancomycin in a pulse dose regimen for 21 days (125 mg every third day).[133] B4 The results of these two observational studies are suggestive that these strategies may be effective, and a randomized trial would be of interest.

Other antibiotics

No randomized controlled trials of teicoplanin, bacitracin, or rifampin have been performed in patients with recurrent CDAD[134] Adjunctive intracolonic vancomycin has been tried in a case series of nine patients (three of whom had recurrent CDAD) with an 8% cure rate, but this approach has not been tested in a randomized controlled trial.[98]

Probiotics

Probiotics have been used in attempts to prevent recurrent CDAD episodes. Probiotics are postulated to provide replacement microflora for those bacteria that have been disrupted by antibiotics or other risk factors, to stimulate the immune response or the production of enzymes that degrade pathogenic toxins, or to provide simple barriers that block attachment sites in the colon.[61]

There have been two double blind randomized controlled trials of *S. boulardii* and antibiotics for patients with recurrent CDAD (see Table 18.2). In the first trial 168 patients were randomized to receive one of three standard 10-day antibiotic regimens followed by *S. boulardii* or a placebo for 28 days.[125] Three antibiotic regimens were used for 10 days: either high dose vancomycin (2 g/day), low

dose vancomycin (500 mg/day) or metronidazole (1 g/day). Then either *S. boulardii* or placebo (1 g/day for 28 days) was added to the antibiotic treatment. The outcome was the proportion of patients with recurrent *C. difficile* infection in a 2-month period. A significant decrease in recurrences was observed only in patients treated with the high dose vancomycin and *S. boulardii* treatment (recurrent rate 16·7%) compared with patients who received high dose vancomycin and placebo (recurrent rate 50%, *P* = 0·05). Ala The NNT for this regimen (number of patients required to be treated with high dose vancomycin and *S. boulardii*, rather than high dose vancomycin alone to prevent one recurrence of CDAD) is 3. However, *S. boulardii* treatment was not shown to be effective in the patients treated with low dose vancomycin or metronidazole. No serious adverse reactions were noted in any of these patients.

In an earlier study patients were randomized to receive either *S. boulardii* (1 g/day) or a placebo for 28 days combined with vancomycin or metronidazole in various doses selected by the participating physician.[75] Approximately half of the patients were experiencing a recurrent episode of CDAD. Analysis of this subgroup of 60 patients revealed a recurrence rate of 35% in *S. boulardii* treated patients compared with a rate of 65% in patients who received placebo. Ald In this study, vancomycin was not more effective than metronidazole, regardless of the dose or duration of therapy.

Figure 18.2 displays the data from these two randomized controlled trials of various antibiotic regimens with and without *S. boulardii therapy*.[75,125]

Observational studies suggest that *Lactobacillus GG* may be effective,[123,135,136] B4 but no randomized controlled trials have been reported for this or other probiotic agents.

Fecal enemas

In an effort to replace the microflora disrupted by recurrent CDAD and antibiotic treatments, there have been several case reports describing the use of fecal enemas prepared from normal stools in patients with recurrent CDAD.[137–140] B4 No randomized placebo-controlled trials have been performed. Whole-bowel irrigation has also been added to antibiotic therapy in one case in an effort to "flush out" pathogenic toxins, but no randomized controlled trials have been reported.[141]

Immunoglobulin

Although the use of immunoglobulin for patients with recurrent CDAD has been reported in the literature in small case series or case reports,[142–144] no randomized controlled trials have been done. C5

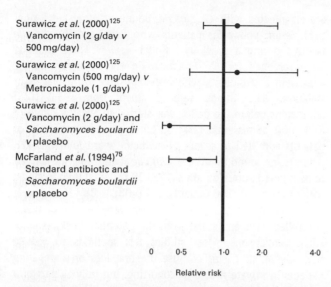

Figure 18.2 Point estimates (black circles) and 95% confidence limits for the risk of recurrence in patients with recurrent *Clostridium difficile*-associated disease by antibiotic treatment from multivariate analysis in randomized controlled trials. Standard antibiotic was physician's choice of vancomycin or metronidazole (dose not regulated by study protocol)

Cholestyramine or other anion binding medication

Cholestyramine binds vancomycin as well as the toxins of *C. difficile* and its use may lead to suboptimal levels of antibiotic,[11] but no randomized controlled trials have been carried out.[145] C5

Prevention

Infection control

The importance of infection control for the prevention and control of nosocomial infections leading to CDAD and recurrent CDAD has been well documented in the literature.[11,69] Microbiologic studies documenting that 48–56% of clinical recurrences are reinfections with a different strain of *C. difficile*, emphasize the importance of disrupting the nosocomial acquisition of new strains of *C. difficile* in the hospital environment.[17,49,146] The most important strategy for prevention of CDAD is to interrupt the horizontal transmission of *C. difficile*. Five infection control practices have been investigated: (i) environmental disinfection of contaminated surfaces or fomites, and medical equipment or use of disposable instruments; (ii) reduction of hand carriage by hospital care personnel; (iii) isolation or cohorting of infected patients; (iv) treatment of asymptomatic carriers; and (v) a multidisciplinary approach using a

combination of the above strategies. None of these infection control practices has been evaluated in randomized controlled trials. Most of the practices have been evaluated by comparing infection rates in hospitals before and after the introduction of the experimental intervention or by comparing the rates between wards where the intervention has or has not been introduced.

Environmental disinfectants

Contamination of environmental surfaces by *C. difficile* and its spores presents an extremely challenging problem for hospitals. The spores of *C. difficile* can persist on surfaces or fomites for months and are not susceptible to normal room cleaning agents. Patients who are carriers of *C. difficile* shed the spores on to a wide variety of hospital surfaces.[4,50,69,147–149] Several reviews have presented evidence that cleaning with an effective disinfectant has resulted in lower rates of nosocomial CDAD.[6,69,70] B4 Three intervention studies have shown significant reductions in rates of nosocomial *C. difficile* after environmental surfaces were adequately disinfected and cleaned. Mayfield *et al.* changed the type of room disinfectant used (to 1:10 hypochlorite solution) in rooms occupied by 4252 bone marrow transplant patients and documented a reduction in the incidence of CDAD from 8·6 cases/1000 patient days before to 3·3 cases/1000 patient days after the intervention was introduced (hazard ratio 0·37, 95% CI 0·19 to 0·74).[150] B2 No decrease in the incidence of CDAD was noted in control wards where the new disinfectant was not used. Struelens *et al.* found that the frequency of environmental positive isolation of *C. difficile* fell significantly from 13% to 3% ($P = 0.04$) after daily room disinfection (0·03% glutaraldehyde and 0·04% formaldehyde solution) was introduced and there was a concurrent decrease in the incidence of CDAD cases.[151] B4 During an outbreak of CDAD Kaatz *et al.* demonstrated a fall in the isolation rate of *C. difficile* from 31·4 % to 0·6 % and a halt in the development of new cases after the introduction of a phosphate buffered hypochlorite solution to disinfect hospital room surfaces.[152] B4

Disinfection of medical equipment

Medical equipment that is used for patients infected with CDAD may become a source of new infection if not properly cleaned. Fiberoptic endoscopes have been shown to be a source of *C. difficile*, but two studies found that exposure to 2% alkaline glutaraldehyde for 5 minutes resulted in 99% killing of *C. difficile* on the surfaces.[149,153] C5 However, neither of these studies used a control group and they were not designed to document whether the disinfection procedure resulted in fewer cases of CDAD. Brooks *et al.* showed that the use of single-use disposable thermometers to replace electronic rectal thermometers, of which 21% had tested positive for *C. difficile*, reduced the incidence of *C. difficile*-associated diarrhea from 2·71/1000 patient days to 1·76/1000 patient days (*P* < 0·05) in an acute care hospital.[154] B4 A significant reduction of CDAD was also observed at a skilled nursing facility at the same time. This study suffers from the weaknesses of "before and after" comparisons, compared with the results of parallel group randomized trials, but suggests that this intervention may be useful.

Handwashing and disinfection

Nosocomial *C. difficile* is frequently transmitted via the hands of hospital care personnel, and visitors to other patients.[4,91] Interventions designed to disrupt this method of transmission have included handwashing with disinfectants instead of non-disinfectant soaps, training programs on the importance of proper handwashing techniques, and the use of disposable gloves.[52,155] In one prospective study, handwashing with 4% chlorhexidine gluconate resulted in a significantly lower isolation frequency of *C. difficile* on the hand surfaces of tested hospital personnel (14%, *P* = 0·002) compared to an isolation rate of 88% when non-disinfectant soap was used.[4] B2 Currently, newer enteric precaution policies have established the use of vinyl disposable gloves. Three studies have documented that the use of gloves reduces the rate of *C. difficile* isolation on the hands of healthcare personnel. In a prospective study of 42 healthcare workers (doctors, nurses, physical therapists), the use of disposable gloves during the care of infected CDAD patients reduced the isolation of the hand carriage of *C. difficile* from 58% to zero.[4] Johnson *et al.* conducted a controlled trial of the effectiveness of an educational program involving the use of disposable gloves in four hospital wards.[52] The incidence of CDAD fell from 7·7/1000 patient discharges before the program was started to 1·5/1000 during the 6-month intervention (*P* = 0·01) in the two wards in which the program was introduced while there was no decrease in CDAD on the two control wards. B2 Bettin *et al.* seeded 10 volunteers with *C. difficile* and found that *C. difficile* counts were significantly lower on gloved hands compared to bare hands, regardless of the type of handwashing agent used.[155] However, the effectiveness of limiting nosocomial spread of *C. difficile* by handwashing alone or by the use of gloves as the sole control policy has not been tested in randomized controlled trials.

Isolation or cohorting practices

Both symptomatic and asymptomatic infected patients have been shown to increase the risk of nosocomial spread of *C. difficile*. One control policy that has been tested is the isolation of the patient from the pool of susceptible uninfected patients by using private rooms, or by cohorting patients who

are all infected with *C. difficile*. Boone *et al.* tested a new readmission policy for patients who had been *C. difficile* positive during a previous hospital stay.[156] These patients were screened for *C. difficile* toxin shortly before or on admission and patients who tested positive were placed in isolation. The attack rate declined from 13·3/1000 admissions before the policy was started to an attack rate of 8·7/1000 admissions. B4 Another prospective study of patients admitted to a general medicine ward followed 428 patients and found that the *C. difficile* acquisition rate tended to be higher in double rooms (17/100 patients) than in single patient rooms (7/100 patients, *P* = 0·08).[4] B4 However, it should be noted that these studies were not randomized controlled trials and suffer from the potential weaknesses of such comparisons. Most studies test methods to reduce transmission of *C. difficile* use the practices of segregating patients in private rooms or cohorting, but only as part of a multiple intervention approach rather than as an independent control policy.

Treatment of asymptomatic carriers

Asymptomatic carriers of *C. difficile* have been shown to be a source of new nosocomial cases of CDAD. In order to control the spread of *C. difficile*, a policy of treating asymptomatic carriers has been tested by several investigators. However, treatment of asymptomatic carriers has not been found to reduce the incidence of CDAD and has not been shown to reduce the frequency of nosocomial outbreaks.[157] B4 Bender *et al.* demonstrated that treatment of carriers with metronidazole was ineffective for reducing the incidence of new CDAD cases at a chronic care facility.[158] B4 Delmee *et al.* showed a reduction in CDAD frequency in patients on a leukemia unit from 16·6% to 3·6% after all symptomatic and asymptomatic patients carrying *C. difficile* were treated with vancomycin.[159] B4 However, this study was not a randomized controlled trial. Johnson *et al.* treated 30 asymptomatic carriers of *C. difficile* in a randomized placebo-controlled trial. The patients received either vancomycin (1 g/day), metronidazole (1 g/day) or placebo for 10 days.[87] The observed *C. difficile* carriage rates in vancomycin, metronidazole or placebo-treated patients were 10%, 70% and 80%, respectively (*P* = 0·02). Recurrence rates at the end of the 2-month follow up period were significantly higher in the vancomycin group (67%) than in the placebo group (11%, *P* < 0·05). A1d Although there are few randomized controlled trials on the treatment of asymptomatic carriers, this policy does not seem warranted on the basis of available evidence.

Multiple intervention practices

A multiple intervention infection control policy that included isolation of *C. difficile* positive patients, a monthly

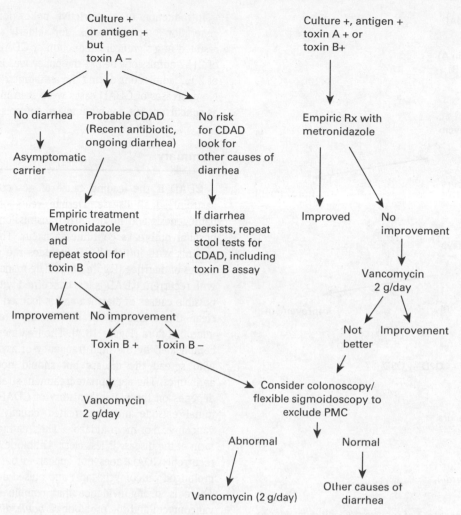

Figure 18.3 Management of an initial episode of *Clostridium difficile*-associated disease. PMC, pseudomembranous colitis

educational program (handwashing, use of gloves, enteric precaution procedures), environmental disinfection and aggressive surveillance was tested at an acute care hospital that had a problem with *C. difficile* cases.[160] The number of CDAD cases fell from 155 to 67 cases per year after this program was introduced, and the reduced incidence of cases was sustained during a 7-year period. B4 Struelens *et al.* also showed significant reduction in new CDAD cases from 1·5 cases/1000 discharges to 0·3/1000 discharges (*P* < 0·05) after the introduction of a control program consisting of intensive screening for *C. difficile*, early enteric isolation precautions, rapid treatment of CDAD cases with vancomycin and room disinfection.[151] B4 Brown *et al.* reported that control practices including rapid patient isolation, treatment of CDAD cases and antibiotic restriction resulted in a decline of CDAD incidence at their hospital from 2·2/100 to 0·7/100.[64] B4 Several reviews have presented the evidence that multidisciplinary infection control programs have

resulted in lower rates of nosocomial CDAD,[6,69,70] but no randomized controlled trials have been carried out.

Antibiotic control policies

Antibiotic control policies have become increasingly popular to control costs and the development of antibiotic resistant strains and epidemics of nosocomial *C. difficile* disease.[162,163] During an outbreak at a tertiary care university hospital age over 65 years, intensive care unit stay, gastrointestinal procedures and antibiotic use greater than 10 days were identified as risk factors for CDAD. The isolation and treatment of suspected cases and formulary restriction of clindamycin and metronidazole therapy for anaerobic infections were associated with a decrease in attack rate from 2·25% at the end of 1987 to 0·74% by the second half of 1988.[64] B4 Three separate studies at Veterans Affairs (VA) hospitals documented the control of epidemics by restriction

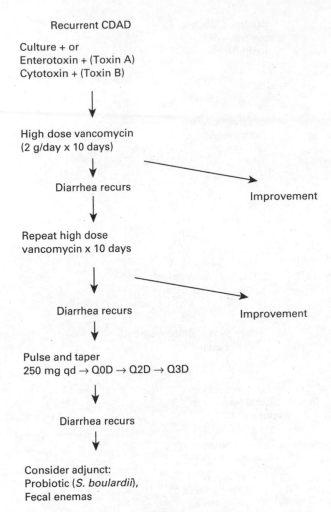

Recurrent CDAD

Culture + or
Enterotoxin + (Toxin A)
Cytotoxin + (Toxin B)

↓

High dose vancomycin
(2 g/day x 10 days)

↓

Diarrhea recurs → Improvement

↓

Repeat high dose
vancomycin x 10 days

↓

Diarrhea recurs → Improvement

↓

Pulse and taper
250 mg qd → Q0D → Q2D → Q3D

↓

Diarrhea recurs

↓

Consider adjunct:
Probiotic (*S. boulardii*),
Fecal enemas

Figure 18.4 Management of recurrent *Clostridium difficile*-associated disease. CDAD, *Clostridium difficile*-associated disease; q/Q, every; d/D, day

of clindamycin use. One study from Tucson identified a five-fold increase in *C. difficile* cases, over half of which were associated with a single strain. Antibiotic use was analyzed, and subsequent restriction of the use of clindamycin was associated with a decrease in infection rates.[21] B4 A later study at another VA medical center showed a prompt reduction in CDAD cases following the introduction of a policy of restricted clindamycin use. Additional observations were that the hospital saved money even though some more expensive antibiotics were used, and bacterial isolates showed a return of clindamycin susceptibility.[161] A third study documented decrease in CDAD following removal of multiple antibiotics from the formulary.[162] B4

Finally, in an elderly care unit, CDAD rates dropped following the introduction of a restrictive antibiotic policy that specifically targeted a reduction in the use of cefuroxime, with replacement by penicillin, trimethoprim or gentamicin as an alternative.[163] B4

Introduction of a restrictive policy for injectable third-generation cephalosporins for elderly medical patients resulted in a significant reduction of CDAD cases from 4·5% of 2157 admissions before the policy was introduced to 2·2% of 2037 admissions during the antibiotic restriction policy.[164] No decreases of CDAD cases were seen in other wards used as concurrent but not randomized controls. B2

Summary

CDAD is the leading cause of nosocomial outbreaks of gastrointestinal disease. Despite years of research on the pathogenesis and nosocomial transmission of this organism, hospital outbreaks continue to occur. The management of patients with initial CDAD includes the exclusion of other causes of diarrhea (Figure 18.3). The management of patients with recurrent CDAD is less concerned with identifying other possible causes of diarrhea and is focused more on efforts to clear the toxins of *C. difficile* and restore the normal microbial flora (Figure 18.4). The treatment of this disease is complicated by the high frequency of asymptomatic carriers who spread the disease but should not be treated with antibiotics. The appropriate treatment strategy for the disease depends on the patient's history of CDAD. Patients with an initial episode may be treated equally well with either vancomycin or metronidazole. The treatment of the recurrent form of the disease is less clear. Antibiotic treatment alone for recurrent CDAD does not appear to be effective, although prolonged vancomycin taper and pulsed doses show promise. There is strong evidence that combination therapy using vancomycin and the probiotic *S. boulardii* is also an effective strategy. More randomized trials are needed to assess other types of antibiotics for the treatment of initial CDAD and other types of probiotics for recurrent CDAD.

References

1 Burdon DW. *Clostridium difficile*: the epidemiology and prevention of hospital-acquired infection. *Infection* 1982; **10**:203–4.

2 Wüst J, Sullivan NM, Hardegger U, Wilkins TD. Investigation of an outbreak of antibiotic-associated colitis by various typing methods. *J Clin Microbiol* 1982;**16**:1096–101.

3 Tabaqchali S, O'Farrell S, Holland D, Silman R. Typing scheme for *Clostridium difficile*: its application in clinical and epidemiological studies. *Lancet* 1984;**i**:935–8.

4 McFarland LV, Mulligan ME, Kwok RYY, Stamm WE. Nosocomial acquisition of *Clostridium difficile* infection. *N Engl J Med* 1989;**320**:204–10.

5 Bowen KE, McFarland LV, Greenberg RN, Ramsey MM, Record KE, Svenson J. Isolation of *Clostridium difficile* at a university hospital: a two-year study. *Clin Infect Dis* 1995;**20**(Suppl 2):S261–262.

6   McFarland LV. Nosocomial acquisition and risk factors for *Clostridium difficile* disease. In: Rambaud JC, LaMont JT (eds). *Updates on Clostridium difficile.* Paris: Springer-Verlag, 1996.

7   Shek FW, Stacey BSF, Rendell J, Hellier MD, Hanson PJV. The risk of *Clostridium difficile*: the effect of length of stay, patient age and antibiotic use. *J Hosp Infect* 2000;**45**: 235–7.

8   Feldman RJ, Kallich M, Weinstein MP. Bacteremia due to *Clostridium difficile*: case report and review of extraintestinal *C difficile* infections. *Clin Infect Dis* 1995;**20**:1560–2.

9   Pron B, Merckx J, Touzet P *et al.* Chronic septic arthritis and osteomyelitis in a prosthetic knee joint due to *Clostridium difficile. Eur J Clin Microb Infect Dis* 1995;**14**: 599–601.

10 Lowenkron SE, Waxner J, Khullar P, Ilowite JS, Niederman MS, Fein AM. *Clostridium difficile* infection as a cause of severe sepsis. *Intensive Care Med* 1996;**22**:990–4.

11 Fekety R. Guidelines for the diagnosis and management of *Clostridium difficile*-associated diarrhea and colitis. *Am J Gastroenterol* 1997;**92**:739–50.

12 Qualman SJ, Petric M, Karmali MA, Smith CR, Hamilton SR. *Clostridium difficile* invasion and toxin circulation in fatal pediatric pseudomembranous colitis. *Am J Clin Pathol* 1990;**94**:410–6.

13 Walley T, Milson D. Loperamide related toxic megacolon in *Clostridium difficile* colitis [Letter]. *Postgrad Med J* 1990; **66**:582.

14 Gravisse J, Bernaud G, Hanau-Bercot B *et al. Clostridium difficile* brain empyema after prolonged intestinal carriage. *J Clin Microbiol* 2003;**41**:509–11.

15 Fekety R, McFarland LV, Surawicz CM, Greenberg RN, Elmer GW, Mulligan ME. Recurrent *Clostridium difficile* diarrhea: characteristics of and risk factors for patients enrolled in a prospective, randomized, double-blinded trial. *Clin Infect Dis* 1997;**24**:324–33.

16 McFarland LV, Surawicz CM, Rubin M, Fekety R, Elmer GW, Greenberg RN. Recurrent *Clostridium difficile* disease: epidemiology and clinical characteristics. *Infect Control Hosp Epidemiol* 1999;**20**:43–50.

17 Barbut F, Richard A, Hamadi K, Chomette V, Burghoffer B, Petit JC. Epidemiology of recurrences or reinfections of *Clostridium difficile*-associated diarrhea. *J Clin Microbiol* 2000;**38**:2386–8.

18 Kyne L, Merry C, O'Connell B, Kelly A, Keane C, O'Neill D. Factors associated with prolonged symptoms and severe disease due to *Clostridium difficile. Age Ageing* 1999;**28**: 107–13.

19 Riley TV, Bowman RA, Carroll SM. Diarrhoea associated with *Clostridium difficile* in a hospital population. *Med J Aust* 1983;**1**:166–9.

20 Yablon SA, Krotenberg R, Fruhmann K. *Clostridium difficile*-related disease: evaluation and prevalence among inpatients with diarrhea in two freestanding rehabilitation hospitals. *Arch Phys Med Rehabil* 1993;**74**:9–13.

21 Pear SM, Williamson TH, Bettin KM, Gerding DN, Galgiani JN. Decrease in nosocomial *Clostridium difficile*-associated diarrhea by restricting clindamycin use. *Ann Intern Med* 1994;**120**:272–7.

22 Samore MH, DeGirolami PC, Tlucko A, Lichtenberg DA, Melvin ZA, Karchmer AW. *Clostridium difficile* colonization and diarrhea at a tertiary care hospital. *Clin Infect Dis* 1994;**18**:181–7.

23 Barbut F, Corthier G, Charpak Y *et al.* Prevalence and pathogenicity of *Clostridium difficile* in hospitalized patients. A French multicenter study. *Arch Intern Med* 1996;**156**:1449–54.

24 Hirschhorn LR, Trnka Y, Onderdonk A, Lee M-LT, Platt R. Epidemiology of community-acquired *Clostridium difficile*-associated diarrhea. *J Infect Dis* 1994;**169**:127–33.

25 Levy DG, Stergachis A, McFarland L, *et al.* Antibiotics and *Clostridium difficile* diarrhea in the ambulatory care setting. *Clin Ther* 2000;**22**:91–102.

26 Alfa MJ, Kabani A, Lyerly D *et al.* Characterization of a toxin A-negative, toxin B-positive strain of *Clostridium difficile* responsible for a nosocomial outbreak of *Clostridium difficile*-associated diarrhea. *J Clin Microbiol* 2000;**38**: 2706–14.

27 Cohen SH, Tang YJ, Rahmani D, Silva J. Persistence of an endemic (toxigenic) isolate of *Clostridium difficile* in the environment of a general medicine ward. *Clin Infect Dis* 2000;**30**:952–4.

28 Johnson S, Samore MH, Farrow KA *et al.* Epidemics of diarrhea caused by a clindamycin-resistant strain of *Clostridium difficile* in four hospitals. *N Engl J Med* 1999; **341**:1645–51.

29 Kato H, Kato N, Watanabe K *et al.* Analysis of *Clostridium difficile* isolates from nosocomial outbreaks at three hospitals in diverse areas of Japan. *J Clin Microbiol* 2001; **39**:1391–5.

30 Mody LR, Smith SM, Dever LL. *Clostridium difficile*-associated diarrhea in a VA Medical Center: clustering of cases, association with antibiotic usage and impact on HIV-infected patients. *Infect Control Hosp Epidemiol* 2001; **22**:42–5.

31 Nath SK, Thornley JH, Kelly M *et al.* A sustained outbreak of *Clostridium difficile* in a general hospital: persistence of a toxigenic clone in four units. *Infect Control Hosp Epidemiol* 1994;**15**:382–9.

32 Samore MH, Venkataraman L, DeGirolami PC, Arbeit R, Karchmer A. Clinical and molecular epidemiology of sporadic and clustered cases of nosocomial *Clostridium difficile* diarrhea. *Am J Med* 1996;**100**:32–40.

33 Gerding DN. Treatment of *Clostridium difficile*-associated diarrhea and colitis. *Curr Top Microbiol Immunol* 2000; **250**:127–39.

34 Crabtree TD, Pelletier SJ, Gleason TG, Pruett TL, Sawyer RG. Clinical characteristics and antibiotic utilization in surgical patients with *Clostridium difficile*-associated diarrhea. *Am Surg* 2000;**66**:507–12.

35 Bradbury AW, Barrett S. Surgical aspects of *Clostridium difficile* colitis. *Br J Surg* 1997;**84**:150–9.

36 Simor AE, Yake SL, Tsimidis K. Infection due to *Clostridium difficile* among elderly residents of a long-term-care facility. *Clin Infect Dis* 1993;**17**:672–8.

37 Walker KJ, Gilliland SS, Vance-Bryan K *et al. Clostridium difficile* colonization in residents of long-term care facilities: prevalence and risk factors. *J Am Geriatr Soc* 1993;**41**: 940–6.

38 Brandt LJ, Kosche KA, Greenwald DA, Berkman D. *Clostridium difficile*-associated diarrhea in the elderly. *Am J Gastroenterol* 1999;**94**:3263–6.

39 Dharmarajan TS, Sipalay M, Shyamsundar R, Norkus EP, Pitchumoni CS. Co-morbidity, not age predicts adverse outcome in *Clostridium difficile* colitis. *World J Gastroenterol* 2000;**6**:198–201.

40 Settle CD, Wilcox MH, Fawley N, Corrado OK, Hawkey PM. Prospective study of the risk of *Clostridium difficile* diarrhea in elderly patients following treatment with cefotaxime or piperacillin-tazobactam. *Aliment Pharmacol Ther* 1998;**12**:1217–23.

41 Langley JM, LeBlanc JC, Hanakowski M, Goloubeva O. The role of *Clostridium difficile* and viruses as causes of nosocomial diarrhea in children. *Infect Control Hosp Epidemiol* 2002;**23**:660–4.

42 McFarland LV, Brandmarker SA, Guandalini S. Pediatric *Clostridium difficile*: a phantom menace or clinical reality? *J Pediatr Gastroenterol Nutr* 2000;**31**:220–31.

43 Kim K, DuPont HL, Pickering LK. Outbreaks of diarrhea associated with *Clostridium difficile* and its toxin in day-care centers: evidence of person-to-person spread. *J Pediatr* 1983;**102**:376–82.

44 Pulvirenti J, Gerding DN, Nathan C *et al.* Difference in the incidence of *Clostridium difficile* among patients infected with human immunodeficiency virus admitted to a public hospital and a private hospital. *Infect Control Hosp Epidemiol* 2002;**23**:641–7.

45 Gorschluter M, Glasmacher A, Hahn C *et al. Clostridium difficile* infection in patients with neutropenia. *Clin Infect Dis* 2001;**33**:786–91.

46 Chakrabarti S, Lees A, Jones SG, Milligan DW. *Clostridium difficile* infection in allogeneic stem cell transplant recipients is associated with severe graft-versus-host disease and non-relapse mortality. *Bone Marrow Transplant* 2000; **26**:871–6.

47 McFarland LV, Surawicz CM, Greenberg RN *et al.* Possible role of cross-transmission between neonates and mothers with recurrent *Clostridium difficile* infections. *Am J Infect Control* 1999;**27**:301–3.

48 Mekonen ET, Gerding DN, Sambot SP *et al.* Predominance of a single restriction endonuclease analysis group with intrahospital subgroup diversity among *Clostridium difficile* isolates at two Chicago hospitals. *Infect Control Hosp Epidemiol* 2002;**23**:648–52.

49 Johnson S, Adelmann A, Clabots CR, Peterson LR, Gerding DN. Recurrences of *Clostridium difficile* diarrhea not caused by the original infecting organism. *J Infect Dis* 1989; **159**:340–1.

50 Mulligan ME, Rolfe RD, Finegold SM, George WL. Contamination of a hospital environment by *Clostridium difficile*. *Curr Microbiol* 1979;**3**:173–5.

51 Chang VT, Nelson K. The role of physical proximity in nosocomial diarrhea. *Clin Infect Dis* 2000;**31**:717–22.

52 Johnson S, Gerding DN, Olson MM *et al.* Prospective, controlled study of vinyl glove use to interrupt *Clostridium difficile* nosocomial transmission. *Am J Med* 1990;**80**: 137–40.

53 Clabots CR, Johnson S, Olson MM, Peterson LR, Gerding DN. Acquisition of *Clostridium difficile* by hospitalized patients: evidence for colonized new admissions as a source of infection. *J Infect Dis* 1992;**166**:561–7.

54 Siemann M, Koch-Dorfler M, Rabenhorst G. *Clostridium difficile*-associated diseases. The clinical courses of 18 fatal cases. *Intensive Care Med* 2000;**26**:416–21.

55 Klipfel AA, Schein M, Fahoum B *et al.* Acute abdomen and *Clostridium difficile* colitis: still a lethal combination. *Dig Surg* 2000;**17**:160–3.

56 Kofsky P, Rosen L, Reed J, Tolmie M, Ufberg D. *Clostridium difficile* – a common and costly colitis. *Dis Colon Rectum* 1991;**34**:244–8.

57 Al-Eidan FA, McElnay JC, Scott MG, Kearney MP. *Clostridium difficile*-associated diarrhea in hospitalised patients. *J Clin Pharm Ther* 2000;**25**:101–9.

58 Kyne L, Hamel MB, Polavaram R, Kelly CP. Health care costs and mortality associated with nosocomial diarrhea due to *Clostridium difficile*. *Clin Infect Dis* 2002;**34**:346–53.

59 McFarland LV, Surawicz CM, Stamm WE. Risk factors for *Clostridium difficile* carriage and *C. difficile*-associated diarrhea in a cohort of hospitalized patients. *J Infect Dis* 1990;**162**:678–84.

60 Eriksson S, Aronsson B. Medical implications of nosocomial infection with *Clostridium difficile*. *Scand J Infect Dis* 1989;**21**:733–4.

61 McFarland LV. Normal flora: diversity and functions. microbial ecology in health and disease. 2000;**12**:193–207.

62 Safdar N, Maki DG. The communality of risk factors for nosocomial colonization and infection with antimicrobial-resistant *S. aureas*, *Enterococcus*, gram-negative bacilli, *Clostridium difficile* and *Candida*. *Ann Intern Med* 2002; **136**:834–44.

63 Bignardi GE. Risk factors for *Clostridium difficile* infection. *J Hosp Infect* 1998;**40**:1–15.

64 Brown EB, Talbot GH, Axelrod P, Provencher M, Hoegg C. Risk factors for *Clostridium difficile* toxin-associated diarrhea. *Infect Control Hosp Epidemiol* 1990;**11**:283–90.

65 Gerding DN, Olson MM, Peterson LR *et al. Clostridium difficile*-associated diarrhea and colitis in adults. A prospective case–controlled epidemiologic study. *Arch Intern Med* 1986;**146**:95–100.

66 Lai KK, Melvin ZS, Menard MJ, Kotilainen HR, Baker S. *Clostridium difficile*-associated diarrhea: epidemiology, risk factors, and infection control. *Infect Control Hosp Epidemiol* 1997;**18**:628–32.

67 Nelson DE, Auerbach SB, Baltch AL *et al.* Epidemic *Clostridium difficile*-associated diarrhea: role of second- and third-generation cephalosporins. *Infect Control Hosp Epidemiol* 1994;**15**:88–94.

68 Kyne L, Sougioultzis S, McFarland LV, Kelly CP. Underlying disease severity as a major risk factor for nosocomial *Clostridium difficile* diarrhea. *Infect Control Hosp Epidemiol* 2002;**23**:653–9.

69 Gerding DN, Johnson S, Peterson LR, Mulligan ME, Silva J Jr. *Clostridium difficile*-associated diarrhea and colitis. *Infect Control Hosp Epidemiol* 1995;**16**:459–77.

70 Johnson S, Gerding DN. *Clostridium difficile*-associated diarrhea. *Clin Infect Dis* 1998;**26**:1027–36.

71 Shim JK, Johnson S, Samore MH, Bliss DZ, Gerding DN. Primary asymptomatic colonization by *Clostridium difficile* is associated with a decreased risk of subsequent *Clostridium difficile* diarrhea. *Lancet* 1998;**351**:633–6.

72 Tal S, Gurevich A, Guller V, Gurevich I, Berger D, Levi S. Risk factors for recurrence of *Clostridium difficile*-associated diarrhea in the elderly. *Scand J Infect Dis* 2002;**34**:594–7.

73 Zimmerman RK. Risk factors for *Clostridium difficile* cytotoxin-positive diarrhea after control for horizontal transmission. *Infect Control Hosp Epidemiol* 1991;**12**: 96–100.

74 Do AN, Fridkin SK, Yechouron S *et al.* Risk factors for early recurrent *Clostridium difficile*-associated disease. *Clin Infect Dis* 1998;**26**:954–9.

75 McFarland LV, Surawicz CM, Greenberg RN *et al.* A randomized placebo-controlled trial of *Saccharomyces boulardii* in combination with standard antibiotics for *Clostridium difficile* disease. *JAMA* 1994;**271**:1913–18.

76 Siegel DL, Edelstein PH, Nachamkin I. Inappropriate testing for diarrheal diseases in the hospital. *JAMA* 1990;**263**: 979–82.

77 Yannelli B, Gurevich I, Schoch P, Cunha BA. Yield of stool cultures, ova and parasite tests, and *Clostridium difficile* determinations in nosocomial diarrheas. *Am J Infect Control* 1988;**16**:246–9.

78 De Girolami PC, Hanff PA, Eichelberger K *et al.* Multicenter evaluation of a new enzyme immunoassay for detection of *Clostridium difficile* enterotoxin A. *J Clin Microbiol* 1992; **30**:1085–8.

79 Borriello SP, Vale T, Brazier JS, Hyde S, Chippeck E. Evaluation of a commercial enzyme immunoassay kit for the detection of *Clostridium difficile* toxin A. *Eur J Clin Microbiol Infect Dis* 1992;**11**:360–3.

80 Doern GV, Coughlin RT, Wu L. Laboratory diagnosis of *Clostridium difficile*-associated gastrointestinal disease: comparison of a monoclonal antibody enzyme immunoassay for toxins A and B with a monoclonal antibody enzyme immunoassay for toxin A only and two cytotoxicity assays. *J Clin Microbiol* 1992;**30**:2042–6.

81 Lozeniewski A, Rabaud C, Dotto E *et al.* Laboratory diagnosis of *Clostridium difficile*-associated diarrhea and colitis: usefulness of Premier Cytoclone A + B enzyme immunoassay for combined detection of stool toxins and toxigenic *C. difficile* strains. *J Clin Microbiol* 2001, 39:1996–8.

82 Landry ML, Topal J, Ferguson D *et al.* Evaluation of Biosite triage *Clostridium difficile* panel for rapid detection of *Clostridium difficile* in stool samples. *J Clin Microbiol* 2001;**39**:1855–8.

83 Alfa MJ, Swan B, VanDekerkhove B, Pang P, Harding GK. The diagnosis of *Clostridium difficile* associated diarrhea: comparison of Triage *C. difficile* panel, EIA for Tox A/B and cytotoxin assays. *Diagn Microbiol Infect Dis* 2002;**43**: 257–63.

84 Vanpoucke H, DeBaere T, Claeys G, *et al.* Evaluation of six commercial assays for the rapid detection of *Clostridium difficile* toxin and/or antigen in stool specimens. *Clin Microbiol Infect* 2001;**7**:55.

85 Yucesoy M, McCoubrey J, Brown R *et al.* Detection of toxin production in *Clostridium difficile* strains by three different methods. *Clin Microbiol Infect* 2002;**8**:413.

86 Manabe YD, Vientz JM, Moore RD *et al.* *Clostridium difficile* colitis: an efficient clinical approach to diagnosis. *Ann Intern Med* 1995;**123**:835–40.

87 Johnson S, Homann SR, Bettin KM *et al.* Treatment of asymptomatic *Clostridium difficile* carriers (fecal excretors) with vancomycin or metrodindazole. A randomized, placebo-controlled trial. *Ann Infect Med* 1992;**15**:297–302.

88 Zimmermann MJ, Bak A, Sutherland LR. Review article: treatment of *Clostridium difficile* infection. *Aliment Pharmacol Ther* 1997;**11**:1003–12.

89 Wenisch C, Parschalk B, Hasenhündl M, Hirschl AM, Graninger W. Comparison of vancomycin, teicoplanin, metronidazole, and fusidic acid for the treatment of *Clostridium difficile*-associated diarrhea. *Clin Infect Dis* 1996;**22**:813–18.

90 Teasley DG, Gerding DN, Olson MM *et al.* Prospective randomised trial of metronidazole versus vancomycin for *Clostridium difficile*-associated diarrhoea and colitis. *Lancet* 1983;**2**:1043–6.

91 De Lalla F, Nicolin R, Rinaldi E *et al.* Prospective study of oral teicoplanin versus oral vancomycin for therapy of pseudomembranous colitis and *C. difficile*-associated diarrhea. *Antimicrob Agents Chemother* 1992;**36**:2192–6.

92 Fekety R, Silva J, Kauffman C, Buggy B, Deery HG. Treatment of antibiotic-associated *Clostridium difficile* colitis with oral vancomycin: comparison of two dosage regimens. *Am J Med* 1989;**86**:15–19.

93 Dudley MN, McLaughlin JC, Carrington G, Frick J, Nightingale CH, Quintiliani R. Oral bacitracin vs vancomycin therapy for *Clostridium difficile*-associated diarrhea. A randomized double-blind trial. *Arch Intern Med* 1986;**146**:1101–4.

94 Young GP, Ward PB, Bayley N *et al.* Antibiotic-associated colitis due to *Clostridium difficile*: double-blind comparison of vancomycin with bacitracin. *Gastroenterology* 1985;**89**: 1038–45.

95 Mogg GA, George RH, Youngs D *et al.* Randomized controlled trial of colestipol in antibiotic-associated colitis. *Br J Surg* 1982;**69**:137–9.

96 Keighley MRB, Burdon DW, Arabi Y *et al.* Randomised controlled trial of vancomycin for pseudomembranous colitis and postoperative diarrhoea. *BMJ* 1978;**2**:1667–9.

97 Olson MM, Shanholtzer CJ, Lee JT Jr, Gerding DN. Ten years of prospective *Clostridium difficile*-associated disease surveillance and treatment at the Minneapolis VA Medical Center, 1982–1991. *Infect Control Hosp Epidemiol* 1994; **15**:371–81.

98 Apisarnthanarak A, Razavi B, Mundy LM. Adjunctive intracolonic vancomycin for severe *Clostridium difficile* colitis: case series and review of the literature. *Clin Infect Dis* 2002;**35**:690–6.

99 Sanchez JL, Gerding DN, Olson MM *et al.* Metronidazole susceptibility in *Clostridium difficile* isolates recovered from cases of *C. difficile*-associated disease treatment failures and successes. *Anaerobe* 1999;**5**:201–4.

100 Peláez T, Alcála R, Alonso M *et al.* Reassessent of *Clostridium difficile* susceptibility to metronidazole and vancomycin. *Antimicrob Agents Chemother* 2002;**46**:1647–50.

101 Friedenberg F, Fernandez A, Kaul V, Niami P, Levine GM. Intravenous metronidazole for the treatment of *Clostridium difficile* colitis. *Dis Colon Rectum* 2001;**44**:1176–80.

102 Tedesco FJ. Bacitracin therapy in antibiotic-associated pseudomembranous colitis. *Dig Dis Sci* 1980;**10**:783–4.

103 Chang TW, Gorbach SL, Bartlett JG, Saginur R. Bacitracin treatment of antibiotic-associated colitis and diarrhea caused by *Clostridium difficile* toxin. *Gastroenterology* 1980;**78**:1584–6.

104 Taylor NS, Bartlett JG. Binding of *Clostridium difficile* cytotoxin and vancomycin by anion-exchange resins. *J Infect Dis* 1980;**141**:92–7.

105 Havenaar R, Huis I, Veld JHS. Probiotics: a general view. In: BJB Wood, ed. *The Lactic Acid Bacteria in Health and Disease*. Amsterdam: Elsevier, 1992.

106 Siitonen S, Vapaatalo H, Salminen S *et al.* Effect of *Lactobacillus GG* yoghurt in prevention of antibiotic associated diarrhoea. *Ann Med* 1990;**22**:57–9.

107 Arvola T, Laiho K, Torkkeli S *et al.* Prophylactic *Lactobacillus GG* reduces antibiotic associated diarrhea in children with respiratory infections: a randomized study. *Pediatrics* 1999;**104**:1121–2.

108 Vanderhoof JA, Whitney DB, Antonson Dl, Hanner TL, Lupo JV, Young RJ. *Lactobacillus GG* in prevention of antibiotic-associated diarrhea in children. *J Pediatr* 1999;**135**:564–8.

109 Armuzzi A, Cremonini F, Ojetti V *et al.* Effect of *Lactobacillus GG* supplementation on antibiotic-associated gastrointestinal side effects during *Helicobacter pylori* eradication therapy: a pilot study. *Digestion* 2001;**63**:1–7.

110 Thomas MR, Litin SC, Osmon DR, Corr AP, Weaver Al, Lohse CM. Lack of effect of *Lactobacillus GG* on antibiotic-associated diarrhea: a randomized, placebo-controlled trial. *Mayo Clin Proc* 2001;**76**:883–9.

111 Gotz V, Romankiewicz JA, Moss J, Murray HW. Prophylaxis against ampicillin-associated diarrhea with a lactobacillus preparation. *Am J Hosp Pharm* 1979;**36**:754–7.

112 Tankanow RM, Ross MB, Ertel IJ *et al.* A double-blind, placebo-controlled study of the efficacy of Lactinex in the prophylaxis of amoxicillin-induced diarrhea. *Ann Pharmacother* 1990;**24**:382–4.

113 Clements ML, Levine MM, Ristaino PA *et al.* Exogenous lactobacilli fed to man – their fate and ability to prevent diarrhoeal disease. *Prog Food Nutr Sci* 1983;**7**:29–37.

114 Wunderlich PF, Braun L, Fumagalli I *et al.* Double-blind report on the efficacy of lactic acid-producing enterococcus SF68 in the prevention of antibiotic-associated diarrhoea and in the treatment of acute diarrhoea. *J Int Med Res* 1980;**17**:333–8.

115 Borgia M, Sepe N, Brancato V, Borgia B. A controlled clinical study on *Streptococcus faecium* preparation for the prevention of side reactions during long-term antibiotic treatments. *Curr Ther Res* 1982;**31**:266–71.

116 Colombel JF, Cortot A, Neut C *et al.* Yoghurt with *Bifidobacterium longum* reduces erythomycin-induced gastrointestinal effects [Letter]. *Lancet* 1987;**2**:43.

117 Adam J, Barret C, Barret-Bellet A *et al.* Essai's cliniques contrôlés en double insu de l'ultra-levure lyophilisée. Étude multicentrique par 25 medecins de 388 cas. *Gaz Med Fr* 1977;**84**:2072–81.

118 Surawicz CM, McFarland LV, Elmer G, Chinn J. Treatment of recurrent *Clostridium difficile* colitis with vancomycin and *Saccharomyces boulardii*. *Am J Gastroenterol* 1989;**84**:1285–7.

119 McFarland LV, Surawicz CM, Greenberg RN, *et al.* Prevention of β-lactam-associated diarrhea by *Saccharomyces boulardii* compared with placebo. *Am J Gastroenterol* 1995;**90**:439–48.

120 Bleichner G, Blehaut H, Mentec H *et al. Saccharomyces boulardii* prevents diarrhea in critically ill tube-fed patients. A multicenter, randomized, double-blind, placebo-controlled trial. *Intensive Care Med* 1997;**23**:517–23.

121 Lewis SJ, Potts LF, Barry RE. The lack of therapeutic effect of *Saccharomyces boulardii* in the prevention of antibiotic-related diarrhoea in elderly patients. *J Infect* 1998;**36**:171–4.

122 Cremonini F, Di Caro S, Covino M *et al.* Effect of different probiotic preparations on anti-*Helicobacter pylori* therapy-related side effects: a parallel group, triple blind, placebo-controlled study. *Am J Gastroenterol* 2002;**97**:2744–9.

123 Biller JA, Katz AJ, Flores AF, Buie TM, Gorbach SL. Treatment of recurrent *Clostridium difficile* colitis with *Lactobacillus GG*. *J Pediatr Gastroenterol Nutr* 1995;**21**:224–6.

124 Seal D, Borriello SP, Barclay F *et al.* Treatment of relapsing *Clostridium difficile* diarrhoea by administration of a non-toxigenic strain. *Eur J Clin Microbiol* 1987;**6**:51–3.

125 Surawicz CM, McFarland LV, Greenberg RN *et al.* The search for a better treatment for recurrent *Clostridium difficile* disease: use of high-dose vancomycin combined with *Saccharomyces boulardii*. *Clin Infect Dis* 2000;**31**:1012–17.

126 Cleary RK, Grossmann R, Fernandez FB *et al.* Metronidazole may inhibit intestinal colonization with *Clostridium difficile*. *Dis Colon Rectum* 1998;**41**:464–7.

127 Levett PN. Time-dependent killing of *Clostridium difficile* by metronidazole and vancomycin. *J Antimicrob Chemother* 1991;**27**:55–62.

128 Bolton RP, Culsaw MA. Fecal metronidazole concentrations during oral and intravenous therapy for antibiotic-associated colitis due to *Clostridium difficile*. *Gut* 1986;**27**:1169–72.

129 Walters BAJ, Roberts R, Stafford R, Seneviratne E. Recurrence of antibiotic associated colitis: endogenous persistence of *C. difficile* during vancomycin therapy. *Gut* 1983;**24**:206–12.

130 Larson HE, Borriello SP. Quantitative study of antibiotic-induced susceptibility to *Clostridium difficile* enterocecitis in hamsters. *Antimicrob Agents Chemother* 1990;**34**:1348–53.

131 Nair S, Yadav D, Corpuz M, Pitchumoni CS. *Clostridium difficile* colitis: factors influencing treatment failure and relapse – a prospective evaluation. *Am J Gastroenterol* 1998;**93**:1873–6.

132 McFarland LV, Elmer GW, Surawicz CM. Breaking the cycle: treatment strategies for 163 cases of recurrent *Clostridium difficile* disease. *Am J Gastroenterol* 2002;**97**:1769–75.

133 Tedesco FJ, Gordon D, Fortson WC. Approach to patients with multiple relapses of antibiotic-associated pseudo-membranous colitis. *Am J Gastroenterol* 1985;**80**:867–8.

134 Buggy BP, Fekety R, Silva J Jr. Therapy of relapsing *Clostridium difficile*-associated diarrhea and colitis with the combination of vancomycin and rifampin. *J Clin Gastroenterol* 1987;**9**:155–9.

135 Bennett RG, Gorbach SL, Goldin R, Chang T. Treatment of relapsing *Clostridium difficile* diarrhea with *Lactobacillus GG*. *Nutr Today* 1996;**31**:S35–S38.

136 Gorbach SL, Chang T, Goldin B. Successful treatment of relapsing *Clostridium difficile* colitis with *Lactobacillus GG*. *Lancet* 1987;**2**:1519.

137 Bowden TA, Mansberger AR, Lykins LE. Pseudo-membraneous enterocolitis: mechanism for restoring floral homeostasis. *Am Surg* 1981;**47**:178–83.

138 Persky SE, Brandt LJ. Treatment of recurrent *Clostridium difficile*-associated diarrhea by administration of donated stool directly through a colonoscope. *Am J Gastroenterol* 2000;**95**:3283–5.

139 Schwan A, Sjolin S, Trottestam U, Aronsson B. Relapsing *Clostridium difficile* enterocolitis cured by rectal infusion of normal faeces. *Scand J Infect Dis* 1984;**16**:211–15.

140 Tvede M, Rask-Madsen J. Bacteriotherapy for chronic relapsing *Clostridium difficile* diarrhoea in six patients. *Lancet* 1989;**I**:1156–60.

141 Liacouras CA, Piccoli DA. Whole-bowel irrigation as an adjunct to the treatment of chronic, relapsing *Clostridium difficile* colitis. *J Clin Gastroenterol* 1996;**22**:186–9.

142 Beales ILP. Intravenous immunoglobulin for recurrent *Clostridium difficile* diarrhoea. *Gut* 2002;**51**:455–458.

143 Hassett J, Meyers S, McFarland LV, Mulligan ME. Recurrent *Clostridium difficile* infection in a patient with selective IgG1 deficiency treated with intravenous immune globulin and *Saccharomyces boulardii*. *Clin Infect Dis* 1995;**20**: S266–8.

144 Leung DY, Kelly CP, Boguniewicz M, Pothoulakis C, LaMont JT, Flores A. Treatment with intravenously administered gamma globulin of chronic relapsing colitis inducted by *Clostridium difficile* toxin. *J Pediatr* 1991;**118**:633–7.

145 Ariano RE, Zhanel GG, Harding GKM. The role of anion-exchange resins in the treatment of antibiotic-associated pseudomembranous colitis. *Can Med Assoc J* 1990;**142**:1049–51.

146 Wilcox MH. Treatment of *Clostridium difficile* infection. *J Antimicrob Chemother* 1998;**41**(Suppl C):41–6.

147 Malamou-Ladas H, Farrell SO, Nash JO, Tabaqchali S. Isolation of *Clostridium difficile* from patients and the environment of hospital wards. *J Clin Pathol* 1983;**6**:88–92.

148 Fekety R, Kim KH, Brown D, Batts DH, Cudmore M, Silva J. Epidemiology of antibiotic-associated colitis: isolation of *Clostridium difficile* from the hospital environment. *Am Med* 1981;**70**:906–8.

149 Rutala WA, Gergen MF, Weber DJ. Inactivation of *Clostridium difficile* spores by disinfectants. *Infect Control Hosp Epidemiol* 1993;**14**:36–9.

150 Mayfield JL, Leet T, Miller J, Mundy LM. Environmental control to reduce transmission of *Clostridium difficile*. *Clin Infect Dis* 2000;**31**:995–1000.

151 Struelens MJ, Maas A, Nonhoff C *et al*. Control of nosocomial transmission of *Clostridium difficile* based on sporadic case surveillance. *Am J Med* 1991;**91**(Suppl 3B):138–44.

152 Kaatz GW, Gitlin SD, Schaberg DR *et al*. Acquisition of *Clostridium difficile* from the hospital environment. *Am J Epidemiol* 1988;**127**:1289–94.

153 Hughes CE, Gebhard RL, Peterson LR, Gerding DN. Efficacy of routine fiberoptic endoscope cleaning and disinfection for killing *Clostridium difficile*. *Gastrointest Endosc* 1986;**32**:7–9.

154 Brooks SE, Veal RO, Kramer M, Dore L, Schupf N, Adachi M. Reduction in the incidence of *Clostridium difficile*-associated diarrhea in an acute care hospital and a skilled nursing facility following replacement of electronic thermometers with single-use disposables. *Infect Control Hosp Epidemiol* 1992;**13**:98–103.

155 Bettin K, Clabots C, Methie P, Willard K, Gerding DN. Effectiveness of liquid soap vs chlorhexidine gluconate for the removal of *Clostridium difficile* from bare hands and gloved hands. *Infec Control Hosp Epidemiol* 1994;**15**:697–702.

156 Boone N, Eagan JA, Gillern P, Armstrong D, Sepkovitz KA. Evaluation of an interdisciplinary re-isolation policy for patients with previous *Clostridium difficile* diarrhea. *Am J Infect Control* 1998;**26**:584–7.

157 Kerr RB, McLaughlin DI, Sonnenberg LW. Control of *Clostridium difficile* colitis outbreak by treating asymptomatic carriers with metronidazole. *Am J Infect Control* 1990;**18**:332–3.

158 Bender BS, Bennett RG, Laughon B *et al*. Is *Clostridium difficile* endemic in chronic-care facilities? *Lancet* 1986;**2**:11.

159 Delmee M, Vandercam B, Avesani V, Michaux JL. Epidemiology and prevention of *Clostridium difficile* infections in a leukemia unit. *Eur J Clin Microbiol* 1987;**6**:623–7.

160 Zafar AB, Gaydoes LA, Furlong WB, Guygen MH, Mennonna PA. Effectiveness of infection control program in controlling nosocomial *Clostridium difficile*. *Am J Infect Control* 1998;**26**:588–93.

161 Climo MW, Isreal DS, Wong ES, Williams D, Courdon P, Markowitz SM. Hospital-wide restriction of clindamycin: effect on the incidence of *Clostridium difficile*-associated diarrhea and cost. *Ann Intern Med* 1998;**128**:989–95.

162 Ho M, Yang D, Wyle FA, Mulligan ME. Increased incidence of *Clostridium difficile*-associated diarrhea following decreased restriction of antibiotic use. *Clin Infect Dis* 1996;Suppl 1:S102–106.

163 McNulty C, Logan M, Donald IP *et al*. Successful control of *Clostridium difficile* infection in an elderly care unit through use of a restrictive antibiotic policy. *J Antimicrob Chemother* 1997;**40**:707–711.

164 Ludlam H, Brown N, Sule O, Redpath C, Coni N, Owen G. An antibiotic policy associated with reduced risk of *Clostridium difficile*-associated diarrhea. *Age Ageing* 1999;**28**:578–80.

19 Ogilvie's syndrome

Michael D Saunders, Michael B Kimmey

Introduction

Acute colonic pseudo-obstruction (ACPO), also referred to as Ogilvie's syndrome,[1] is a clinical condition with symptoms, signs and radiographic appearance of acute large bowel obstruction without a mechanical cause. ACPO occurs most often in hospitalized or institutionalized patients with serious underlying medical and surgical conditions. ACPO is an important cause of morbidity and mortality. The mortality rate is estimated at 40% when ischemia or perforation occurs.[2] Early detection and prompt appropriate management are critical to minimizing morbidity and mortality.

Pathogenesis

The pathogenesis of ACPO is not completely understood but likely results from an alteration in the autonomic regulation of colonic motor function.[3] Colonic pseudo-obstruction was first described in 1948 by Sir Heneage Ogilvie, who reported two patients with chronic colonic dilation associated with malignant infiltration of the celiac plexus.[1] Ogilvie attributed the syndrome to sympathetic deprivation. A better understanding of the autonomic nervous system in the gut has modified this hypothesis. The parasympathetic nervous system increases contractility, whereas the sympathetic nerves decrease motility.[3] An imbalance in autonomic innervation, produced by a variety of factors, leads to excessive parasympathetic suppression or sympathetic stimulation. The result is colonic atony and pseudo-obstruction.

Multiple predisposing factors or conditions have been associated with ACPO (Table 19.1). In a large retrospective series of 400 patients, the most common predisposing conditions were non-operative trauma (11·3%), infections (10%), and cardiac disease (10%).[2] Cesarean section and hip surgery were the most common surgical procedures, with the onset of the syndrome occurring post-operatively at an average of 4·5 days. In another retrospective analysis of 48 patients, the spine or retroperitoneum had been traumatized or manipulated

Table 19.1 Predisposing conditions associated with acute colonic pseudo-obstruction – an analysis of 400 cases[a]

Condition	No. of patients	Proportion (%)
Trauma (non-operative)	45	11·3
Infection (pneumonia, sepsis most common)	40	10·0
Cardiac (myocardial infarction, heart failure)	40	10·0
Obstetrics/gynecology	39	9·8
Abdominal/pelvic surgery	37	9·3
Neurologic	37	9·3
Orthopedic surgery	29	7·3
Miscellaneous medical conditions (metabolic, cancer, respiratory failure, renal failure)	128	32
Miscellaneous surgical conditions (urologic, thoracic, neurosurgery)	47	11·8

[a]Associated conditions in approximately 400 patients, reported by Vanek and Al-Salti.[2] Some patients had more than one associated condition.

in 52%.[4] Over half the patients were receiving narcotics, and electrolyte abnormalities were present in approximately two-thirds. Thus, multiple metabolic, pharmacologic, or traumatic factors appear to alter the autonomic regulation of colonic function resulting in pseudo-obstruction.

Clinical features

The clinical features of ACPO include abdominal distension, abdominal pain (80%), and nausea and/or vomiting (60%).[2] Passage of flatus or stool is reported in up to 40% of patients. There is no significant difference in symptoms of patients with ischemic or perforated bowel, except for a higher incidence of fever.[2] On examination, the abdomen is tympanitic and bowel sounds are typically present. Fever, marked abdominal tenderness and leukocytosis are more common in patients with ischemia or perforation but also occur in those who have not developed these complications.[2]

The diagnosis of ACPO is confirmed by plain abdominal radiographs, which show varying degrees of colonic dilatation (Figure 19.1). Air fluid levels and dilatation can also be seen in the small bowel. Typically, the right colon and cecum show the most marked distension, and cut-offs at the splenic flexure are common. This distribution of colonic dilation may be caused by the different origins of the proximal and distal parasympathetic nerve supply to the colon.[3] A water soluble contrast enema should be obtained to exclude mechanical obstruction if gas and distension are not present throughout all colonic segments including the rectum and sigmoid colon.

Keys to management of ACPO include (i) early recognition and diagnosis, (ii) evaluation to exclude mechanical obstruction or other causes of pseudo-obstruction (such as *Clostridium difficile* colitis[5]), (iii) assessment for signs of ischemia or perforation which would warrant urgent surgical intervention, and (iv) initiation of appropriate treatment measures.

Management

Treatment options for ACPO include appropriate supportive measures, medical therapy, colonoscopic decompression, and surgery. Despite extensive literature documenting the clinical features of ACPO, there are very few randomized controlled clinical trials on the treatment of this condition, and most evidence for efficacy of treatments comes from uncontrolled studies.

Supportive therapy

Supportive therapy (Box 19.1) should be instituted in all patients as it appears to be successful as the primary treatment in the majority of patients.[6] B4 Patients are given

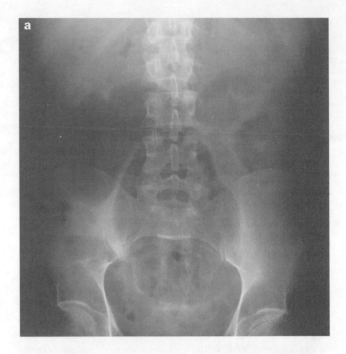

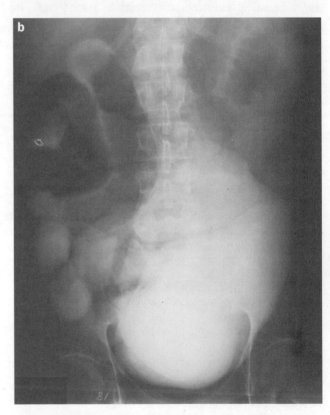

Figure 19.1 Abdominal radiographs of a patient with acute colonic pseudo-obstruction. (a) The plain abdominal film shows marked dilatation, especially of the right colon. In addition, moderate small bowel dilatation is present. (b) A water soluble contrast enema was obtained excluding mechanical obstruction

---

Box 19.1 Supportive therapy for acute colonic pseudo-obstruction

- Nil per os
- Correct fluid and electrolyte imbalances
- Nasogastric tube suction
- Rectal tube to gravity drainage
- Limit offending medications (especially narcotics)
- Frequent position changes, ambulate if possible

---

nothing by mouth. Intravenous fluids are administered and electrolyte imbalances are corrected. Nasogastric suction is provided to limit swallowed air from contributing further to colonic distension. A rectal tube should be inserted and attached to gravity drainage. Medications that can adversely affect colonic motility, such as opiates, anti-cholinergics, and calcium channel antagonists are discontinued if possible. Ambulation and mobilization of patients are encouraged. The knee–chest position with hips held high has been advocated as aiding in evacuation of colonic gas.[7] None of these supportive measures has been studied in a randomized trial. C5

The reported success of supportive management is variable with pooled rates from several retrospective series of approximately 85%.[6,8–12] In these combined series, 111 patients were treated conservatively, of which 95 (86%) had resolution of the pseudo-obstruction. B4 Sloyer *et al.* reported outcomes of 25 cancer patients with ACPO (mostly non-gastrointestinal malignancies).[6] The mean cecal diameter was 11·7 cm (range 9–18 cm). Of the 24 patients treated conservatively, 23 (96%) improved by clinical and radiologic criteria with the median time to improvement of 1·6 days (mean 3 days). There were no perforations or ACPO-related deaths. The authors concluded that early endoscopic or surgical decompression is not necessary in patients with ACPO. B4 In another recent retrospective series of 151 patients reported by Loftus *et al.*, 117 (77%) had spontaneous resolution of ACPO with conservative treatment.[13] B4 These studies demonstrate that the initial management of ACPO should be directed towards eliminating or reducing the factors known to contribute to the problem.

Patient outcome

The clinical dilemma facing the clinician caring for a patient with ACPO is whether to treat the patient with conservative measures and close observation versus proceeding with medical or endoscopic decompression of the dilated colon. The outcome of patients with ACPO is determined by multiple factors. The severity of the underlying illness appears to exert the greatest influence on patient outcome. ACPO often afflicts debilitated patients, which explains the significant morbidity and mortality even with successful treatment of the colonic dilatation. Other factors

that appear to influence outcome are increasing age, maximal cecal diameter, delay in decompression and status of the bowel.[2] The risk of spontaneous colon perforation in ACPO is low but clearly exists. Rex reviewed all available reports in the literature and estimated the risk of spontaneous perforation to be approximately 3%.[14] The mortality rate in ACPO is approximately 40% when ischemia or perforation are present, compared with 15% in patients with viable bowel.[2] Retrospective analyses of patients with ACPO[2,12] have attempted to identify clinical factors that predict which patients are more likely to have complications such as ischemia or perforation. The risk of colonic perforation has been reported[2] to increase with cecal diameter greater than 12 cm and when distension has been present for more than 6 days.[12] In the large series reported by Vanek and Al-Salti, no cases of perforation were seen when the cecal diameter was less than 12 cm.[2] However, at diameters greater than 12 cm, there was no clear relationship between risk of ischemia or perforation and the size of the cecum. The duration and progression of colonic distension may be more important. Johnson and Rice reported a mean duration of distension of 6 days in patients who perforated compared with 2 days in those who did not.[12] A two-fold increase in mortality occurs when cecal diameter is greater than 14 cm and a five-fold increase when delay in decompression is greater than 7 days.[2] Thus, the decision to intervene with medical therapy, colonoscopy or surgery is dictated by the patient's clinical status. On the basis of the limited available evidence patients with marked cecal distension (> 10 cm) of significant duration (> 3–4 days) and those not improving after 24–48 hours of supportive therapy are considered to be candidates for further intervention. B4 In the absence of signs of ischemia or perforation, medical therapy with neostigmine should be considered the initial therapy of choice.

Medical therapy

Neostigmine

The only randomized controlled trial of an intervention for ACPO involves the use of neostigmine.[15] Neostigmine, a reversible acetylcholinesterase inhibitor, indirectly stimulates muscarinic receptors, thereby enhancing colonic motor activity, inducing colonic propulsion and accelerated transit.[16] The rationale for using neostigmine stems from the imbalance in autonomic regulation of colonic function that is proposed to occur in ACPO. Neostigmine was first used for manipulation of the autonomic innervation to the gastrointestinal tract by Neely and Catchpole over 30 years ago in studies on small bowel paralytic ileus.[17] Neostigmine, administered intravenously, has a rapid onset (1–20 minutes) and short duration (1–2 hours) of action.[18] The elimination half-life

Table 19.2 Neostigmine for colonic decompression in patients with acute colonic pseudo-obstruction

Study	No. of patients	Design	Dose	Decompression	Recurrence
Ponec *et al.* (1999)[15]	21 (neostigmine 11, placebo 10)	RCT; (OL in non-responders)	2·0 mg IV over 3–5 min	Neostigmine 10/11 in RCT; 17/18 total; placebo 0/10	2
Hutchinson and Griffiths (1992)[20]	11	OL	2·5 mg IV in 1 min	8/11	0
Stephenson *et al.* (1995)[21]	12	OL	2·5 mg IV over 1–3 min	12/12 (2 patients required 2 doses)	1
Turegano-Fuentes *et al.* (1997)[22]	16	OL	2·5 mg IV over 60 min	12/16	0
Trevisani *et al.* (2000)[23]	28	OL	2·5 mg IV over 3 min	26/28	0
Paran *et al.* (2001)[24]	11	OL	2·5 mg IV over 60 min	10/11 (2 patients required 2 doses)	0
Abeyta *et al.* (2001)[25]	8	Retrospective	2·0 mg IV	6/8 (2 patients required 2 doses)	0
Loftus *et al.* (2002)[13]	18	Retrospective	2·0 mg IV	16/18	5

RCT, randomized controlled trial; OL, open label trial; IV, intravenous

averages 80 minutes, but is more prolonged in patients with renal insufficiency.[19]

A randomized double blind placebo-controlled trial evaluated neostigmine in patients with ACPO with a cecal diameter of > 10 cm and no response to 24 hours of conservative therapy.[15] Exclusion criteria were suspected ischemia or perforation, pregnancy, severe active broncho-spasm, cardiac arrhythmias and renal failure. Patients were randomized to receive neostigmine, 2 mg, or saline by intravenous infusion over 3–5 minutes. The primary endpoint was the clinical response to infusion, defined as a prompt reduction in abdominal distension by physical examination. Secondary endpoints included the change in measurements of colonic diameter on radiographs and abdominal girth. Patients not responding within 3 hours to initial infusion were eligible for open label neostigmine. A clinical response was observed in 10 of 11 patients (91%) randomized to receive neostigmine compared to 0 of 10 receiving placebo. Ald The median time to response was 4 minutes. Median reduction in cecal diameter (5 cm *v* 2 cm) and abdominal girth (7 cm *v* 1 cm) were significantly reduced in neostigmine-treated patients. Open label neostigmine was administered to eight patients who failed to respond to the initial infusion (seven placebo, one neostigmine), and all had prompt decompression. Of the 18 patients who received neostigmine, either initially or during open label treatment, 17 (94%) had a clinical response. The recurrence rate of colonic distension after neostigmine decompression was low (11%). The most common adverse effects observed with neostigmine were mild abdominal cramping and excessive salivation. Symptomatic bradycardia requiring atropine occurred in two of 19 patients.

There are also several uncontrolled observational studies supporting the use of neostigmine in this condition.[13,20–25] Collectively, rapid decompression of colonic distension was observed in 88% of patients with a recurrence rate of 7% (Table 19.2). B4 The cost of neostigmine is minimal, with a 2 mg ampoule for parenteral use costing only US$3.[15] The cost to the patient after storage and handling fees are included is approximately US$15.

Although neostigmine was associated with a favorable safety profile in the reported clinical trials, caution should be used when administering the medication. Neostigmine should be administered with the patient kept supine in bed with continuous electrocardiographic monitoring, physician assessment and measurement of vital signs for 15–30 minutes following administration.[15] Contraindications to its use include mechanical bowel obstruction, presence of ischemia or perforation, pregnancy, uncontrolled cardiac arrhythmias, severe active bronchospasm, and renal insufficiency.

Thus, neostigmine appears to be an effective, safe and inexpensive method of colonic decompression in ACPO. The published data support its use as the initial therapy of choice for patients not responding to conservative therapy if there are no contraindications to its use. Ald, B4 In patients with only a partial response or recurrence after an initial infusion, a repeated dose is reasonable and often successful. If the patient fails to respond after two doses, proceeding with colonoscopic decompression is advised.

Other medications

There are only anecdotal reports using other prokinetic agents in ACPO, and their use for the treatment of this

Table 19.3 Observational studies of colonoscopic decompression in acute colonic pseudo-obstruction

Study	No. of patients	Successful initial decompression (%)	Overall colonoscopic success (%)	Complications
Nivatvongs *et al.* (1982)[31]	22	68	73	< 1 % (no perforations)
Strodel *et al.* (1983)[32]	44	61	73	2 % (1 perforation)
Bode *et al.* (1984)[33]	22	68	77	4·5 % (1 perforation)
Jetmore *et al.* (1992)[4]	45	84	36	< 1 % (no perforations)
Geller *et al.* (1996)[34]	41	95	18	2 % (2 perforations)

condition cannot be recommended. Erythromycin, a motilin receptor agonist, has been reported to be successful in treating patients in a few case reports.[26,27] Armstrong *et al.* reported decompression in two patients with ACPO with oral erythromycin (500 mg four times daily) for 10 days.[26] In another report, one patient had resolution of ACPO after 3 days of intravenous erythromycin therapy.[27] Cisapride, a partial 5-HT$_4$-receptor agonist, has also been employed with some success in patients with ACPO.[28] However, this agent is no longer available for use in the USA and Canada due to class III antiarrhythmic properties. Second generation 5-HT$_4$ partial receptor agonists, such as tegaserod, may be more active at the colonic level than cisapride.[29] C5 However, data evaluating these agents in ACPO are not available.

Endoscopic decompression

Colonoscopic decompression may be required in patients with persistent, marked colonic dilatation that has failed to respond to supportive therapy and neostigmine or when neostigmine is contraindicated. There is no well-defined standard of care regarding the use of colonoscopy in ACPO.[7] Colonoscopic decompression appears to be beneficial in ACPO, but it is associated with a greater risk of complications, is not completely effective and can be followed by recurrence.[30] B4 Colonoscopy is done to prevent bowel ischemia and perforation. It should not be done if these complications have already developed.

Colonoscopy in ACPO is a technically difficult procedure and should be carried out by experts. Oral laxatives and bowel preparations should not be administered prior to colonoscopy. Air insufflation should be minimized and the entire colon need not be examined. Prolonged attempts at cecal intubation are not necessary because reaching the hepatic flexure usually appears to be effective. Gas should be aspirated and the viability of the mucosa assessed during slow withdrawal of the endoscope. A tube for decompression should be placed in the right colon with the aid of a guidewire and fluoroscopic guidance. Commercially available, single use, over-the-wire colon decompression tubes are available. The guidewires for these kits are quite flexible (0·035 inches (0·89 mm)) and must be watched under fluoroscopy during

advancement and endoscopic withdrawal to minimize loops from forming and ensure placement into the right colon.

The efficacy of colonoscopic decompression has not been established in randomized trials. Successful colonoscopic decompression has been reported in many retrospective case series, now totaling many hundreds of patients.[4,31–34] B4 Table 19.3 summarizes the larger reported series of colonoscopic decompression in ACPO. Rex reviewed the available literature of patients with ACPO treated with colonoscopy.[30] Successful initial decompression, determined by a reduction in radiographically measured cecal diameter was observed in 69% of 292 patients. Forty percent of patients treated without decompression tube placement had at least one recurrence, requiring an additional colonoscopy. Thus, an initial decompression colonoscopy without tube placement can be considered to be definitive therapy for less than 50% of patients.[30] To improve the therapeutic benefit, decompression tube placement at the time of colonoscopy is strongly recommended. The value of decompression tubes has not been evaluated in controlled trials, but anecdotal evidence suggests that they may lower the recurrence rate. In the series reported by Geller *et al.*, the overall clinical success of colonoscopic decompression was 88%. However, in procedures where a decompression tube was not placed the clinical success was poor (25%).[34] Tube placement is not, however, completely effective in preventing recurrences. Decompression colonoscopy has a reported colonic perforation rate of approximately 3%,[34] a figure that is much higher than is reported in patients without ACPO.

Surgical therapy

Grade C Surgical management is reserved for patients with signs of colonic ischemia or perforation or for those who fail endoscopic and pharmacologic treatment. Surgical intervention is associated with significant morbidity and mortality, probably related to the severity of the underlying medical conditions in this group of patients. In the large retrospective series reported by Vanek and Al-Salti, 179 patients underwent surgery for ACPO with resulting morbidity and mortality rates of 30% and 6%, respectively.[2] B4 The type of surgery depends on the status of the bowel.

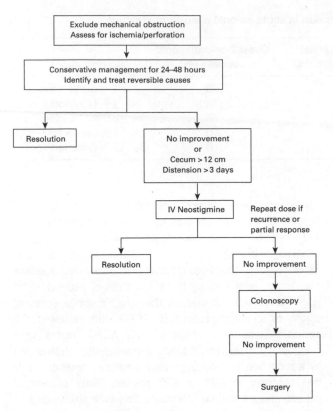

Figure 19.2 Algorithm for suggested management for acute colonic pseudo-obstruction. IV, intravenous

Without perforated or ischemic bowel, cecostomy is the procedure of choice because the success rate is high, morbidity is relatively low and the procedure can be carried out under local anesthesia.[2] Alternatively, percutaneous cecostomy through a combined endoscopic-radiologic approach can be considered in high surgical risk patients.[35,36] C5 In cases of ischemic or perforated bowel, segmental or subtotal colonic resection is indicated, with either exteriorization or primary anastomosis.

Clinical guidelines

An evidence-based guideline for the treatment of ACPO was recently published by the American Society for Gastrointestinal Endoscopy.[7] The guidelines recommend conservative therapy as the initial preferred management, based on observational studies only. Potentially contributory metabolic, infectious and pharmacologic factors should be identified and corrected. Active intervention is indicated for patients at risk of perforation and/or failing conservative therapy. Neostigmine is effective for the majority of patients. A1a, B4 Colonic decompression is the initial invasive procedure of choice for patients who fail neostigmine therapy

or for whom this drug is contraindicated. B4 Surgical decompression should be reserved for patients with peritonitis or perforation and for those who fail endoscopic and medical therapy. B4 A proposed algorithm for the management of ACPO is detailed in Figure 19.2.

Summary

ACPO is a syndrome of massive dilatation of the colon without mechanical obstruction that results from an imbalance in the autonomic control of the colon. Evaluation involves exclusion of mechanical obstruction and assessing for signs of ischemia or perforation. Appropriate management includes supportive measures and selective use of neostigmine and colonoscopic decompression. Neostigmine is the only therapy for ACPO proved to be efficacious in a randomized controlled trial. Patient outcome is determined by the severity of the predisposing illness, patient age, maximal cecal diameter, duration of colonic distension and viability of the bowel. Of these factors affecting outcome, the latter three are amenable to intervention. Thus, early recognition and management are critical to minimizing morbidity and mortality.

References

1 Ogilvie WH. Large intestine colic due to sympathetic deprivation: A new clinical syndrome. *BMJ* 1948;**2**:671–3.

2 Vanek VW, Al-Salti M. Acute pseudo-obstruction of the colon (Ogilvie's syndrome). An analysis of 400 cases. *Dis Colon Rectum* 1986;**29**:203–10.

3 Dorudi S, Berry AR, Kettlewell MGW. Acute colonic pseudo-obstruction. *Br J Surg* 1992;**79**:99–103.

4 Jetmore AB, Timmcke AE, Gathright Jr BJ *et al*. Ogilvie's syndrome: colonoscopic decompression and analysis of predisposing factors. *Dis Colon Rectum* 1992;**35**:1135–42.

5 Sheikh RA, Yasmeen S, Pauly MP *et al*. Pseudomembranous colitis without diarrhea presenting clinically as acute intestinal pseudo-obstruction. *J Gastroenterol* 2001;**36**: 629–32.

6 Sloyer AF, Panella VS, Demas BE *et al*. Ogilvie's syndrome. Successful management without colonoscopy. *Dig Dis Sci* 1988;**33**:1391–6.

7 Eisen GM, Baron TH, Dominitiz JA *et al*. Acute colonic pseudo-obstruction. *Gastrointest Endosc* 2002;**56**:789–92.

8 Wandeo H, Mathewson C, Conolly B. Pseudo-obstruction of the colon. *Surg Gynecol Obstet* 1971;**133**:44.

9 Meyers MA. Colonic ileus. *Gastrointest Radiol* 1977;**2**: 37–40.

10 Bachulis BL, Smith PE. Pseudo-obstruction of the colon. *Am J Surg* 1978;**136**:66–72.

11 Baker DA, Morin ME, Tan A *et al*. Colonic ileus: indication for prompt decompression. *JAMA* 1979;**241**:2633–4.

12 Johnson CD, Rice RP. The radiographic evaluation of gross cecal distention. *Am J Radiol* 1985;**145**:1211–17.

13 Loftus CG, Harewood GC, Baron TH. Assessment of predictors of response to neostigmine for acute colonic pseudo-obstruction. *Am J Gastroenterol* 2002;**97**:3118–22.

14 Rex DK. Acute colonic pseudo-obstruction (Ogilvie's syndrome). *Gastroenterology* 1994;**2**:223–8.

15 Ponec RJ, Saunders MD, Kimmey MB. Neostigmine for the treatment of acute colonic pseudo-obstruction. *N Engl J Med* 1999;**341**:137–41.

16 Law NM, Bharucha AE, Undale AS *et al.* Cholinergic stimulation enhances colonic motor activity, transit, and sensation in humans. *Am J Physiol Gastrointest Liver Physiol* 2001;**281**:G1228–37.

17 Neely J, Catchpole B. Ileus: The restoration of alimentary-tract motility by pharmacologic means. *Br J Surg* 1971;**58**: 21–8.

18 Aquilonius SM, Hartvig P. Clinical pharmacokinetics of cholinesterase inhibitors. *Clin Pharmacokinet* 1986;**11**: 236–49.

19 Cronnelly R, Stanski DR, Miller RD *et al.* Renal function and the pharmacokinetics of neostigmine in anesthetized man. *Anesthesiology* 1979;**51**:222–6.

20 Hutchinson R, Griffiths C. Acute colonic pseudo-obstruction: a pharmacologic approach. *Ann R Coll Surg Engl* 1992;**74**:364–7.

21 Stephenson BM, Morgan AR, Salaman JR *et al.* Ogilvie's syndrome: a new approach to an old problem. *Dis Colon Rectum* 1995;**38**:424–7.

22 Turegano-Fuentes F, Munoz-Jimenez F, Del Valle-Hernandez E *et al.* Early resolution of Ogilvie's syndrome with intravenous neostigmine. A simple, effective treatment. *Dis Colon Rectum* 1997;**40**:1353–7.

23 Trevisani GT, Hyman NH, Church JM. Neostigmine: safe and effective treatment for acute colonic pseudo-obstruction. *Dis Colon Rectum* 2000;**43**:599–603.

24 Paran H, Silverberg D, Mayo A *et al.* Treatment of acute colonic pseudo-obstruction with neostigmine. *J Am Coll Surg* 2000;**190**:315–18.

25 Abeyta BJ, Albrecht RM, Schermer CR. Retrospective study of neostigmine for the treatment of acute colonic pseudo-obstruction. *Am Surg* 2001;**67**:265–8.

26 Armstrong DN, Ballantyne GH, Modlin IM. Erythromycin for reflex ileus in Ogilvie's syndrome. *Lancet* 1991;**337**: 378.

27 Bonacini M, Smith OJ, Pritchard T. Erythromycin as therapy for acute colonic pseudo-obstruction (Ogilvie's syndrome). *J Clin Gastroenterol* 1991;**13**:475–6.

28 MacColl C, MacCannell KL, Baylis B *et al.* Treatment of acute colonic pseudo-obstruction (Ogilvie's syndrome) with cisapride. *Gastroenterology* 1990;**98**:773–6.

29 Camilleri M. Review article: tegaserod. *Aliment Pharmacol Ther* 2001;**15**:277–289.

30 Rex DK. Colonoscopy and acute colonic pseudo-obstruction. *Gastrointest Endosc Clin North Am* 1997;**7**: 499–508.

31 Nivatvongs S, Vermeulen FD, Fang DT. Colonoscopic decompression of acute pseudo-obstruction of the colon. *Ann Surg* 1982;**196**:598–600.

32 Strodel WE, Nostrant TT, Eckhauser FE *et al.* Therapeutic and diagnostic colonoscopy in non-obstructive colonic dilatation. *Ann Surg* 1983;**19**:416–21.

33 Bode WE, Beart RW, Spencer RJ *et al.* Colonoscopic decompression for acute pseudo-obstruction of the colon (Ogilvie's syndrome): report of 22 cases and review of the literature. *Am J Surg* 1984;**147**:243–5.

34 Geller A, Petersen BT, Gostout CJ. Endoscopic decompression for acute colonic pseudo-obstruction. *Gastrointest Endosc* 1996;**44**:144–50.

35 vanSonnenberg E, Varney RR, Casola G *et al.* Percutaneous cecostomy for Ogilvie's syndrome: laboratory observations and clinical experience. *Radiology* 1990;**175**:679–82.

36 Chevallier P, Marcy PY, Francois E *et al.* Controlled transperitoneal percutaneous cecostomy as a therapeutic alternative to the endoscopic decompression for Ogilvie's syndrome. *Am J Gastroenterol* 2002;**97**:471–4.

20 Gallstone disease

Calvin HL Law, Dana McKay, Véd R Tandan

Introduction

Surgical therapy for gallstones can be associated with morbidity and mortality which has led to debate on its use, especially in asymptomatic and mildly symptomatic patients. Advancements in minimally invasive and endoscopic techniques have the potential to improve surgical outcomes. The development of these techniques makes it imperative to understand the current evidence concerning the benefits and risks of surgical therapy for gallstone disease and its complications.

Elective cholecystectomy

Asymptomatic cholelithiasis in the general population

There are no controlled trials comparing prophylactic surgery with expectant management in asymptomatic patients with cholelithiasis. However, a number of cohort studies have been done to assess the probability of developing biliary pain and biliary complications in asymptomatic persons with gallstones.

Through the 1980s, a series of cohort studies were conducted by Gracie and Ransohoff,[1] McSherry et al.[2] and Freidman et al.[3,4] Gracie's study had complete follow up on 123 persons for 11–24 years. The cumulative probability of the development of biliary pain was 10% at 5 years, 15% at 10 years, and 18% at 20 years. However, the fact that 89% of the study population were white American males, and all were faculty members of the University of Michigan, limits the generalizability of this study. McSherry's study retrospectively identified 135 patients with asymptomatic cholelithiasis who were subscribers to the Health Insurance Plan of Greater New York, a mainly middle-income population of diverse ethnic origin. Over a mean follow up of 46 months, 10·4% of patients developed symptoms, yielding a 2·7% annual rate of developing symptoms. Similarly, Friedman followed 123 ethnically diverse patients with asymptomatic gallstones in the Kaiser Permanente Medical

Care Program (San Francisco) for 16–25 years. There was a 3–4% annual rate of biliary events in the initial 10 years, and a 1–2% annual rate in the following 10 years. At 5 years, 18% of patients had developed biliary symptoms. One death was attributable to cholangitis secondary to gallstones. A more detailed explanation of Gracie's data revealed that three patients eventually experienced biliary complications (2·4% of the population), but all of these had presented with pain before the complication. In McSherry's study, 10% of the population eventually developed symptoms and 71% of these patients had biliary colic as their only indication for elective cholecystectomy. Although the remaining patients had biliary complications prior to surgery (3% of the study population), it is unclear if they presented with pain first. Overall these studies yield an estimate of an annual rate of 1–2% of symptom development, and provide evidence that 90% of patients will present with pain prior to developing a biliary complication. Only 10% of patients will present with a biliary complication as the first manifestation of their biliary tract disease.[4]

The Group for Epidemiology and Prevention of Cholelithiasis (GREPCO) in Italy prospectively followed 118 patients with asymptomatic cholelithiasis.[5] The cumulative probability of developing biliary colic was 12% at 2 years, 17% at 4 years and 26% at 10 years. The cumulative probability of biliary complications was 3% at 10 years. One patient died of gallbladder carcinoma. This represents a higher rate of symptoms, but not a higher rate of complications than the studies from the 1980s.

Ransohoff et al. performed a decision analysis[6,7] on data first published by Gracie.[1] Using cholecystectomy mortality figures up to 1983, they found prophylactic cholecystectomy slightly decreased survival. The economic analysis did not favor prophylactic cholecystectomy.

In 2001, Mentes et al. evaluated the gastrointestinal quality of life of 37 patients with symptomatic cholelithiasis and 30 patients with asymptomatic cholelithiasis before and after cholecystectomy.[8] They found that uncomplicated laparoscopic cholecystectomy improved quality of life significantly in both groups, but had a larger impact on the symptomatic gallstone group. However, any conclusions regarding improvements of quality of life in the asymptomatic group must be tempered by the fact that only uncomplicated, uneventful cholecystectomies were included, which is not a reflection of true practice.

Considering the current evidence, expectant management rather than prophylactic cholecystectomy is indicated for the typical patient with asymptomatic gallstones. However, certain populations who are more at risk for complications of gallstone disease should be considered separately.

Asymptomatic cholelithiasis in diabetic patients

More liberal thresholds for elective cholecystectomy in asymptomatic diabetic patients have been suggested,[9] based on early evidence suggesting a higher incidence of gallstone disease and biliary complications, and poorer outcomes for emergency surgery for biliary complications. Only Grade B evidence is available, which supports expectant management of asymptomatic cholelithiasis in this population rather than a more aggressive approach.

In 1952, Lieber studied 26 895 autopsies, revealing an overall incidence of cholelithiasis of 11·6%; among diabetic patients the rate of cholelithiasis was 30·2%.[10] Since then, the belief that cholelithiasis is more common in diabetic patients has become widely accepted.[11] More recently, Chapman reviewed 308 diabetic patients and 318 non-diabetic controls.[12] The incidence of cholelithiasis was higher in the diabetic population (32·7% v 20·8%, $P < 0.001$). However, when the data were subjected to multivariate analysis, diabetes did not correlate strongly with the incidence of cholelithiasis, except in a subgroup of females with non-insulin dependent diabetes.

Del Favero prospectively studied the natural history of cholelithiasis in diabetes by following a cohort of 47 diabetic patients with asymptomatic cholelithiasis.[13] After 5 years, seven patients (15%) had developed symptoms or complications. Of this group, five had presented with pain as their first symptom. One patient presented with cholecystitis and one with jaundice. These data compare favorably with the data available from studies of the general population.

Higher complication rates with emergency surgery for biliary complications in diabetic patients have been observed. Hickman *et al.* studied 72 diabetic patients who underwent cholecystectomy for cholecystitis and matched them for age, sex and date of operation with 72 non-diabetic patients.[14] Morbidity for the diabetic patients was 38·9% compared with 20·8% in the non-diabetic population. Mortality in the diabetic population was 4·2%, compared with zero in the control population and was attributed to sepsis. The septic complication rate was higher in the diabetic (19·4%) than in the non-diabetic group (6·9%). This higher rate was maintained whether the diabetic patients had concurrent medical illness or not.

The apparent higher incidence of cholelithiasis in diabetic patients is likely related to factors other than the diabetes itself. The natural history of asymptomatic cholelithiasis in diabetic patients appears to be similar to that in the general population. Nevertheless, diabetic patients who have biliary complications may have increased morbidity with emergency cholecystectomy, though this has not been well studied to date. Individualized considerations such as concurrent illness must be considered in deciding whether to recommend prophylactic cholecystectomy in this population, and recommendations have to be made without good supporting evidence.

Asymptomatic cholelithiasis and the risk of cancer

Autopsy data have provided evidence that greater than 80% of patients with gallbladder cancer have concomitant cholelithiasis. Maringhini *et al.* followed 2583 patients with known gallstones.[15] Only five patients (0·2%) developed gallbladder carcinoma. In the previously discussed cohorts of patients with asymptomatic cholelithiasis,[1–4] only one patient from a total of 499 patients followed for up to 25 years was found to have gallbladder carcinoma.

The incidence of gallbladder cancer varies widely in different populations, even in the presence of gallstone disease. Lowenfels *et al.* reported a case–control study of 131 patients with gallbladder carcinoma and 2399 patients without gallbladder carcinoma.[16] The 20-year cumulative risk for gallbladder cancer ranged from 0·13% in black males to 1·5% in native American females. The authors calculated that 769 cholecystectomies were required to prevent one gallbladder cancer in a low risk population. However, only 67 cholecystectomies would be necessary to prevent one gallbladder malignancy in a high risk population. B3

Patients with gallstones greater than 3 cm may be at risk for the development of gallbladder carcinoma. Diehl reported this in a case–control study in 1983[17] and the study by Lowenfels confirmed this observation in 1989.[18] These studies provided evidence for a 9–10-fold increase in relative risk of developing gallbladder carcinoma for patients with stones greater than 3 cm in diameter compared to patients with stones less than 1 cm in diameter.

Grade B evidence supports the view that the risk of developing gallbladder cancer may be higher in patients with cholelithiasis. However, the increased risk appears to be insufficient to support a recommendation for prophylactic cholecystectomy. Although some subsets of the population (especially native American females) and patients with stones greater than 3 cm may be at sufficient risk to justify prophylactic cholecystectomy, further evidence would be needed to support a firm recommendation. B3, B4

Porcelain gallbladder and risk of gallbladder cancer

Early case reports and small series initially indicated a correlation between porcelain gallbladder and carcinoma, which guided a recommendation for surgical therapy. However, more relevant information has only recently been published. A retrospective assessment by Towfigh *et al.*[19] examined 10 741 gallbladder specimens. Only 15 (0·14%) were porcelain gallbladders. All porcelain gallbladder specimens demonstrated chronic cholecystitis and partial calcification of the gallbladder wall and nine had cholelithiasis (60%). During this same period, 88 (0·82%) patients developed gallbladder cancer, none of whom showed calcification of the gallbladder wall. From these data, the authors challenged the link between porcelain gallbladder and gallbladder cancer. However, further insight may be gained from a study by Stephen and Berger.[20] This study reported data on 25 900 gallbladder specimens of which 150 cases of gallbladder cancer and 44 cases of porcelain gallbladder (defined as the presence of wall calcifications) were identified. This study demonstrated that there are two types of wall calcification – diffuse *intramural* calcification and selective *mucosal* calcification. Gallbladder cancer was found in 7% of cases with selective mucosal calcification, but no case of gallbladder cancer was identified in the specimens with diffuse intramural calcification. Thus, conflicting data in the past may be attributable to misclassification. However, in the preoperative setting, it may be difficult to distinguish these types of calcifications with standard imaging modalities. There are no studies beyond scattered, single case reports examining the efficacy of imaging modalities in distinguishing the types of porcelain gallbladder as defined by Stephen's study[20] and the low incidence of this disease makes future study difficult. Therefore, the authors still recommend open cholecystectomy for patients with porcelain gallbladder, especially in whom there is incomplete calcification of the gallbladder wall. C5

Symptomatic cholelithiasis

Grade B evidence supports the current approach to patients with symptomatic cholelithiasis. Patients with uncomplicated biliary colic should be offered surgery as an option to controlling symptoms. Patients with complications of cholelithiasis should have surgery to prevent further complications. The previously discussed natural history studies of McSherry *et al.*[2] and Friedman *et al.*[3] included a group of patient with symptomatic cholelithiasis. Additional data are also available from the National Cooperative Gallstone Study (NCGS).[21,22] McSherry followed 556 patients with symptomatic cholelithiasis.[2] During an average follow up of 83 months, 169 (30%) of patients reported worsening or continued severe symptoms, 9 (1·6%) patients developed jaundice, and 47 (8·5%) patients developed cholecystitis. These data indicate a 4·3% annual rate of worsening or persistently severe symptoms and a 1·5% annual rate of biliary complications arising from symptomatic cholelithiasis. Friedman followed 298 patients with mild or non-specific symptoms and cholelithiasis for 16–25 years.[3,4] The annual rate of developing cholecystitis or jaundice was 1%.

The NCGS was designed as a double blind, randomized controlled trial of chenodiol.[21,22] The group of patients who had received placebo provided another opportunity to study the natural history of symptomatic cholelithiasis. Seventy-seven patients presented with worsening symptoms of biliary colic or prolonged biliary pain during 2 years of follow up. Seven patients "required cholecystectomy" during the follow up which represents a 34% annual incidence of "requiring a cholecystectomy". The patients with symptomatic cholelithiasis in these studies did not suffer any greater mortality during the follow up period than was experienced by patients in the asymptomatic population.

The rate of complications secondary to symptomatic cholelithiasis appears to be higher than that in patients with asymptomatic cholelithiasis. Recurrent or worsening symptoms may develop but there is no increased mortality from observation, at least in the short term. Therefore, "the subjective experience of the patient should be the principal determinant of whether and when the procedure should be performed". Early surgical treatment is indicated once cholelithiasis is complicated by acute cholecystitis, choledocholithiasis or cholangitis.

Elective laparoscopic versus open cholecystectomy

Laparoscopic cholecystectomy is now considered standard of care for elective cholecystectomy. This was "accepted" despite the lack of any evidence from a randomized controlled trial comparing standard open cholecystectomy and standard laparoscopic cholecystectomy. Nonetheless, laparoscopic cholecystectomy has had a significant impact on the management of gallstone disease as evidenced by increasing rates of elective cholecystectomy since its introduction in the 1980s.[23,24]

Evidence from four randomized controlled trials comparing elective laparoscopic cholecystectomy and mini-laparotomy cholecystectomy is available[25–28] (Table 20.1). A1c There is no statistically significant difference in the incidence of biliary tract injuries, although in McMahon *et al.*'s study,[26] the only major biliary injury occurred in the laparoscopic group. Quality of life data were obtained by both Barkun *et al.*[25] and McMahon *et al.*[26] The laparoscopic group experienced a faster improvement in quality of life, but

Table 20.1 Randomized controlled trials of laparoscopic cholecystectomy (LC) and mini-cholecystectomy (MC)

		Study		
		Barkun et al.[25]	McMahon et al.[26]	McGinn et al.[27]
No. of patients	LC	37	151	155
	MC	25	148	155
Operative time (minutes)	LC	85·9	57*	74*
	MC	73·1	71*	50*
Conversion to standard open cholecystectomy	LC	1 (3%)	15 (10%)	20 (13%)
	MC	0 (0%)	14 (10%)	6 (4%)
Time to oral intake	LC	1·1 days*	N/A	N/A
	MC	1·7 days*	N/A	N/A
Hospital stay (days)	LC	3*	2*	2[a]
	MC	4*	4*	3[a]
Non-biliary complications	LC	1 (3%)	30 (20%)[b]	12 (7·7%)*
	MC	1 (4%)	26 (17%)[b]	2 (1·3%)*
Biliary complications	LC	0 (0%)	5 (3%)[c]	1 (0·6%)
	MC	1 (4%)	3 (2%)[c]	2 (1·3%)
Mortality	LC	0 (0%)	0 (0%)	1 (0·6%)
	MC	0 (0%)	1 (0·7%)	0 (0%)

N/A, data not available.

*Indicates differences reached statistical significance.

[a]This was statistically significant but did not include patients who were converted to standard cholecystectomy. If included, there was no statistical difference in length of hospital stay.

[b]Total complications.

[c]This included 1 (0·7%) major biliary injury in the LC group and no major biliary injuries in the MC group.

the two treatment groups were equal in this respect at 3 months. Similarly, there was better satisfaction with scarring in the laparoscopic group, but both groups were equally satisfied with their result at 3 months. The data from Majeed revealed no difference in time off work or time to return to full activity.[28] A cost minimization economic analysis was carried out by McMahon.[26] Laparoscopic cholecystectomy was more costly after considering both perioperative and hospitalization costs (£1486 compared with £1090, $P < 0.001$).

Further data comparing laparoscopic to open cholecystectomy are available from the meta-analysis of Shea *et al.* of the outcomes of 78 747 patients undergoing laparoscopic cholecystectomy and 12 973 patients undergoing open cholecystectomy.[29] Mortality rates were lower for laparoscopic cholecystectomy than for open cholecystectomy, while common bile duct injury was higher for laparoscopic cholecystectomy than for open cholecystectomy. The data for common bile duct injury were reanalyzed by group-level logistic regressions to identify the differences in rates among the studies. A pattern of infrequent common duct injury in early studies, an increased incidence in studies initiated in early 1990, followed by a subsequent decrease in rate was

revealed. However, the data were quite variable in terms of reporting of results and length of follow up. The authors conceded, "there are still some considerable uncertainties that need to be addressed by better-designed studies and more complete reporting".

Considering the current evidence, in the elective setting, laparoscopic cholecystectomy appears to be as safe as open cholecystectomy and may provide short-term improvement in quality of life. Ala, C There is a lack of convincing evidence of its touted beneficial effects on length of stay, recovery time or economics (hospital or societal). However, the general acceptance of laparoscopic cholecystectomy as the standard of care as well as public demand for minimally invasive surgery will prevent a future randomized controlled trial that may definitively answer these questions.

Further issues in elective laparoscopic cholecystectomy

With the advent of the laparoscopic cholecystectomy, there has been a move towards ambulatory surgery. Grade A evidence from two randomized trials which compared outpatient to inpatient laparoscopic cholecystectomy are available.[30,31] Exclusion criteria included American Society of Anesthesiologists (ASA) III/IV, patients less that 18 and more than 70 years old, lack of a capable caregiver at home and complicated cholelithiasis (common bile duct stones or acute cholecystitis). The degree of pain, readmission and complication rates was the same in both groups. Late complications such as bile leaks became evident several days later and there was no benefit from 24-hour admission. Keulemans *et al.* found that 92% of the outpatients preferred outpatient care to clinical observation.[31] In summary, outpatient laparoscopic cholecystectomy is a safe and feasible option for selected patients (defined by the exclusion criteria in the randomized trials). Alc

A newer technique called "mini-laparoscopic cholecystectomy" has recently been reported. This technique entails the use of even smaller diameter instruments (2–3 mm) and smaller laparoscopic cameras (5 mm) to allow for a near scar-less operation. Evidence comparing mini-laparoscopic cholecystectomy and conventional laparoscopic cholecystectomy is available from four randomized controlled trials.[32–35] Alc Chea *et al.*[32] and Bisgaad *et al.*[33] demonstrated that mini-laparoscopic cholecystectomy resulted in less pain (visual analog scale) than was the case for conventional laparoscopic cholecystectomy. Sarli *et al.* confirmed this observation and also showed that the group with mini-laparoscopy required fewer injections of analgesic.[35] Mini-laparoscopic cholecystectomy was found to result in less scar when compared to laparoscopic cholecystectomy (total scar length: 17 mm *v* 25 mm; $P < 0.001$)[32] and more patients expressed satisfaction with cosmesis in the mini-laparoscopy group.[34,35] It is noted however, that in all current studies examining mini-laparoscopy the procedures were carried out by expert hands and no data that can be generalized to the whole population of surgeons and patients have yet been presented. This technique may have a steep learning curve for some surgeons and is currently carried out predominantly by experts in laparoscopy.

Acute cholecystitis

Acute cholecystitis, inflammation secondary to obstruction of the cystic duct, is the most common complication of cholelithiasis. There is little disagreement that the treatment of acute cholecystitis should involve cholecystectomy. The areas of controversy are the timing of cholecystectomy and to a lesser degree the use of laparoscopic cholecystectomy versus open cholecystectomy. Acute cholecystitis was previously considered to be a contraindication to laparoscopic cholecystectomy. Growing surgeon comfort and expertise with laparoscopic cholecystectomy has resulted in this

technique becoming the treatment of choice for acute cholecystitis.

In the pre-laparoscopic era, the question of early versus delayed cholecystectomy was heavily debated. Evidence from five randomized trials carried out in the 1970s and 1980s is available.[36–40] Alc These studies demonstrated that cholecystectomy could be carried out in the acute stage with shorter hospital stay, decreased mortality and fewer operative complications (Table 20.2).

The introduction of laparoscopic cholecystectomy caused a movement to return to delayed cholecystectomy for acute cholecystitis. This movement arose because laparoscopic cholecystectomy was considered to be associated with more complications and an increased risk of common bile duct injuries than interval laparoscopic cholecystectomy after the resolution of the acute episode. Grade A evidence from three randomized controlled trials[41–43] on early versus delayed laparoscopic cholecystectomy is available (Table 20.3). Once again, the data show that early cholecystectomy, even if carried out with the laparoscopic approach, is safe and better for patients in terms of shorter illness and hospital stay compared with delayed surgery.

Evidence regarding laparoscopic versus open cholecystectomy for acute cholecystitis is available from two randomized trials.[44,45] Alc The results are summarized in Table 20.4. The laparoscopic approach did not increase mortality or morbidity compared with the open approach and offered the benefit of shorter hospital stay. Both studies found that the rate of conversion to the open procedure was slightly higher than the average observed in elective cholecystectomy series.

Considering the current evidence, acute cholecystitis should be treated with early (48–72 hours) laparoscopic cholecystectomy with a reasonable threshold for conversion to open surgery.

Gallstone pancreatitis

Early endoscopic retrograde cholangiopancreatography

Evidence from three randomized controlled trials on early endoscopic retrograde cholangiopancreatography (ERCP) with stone extraction versus conservative therapy as a treatment for biliary pancreatitis is available.[46–48] Alc In patients with severe pancreatitis or with evidence of biliary obstruction or cholangitis, early ERCP within 72 hours of presentation probably decreases morbidity and mortality rates. In patients without these criteria, early ERCP has no benefit and may in fact increase morbidity and mortality. Therefore, patients must be carefully selected for early ERCP. (See Chapter 21 for further discussion.)

Table 20.2 Randomized controlled trials comparing early versus delayed open cholecystectomy for acute cholecystitis

		Study			
		McArthur *et al.*[36]	Lahtinen *et al.*[37a]	van der Linden *et al.*[38a]	Jarvinen and Hastbacka[39]
No. of patients	Early	15	47	70	80
	Delayed	13	44	58	75
Operative time (minutes)	Early	N/A	76·7	N/A[b]	93
	Delayed	N/A	98·0	N/A[b]	85
Hospital stay (days)	Early	13·1	13·0	10·1	10·7
	Delayed	24·2	25·0	10·9 + 8[c]	18·2
Biliary complications	Early	1 (6·7%)	1 (2·1%)	0	3 (3·8%)
	Delayed	0	3 (6·8%)	0	2 (2·7%)
Non-biliary complications	Early	3 (20%)	12 (25·5%)	10 (14·3%)	11 (13·8%)
	Delayed	5 (38·4%)	16 (36·4%)	2 (3·4%)	13 (17·3%)
Mortality	Early	0	0	0	0
	Delayed	0	4 (9·1%)	0	1 (1·3%)
Failure of delayed treatment[d]		3 (23·1%)	7 (15·9%)	0	10 (13·3%)

N/A, data not available

[a]Also showed decreased insurance payments (for time off work) for the patients treated with early cholecystectomy.

[b]No average or mean time for surgery was given but the distributions of operative times were similar.

[c]The mean stay for initial conservative management was 10·9 days followed by a mean stay of 8·0 days at the time of the delayed cholecystectomy.

[d]Patients randomized to conservative treatment initially who failed and required urgent cholecystectomy.

Preoperative endoscopic retrograde cholangiopancreatography versus cholecystectomy with cholangiogram

Gallstone pancreatitis is considered to be an indication for imaging the biliary tree with either ERCP or intraoperative cholangiogram (IOC). Due to the possibility of common bile duct (CBD) stones, no studies have evaluated cholecystectomy without imaging the biliary tree. Seven observational studies,[49–55] two with controls, have assessed the optimal approach to imaging the biliary tree following an attack of gallstone pancreatitis. Gallstone pancreatitis does not appear to be a strong predictor of CBD stones without evidence of a dilated CBD, persistently abnormal alkaline phosphatase or bilirubin, or evidence of cholangitis. Patients with these features may be considered for preoperative ERCP. C5 In one retrospective study,[49] the incidence of procedure-induced pancreatitis was 19% in the ERCP group and 6% in the surgical/IOC group. The other retrospective study demonstrated similar results with pancreatic-biliary complications in 24% of the ERCP group and 6% of the surgical/IOC group.[55] The data suggest that preoperative ERCP may in fact increase overall morbidity compared with cholecystectomy with IOC, further supporting the approach of selective ERCP in this group of patients. C5

Timing of surgery

A number of studies have evaluated early versus delayed cholecystectomy in patients with gallstone pancreatitis. Burch

et al. evaluated patients who underwent surgery after recovering from acute pancreatitis either during the same hospital admission or following discharge and scheduling for elective surgery.[56] Although surgical complication rates were the same in both groups, total hospital stay was significantly longer in the delayed surgery group (14 *v* 17 days, *P* = 0·01). Furthermore, in the delayed group only 60% returned for surgery and 29% of the original cohort required emergency treatment for recurrent pancreatitis or biliary disease before elective surgery. Kelly *et al.* randomized patients to early (less than 48 hours) and delayed (more than 48 hours) surgery.[57] With early surgery the morbidity and mortality rates were 30·1% and 15·1%, as compared with 5·1 and 2·4% in the delayed group (*P* < 0·005). A1c When patients were stratified for disease severity based on Ranson's criteria, the differences in morbidity and mortality rates between early and delayed surgery were not statistically significant in patients with three or fewer Ranson's criteria. In patients with severe pancreatitis (more than three Ranson's criteria), the differences remained significant.

Grade B/C evidence has recently been published[58,59] examining the issue of whether cholecystectomy is even necessary after successful ERCP with endoscopic sphincterotomy (ES) and clearance of bile duct stones. Kaw *et al.* followed patients prospectively to compare outcome after laparoscopic cholecystectomy and ERCP with ES or ERCP and ES alone.[58] During follow up, there was no significant difference in biliary complications or procedure-related complications. They

Table 20.3 Randomized controlled trials comparing early versus delayed laparoscopic cholecystectomy for acute cholecystitis

		Study	
		Lo *et al.*[41]	Lai *et al.*[42]
No. of patients	Early	45	53
	Delayed	41	51
Operative time	Early	135	122·8
(minutes)	Delayed	105	106·6
Conversion	Early	5 (11%)	(21%)
	Delayed	9 (23%)	(24%)
Hospital stay	Early	6	7·6
(days)	Delayed	11	11·6
Biliary	Early	1 (2·2%)	
complications	Delayed	3 (7·3%)	
Non-biliary	Early	5	(11·1%)
complications	Delayed	9 (22·0%)	
Mortality	Early	0	
	Delayed	0	
Failure of delayed treatment[a]			8 (19·5%)

[a]Patients randomized to conservative treatment initially who failed and required urgent cholecystectomy

Table 20.4 Randomized controlled trials comparing open (OC) versus laparoscopic (LC) cholecystectomy for acute cholecystitis

		Study	
		Kiviluoto *et al.*[44]	Lujan *et al.*[45]
No. of patients	OC	31	110
	LC	32	114
Operative time	OC	99·8	77
(minutes)	LC	108·2	88
Conversion	LC (only)	5 (16%)	17 (15%)
Hospital stay	OC	6	8·1
(days)	LC	4	3·3
Biliary	OC	0	1 (0·9%)
complications	LC	0	4 (3·5%)[a]
Non-biliary	OC	7 (minor) (23%)	28 (25·5%)
complications		6 (major) (19%)	
	LC	1 (minor) (3%)	14 (12·3%)
Mortality	OC	0	0
	LC	0	0

[a]Two out of four were retained common bileduct stones

concluded that laparoscopic cholecystectomy should only be attempted in patients with overt biliary symptoms and not for the prevention of gallstone pancreatitis. Kwon *et al.* found that only 4.8% of patients required a cholecystectomy for biliary complications at an average of 18·4 months following ERCP and ES.[59] This issue should be examined further by randomized controlled trials, but at this point there is no clear evidence that biliary complications can be completely avoided by ERCP and ES alone. In addition, these data conflict with Grade A evidence from studies looking at CBD stones (see below).

Based on these data, it is recommended that patients with acute severe gallstone pancreatitis undergo cholecystectomy following resolution of the acute episode but during the initial hospital stay. Patients with mild to moderate pancreatitis (three or fewer Ranson's criteria) can be considered for early laparoscopic cholecystectomy. Alc, C5

Choledocholithiasis

CBD stones may be identified by many different modalities including laparoscopic and open intraoperative cholangiogram, ERCP, laparoscopic ultrasound and magnetic resonance cholangiopancreatography (MRCP). Once CBD stones are identified, most surgeons agree that they should be removed, since stones left in the CBD may cause subsequent biliary complications including obstructive jaundice, pancreatitis and cholangitis.

See Chapter 21 for further discussion.

The surgical method for identifying CBD stones is operative cholangiography. However, the choice of routine versus selective cholangiography remains somewhat controversial.[60–62] In a review of 2043 patients[60] undergoing routine laparoscopic operative cholangiography, the incidence of unsuspected CBD stones was 2·8%. On the other hand, a smaller series[61] identified a 26% rate of what was felt to be clinically significant retained or recurrent stones found at operative cholangiography after a clear preoperative ERCP. The authors argued that routine operative cholangiography should be performed. However, on reviewing the literature,[60] only 0·30% of patients not undergoing operative cholangiography will ever become symptomatic. In order to better use resources, other studies have attempted to determine criteria for selective operative cholangiography. Borjeson *et al.*[62] proposed criteria that included: normal liver function tests, CBD diameter < 10 mm and no history of gallstone pancreatitis or jaundice.[62] One hundred and fifty-five patients who met these criteria were followed prospectively after laparoscopic cholecystectomy for a mean follow up of 26 months. No patients had retained CBD stones during the follow up period. Although none of these data provides Grade A evidence, the literature suggests that selective operative cholangiography is justified.

Once CBD stones are identified, there are three approaches to the management: open common bile duct exploration (OCBDE), ERCP and sphincterotomy, and laparoscopic common bile duct exploration (LCBDE).

Five randomized trials (Grade A) have compared OCBDE with ERCP in the management of CBD stones.[63–67] In the two smaller trials,[64,65] with 52 and 34 patients respectively, no differences in morbidity or mortality were seen. OCBDE was more successful at clearing stones than ERCP in one study (88% *v* 65%).[64] The two larger studies, with 228 and 120 patients respectively,[63,66] demonstrated statistically significant increases in morbidity with ERCP, with the latter study[66] also showing an increase in mortality with ERCP. Alc The fifth study[67] (*n* = 83) also demonstrated a trend to increased morbidity with ERCP, but the difference was not statistically significant.

Evidence from three randomized trials comparing LCBDE and ERCP showed no difference in morbidity and mortality between the two approaches.[68–70] Alc One trial[69] demonstrated a statistically significant decrease in hospital stay for LCBDE (1 day *v* 3·5 days) and another demonstrated a similar trend that was not statistically significant.[70] It should be noted that the rates of complications with ERCP in these studies were relatively high (11–28%). More recent studies demonstrate a much lower complication rate. Freeman *et al.*[71] reported a complication rate of only 4·9% among 2347 ERCPs. Similarly, Masci *et al.*[72] reported a series of 2444 ERCPs where the rate of complications was only 4·95% (pancreatitis in 1·8%, hemorrhage in 1·13%, cholangitis in 0·57%, perforation in 0·57% and death in 0·12%).

Grade A evidence regarding timing of surgery for choledocholithiasis following ERCP is available in the randomized trial reported by Boerma *et al.*[73] These authors randomized patients who underwent ERCP and stone extraction with proven gallbladder stones to a "wait and see" policy or to laparoscopic cholecystectomy after ERCP. In the wait and see group, 47% had recurrent biliary symptoms compared with 2% of laparoscopic cholecystectomy patients. The conversion rate to open surgery in patients allocated to wait and see was 55% compared with 23% in the laparoscopic group. Also morbidity was increased in the wait and see group (32% *v* 14%) as was length of stay (9 *v* 7 days). Alc

Conflicting data with respect to the outcomes observed in these studies may be explained in part by variation in operator expertise. LCBDE and ERCP are highly operator-dependent techniques with a steep learning curve. The approach to CBD stones should be individualized and based on the type of expertise available at each institution. However, patients presenting with choledocholithiasis should be expedited to undergo cholecystectomy to avoid further biliary complications and potentially increased morbidity at emergent cholecystectomy.

References

1 Gracie WA, Ransohoff DF. The natural history of silent gallstones: the innocent gallstone is not a myth. *N Engl J Med* 1982;**307**:790–800.

2 McSherry CK, Ferstenberg H, Calhoun WF *et al.* The natural history of diagnosed gallstone disease in symptomatic and asymptomatic patients. *Ann Surg* 1985;**202**:59–63.

3 Friedman GD, Raviola CA, Fireman B. Prognosis of gallstones with mild or no symptoms: 25 years of follow up in a health maintenance organization. *J Clin Epidemiol* 1989;**42**:127–36.

4 Friedman GD. Natural history of asymptomatic and symptomatic gallstones. *Am J Surg* 1993;**165**:399–404.

5 Attili AF, De Santis A, Capri R *et al.* The natural history of gallstones; the GREPCO experience. The GREPCO Group. *Hepatology* 1995;**21**:655–60.

6 Ransohoff DF, Gracie WA. Treatment of gallstones. *Ann Intern Med* 1993;**119**:606–19.

7 Ransohoff DF, Gracie WA, Wolfenson LB *et al.* Prophylactic cholecystectomy or expectant management for silent gallstone? A decision analysis to assess survival. *Ann Intern Med* 1983;**99**:199–204.

8 Mentes BB, Akin M, Irkorucu O *et al.* Gastrointestinal quality of life in patients with symptomatic or asymptomatic cholelithiasis before and after cholecystectomy. *Surg Endosc* 2001;**15**:1267–72.

9 Gibney EJ. Asymptomatic gallstones. *Br J Surg* 1990;**77**:368–72.

10 Lieber MM. The incidence of gallstones and their correlation with other diseases. *Ann Surg* 1952;**135**:394–405.

11 Ikard RW. Gallstones, cholecystitis and diabetes. *Surg Gynecol Obstet* 1990;**171**:528–32.

12 Chapman BA, Wilson IR, Frampton CM *et al.* Prevalence of gallbladder disease in diabetes mellitus. *Dig Dis Sci* 1996;**41**:2222–8.

13 Del Favero G, Meggiato CA, Volpi A *et al.* Natural history of gallstones in non-insulin dependent diabetes mellitus. A prospective 5-year follow up. 1994;**219**:275–80.

14 Hickman MS, Schwesinger WH, Page CP. Acute cholecystitis in the diabetic. A case–control study of outcome. *Arch Surg* 1988;**123**:409–11.

15 Maringhini A, Moreau JA, Melton LJ *et al.* Gallstones, gallbladder cancer and other gastrointestinal malignancies; an epidemiologic study in Rochester, Minnesota. *Ann Intern Med* 1987;**107**:30–5.

16 Lowenfels AB, Lindstron CG, Conway MJ *et al.* Gallstones and risk of gallbladder cancer. *J Natl Cancer Inst* 1985;**75**:77–80.

17 Diehl AK. Gallstone size and the risk of gallbladder cancer. *JAMA* 1983;**250**:2323–6.

18 Lowenfels AB, Walker AM, Althaus DP *et al.* Gallstone growth, size, and risk of gallbladder cancer: an interracial study. *Int J Epidemiol* 1989;**18**:50–4.

19 Towfigh S, McFadden DW, Cortina GR *et al.* Porcelain gallbladder is not associated with gallbladder carcinoma. *Am Surg* 2001;**67**:7–10.

20 Stephen AE, Berger DL. Carcinoma in the porcelain gallbladder: a relationship revisited. *Surgery* 2001;**129**:699–703.

21 Thistle JL, Cleary PA, Lachin JM *et al.* The natural history of cholelithiaisis: the National Cooperative Gallstone Study. *Ann Intern Med* 1984;**101**:171–5.

22 Way LW. The National Cooperative Gallstone study and chenodiol. *Gastroenterology* 1983;**84**:648–51.

23 Wetter LA, Way LW. Surgical therapy of gallstone disease. *Gastroenterol Clin North Am* 1991;**20**:157–69.

24 Steinle EW, VanderMolen RL, Silbergleit A *et al.* Impact of laparoscopic cholecystectomy on indications for surgical treatment of gallstones. *Surg Endosc* 1997;**11**:933–5.

25 Barkun JS, Barkum AN, Sampalis JS *et al.* Randomised controlled trial of laparoscopic versus mini cholecystectomy. *Lancet* 1992;**340**:116–19.

26 McMahon AJ, Russell, IT, Baxter JN. Laparoscopic versus minilaparotomy cholecystectomy: a randomised trial. *Lancet* 1994;**343**:135–8.

27 McGinn FP, Miles AJ, Ulgalow M *et al.* Randomized trial of laparoscopic cholecystectomy and mini-cholecystectomy. *Br J Surg* 1995;**82**:1347–77.

28 Majeed AW, Troy G, Nicholl JP *et al.* Randomised, prospective, single blind comparison of laparscopic versus small incision cholecystectomy. *Lancet* 1996:**347**;989–94.

29 Shea JA, Healey MJ, Berlin JA *et al.* Mortality and complications associated with laparoscopic cholecystectomy. A meta-analysis *Ann Surg* 1996;**224**:690–720.

30 Curet MJ, Contreras M, Weber DM *et al.* Laparoscopic cholecystectomy: outpatient versus inpatient management. *Surg Endosc* 2002;**16**:453–7.

31 Keulemans Y, Eshuis J, de Haes H, de Wit LT, Gouma DJ. Laparoscopic cholecystectomy: day-care versus clinical observation. *Ann Surg* 1998;**228**:734–40.

32 Cheah WK, Lenzi JE, So JBY *et al.* Randomized trial of needlescopic versus laparoscopic cholecystectomy. *Br J Surg* 2001;**88**:45–7.

33 Bisgaard T, Klarskov B, Trap R *et al.* Microlaparoscopic versus conventional laparoscopic cholecystectomy. A prospective randomized double blind trial. *Surg Endosc* 2002;**16**:458–64.

34 Schwenk W, Neudecker J, Mall J, Bohm B, Muller JM. Prospective randomized blinded trial of pulmonary function, pain, and cosmetic results after laparoscopic vs. microlaparoscopic cholecystectomy. *Surg Endosc* 2000;**14**:345–8.

35 Sarli L, Iusco D, Gobbi S, Porrini C, Ferro M, Roncoroni L. Randomized clinical trial of laparoscopic cholecystectomy performed with mini-instruments. *Br J Surg* 2003;**90**:1345–8.

36 McArthur P, Cuschieri A, Sells RA *et al.* Controlled clinical trial comparing early with interval cholecystectomy for acute cholecystitis. *Br J Surg* 1975;**62**:850–2.

37 Lahtinen J, Alhava EM, Aukee S. Acute cholecystitis treated by early and delayed surgery. A controlled clinical trial. *Scand J Gastroenterol* 1978;**13**:673–8.

38 van der Linden W, Sunzel H. Early versus delayed operation for acute cholecystitis. A controlled clinical trial. *Am J Surg* 1970;**120**:7–13.

39 Jarvinen HJ, Hastbacka J. Early cholecystectomy for acute cholecystitis: a prospective randomized study. *Ann Surg* 1980;**191**:501–5.

40 Norrby S, Herlin P, Holmin T *et al.* Early or delayed cholecystectomy in acute cholecystitis? A clinical trial. *Br J Surg* 1983;**70**:163–5.

41 Lo CM, Liu Cl, Fan ST *et al.* Prospective randomized study of early versus delayed laparoscopic cholecystectomy for acute cholecystitis. *Ann Surg* 1998;**227**:461–7.

42 Lai PB, Kwong KH, Leung KL *et al.* Randomized trial of early versus delayed laparosclopic cholecystectomy for acute cholecystitis. *Br J Surg* 1998;**85**:764–7.

43 Chandler CF, Lane JS, Ferguson P, Thompson JE, Ashley SW. Prospective evaluation of early versus delayed laparoscopic cholecystectomy for treatment of acute cholecystitis. *Am Surg* 2000;**66**:896–900.

44 Kiviluoto T, Siren J, Luukkonen P *et al.* Randomised trial of laparoscopic versus open cholecystectomy for acute and gangrenous cholecystitis. *Lancet* 1998;**351**:321–5.

45 Lujan JA, Parilla P, Robles R *et al.* Laparoscopic cholecystectomy vs open cholecystectomy in the treatment of acute cholecystitis: a prospective study. *Arch Surg* 1998;**133**:173–5.

46 Neoptolemos JP, Carr-Locke DL, London NJ *et al.* Controlled trial of urgent endoscopic retrograde cholangiopancreatography and endoscopic spincterotomy versus conservative treatment for acute pancreatitis due to gallstones. *Lancet* 1988;**2**:979–83.

47 Fan ST, Lai EC, Mok FP *et al.* Early treatment of acute biliary pancreatitis by endoscopic papillotomy. *N Engl J Med* 1993;**328**:228–32.

48 Folsch UR, Nitsche R, Ludtke R *et al.* Early ERCP and papillotomy compared with conservative treatment for acute biliary pancreatitis. The German Study Group on Acute Biliary Pancreatitis. *N Engl J Med* 1997;**336**:237–42.

49 Sees DW, Martin RR. Comparison of preoperative endoscopic retrograde cholangiopancreatography and laparoscopic cholecystectomy with operative management of gallstone pancreatitis. *Am J Surg* 1997;**174**:719–22.

50 Lin G, Halevy A, Girtler O, Gold-Deutch R, Zisman A, Scapa E. The role of endoscopic retrograde cholangiopancreatography in management of patients recovering from acute biliary pancreatitis in the laparoscopic era. *Surg Endosc.* 1997;**11**:371–5.

51 Robertson GS, Jagger C, Johnson PR, Rathbone BJ, Wicks AC, Lloyd DM, Veitch PS. Selection criteria for preoperative endoscopic retrograde cholangiopancreatography in the laparoscopic era. *Arch Surg* 1996;**131**:89–94.

52 Scapa E. To do or not to do an endoscopic retrograde cholangiopancreatography in acute biliary pancreatitis? *Surg Laparosc Endosc* 1995;**5**:453–4.

53 de Virgilio C, Verbin C, Chang L, Linder S, Stabile BE, Klein S. Gallstone pancreatitis. The role of preoperative endoscopic retrograde cholangiopancreatography. *Arch Surg* 1994;**129**:909–12.

54 Leitman IM, Fisher ML, McKinley MJ, Rothman R, Ward RJ, Reiner DS, Tortolani AJ. The evaluation and management of known or suspected stones of the common bile duct in the era of minimal access surgery. *Surg Gynecol Obstet* 1993;**176**:527–33.

55 Srinathan SK, Barkun JS, Mehta SN, Meakins JL, Barkun AN. Evolving management of mild-to-moderate gallstone pancreatitis. *J Gastrointest Surg* 1998;**2**:385–90.

56 Burch JM, Feliciano DV, Mattox KL, Jordan GL Jr. Gallstone pancreatitis. The question of time. *Arch Surg* 1990;**125**: 853–9.

57 Kelly TR, Wagner DS, Kelly TR, Wagner DS. Gallstone pancreatitis: a prospective randomized trial of the timing of surgery. *Surgery* 1988;**104**:600–5.

58 Kaw M, Al-Antably Y, Kaw P. Management of gallstone pancreatitis: cholecystectomy or ERCP and endoscopic sphincterotomy. *Gastrointest Endosc* 2002;**56**:61–5.

59 Kwon SK, Lee BS, Kim NJ, Lee HY, Chae HB, Youn SJ, Park SM. Is cholecystectomy necessary after ERCP for bile duct stones in patients with gallbladder *in situ? Korean J Intern Med* 2001;**16**:254–9.

60 Snow LL, Weinstein LS, Hannon JK *et al.* Evaluation of operative cholangiography in 2043 patients undergoing laparoscopic cholecystectomy. A case for the selective operative cholangiogram. *Surg Endosc* 2001;**15**:14–20.

61 Edye M, Dalvi A, Canin-Endres J *et al.* Intraoperative cholangiography is still indicated after preoperative endoscopic cholangiography for gallstone disease. *Surg Endosc* 2002;**16**:799–802.

62 Borjeson J, Liu SK, Jones S, Matolo NM. Selective intraoperative cholangiography during laparoscopic cholecystectomy: how selective? *Am Surg* 2000;**66**:616–18.

63 Neoptolemos JP, Carr-Locke DL, Fossard DP. Prospective randomised study of preoperative endoscopic sphincterotomy versus surgery alone for common bile duct stones. *BMJ (Clin Res Ed)* 1987;**294**:470–4.

64 Stain SC, Cohen H, Tsuishoysha M, Donovan AJ. Choledocholithiasis. Endoscopic sphincterotomy or common bile duct exploration. *Ann Surg* 1991;**213**:627–33.

65 Stiegmann GV, Goff JS, Mansour A, Pearlman N, Reveille RM, Norton L. Precholecystectomy endoscopic cholangiography and stone removal is not superior to cholecystectomy, cholangiography, and common duct exploration. *Am J Surg* 1992;**163**:227–30.

66 Suc B, Escat J, Cherqui D, Fourtanier G, Hay JM, Fingerhut A, Millat B. Surgery vs endoscopy as primary treatment in symptomatic patients with suspected common bile duct stones: a multicenter randomized trial. French Associations for Surgical Research. *Arch Surg* 1998;**133**:702–8.

67 Hammarstrom LE, Holmin T, Stridbeck H, Ihse I. Long-term follow up of a prospective randomized study of endoscopic versus surgical treatment of bile duct calculi in patients with gallbladder *in situ. Br J Surg* 1995;**82**:1516–21.

68 Sgourakis G, Karaliotas K. Laparoscopic common bile duct exploration and cholecystectomy versus endoscopic stone extraction and laparoscopic cholecystectomy for choledocholithiasis. A prospective randomized study. *Minerva Chir* 2002;**57**:467–74.

69 Rhodes M, Sussman L, Cohen L, Lewis MP. Randomised trial of laparoscopic exploration of common bile duct versus postoperative endoscopic retrograde cholangiography for common bile duct stones. *Lancet* 1998;**351**:159–61.

70 Cuschieri A, Croce E, Faggioni A *et al.* EAES ductal stone study. Preliminary findings of multi-center prospective randomized trial comparing two-stage vs single-stage management. *Surg Endosc* 1996;**10**:1130–5.

71 Freeman ML, Nelson DB, Sherman S *et al.* Complications of endoscopic biliary sphincterotomy. *N Engl J Med* 1996; **335**:909–18.

72 Masci E, Toti G, Mariani A *et al.* Complications of diagnostic and therapeutic ERCP: a prospective multicenter study. *Am J Gastroenterol* 2001;**96**:417–23.

73 Boerma D, Rauws EAJ, Keulemans YCA *et al.* Wait-and-see policy or laparoscopic cholecystectomy after endoscopic spincterectomy for bile duct stones: a randomized trial. *Lancet* 2002;**360**:761–5.

21 Acute pancreatitis

Jonathon Springer, Hillary Steinhart

Introduction

Acute pancreatitis is a common admission diagnosis on gastroenterology and general surgical services. It is an inflammatory condition of the pancreas characterized clinically by abdominal pain and elevated levels of pancreatic enzymes in the blood. The incidence of acute pancreatitis in England, Denmark and the USA varies from 4·8 to 24·2 per 100 000 patients.[1] However, estimates of incidence are inaccurate because the diagnosis of mild disease may be missed, and death may occur before diagnosis in 10% of patients with severe disease.[2]

The term acute pancreatitis encompasses a wide spectrum of clinical and pathological findings arising from many different causes. Gallstones and chronic alcohol abuse account for 75% of cases in the USA. No obvious etiology is identifiable in approximately 30% of patients with acute pancreatitis. Uncommon causes include biliary sludge and microlithiasis, hypertriglyceridemia, hypercalcemia, drugs, infection and trauma. Despite extensive research in the area, the underlying pathophysiology of acute pancreatitis still remains speculative.

Most patients with acute pancreatitis will have a mild form and ultimately follow a benign clinical course but up to 20% will develop severe pancreatitis with all its inherent morbidity and risk of mortality. Despite the many advances in the treatment and diagnosis of acute pancreatitis, the mortality rate remains between 5% and 15%.[3]

Unfortunately, acute pancreatitis generally has an unpredictable course and prognosis. Most attacks of acute pancreatitis are mild with recovery occurring within 5–7 days. In contrast, severe necrotizing pancreatitis is associated with a high rate of complications and significant mortality. This has prompted a search for the ideal prognostic tools (single or multiple laboratory or clinical variables) that might predict severe disease and morbid complications early in the course when potential therapeutic interventions may alter the natural history. However, the variable nature of the disease, its many different causes, and potential complications make it a difficult disease to treat and one for which a universally effective treatment is unlikely to be achievable. At the present time there is no single, simple, universally accepted prognostic instrument or treatment protocol for those with acute pancreatitis.

This chapter will critically review the evidence available from the literature that examines the use of various prognostic instruments and the medical, surgical and endoscopic treatment options available for acute pancreatitis.

A review of the literature was conducted after carrying out a computerized search of the MEDLINE database for the years 1974 to 2003. The search included all English language articles indexed under the MeSH heading "pancreatitis" and the text words "acute pancreatitis". Review articles and articles of special interest in the area were reviewed and their bibliographies were searched for additional references. The articles dealing with prognosis or treatment of acute pancreatitis were then critically reviewed but a formal meta-analysis was not conducted.

Prognosis

Some patients with acute pancreatitis may go on to develop life-threatening complications while others will have a brief illness and recover uneventfully. It is important to be able to accurately identify which patients are at greater risk for potential complications including death if an efficient and effective use of resources is to be achieved. Most studies have suggested that a basic clinical assessment at the time of admission is quite poor for identifying these patients.[4–6] Corfield *et al.* found in their prospective study of 418 patients that 60% who went on to develop severe pancreatitis were not predicted to do so by a basic clinical assessment at the time of admission.[5] With this knowledge in mind, various methods have been used in an attempt to predict the severity of acute pancreatitis. This has included the use of multiple clinical scoring systems, individual laboratory tests, invasive procedures (peritoneal tap), and imaging techniques (CT scanning). However, none of these prognostic tools are both highly sensitive and specific and therefore have limited application for the individual patient. We will review some of the variables that have been investigated more extensively and shown some promise.

Multiple variable scoring systems

Ranson's criteria, the Glasgow score, and the APACHE-II score are three common clinical scoring systems used to predict the severity of acute pancreatitis. Ranson's criteria is the most widely used clinical scoring system for the prediction of severity (Table 21.1). Ranson's initial study was retrospective, looked at 43 variables in 100 patients and identified 11 variables with prognostic capabilities.[7] The presence of three or more clinical signs predicted a significant risk of death or severe illness. These findings were weakened by the retrospective nature of the study and the disproportionately large number of variables studied for the sample size. However, Ranson's criteria were subsequently validated by several large studies (Table 21.2).[8–14] Drawbacks associated with the use of Ranson's criteria include the 48-hour observation period required for a prediction to be made, the maximum "one time" assessment and its original derivation from a population of patients with mostly alcoholic pancreatitis. It is also cumbersome to remember all the criteria and often some of the laboratory tests required to establish the score are not done routinely for these patients.

The Glasgow criteria were created because of the concern that Ranson's criteria were formulated on a population of mostly alcoholic pancreatitis and, as a result, might not hold the same prognostic value in other populations.[15] The Glasgow criteria have subsequently been modified on several occasions but the comparative studies have shown no added benefit of one scoring system over the other. The Glasgow criteria include nine clinical variables but still require 48 hours of observation and do not allow for continuous monitoring. The sensitivity and specificity are comparable to Ranson's criteria and have been reported to be 55–85% and 75–90%, respectively.[7–9,12,14,16,17]

More recently, the APACHE-II scoring system has been used as a prognostic index in acute pancreatitis because of the perceived limitations of the Glasgow and Ranson scoring systems. Unlike the other scoring systems, it allows early assessment of prognosis and continuous monitoring and reassessment. Comparative studies have shown that an APACHE-II score > 5 or a peak score > 9 provides operating characteristics similar to or slightly better than the other multiple variable scoring systems.[9,12] The operating characteristics for the APACHE II score are shown in Table 21.3.

There are several problems with the studies that have examined the use of scoring systems as a prognostic tool in acute pancreatitis. The retrospective nature of some studies or the lack of consecutive accrual of study patients in

Table 21.1 Ranson's criteria for prediction of severity of acute pancreatitis

	Non-gallstone pancreatitis	Gallstone pancreatitis
On admission		
Age (years)	>55	>70
WBC (per mm³)	>16 000	>18 000
LDH (IU/l)	>200	>400
AST (IU/l)	>350	>250
Within 48 hrs		
Hct decreases (%)	>10	
BUN increases (mg/dl)	>5	>2
Calcium (mmol/l)	<2·0	<2·0
Po_2 (mmHg)	<60	–
Base deficit (mmol/l)	>4	>5
Fluid (l)(I – O)	>6	>4

WBC, white blood cells; LDH, lactose dehydrogenase; AST, aspartate aminotransferase; Hct, hematocrit; BUN, blood urea nitrogen; Po_2, partial pressure of oxygen; I – O, in – out

prospective trials may lead to selection bias but likely does not impact the results significantly. However, the lack of complete data in some studies makes interpretation of the results very difficult. Finally, the differences in the definition of severe pancreatitis make comparison between trials questionable. The definition of severe pancreatitis as major organ failure biases the prognostic ability of an APACHE-II score and inflates its accuracy because the calculation of the score is directly dependent on inclusion of at least part of the endpoint. Overall, these scoring systems are helpful but only provide a slight improvement from a basic clinical assessment at 48 hours. In general, they do not adequately identify patients at risk of severe pancreatitis (low positive predictive value) but can identify those patients who experience only mild pancreatitis (high negative predictive value).[17]

More recently, the Hong Kong criteria were formulated in an attempt to simplify the previous prognostic scoring systems. Fan *et al.* have shown that a urea level above 7·4 mmol/l and blood glucose level above 11·0 mmol/l predicted severity of disease with a sensitivity of 79% and a specificity of 67%.[18] However, their results were not reproduced by Heath and Imrie who compared the Hong Kong criteria with the Glasgow criteria in 125 European patients and found a sensitivity of only 33% and a specificity of 86%, much lower than the operating characteristics for the Glasgow criteria.[19] This discrepancy may be explained by differences in study populations but this characteristic limits its general application.

Table 21.2   Studies validating the prognostic ability of Ranson's criteria

Reference	Sample size	Endpoint	Sensitivity (%)	Specificity (%)	Criticisms
Ranson et al.[7]	100	Death/ICU stay >7 days	46	99	See text
Ranson et al.[8]	200	Death/ICU stay >7 days	96	92	Endpoint subjective
Larvin and McMahon[6]	290	OF/PC	75	68	
McMahon et al.[4]	79	14-day hospitalization OF/PC	82	79	
Wilson et al.[9]	160	OF/PC/D	87	71	
Gross et al.[10]	75	D/Comp ≥ 2	PPV 80	NPV 68	
Dominguez-Munoz et al.[11]	182	D/OF/PC	77	70	
Agarwal and Pitchumoni[12]	76	OF/PC	40	90	Retrospective, Ranson's > 2
Banks et al.[13]	75		74	71	
Wilson et al.[14]	72		88	79	

D, death; PC, pancreatic collection, OF, organ failure; ICU, intensive care unit; PPV, positive predictive value; NPV, negative predictive value

Table 21.3   Prognostic ability of APACHE II score for in acute pancreatitis

Reference	Sample size	Endpoint	Sensitivity (%)	Specificity (%)	Criticisms
Larvin and McMahon[6]	290	OF/PC	63 (0 hour) 75 (48 hours)	81 (0 hour) 92 (48 hours)	Variable dependent on endpoint
Wilson et al.[9]	160	PC/OF/D	95 (>5) 82 (>9)	54 (>5) 74 (>9)	

For abbreviations see Table 21.2.

Computed tomography

The limited usefulness of the scoring systems and the cumbersome nature of calculating them has stimulated further investigation into other potential tools. Contrast enhanced computed tomography (CT) scanning has been investigated extensively because of its ability to identify local complications (pseudocyst, abscess, phlegmon, peripancreatic fluid) and necrotizing pancreatitis, both of which are thought to lead to increased morbidity and mortality.[20–26] The sensitivity and specificity of CT findings for the prediction of severe pancreatitis from several prospective studies is shown in Table 21.4. Although the presence of necrosis did correlate with a more complicated course, the extent of necrosis did not provide any additional prognostic value. Unfortunately, comparison between studies is problematic because of the lack of a standardized CT staging system, variations in the definitions of clinical disease severity, dissimilar inclusion criteria and the timing of the CT scan. However, based on the

evidence available, contrast enhanced CT scans which can detect pancreatic necrosis and local complications, can serve a valuable role in the management of these patients but the exact timing of the scan remains controversial. It is probably best done between 48 and 96 hours after onset of the symptoms in patients without improvement.

Peritoneal tap

The color and volume of peritoneal fluid obtained by means of percutaneous drainage from a patient shortly after diagnosis have been shown to predict the severity of pancreatitis to the same extent as non-invasive techniques but also provide information on possible alternative diagnoses (for example bowel perforation).[27] However, the procedure is invasive and carries a 0·8% risk of complications.[27] The operating characteristics of a peritoneal tap for prognosis in acute pancreatitis are shown in Table 21.5. The application of

Table 21.4 Prognostic ability of computed tomography in acute pancreatitis

Reference	Sample size	Endpoint	Sensitivity (%)	Specificity (%)	Criticisms
Balthazar *et al.*[20] Grade D+E	83	PC/D	89	71	
Balthazar *et al.*[21] Grade D+E	88	PC/D	90	73	
Hjelmqvist *et al.*[22]	47	PC/14-day hospitalization	71	80	
London *et al.*[23]	32	D/PC/20-day hospitalization	83	65	Selection bias, criteria
London *et al.*[24]	126	D/PC	71	77	
Clavien *et al.*[25]	176	D/PC	66	97	
Puolakkainen[26]	88		66	100	

For abbreviations see Table 21.2.

Table 21.5 Prognostic ability of peritoneal tap in acute pancreatitis

Reference	Sample size	Endpoint	Sensitivity (%)	Specificity (%)	Criticisms
McMahon *et al.*[4] (10ml)	79	14-days hospitalization PC/OF/D	72	95	Selection bias, 68 patients excluded for mild disease
Corfield *et al.*[5]	253		53		
Mayer and McMahon[27]	231		60	87	

For abbreviations see Table 21.2.

the results of these studies and their interpretation are hindered by the selection criteria used for inclusion. Patients selected for the procedure tended to be those with more severe disease because of the invasive nature of the procedure. Thus, a broad spectrum of disease severity and presentations were not assessed.

Individual laboratory tests

In an attempt to simplify the prognostic indices and provide a non-invasive early assessment of disease severity, many studies have examined individual laboratory tests. Only tests that have been studied extensively or shown some promise in this area will be reviewed below.

C-reactive protein (CRP) is an acute phase reactant that rises in many inflammatory conditions including acute pancreatitis. CRP rises steadily in relation to severity, is inexpensive to measure and testing is readily available. However, CRP takes 48 hours to become significantly elevated and it is unclear if it accurately predicts necrosis. Several studies have measured CRP in acute pancreatitis and found a correlation between the level of CRP and the severity.[28–37] The operating characteristics are shown in

Table 21.6. Most studies are comparable since the cut-off level used and study designs were similar. These results suggest that, as a single test, CRP provides a prognostic capability equal to or better than all the prognostic tools previously studied without significant cost or morbidity.

α_2Microglobulin, $\alpha_1$antitrypsin, and methemalbumin have been extensively investigated but have not been found to confer any additional benefit over clinical assessment or multiple scoring systems.[38,39]

More recently, PMN elastase, an acute phase reactant released by granulocytes during inflammatory processes, has been explored for its potential to identify those patients at risk of developing severe pancreatitis. It has shown the most promise in this regard with sensitivity and specificity in the range of 82–93% and 82–99%, respectively when measured 24 hours *after* the onset of the disease. This may provide improved and earlier prognostic information than multiple scoring systems. The operating characteristics are shown in Table 21.7.

Several other laboratory tests, including phospholipase A_2, tumor necrosis factor, complement levels, trypsinogen activated peptide, and pancreatitis-associated protein have all been investigated but none have provided significant prognostic ability or adequate reproducibility.

Table 21.6   Prognostic ability of C-reactive protein test in acute pancreatitis

Reference	Sample size	End point	Sensitivity (%)	Specificity (%)	Criticisms
Buchler et al.[28]	35	NP	95		No clinical endpoint, no data shown
Puolakkainen[26] (140 mg/l)	88	D/C	100	81	
Puolakkainen et al.[30]	53	D/Hemorrhagic pancreatitis	15/17	100	
Gross et al.[10]	75	D/≥+2 complications	PPV 73	NPV 73	Endpoint broad
Leser et al.[33]	50	D/≥+2 complications	83	62	
Paajanen et al.[32]	77	D/complication	84	71	
Dominguez-Munoz et al.[11] (60, 70mg/l)	182	D/PC/OF	63 (24 hours) 73 (48 hours)	65 (24 hours) 71 (48 hours)	Cut-off different than most studies
Viedma et al.[34]	80	D/PC/systemic complications	Discrim function		Non-consecutive
Kaufman et al.[35]	25	AP > 25	90	86	Inclusion = ICU
Hedstrom et al.[36]	110	OF/D/PC	95	11	
Wilson et al.[14] (210 mg/l)	72	D/C	83	85	
Leese et al.[29] (150 mg/l)	198	D/C	70 (72 hours)	71 (72 hours)	
Kemppainen et al.[37]	147	PC/OF/RC/AP	60	92	
Gudgeon et al.[31]	55	D/C	60	75	

NP, normal protein AP, acute pancreatitis, ICU, intensive care unit; for other abbreviations see Table 21.2.

Table 21.7   Prognostic ability of PMN elastase test in acute pancreatitis

Reference	Sample size	Endpoint	Sensitivity (%)	Specificity (%)
Gross et al.[10]	75	D/C ≥ 2	81	82
Dominguez-Munoz et al.[11]	182	D/PC/OF	93 (24 hours)	99 (24 hours)
Viedma et al.[34]	80	D/PC/Systemic complications	84	N/A

N/A, not applicable. For other abbreviations see Table 21.2.

Summary

At this point, no single laboratory test can be advocated as the only method of assessing prognosis in acute pancreatitis. The two laboratory tests with the greatest promise are CRP and the PMN elastase but their routine clinical use is still limited. Based on the available evidence, an assessment of prognosis tailored to the clinical setting and hospital resources is suggested. A practical approach would be the use of a clinical scoring system in conjunction with PMN elastase and consideration of a contrast enhanced CT scan should the patient's condition not improve within 72–96 hours. However, such a combined approach has not been formally evaluated relative to the predictive value of single modality prognostic approaches.

Treatment

The management of acute pancreatitis continues to evolve as our understanding of the pathophysiology and natural history becomes more complete. The diversity of clinical presentations has prevented the establishment of a standard treatment strategy and hindered the interpretation of clinical research in the area. The management of acute pancreatitis has evolved to include medical, endoscopic and surgical treatment options. This analysis will be restricted to the treatments that have been examined more rigorously. These can be broadly categorized into three main groups according to their therapeutic objectives. The basic goals of treatment strategies are to limit the severity of pancreatic inflammation by inhibiting pancreatic secretion, to interrupt the pathogenesis of complications and to treat the complications when they occur. Most of the medical treatments have focused their effort on limiting the severity of pancreatic inflammation by either reducing pancreatic secretions or inhibiting pancreatic enzymes and the inflammatory cascade.

Supportive measures

The use of nasogastric suction and keeping patients nil per os has been based on the theory of "resting the pancreas" and thereby reducing pancreatic secretions and inflammation. Nasogastric suction raises duodenal pH and reduces secretin release and pancreatic stimulation. However, there has been little clinical evidence to support this practice. Several prospective randomized studies have looked at the use of nasogastric suction and found no significant benefit in morbidity, mortality or length of hospital stay.[40–43] Ald However, most of the studies were very small (< 50 patients) and restricted to patients with alcoholic pancreatitis. Since these patients also had mild pancreatitis and low mortality rates it is unknown whether there might be a benefit in patients with severe pancreatitis. In addition, the small sample sizes create the possibility of a type II error. Certainly those patients with severe nausea or ileus benefit symptomatically from nasogastric suction but the benefits of this modality in improving outcomes remain unproved. Ald

H₂-receptor antagonists

Using the same premise, H_2 blockers have been investigated in the treatment of acute pancreatitis. Several randomized controlled trials have failed to show any clinical benefit[44,45] but once again the patient numbers have generally been small and entry into the studies was restricted to patients with mild to moderate disease severity.

Peptide hormone therapy

Glucagon, calcitonin, and somatostatin and its analog octreotide have also been studied as agents that directly inhibit pancreatic secretion and, as such, might benefit patients with acute pancreatitis. Six randomized controlled trials have examined the use of glucagon and found no significant reduction in morbidity or mortality.[46–51] Ald Although none of the studies showed even a trend towards improved clinical status with the use of glucagon, it should be noted that all the studies were very small (< 30 patients in each arm).

Calcitonin has been examined in two moderate sized (100 patients) randomized double blind placebo-controlled studies.[52,53] Although there was a significant reduction in abdominal pain and serum amylase levels with treatment, the complication and mortality rates were unchanged. Ald

Somatostatin and octreotide are thought to reduce exocrine pancreatic secretions and possess cytoprotective effects and somatostatin has been found to reduce the complications and mortality of acute pancreatitis in animal studies.[54,55] C5 There have been many controlled trials examining the use of somatostatin or octreotide in the treatment of acute pancreatitis with varying results (Table 21.8). Only one study demonstrated a decrease in mortality.[56] Ald Three studies[56–58] have shown a significant decrease in complications with an additional two studies[59,60] showing a trend toward reduced complications. In two studies[56,61] there was a statistically significant decrease in the length of hospitalization. Ald One study[62] reported a more pronounced decrease in serum amylase levels, improvements in pancreatic edema and earlier return to oral intake in the high dose octreotide group (octreotide 0·5 microgram/kg per hour continuous intravenous infusion). However, three of the largest and best designed studies have failed to show any benefit in mortality or morbidity.[63–65] Ald Therefore, based on the available evidence, the routine use of somatostatin or octreotide in the treatment of acute pancreatitis is not recommended.

Protease inhibition

The release of pancreatic enzymes and subsequent autodigestion is one of the postulated mechanisms for the development of acute pancreatitis and a modulator of the severity of the disease. A number of antiprotease agents, including aprotinin, gabexate (Foy), and fresh frozen plasma have thus been investigated.

There have been several studies examining the benefit of aprotinin, a high molecular weight protease inhibitor. However, only three of these were randomized, controlled studies published as full articles.[66] These relatively large studies (~200 patients) found no reduction in morbidity or mortality. Ald An earlier study had suggested a reduction in mortality, particularly in the elderly, but these results have not been reproduced.[67]

Gabexate mesilate, a potent lower molecular weight protease inhibitor thought to enter pancreatic acinar cells and inhibit intracellular proteases has been studied in several randomized controlled trials (Table 21.9).[68–74] Only one study shows a reduction in 7-day and 90-day mortality.[73] Ald One study[70] which compared gabexate with aprotinin in patients with severe pancreatitis (at least two Ranson's criteria), found a reduction in systemic and total complications in those treated with gabexate. However, the study lacked a placebo arm and the treatment groups differed in some important

Table 21.8 Clinical trials of treatment of acute pancreatitis with somatostatin/octreotide

Reference	Sample size	Entry criteria	Endpoint	% Complications (placebo)	% Complications (O or S)	% Mortality (placebo)	% Mortality (O or S)	Criticism
Paran et al.[56]	38	Ranson's ≥3	PC/OF/D/LS	74 (sepsis) 34d (LS)[a]	26 (sepsis) 18d (LS) 46 (S)	6/19	2/19	Unblinded
Planas[58]	50	ICU patients, severe AP	C/surgery/PC/OF	86 (S)	46 (S)	32	38	Unblinded, delayed intervention
Choi et al.[59]	71	AP	D/OF/PC/Lab tests	13/36	5/35	2/36	1/35	Unblinded? follow up
Binder et al.[60]	24	Moderate-severe AP (4/11 criteria)	D/OF/Metabolic complication score	−2.1 score	−1.5 (300 micrograms) 3.0 (600 micrograms) 1.0 (1500 micrograms)	14.8	8.3	Historical controls, unvalidated subject endpoint small numbers
D'Amico et al.[63]	164	AP	D/OF/PC/LS	12	11	8.5	2.4	Complex study design, unblinded
Gjorup et al.[64]	63	AP	Complication/LS	70	58	3	3	Unblinded
Uhl (Binder et al.[60]	302	>3 Ranson's	PC/mortality			16	15,12	
Paran et al.[56]	60	>3 Ranson's, CT	PC, LS, mortality	76, 56	24, 28	80	20	Study not powered properly
Karakoyunlar et al.[62]	43	AP	PC	4.5–13.6	4.5–22.7	4.5	4.5	
Lata et al.[61]	21	AP	LS, free radicals	13.7 (LS)	9.8 (LS)	0	0	Small study
McKay et al.[65]	58	Severe AP, APACHE>5	PC/OF/D	40	54	20	18	Not all had CT abdomen

D, death; PC, pancreatic complication; OF, organ failure[a]; LS, length of hospital stay; O, octreotide; S, somatostatin

Table 21.9   Clinical trials of treatment of acute pancreatitis with gabexate

Study	Study design; intervention	No. of patients	Conclusion
Yang et al.[68]	RCT; gabexate v placebo	42	No benefit
Valderrama et al.[69]	Multicenter RCT; gabexate v placebo	100	No benefit
Pederzoli et al.[70]	RCT; gabexate v aprotinin	182	Reduction in systemic complications
Pezzilli et al.[72]	Prospective open label multicenter; gabexate v gabexate	397	No benefit in higher doses
Chen et al.[73]	RCT; gabexate v placebo	52	Improved short-term survival
Berling et al.[66]	multicenter; RCT gabexate v placebo	48	No benefit
Chen et al.[74]	RCT; gabexate v placebo	26	Reduction in inflammatory mediators
Buchler et al.[71]	Multicenter RCT gabexate v placebo	223	No benefit

RCT, randomized controlled trial

baseline characteristics such as the proportion with necrotizing pancreatitis. Another study evaluated the effect of gabexate mesilate on various inflammatory markers.[74] The results of this study suggest that gabexate mesilate given early in the course of acute pancreatitis lessens the magnitude of changes of inflammatory mediators. Ald

The use of fresh frozen plasma (FFP) to replenish the levels of naturally occurring antiproteases has also been examined. Leese et al. conducted a randomized controlled trial on 202 patients and found no difference in mortality or morbidity between those who received FFP and those who received colloid.[75] Ald

Anti-inflammatory therapy

More recently, as our knowledge of the pathophysiology of acute pancreatitis has evolved, the focus of treatment has changed. Platelet activating factor (PAF), a proinflammatory lipid mediator released by macrophages, neutrophils and endothelial cells, plays a significant role in acute inflammation. There have been three randomized controlled trials which have examined the use of lexipafant, a PAF antagonist, in the treatment of acute pancreatitis.[76–78] Two studies, despite their small size (< 100 patients), found a significant reduction in organ failure scores. This was seen in all patients irrespective of the severity of pancreatitis. Ald The studies were not designed to detect a change in mortality or local complications but a trend toward lower mortality was seen in one of the studies.[77] The third study,[78] a randomized double blind study of 290 patients included endpoints such as pancreatic complications, severity of organ failure, markers of inflammatory response and mortality rate. The study findings were complicated by the fact that 44% of patients had organ failure upon entry into the study. As a result, there was no difference in the primary outcome of pancreatic complications. Furthermore, lexipafant had no effect on new

organ failure. Ala Although there is insufficient evidence presently available to advocate the use of PAF inhibitors, the results to date are sufficiently encouraging as to suggest the importance of further research. If these agents are to have any role it will likely be in reducing the risk of early systemic complications in those patients predicted to have severe disease.

Antibiotics

The close association between infection and increased morbidity and mortality in severe pancreatitis (particularly necrotizing pancreatitis) has led to studies of the use of antibiotic prophylaxis. Initial studies in the early 1970s were disappointing and the concept was dropped until recently. On further review, it was recognized that these early studies were not designed in a manner that could adequately address the effect of antibiotic prophylaxis. The three randomized trials had small sample sizes and all compared ampicillin with placebo.[79–81] The mortality in the control groups was zero, indicating that the study population had mild disease with a negligible risk of pancreatic infection. Given that the incidence of infection in the control groups was only 7%, it would have been virtually impossible to achieve a clinically or statistically significant result with the sample sizes studied. In addition, the choice of antibiotic has now been recognized as inappropriate since ampicillin is not effective against many of the organisms commonly seen in pancreatic infection and since it has poor penetration into pancreatic tissue.

With these considerations in mind further studies of antibiotic therapy have been conducted. Three initial studies have tested the hypothesis that antibiotics prevent pancreatic complications.[82–84] Pederzoli and colleagues randomized 74 patients with necrotizing pancreatitis to receive a 14-day course of imipenem, a broad-spectrum antibiotic with good pancreatic penetration, or placebo within 72 hours of onset.[82]

All pancreatic infections were confirmed microbiologically by tissue culture from aspiration or surgical debridement. The unblinded study found that the incidence of both pancreatic sepsis (30% *v* 12%, *P* < 0·01) and non-pancreatic sepsis (49% *v* 15%, *P* < 0·01) were decreased in patients on imipenem. However, there were no differences in the number of operations for pancreatic sepsis (33% *v* 29%), the incidence of organ failure (39% *v* 29%) or death (12% *v* 7%). Ald

Sainio and colleagues conducted a similar randomized study in Finland comparing cefuroxime (4·5 g/day for 14 days) versus placebo in 60 patients with alcohol-induced necrotizing pancreatitis.[83] The mean Ranson's score was 5·5 and the degree of pancreatic necrosis was over 30% in 80% of the patients. The total number of infectious complications was higher in the placebo group (54 *v* 30, *P* < 0·01) but this was largely due to a higher rate of urinary tract infections (17 *v* 6, *P* = 0·0073). The incidence of pancreatic infections was similar in the two groups (40% *v* 30%). Although the overall incidence of infection was lower in the antibiotic-treated group, there were no differences in length of hospital stay or need for pancreatic drainage or debridement. However, prophylaxis with cefuroxime reduced overall mortality (23% *v* 3%, *P* < 0·03, NNT (number needed to treat) 5). Ald Since three deaths in the placebo group were associated with pancreatic cultures that were positive for *Staphylococcus epidermidis* the authors suggest that cefuroxime may reduce severe infectious complications and prevent secondary *S. epidermidis* infections.

The finding that most bacteria in pancreatic infection are enteric flora has led to the presumption that most such organisms migrate from the intestine by bacterial translocation. Luiten and colleagues[84] conducted a randomized study in 102 patients with severe pancreatitis (Imrie score > 2 or Balthazar grade D or E on CT scan) comparing selective bowel decontamination using topical pharyngeal (paste), rectal (enema) and oral preparations of colistin sulfate, amphotericin, and norfloxacin with placebo. The patients in the treatment arm also received cefotaxime intravenously every 8 hours until cultures of the rectum and pharynx were free of Gram-negative bacteria. The overall mortality was similar in the two groups in an intention to treat analysis (35% *v* 22%, *P* = 0·19). Alc When corrected for disease severity by a multivariate analysis, a modest survival benefit was evident (*P* = 0·048) owing to a reduction in late mortality (> 2 weeks) in the active treatment arm. In addition, pancreatic infections were significantly reduced from 38% to 18% (*P* = 0·03) and Gram-negative infections were reduced from 33% to 8% (*P* = 0·003) with selective decontamination. Alc The results suggest a potential benefit for selective decontamination but should be interpreted with a degree of caution because of the lack of clear difference in mortality in the primary analysis, the unblinded nature of the study, and the fact that intravenous antibiotics were also given, albeit for a short time.

More recently the use of imipenem has been studied in the management of acute pancreatitis complicated by pancreatic necrosis. Olah *et al.* in a two-phase randomized controlled trial studied the outcomes of 89 patients admitted with acute pancreatitis (48 patients randomized into a parenteral group, 41 patients into an enteral group).[85] They have shown that the combination of enteral feeding and imipenem can prevent multiple organ failure in patients with acute pancreatitis. Ald Nordback *et al.* in a single center randomized trial investigated the use of early versus delayed treatment with imipenem on the prevention of pancreatic infection in necrotizing pancreatitis.[86] They randomized 25 patients to receive imipenem early (1·0 g plus cilastin intravenously three times a day within 48 hours of diagnosis) and 33 patients to the control strategy (imipenem when the operative indication was fulfilled). The main endpoint was the indication for necrosectomy due to infection. The authors show a trend towards reduce need for surgery (two (8%) patients in the imipenem group, five (36%) in the control group, *P* = 0·04), and overall major organ failure (seven (25%) in the imipenem group, 25 (76%) in the control group, *P* = 0·0003). Ald Their study is limited because of a low sample size and high dropout rate.

The success of imipenem in randomized controlled trials has resulted in the investigation of both novel as well as older antibiotics. Bassi *et al.* compare the use of imipenem to pefloxacin (a broad spectrum antibiotic with proved pancreatic penetration).[87] Imipenem proved to be significantly more effective in prevention of pancreatic infection (20% *v* 44%). Ald There was no difference in mortality between the two groups. Isenmann *et al.* reported on the use of ciprofloxacin and metronidazole in the management of severe acute pancreatitis.[88] They randomized 56 patients to the placebo arm and 58 patients to the treatment group. Antibiotics were given for at least 11 days. They concluded that treatment with ciprofloxacin and metronidazole does not have a positive effect on mortality (7% treatment, 11% placebo) and infected pancreatic necrosis (17% treatment, 14% placebo). Ald

The recent use of probiotics in the management of various gastrointestinal illnesses prompted Kecskes *et al.* to study the effects of *Lactobacillus plantarum* on patients with acute pancreatitis (defined as plasma amylase > 200 U/l, CRP > 150 mg/l and an Imrie-score ≥ 3).[89] The authors reported a reduction in abscesses (4·5% *v* 30%) in the treated group. Ald They also showed a decreased length of stay (13·7 *v* 21·4 days) in the treated group compared to the group that received placebo.

At this time, the available evidence suggests a potential benefit for antibiotic prophylaxis or selective decontamination in patients with severe pancreatitis and evidence of necrosis. However, larger studies are needed before this treatment can be considered to be standard care. Several questions remain unanswered including the minimum degree of disease severity for which treatment benefit might be expected, and the duration, dose and type of antibiotic to be used. It seems reasonable to use an antibiotic that covers the common enteric flora and penetrates the pancreatic tissue adequately. C5 Imepenem does appear to produce a reduction in pancreatic infections and overall infections. At present, there are not sufficient data to support the use of probiotics in the management of acute pancreatitis.

Nutritional support

Nutritional support in patients with acute pancreatitis is a complex and controversial issue. Most (80%) patients have mild disease and recover over the first 5 days without requiring nutritional support. However, the remaining patients with severe disease often have a protracted course with a combination of decreased oral intake and increased metabolic demand that often leads to a negative nitrogen and energy balance. In order to combat these nutritional problems and to put the pancreas at "rest", parenteral nutrition has been the standard of care for patients with severe pancreatitis despite a paucity of supportive controlled data. Early studies of total parenteral nutrition (TPN) were poorly controlled, non-randomized and often retrospective. Several retrospective studies have suggested that TPN can improve nutritional status without compromising the patients' overall condition.[90,91] B4 These early studies, together with several small case series examining the effect of intravenous nutrients, particularly lipid components, on pancreatic secretion and pancreatitis have concluded that TPN is safe to use in patients with acute pancreatitis.[92–95] More recently the use of TPN in prospective trials in patients with severe acute pancreatitis have been conducted. Two prospective non-randomized studies have suggested that early use of TPN can decrease morbidity and mortality in patients with severe pancreatitis.[96,97] B1 Sitzman and colleagues[96] treated 73 patients with one of three different TPN preparations and found that the mortality rate in the 81% of patients who were able to maintain a positive nitrogen balance was significantly lower than in the 19% who were not (2·5% v 21·4% ($P < 0·01$). The analysis was not controlled for the severity of pancreatitis and, therefore, the interpretation of these results is difficult. Kalfarentzos and colleagues[97] prospectively studied the benefit of TPN in 67 patients according to time of initiation. They found that patients who had TPN started within the first 72 hours had significant reduction in mortality and morbidity in comparison to those who started later in the course of their disease (mortality 13% v 38%, $P < 0·05$, complications 23·6% v 95·6%, $P < 0·01$). B4

Sax and colleagues randomized 54 patients with mild acute pancreatitis to conventional therapy consisting of intravenous fluids, analgesics, antacids and nasogastric suction or to conventional therapy with TPN within the first 24 hours.[98] They found no advantage to early TPN as the number of days to oral intake, duration of hospital stay and number of pancreatic-related complications were similar in both groups, while there was an increase in catheter-related sepsis in the TPN group (10·5% v 1·5%, $P < 0·01$). A1d However, the overall mortality was only 1·8%, reflecting the very mild form of pancreatitis studied. As a result it would have been unlikely to demonstrate a significant improvement in morbidity or mortality in this population with the institution of TPN. Therefore, there remains a paucity of data with which to evaluate the use of TPN in patients with severe pancreatitis.

The failure of earlier studies to clearly demonstrate a clinical benefit with the use of TPN in patients with severe acute pancreatitis led to the investigation of other techniques of nutritional support. The recognition that a significant component of the morbidity and mortality arising from acute pancreatitis is related to sepsis, which is thought to arise from bacterial translocation from the bowel, has led researchers to rethink the dogma of complete bowel rest. One train of thought is that enteral nutrition may maintain bowel wall integrity and reduce bacterial translocation without risking further pancreatic stimulation. C5 The issue of whether or not the enteral infusion of nutrients can successfully put the pancreas to rest remains controversial. Various animal and human studies have shown conflicting results.[99–101] However, pancreatic stimulation appears to be lessened as nutrients are infused more distally in the intestine. It appears that jejunal feeds reduce pancreatic secretion to clinically insignificant levels but do not eliminate pancreatic secretion completely.[100,101] Studies showing that the combination of TPN and nil per os increases intestinal mucosal permeability and bacterial translocation and decreases gastrointestinal immunoglobulin levels have served as further stimulus to re-evaluate the manner in which nutritional supplementation is provided to patients with acute pancreatitis.[102–104]

Until recently, most of the studies in this area have been limited to case series. Initial studies describe the safe use of enteral nutrition in acute pancreatitis. In the case series by Kudst *et al.* 11 patients underwent laparotomy for complications from pancreatitis and had jejunostomy tubes placed at the time.[105] All nine patients who had successful tube placement tolerated feeds without worsening pancreatitis, thus demonstrating that severely ill patients can safely be treated with enteral nutrition. More recently, there have been five randomized controlled studies comparing the use of TPN with enteral nutrition.[106–111] McClave and colleagues[106] conducted the first randomized controlled trial comparing isocaloric and isonitrogenous TEN (total enteral nutrition; Peptamen) via a nasojejunal feeding tube and TPN in 30 patients started within 48 hours of admission. There were no deaths and no differences between the groups in serial pain scores, length of hospital or intensive care unit stay, days to normalization of amylase, days to diet by mouth, serum albumin levels or incidence of nosocomial infection. Ald However, the mean cost of TPN was over four times greater than that for TEN (US$3294 versus US$761, $P < 0.001$). While this study suggested that TEN is safe and less costly than TPN, it included only patients with mild pancreatitis, the group in which a change in outcome is least likely to be appreciated. Kalfarentzos and colleagues[107] evaluated 38 patients with severe acute pancreatitis and randomized them to receive a semi-elemental diet via nasojejunal tube or TPN within 48 hours after admission. TEN was well tolerated without adverse effects on the course of the disease and reduced total and septic complications compared to TPN ($P < 0.05$, mean infections per patient 0.56 *v* 1.35, $P < 0.01$). Ald The cost of nutritional support was also three times higher in those who received parenteral nutrition. This study suggests that early enteral nutrition can provide a greater clinical benefit than TPN for patients with severe pancreatitis. The trial by Windsor and colleagues[108] supports this contention. They randomized 34 consecutive patients to a lipid-based TPN solution or TEN (via a nasojejunal feeding tube in those with severe pancreatitis or per os in those with mild pancreatitis) within 48 hours of presentation. Treatment duration was 1 week and the primary endpoint of the study was the incidence of the systemic inflammatory response syndrome, with sepsis, organ failure, hospital stay and mortality as secondary endpoints. All the patients randomized to the enteral feeding group tolerated this form of nutritional support. The median amount of non-protein energy delivered was 5.02< mJ in the enterally fed patients and 7.52 < mJ in the parenterally fed patients ($P < 0.0004$). However, the nitrogen delivery per patient per day in the two groups was 9.24 g and 9.4 g, respectively and this was not statistically significant. Clinical outcome measures all improved in the enterally fed patients when compared with the parenterally fed patients. Ald However, only the reduction in systemic inflammatory response syndrome (SIRS) was statistically significant with 11 patients in the enterally fed group fulfilling the criteria prior to nutritional support but only two patients meeting the criteria after enteral nutrition ($P < 0.05$). On the other hand, in the parenterally fed group, there was no significant change (12 *v* 10) in the incidence of SIRS. Hospital stay and mortality were not statistically significantly different between the two groups. Abou-Assi *et al.* evaluated the cost effectiveness of nutritional support in patients with acute pancreatitis.[109] After 48 hours those patients who were improving were started on oral feeding. The remaining patients were randomized to receive nasojejunal or parenteral feeding. Outcomes in the three groups were compared with respect to length of hospital stay, duration of feeding, complications and hospital costs. They concluded that hypocaloric enteral feeding is safer and less expensive than parenteral feeding and bowel rest in patients with acute pancreatitis. Duration of feeding was shorter with enteral feeding (6.7 *v* 10.8 days, $P < 0.05$),

and nutrition costs were lower. Metabolic and septic complications were lower in the enterally fed group. Ald Louie *et al.* screened 548 patients and conducted a randomized controlled trial comparing 15 patients on TPN with 10 patients administered TEN in severe pancreatitis combining measures of nutritional support and inflammatory attenuation with a cost effectiveness analysis.[110] CRP levels in TEN patients were reduced by 50% 2.6 days faster than TPN patients ($P = 0.171$). Mortality was 8.3% with all deaths in the TPN group. Ald TEN had an average cost per patient of US$1207 compared with US$1968 for TPN ($P = 0.236$). Their results suggest that TEN is associated with faster attenuation of inflammation with fewer septic complications and is the preferred therapy in term of cost effectiveness.

It also appears that the type of formula determines the degree of pancreatic secretion, with polymeric formula with intact protein and long chain triglycerides producing more secretion than low fat elemental formula.[112,113] Runzi *et al.* have shown that the use of glutamine in a rat model of severe acute pancreatitis stabilizes the mucosal barrier thus allowing for less translocation of intestinal bacteria.[114] C5 This study has prompted the use of glutamine in TPN solutions for the management of acute pancreatitis. Two trials have looked at the effect of the inclusion of glutamine in conventional TPN for patients with acute pancreatitis. Ockenga *et al.* randomized 28 patients with acute pancreatitis either to a standard TPN solution with 1.5 g/kg per bodyweight protein or an isonitrogenous isocaloric TPN which contains 0.3 g/kg/L-alanine-L-glutamine.[115] Patients were assessed for nutritional and inflammatory parameters, infectious complications, length of TPN, length of hospital stay, and cost of TPN. Glutamine was associated with a significant increase of cholinesterase, albumin and lymphocyte count as well as a decrease of CRP compared with standard TPN at day 14. Ald There was a reduced length of TPN (10 *v* 16 days, $P < 0.05$), and a trend toward reduced length of hospital stay. There was no difference in the overall cost of TPN in the two groups. de Beaux *et al.* examined the effect of glutamine administration on lymphocyte proliferation and proinflammatory cytokine release in patients with severe acute pancreatitis.[116] Fourteen patients were randomized to receive either conventional or isocaloric isonitrogenous glutamine supplemented TPN for 7 days. They concluded that there is a trend for the glutamine group to exhibit improved lymphocyte proliferation and reduced proinflammatory cytokine release. Their study was limited by a small sample size that resulted in inadequate power to detect differences between the treatment arms.

The use of nasogastric feeding compared with nasojejunal feeding is being investigated by Eatock *et al.*[117] In a preliminary report these authors have shown that nasogastric feeding is safe, practical and does not exacerbate pain or the acute phase response. This trial suggests that the optimal route of feeding for patients with severe acute pancreatitis is still unclear.

Collectively, these studies suggest that enteral nutrition is safe and at least as efficacious as parenteral nutrition in patients with mild and severe pancreatitis. As the cost is much less and there is a potential for improved clinical outcome, enteral nutrition should supplant parenteral nutrition as the standard of care for patients in whom nutritional support is indicated. However, large-scale trials examining the role of enteral nutrition and different formulations for patients with severe pancreatitis are needed before more specific recommendations can be made. Certainly, it would be reasonable to attempt to provide nutritional supplementation enterally in most patients, using clinical judgment to determine if individual patients are unable to tolerate this method.

Endoscopic retrograde cholangiopancreatography

Several studies have examined the benefit of early endoscopic intervention in patients with pancreatitis of presumed biliary origin in the belief that endoscopic sphincterotomy (ES) and removal of stones impacted in the ampulla of Vater or floating in the common bile duct will reduce subsequent morbidity and mortality.

The first randomized controlled trial of urgent endoscopic retrograde cholangiopancreatography (ERCP) for acute biliary pancreatitis was published in 1988 by Neoptolemos and colleagues.[118] Within 72 hours of presentation they randomized 121 patients, stratified according to disease severity, to undergo ERCP (and ES if appropriate) or to receive conventional treatment. They found a significant reduction in the complication rate, the primary outcome measure of the trial, in ERCP-treated patients (ERCP 17% *v* control 34%, $P = 0.03$, NNT = 6). Ald This difference in morbidity appeared to be accounted for by a difference in the severe disease stratum (ERCP 24% *v* control 61%, $P < 0.01$), while no benefit from the intervention was demonstrated in the mild disease stratum. Although not statistically significant, there was a trend toward reduced mortality in the ERCP group (2% *v* 8%).

In 1993, Fan and colleagues published the results of a randomized controlled trial of early ERCP in 195 patients with acute pancreatitis, approximately two-thirds of whom were eventually considered to have biliary pancreatitis. Patients were randomized within 24 hours of presentation to undergo ERCP (and ES if appropriate) or conventional therapy. Treatment of the latter group included ERCP electively after the acute attack subsided or selectively at an earlier time for those patients whose condition deteriorated.[119] The rate of local or systemic complications (including sepsis), the primary outcome measure of the trial, was 18% in the early ERCP group and 29% in the control group ($P = 0.07$). Ald The mortality rates were 5% and 9%, respectively, but this was not statistically significant.

Subgroup analysis of the results in patients with proved gallstones also revealed that morbidity was significantly reduced in the ERCP group (16% *v* 33%, $P = 0.03$) and there was a trend toward lower mortality (2% *v* 8%, $P = 0.09$). Ala Additional subgroup analysis revealed no significant difference in the local or systemic complications, but the incidence of subsequent biliary sepsis was significantly lower in the ERCP group (0% *v* 13%, $P = 0.001$). The latter results should be interpreted with caution, since it appears that no corrections were applied to the statistical analysis to account for the use of multiple subgroup analyses.

Folsch and colleagues conducted a multicenter study in which they randomized 126 patients with biliary pancreatitis without significant biliary obstruction or cholangitis to early ERCP (within 72 hours) or conventional therapy.[120] Ala Forty-eight percent of the invasive group had biliary stones at ERCP. Eleven percent in the invasive treatment group and 6% in the conservative treatment group died ($P = 0.10$). The overall rate of complications was similar in the two groups but patients in the invasive treatment group appeared to have more severe complications, particularly respiratory failure (12% *v* 4%, $P = 0.03$). These results were not analyzed according to the severity of pancreatitis in the affected patients.

More recently, two meta-analyses have been conducted investigating the role of early ERCP as compared to conservative management in patients with acute biliary pancreatitis. Sheikh *et al.* conducted a Medline search from 1985 to 1997.[121] Five controlled studies were identified. Two were excluded in their analysis. In the remaining three trials ($n = 470$, treated 243, control 227) ERCP and endoscopic sphincterotomy in acute biliary pancreatitis decreased the risk of local complications. The authors were unable to conclude whether there was a mortality benefit. Ala The meta-analysis of Sharma and colleagues included four randomized controlled trials.[122] In 460 treated patients and 374 controls they were able to show that complications occurred in 115/460 treated and 143/374 controls ($P < 0.001$). Death occurred in 24/460 treated patients compared with 34/374 controls ($P < 0.05$). They concluded that ERCP + ES in patients with acute gallstone pancreatitis is safe and reduces morbidity and mortality. Ala

Collectively, these studies suggest that early ERCP is generally a safe procedure in the setting of acute pancreatitis. Patients with severe biliary pancreatitis appear to be more likely to benefit from early intervention.

Surgical management

Early versus delayed surgery for biliary pancreatitis

The surgical management of acute pancreatitis has evolved considerably over the past 30 years. In the 1960s and 1970s early surgical management was considered for the treatment of biliary pancreatitis to remove stones impacted in the distal common bile duct, to remove the gall bladder and stones contained within it, and to resect, debride or drain a necrotic pancreas or fluid collection. However, several uncontrolled retrospective studies[123-125] suggested that early intervention is potentially hazardous and appeared to increase mortality. B4 The observations led to the recommendation that definitive biliary surgery should be avoided until the acute pancreatitis resolves, but done prior to discharge from hospital.[123] Kelly and Wagner confirmed the wisdom of this approach when they conducted a randomized study in 165 patients comparing early definitive biliary surgery (within 48 hours) to delayed surgery (after the pancreatitis subsided 4–10 days later).[126] They found a significant overall reduction in morbidity and mortality in the group who underwent the delayed surgery, with most of the observed benefit derived in those patients with severe pancreatitis, as defined by having more than three Ranson's criteria. In the overall population of patients with mild and severe pancreatitis the morbidity rates were 30% and 5·1% ($P < 0.005$) for the early and delayed surgery groups respectively and the mortality rates were 15·1% and 2·4% ($P < 0.005$). Ala In patients with severe pancreatitis the morbidity rates were 82·6% and 17·6% ($P < 0.001$) for those with early and delayed surgery and the mortality rates were 47·8% and 11%, respectively ($P < 0.025$). From these data the NNT for early surgery to cause one additional death, is approximately 8 overall and approximately 3 for patients with severe pancreatitis. Ala Although these data are convincing, the more widespread use of ERCP since the time that these studies were conducted has shifted this question to the possible benefits of early ERCP and has made the question of a role for early definitive biliary surgery much less relevant. The current recommendation is for cholecystectomy not to be carried out until the acute pancreatitis has subsided. This is based on very strong evidence. It is also recommended that it be done as soon as possible after the pancreatitis has subsided, although the evidence supporting this recommendation is somewhat less convincing.

Peritoneal lavage

More recently, early surgical intervention has been limited to early peritoneal lavage and the treatment of infected pancreatic necrosis or peritonitis. However, there still remains considerable controversy as to the method and timing of surgical intervention in the setting of necrotizing pancreatitis and the use of peritoneal lavage in the non-operative setting. Several small controlled studies have examined the effectiveness of continuous peritoneal lavage. Ranson and colleagues[8] randomized 10 patients with severe pancreatitis to receive continuous lavage for 48–96 hours or standard therapy. They found no statistically significant differences

in the duration of intensive care unit care, rapidity of resumption of oral intake, or duration of hospitalization, although there was a trend favoring lavage for each of these outcomes. Stone and Fabian[127] randomized 70 patients with severe alcoholic pancreatitis to 24 hours of peritoneal lavage or supportive treatment followed by 24 hours of peritoneal lavage for those who worsened. They found a "decided improvement in the over-all condition" in 29/34 patients in the treatment group compared with 13/36 in the control group ($P = 0.001$). However, the method of determining this improvement was not discussed, and the mortality rate was not significantly different between the two groups. In addition, 17/36 patients in the control group were crossed over to peritoneal lavage after worsening in 24 hours, making interpretation of the results problematic. Subsequently, two larger randomized studies by Mayer *et al.*[128] ($n = 91$) and Ihse *et al.*[129] ($n = 39$) have failed to show benefit from peritoneal lavage. Alc Teerenhovi and colleagues[130] randomized 24 patients with necrotizing pancreatitis to undergo lesser sac lavage for 7 days or drainage, following laparotomy and choledochostomy or cholecystostomy. They were unable to identify any benefit for lavage over drainage as the mortality and morbidity were similar in both groups (36% *v* 17% mortality). However, neither group underwent necrosectomy, and the onset of symptoms until operation was 4·1 ± 3·6 days for the lavage group, a pretreatment interval which is much longer than previously advocated for lavage alone. Berling *et al.* coupled the effect of protease inhibition and peritoneal lavage.[131] In their study 26 patients received standard peritoneal lavage while 22 patients received lavage with aprotinin (20 million KIU given over 30 hours). The endpoint was the effect of treatment on the balance between proteases and endogenous antiproteases. They conclude that the addition of aprotinin offers no advantage over standard peritoneal lavage. Ald

All the studies listed above examined short courses of peritoneal lavage with durations less than four days and may have overlooked a beneficial time–response relationship. Therefore, Ranson and Berman[132] randomized 29 patients with severe pancreatitis to long peritoneal lavage (7 days) or short lavage (2 days). They found no statistically significant difference between the groups with respect to either pancreatic sepsis (long lavage 22% *v* short lavage 40%) or death from sepsis (long lavage 0% *v* short lavage 20%). However in the subgroup of patients with five or more prognostic signs, pancreatic sepsis occurred in 30% of the long lavage group versus 57% of the short lavage group and death from sepsis occurred in 0% and 43%, respectively ($P = 0.05$). Ald These promising results must be interpreted with caution since they are the result of *post hoc* subgroup analysis of a rather small trial. However, they suggest that longer duration of peritoneal lavage might benefit those with the most severe forms of acute pancreatitis. Larger studies would be needed to confirm this result before peritoneal lavage can be advocated as part of the standard treatment of severe pancreatitis.

Early pancreatic resection without documented infection

The management of necrotizing pancreatitis in the absence of documented infection remains the most controversial surgical issue in acute pancreatitis. Early pancreatic resection for severe acute pancreatitis has been examined in small retrospective studies that have generally shown high mortality and morbidity.[133] B4 Only two studies have compared resection with alternative forms of management. Kivilaakso and colleagues[134] randomized 35 patients with severe pancreatitis to subtotal pancreatic resection and T tube placement or operative peritoneal lavage and T tube placement for 7–12 days. Twenty-two percent died in the resection group and 47% in the lavage group but this was not statistically significant. A1d The septic complication rate and duration of hospital stay were similar, but 6/14 patients who underwent resection developed diabetes while none did in the lavage group. This study suggested that resection might benefit a select group of patients, but in addition to the lack of a statistically significant result, the study design, without a true control group in which patients were not exposed to the usual surgical risks, prevented any definite conclusions. In addition, the degree of pancreatitis in the randomized patients was not severe with a mean number of prognostic signs of less than four. A second small study by the same group re-examined this question using an improved study design.[135] They randomized 21 patients with severe pancreatitis to non-operative peritoneal lavage or pancreatic resection. There was no statistically significant difference in mortality (27% for resection and 10% for lavage) or in morbidity or hospital stay between the groups. These studies together with the previous retrospective data suggest that early pancreatic resection offers no benefit over non-operative management for severe acute pancreatitis. A1d

Management of infected pancreatic necrosis

While there is considerable controversy regarding the use of surgical management for severe acute pancreatitis without sepsis, there is no disagreement about the need for surgical intervention or drainage for infected necrosis. However, the timing and surgical method in this setting remain controversial. Three main patterns of surgical management of infected necrosis have developed over the past 20 years. They include: conventional treatment with necrosectomy followed by simple drainage of the peripancreatic bed, closed procedures with necrosectomy followed by continuous closed lavage or open management with necrosectomy, and

subsequent scheduled reoperations or continued open abdominal management. The evidence for or against these treatment modalities is based on case series either followed prospectively or retrospectively but there is a paucity of randomized studies.

Warshaw and Gongliang[136] retrospectively reviewed their experience in 45 patients with pancreatic abscesses. Their patients had a 24% mortality rate with conventional treatment and 84% had further complications. Allardyce[137] conducted a retrospective review and found that 14/17 patients with infected necrosis or abscess died with the conventional treatment. Both groups advocated a more aggressive debridement of necrotic tissue and adequate drainage. B4

Wertheimer and Norris[138] reported their results in 10 consecutive patients with persistent infected necrosis treated with necrosectomy and packing with continued open abdominal management in the intensive care unit. Their 20% mortality rate was much lower than expected for the patient population and, as a result, this approach has gained some popularity. Bradley and Allen[139] prospectively followed 27 patients with infected necrosis treated with debridement, open drainage and scheduled reoperation. Mortality was 15% in this group, again lower than expected but no concurrent control group was available for comparison. B4

Necrosectomy with continuous closed lavage has also gained favor over conventional treatment of infected necrosis. Gebhardt and Gall[140] retrospectively reviewed their surgical results for necrotizing pancreatitis and found a mortality of 37% for those treated with necrosectomy, drainage and lavage compared with 54% for those treated earlier in their experience with surgery alone without drainage or lavage. B4 Larvin and colleagues[141] prospectively followed 14 patients with necrotizing pancreatitis who underwent pancreatic debridement, closed drainage and lavage. Their mortality rate was 3/14 with only two patients requiring reoperation. B4 Bassi and colleagues[142] retrospectively reviewed their experience with surgically treated patients with acute and chronic pancreatitis and intra-abdominal sepsis. Fifty-five patients had infected necrosis and were treated with necrosectomy and closed lavage. The mortality rate in this cohort was 24% but the severity of their pancreatitis as represented by a conventional multiple scoring system was not discussed, making interpretation of the results difficult. B4 Finally, Farkas and colleagues[143] retrospectively reviewed their results with necrosectomy and closed lavage for infected necrosis in 123 patients with severe pancreatitis (mean Ranson's score 6·2). Their mortality rate was only 7% with a 17% reoperation rate. However, 46% had another surgical procedures at the time of the necrosecectomy (distal pancreatectomy, splenectomy, colonic resection, cholecystectomy, or sphincteroplasty). Nevertheless, the results of this study, albeit retrospective, suggest a benefit in widespread necrosectomy, lavage with multiple drains, and additional surgery when necessary. Collectively, these studies, although limited by their retrospective study designs and use of historical controls, suggest that the treatment of infected necrosis should involve necrosectomy and long-term lavage or open management instead of the previous conventional surgical management. It is unlikely that large randomized studies of this approach will be undertaken and as a result recommendations are based on the relatively weak evidence which is available.

The high mortality rate and poor surgical outcome of patients with infected necrotic tissue has prompted the investigation of new techniques. Carter *et al.* studied 14 patients with infected necrosis secondary to acute pancreatitis.[144] Four patients underwent sinus tract endoscopy along a drainage tract after prior open necrosectomy. Additional surgery for sepsis was avoided in the four patients managed by sinus tract endoscopy, and none died. B4 Freeny *et al.* carried out percutaneous drainage in 34 patients with acute necrotizing pancreatitis.[145] Sixteen (47%) of the 34 patients were cured with only percutaneous catheter drainage. Sepsis was controlled in 74% of patients, permitting elective surgery for treatment of pancreatic fistula. B4 Gentile *et al.* reported on the use of an absorbable mesh in the management of patients with acute necrotizing pancreatitis.[146] Eleven patients requiring multiple operations had placement of absorbable polyglycolic acid mesh. The placement of mesh provided open drainage of the abdominal cavity and simplified further care by allowing easy abdominal access for repeat drainage procedures. The patients with mesh had a higher rate of fistula formation. Horvath *et al.* carried out laparoscopically assisted retroperitoneal debridement as an adjunct to percutaneous drainage for patients with infected pancreatic necrosis.[147] The study retrospectively analyzed six patients undergoing laparoscopically assisted debridement of the infected pancreatic tissue. In four patients laparoscopically assisted percutaneous drainage was successful. Complications included self-limited enterocutaneous fistula and a small flank hernia. Mann *et al.* described the placement of volumic catheters for fragmentation and extraction of necrotic pancreatic tissue in 26 patients.[148] Twelve patients were healed by the minimally invasive radiologically assisted technique. The advantages of the technique include reduced trauma, no need for general anesthesia, avoidance of complex surgery, and reduced damage to neighboring organs. B4

Summary

Medical management continues to remain the mainstay of treatment for patients with acute pancreatitis. Further research identifying patients at risk for severe pancreatitis at an earlier stage is needed if a dramatic decrease in the mortality rate is to be achieved. Early reduction in the systemic response to pancreatitis might be achieved with pharmacotherapy but this has not been proved to be effective with the agents available to date. Antibiotic prophylaxis is becoming part of the standard therapy for those with necrotizing pancreatitis. Early enteral feeding shows promise and should become the standard method of nutritional supplementation in these patients. The role of tailored enteral feeding with glutamine or probiotics is still being investigated. Early ERCP for those patients with jaundice or cholangitis has proved to be beneficial when used by experienced individuals. The role of peritoneal lavage remains controversial and the patient population who may benefit from this intervention is not well defined. Early pancreatic resection or necrosectomy with closed drainage appears to contribute to increased complications without overall benefit. As such, early surgical management of acute pancreatitis should be limited to those patients with *infected necrosis*. The surgical approach still remains controversial but based on the evidence available widespread necrosectomy and lavage or necrosectomy and open management probably results in better overall outcome than the conventional surgical approach. Novel, less invasive approaches to the management of infected necrosis are still in the investigative stage.

References

1 Go VL, Everhart JE. Pancreatitis. In: Evergart, JE (ed). *Digestive diseases in the United States: Epidemiology and impact.* Philadelphia, Pennsylvania: US Department of Health and Human Services, Public Health Service, National Institutes of Health, National Institute of Diabetes and Digestive and Kidney Diseases. Washington, DC: US Government Printing Office NIH Publication no. 94–1447, 1994, 9.693.

2 Riela A, Zinsmeister, AR, Melton LJ, DiMagno EP. Etiology incidence and survival of acute pancreatitis in Olmstead County, Minnesota. *Gastroenterology* 1991;**100**:A296.

3 Halvorsen FA, Ritland S. Acute pancreatitis in Buskerud County, Norway. Incidence and etiology. *Scand J Gastroenterol* 1996;**31**: 411–14.

4 McMahon MJ, Playforth MJ, Pickford IR. A comparative study of methods for the prediction of severity of attacks of acute pancreatitis. *Br J Surg* 1980;**67**:22–5.

5 Corfield AP, Williamson RCN, McMahon MJ *et al.* Prediction of severity in acute pancreatitis: prospective comparison of three prognostic indices. *Lancet* 1985;**8542**:403–7.

6 Larvin M, McMahon MJ. APACHE-II score for assessment and monitoring of acute pancreatitis. *Lancet* 1989;**2**: 201–5.

7 Ranson JHC, Rifkind KM, Roses DF *et al.* Prognostic signs and the role of operative management in acute pancreatitis. *Surg Gynecol Obstet* 1974;**139**:69–81.

8 Ranson JHC, Rifkind KM, Turner JW. Prognostic signs and nonoperative peritoneal lavage. *Surg Gynecol Obstet* 1976; **143**:209–19.

9 Wilson C, Heath DI, Imrie CW. Prediction of outcome in acute pancreatitis: a comparative study of APACHE II, clinical assessment and multiple factor scoring systems. *Br J Surg* 1990;**77**:1260–4.

10 Gross V, Scholmerich J, Leser HG *et al.* Granulocyte elastase in assessment of severity of acute pancreatitis. *Dig Dis Sci* 1990;**35**:97–105.

11 Dominguez-Munoz JE, Carballo F, Carcia MJ, de Diego JM, Rabago L, de la Morena J. Cilinical usefulness of poymorphonuclear elastase in predicting the severity of acute pancreatitis: results of a multicentre study. *Br J Surg* 1991;**78**:1230–4.

12 Agarwal N, Pitchumoni CS. Simplified prognostic criteria in acute pancreatitis. *Pancreas* 1986;**1**:69–73.

13 Bank S, Wise L, Gersten M. Risk factors in acute pancreatitis. *Radiol Clin North Am* 1989;**78**:637–40.

14 Wilson C, Heads A, Shenkin A, Imrie CW. C-reactive protein, antiproteases and complement factors as objective markers of severity in acute pancreatitis. *Br J Surg* 1989;**76**:177–81.

15 Imrie CW, Benjamin IS, Ferguson JC, Mckay AJ, Mackenzie I, O'Neill J, Blumgart LH. A single-centre double-blind trial of Trasylol therapy in primary acute pancreatitis *Br J Surg* 1978;**65**:337–41.

16 Blamey SL, Imrie CW, O'Neill J *et al.* Prognostic factors in acute pancreatitis. *Gut* 1984;**25**:1340–6.

17 Steinberg WM. Predictors of severity of acute pancreatitis. *Gastroenterol Clin North Am* 1990;**19**:849–61.

18 Fan ST, Lai E, Mok F. Prediction of the severity of acute pancreatitis. *Am J Surg* 1993;**166**:262–9.

19 Heath DI Imrie CW. The Hong Kong Criteria and severity prediction in acute pancreatitis. *Int J Pancreatol* 1994;**15**:1–7.

20 Balthazar EJ, Ranson JHC, Naidich DP, Megibow AJ, Caccavale R, Cooper MM. Acute pancreatitis: prognostic value of CT. *Radiology* 1985;**156**:767–72.

21 Balthazar EJ, Robinson DL, Megibow AJ, Ranson JHC. Acute pancreatitis: value of CT in establishing prognosis. *Radiology* 1990;**174**:331–6.

22 Hjelmqvist B, Wattsgard C, Borgstrom A, Lasson A, Nyman U, Aspelin P, Ohlssohn K. Early diagnosis and classification in acute pancreatitis. *Digestion* 1989;**44**:177–83.

23 London NJM, Leese T, Lavelle JM, Miles K, West KP, Watkin DFL, Fossard DP. Rapid-bolus contrast-enhanced dynamic computed tomography in acute pancreatitis: a prospective study *Br J Surg* 1991;**78**:1452–6.

24 London NJM, Neoptolemos JP, Lavelle J *et al.* Contrast-enhanced abdominal computed tomography scanning and prediction of severity of acute pancreatitis: a prospective study. *Br J Surg* 1989;**76**:268–72.

25 Clavien PA, Hauser H, Meyer P, Rohner A. Value of contrast-enhanced computerized tomograghy in the early diagnosis and prognosis of acute pancreatitis. *Am J Surg* 1988;**155**:457–66.

26 Puolakkainen PA. Early assessment of acute pancreatitis. A comparative study of computed tomography and laboratory tests. *Acta Chir Scand* 1989;**155**:25–30.

27 Mayer AD, McMahon MJ. The diagnostic and prognostic value of peritoneal lavage in patients with acute pancreatitis. *Surg Gynecol Obstet* 1985;**160**:597–612.

28 Buchler M, Malfertheiner P, Schoetensack D, Uhl W, Beger HG. Sensitivity of antiproteases, complement factors and C-reactive protein in detecting pancreatic necrosis. Results of a prospective clinical study. *Int J Pancreatol* 1986;**1**:227–35.

29 Leese T, Shaw D, Holliday M. Prognostic markers in acute pancreatitis: can pancreatic necrosis be predicted? *Ann R Coll Surg Engl* 1988;**70**:227–32.

30 Puolakkainen P, Valtonen V, Paanenen A, Schroder T. C-reactive protein (CRP) and serum phospholipase A2 in the assessment of the severity of acute pancreatitis. *Gut* 1987;**28**:764–71.

31 Gudgeon AM, Heath DI, Hurley P *et al.* Trypsmogen activation peptides assay in the early prediction of severity of acute pancreatitis. *Lancet* 1990;**1**:4–8.

32 Paajanen H, Laato M, Jaakkola M, Pulkki K, Niinikoski J, Nordback I. Serum tumor necrosis factor compared with C-reactive protein in the early assessment of severity of acute pancreatitis. *Br J Surg* 1995;**82**:271–3.

33 Leser HG, Gross V, Scheibenbogen C *et al.* Elevation of serum Interleukin-6 concentration precedes acute-phase response and reflects severity in acute pancreatitis. *Gastroenterology* 1991;**101**:782–5.

34 Viedma JA, Perez-Mateo M, Agullo J, Dominguez JE, Carballo F. Inflammatory response in the early prediction of severity in human acute pancreatitis. *Gut* 1994;**35**:822–7.

35 Kaufmann P, Tilz GP, Lueger A, Demel U. Elevated plasma levels of soluble tumor necrosis factor receptor (sTNFRp60) reflect severity of acute pancreatitis. *Intensive Care Med* 1997;**23**:841–8.

36 Hedstrom J, Sainio V, Kemppainen E *et al.* Serum complex of trypsin 2 and (alpha₁ antitrypsin as diagnostic and prognostic marker of acute pancreatitis: clinical study in consecutive patients. *BMJ* 1996;**313**:333–7.

37 Kemppainen E, Sand J, Puolakkainen P *et al.* Pancreatitis associated protein as an early marker of acute pancreatitis. *Gut* 1996;**39**:675–8.

38 Lankisch PG, Koop H, Otto J, Oberdieck U. Evaluation of methaemalbumin in acute pancreatitis. *Scand J Gastroenterol* 1978;**13**:975–8.

39 Lankisch PG, Schirren CA, Otto J. Methemalbumin in acute pancreatitis: an evaluation of its prognostic value and comparison with multiple prognostic paramaters. *Am J Gastroenterol* 1989;**84**:1391–5.

40 Loiudice TA, Lang J, Mehta H, Banta L. Treatment of acute alcoholic pancreatitis: the role of cimetidine and nasogastric suction. *Am J Gastroenterol* 1984;**79**:553–8.

41 Naeije R, Salingret E, Clumeck N, De Troyer A, Devis G. Is nasogastric suction necessary in acute pancreatitis? *BMJ* 1978;**2**:659–60.

42 Levant JA, Secrist D, Resin H *et al.* Nasogastric suction in the treatment of alcoholic pancreatitis. *JAMA* 1974;**229**:51–2.

43 Lange P, Pedersen T. Initial treatment of acute pancreatitis. *Surg Gynecol Obstet* 1983;**157**:332–4.

44 Broe PJ, Zinner MJ, Cameron JL. A clinical trial of cimetidine in acute pancreatitis. *Surg Gynecol Obstet* 1982;**154**:13–6.

45 Meshkinpour H, Molinaari MD, Gardner L, Berk JE, Hoehler FK. Cimetidine in the treatment of acute alcoholic

pancreatitis: a radomized,double blind study. *Gastroenterology* 1979;**77**:687–90.

46 Waterworth MW, Barbezat GO, Bank S. Glucagon in treatment of acute pancreatitis. *Lancet* 1974;**1**:231.

47 Medical Research Council of the United Kingdom. Death from acute pancreatitis: multicentre trial of glucagon and aprotinin. *Lancet* 1977;**2**:632–5.

48 Olazabal A, Fuller R. Failure of glucagon in the treatment of alcoholic pancreatitis. *Gastroenterology* 1978;**74**:489–91.

49 Durr HK, Maroske D, Zelder O, Bode JC. Glucagon therapy in acute pancreatitis. Report of a double blind trial. *Gut* 1978;**19**:175–9.

50 Debas HT, Hancock RJ, Soon-Shiong P, Smythe HA, Cassim MM. Glucagon therapy in acute pancreatitis: prospective randomized double blind study. *Can J Surg* 1980;**23**: 578–80.

51 Kronborg O, Bulow S, Jowrgensen PM, Svendsen LB. A randomized double-blind trial of glucagon in treatment of first attack of severe acute pancreatitis without associated biliary disease. *Am J Gastroenterol* 1980;**73**:423–5.

52 Goebell H, Ammann R, Herfarth CH *et al.* A double-blind trial of synthetic salmon calcitonin in the treatment of acute pancreatitis. *Scand J Gastroenterol* 1979;**14**:881–9.

53 Paul F, Ohnhaus E, Hesch RD. Einfluss von salmcalcitonin auf der verlauf der akuten pancreatitis. *Dtsch Med Wochenschr* 1979;**104**:615–22.

54 Schwedes M, Althoff PM, Klempa L. Effects of somatostatin on bile induced acute haemorrhagic pancreatitis in the dog. *Horm Metab Res* 1979;**11**:655–61.

55 Baxter JN, Jenkins SA, Day DW, Roberts NB. Effects of somatostatin and a long acting somatostatin analogue on the prevention and treatment of experimentally induced acute pancreatitis in the rat. *Br J Surg* 1985;**72**:382–5.

56 Paran H, Mayo A, Paran D *et al.* Octreotide treatment in patients with severe acute pancreatitis. *Dig Dis Sci* 2000; **45**:2247–51.

57 Paran H, Neufeld D, Mayo A *et al.* Preliminary report of a prospective randomized study of octreotide in the treatment of severe acute pancreatitis. *J Am Coll Surg* 1995;**182**: 121–4.

58 Planas M, Perez A, Iglesia R, Porta I, Masclans JR, Bermejo B. Severe acute pancreatitis: treatment with somatostatin. *Intensive Care Med* 1998;**24**:37–9.

59 Choi TK, Mok F, Zhan WH, Fan ST, Lai ECS, Wong J. Somatostatin in the treatment of acute pancreatitis: a prospective randomized controlled trial. *Gut* 1989;**30**: 223–7.

60 Binder M, Uhl W, Friess H, Malfertheiner P, Buchler MW. Octreotide in the treatment of acute pancreatitis: results of a unicenter prospective trial with three different octreotide dosages. *Digestion* 1994;**55**(S1):20–3.

61 Lata J, Dite P, Julinkova K, Precechtelova M, Prasek J. [Effect of octreotide on the clinical course of acute pancreatitis and levels of free oxygen radicals and antioxidants]. *Vnitr Lek* 1998;**44**:524–7.

62 Karakoyunlar O, Sivrel E, Tanir N, Denecli AG. High dose octreotide in the management of acute pancreatitis. *Hepatogastroenterology* 1999;**46**:1968–72.

63 D'Amico D, Favia G, Biasiato R *et al.* The use of somatostatin in acute pancreatitis: results of a multicenter trial. *Hepatogastroenterology* 1990;**37**:92–8.

64 Gjorup I, Roikjaer O, Andersen B *et al.* A double-blinded multicenter trial of somatostatin in the treatment of acute pancreatitis. *Surg Gynecol Obstet* 1992;**175**:397–400.

65 McKay C, Baxter J, Imrie C. A randomized, controlled trial of octreotide in the management of patients with acute pancreatitis. *Int J Pancreatol* 1997;**21**:13–19.

66 Berling R, Borgstrom A, Ohlsson K. Peritoneal lavage with aprotinin in patients with severe acute pancreatitis. Effects on plasma and peritoneal levels of trypsin and leukocyte proteases and their major inhibitors. *Int J Pancreatol* 1998;**24**:9–17.

67 Trapnell JE, Rigby CC, Talbot CH, Duncan EH. A controlled trial of trasylol in the treatment of acute pancreatitis. *Br J Surg.* 1974;**61**:177–82.

68 Yang CH, Chang-Chien CS, Liaw YF. Controlled trial of protease inhibitor gabexelate mesilate (FOY) in the treatment of acute pancreatitis. *Pancreas* 1987;**2**:698–700.

69 Valderrama R, Perez-Mateo M, Navarro S *et al.* Multicenter double-blind trial of gabexate mesylate (FOY) in unselected patients with acute pancreatitis. *Digestion* 1992;**51**: 65–70.

70 Pederzoli P, Cavallini G, Falconi M, Bassi C. Gabexate mesilate *v* aprotinin in human acute pancreatitis (GA.ME.P.A.). *Int J Pancreatol* 1993;**14**:117–24.

71 Buchler M, Malfertheiner P, Uhl W *et al.*, and the German Pancreatitis Study Group.Gabexate mesilate in human acute pancreatitis. *Gastroenterology* 1993;**104**:1165–70.

72 Pezzilli R, Miglioli M. Multicentre comparative study of two schedules of gabexate mesilate in the treatment of acute pancreatitis. Italian Acute Pancreatitis Study Group. *Dig Liver Dis* 2001;**33**:49–57.

73 Chen HM, Chen JC, Hwang TL, Jan YY, Chen MF. Prospective and randomized study of gabexate mesilate for the treatment of severe acute pancreatitis with organ dysfunction. *Hepatogastroenterology* 2000;**47**:1147–50.

74 Chen HM, Chen MF, Hwang TL, Jan YY, Chen JC. Gabexate mesilate promotes neutrophil apoptosis and attenuates serum cytokines alterations in human acute pancreatitis. *Gastroenterology* 2000;**118**(Suppl 2):A1043.

75 Leese T, Holliday M, Heath D, Hall AW, Bell PRF. Multicentre clinical trial of low volume fresh frozen plasma therapy in acute pancreatitis. *Br J Surg* 1987;**74**:907–11.

76 Kingsnorth AN, Galloway SW, Formela LJ. Randomized, double-blind phase II trial of lexipafant, a platelet-activating factor antagonist, in human acute pancreatitis. *Br J Surg* 1995;**82**:1414–20.

77 Mckay CJ, Curran F, Sharples C, Baxter JN, Imrie CW. Prospective placebo-controlled randomized trial of lexipafant in predicted severe acute pancreatitis. *Br J Surg* 1997;**84**:1239–43.

78 Johnson CD, Kingsnorth AN, Imrie CW *et al.* Double blind, randomised, placebo controlled study of a platelet activating factor antagonist, lexipafant, in the treatment and prevention of organ failure in predicted severe acute pancreatitis. *Gut* 2001;**48**:62–9.

79 Craig RM, Dordal E, Myles L. The use of ampicillin in acute pancreatitis. *Ann Intern Med* 1975;**83**:831–2.

80 Howes R, Zuidema GD, Cameron JL. Evaluation of prophylactic antibiotics in acute pancreatitis. *J Surg Res* 1975;**18**:197–200.

81 Finch WTK, Sawyers JL, Schenker S. A prospective study to determine the efficacy of antibiotics in acute pancreatitis. *Ann Surg* 1976;**183**:667–71.

82 Pederzoli P, Bassi C, Vesentini S, Campedelli A. A randomized multicenter clinical trial of antibiotic prophlaxis of septic compications on acute necrotizing pancreatitis with imipenem. *Surg Gynecol Obstet* 1993;**176**:480–3.

83 Sainio V, Kemppainen E, Puolakkainen P *et al.* Early antibiotic treatment in acute necrotising pancreatitis. *Lancet* 1995;**346**:663–7.

84 Luiten EJT, Hop WCJ, Lange JF, Bruining HA. Controlled clinical trial of selective decontamination for the treatment of severe acute pancreatitis. *Ann Surg* 1995;**222**:57–65.

85 Olah A, Pardavi G, Belagyi T, Nagy A, Issekutz A, Mohamed GE. Early nasojejunal feeding in acute pancreatitis is associated with a lower complication rate. *Nutrition* 2002;**18**:259–62.

86 Nordback I, Sand J, Saaristo R, Paajanen H. Early treatment with antibiotics reduces the need for surgery in acute necrotizing pancreatitis – a single-center randomized study. *J Gastrointest Surg* 2001;**5**:113–18: discussion 118–20.

87 Bassi C, Falconi M, Talamini G *et al.* Controlled clinical trial of pefloxacin versus imipenem in severe acute pancreatitis. *Gastroenterology* 1998;**115**:1513–17.

88 Isenmann R, Ruenzi M, Kron M, Goebell H, Beger HG. Prophylactic antibiotics in severe acute pancreatitis. Results of a double-blind, placebo-controlled multicenter trial. *Gastroenterology* 2003;**124**(Suppl 1):A32.

89 Kecskes G, Belagyi T, Olah A. Early jejunal nutrition with combined pre- and probiotics in acute pancreatitis – prospective, randomized, double-blind investigations. *Magy Seb* 2003;**56**:3–8.

90 Van Gossum A, Lemoyne M, Greig PD, Jeejeebhoy KN. Lipid-associated total parenteral nutrition in patients with severe acute pancreatitis. *World J Surg* 1988;**12**:250–5.

91 Robin AP, Campbell R, Palani CK, Liu K, Donahue PE, Nyhus LM. Total parenteral nutrition in severe pancreatitis: clinical experience with 156 patients. *World J Surg* 1990;**14**:572–9.

92 Buch A, Buch J, Carlsen A *et al.* Hyperlipidemia and pancreatitis. *World J Surg* 1980;**4**:307–14.

93 Silberman H, Dixon NP, Eisenberg D. The safety and efficacy of a lipid-based system of parenteral nutrition in acute pancreatitis. *Am J Gastroenterol* 1982;**77**:494.

94 Grant JP, James S, Grabowski V *et al.* Total parenteral nutrition in pancreatic disease. *Ann Surg* 1984;**200**:627.

95 Leibowitz AB, O'Sullivan P, Iberti TJ. Intravenous fat emulsions and the pancreas: A review. *Mt Sinai J Med* 1992;**59**:38–42.

96 Sitzman JV, Steinborn PA, Zinner MJ, Cameron JL. Total parental nutrition and alternate energy substrates in the treatment of severe acute pancreatitis. *Surg Gynecol Obstet* 1989;**168**:311–17.

97 Kalfarentzos FE, Karavias DD, Karatzas TM, Alevizatos BA, Androulakis JA. Total parenteral nutrition in severe acute pancreatitis. *J Am Coll Nutr* 1991;**10**:156–62.

98 Sax HC, Warner BW, Talamini MA *et al.* Early total parenteral nutrition in acute pancreatitis: lack of beneficial effects. *Am J Surg* 1987;**153**:117–24.

99 DiMagno EP, Vay LW, Summerskill HJ. Intraluminal and postabsorptive effects of amino acids on pancreatic enzyme. *J Lab Clin Med* 1971;**82**:241–8.

100 Ragins H, Levenson SM, Singer R, Stamford W, Seifter E. Intrajejunal administration of an elemental diet at neutral pH avoids pancreatic stimulation. *Am J Surg* 1973;**126**:606–14.

101 Keith RG. Effect of a low fat elemental diet on pancreatic secretion during pancreatitis. *Surg Gynecol Obstet* 1980; **151**:337–43.

102 Alverdy JC, Aoys E, Moss GS. Total parenteral nutrition promotes bacterial translocation from the gut. *Surgery* 1988;**104**:185–90.

103 Purandare S, Offenbartl K, Westerom B *et al.* Increased permeability to fluorescein isothiocyanate-dextran after total parenteral nutrition in the rat. *J Gastroenterol* 1989; **24**:678–82.

104 Li J, Gocinski Bj, Henken B *et al.* Effects of parenteral nutrition on gut-associated lymphoid tissue. *J Trauma* 1995;**39**:44–52.

105 Kudsk KA, Campbell SM, O'Brien T *et al.* Postoperative jejunal feedings following complicated pancreatitis. *Nutr Clin Pract* 1990;**5**:14–17.

106 McClave, SA, Greene LM, Snider HL *et al.* Comparison of the safety of early enteral vs parenteral nutrition in mild acute pancreatitis. *Am J Gastroenterol* 1997;**21**: 14–20.

107 Kalfarentzos FE, Kehagias J, Mead N, Kokkinis K, Gogos CA. Enteral nutritition is superior to parenteral nutrition in severe acute pancreatitis: results of randomized prospective trial. *Br J Surg* 1997;**84**:1665–9.

108 Windsor ACJ, Kanwar S, Li AGK *et al.* Compared with parenteral nutrition, enteral feeding attenuates the acute phase response and improves disease severity in acute pancreatitis. *Gut* 1998;**42**:431–5.

109 Abou-Assi S, Craig K, O'Keefe SJ. Hypocaloric jejunal feeding is better than total parenteral nutrition in acute pancreatitis: results of a randomized comparative study. *Am J Gastroenterol* 2002;**97**:2255–62.

110 Louie B, Noseworthy T, Hailey D, Gramlich L, Jacobs P, Warnock G. A randomized controlled trial and cost effectiveness analysis of enteral vs. parenteral nutrition in severe pancreatitis. *Gastroenterology* 2002;**122**(Suppl 1): A369.

111 Abou-Assi SG, Craig K, O'Keefe SJ. Prospective randomized trial of jejunal (EN) and intravenous (TPN) feeding in the management of acute pancreatitis (AP). *Gastroenterology* 2001;**120**(Suppl 1): A469.

112 Cassim MM, Allardyce DB. Pancreatic secretion in response to jejunal feeding of elemental diet. *Ann Surg* 1974;**180**:228–31.

113 Grant JP, Davey-McCrae J, Snyder PJ. Effect of enteral nutrition on human pancreatic secretions. *Nutrition* 1987; **11**:302–4.

114 Runzi M, Schneider A, Lohr M, Adam U, Liebe S. Incentive for rethinking – early enteral nutrition in patients with pancreatitis. *Z Gastroenterol* 1999;**37**:317–20.

115 Ockenga J, Borchert K, Rifai K, Manns MP, Bischoff SC. A randomised, controlled trial of glutamine supplementation in gastroenterological patients scheduled for parenteral nutrition. *Gastroenterology* 2000;**118**(Suppl 2):A775.

116 de Beaux AC, O'Riordain MG, Ross JA, Jodozi L, Carter DC, Fearon KC. Glutamine-supplemented total parenteral nutrition reduces blood mononuclear cell interleukin-8 release in severe acute pancreatitis. *Nutrition* 1998;**14**: 261–5.

117 Eatock FC, Chong PS, Menezes N, Imrie CW, McKay CJ, Carter R. Nasogastric feeding in severe acute pancreatitis is safe and avoids the risks associated with the nasojejunal route: a randomised controlled trial. *Gastroenterology* 2001;**120**(Suppl 1):A469.

118 Neoptolemos JP, London NJ, James D, Carr-locke DL, Bailey IA, Fossard DP. Controlled trial of urgent endoscopic retrograde cholangiopancreatography and endoscopic sphincterotomy versus conservative treatment for acute pancreatitis due to gallstones. *Lancet* 1988;**2**:979–83.

119 Fan ST, Lai ECS, Mok FPT, Lo C-M, Zheng S-S, Wong J. Early treatment of acute biliary pancreatitis by endoscopic papillotomy. *N Engl J Med* 1993;**328**:228–32.

120 Folsch UR, Nitsche R, Ludtke R, Hilgers RA, Creutzfeldt W, German Study Group on Acute Biliary Pancreatitits. Early ERCP and papillotomy compared with conservative treatment for acute biliary pancreatitis. *N Engl J Med* 1997;**336**:237–42.

121 Sheikh AM, Warshafsky S, Wolf DC, Lebovics E. Role of early ERCP and sphincterotomy in the management of acute pancreatitis [Abstract]. *Surgery* 2000;3390.

122 Sharma VK, W Howden, W. Meta-analysis of randomized, controlled trials of endoscopic retrograde cholangiography (ERC) and endoscopic sphincterotomy (ES) in acute pancreatitis due to gallstones. *Am J Gastroenterol* 1999; **94**:3211–14.

123 Ranson JHC. The timing of biliary surgery in acute pancreatitis. *Ann Surg* 1978;**189**:654–62.

124 Kelly TR. Gallstone pancreatitis: the timing of surgery. *Surgery* 1980;**88**:345–50.

125 Osborne DH, Imrie CW, Carter DC. Biliary surgery in the same admission for gallstone-associated acute pancreatitis. *Br J Surg* 1981;**68**:758–61.

126 Kelly TR, Wagner DS. Gallstone pancreatitis: a prospective randomized trial of the timing of surgery. *Surgery* 1988; **104**:600–5.

127 Stone HH, Fabian TC. Peritoneal dialysis in the treatment of acute alcoholic pancreatitis. *Surg Gynecol Obstet* 1980;**150**:878–82.

128 Mayer AD, McMahon MJ, Corfield AP *et al.* Controlled clinical trial of peritoneal lavage for the treatment of severe acute pancreatitis. *N Engl J Med* 1985;**312**:399–404.

129 Ihse I, Evander A, Holmberg JT, Gustafson I. Influence of peritoneal lavage on objective prognostic signs in acute pancreatitis. *Ann Surg* 1986;**204**:122–27.

130 Teerenhovi O, Nordback I, Eskola J. High volume lesser sac lavage in acute necrotizing pancreatitis *Br J Surg* 1989; **76**:370–3.

131 Berling R, Borgstrom A, Ohlsson K. Peritoneal lavage with aprotinin in patients with severe acute pancreatitis. Effects on plasma and peritoneal levels of trypsin and leukocyte proteases and their major inhibitors. *Int J Pancreatol* 1998; **24**:9–17.

132 Ranson JHC, Berman RS. Long peritoneal lavage decreases pancreatic sepsis in acute pancreatitis. *Ann Surg* 1990; **211**:708–16.

133 Alexandre JH, Guerrari MT. Role of total pancreatectomy in the treatment of necrotizing pancreatitis. *World J Surg* 1981;**5**:369–77.

134 Kivilaakso E, Lempinen M, Makelainen A, Nikki P, Schroder T. Pancreatic resection versus peritoneal lavation for acute fulminant pancreatitis. *Ann Surg* 1984;**199**: 426–31.

135 Schroder T, Sainio V, Kivisaari L, Puolakkainen P, Kivilaakso E, Lempinen M. Pancreatic resection versus peritoneal lavage in acute necrotizing pancreatitis. *Ann Surg* 1991;**214**:663–6.

136 Warshaw AL, Gongliang J. Improved survival in 45 patients with pancreatic abscess. *Ann Surg* 1985;**202**:408–15.

137 Allardyce DB. Incidence of necrotizing pancreatitis and factors related to mortality. *Am J Surg* 1987;**154**:295–9.

138 Wertheimer MD, Norris CS. Surgical management of necrotizing pancreatitis. *Arch Surg* 1986;**121**:484–7.

139 Bradley EL, Allen K. A prospective longitudinal study of observation versus surgical intervention in the management of necrotizing pancreatitis. *Am J Surg* 1991; **161**:19–24.

140 Gebhardt C, Gall FP. Importance of peritoneal irrigation after surgical treatment of hemorrhagic, necrotizing pancreatitis. *World J Surg* 1981;**5**:379–85.

141 Larvin M, Chalmers AG, Robinson PJ, McMahon MJ. Debridement and closed cavity irrigation for the treatment of pancreatic necrosis. *Br J Surg* 1989;**76**:465–71.

142 Bassi C, Vesentini S, Nifosi F, Girelli R, Falconi M, Elio A, Pederzoli P. Pancreatic abscess and other pus-haboring collections related to pancreatitis: a review of 108 cases. *World J Surg* 1990;**14**:505–12.

143 Farkas G, Marton J, Mandi Y, Szederkenyi E. Surgical strategy and management of infected pancreatic necrosis. *Br J Surg* 1996;**83**:930–3.

144 Carter CR, McKay CJ, Imrie CW. Percutaneous necrosectomy and sinus tract endoscopy in the management of infected pancreatic necrosis: an initial experience. *Ann Surg* 2000;**232**:175–80.

145 Freeny PC, Hauptmann E, Althaus SJ, Traverso LW, Sinanan M. Percutaneous CT-guided catheter drainage of infected acute necrotizing pancreatitis: techniques and results. *AJR Am J Roentgenol* 1998;**170**:969–75.

146 Gentile AT, Feliciano PD, Mullins RJ, Crass RA, Eidemiller LR, Sheppard BC. The utility of polyglycolic acid mesh for abdominal access in patients with necrotizing pancreatitis. *J Am Coll Surg* 1998;**186**:313–18.

147 Horvath KD, Kao LS, Ali A, Wherry KL, Pellegrini CA, Sinanan MN. Laparoscopic assisted percutaneous drainage of infected pancreatic necrosis. *Surg Endosc* 2001;**15**: 677–82.

148 Mann S, Gmeinwieser J, Schmidt J, Zirngibl H, Jauch KW. Possibilities and limits of interventional therapy in necrotizing pancreatitis. *Zentralbl Chir* 2001;**126**:15–22.

22 Obesity

Jarol Knowles

Introduction

Obesity is a worldwide epidemic, and a patient with medical problems stemming from obesity will be encountered with increasing frequency in the career of a practicing physician. Obesity is the result of sustained positive energy balance, and the current obesity epidemic is the result of interactions between genes and the environment (i.e. diet and exercise habits) as well as metabolic, social, behavioral and psychological factors.

This chapter will focus on obesity as it relates to gastrointestinal disease. Obesity is associated with metabolic complications (hypertension, diabetes, hyperlipidemia, etc.), and those interested in the common comorbidities associated with obesity are referred to an excellent review by Pi-Sunyer.[1]

For the gastroenterologist, obesity provides multiple challenges related to diagnosis and treatment. Obesity is associated with higher rates of gastroesophageal reflux symptoms, gallstones, cancer and fatty infiltration of the liver. There is a high prevalence of gastrointestinal symptoms in obese patients who indulge in binge eating, and binge eating is often undisclosed by these patients. The gastroenterologist is also faced with specific diagnostic challenges in the abdominal examination of obese patients. Common landmarks in the abdomen of these patients are not palpable, and proper examination requires more expensive and invasive testing.

Obesity is a chronic disease and a chronic disease model should be undertaken in treatment. Since dieting is associated with a high failure rate, physicians are hesitant to recommend it as a treatment for improving obesity comorbidities. However, physicians can effect behavioral change that can lead to successful weight loss if they maintain an empathetic attitude. Concerning obese patients, gastroenterologists would be well-advised to:

- develop techniques to motivate positive health behaviors
- understand the common presenting features of obesity
- know the current medications for obesity
- know how to refer patients appropriately.

The current obesity epidemic and the problems it can cause in the diagnosis and treatment of the obese patient make it essential that today's gastroenterologist understands the associations between gastrointestinal disease and obesity as well as the evidence supporting this association.

Definition

Obesity is defined as an excess of fat in the body, that increases body weight beyond physical and skeletal requirements. Because total body fat is difficult to measure except in research protocols, obesity is determined by the body mass index (BMI). BMI is defined as weight divided by height squared ($weight/height^2$) and reflects body fat. A short person carries weight differently than a tall person making comparisons of weight between two individuals in a population difficult. The BMI is a concept of weight that estimates the degree of body fat independent of height, sex or ethnicity. Since increasing BMI is associated with increasing risks for comorbidities, every physician should be familiar with the common cut-off points. These are presented in Box 22.1.

Box 22.1 Weight classification: body mass index (BMI)

Underweight	< 18.5
Normal	18.5–24.9
Overweight	25.0–29.9
Obesity, class I	30.0–34.9
Obesity, class II	35.0–39.9
Obesity, class III	> 40.0

Epidemiology

Worldwide, around 250 million people are obese, and the World Health Organization has estimated that 300 million people will be obese in 2025.[2] The prevalence rates for overweight and obese people are highest in the Middle East, central and eastern Europe, and North America.[3] Special populations (Native American tribes, American Pacific Islanders) have obesity rates approaching 80%.[4] The US National Health and Nutrition Examination Surveys, which survey people across the USA, showed a marked increase in obesity in the first survey cycle in 1960–1961 and the third cycle in 1988–1994. Currently, approximately 30% of the US population has a BMI greater than 30 kg/m².[5]

The epidemic of obesity is a worldwide phenomenon affecting industrialized as well as non-industrialized nations. Global availability of cheap vegetable oils and fats has resulted in a greatly increased fat consumption in low-income nations. Consumption of carbohydrates has also increased worldwide, with a marked increase in soft drink consumption in the developing world.[6] Recent economic analysis of the obesity epidemic suggests that industrialization and the conveniences and inactive lifestyle that come with it play a major role in promoting obesity.

The rates for obesity are higher for women than for men in most countries, with a greater BMI distribution being seen in women. The obesity epidemic is not confined to adults, children also are affected. Worldwide, 22 million children under the age of 5 years are overweight. In the USA, the prevalence of overweight children has doubled in the past three decades. The prevalence of overweight children is even higher in African-American and Hispanic communities. Nearly 22% of children who are African-American or Hispanic are overweight. The majority of obese adults with class III obesity (those with a BMI > 40 kg/m²) developed obesity in childhood or adolescence.

Etiology

Evidence for genetic causes

A role for genetics in the tendency to gain weight is supported by data from familial studies. Correlations of obesity among first-degree relatives generally range from 0·20 to 0·30 and studies in identical (monozygotic) twins show a correlation of 0·60 to 0·70.[7] Adoption studies (twins raised apart) have shown that adoptees tend to resemble their biological relatives rather than their adopted families in body composition.

Genetics may also influence the effect of exercise on body weight. In twin studies, Bouchard *et al.* showed that the effect of exercise may be influenced by genetic differences between individuals.[8] In their studies, there was a 6·8-fold greater change in body weight between pairs than within pairs of twins who were engaging in the same type and amount of physical activity.[8]

With the discovery of the leptin gene in 1994, enthusiasm abounded for a genetic cause for obesity.[9] It is now known that obesity is controlled by several genes with gene–gene and gene–environment interactions playing crucial roles. As of 2002, there have been more than 250 genes, genetic markers or chromosomal regions identified that are associated with obesity.[10]

Evidence for dietary causes

Population-based dietary intake studies showed a decrease in average daily fat intake from 41% in 1976 to 36·6% in 1991.[11] Yet, in this same time period the prevalence of obesity increased, suggesting that something other than fat intake has contributed to the rise in obesity. Food disappearance data (a measure of the flow of raw and semiprocessed food commodities through the US marketing system) has shown an increase in consumption. Over the past 30 years, each American consumed, on average:

- 39 kg (86 lbs) more of commercially grown vegetables
- 26·8 kg (59 lbs) more of grain products
- 25·9 kg (57 lbs) more of fruit
- 16·3 kg (36 lbs) more of caloric sweeteners
- 10·9 kg (24 lbs) more of total red meat, poultry and fish (boneless, trimmed equivalent)
- 8·2 kg (18 lbs) more of cheese
- 7·3 kg (16 lbs) more of added fats and oils
- 15·1 l (4 gallons) more of beer
- 54 fewer eggs
- 30·3 l (8 gallons) less of coffee
- 30·3 l (8 gallons) less of milk.

These data (1970–1999 USDA data)[12] are neither a direct measure of actual consumption nor of the quantity of food actually ingested, but they have the advantage of avoiding the problems implicit in consumer survey data. Neilsen and Popkin examined portion-size changes in consumer surveys from 1977 to 1996 and found that food portion sizes increased both inside and outside the home for all categories except pizza.[13] These data have given rise to the concept of a toxic environment that "pervasively surrounds [Americans] with inexpensive, convenient foods high in both fat and calories".[14] In an effort to understand appetite control mechanisms and food choices, Rolls and colleagues have done elegant double blind feeding studies in various populations. These studies revealed that people eat more when they are served larger portion sizes, choose high fat foods, and are unaware of the energy density of dietary intake.[15] Modern industrialized society makes eating food practically effortless. Drive-up windows, 24-hour food service, and increased portion sizes make spending time and energy preparing food a thing of the past. Today's society enables us to eat food that is easily available, inexpensive and energy dense.

Evidence for sedentary lifestyle

Modern conveniences and energy-saving devices such as automobiles, washing machines, elevators, computers and remote controls have all contributed to a decrease in total energy expenditure. Few studies have quantified sedentary activities as they relate to obesity making it difficult to assess the relationship between sedentary lifestyle and obesity. The majority of studies measure physical activity levels by self-report, observation, pedometer or accelerometer. There are few studies that document the absence of physical activity and weight changes. Inferences have been made from the absence of active physical activities (occupational and recreational) and these show that decreased activity correlates with time watching television and increased car ownership. In two evidence-based reviews, DePietro[16] and Jebb and Moore[17] report that low levels of activity are associated with obesity.

Energy expended during physical activity is highly variable, and it is the component of total energy expenditure over which an individual has the most control. It may represent 15–50% of the total 24-hour energy expended depending on the activity of the individual. Increasing intensity and duration of activity will increase energy expenditure.

Evidence for psychological causes

Obese people are particularly vulnerable to symptoms of low self-esteem and depression when they fail to measure up to the thin ideal promoted by the media. Healthcare providers should be aware of the possibility of depressive symptoms in obese patients, and they should also be careful to avoid stereotyping their obese patients with specific personality disorders that they think may be responsible for their obesity. More than likely, poor self-esteem and discrimination influence mood disorders in obese patients. Discrimination has been reported in employment[18,19] housing[20] and college admissions.[21] In a 7-year follow up study of the National Longitudinal Survey of Labor Market Experience, Gortmaker *et al.* showed that women who were overweight as adolescents were 20% less likely to be married and had a 10% higher rate of poverty than normal weight adolescent girls who had other chronic illness.[22] Men were 11% less likely to be married when they were overweight as adolescents compared with normal weight boys who had other chronic illness.[22] It is generally thought that obese individuals suffer emotionally from cultural bias, negative attitudes, and discrimination.

In addition to low self-esteem, discrimination, and depression, obese people have a higher prevalence of two distinct eating disorders: binge-eating syndrome and night-eating syndrome. Obesity is associated with a two-fold increase in the prevalence of binge eating, with similar rates found among black women, white women and white men.[23] The key features that distinguish binge eating from overeating is a feeling of loss of control while consuming an amount of food which is larger than most people would eat. Relative to obese patients who do not binge eat, binge eaters have higher BMIs as well as higher rates of comorbid depression and anxiety. Across three studies, the average depression score among patients with binge-eating disorder was in the mild depressive range.[24] Among bariatric surgery patients, the prevalence of preoperative binge eating ranges from 13% to 49%.[25]

Night-eating syndrome, first recognized by Stunkard in 1955, has not been systematically evaluated until recently. It is defined by ingestion of 50% of the daily caloric intake after the evening meal, awakening at least once a night for three nights a week to eat and morning anorexia. In class III obese patients, the prevalence of night-eating syndrome may be as high as 26%.[26] Birketvedt *et al.* conducted two studies that examined the behavioral and neuroendocrine characteristics of individuals in this population and compared them with sex, age and weight-matched controls.[27] Participants who had night-eating syndrome consumed less than control participants until 11:00 pm, after which their intake exceeded the control participants' intake, with a cumulative intake of 4000 KJ above the control group in a 24-hour period.

Evidence for drug causes

There are numerous medications that contribute to weight gain as shown in Box 22.2. Change in weight was a major concern in the Diabetes Control and Complications Trial (DCCT). In this study, intensive treatment with insulin (three or more daily injections or continuous subcutaneous infusion) increased the risk of becoming overweight by 73% when compared with less intensive diabetic therapy.[28] Tricyclic antidepressants and the selective serotonin reuptake inhibitors are associated with varying degrees of weight gain; the type, dose and duration of therapy influence the degree of

---

Box 22.2 Selected medications that can cause weight gain

- Psychotropic medications

   Tricyclic antidepressants
   Monoamine oxidase inhibitors
   Specific selective serotonin reuptake inhibitors
   Atypical antidepressants
   Lithium
   Specific anticonvulsants

- β-adrenergic receptor blockers
- Diabetes medications

   Insulin
   Sulfonylureas
   Thiazolidinediones

- Highly active antiretroviral therapy
- Tamoxifen
- Steroid hormones

   Glucocorticoids
   Progestational steroids

weight gain. Bupropion, a dopamine agonist, is an atypical antidepressant that does not appear to induce weight gain. The lack of stimulation of norepinephrine and serotonin pathways appear to be responsible for this difference in effect.

Effects of obesity: clinical features

Gastro-esophageal reflux disease

Symptomatic esophagitis is common in obese patients. Obesity causes an increased incidence of hiatal hernia which impairs acid clearance from the esophagus and the crural diaphragm's function as a sphincter. The increased intra-abdominal pressure associated with obesity results in cephalad displacement of the lower esophageal sphincter (LES).[29] One population-based, cross-sectional study of 1524 people in Olmstead County, Minnesota showed a prevalence of gastro-esophageal reflux disease (GERD) in 69% of participants with a BMI greater than 30 kg/m².[30] These findings were replicated by Ruhl and Everhart who showed that hospitalization rates for any esophageal-related condition were higher as BMI increased.[31] Each 5-unit increase in BMI was associated with a 1·22-increased hazard of developing GERD.

The strongest data to suggest a relationship between GERD and obesity comes from studies using objective measurements such as manometry and ambulatory pH monitoring. In a study reported by Fisher *et al.*, 24-hour pH monitoring of 30 class III obese patients with a mean BMI of 51·5 kg/m² showed that 50% of these subjects complained of GERD symptoms and 37% had objective evidence of GERD by pH monitoring.[32] Neither BMI nor body weight correlated with LES pressure or length, upper esophageal sphincter pressure or length, or esophageal body peristalsis or maximum pressure. Three observational studies failed to show a relationship between observed weight or BMI and abnormal 24-hour pH monitoring values.[33–35] The differences between observational studies and studies using objective measurements may be a result of the analyses: BMI correlates with abnormal pH monitoring when subjects are grouped according to abnormal pH monitoring results. When researchers tried to model the degree of obesity with the pH monitoring result, BMI and abnormal pH monitoring did not correlate. Despite the differences in statistical analyses in these small prospective studies, it is clear that not all obese patients with symptoms of reflux have objective evidence of GERD.

Treatment options for those with GERD include weight loss, histamine H₂-receptor antagonists, proton pump inhibitors and bariatric surgery. Only two prospective studies documenting the role of weight loss to improve GERD symptoms have been published. In one study, weight loss improved symptoms of GERD.[36] B4 In another study, pH monitoring showed that there was no reduction in reflux despite an average weight loss of 10 kg.[37] B4 The histamine H₂-receptor antagonists have been shown to be efficacious in obese patients. Pharmacokinetic studies in obese patients using cimetidine and ranitidine demonstrate that dosing should be calculated according to patients' ideal body weight and not their actual weight. The safety and efficacy of the proton pump inhibitors has not been studied in this population. The Roux-en-Y gastric bypass has been shown to be very effective for improving GERD symptoms.[38,39] B4

Gallstones

The prevalence of gallstones in patients in the Women's Health Study and Health Professionals Study was 7·8% among women and 3·5% among men over a 10-year period. These studies showed that the risk of developing gallstones increased with the severity of obesity.[40,41] The risk factors for symptomatic gallstone disease are female sex (relative risk (RR) 8·8, $P < 0.003$), obesity (BMI > 30, RR 3·7, $P < 0.001$), age greater than 50 years (RR 2·5, $P < 0.001$), and a positive family history of previous cholecystectomy in a first-degree family member (RR 2·2, $P < 0.01$). In a family study of 1038 individuals who participated in the *MRC-OB* genes project, the additive genetic heritability of symptomatic gallstones was 29% ($P < 0.02$).[42] Additionally, weight loss is a strong predictor of developing gallstones, especially in women.[43] In several studies, approximately 11–28% of obese patients who severely restricted their dietary intake[44–46] and 27–43% of patients who underwent bariatric surgery developed gallstones within a period of 1–5 months after initiating their treatment.[47,48] The relative risk for cholecystectomy associated with weight cycling is 1·68 and is independent of attained relative body weight.[41]

Rate of weight loss influences the development of gallstones. In a 1995 meta-analysis of published studies evaluating the risk of gallstone formation during active weight loss, Weinsier *et al.* demonstrated an increasing risk of gallstone formation at rates of weight loss above 1·5 kg per week.[49]

Irritable bowel syndrome

Obesity is associated with an increased prevalence of irritable bowel syndrome (IBS) although there has been very little research done in this area. In a case–control study, Crowell *et al.* examined 119 obese binge eaters (BMI > 30 kg/m²) and 77 normal weight binge eaters. They found that obesity was associated with more frequent constipation, diarrhea, straining and flatus.[50] Another report demonstrated that abdominal bloating is more frequent in those with recent weight gain.[51] In a case–control study with co-twin control design, Svedburg *et al.* examined the association of IBS with obesity in 850 Swedish twin pairs and found an association (odds ratio (OR) 2·6, CI 1·0 to 6·4).[52] Additionally, obese binge eaters reported two to four times more upper gastrointestinal symptoms (nausea, vomiting, and bloating) than normal controls or obese non-binge eaters ($P < 0.001$). Obese binge eaters reported more lower gastrointestinal symptoms (abdominal pain and dyschezia) than normal-weight controls ($P < 0.05$).[49]

Weight reduction appears to improve symptoms of IBS, especially in morbidly obese persons. In a recent abstract, morbidly obese patients who underwent Roux-en-Y gastric bypass had significant improvement according to a gastrointestinal symptom questionnaire after weight loss.[53] B4 Therefore, weight loss may be suggested as a treatment for obese patients who have IBS, but further studies will be needed to clarify the relationship between IBS symptoms and the psychosocial aspects of improved self-esteem associated with weight loss in this patient population.

Non-alcoholic steatohepatitis

Steatosis is found in 60–70% of obese adults and progression to liver cell injury on liver biopsy is found in 18·5% of obese individuals and 2·7% of normal weight individuals on autopsy studies.[54] Among 75 patients undergoing bariatric surgery with a mean BMI 57 kg/m², 84% of patients had steatosis and 8% had fibrosis or cirrhosis.[55] In 181 patients with a mean BMI 47 kg/m², 91% of patients had non-alcoholic fatty infiltration of the liver and 10% had fibrosis.[56] The risk of progression to cirrhosis correlates with the initial histology. In a long-term follow up study of 132 patients with steatosis on initial biopsy, cirrhosis developed in only 4%. If there was balloon degeneration and Mallory's hyaline bodies on initial biopsy, after 18 years of follow up 26% of patients had developed cirrhosis.[57] In case series, 10% weight reduction is associated with normalization of alanine aminotransferase (ALT).[58–62] In an obese patient, liver biopsy is recommended if any of the following is true:

- the AST:ALT ratio is greater than 1
- the ALT is twice normal
- there is evidence of metabolic syndrome
- there is the persistent elevation of liver function test scores despite weight loss.

Cancer

The risk of cancer is increased in obese individuals, with 33% more cases of cancer seen in the obese population than the general population.[63] Increased cancer rates associated with obesity have been noted for renal cell, gallbladder, colon, brain, endometrial, ovarian and cervical cancer, and lymphoma. Twice as many women with a BMI greater than 29 kg/m² had distal colon cancer than women with a BMI less than 21 kg/m². The causal factors associates with the increase in gallbladder cancer risk are controversial, but possibilities that are diet related include caloric intake, increased fat intake, decreased fiber intake and hormonal milieu.

Vomiting

Vomiting is not usually considered a comorbidity associated with obesity, but it deserves mention because it is a symptom that is sometimes disclosed during the gastrointestinal evaluation. Bulimia nervosa is common in obese individuals, and it is often associated with binge eating. Russell introduced the diagnosis of bulimia nervosa in 1979.[64] Bulimia nervosa is characterized by recurrent binge eating and extreme weight-control behavior such as self-induced vomiting, strict dieting and the misuse of laxatives. The DSM IV criteria for bulimia nervosa require that an individual binges and purges twice a week for 3 months. The prevalence of bulimia and binge eating varies according to the sample assessed. In a school-based sample of 4746 boys and girls in public middle and high schools in Minnesota (Project EAT – Eating Among Teens), 17·3% of girls and 7·8% of boys reported objective overeating in the last year before the survey.[65] Overeating was associated with suicide risk; more than a quarter of girls (28·6%) and boys (27·8%) who had met the criteria for binge-eating syndrome reported that they had attempted suicide. Dieting, chronic restrained eating and excessive exercise may be important triggers for binge eating and bulimia nervosa. Since bulimia and binge eating are surreptitious methods to control weight, they are often undisclosed by patients. In patients who are obese and have a history of vomiting, the diagnosis of bulimia nervosa should be considered. Referral to a psychiatric program with therapists skilled in the therapy of eating disorders is the most appropriate treatment. C5

Patients recovering from Roux-en-Y gastric bypass surgery often experience vomiting. The prevalence of vomiting after Roux-en-Y gastric bypass varies between 1% and 68%. In a review of a long-term (13–15-year) follow up of a cohort of 100 patients who underwent gastric bypass for morbid obesity, Mitchell *et al.* found that 68% of the patients complained of continued vomiting.[66] In contrast, Balsiger *et al.* reported that only 1% of patients complained of persistent vomiting 3 years after Roux-en-Y gastric bypass.[67] It appears that preoperative diagnosis of binge-eating disorder and a multidisciplinary team approach to the postoperative management of these patients affects the prevalence of postoperative vomiting. B4 The prevalence of stricture at the gastrojejunal anastomosis is approximately 2% of cases after Roux-en-Y gastric bypass. Persistent vomiting should be evaluated with endoscopy and possible dilatation.

Chronic vomiting and gastroparesis is also seen in some patients with type 2 diabetes mellitus-associated obesity.

Gastroparesis is usually seen in severe type 1 diabetic patients, but it may be seen in up to 30% of patients with type 2 diabetes.[68] Chronic hyperglycemia alone has adverse effects on gastric emptying activity with a prolongation of the lag phase.[69] Although weight loss is the classic presentation of gastroparesis, obesity and type 2 diabetes without evidence of weight loss is increasingly common in patients with a diagnosis of gastroparesis. An improvement in glucose control combined with a low-fat diet (< 40 g/day) is advised for treatment since lipids slow gastric emptying rates.[70]

Depression

Depression is a common diagnosis in obese patients with unexplained physical symptoms. These patients often attribute depressed moods to their excess weight rather than recognizing that depression or anxiety may have triggered their overeating. ("Doctor, I know my depression is related to my weight, but I still have this belly pain"). In a systematic review of the evidence that links obesity with depression, no clear relationship could be determined. In cross-sectional studies, depression has been associated with a high BMI. In face to face interviews with individuals in more than 42 000 households, the 1992 National Longitudinal Alcohol Epidemiologic Survey (NLAES) showed a U-shaped relationship between depression and weight, with relatively high and low BMI values associated with an increased probability of major depression.[71] Prospective longitudinal studies are required to determine the relative risk (RR) of depression in obese patients, but these types of studies are rare. In one prospective study controlling for mental health problems at baseline, there was an increased RR of depression in obese patients followed for 5 years.[72]

Diagnosis

See Table 22.1 which gives an overview of the treatments suggested for the various categories of BMI in the National Institutes for Health (NIH) publication *A Practical Guide: Identification, Evaluation, and Treatment of Overweight and Obesity in Adults*.[73]

Treatment

Controlling intake and increasing activity (dieting and exercise) are very difficult, and it is important for physicians to understand that some patients may have to do much more than others to maintain a healthy weight. There are windows of opportunity when radical behavior changes seem to be effective interventions. For example, after a diagnosis of diabetes or myocardial infarction, patients are often highly

Table 22.1 Guide for selecting obesity treatment[73]

Treatment	BMI category (kg/m^2)				
	25–26·9	27–29·9	30–34·9	35–39·9	≥ 40
Diet, exercise, behavior treatment	+	+	+	+	+
Pharmacotherapy		With comorbidities	+	+	+
Surgery				With comorbidities	+

motivated to undertake behavioral changes. Unfortunately, the amount of weight loss by non-surgical approaches rarely surpasses 15% from baseline weight. It is important that physicians not take non-adherence to their suggestions personally and criticize patients when they don't achieve their weight goals. After validating the difficulties that their patients face, it is important for physicians to focus on identifying obstacles and help their patients form a plan to succeed in future attempts at weight loss.

Evidence for dietary treatment

An evidence-based review of the effectiveness of diet interventions in the treatment of obesity is limited by several factors. The most important factor is the lack of blinded studies in diet interventions. It is very difficult to blind participants in a weight loss trial since changes in diet are readily noticed. Additionally, it is difficult for the study investigators to be blinded to the intervention. Randomization is another factor that is difficult to achieve in weight loss studies since the issues of consent and compliance may be more difficult to achieve than is the case for some interventions. Since there is no gold standard for comparison with the intervention, diet interventions tend to compare low fat, low carbohydrate, low calorie or high protein at different percentages within the diet.

The evidence-based review of dietary interventions is severely limited by methodological factors. There is a wide variety among prescribed diets and true control groups are often lacking. Dietary interventions often include or are compared with a combination of exercise and behavior interventions that vary with respect to intensity and frequency of follow up visits. Additionally, a change in weight often results from a change in activity, behavior, or both, and these may be difficult to measure. The overall attrition rate in weight loss studies has been estimated to be 50%, severely limiting analysis of long-term success. The majority of diet studies do not use intention to treat analysis, and when they do include this analysis they often employ the last known weight during participation as the endpoint. This method of

Table 22.2 Summary of studies of low carbohydrate dietary interventions for obesity

Author	Diet	Length	Enrolled	Completed	Weight loss	P	Comments
Sondike et al.[74]	LC v LF	12 weeks	39	30	9·9 ± 9·3 kg v 4·1 ± 4·9 kg	<0·05	Mean age = 15 years Significant reduction of LDL-cholesterol on LF diet, no change on LC diet
Samaha et al.[83]	LC v LF	6 months	132	79	5·8 ± 8·6 kg v 1·9 ± 4·2 kg	<0·002	Significant reduction of TG on LC diet
Foster et al.[84]	LC v LF	12 months	63	37	4·4 ± 6·7% v 2·5 ± 6·3%	Not significant	Weight loss measured in percent of body weight Subjects on the low carbohydrate diet lost significantly more weight than the subjects on the conventional diet at 3 months (P = 0·002) and 6 months (P = 0·03)

LC, low carbohydrate diet; LF, low fat diet; LDL, low density lipoprotein; TG, triglycerides

analysis overestimates the true long-term weight loss. Despite the limitations in dietary intervention studies, a recent review of long-term outcomes of obesity showed a 15% success rate among 2131 patients followed for 5 years.[74] The reported prevalence of people trying to lose weight in a community-based survey was 28·8% for men and 43·6% for women.[75]

Several low cost strategies can be effective in achieving weight loss. Weight Watchers and TOPS (Take Off Pounds Sensibly) are usually rated highly by patients because of low cost and good social support. Meal replacements (liquid formulations, meal replacement bars) have an advantage in a busy lifestyle. Because the portions are controlled, the caloric content is known. Meal replacements are useful for patients who need structured portion control. In a study that randomized patients to meal replacements or an energy restricted diet over a 28-month period, the meal replacement group had superior weight loss (10% v 4% weight loss).[76] Alc

In a meta-analysis of 12 controlled trials that evaluated the effect of an *ad libitum* low fat diet on daily energy intake, Astrup et al. found that daily energy intake was decreased by 10·8%.[77] The data show that decreasing dietary fat was directly associated with a decrease in body weight. Changes in percent dietary fat were also highly correlated with changes in energy intake. For every 1% decrease in energy from fat, there was a corresponding 0·28 kg weight loss.[78]

Despite the strong data to support lowering dietary fat, recent evidence from a systematic review[79] suggests that low fat diets are no better than other types of weight-reducing diets in achieving and maintaining weight loss over a 12–18-month period. Over 3000 citations were reviewed and only six trials were found that met the inclusion criteria for randomization, blinding, and intention to treat analysis. Additionally, within the six trials, dropouts and withdrawals varied from 11% to 40%. Furthermore, only one study showed a significant improvement in serum lipids with a low-fat diet. The authors conclude that fat-restricted diets are no better than calorie-restricted diets in achieving weight loss in overweight people. Ala

The lack of evidence supporting the role of low-fat diets in achieving weight loss or improvement in co-morbidities associated with obesity coincides with a shift in philosophy within the nutrition community. Recent recommendations from both the US Department of Agriculture (Dietary Guidelines),[80] and the National Heart Lung and Blood Institute(NHLBI) of the NIH (Clinical Guidelines)[81] recommend a decrease in total caloric intake, including reducing portions sizes, to achieve weight loss. Greater weight loss and improvement in serum lipids has recently been reported with a low carbohydrate/high fat diet (Atkins-type diet), suggesting that the role of dietary fat requires re-evaluation. Three randomized controlled trials[82–84] have been published (Table 22.2). Alc The only study that followed patients for 12 months reported no significant difference in weight loss when compared to a low fat diet.[84] It should be noted that the dropout rate was significant in all the studies, making it difficult to establish clear recommendations.

Evidence for exercise treatment

The current public health recommendation for physical activity is for individuals to participate in 30 minutes of moderately intense physical activity on most days of the week.[85] Despite the importance of physical activity, there is little evidence that exercise alone will produce weight loss. A meta-analysis of weight loss studies found that aerobic exercise programs produce weight loss of 2·9 kg over

21 weeks, compared with 11 kg weight loss from 15 weeks of caloric restriction.[86] Alc The reason that people do not lose weight with increased exercise alone is because they usually also increase their food intake. Therefore, exercise combined with energy restriction is recommended based on the rationale that physical activity will result in an increase in total energy expenditure. C5

Evidence-based analysis of the studies using exercise as an adjunct to either diet or behavior therapy is limited by the wide variety of protocols used. These studies use a variety of parameters to measure the efficacy of exercise treatment (individual variation in response, exercise duration, exercise intensity, lifestyle activities, and type of exercise) and this variability limits comparability. Individual studies provide the basis for the recommendations for the population, since combining these heterogeneous studies is difficult. Documentation of factors such as previous weight loss attempts, smoking status, change in body composition, and changes in lifestyle activities is often missing. The quantification of diet and physical activity is biased in favor of underreporting dietary intake and overreporting physical activity.[87] Despite the methodological problems that plague this area of study, Jebb *et al.* reviewed several studies on the relationship between physical activity and body weight and found that there is clear evidence that low levels of physical activity are associated with an increased risk of weight gain and obesity.[17]

The amount of exercise required to improve fitness may be different from the amount of exercise recommended to achieve optimal health or prevent death. There is a striking difference in the relative risk of cardiovascular disease and all-cause mortality between the fit and unfit. In the Nurses Health Study, the relative risk of death increased with an increase in BMI, with a four-fold relative risk of death from cardiovascular disease in non-smoking women with a BMI greater than 32 kg/m[2].[88] In obese individuals with a BMI greater than 25 kg/m^2, the relative risk of death was 1·25 in the fit and 4·0 in the unfit.[89] It appears that exercise intensity can affect cardiorespiratory fitness but not change body composition or body weight.[90] B2

Exercise has a powerful effect on insulin sensitivity. Obese individuals with type 2 diabetes mellitus had an increase in insulin sensitivity following low intensity bicycle riding.[91] In non-obese, insulin-resistant relatives of type 2 diabetic patients, moderate intensity exercise led to a 40% increase in insulin sensitivity.[92] The Diabetes Prevention Program found that intensive exercise in combination with a change in diet could lower the risk of progressing to diabetes by 58% when compared to metformin or placebo.[93] Ald

Despite recommendations of exercise for prevention of weight gain and improvement of cardiovascular fitness and insulin sensitivity, the major challenge is adoption of a regular exercise pattern. Recent studies on the effectiveness of intermittent exercise (multiple 10–15 minute exercise sessions daily) suggest that intermittent exercise is a successful strategy for increasing the adoption of exercise in overweight individuals who are sedentary.[94] B4 The long-term cumulative effect of small changes in activity level can be beneficial. By walking about 2000 extra steps a day, 100 extra calories can be burned a day. It appears that the key factor that explains the relationship between exercise and weight is the adoption of an active lifestyle to prevent weight gain and weight regain. Evidence from the National Weight Control Registry, which is a collection of data on 1047 individuals who lost at least 30 pounds (13·6 kg) and maintained that loss for at least 1 year, supports this claim. In an analysis of successful weight maintainers, 1 hour or more of moderate to vigorous physical activity per day was the factor that led to a successfully maintained weight loss over an average of 6·9 years.[95] B2

Evidence for psychological treatment

Behavior therapy in the treatment of obese patients includes strategies used to modify eating and activity patterns. Early studies using behavior therapy addressed questions of types of behavioral treatment, and length of treatment, and were often compared to conventional low calorie diets. From these studies, a typical behavioral program, incorporates a 1200 kcal/day diet, includes 6 months of weekly meetings and key components of self-monitoring (daily records of food intake and physical activity), stimulus control strategies, problem solving, preplanning and relapse prevention. On average, these studies showed that participants in behavior treatment lost 10% of their body weight after 1 year.[96] B4 Weight re-gain has been noted as a problem, and behavior programs now include a longer follow up period, averaging 18 months. Maintaining contact with participants improves long-term weight control.[97] With longer follow up, weight maintenance has improved with reported sustained weight loss of 62% of initial weight loss.[98] B4

Table 22.3 lists recent randomized controlled trials of various therapies (intensive lifestyle counseling, nutrient-density diet behavioral modification, counseling-based, skill-building, problem solving, cognitive behavioral body image therapy, family-based treatment, sibutramine plus family-based, behavioral weight control, etc).[93,99–113] The majority of these trials focus on children and adolescents, suggesting that efforts at the prevention of weight gain in childhood are a priority. The failure of most of these trials to demonstrate statistically significant benefits from these interventions may be because they lack statistical power but it is also true that behavior is complex and difficult to change. The strongest argument for including behavior therapy in the treatment of obesity comes from the Diabetes Prevention Program. In this trial, 3234 non-diabetic persons with elevated fasting and post-load plasma glucose concentrations were randomized to metformin or lifestyle intervention or placebo with a follow

Table 22.3 Randomized controlled trials of behavioural treatment of obesity

Authors	Behaviour intervention	Participants	Length of study	Comments
Robinson et al.[99]	After-school dance program v newsletters, health education lectures	61 8–10-year-old African-American girls and their parents'/guardians	12 weeks	Treatment group: lower BMI (adjusted difference = −0·32 kg/m², 95% CI −0·77 to 0·12; significantly reduced household television viewing (d = 0·73, P = 0.007)
Story et al.[100]	After-school program increasing physical activity and healthy eating v program unrelated to nutrition and physical activity	54 African-American girls, 8–10 years of age, and their parents'/caregivers	12 weeks	BMI did not differ between the treatment groups
Beech et al.[101]	Interactive weekly group sessions child-targeted program v parent-targeted program	60 African-American girls aged 8–10 years and their parents'/caregivers	12 weeks	Trend toward reduced BMI and waist circumference
Baranowski et al.[102]	4-week summer day camp, followed by a special 8-week home internet intervention for the girls and their parents v similar intervention without Fun, Food, and Fitness Project	35 8-year-old African-American girls and their parents or caregivers	12 weeks	No significant differences in BMI between treatment and control group girls
Tate et al.[103]	Basic internet weight loss program alone v with the addition of behavioral counseling via e-mail (e-counseling) to individuals at risk of type 2 diabetes	92 overweight adults	1 year	Behavioral e-counseling group lost more mean weight than the basic internet group −4·4 v −2·0 kg, P = 0·04)
Berkowitz et al.[104]	Sibutramine plus family-based, behavioral weight control program v placebo plus family-based, behavioral weight control program	82 adolescents aged 13–17 years	6 months, followed by open-label treatment during months 7–12	Significantly more weight loss in the sibutramine group compared with placebo (7·8 kg v 3·2 kg)
Rameriz and Rosen[105]	Weight control v weight control plus cognitive behavioral body image therapy	65 obese men and women	16 week intervention followed by 1-year follow up weight	Weight loss and maintenance were equivalent between groups
Kaukua et al.[106]	VLED and behaviour modification v no intervention in the control group.	38 obese men	8 months with 10 weeks on VLED and 17 behaviour modification visits	Treatment group showed significant weight loss 13·9 (7·8)% of baseline weight v no change in control group
Katz et al.[107]	Individualized office-based counseling-based intervention v group-based skill-building intervention	80 obese women	6 months	Counselling-based group weight loss was superior to skill-building group 3·9 kg (8·8 lb) v 1·7 kg (3·8 lb)

(Continued)

Table 22.3 (Continued)

Authors	Behaviour intervention	Participants	Length of study	Comments
Raynor et al.[108]	Behavior modification intervention emphasizing diet nutrient-density in group and individual sessions v group sessions (control)	31 families with an obese 8–12-year-old child	12 months	Significant decreases in percent overweight in children and parents in behavior modification group v control (−10·0% in children; 6·7% in parent v 8·0% in children, 5·3% in parents)
Saelens et al.[109]	Behavioural weight control intervention v a single session of physician weight counseling	44 overweight adolescents	4-month behavioral weight control program initiated in a primary care setting and extended through telephone and mail contact	Treatment group reduced their BMI Z score v control ($P < 0.04$). No significant changes in the secondary outcomes of total energy or dietary fat intake, physical activity, sedentary behavior, or problematic eating and weight-related behaviors or beliefs
Goldfield et al.[110]	Family-based behavioural treatment of both group and individualized treatment v group treatment only	31 families with obese children	12 months	No significant difference in weight loss between groups but group intervention was significantly more cost-effective
Mayer-Davis et al.[111]	Intensive lifestyle (reduced fat and calorie intake and increased activity) v intensive lifestyle plus ongoing formal evaluation for continuous quality improvement.	23 obese women with type 2 diabetes living in rural, medically under-seved communities	8 weeks	No difference between groups, the addition of formal evaluation did not result in improved outcomes.
Faith et al.[112]	TV viewing contingent on pedaling a stationary cycle ergometer v TV viewing not contingent on pedaling for control participants.	10 obese children	12 weeks	Experimental group showed significantly greater reductions in total body fat and percent leg fat
Epstein et al.[113]	Family-based behavioural weight control program with 3 arms: problem solving taught to parent and child, problem solving taught to child, or standard family-based treatment.	62 families stratified by sex and degree of child and parental obesity	6 month intervention with 2 year follow up weight	Significant weight loss in child only and standard family treatment compared to parent and child group
Knowler and Nathan[93]	Metformin (850 mg twice daily), or a lifestyle-modification program or placebo	3234 non-diabetic persons with elevated fasting and post-load plasma glucose concentrations	2·8 years	The incidence of diabetes was 11·0, 7·8, and 4·8 cases per 100 person-years in the placebo, metformin and lifestyle groups, respectively. The lifestyle intervention reduced the incidence by 58% (95% CI 48 to 66%) and metformin by 31% (95% CI 17 to 43%), as compared with placebo; the lifestyle intervention was significantly more effective than metformin

BMI, body mass index; VLED, very-low-energy diet

Table 22.4 Anti-obesity agents: how they work

Agents	Releasing agent			Reuptake inhibitor			Selective lipase inhibitor
	5-HT	NE	DA	5-HT	NE	DA	
Dexamphetamine		+++	+++				
Phentermine		+++	+++				
Sibutramine				+++	+++	+	
Orlistat							+++

5-HT = serotonin; NE = noradrenaline; DA = dopamine

Ann Intern Med 1993;**119**(7 pt 2):707–13 PharmacoEconomics 1994;**5**(suppl1):181–32 Prog Neuropsychopharmacol Biol Psychiatry 1988;**12**:575–84 Int J Obes Relat Metab Disord 1995;**19**:221 Psychopharmacology (Berl) 1992;**107**:303

up of 2·8 years.[93] Subjects randomized to the lifestyle intervention underwent 24 weeks of personal counseling with the goal of decreasing caloric intake by 700 kcal/day and increasing physical activity to 150 minutes per week, followed by monthly follow up visits. At 3 years, the lifestyle intervention had lost 4% of body weight and there was a 58% risk reduction for the development of diabetes. A1d These results favored lifestyle intervention so profoundly, that the trial was discontinued a year earlier than expected. This study is often quoted as the rationale for including behavior modification in the treatment of obesity. Further studies are needed to determine the appropriate style of behavior therapy for specific subgroups of patients.

Binge eating is often treated with either cognitive behavior therapy (focusing on treating the eating disorder and associated cognitive disturbances) or interpersonal therapy (focusing on achieving interpersonal change). In a randomized controlled trial of 220 subjects with binge eating comparing 20 sessions of cognitive behavior therapy versus interpersonal therapy, 45% of those treated with cognitive behavior therapy had stopped binging, compared to 8% in the interpersonal therapy group.[114] A1d At 12 months follow up, both treatments were equally effective in reducing binge eating due to relapse in the cognitive behavior therapy group and continued improvement in the interpersonal therapy group.[114] However, despite an improvement in the episodes of binge eating with both types of behavior therapy, no significant weight loss was seen.[115] Recently, a 14-week, double blind trial comparing topiramate to placebo, showed topiramate was associated with a significant reduction in binge frequency, binge day frequency, BMI and weight.[116] A1d Binge eating is a complex psychological illness and further studies are needed to define appropriate therapy in obesity.

Combining behavioral treatment with antidepressants has been found to improve symptoms and decrease body weight.[117–119] However, trials with antidepressants have been short, lasting 6–9 weeks and symptoms have recurred upon medication withdrawal. B4 Long-term use of antidepressants for the treatment of binge eating occurs in clinical practice, but there are no clinical trials to support its use.

Evidence for adjunctive pharmacotherapy

Weight loss medications are indicated for patients with a BMI greater than 30 kg/m^2 (27 kg/m^2 with comorbidities) who have not achieved weight loss with lifestyle changes. The approved antiobesity medications are listed in Table 22.4.

One study has shown that sibutramine has helped obese patients on a 4-week very-low-calorie diet maintain their weight loss for a period of 12 months.[120] Predictors of an effective response with the use of sibutramine include the following:

- a history of successful weight loss with lifestyle change alone
- a patient who struggles with recognition of signals for hunger and fullness
- a patient who admits to feelings of a lack of control over food intake.

In the STORM trial (Sibutramine Trial in Obesity Reduction and Maintenance) 605 patients were followed for 24 months. Eighty-two percent of the patients on sibutramine achieved at least a 5% weight reduction and were able to maintain it for 18 months compared to 16% of patients on placebo (odds ratio 4·64, absolute risk reduction 0·66, number needed to treat 2, $P < 0·001$).[121] A1d Of note, the dropout rate was similar to other randomized controlled trials in the obesity field – 42% in the sibutramine group, 50% in the placebo group.

The drug orlistat has also been shown to be an effective obesity medication. Orlistat works by inhibiting absorption of approximately 30% of dietary fat from the small intestine. The following group of patients have a superior response to orlistat:

Table 22.5   Anti-obesity drugs under development

- Phase III drugs

  - Ciliary neurotrophic factor (Axokine)
  - Cannabinoid CB1 agonist (Rimonabant)

- Various clinical stages

  - Topiramate (Topimax)
  - Bupropion (Wellbutrin)
  - Beta-3 agonists

(plus about 50 other compounds in pre-clinical or unknown stages of development)

- those with an inability to identify hidden fat in foods
- those with significant restaurant eating
- those seeking negative reinforcement.

In a double blind randomized controlled trial of obese patients with orlistat 120 mg (three times a day) or placebo for 1 year in conjunction with the hypocaloric diet (600 kcal/day deficit), Sjostrom *et al.* found the orlistat group lost a greater proportion of body weight than the placebo group (10·2% *v* 6·1%; least squared means (LSM) difference 3·9 kg, $P < 0·001$).[122]

The pharmacological treatment of obesity receives substantial attention from research and development. It is estimated that the annual market for obesity treatments in the USA ranges from US$735·5 million to US$1·23 billion. Drugs presently being evaluated in pre-clinical or unknown stages of development are presented in Table 22.5.

Evidence for complementary and alternative medicine

In the USA alone, health clubs, diet centers, low fat, and low carbohydrate snacks fuel a US$33 billion per year weight control industry.[123] There is no good evidence (well-designed randomized controlled trials) to support a magic bullet for weight loss despite the mass marketing of several over-the-counter complementary and alternative medicine (CAM) products that claim there is. However, it is not hard to see why despondent obese patients might grasp at a quick fix for their weight problems.

Table 22.6 provides a summary of systematic reviews of some of the most popular CAM products on the market today. Ephedra (sometimes called Ma Huang) was the active ingredient in some of the most popular CAM products that claim to promote weight loss. On 30 December 2003, the US Food and Drug Administration issued a consumer alert prohibiting use of Ephedra alkaloids.

Evidence for a surgical approach

Currently surgery is only recommended for obese patients with a BMI greater than 40 kg/m^2 or obese patients with a BMI greater than 35 kg/m^2 with comorbidities. The ability to comply with long-term lifestyle change is a requirement. Although there are many surgical procedures available for the morbidly obese patient, three surgical procedures are used most commonly: the Roux-en-Y gastric bypass, laparoscopic gastric banding, and biliopancreatic diversion. The advantages of carrying out the procedure laparoscopically are smaller scars, quicker recovery, and fewer wound problems. The advantage of any gastric surgery procedure is the sustained weight loss, and the dramatic decrease in comorbidities associated with obesity.

Roux-en-Y gastric bypass is considered the gold standard with well reported safety and efficacy.[126] Pories *et al.* have established the long-term benefits of the Roux-en-Y gastric bypass with an average, sustained weight loss of 45·4 kg (100 lb)[127,128] B4   This surgical procedure creates a 30 ml pouch that empties directly into the jejunum by an anastomosis, thus bypassing the duodenum. This technique induces weight loss by combining restricted intake and a moderate degree of malabsorption. The gastric pouch is separated from the excluded part of the stomach by stapling, and drained through a relatively large stoma directly into a jejunal loop in a Roux-en-Y arrangement. Thus, one limb of a Y-shaped reconstruction of jejunum allows the drainage of the gastric pouch, while the bile and pancreatic juice are evacuated by the second limb of the Y structure. Since hypertonic contents of the stomach rapidly enter the small bowel, patients frequently experience a dumping syndrome consisting of weakness and sweating after a carbohydrate-rich meal. This may obviously discourage them from consuming sweet foods; hence the opinion that this type of gastrojejunal surgery is particularly indicated for obese patients considered as "sweet eaters". It should be stressed, however, that by bypassing the duodenum, this kind of surgery may cause malabsorption of iron and calcium, increasing the risk of anemia, osteoporosis and hip fracture.[129]

Roux-en-Y gastric bypass purports low mortality and morbidity rates for morbidly obese patients. Data from the International Bariatric Surgery Registry of over 25 000 patients undergoing bariatric surgery of all types reports a death rate at 0·3% and a total postoperative morbidity of 7%.[130] With the introduction of laparoscopic technique for Roux-en-Y gastric bypass, risks associated with this surgery decreased dramatically. In reported series, operative mortality ranges between 0% and 1·5%,[131,132] and the overall incidence of major complications, including anastomotic leaks, pulmonary embolus and bowel occlusions, is between 0·6%[133] and 6%.[134] B4

A particular form of gastric bypass, referred to as biliopancreatic diversion, introduced in 1968 by Scopinaro, was designed to bypass a large part of the intestine with a

Table 22.6 Overview of complementary and alternative medicines for treatment of obesity

Product	Proposed mechanism of action	Efficacy evidence	Safety evidence	Reference
Chitosan	Blocks fat absorption	Does not appear to reduce body weight	Has not been studied	Crit Rev FS Nutr 2001;**41(1)**:1–28; 6 studies reviewed
Chromium	Increases insulin sensitivity and decreases circulating insulin	Majority of all studies done do not support a beneficial effect	Case report of suspected chromium picolinate-induced rhabdolysis from ingestion of 6–24 times the daily required allowance	same as above; 11 studies reviewed
DHEA	Thermogenic effect. Stimulates levels of cholecystokinin	Very small database, 1 RCT suggests benefit in normal weight subjects. Should be repeated in larger study	Cases of adverse events reported	same as above, 1 study
HCA (hydroxycitric acid) herbal compound in *Garcinia cambogia*	Increased rate of hepatic glycogen synthesis	Rigorous studies do not support efficacy	No adverse effects in short-term studies, longer studies needed	same as above and Jama 1998;**280(18)**: 1596–1600; 9 studies evaluated
Pyruvate	Increased thermogenesis	Results not clear	No safety issues so far but more studies needed	same as 1; 5 studies reviewed

DHEA, dihydroeipandrosterone.
RCT, randomized controlled trial

concomitant resection of the excluded part of the stomach to decrease the risk of gastric ulcer. While the volume of the remaining gastric pouch is much larger than in other procedures, and may vary from 200 ml to 500 ml, the loss of weight is essentially due to intestinal malabsorption. This procedure seems very effective in terms of loss of weight, but it frequently induces protein malnutrition and other metabolic complications. It is, therefore, not surprising that the extent of weight loss after this kind of surgery is proportional to the length of the intestinal bypass and, thus, to the severity of malabsorption and risks of late complications.

The LapBand is a silastic ring that forms a small gastric pouch and can be removed when weight loss has been achieved. LapBand adjustable gastric banding device was approved by the Food and Drug Administration in 2001.[135] The procedure is less invasive than the Roux-en-Y gastric bypass, and has a lower postoperative mortality rate. Unfortunately, the morbidity rate is higher, and the degree of weight loss is less than is observed with the Roux-en-Y gastric bypass. B4 In a review of 500 cases,[136] 10·4% had complications requiring an abdominal reoperation. Forty-nine underwent a reoperation for minor complications: slippage (*n* = 43, incisional hernias (*n* = 3), and reconnection of the catheter (*n* = 3). Three patients underwent a reoperation for major complications: gastroesophageal perforation (*n* = 2) and gastric necrosis (*n* = 1). Seven patients had pulmonary complications and 36 patients experienced minor problems related to the access port. Despite its complication rate, it is a very popular procedure due to its ease of insertion and its ability to achieve weight loss.

References

1 Pi-Sunyer FX. The obesity epidemic: pathophysiology and consequences of obesity. *Obes Res* 2002;**10**(Suppl 2): 97S–104S.

2 WHO1998. *Life in the 21st Century – A Vision for All.* The World Health Rep. Geneva, Switzerland: World Health Organization.

3 James PT, Leach R, Kalamara E, Shayeghi M. The worldwide obesity epidemic. *Obes Res* 2001;**9**(Suppl 4):228S–233S.

4 Caballero B. Introduction 2001 Symposium Obesity in developing countries biological and ecological factors. *J Nutr* 2001;**131**:866S–870S.

5 Flegal KM, Carroll MD, Ogden CL, Johnson CL. Prevalence and trends in obesity among US adults, 1999–2000. *JAMA* 2002;**288**:1723–7.

6 Popkin BM, Lu B, Zhai F. Understanding the nutrition transition: measuring rapid dietary changes in transitional countries. *Public Health Nutr* 2002;**5**:947–53.

7   Price RA, Gottesman II. Body fat in identical twins reared apart: roles for genes and environment. *Behav Genet* 1991;**21**:1–7.

8   Bouchard CA, Tremblay A, Despres JP. The response to exercise with constant energy intake in identical twins. *Obes Res* 1994;**5**:400–10.

9   Halaas JL, Gajiwala KS, Maffei M *et al.* Weight-reducing effects of the plasma protein encoded by the obese gene. *Science* 1995;**269**:543–6.

10 Chagnon YC, Rankinen T, Snyder EE, Weisnagel SJ, Parusse L, Bouchard C. The human obesity gene map: the 2002 update. *Obes Res* 2003;**11**:313–67.

11 Heini AF, Weinsier RL. Divergent trends in obesity and fat intake patterns: the American paradox. *Am J Med* 1997; **102**:259–64.

12 Putnam J, Allshouse J. Per Capita food supply trends: progress towards dietary guidelines. Food and Rural Economics Division, Economic Research Service, USDA, Washington, DC, 2002.

13 Nielsen SJ, Popkin BM. Patterns and trends in food portion sizes, 1977–1998. *JAMA* 2003;**289**:450–3.

14 Wadden TA, Brownell KD, Foster GD. Obesity: responding to the global epidemic. J Consult Clin Psychol 2002;**70**:510–25.

15 Kral TV, Roe LS, Rolls BJ. Does nutrition information about the energy density of meals affect food intake in normal-weight women? *Appetite* 2002;**39**:137–45.

16 DePietro L, Physical activity in the prevention of obesity: current evidence and research issues. *Med Sci Sports Exerc* 1999;**31**:S452–546.

17 Jebb, SA, Moore MS. Contribution of a sedentary lifestyle and inactivity to the etiology of overweight and obesity: current evidence and research issues. *Med Sci Sports Exerc* 1999;**31**:S534.

18 Allon, N. The stigma of overweight in everyday life. In: Wolman B (ed). *Psychological aspects of obesity: A handbook.* New York: Van Nostrand Reinhold, 1982.

19 Larkin JE, Pines HA. No fat persons need apply. *Social Work Occupations* 1979;**6**:312–27.

20 Karris L. Prejudice against obese renters. *J Social Psychol* 1977;**101**:159–60.

21 Canning H, Mayer J. Obesity – its possible effects on college admissions. *N Eng J Med* 1966;**275**:1172–4.

22 Gortmaker A, Must A, Perrin JM, Sobol AM, Dietz WH. Social and economic consequences of overweight in adolescence and young adulthood. *N Engl J Med* 1993;**329**:1008–12.

23 Smith DE, Marcus MD, Lewis CE, Fizgibbon M, Schreiner P. Prevalence of binge eating disorder, obesity, and depression in a biracial cohort of young adults. *Ann Behav Med* 1998;**20**:227–32.

24 Wadden TA, Womble LG, Stunkard AJ, Anderson DA. Psychosocial consequences of obesity and weight loss. In: Wadden TA, Stunkard AJ (eds). *Handbook of Obesity Treatment.* New York: Guilford Press, 2002.

25 Powers PS, Perez A, Boyd F, Rosemurgy A. *Int J Eating Disord* 1999;**25**:293–300.

26 Rand CS, Macgregor AM, Stunkard AJ. The night eating syndrome in the general population and among post-operative obesity surgery patients. *Int J Eating Disord* 1997;**22**:65–9.

27 Birketvedt GS, Florholmen J, Sundsfjord J *et al.* Behavioral and neuroendocrine characteristics of the night-eating syndrome. *JAMA* 1999;**282**:657–63.

28 Anonymous. Weight gain associated with intensive therapy in the diabetes control and complications trial. The DCCT Research Group. *Diabetes Care* 1988;**11**:567–73.

29 Farrow DC, Vaughan TL, Sweeney C *et al.* Gastroesophageal reflux disease, use of H_2 receptor antagonists, and risk of esophageal and gastric cancer. *Cancer Causes Control* 2000;**11**:231–8.

30 Locke GR III, Talley NJ, Fett SL *et al.* Risk factors associated with symptoms of gastroesophageal reflux. *Am J Med* 1999;**106**:642–9.

31 Ruhl CE, Everhart JE. Overweight, but not high dietary fat intake, increases risk of gastroesophageal reflux disease hospitalization: the NHANES 1 Epidemiologic Followup Study. *Ann Epidemiol* 1999;**9**:424–35.

32 Fisher BL, Pennathur A, Mutnick JL, Little AG. Obesity correlates with gastroesophageal reflux. *Dig Dis Sci* 1999; **44**:2290–4.

33 O'Brien, TF Jr, Stop EM. Lower esophageal sphincter pressure (LESP) and esophageal function in obese humans. *J Clin Gastroenterol* 1980;**2**:145–8.

34 Beauchamp G. Gastroesophageal reflux and obesity. *Surg Clin North Am* 1983;**63**:869–76.

35 Lundell L, Ruth M, Sandberg N *et al.* Does massive obesity promote abnormal gastroesophageal reflux. *Dig Dis Sci* 1995;**40**:1632.

36 Murray FE, Ennis J, Lennon JR, Crowe JP. Management of reflux oesophagitis: role of weight loss and cimetidine. *Ir J Med Sci* 1991;**160**:2–4.

37 Kjellin A, Ramel S, Rossner S, Thor K. Gastroesophageal reflux in obese patients is not reduced by weight reduction. *Scand J Gastroenterol* 1996;**31**:1047–51.

38 Jones KB Jr. Roux-en-Y gastric bypass: an effective antireflux procedure in the less than morbidly obese. *Obes Surg* 1998;**8**:35–8.

39 Smith SC, Edwards CB, Goodman GN. Symptomatic and clinical improvement in morbidly obese patients with gastroesophageal reflux disease following Roux-en-Y gastric bypass. *Obes Surg* 1997;**7**:479–84.

40 Field AE, Coakley EH, Must A *et al.* Impact of overweight on the risk of developing common chronic diseases during a 10-year period. *Arch Intern Med* 2001;**161**:1581–6.

41 Stampfer MJ, Maclure KM, Colditz GA, Manson JE, Willett WC. Risk of symptomatic gallstones in women with severe obesity. *Am J Clin Nutr* 1992;**55**:652–8.

42 Nakeeb A, Comuzzie AG, Martin L *et al.* Gallstones: genetics versus environment. *Ann Surg* 2002;**235**:842–9.

43 Maclure KM, Hayes KC, Colditz GA, Stampfer MJ, Speizer FE, Willett WC. Weight, diet, and the risk of symptomatic gallstones in middle-aged women. *N Engl J Med* 1989;**321**: 563–9.

44 Yang H, Petersen GM, Roth MP, Schonfield LJ, Marks JW:. Risk factors for gallstone formation during rapid loss of weight. *Dig Dis Sci* 1992;**37**:912–18.

45 Broomfield PH, Chopra R, Sheinbaum RC *et al.* Effects of ursodeoxycholic acid and aspirin on the formation of

lithogenic bile and gallstones during loss of weight. *N Engl J Med* 1988;**319**:1567–72.

46 Liddle RA, Goldstein RB, Saxton J. Gallstone formation during weight reduction dieting. *Arch Intern Med* 1989; **149**:1750–3.

47 Shiffman ML, Sugerman HJ, Kellum JM, Brewer WH, Moore EW. Gallstone formation after rapid weight loss: a prospective study in patients undergoing gastric bypass surgery for treatment of morbid obesity. *Am J Gastroenterol* 1991;**86**:1000–5.

48 Wattchow DA. Prevalence and treatment of gallstones after gastric bypass surgery for morbid obese. *Br J Med* 1983; **286**:763–4.

49 Weinsier RL, Wilson LJ, Lee J. Medically safe rate of weight loss for the treatment of obesity: a guideline based on risk of gallstone formation. *Am J Med* 1995;**98**:115–17.

50 Crowell MD, Cheskin LJ, Musial F. Prevalence of gastrointestinal symptoms in obese and normal weight binge eaters. *Am J Gastroenterol* 1994;**89**:387–91.

51 Sullivan SN, A prospective study of unexplained visible abdominal bloating. *NZ Med J* 1994;**107**:428–30.

52 Svedberg P, Johansson S, Wallander MA, Hamelin B, Pedersen NL. Extra-intestinal manifestations associated with irritable bowel syndrome: a twin study. *Aliment Pharmacol Ther* 2002;**6**:975–83.

53 Clements RH, Foster A, Richards WO *et al.* Gastrointestinal symptoms are more intense in morbidly obese patients and are improved with laprascopic Roux-en-Y Gastric Bypass [Abstract]. *Obes Surg* 2002;**12**:201.

54 Wanless IR, Lentz JS. Fatty liver hepatitis (steatohepatitis) and obesity: an autopsy study with analysis of risk factors. *Hepatology* 1990;**12**:1106–10.

55 Gholam PM, Kotler DP, Flancbaum LJ. Liver pathology in morbidly obese patients undergoing Roux-en-Y gastric bypass surgery. *Obes Surg* 2002;**12**:49–51.

56 Crespo J, Fernandez-Gil P, Hernandez-Guerra M *et al.* Are there predictive factors of severe liver fibrosis in morbidly obese patients with non-alcoholic steatohepatitis?. *Obes Surg* 2001;**11**:254–7.

57 Matteoni CA, Younossi ZM, Gramlich T, Boparai N, Liu YC, McCullough AJ. Nonalcoholic fatty liver disease: a spectrum of clinical and pathological severity. *Gastroenterology* 1999;**116**:1413–19.

58 Luyckx FH, Desaive C, Thiry A *et al.* Liver abnormalities in severely obese subjects: effect of drastic weight loss after gastroplasty. *Int J Obes Relat Metab Disord* 1998;**22**: 222–6.

59 Andersen T, Gluud C, Franzmann MB, Christoffersen P. Hepatic effects of dietary weight loss in morbidly obese subjects. *J Hepatol* 1991;**12**:224–9.

60 Palmer M, Schaffner F. Effect of weight reduction on hepatic abnormalities in. *Gastroenterology* 1990;**99**:1408–13.

61 Eriksson S, Eriksson KF, Bondesson L. Nonalcoholic steatohepatitis in obesity: a reversible condition. *Acta Med Scand* 1986;**220**:83–8.

62 Ueno T, Sugawara H, Sujaku K *et al.* Therapeutic effects of restricted diet and exercise in obese patients with fatty liver. *J Hepatol* 1997;**27**:103–7.

63 Wolk A, Gridley G, Svensson M, Nyren O, McLaughlin JK, Fraumeni JF, Adam HO. A prospective study of obesity and cancer risk (Sweden). *Cancer Causes Contr* 2001;**12**:13–21.

64 Russell GFM. Bulimia nervosa: an ominous variant of anorexia nervosa. *Psychol Med* 1979;**9**:429–448.

65 Ackard DM, Neumark-Sztainer D, Story M, Perry C. Overeating among adolescents: prevalence and associations with weight-related characteristics and psychological health. *Pediatrics* 2003;**111**:67–74.

66 Mitchell JE, Lancaster KL, Burgard MA *et al.* Long-term follow-up of patients' status after gastric bypass. *Obes Surg* 2001;**1**:464–8.

67 Balsiger BM, Kennedy FP, Abu-Lebdeh HS *et al.* Prospective evaluation of Roux-en-Y gastric bypass as primary operation for medically complicated obesity. *Mayo Clin Proc* 2000;**75**:673–80.

68 Horowitz M, Harding PE, Maddox AF *et al.* Gastric and oesophageal emptying in patients with type 2 (non-insulin-dependent) diabetes mellitus. *Diabetologia* 1989;**32**:151–9.

69 Schvarcz E, Palmér M, Åman J, Horowitz M, Stridsberg M, Berne C. Physiological hyperglycemia slows gastric emptying in normal subjects and patients with insulin-dependent diabetes mellitus. *Gastroenterology* 1997;**113**:60–6.

70 Nilsson P-H. Diabetic gastroparesis: A review. *J Diabetes Complications* 1996;**10**:113–22.

71 Carpenter KM, Hasin DS, Allison DB, Faith MS. Relationships between obesity and DSM-IV major depressive disorder, suicide ideation, and suicide attempts: results from a general population study. *Am J Public Health* 2000;**90**:251–7.

72 Roberts RE, Strawbridge WJ, Deleger S, Kaplan GA. Are the fat more jolly?. *Ann Behav Med* 2002;**24**:169–80.

73 National Institutes for Health. *A Practical Guide: Identification, Evaluation, and Treatment of Overweight and Obesity in Adults.* NIH publication no. 00-4084. Bethesda, Maryland: NIH, 2000.

74 Ayyad C, Anderson T. Long-term efficacy of dietary treatment of obesity: a systematic review of studies published between 1931 and 1999. *Obes Rev* 2000;**1**:113–19.

75 Serdula MK, Mokdad AH, Williamson DF, Galuska DA, Mendlein JM, Heath GW. Prevalence of attempting weight loss and strategies for controlling weight. *JAMA* 1999;**282**: 1353–8.

76 Ditschuneit HH, Flechtner-Mors M, Johnson TD, Adler G. Metabolic and weight loss effects of a long-term dietary intervention in obese patients. *Am J Clin Nutr* 1999;**69**: 198–204.

77 Astrup A, Grunwald GK, Melanson EL *et al.* The role of low-fat diets in body weight control: a meta-analysis of ad labium dietary intervention studies. *Int J Obes* 2000;**24**: 1545–52.

78 Yu-Poth S, Zhao G, Etherton T *et al.* Effects of the national Cholesterol Education Programs Step I and Step II dietary intervention programs on cardiovascular disease risk factors: a meta-analysis. *Am J Clin Nutr* 1999;**69**:6323–646.

79 Pirozzo S, Summerbell C, Cameron C, Glasziou P. Advice on low-fat diets. In: Cochrane Collaboration. *Cochrane Library* Oxford:Update Software, 2002;4.

80 Dietary Guidelines Advisory Committee. *Report of the Dietary Guidelines Advisory Committee on the Dietary Guidelines for Americans, 1995.* Washington DC: US Dept of Agriculture, Agricultural Research Services, 1995.

81 National Institutes of Health, National Heart, Lung, and Blood Institute, Obesity Education Initiative. *Clinical Guidelines on the Identification, Evaluation, and Treatment of Overweight and Obesity in Adults.* Bethseda Maryland: NIH, 1998.

82 Sondike SB, Copperman N, Jacobson MS. Effects of a low-carbohydrate diet on weight loss and cardiovascular risk factors in overweight adolescents. *J Pediatr* 2003;**142**:253–8.

83 Samaha FF, Iqbal N, Seshadri P *et al.* A low-carbohydrate as compared with a low-fat diet in severe obesity. *N Engl J Med* 2003;**348**:2074–81.

84 Foster GD, Wyatt HR, Hill JO, Mcguckin BG, Brill C, Mohammed S, Szapary PO, Rader DJ, Edman JE, Klein S, MD. A randomized trial of a low-carbohydrate diet for obesity. *N Engl J Med* 2003;**348**:2082–90.

85 Pate RR, Pratt SN, Blair S *et al.* Physical activity and public health: a recommendation from the Centers of Disease Control and Prevention and the American College of Sports Medicine. *JAMA* 1995;**273**:402–7.

86 Miller WC, Kocega DM, Hamilton EJ. A meta-analysis of the past 25 years of weight loss research using diet, exercise or diet plus exercise intervention. *Int J Obes* 1997;**21**:941–7.

87 Lichtman SW, Pisarska K, Berman E, *et al.* Discrepancy between self-reported and actual caloric intake and exercise in obese subjects. N Eng. J, Med. 1993;**327**:1893–1898.

88 Manson JE, WC, Willett, MJ, Stampfer *et al.* Body weight and mortality among women. *N Engl J Med* 1995; **333**:677–85.

89 Lee CD, Blair SN, Jackson AS. Cardiorespiratory fitness, body compositon, and all-cause and cardiovascular disease mortality in men. *Am J Clin Nutr* 1999;**69**:373–80.

90 Duncan JJ, Gordon NF, Scott CB. Women walking for health and fitness: how much is enough? *JAMA* 1991;**266**:3295–9.

91 Usui K. *Diabetes Res Clin Pract* 1998;**41**:57.

92 Perseghin G, Price TB, Peterson KF *et al.* Increased glucose transport – phosphorylation and muscle glycogen synthesis after exercise training in insulin resistant subjects. *N Eng J Med* 1996;**335**:1337–62.

93 Knowler WC, Nathan DM. Diabetes Prevention Program Research Group. Reduction in the incidence of type 2 diabetes with lifestyle intervention or metformin. *N Eng J Med* 2002;**346**:393–403.

94 Jakicic JM, Wing RR, Butler BA, Robertson RJ. Prescribing exercise in multiple short bouts versus one continuous bout: effects on adherance, cardiorespiratory fitness, and weight loss in overweight women. *Int J Obes* 1995;**19**:893–901.

95 McGuire MT, Wing RR, Klem ML, Seagle HM, Hill JO. Long term maintenance of weight loss: Do people who lose weight through various weight loss methods use different behaviors to maintain their weight? *Int J Obes* 1998;**22**: 572–7.

96 Wing RR. Behavioral approaches to the treatment of obesity. In: Bray G, Bouchard C, James WPT (eds). *Handbook of Obesity.* New York: Marcel Dekker, 1998.

97 Perri MG, McAdoo WG, McAllister DA. Effects of peer support and therapist contact on long-term weight loss. *J Consult Clin Psychol* 1987;**55**:615–17.

98 Wing RR. Behavioral weight control. In: Wadden TA, Stunkard AJ (eds). *Handbook of Obesity Treatment.* New York: Guilford Press, 2002.

99 Robinson TN, Killen JD, Kraemer HC *et al.* Dance and reducing television viewing to prevent weight gain in African-American girls: the Stanford GEMS pilot study. *Ethnicity Dis* 2002;**13**(1 Suppl 1):S65–77.

100 Story M, Sherwood NE, Himes JH *et al.* An after-school obesity prevention program for African-American girls: the Minnesota GEMS pilot study. *Ethnicity Dis* 2003; **13**(1 Suppl 1):S54–64.

101 Beech BM, Klesges RC, Kumanyika SK *et al.* Child- and parent-targeted interventions: the Memphis GEMS pilot study. *Ethnicity Dis* 2003;**13**(1 Suppl 1):S40–53.

102 Baranowski T, Baranowski JC, Cullen KW *et al.* The Fun, Food, and Fitness Project (FFFP): the Baylor GEMS pilot study. *Ethnicity Dis* 2003;**13**(1 Suppl 1):S30–9.

103 Tate DF, Jackvony EH, Wing RR. Effects of internet behavioral counseling on weight loss in adults at risk for type 2 diabetes: a randomized trial. *JAMA* 2003;**289**:1833–6.

104 Berkowitz RI, Wadden TA, Tershakovec AM. Cronquist JL. Behavior therapy and sibutramine for the treatment of adolescent obesity: a randomized controlled trial [Comment]. *JAMA* 2003;**289**:1805–12.

105 Ramirez EM, Rosen JC. A comparison of weight control and weight control plus body image therapy for obese men and women. *J Consult Clin Psychol* 2001;**69**:440–6.

106 Kaukua J, Pekkarinen T, Sane T, Mustajoki P. Health-related quality of life in WHO class II-III obese men losing weight with very-low-energy diet and behaviour modification: a randomised clinical trial. *Int J Obes Relat Metab Disord* 2002;**26**:487–95.

107 Katz DL, Chan W, Gonzalez M *et al.* Technical skills for weight loss: preliminary data from a randomized trial. *Prev Med* 2002;**34**:608–15.

108 Raynor HA, Kilanowski CK, Esterlis I, Epstein LH. A cost-analysis of adopting a healthful diet in a family-based obesity treatment program. *J Am Dietetic Assoc* 2002; **102**:645–56.

109 Saelens BE, Sallis JF, Wilfley DE, Patrick K, Cella JA, Buchta R. Behavioral weight control for overweight adolescents initiated in primary care. *Obes Res* 2002; **10**:22–32.

110 Goldfield GS, Epstein LH, Kilanowski CK, Paluch RA, Kogut-Bossler B. Cost-effectiveness of group and mixed family-based treatment for childhood obesity. *Int J Obes Relat Metab Disord* 2001;**25**:1843–9.

111 Mayer-Davis EJ, D'Antonio A, Martin M, Wandersman A, Parra-Medina D, Schulz R. Pilot studies of strategies for effective weight management in type 2 diabetes: Pounds Off With Empowerment (POWER). *Fam Community Health* 2001;**24**:27–35.

112 Faith MS, Berman N, Heo M *et al.* Effects of contigent television on physical activity and television viewing in obese children. *Pediatrics* 2001;**107**:1043–8.

113 Epstein LH, Paluch RA, Gordy CC, Saelens BE, Ernst MM. Problem solving in the treatment of childhood obesity. *J Consult Clin Psychol* 2000;**68**:717–21.

114 Agras WS, Walsh T, Fairburn CG, Wilson GT, Kraemer HC. A multicenter comparison of cognitive-behavioral therapy and interpersonal psychotherapy for bulimia nervosa. *Arch Gen Psychiatry* 2000;**57**:459–66.

115 Wadden TA, Foster GD, Letizia KA. Response of obese binge eaters to treatment by behavior therapy combined with very low calorie diet. *J Consult Clin Psychol* 1992;**60**:808–11.

116 McElroy SL, Arnold LM, Shapira NA *et al.* Topiramate in the treatment of binge eating disorder associated with obesity: a randomized, placebo-controlled trial. *Am J Psychiatry* 2003;**160**:255–61.

117 Hudson JI, McElroy SL. Fluvoxamine in the treatment of binge-eating disorder: a multicenter placebo-controlled double blind trial. *Am J Psychiatry* 1998;**155**:1756–62.

118 McElroy SL, Casuto LS. Placebo controlled trial of sertraline in the treatment of binge eating disorder. *Am J Psychiatry* 2000;**157**:1004–6.

119 Applinario JC, Godoy-Matos A. An open-label trial of sibutramine in obese patients with binge eating disorder. *J Clin Psychiatry* 2002;**63**:28–30.

120 Apfelbaum M, Vague P, Ziegler O *et al.* Long-term maintenance of weight loss after a very-low-calorie-diet: a randomized blinded trial of the efficacy and tolerability of sibutramine. *Am J Med* 1999;**106**:179–84.

121 James WP, Astrup A, Finer N *et al.* Effect of sibutramine on weight maintenance after weight loss: a randomised trial. STORM Study Group. Sibutramine Trial of Obesity Reduction and Maintenance. *Lancet* 2000;**356**:2119–25.

122 Sjostrom L, Rissanen A, Andersen T *et al.* Randomised placebo-controlled trial of orlistat for weight loss and prevention of weight regain in obese patients. European Multicentre Orlistat Study Group. *Lancet* 1998;**352**:167–72.

123 Institute of Medicine Annual Meeting 2000: Obesity. Institute of Medicine, Washington, DC.

124 Shekelle PG, Hardy ML, Morton SC *et al.* Efficacy and safety of ephedra and ephredrine for weight loss and athletic performance: a meta analysis. *JAMA* 2002;**289**:1537–45.

125 Haller CA, Benowitz MD. Adverse cardiovascular and central nervous system events associated with dietary supplements containing ephedra alkaloids. *N Engl J Med* 2000;**343**:1833–8.

126 Kral JG. Overview of surgical techniques for treating obesity. *Am J Clin Nutr* 1992;**55**(Suppl):552S–5S.

127 Pories, WJ, MacDonald KG, Morgan EJ *et al.* Surgical treatment of obesity and its effect on diabetes: 10-y follow-up. *Am J Clin Nutr* 1992;**55**:582S–585S.

128 DeMaria EJ, Sugerman HJ, Kellum JM *et al.* Results of 281 consecutive total laparoscopic Roux-en-Y gastric bypasses with a linear stapled gastrojejunostomy to treat morbid obesity. *Ann Surg* 2002;**235**:640–5.

129 Workshop on Research Considerations in Obesity Research. Sponsored by the National Institutes of Health and the American Society for Bariatric Surgery. Bethesda, Maryland: Lister Hill Center, National Institutes of Health, 4–5 June 2001.

130 Rationale for the Surgical Treatment of Morbid Obesity. www.asbs.org Updated 29 November 2001.

131 Smith SC, Goodman GN, Edwards CB. Roux-en-Y gastric bypass. A 7-year retrospective review of 3,855 patients. *Obes Surg* 1995;**5**:314–18.

132 MacLean LD, Rhode BM, Sampalis J *et al.* Results of the surgical treatment of obesity. *Am J Surg* 1993;**165**:155–60.

133 Linner JH. Comparative effectiveness of gastric bypass and gastroplasty: a clinical study. *Arch Surg* 1982;**117**:695–700.

134 Griffen WO, Bivins BA, Bell RM *et al.* Gastric bypass for morbid obesity. *World J Surg* 1981;**5**:817–822.

135 Lap-Band. Adjustable gastric band system report of safety and effectiveness data. US Federal Drug Agency Center for Devices and Radiological Health NDA, 2001; www.fda.gov/cdrh/pdf/P000008b.pdf

136 Zinzindohoue F, Chevallier JM, Douard R *et al.* Laparoscopic gastric banding: a minimally invasive surgical treatment for morbid obesity: prospective study of 500 consecutive patients. *Ann Surg* 2003;**237**:1–9.

23 Hepatitis C

Patrick Marcellin

Introduction

Hepatitis C is a relatively common disease. An estimated 3% of the world population is chronically infected with hepatitis C virus (HCV), and in Western countries HCV accounts for approximately 20% of cases of acute hepatitis and 70% of cases of chronic hepatitis.[1,2] Chronic hepatitis C is a major cause of cirrhosis and hepatocellular carcinoma. Moreover, HCV-related endstage liver disease is the most frequent indication for liver transplantation.

Hepatitis C is characterized by its propensity to chronicity. Since chronic hepatitis C is generally silent, its diagnosis is often fortuitous. Systematic screening should be recommended in subjects who have a history of blood transfusion or intravenous drug addiction. The enzyme-linked immunosorbent assay (ELISA) is the appropriate test for screening. In ELISA positive subjects, the presence of chronic infection is established by the detection of serum HCV RNA. A liver biopsy is recommended in patients who are HCV RNA positive with increased alanine transaminase (ALT) levels in order to assess the severity of the liver disease and determine whether there is an indication for therapy. Combination with pegylated interferon and ribavirin is now standard, which results in a sustained response in approximately 45% (genotype 1) and 80% (genotype 2 and 3) of patients. Genotyping of the virus is useful to assess the probability of sustained response and to determine the appropriate duration of combination therapy.

Acute hepatitis

HCV is mainly transmitted by blood. Post-transfusion acute hepatitis has almost disappeared and most subjects are now infected by intravenous drug use. The average incubation period is 7–8 weeks.[3] Prodromic symptoms are rare. Acute hepatitis C is icteric in a minority of cases (20%) and anicteric with no or few symptoms in most cases (80%). Symptoms are non-specific (malaise, nausea, and right upper quadrant pain followed by dark urine and jaundice) and similar to those in other types of acute viral hepatitis. Thus, the clinical diagnosis of acute hepatitis C is rarely made and the diagnosis is based on the presence of viral markers. Severe acute hepatitis is rare and whether fulminant hepatitis is caused by HCV is controversial.[4] When it is clinically apparent, the illness generally lasts for 2–12 weeks.

The first marker of HCV infection is serum HCV RNA detectable by polymerase chain reaction (PCR), as early as 1 week after exposure.[5–7] Anti-HCV antibodies become detectable at the acute phase of hepatitis in most cases but in some cases seroconversion is delayed up to several weeks. Serum alanine aminotransferase (ALT) levels begin to increase shortly before clinical symptoms appear. Peak levels are generally mildly or moderately increased, less than in acute hepatitis A or B.

In 15% of patients, hepatitis resolves spontaneously, serum ALT levels return to normal and serum HCV RNA becomes undetectable; anti-HCV antibodies remain detectable for many years. In 85% of patients, chronic infection develops and serum ALT levels can either normalize or remain elevated.[3,8,9] However, serum HCV RNA remains detectable, with the exception of a transient period of being negative in some cases.

Chronic hepatitis

There are three patterns of chronic hepatitis C: chronic hepatitis with normal serum ALT, mild chronic hepatitis and moderate to severe chronic hepatitis.

Chronic hepatitis with normal ALT level

About 25% of patients with chronic HCV infection have normal serum ALT levels despite detectable HCV RNA in serum.[10–15] These patients are often identified after donating blood or by systematic screening. The definition of this patient population includes presence of anti-HCV antibodies, HCV RNA, and persistently normal ALT levels (measured at least three times in 6 months). These patients are usually asymptomatic and histological lesions in the liver are generally mild.[2,16] Virological features (genotype and viral load) do not seem to be different in these patients as compared with those with increased serum ALT levels.[17,18] The long-term outcome of this group of patients is not known. Monitoring is recommended, but the prognosis is probably good.[19] A liver biopsy is not recommended for these patients.

Mild chronic hepatitis

About 50% of patients have mild liver disease with detectable serum HCV RNA and mildly elevated or fluctuating serum ALT levels. These patients are usually asymptomatic but may complain of fatigue. Liver histology shows mild necroinflammatory lesions and no or mild fibrosis. This type of chronic hepatitis C generally progresses very slowly and the long-term risk of developing cirrhosis is low. However, a minority of these patients may eventually develop more progressive liver disease.[2]

Moderate to severe chronic hepatitis

About 25% of patients have moderate to severe chronic hepatitis. These patients are difficult to distinguish from those with mild chronic hepatitis. Clinically, most are asymptomatic: the intensity of fatigue, if present, is not correlated with the severity of liver disease. Clinical examination is generally normal. Although these patients generally have higher serum ALT levels, the serum ALT level is not a good prognostic factor on an individual basis. Increased serum γ-glutamyl-transpeptidase, ferritin or γ-globulin levels, or thrombocytopenia usually indicate severe liver disease but are not always present, i.e. they are *fairly* specific but not *highly* specific markers of severity. Ultrasonographic abnormalities are useful when present. However, a liver biopsy is the most accurate way to distinguish mild from moderate or severe chronic hepatitis and thus assess the prognosis. Liver histology shows marked necroinflammatory lesions and extensive fibrosis (or unexpected cirrhosis). This pattern of chronic hepatitis is more common in older patients and in those with aggravating factors such as alcohol or immune deficiency. These patients have a high risk of developing cirrhosis in 5–10 years.[2,9]

Cirrhosis and hepatocellular carcinoma

HCV-related cirrhosis may be silent for many years. Thus, asymptomatic cirrhosis is often discovered at liver biopsy. In other cases, cirrhosis is diagnosed because of a complication (variceal hemorrhage, ascites, jaundice or hepatocellular carcinoma). Clinical examination, ultrasonography and biochemistry may help to predict the presence of cirrhosis.

Box 23.1 Extra-hepatic manifestations of hepatitis C

	Evidence of association
● Mixed cryoglobulinemia	+++
● Glomerulonephritis	+++
● Porphyria cutanea tarda	+
● Low grade malignant lymphoma	+
● Autoimmune thyroiditis	±
● Lichen planus	±
● Sjögren's syndrome	−
● Aplastic anemia	−
● Polyarteritis nodosa	−
● Erythema nodosum	−
● Idiopathic pulmonary fibrosis	−

In patients with HCV-related cirrhosis, mortality related to portal hypertension, hepatic failure or hepatocellular carcinoma is 2–5% per year. Endstage HCV-related cirrhosis is the most common indication for liver transplantation.[2] The incidence of hepatocellular carcinoma is high (3–4% per year).[20] Hepatocellular carcinoma generally occurs in patients with cirrhosis; it is exceptional in patients without cirrhosis. Although the rationale for systematic surveillance with ultrasonography and α-fetoprotein has not been not clearly demonstrated, it is usually recommended in patients with cirrhosis.[20]

Extrahepatic manifestations

Many extrahepatic manifestations have been described in association with HCV infection.[21,22] Some are well documented, while others may be fortuitous (Box 23.1).

The disorder which is most clearly, and most frequently, associated with HCV is mixed cryoglobulinemia.[23,24] Although detectable cryoglobulinemia is common in chronic hepatitis C (30–40%), it is usually asymptomatic. The clinical syndrome of cryoglobulinemia with arthralgias, Raynaud's disease, and purpura is rare (less than 1%). Glomerulonephritis or neuropathy are rare but may be severe.

Treatment

The goal of therapy in patients with chronic hepatitis C is to inhibit viral replication in order to decrease the activity of the liver disease. Decreased activity is believed to be associated with a decreased risk of occurrence of cirrhosis and therefore the risk of hepatocellular carcinoma.[25] In the past 10 years, efficacy of therapy of chronic hepatitis C has dramatically improved from less than 10% to more than 50%.

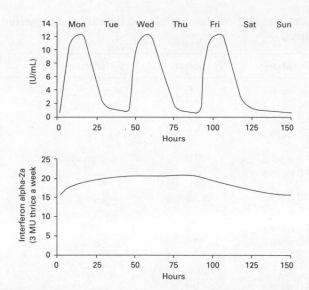

Figure 23.1 Plasma concentration of standard interferon (here interferon alpha-2a) administered by subcutaneous injections, three times per week, shows peaks followed by troughs of concentration. Conversely, the concentration obtained with pegylated interferon (here pegylated interferon alpha-2a) administered by subcutaneous injections, once a week, is more stable and prolonged

Interferon alpha

In chronic hepatitis C, the antiviral effect of interferon (IFN) has been well demonstrated, with a rapid decrease of serum HCV RNA within the first weeks of therapy, with a parallel decrease in serum ALT levels.[26] B4 Treatment efficacy is defined by a sustained virological response demonstrated by undetectable serum HCV RNA with a sensitive method, 6 months after treatment is stopped. A sustained virological response is generally associated with a sustained biochemical response (sustained normalization of serum ALT levels).[27,28] B4 In more than 95% of cases, this response lasts with no relapse later on, and it is accompanied by a gradual improvement in histologic liver lesions that in certain cases, completely disappear.[28] Although some studies have shown that HCV RNA is undetectable in the liver of patients with a sustained virological response 2–5 years after treatment,[28] the eradication of the HCV infection has not been entirely proved and the benefit on survival, although probable, has not been firmly established.

Since the first study carried out with standard IFN in 1986,[29] several controlled studies have provided a reference treatment protocol of 3 million units (MU), three times a week for 12 months.[25] This protocol resulted in a sustained virological response in about 15% of cases. The administration of higher doses of IFN or extending the duration of treatment did not increase the effectiveness of treatment and was accompanied by increased intolerance to treatment.[30,31]

Combination of interferon alpha with ribavirin

A major improvement occurred in 1998 with treatment combining IFN with ribavirin. Indeed, two large controlled studies confirmed that this therapeutic protocol administered for 24 or 48 weeks (according to the HCV genotype and baseline serum HCV RNA level) resulted in a sustained virological response rate (around 40%) that was significantly greater than that with IFN alone[32,33] (Table 23.1). Ala As a result, this combination became the treatment of choice for chronic hepatitis C, and it was recommended in the statement of the European Association for the Study of the Liver (EASL) International Consensus Conference on Hepatitis C held in Paris in 1999.[34]

Combination of pegylated interferon with ribavirin

More recently, the efficacy of treatment has improved even more with the replacement of standard IFN by IFN conjugated with polyethylene glycol (PEG IFN). This new form of IFN reduces elimination of IFN by the kidneys, thus significantly increasing its half-life and resulting in more stable plasma concentrations of IFN that last 1 week (Figure 23.1). Moreover, pegylation reduces the immunogenicity of the protein (reduction of the production of anti-IFN antibodies). Finally the number of injections has been reduced from thrice weekly to once weekly because of improved pharmacokinetics, which is obviously more comfortable for the patient.

Two PEG IFNs which differ in the quality and quantity of conjugated PEG to IFN have been evaluated in patients with chronic hepatitis C: 12 kD of linear PEG for IFN alpha-2b and 40 kD ramified PEG for IFN alpha-2a. In both cases PEG IFNs have been shown to be twice as effective overall than the corresponding non-pegylated IFNs[35,36] (see Table 23.1). Ala Most importantly, the combination of these agents with ribavirin increased the efficacy of combination therapy and resulted in a sustained average virological response rate of 55%, which has been the best result obtained in the treatment of hepatitis C.[37,38] Ala

A recent randomized controlled study of the combination of PEG IFN alpha-2a and ribavirin showed that the optimal regimens were 24 weeks of therapy with a 800 mg daily dose of ribavirin in patients with genotype 2 or 3 and 48 weeks with a 1000 mg or 1200 mg daily dose of ribavirin (according to weight more or less than 75 kg) in patients with genotype 1 (see Figure 23.2).[39] Ala These therapeutic schedules have been recommended by the French and the US consensus conferences held in 2002.[40–42]

Specific subgroups of patients

In the large clinical trials that were described above, the patients were selected according to strict criteria. As a result,

Table 23.1 Main randomized controlled studies of combinations of standard interferon (IFN) and ribavirin and pegylated interferon (PEG IFN) with ribavirin in patients with chronic hepatitis C

Protocol	Dose	Duration	Response %	Reference
IFN alpha 2b	3 MU TIW	24 weeks	6	McHutchison et al.[33]
IFN alpha 2b + ribavirin	3 MU TIW 1000–1200 mg	24 weeks	33	Poynard et al.[32]
IFN alpha 2b	3 MU TIW	48 weeks	16	
IFN alpha 2b + ribavirin	3 MU 1000–1200 mg	48 weeks	41	
IFN alpha-2a	6 MU then 3 MU	48 weeks	19	Zeuzem et al.[35]
PEG IFN alpha-2a	180 micrograms/week	48 weeks	39	
IFN alpha-2b	3 MU	48 weeks	12	Lindsay et al.[36]
PEG IFN alpha-2b	1 kg/week	48 weeks	25	
IFN alpha-2b + ribavirin	3 MU 1000–1200 mg	48 weeks	47	Manns et al.[37]
PEG IFN alpha-2b + ribavirin	1·5 kg/week then 0·5 kg/week 1000–1200 mg/day	48 weeks	47	
PEG IFN alpha-2b + ribavirin	1·5 kg/week 800 mg/day	48 weeks	54	
IFN alpha-2b + ribavirin	3 MU 1000–1200 mg/day	48 weeks	44	Fried et al.[38]
PEG IFN alpha-2a	180 micrograms/week	48 weeks	29	
PEG IFN alpha-2a + ribavirin	180 micrograms/week 1000–1200 mg/day	48 weeks	56	

MU, Million Units; TIW, three times a week

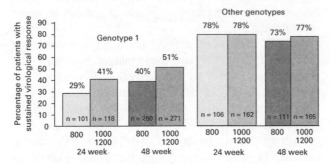

Figure 23.2 Sustained virological response rates according to the dose of ribavirin and the duration of treatment in patients with genotype 1 and in patients with genotype non-1.[39] All patients (four treatment arms) received the same dose of pegylated interferon alpha-2a (180 micrograms every week) and 800 mg or 1000/1200 mg ribavirin

treatment efficacy has not been clearly established for a certain number of large, or severely ill patient subgroups who have not been included in controlled studies.

One important group is patients who did not respond to initial treatment with interferon alone or with the combination of standard IFN with ribavirin. Preliminary data suggest that re-treatment with the combination of PEG IFN with ribavirin is effective in those who had received IFN therapy (around 40% sustained virological response) and is not effective in those who have received combination therapy

(around 10% sustained virological response). Some studies suggest that the triple therapy combining interferon, ribavirin and amantadine could be effective in these patients.[43] B4 However, these results must be confirmed in larger ongoing controlled studies.

Another specific group is patients with cirrhosis. In these patients, combination therapy of PEG IFN with ribavirin gives a lower but clinically useful rate of sustained virological response (around 40%). Some studies have suggested that treatment with IFN nevertheless reduces the risk of the complications of cirrhosis, in particular, hepatocellular carcinoma.[44] A1c However, this hypothesis is controversial, and other studies did not show any significant difference between treated and untreated patients.[45] B4 Although antiviral therapy is probably beneficial in patients who respond to treatment, the potential benefit in non-responder patients has not been shown.[46] There are ongoing controlled prospective studies to evaluate the benefits of maintenance therapy with PEG IFN alone in patients with cirrhosis.

In patients with normal serum ALT levels, the response rate to IFN monotherapy does not seem to be different from that observed in other patients. The efficacy of combined therapy (PEG IFN and ribavirin) is under evaluation. Currently, in these patients, who generally have mild liver lesions and a very slow progression of the liver disease, treatment is generally not recommended.[16,40–42]

Finally, when the diagnosis of HCV infection is made at the acute stage, it has been clearly established that treatment (only IFN alone has been evaluated) reduces the risk of progression to chronic hepatitis[47] (approximately 50% instead of 80%). An especially high response rate (98%) was reported in a selected population of patients with a more intensive treatment regimen with a daily dosing of IFN.[48] B4 Combination therapy has not yet been evaluated in this group.

In patients with chronic hepatitis C and human immunodeficiency virus (HIV) coinfection, the progression to cirrhosis is more rapid and more frequent.[49] Small studies showed that the response rates to therapy are lower than those usually observed in HIV negative patients.[50] B4 Large randomized controlled trials of the combination of PEG IFN with ribavirin are in progress. Serious complications possibly due to the mitochondrial toxicity of ribavirin have recently been described. These complications are stimulated by interactions between ribavirin and certain antiretroviral agents (zidovudine and stavudine).

Liver transplantation

Chronic hepatitis C is the main indication for (approximately 30%) liver transplantation in the USA and Europe. Transplantation can be justified by the presence of decompensated cirrhosis, hepatocellular carcinoma or a combination of both. The results of transplantation are basically limited by the nearly constant recurrence of HCV infection in the graft, as shown by detectable HCV RNA in serum an average of 2 weeks after transplantation.[51] Although the 5-year survival rate of these patients is comparable to transplantation for other liver diseases, recent studies have shown that their long-term prognosis is poorer and that there is an increased incidence of cirrhosis in these grafts, for reasons that are not yet clearly understood. At present the tendency is to reduce immunosuppressive treatments as quickly as possible, as they may be one of the main factors associated with progression of chronic hepatitis C in the graft. Preliminary studies suggest that standard combination therapy may be effective but is not well tolerated in these patients.[52] B4 Studies on the combination of PEG IFN and ribavirin are in progress.

Factors predictive of response to treatment

The probability of a sustained virological response to treatment essentially depends upon the genotype. Younger age, female sex, the absence of or minimal fibrosis and low viral load are also associated with a better rate of response but to a lesser extent. Unfortunately, genotype 1 (1a or 1b) which is associated with a poor response to treatment is the most frequent genotype in Europe and the USA and is present in 60–80% of the cases depending on the country. Likewise in most Western countries, such as in France this genotype is the most frequent (57% of cases), while genotypes 2 and 3 which are associated with a good response to treatment are less frequent (11% and 22% of patients, respectively).[53]

Treatment with IFN alone resulted in an overall long-term response in 30% of patients with genotypes 2 and 3 but in only 5% of those with genotype 1 (1a or 1b).[54] With standard combination therapy, the sustained virological response rate is twice as high (60% for genotypes 2 or 3 whatever the viral load), and increases to 35% in patients with genotype 1 and a low viral load (defined as less than 2 million RNA viral copies/ml).[32,33] A1c The duration of treatment (12 months) only affects the sustained virological response in patients with genotype 1 and a high viral load.[34]

In patients infected with HCV genotype 1, combination therapy of PEG IFN alpha-2a or 2b is more effective than the combination of standard IFN alpha-2a or 2b with ribavirin[37,38] A1c (see Table 23.1). In patients with genotype 2 or 3, results of studies on combination therapy with PEG IFNs are contradictory: combination therapy with PEG IFN alpha-2b is not significantly more effective[37]; combination therapy with PEG IFN alpha-2a is significantly more effective.[37,38] A1c

Early virological response defined by the early disappearance of detectable HCV RNA in serum during treatment is the best predictive factor of a sustained virological response. This was shown in early studies with IFN alone,[30] then with the combination with standard interferon.[34] This has been confirmed in recent studies with pegylated combination.[37,38] Thus, it would seem that treatment can be discontinued after 12 weeks of treatment if the serum HCV RNA level has decreased by less than 2 log since the probability of a sustained virological response in these cases is approximately 0–3%.[38]

Adverse effects

Adverse effects of IFN alpha

During treatment, the quality of life is impaired.[55] The main adverse effects of IFN alpha are flu-like symptoms, that are usually moderate and can be controlled with paracetamol.[56,57] Nevertheless, these symptoms may be more severe and require a reduction in the dose and rarely discontinuation of treatment. Treatment may also be discontinued in rare cases of severe depression (with risk of suicide) and thyroid disorders. Treatment needs to be stopped in less than 10% of cases overall.

Tolerance to treatment with PEG IFN alone is globally comparable to tolerance to standard IFN.[35,36] A1a There is no difference in the frequency of severe adverse effects, in particular psychiatric ones. Flu-like symptoms, inflammatory skin reactions at the injection site and neutropenia are slightly more frequent. Tolerance to combination therapy with PEG

IFNs is basically similar to that of standard combination therapy. Although the dose must be reduced slightly more frequently (42% of cases compared with 34%), the rates of discontinuation of treatment are similar (14% and 13%, respectively).[37,38]

Adverse effects of ribavirin

The main side effect of ribavirin is hemolytic anemia which is related to direct toxicity on the red cells. It is responsible for a mean decrease of 3 g/dl occurring usually during the first month of treatment.[32,33,37,38] Ala This anemia may require decreasing the dose (rarely discontinuation) of ribavirin in approximately 20% of patients. A cardiac assessment is recommended in patients older than 50 years prior to therapy. Because of the teratogenic potential, both women of childbearing potential and their partners must use an effective contraceptive.

Indications for treatment

In patients with acute hepatitis C, treatment is indicated since it significantly reduces the risk of progression to chronic hepatitis.

In patients with chronic hepatitis C, the decision to treat should be based on various parameters including the age of the patient, the risk of developing cirrhosis, the chances of response, any other medical circumstances that might reduce the patient's life expectancy or contraindications to the use of interferon or ribavirin. Moreover, the side effects and quality of life during treatment must be taken into account.

The indications are based mainly on the stage and the risk of progression of fibrosis which are determined by the results of a liver biopsy.[40–42,58,59] Thus the risk–benefit ratio for treatment seems to be positive in patients with severe or moderate chronic hepatitis C, while it has not been proved in patients with mild chronic hepatitis C. The genotype is very helpful for evaluating the probability of a sustained virological response to treatment.

Naive patients (patients who have never been treated) should be treated with the combination of PEG IFN and ribavirin. Patients with contraindications or who do not tolerate ribavirin can be treated with PEG IFN alone.

Recent consensus conferences have recommended 24 weeks of therapy with a 800 mg daily dose of ribavirin in patients with genotype 2 or 3 and 48 weeks of therapy with a daily dose of ribavirin of 1000 mg or 1200 mg according to weight (more or less than 75 kg) in patients with genotype 1.[40–42]

New strategies

Despite the major progress made in research on hepatitis C in the last ten years, numerous questions remain both on the understanding of the pathogenesis of the disease and the treatment of hepatitis C.[60,61] First, further knowledge concerning the natural history of HCV infection is necessary and the prognostic factors must be precisely defined, requiring studies with large cohorts. Ideally, procedures that are less invasive than liver biopsy, such as blood markers of fibrosis should be developed to evaluate the severity of liver damage. The influence of factors such as age, sex and alcohol should be more clearly determined and other as yet unknown but potentially important factors should be investigated.[59] One of the most urgent problems is to understand the mechanisms that favor the fibrogenesis and carcinogenesis associated with chronic hepatitis C.

The second problem is to improve treatment efficacy. Although the combination of PEG IFN with ribavirin is obviously an important step forward, the results are still unsatisfactory with roughly 45% of non-responders overall and 55% non-responders among patients with genotype 1. Better use of existing drugs will probably not significantly improve response rates. The development of new molecules is therefore necessary, such as inhibitors of viral enzyme (protease, helicase and polymerase).[61] Such molecules are currently in phase I and II studies. However, it will be many years before these drugs are available for the treatment of patients with chronic hepatitis C, most probably in combination as in current antiretroviral therapy.

An innovative therapeutic approach is based on antisense oligonucleotides developed to specifically hybridize to viral RNA and thus inhibit HCV replication. Another molecular approach involves the use of ribozymes (ribonucleic acids with an enzymatic action).

Finally, the major long-term goal is to develop vaccines, but there are several major scientific and practical problems that need to be overcome[61,62]: (i) the great variability of viral proteins; (ii) the lack of an animal model of HCV infection except for the chimpanzee; and (iii) the lack of an effective *in vivo* system of replication (the replicon system currently available is an artificial system the results of which cannot be extrapolated to clinical effects). The development of animal models and *in vivo* cultures are a major challenge. Results in the chimpanzee have shown that the proteins of the recombinant envelope may cause an antibody response and a response of T CD4 cells. Nevertheless, candidates for a preventive vaccine are still probably far off, while in the nearer future therapeutic vaccines are probably a more realistic possibility.

Conclusion

Hepatitis C is a major public health problem. An increase in the incidence of cirrhosis and hepatocellular carcinoma linked to HCV is expected in the next 10 years. Large scale surveillance and improved treatment are necessary to slow or stop the progress of liver disease in infected individuals. For this, major efforts are necessary to improve the efficacy and reduce the costs of treatment, so that a greater number of patients can receive better care worldwide.

References

1 Alter MJ. Epidemiology of hepatitis C in the West. *Semin Liver Dis* 1995;**15**:5–14.

2 Marcellin P. Hepatitis C: the clinical spectrum of the disease. *J Hepatol* 1999;**31**(Suppl 1):9–16.

3 Dienstag JL. NANB hepatitis I. Recognition, epidemiology and clinical features. *Gastroenterology* 1993;**85**:439–62.

4 Hoofnagle JH, Carithers RL, Shapiro C *et al.* Fulminant hepatic failure: summary of a workshop. *Hepatology* 1995;**21**:240–52.

5 Farci P, Alter HJ, Wong D *et al.* A long-term study of hepatitis C virus replication in non-A, non-B hepatitis. *N Engl J Med* 1991;**325**:98–104.

6 Puoti M, Zonaro A, Ravaggi A *et al.* Hepatitis C virus RNA and antibody response in the clinical course of acute hepatitis C infection. *Hepatology* 1992;**16**:877–81.

7 Hino K, Sainokami S, Shimoda K *et al.* Clinical course of acute hepatitis C and changes in HCV markers. *Dig Dis Sci* 1994;**39**:19–27.

8 Alter HJ, Purcell RH, Shih JW *et al.* Detection of antibody to hepatitis C virus in prospectively followed transfusion recipients with acute and chronic non-A, non-B hepatitis. *N Engl J Med* 1989;**321**:1494–500.

9 Mattsson L, Sönnerborg A, Weiland O. Outcome of acute symptomatic non-A, non-B hepatitis: a 13-year follow-up study of hepatitis C virus markers. *Liver* 1993;**13**:274–8.

10 Esteban JI, Lopez-Talavera JC, Genescà J *et al.* High rate of infectivity and liver disease in blood donors with antibodies to hepatitis C virus. *Ann Intern Med* 1991;**115**:443–9.

11 Alberti A, Morsica G, Chemello L *et al.* Hepatitis C viremia and liver disease in symptom-free individuals with anti-HCV. *Lancet* 1992;**340**:697–8.

12 Prieto M, Olaso V, Verdu C *et al.* Does the healthy hepatitis C virus carriers state really exist? An analysis using polymerase chain reaction. *Hepatology* 1995;**22**:413–17.

13 Shakil AO, Conry-Cantilena C, Alter HJ *et al.* Volunteer blood donors with antibody to hepatitis C virus: clinical, biochemical, virologic and histologic features. *Ann Intern Med* 1995;**123**:330–7.

14 Serfaty L, Nousbaum JB, Elghouzzi MH *et al.* Prevalence, severity, and risk factors of liver disease in blood donors positive in a second-generation anti-hepatitis C virus screening test. *Hepatology* 1995;**21**:725–9.

15 Conry-Cantilena C, Van Raden M, Gibble J *et al.* Routes of infection, viremia, and liver disease in blood donors found to have hepatitis C infection. *N Engl J Med* 1996;**334**:1691–6.

16 Marcellin P, Lévy S, Erlinger S. Therapy of hepatitis C:patients with normal aminotransferase levels. *Hepatology* 1997;**26**(Suppl. 1):133S–137S.

17 Martinot-Peignoux M, Marcellin P, Gournay J *et al.* Detection and quantitation of serum hepatitis C virus (HCV) RNA by branched DNA amplification in anti-HCV positive blood donors. *J Hepatol* 1994;**20**:676–8.

18 Silini E, Bono F, Cividini A *et al.* Differential distribution of hepatitis C virus genotypes in patients with and without liver function abnormalities. *Hepatology* 1995;**21**:285–290.

19 Martinot-Peignoux M, Boyer N, Cazals-Hatem D *et al.* Prospective study on anti-hepatitis C virus-positive patients with persistently normal serum alanine transaminase with or without detectable serum hepatitis C virus RNA. *Hepatology* 2001;**34**:1000–5.

20 Bruix J, Sherman M, Llovet JM *et al.* Clinical management of hepatocellular carcinoma: conclusions of the Barcelona-2000 EASL Conference. *J Hepatol* 2001;**35**:421–30.

21 Marcellin P, Benhamou JP. Autoimmune disorders associated with hepatitis C. In: Boyer JL, Ockner RK (eds). *Progress in Liver Diseases*. Volume XIII. Philadelphia: WB Saunders, 1995.

22 Koff RS, Dienstag JL. Extrahepatic manifestations of hepatitis C and the association with alcohol liver disease. *Semin Liver Dis* 1995;**15**:101–9.

23 Pawlotsky JM, Ben Hayia M, André C *et al.* Immunological disorders in C virus chronic active hepatitis: a prospective case–control study. *Hepatology* 1994;**19**:841–8.

24 Lunel F, Musset L, Franjeul L *et al.* Cryoglobulinemia in chronic liver diseases: role of hepatitis C virus and liver damage. *Gastroenterology* 1994;**106**:1291–300.

25 Hoofnagle JH, Di Bisceglie AM. The treatment of chronic viral hepatitis. *N Engl J Med* 1997;**226**:347–56.

26 Neumann AU, Lam NP, Dahari H *et al.* Hepatitis C viral dynamics *in vivo* and the antiviral efficacy of interferon-a therapy. *Science* 1998;**282**:103–7.

27 Chemello L, Cavalletto L, Casarin C *et al.* Persistent hepatitis C viremia predicts late relapse after sustained response to interferon-a in chronic hepatitis C. *Ann Intern Med* 1996;**124**:1058–60.

28 Marcellin P, Boyer N, Gervais A *et al.* Long term histologic improvement and disappearance of intra hepatic HCV RNA after alpha interferon therapy in patients with chronic hepatitis C. *Ann Intern Med* 1997;**127**:875–81.

29 Hoofnagle JH, Mullen KD, Jones DB *et al.* Treatment of chronic non-A, non-B hepatitis with recombinant human alpha interferon: a preliminary report. *N Engl J Med* 1986;**315**:1575–8.

30 Marcellin P, Pouteau M, Martinot-Peignoux M *et al.* Lack of benefit of escalating dosage of interferon alpha in patients with chronic hepatitis C. *Gastroenterology* 1995;**109**:156–65.

31 Shiffman ML. Use of high-dose interferon in the treatment of chronic hepatitis C. *Semin Liver Dis* 1999;**19**(Suppl 1):25–33.

32 Poynard T, Marcellin P, Lee SS *et al.* Randomised trial of interferon a2b plus ribavirin for 48 weeks or for 24 weeks versus interferon a2b plus placebo for 48 weeks for treatment of chronic infection with hepatitis C virus. *Lancet* 1998;**352**:1426–32.

33 McHutchison JG, Gordon SC, Schiff ER *et al.* Interferon alpha-2b alone or in combination with ribavirin as initial treatment for chronic hepatitis C. *N Engl J Med* 1998;**339**:1485–92.

34 EASL International Consensus Conference on Hepatitis C. Consensus Statement. *J Hepatol* 1999;**30**:956–61.

35 Zeuzem S, Feinman SV, Rasenack J *et al.* Peginterferon alpha-2a in patients with chronic hepatitis C. *N Engl J Med* 2000;**343**:1666–72.

36 Lindsay KL, Trépo C, Heintges T *et al.* A randomized, double-blind trial comparing pegylated interferon alpha-2b to interferon alpha-2b as initial treatment for chronic hepatitis C. *Hepatology* 2001;**34**:395–403.

37 Manns MP, McHutchison JG, Gordon S *et al.* Peginterferon alpha-2b plus ribavirin compared with IFN-2b plus ribavirin for initial treatment of chronic hepatitis C: a randomised trial. *Lancet* 2001;**358**:958–65.

38 Fried MW, Shiffman ML, Reddy RK *et al.* Peginterferon alpha-2a plus ribavirin for chronic hepatitis C virus infection. *N Engl J Med* 2002;**347**:975–82.

39 Hadziyannis SJ, Sette H, Morgan TR *et al.* Peginterferon alpha-2a (40 kilodaltons) and ribavirin combination therapy in chronic hepatitis C: randomized study of the effect of treatment duration and ribavirin dose. *Ann Intern Med* 2004 (in press).

40 French Consensus Conference Treatment of Hepatitis C. Guidelines. *Gastroenterol Clin Biol* 2002;**26**:B312–B320.

41 Lerebours E, Marcellin P, Dhumeaux D. Treatment of hepatitis C: the French Consensus 2002. *Gut* 2003;**52**:1784–7.

42 National Institutes of Health Consensus Development Conference Statement: management of hepatitis C:2002. *Hepatology* 2002;**36**(Suppl 1):S3–S21.

43 Brillanti S, Levantesi F, Masi L *et al.* Triple antiviral therapy as a new option for patients with interferon nonresponsive chronic hepatitis C. *Hepatology* 2000;**32**:630–4.

44 Nishiguchi S, Kuroki T, Nakatani S *et al.* Randomised trial of effects of interferon-α on incidence of hepatocellular carcinoma in chronic active hepatitis C with cirrhosis. *Lancet* 1995;**346**:1051–5.

45 Fattovich G, Giustina G, Degos F *et al.* Morbidity and mortality in compensated cirrhosis type C: a retrospective follow-up study of 384 patients. *Gastroenterology* 1997;**112**:463–72.

46 Yoshida H, Shiratori Y, Moriyama M *et al.* Interferon therapy reduces the risk for hepatocellular carcinoma: national surveillance program of cirrhotic and noncirrhotic patients with chronic hepatitis C in Japan. *Ann Intern Med* 1999;**131**:174–81.

47 Alberti A, Boccato S, Vario Alessandro *et al.* Therapy of acute hepatitis C. *Hepatology* 2002;**36**(Suppl 1):S195–S200.

48 Jaeckel E, Cornberg M, Wedemeyer H *et al.* Treatment of acute hepatitis C with interferon alpha-2b. *N Engl J Med* 2001;**345**:1452–7.

49 Di Martino V, Rufat P, Boyer N *et al.* The influence of human immunodeficiency virus coinfection on chronic hepatitis C in injection drug users: a long-term retrospective cohort study. *Hepatology* 2001;**34**:1193–9.

50 Thomas DL. Hepatitis C and human immunodeficiency virus infection. *Hepatology* 2002;**36**(Suppl 1):S201–S209.

51 Féray C, Caccamo L, Alexander GJM *et al.* European collaborative study on factors influencing outcome after liver transplantation for hepatitis C. *Gastroenterology* 1999;**11**:619–25.

52 Bizollon T, Palazzo U, Ducerf C *et al.* Pilot study of the combination of alpha interferon and ribavirin as therapy of recurrent hepatitis C after liver transplantation. *Hepatology* 1997;**26**:500–4.

53 Martinot-Peignoux M, Roudot-Thoraval F, Mendel I *et al.* Hepatitis C virus genotypes in France: relationship with epidemiology, pathogenicity and response to interferon therapy. *J Viral Hepatitis* 1999;**6**:435–43.

54 Martinot-Peignoux M, Boyer N, Pouteau M *et al.* Predictors of sustained response to alpha interferon therapy in chronic hepatitis C. *J Hepatol* 1998;**29**:214–23.

55 Foster GR. Hepatitis C virus infection: side effects and quality of life. *J Hepatol* 1999;**31**(Suppl 1):250–4.

56 Dusheiko G. Side effects of alpha interferon in chronic hepatitis C. *Hepatology* 1997;**26**(Suppl 1):112S–121S.

57 Gervais A, Boyer B, Marcellin P. Tolerability of treatments for viral hepatitis. In: *Drug Safety.* Auckland: Adis International Ltd, 2001;**24**:375–84.

58 Seeff LB. Natural history of chronic hepatitis C. *Hepatology* 2002;**36**(Suppl 1):S35–S46.

59 Marcellin P, Asselah T, Boyer N. Fibrosis and disease progression in hepatitis C. *Hepatology* 2002;**36**(Suppl 1): S47–S56.

60 Boyer N, Marcellin P. Pathogenesis, diagnosis and management of hepatitis C. *J Hepatol* 2000;**32**(Suppl 1): 98–112.

61 McHutchison JG, Patel K. Future therapy of hepatitis C. *Hepatology* 2002;**36**(Suppl 1):S245–S245.

62 Abrignani S, Houghton M, Hsu HH. Perspective for a vaccine against hepatitis C virus. *J Hepatol* 1999;**31**:259–63.

24 Hepatitis B

Piero Almasio, Calogero Cammà, Vito Di Marco, Antonio Craxì

Background

Hepatitis B virus (HBV) infection, together with hepatitis C and alcohol abuse, is among the leading causes of cirrhosis and hepatocellular carcinoma (HCC) worldwide.[1,2] It thus represents a relevant cause of morbidity and mortality,[3–5] and induces substantial direct and indirect social costs. Effective treatment of HBV-related conditions would significantly reduce the global burden of chronic liver disease.

Interferon (IFN) alpha has been the mainstay of therapy for chronic hepatitis B since the early 1980s. Meta-analyses[6–9] of randomized clinical trials (RCTs) conclusively prove its effectiveness in normalizing alanine aminotransferases (ALT) and clearing HBeAg and HBV-DNA from blood in 25–40% of patients treated. A1d No definite data are available from these reviews on improvement of liver histology. Standardized response criteria have been set by the use of these "surrogate" markers of cure,[10,11] on the ground of clinical and biological plausibility. "True" disease endpoints (i.e. progression to cirrhosis, to HCC and death) cannot usually be assessed in short-term trials of IFN due to the slow natural course of chronic hepatitis B. Since RCTs of IFN for chronic hepatitis B have been mostly carried out with patients without advanced fibrosis or cirrhosis, the generalizability of results to the whole spectrum of individuals with chronic liver disease due to HBV is questionable. Since IFN is in widespread use as the first-line therapy for chronic hepatitis B,[1,2,10,11] no additional prospective cohort studies on the course of untreated disease will be feasible. Long-term retrospective or prospective studies to evaluate the benefits of IFN therapy on true endpoints, i.e. prevention of cirrhosis, liver failure, HCC and death, will also be difficult to carry out due to the prolonged and slow course of the disease.

Recently, two nucleoside/nucleotide drugs that specifically block the HBV-DNA polymerase enzyme activity have been approved for treating patients with chronic HBV infection: lamivudine and adefovir. Both, when compared to IFN alpha, are less expensive and better tolerated, but their long-term efficacy is limited by inability to obtain sustained viral suppression after withdrawal. Prolonging the administration of lamivudine beyond 1 year of therapy causes the emergence of lamivudine-resistant HBV mutants at a yearly rate of 15–20%. B4

Other drugs, such as entecavir, emtricitabine (FTC), clevudine (L-FMAU) and β-L-nucleosides (LdT) currently undergoing phase II and III evaluation as potential anti-HBV treatments have been suggested either for monotherapy or for combination with IFN. Initial results suggest that these newest antiviral compounds, even if endowed with a strong antiviral effect, cannot by themselves eradicate HBV infection. Phase III studies of combination therapy using IFN and nucleoside/nucleotide analogs are ongoing.

The aim of this evidence-based review[12] is to appraise and update the evidence available for drugs which are currently on the market in order to estimate the effectiveness of antiviral therapy on both "surrogate markers" of response and long-term benefit.

Evaluation of available evidence

What effects has interferon therapy of chronic hepatitis B on "surrogate" markers of response?

HBeAg positive chronic hepatitis B

We have reviewed 24 RCTs[13–35] recovered by Medline search (1985–2002) which compared IFN to no treatment in adult patients with chronic hepatitis B due to wild type (HBeAg positive HBV) (Table 24.1). The 24 RCTs included a total of 1301 patients, 444 not receiving any active treatment. Overall, IFN treatment had a favorable, statistically significant effect on all four endpoints in comparison with no treatment. Meta-analysis showed the following risk differences, all in favor of IFN: A1a

- persistent ALT normalization (Figure 24.1): + 26·2% (95% CI 18·3 to 34·0%, $P < 0.00001$); NNT (numbers needed to treat) 4
- clearance of HBeAg (Figure 24.2): + 24·3% (95% CI 8·3 to 30·4%, $P < 0.00001$); NNT 4
- sustained loss of HBV-DNA (Figure 24.3): + 23·4% (95% CI 17·9 to 28·8%, $P < 0.00001$); NNT 4
- clearance of HBsAg (Figure 24.4): + 5·6% (95% CI 3·5 to 7·6%, $P < 0.00001$); NNT 18.

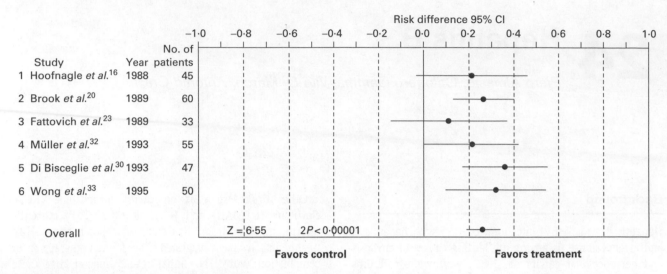

Figure 24.1 Meta-analysis of interferon therapy for HBeAg positive chronic hepatitis B: effect of treatment, measured as risk difference, on sustained ALT (alanine aminotransferase) normalization

The amount of IFN used was clearly an important factor in determining effectiveness. Subjects receiving a total dose of < 200 MU did not show statistically significant benefit (odds ratio (OR) 1·37, 95% CI 0·95 to 1·98) with respect to HBeAg clearance compared with controls, while those who received > 200 MU showed significant benefit (OR 2·05, 95% CI 1·5 to 2·78).[36,37] Ala

Overall experience suggests that the optimal cost-effectiveness ratio as judged by surrogate endpoints is reached by treating HBeAg positive patients with 9–10 MU IFN three times weekly for 4–6 months. Predictive factors of a favorable response are[8,9,25,28,29,38,39]

- low serum HBV-DNA (< 100 pg/ml)
- low amounts of HBcAg in the liver
- high levels of ALT
- high Hepatitis Activity Index (HAI) grade at biopsy
- infection in adult age and/or a history of acute hepatitis
- non-Asian ethnic origin.

An alternative approach to chronic HBV infection is based on the induction of a brief period of immunosuppression by steroids,[40,41] then a withdrawal to provoke an abrupt ALT elevation due to the host immune reconstitution, and a subsequent decline of HBV-DNA. IFN administration is then started 2–4 weeks after stopping steroids. The sequential regimen has been studied in some RCTs and the results have been pooled in a meta-analysis.[42] The overall rate of HBeAg loss in seven RCTs was comparable between the prednisone-IFN and IFN monotherapy groups (41% *v* 35%, OR 1·20, 95% CI 0·8 to 1·7). Similar results were observed for sustained ALT normalization (44·5% *v* 38%, OR 1·19, 95% CI 0·6 to 2·0). Ala Analysis of HBeAg clearance stratifying the patients according to pretreatment ALT levels showed that

prednisone-IFN treated cases had a significantly higher proportion of clearance (47·9% *v* 18·4%, *P* < 0·01) only when ALT levels were low before starting therapy. Even if there may be an advantage in pretreatment with steroids of this subset of patients, this potential benefit must be balanced against the risk of flare of liver disease after steroid withdrawal. A severe, sometimes fatal "seroconversion hepatitis" has been reported in subjects with pre-existing cirrhosis.[43,44]

Few RCTs were planned to assess the effects of IFN on liver histology. In these RCTs,[19,21,22,27] histologic improvement was observed. Ald However, the histologic approach to the evaluation of IFN response in chronic hepatitis B has several important limitations and sources of bias.

- The histological picture of chronic hepatitis B is mild to moderate in most cases. Therefore, the relatively small change induced by IFN can be difficult to assess with accuracy and reliability.
- Many factors might influence the interpretation of histology: inconsistency in the definition of pathological features, technical processing of the specimens, sampling variation.
- None of the trials reported a preliminary assessment of the intra/interobserver variations inherent to the semiquantitative evaluation of histological lesions. This can be a particularly important source of bias in cooperative studies, or in studies where the biopsy specimens were observed by different pathologists.
- The biopsy specimens reflect just one timepoint in a long-term dynamic process, developing at variable speed.

Taking these limitations into account, we regard the IFN-induced histologic changes reported as an approximate,

Table 24.1 Randomized controlled trials of interferon (IFN) treatment of HBeAg positive chronic hepatitis B

Study	Year	Patients	Schedule	Total dose	Type of IFN
Alexander et al.[13]	1987	46	10 MU/m² TIW for 6 months	720 MU	Lymphoblastoid
Carreño et al.[14]	1987	20	5·5 MU/m² IM daily for 3 weeks then twice weekly for 6 months	380 MU/m²	r-IFN α-2c
McDonald et al.[15]	1987	41	2·5, 5, 10 MU/m² IM TIW for 6 months	180, 360, 720 MU	r-IFN α-2a
Hoofnagle et al.[16]	1988	45	5 MU daily or 10 MU every other day for 4 months	560 MU	r-IFN α-2b
Lok et al.[17]	1988	72	2·5, 5, 10 MU/m² IM TIW for 6 months	180, 360, 720 MU	r-IFN α-2a
Porres et al.[18]	1988	24	2·5, 5, 10 MU/m² IM TIW for 6 months	180, 360, 720 MU	r-IFN α-2a
Pastore et al.[19]	1988	28	0·07 to 0·10 MU/kg IM daily for 1 month then twice weekly for 2 months	2·52–3·6 MU/kg	Leukocyte
Brook et al.[20]	1989	60	10 MU/m² TIW IM for 6 months	720 MU	r-IFN α-2a
Brook et al.[21]	1989	71	2·5, 5, 10 MU/m² IM TIW for 6 months	180, 360, 720 MU	r-IFN α-2a
Saracco et al.[22]	1989	64	5 MU/m² IM TIW for 6 months	360 MU	Lymphoblastoid
Fattovich et al.[23]	1989	33	4·5 MU IM TIW for 4 months	216 MU	r-IFN α-2a
Müller et al.[24]	1990	58	3 MU SC TIW for 4 months	144 MU	r-IFN α-2b
Perrillo et al.[25]	1990	125	1 or 5 MU, SC daily for 4 months	112 or 560 MU	r-IFN α-2b
Williams et al.[26]	1990	30	2·5, 5, 10 MU/m² IM TIW for 6 months	180, 360, 720 MU	r-IFN α-2a
Waked et al.[27]	1990	40	5 MU/m² SC 3 or 7 times weekly for 4 months	240 or 560 MU/m²	r-IFN α-2b
Realdi et al.[28]	1990	79	4·5 MU IM TIW for 4 months	216 MU	r-IFN α-2a
Lok et al.[29]	1992	34	10 MU SC TIW for 4 months	480 MU	r-IFN α-2b
Lok et al.[29]	1992	41	10 MU SC TIW for 4 months	480 MU	r-IFN α-2b
Di Bisceglie et al.[30]	1993	47	10 MU SC TIW for 4 months	480 MU	r-IFN α-2b
Bayraktar et al.[31]	1993	35	5 MU TIW SC for 6 months	360 MU	r-IFN α-2b
Müller et al.[32]	1993	55	3 MU SC TIW for 4 months	144 MU	r-IFN α-2b
Wong et al.[33]	1995	50	10 MU/m² TIW for 3 months	360 MU	r-IFN α-2
Sarin et al.[34]	1996	41	3 MU SC TIW for 4 months	144 MU	r-IFN α-2b
Janssen et al.[35]	1999	162	10 MU SC TIW for 4 or 8 months	480 or 960 MU	r-IFN α-2b

IM, intramuscular; SC, subcutaneous

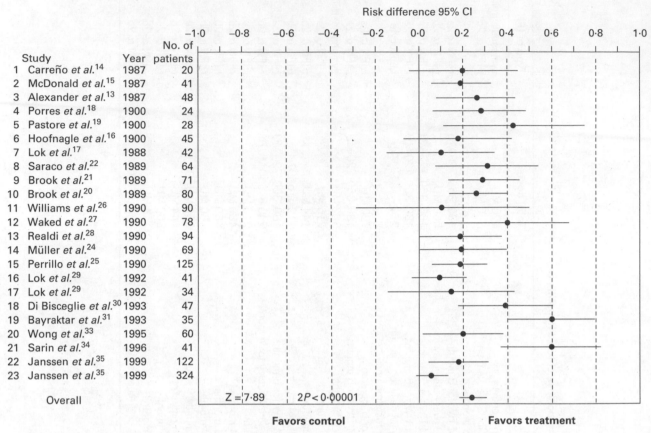

Figure 24.2 Meta-analysis of interferon therapy for HBeAg positive chronic hepatitis B: effect of treatment, measured as risk difference, on HBeAg clearance

although important, indication of treatment effect, rather than a precise quantitative estimate. Significant histological improvement was usually observed among patients who normalized ALT and cleared serum HBV-DNA, but complete healing of liver lesions was only seen among subjects rebiopsied many years after seroconversion. Many of these patients had also lost serum HBsAg.

HBeAg negative chronic hepatitis B

Data on the efficacy of IFN therapy in HBeAg negative chronic hepatitis B are scanty, the results of published RCTs remain inconsistent and the overall assessment of benefit is difficult. The drawing of firm conclusions based on the results of these studies is hampered by the small sample size and by the heterogeneity in the baseline severity of patients and in the schedule of treatment. Treatment efficacy on HBV-DNA clearance and sustained ALT normalization was evaluated in a second meta-analysis of seven RCTs[45–51] enrolling only patients infected by the HBe minus mutant. Five RCTs compared IFN regimens with non-active treatment; two trials compared different doses of IFN. We combined the results of the IFN arms of these two trials and made a single pair-wise comparison with the overall control rate of the other five

RCTs. All the RCTs were carried out in centers in the Mediterranean area, indirectly confirming the high geographical prevalence of this mutation. Pooled data from the seven studies (Figure 24.5), totaling 301 patients, showed a significant effect of IFN therapy on the combined outcome of suppression of HBV replication and reduction of necroinflammation (absolute risk difference + 21%, 95% CI 6·8 to 35%, *P* < 0·003). Ala

What are the long-term benefits of interferon treatment for chronic hepatitis B?

HBeAg positive chronic hepatitis B

We critically reviewed and combined data from 12 studies (11 prospective and one retrospective) which included a total of 1952 patients, 1187 not receiving active treatment (Table 24.2).[52–63] Length of follow-up ranged from 2·1 to 8·9 years (mean 6·1 years).

Meta-analysis showed the following results:

- loss of HBsAg (Figure 24.6): treated 11·4% (95% CI 9·1 to 13·7%), controls 2·6% (95% CI 1·8 to 3·4%), RD 8·8%, NNT 11 Ala

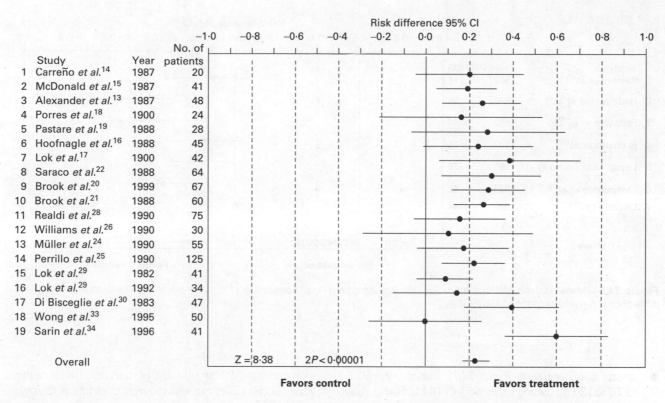

Figure 24.3 Meta-analysis of interferon therapy for HBeAg positive chronic hepatitis B: effect of treatment, measured as risk difference, on sustained loss of HBV-DNA

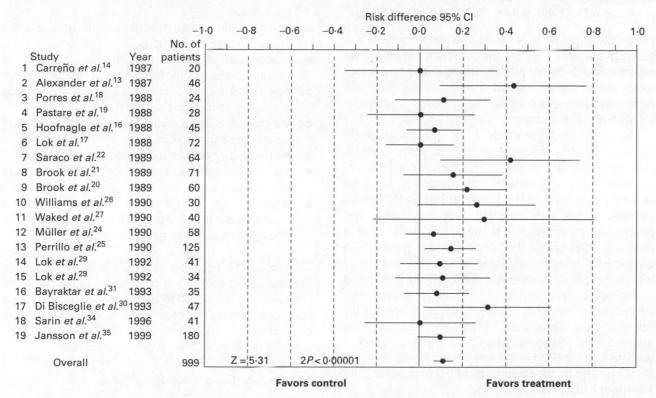

Figure 24.4 Meta-analysis of interferon therapy for HBeAg positive chronic hepatitis B: effect of treatment, measured as risk difference, on loss of HBsAg

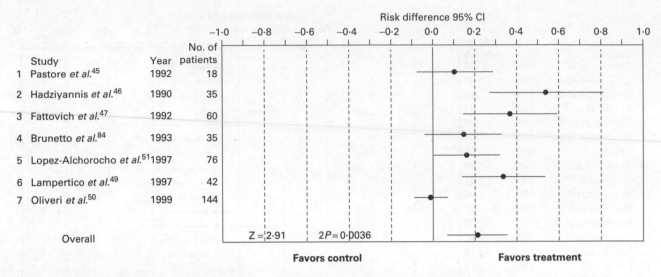

Figure 24.5 Meta-analysis of IFN therapy for HBeAg negative chronic hepatitis B: effect of treatment, measured as risk difference, on sustained loss of HBV-DNA

- disease decompensation (Figure 24.7): treated 9·9% (95% CI 7·7 to 12·1%), controls 13·3% (95% CI 10·1 to 16·4%) Ala
- development of HCC (Figure 24.8): treated 1·9% (95% CI 0·8 to 3·0%), controls 3·16% (95% CI 1·8 to 4·5%) Ala
- liver-related death (Figure 24.9): treated 4·9% (95% CI 3·3 to 6·5%), controls 8·7% (95% CI 6·1 to 11·3%). Ala

The rate of clearance of HBsAg in untreated patients was generally low, and a statistically significant advantage was observed for IFN-treated patients. HBsAg clearance was seen mostly among subjects infected as adults, among those with more active disease at onset, and on average 2–4 years after HBeAg/HBV-DNA clearance.

Data on the protective effects of IFN against development of HCC are less encouraging: studies show a strong heterogeneity, which makes the reliability of conclusions of individual studies questionable. Thus, there is no firm basis on which to recommend IFN to prevent HCC in HBV-related cirrhosis. It has been suggested from retrospective and prospective studies that IFN treatment might have a protective effect against HCC development in patients with chronic HBV infection independently from viral clearance or resolution of necroinflammation.[64] B4 Obviously, IFN-induced viral clearance remains a major outcome for patients with HBV-related chronic liver disease and indirectly reduces the risk of cancer. Some cases of HBV-associated HCC are observed in the absence of cirrhosis (mostly young males with perinatal infection), and have a very aggressive clinical course. No information on the effectiveness of IFN in preventing this subtype of HCC is available currently.

All the data on disease events (i.e. liver decompensation and HCC) and on liver-related mortality coming from studies

with prolonged follow up must be considered with caution, since possible biases can lead to errors in estimates through:

- data collected from both prospective and retrospective studies conducted in tertiary care centers with limited generalizability
- lack of randomization reducing the internal and the external validity of the studies
- heterogeneity of patients enrolled, both in respect of clinical and demographic features and of possible cofactors
- slow and prolonged course of the disease not allowing assembly of an inception cohort
- few clinically relevant events, relatively small numbers of patients and duration of follow up less than 8–10 years
- high mortality from non-hepatic causes
- selection and increased surveillance for cases with more severe disease and unfavorable course
- progressive shift over the years of the global spectrum of the disease due to intervening factors (e.g. new diagnostic tests and screening programs, new treatments).

Overall, IFN treatment had a favorable, statistically significant effect only on loss of HBsAg in comparison to no treatment. In contrast, IFN treatment has failed to show statistically significant effects on disease decompensation, development of HCC and liver-related death, although favorable trends for all these points are observed.

HBeAg negative chronic hepatitis B

There have been controversies about the long-term benefit of IFN therapy in the HBeAg negative form of chronic

Table 24.2 Long-term follow up of interferon (IFN)-treated and untreated patients with HBeAg positive chronic hepatitis B

Study	Year	Follow up (years)	Race (Asian/White)	Age (mean years)	HBsAg loss		Decompensation		HCC		Death	
					IFN	Control	IFN	Control	IFN	Control	IFN	Control
Niederau et al.[52]	1996	4·2	W		10/103	0/53	16/103	13/53	NR	NR	6/103	3/53
Lin et al.[53]	1999	7	A	32	0/67	0/34	6/67	5/34	1/67	4/34	1/67	4/34
Fattovich et al.[54]	1997	7·2	W	46	11/40	5/50	6/40	11/50	4/40	6/50	8/40	15/50
Di Marco et al.[55]	1999	7·8	W	33·5	4/39	0/54	8/39	11/54	NR	NR	3/39	8/54
Yuen et al.[56]	2001	8·9	A	27·5	5/208	1/203	4/208	2/203	5/208	0/203	2/208	0/203
Chen et al.[57]	1999	5	W	>18	3/13	0/11	NR	NR	NR	NR	NR	NR
Evans et al.[58]	1997	2·1	A	5–50		2/49	NR	NR	NR	NR	NR	NR
Korenman et al.[59]	1991	4·4	W	40	13/64		NR		NR		NR	
Lok et al.[60]	1993	6	A	19–46	2/128		3/128		0/128		1/120	
Lau et al.[61]	1997	6·7	W	41·5	34/103		24/103		0/103		12/103	
Fattovich et al.[62]	2000	5·5	W	47		NR	11/45	NR	3/45		9/45	
Hsu et al.[63]	2002	8·6	A	32	12/283		NR			6/283		NR

NR, not reported; HCC, hepatocellular carcinoma

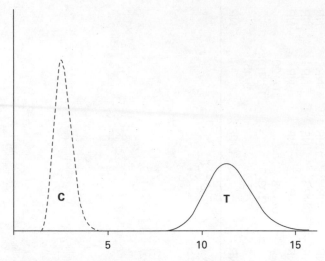

Figure 24.6 Probability distribution of the loss of HBsAg rate in HBeAg positive chronic hepatitis B from interferon-treated (T) patients and controls (C). Data from cohort studies

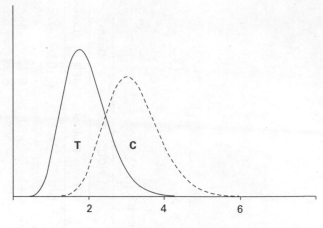

Figure 24.8 Probability distribution of rate of development of hepatocellular carcinoma in HBeAg positive chronic hepatitis B from interferon-treated (T) patients and controls (C). Data from cohort studies

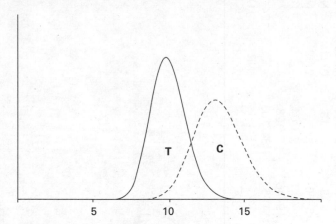

Figure 24.7 Probability distribution of disease decompensation rate in HBeAg positive chronic hepatitis B from interferon-treated (T) patients and controls (C). Data from cohort studies

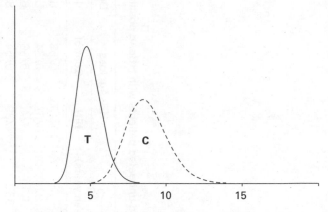

Figure 24.9 Probability distribution of rate of liver-related mortality in HBeAg positive chronic hepatitis B from interferon-treated (T) patients and controls (C). Data from cohort studies

hepatitis B. Differences in the baseline severity of illness in the population of the studies, in the length of follow up, in the type and the frequency of post-treatment monitoring, and in the treatment regimens limit the assessment of the impact of IFN therapy on the course of the disease. Overall, the three cohort studies[65-67] with a length of follow up ranging from 2 to 7 years showed that the response appeared to be less durable at long-term follow up compared to HBeAg positive cases and that relapse can occur even years after therapy. The rate of HBsAg loss ranged from 4·5% to 13%. B2

Interferon: summary

The available evidence from RCTs or cohort studies of IFN alpha treatment for chronic hepatitis B is sufficient to conclude that:

- in patients with HBeAg positive chronic hepatitis IFN therapy significantly improves clearance of HBeAg (NNT 4) and loss of HBV-DNA (NNT 4) compared with no treatment
- in patients with HBeAg negative chronic hepatitis less than 20% of subjects who have achieved an end-of-treatment virological response after a course of IFN, maintain a sustained virological response
- The rate of clearance of HBsAg is significantly higher in the IFN-treated than in untreated patients. The magnitude of the overall effect is small but clinically relevant (NNT 18)
- There is no clear evidence of a protective effect of IFN against HCC
- IFN treatment may help to delay or prevent disease decompensation and liver-related deaths, but further large studies are needed to determine this point.

Effects of nucleoside/nucleotide analogs on "surrogate" markers of response

Lamivudine

Evidence of effectiveness from phase II and phase III randomized trials is now available in the literature for some of the nucleoside/nucleotide analogs. Most of these drugs are used by the oral route and display a powerful inhibitory effect on the HBV-DNA polymerase.[68] Their action is often jeopardized by the appearance of mutations in specific regions of the polymerase-encoding HBV gene (so-called YMDD mutant and others).[69–71] These mutants, which often display cross-insensitivity to drugs[72] cause reappearance of high level viral replication but tend to subside after stopping lamivudine.

The original observations on the anti-HBV efficacy of lamivudine came from the treatment of HIV-infected subjects who were also HBsAg positive.[73–76] B4 Effectiveness of lamivudine in dramatically reducing HBV replication has been exploited also in subjects with iatrogenic immune suppression, mostly recipients of organ transplants[77–92] or patients receiving antineoplastic chemotherapy.[93–105] B4

The great majority of published clinical studies of lamivudine in immunocompetent HBV patients[106–133] are pilot or dose-finding trials, or pharmacokinetic and virological studies, without appropriate control groups. The optimal dosage, found by a dose-ranging study[115] and confirmed by an RCT,[127] is 100 mg daily. Only a minority, published as full papers, are clinical trials with an appropriate control group.[114,115,127,134–136] We have analyzed the results of these RCTs all of which included patients with HBeAg positive chronic hepatitis but one of which[132] employed different doses (25–300 mg daily) of lamivudine for periods of 4 weeks to 1 year. At the end of treatment the rate of HBeAg seroconversion (defined as loss of HBeAg and appearance of anti-HBe) ranged from 0 to 19%. Alc The probability of response, in terms of ALT normalization under lamivudine, was between 41% and 72%; similar rates were observed in terms of sustained suppression of HBV-DNA after 52 weeks (range 44–60%). The durability of HBeAg seroconversion beyond 52 weeks was evaluated in several papers[137–140] and all these studies reporting a sufficient follow up (up to 3 years) showed a relapse rate ranging from 36% to 57·4% with highest rates of relapse in Asiatic patients. The identified predictors of virological relapse were older age, male sex and low levels of ALT. However, not all virological relapses result in clinically important hepatitis.

The only published RCT including patients with anti-HBe positive chronic hepatitis used a regimen of 52 weeks of therapy with lamivudine.[136] At the end of this period 35 of 54 (65%) treated patients had undetectable serum HBV-DNA Ald This finding was paralleled with histological changes in paired biopsies that showed improvement in 42% of patients. However, in this clinical setting there are two major problems with lamivudine treatment: the occurrence of YMDD mutants under therapy and the stability of viral suppression after drug discontinuation.

In a cumulative analysis of two studies of long-term lamivudine monotherapy[141] 32 out of 73 virological responders (44%) experienced viral breakthroughs within a median of 15 months, almost always related to YMDD appearance. Appearance of the YMDD mutant was associated with an ALT relapse in 30–70% of cases, and usually both the YMDD mutant and the ALT peak subside rapidly upon stopping lamivudine. The efficacy of lamivudine to inhibit HBV replication seems limited only to the period of drug exposure. B4 In fact one paper[132] showed that only two out of 15 anti-HBe positive patients treated with lamivudine had a sustained virological and biochemical response after 52 weeks of treatment.

The inability of lamivudine to induce a sustained virological and biochemical response has led to evaluation of combination therapy. The combination with IFN has been tested only in two RCTs both in patients with HBeAg positive chronic hepatitis.[142,143] Overall 49 out of 151 (32·5%) patients treated with combination therapy seroconverted after 52 weeks of treatment, a response rate significantly higher ($P < 0·005$) than the 29 seroconversions in 157 patients (18·5%) obtained with lamivudine alone. There are as yet no firm data available to prove an increase in effectiveness over treatment with lamivudine alone. Alc Only one non-randomized study has been done in patients with precore mutant chronic hepatitis B.[144] B4 Twenty-nine patients were treated with combination therapy for 52 weeks and at the end of this period 93% of patients showed a biochemical and virological response. However this effect was not maintained during follow up since only four subjects did not relapse. These figures are very similar to those observed in subjects treated with monotherapy.

There is experimental evidence[145,146] to suggest that the appearance of lamivudine-induced HBV mutants may be circumvented by the use of other nucleoside analogs. The potential benefits of this substitution has not yet been evaluated in clinical trials. Concerns have been raised about the possibility of enhanced toxicity.

Lamivudine is registered in the USA and in Europe as an antiviral active against HBV.

Lamivudine: summary

Available evidence is sufficient to draw the following conclusions.

- HBeAg positive immunocompetent patients with raised ALT should receive IFN as a first-line drug, and lamivudine or adefovir as a second-line drug only when IFN has failed and there is histological evidence of progressive disease. If the patient has severe decompensated liver disease, the risk of a sero-conversion flare with worsening liver function following IFN needs to be considered as an indication for lamivudine or adefovir.

- HBeAg positive patients with normal or mildly raised ALT should be treated only if there is histological evidence of progressive disease and should receive lamivudine or adefovir as a first-line drug, switching from lamivudine to adefovir if there is an HBV-DNA breakthrough under therapy.
- HBeAg negative, HBV-DNA positive patients can receive IFN, lamivudine or adefovir as first-line therapy. IFN should be given for 24 months. Lamivudine and adefovir should be continued over an undefined extended period of time (24 or more months).
- Lamivudine is effective in reducing and sometimes clearing HBV replication in heavily immunosuppressed patients and can be safely administered to patients with advanced liver disease.
- Long-term clinical effectiveness of lamivudine is still unproved.

Adefovir dipivoxyl

Adefovir dipivoxyl, a nucleotide analog, has been recently approved in the USA for therapy of chronic hepatitis B. This agent has a potent *in vitro* and *in vivo* effect against herpes virus, retroviruses and hepadnaviruses. Adefovir dipivoxyl, given orally at a dose of 10 mg daily, inhibits both the wild type and lamivudine-resistant HBV strains with an excellent safety profile. Renal tubular damage has been observed when prolonged treatment with higher doses has been given. Up to now, no evidence of HBV resistance to adefovir dipivoxyl has been detected, and this constitutes one of its main advantages over lamivudine as it permits longer duration of therapy and also its use as rescue therapy for lamivudine-resistant HBV strains. Two phase III multicenter RCTs, one in HBeAg positive[147] and one in HBeAg negative patients[148] have recently been published. In the study by Marcellin *et al.*,[147] 1515 patients worldwide with HBeAg positive chronic hepatitis B (HBV-DNA $< 1 \times 10^6$ copies/ml) were randomized to receive 10–30 mg of adefovir or placebo for 48 weeks. Most of them were treatment naive, since only 123 had been previously treated with IFN alpha. The observed reduction of HBV-DNA levels expressed as log copies/ml was 4·76 with 30 mg versus 3·52 with 10 mg of adefovir, in both cases a significantly greater suppression than was observed with placebo. Ald The rates of biochemical and histological improvement were comparable for the two adefovir regimens (59% *v* 53% and 55 *v* 48%, respectively). HBeAg seroconversion, although significantly more common in patients receiving adefovir (12% at 30 mg,14% at 10 mg) than in the control group (6%, $P = 0.049$ and 0·01, respectively), was relatively uncommon. No adefovir-associated resistance mutations were identified in the HBV-DNA polymerase gene. Mild

nephrotoxicity was observed with the 30 mg regimen, and thus 10 mg was considered to be the best regimen.

Patients with chronic HBeAg negative, HBV-DNA positive chronic hepatitis were studied in a multicenter trial by Hadziyannis *et al.*,[148] comparing the efficacy of 10 mg of adefovir daily for 48 weeks with placebo. Viral suppression, as measured by undetectable HBV-DNA levels, was obtained in 51% of patients on adefovir versus none in the placebo group. Ald The median HBV-DNA level of adefovir-treated patients at 48 weeks (3·91 log copies/ml) was lower than with placebo (1·35 log copies/ml, $P < 0.001$). HBsAg seroconversion was never achieved. Histology was significantly in the adefovir group, (adefovir 64%, placebo 33%) and ALT levels normalized more frequently (adefovir 72%, placebo 29%).

Remarkably, both studies do not give follow up information beyond the 48 weeks of therapy. Thus the ultimate effectiveness in terms of stable HBeAg seroconversion (for HBeAg positive patients), sustained HBV suppression (for HBeAg negative patients) and more importantly reduction of progression of HBV-related liver disease in the long term remain to be assessed.

In both studies, YMDD or other repetitive mutations in the HBV polymerase region were not observed with either dose of adefovir during the 48 weeks of treatment. Further follow up of patients on long-term therapy will assess the actual safety of adefovir in this respect. No cross-resistance with lamivudine has been reported to date.

European consensus conference on Hepatitis B

Detailed reviews on pathogenesis, natural course prognosis, epidemiology, vaccination, as well as therapeutic strategies in standard and special patient groups are available from the September 2002 International Consensus Conference.[149]

Conclusions

Data from studies of natural history and RCTs or non-randomized studies of antiviral treatment provide sufficient evidence to make the following conclusions.

- The natural history of chronic hepatitis B is variable, according to phenotypic and ethnic background, and is also influenced by viral coinfections and toxic cofactors. At least 20% of patients develop clinically significant liver disease in the long term.
- Presence of markers of HBV replication and of continuing liver necroinflammation predict an adverse outcome.
- IFN therapy results in stable clearance of HBeAg in 25% of all patients chronically infected by wild type HBV, but only rarely results in HBsAg clearance.

- IFN therapy results in stable clearance of HBV-DNA in 25% of all patients chronically infected by HBe minus HBV.
- Lamivudine and adefovir are effective in clearing HBV-DNA and normalizing ALT during therapy in 65% of patients, but the long-term effectiveness of these agents is unknown.
- There is no acceptable evidence for a protective effect of IFN against development of HCC in HBV-related cirrhosis.

References

1 Lok AS, McMahon BJ. Chronic hepatitis B. *Hepatology* 2001;**34**:1225–41.

2 Lok AS, Heathcote J, Hoofnagle JH. Management of hepatitis B: 2000 – Summary of a workshop. *Gastroenterology* 2001;**120**:1828–53.

3 Liaw YF, Tai DI, Chu CM, Chen TJ. The development of cirrhosis in patients with chronic type B hepatitis: a prospective study. *Hepatology* 1988;**8**:493–6.

4 De Jongh FE, Janssen HLA, De Man RA, Hop WCJ, Schalm SW, Van Blankenstein M. Survival and prognostic indicators in hepatitis B surface antigen-positive cirrhosis of the liver. *Gastroenterology* 1992;**103**:1630–5.

5 Fattovich G, Giustina G, Schalm SW *et al.* Occurrence of hepatocellular carcinoma and decompensation in western European patients with cirrhosis type B. *Hepatology* 1995; **21**:77–82.

6 Craxì A, Di Bona D, Cammà C. Interferon-α for HBeAg-positive chronic hepatitis B. *J Hepatol* 2003 (in press).

7 Wong JB, Koff RS, Tiné F, Pauker SG. Cost-effectiveness of interferon-alpha 2b treatment for hepatitis B e antigen-positive chronic hepatitis B. *Ann Intern Med* 1995;**122**:664–75.

8 Tiné F, Liberati A, Craxì A, Almasio P, Pagliaro L. Interferon treatment in patients with chronic hepatitis B: a meta-analysis of the published literature. *J Hepatol* 1993;**18**:154–62.

9 Wong DK, Cheung AM, O'Rourke K, Naylor CD, Detsky AS, Heathcote J. Effect of alpha-interferon treatment in patients with hepatitis B e antigen-positive chronic hepatitis B. A meta-analysis. *Ann Intern Med* 1993;**119**:312–23.

10 Evans AA, London WT. Interferon for chronic hepatitis B. *Ann Intern Med* 1996;**124**:276.

11 Carithers RL Jr. Effect of interferon on hepatitis B. *Lancet* 1998;**351**:157.

12 Lau J, Ioannidis JP, Schmid CH. Quantitative synthesis in systematic reviews. *Ann Intern Med* 1997;**127**:820–6.

13 Alexander GJ, Brahm J, Fagan EA, Smith HM, Daniels HM, Eddleston AL, Williams R. Loss of HBsAg with interferon therapy in chronic hepatitis B virus infection. *Lancet* 1987;**8550**:66–9.

14 Carreño V, Porres JC, Mora I *et al.* A controlled study of treatment with recombinant interferon alpha in chronic hepatitis B virus infection: induction and maintenance schedules. *Antiviral Res* 1987;**3**:125–37.

15 McDonald JA, Caruso L, Karayiannis P, Scully LJ *et al.* Diminished responsiveness of male homosexual chronic hepatitis B virus carriers with HTLV-III antibodies to recombinant alpha-interferon. *Hepatology* 1987;**7**:719–23.

16 Hoofnagle JH, Peters M, Mullen KD *et al.* Randomized, controlled trial of recombinant human alpha-interferon in patients with chronic hepatitis B. *Gastroenterology* 1988;**95**:1318–25.

17 Lok AS, Lai CL, Wu PC, Leung EK. Long-term follow-up in a randomised controlled trial of recombinant alpha 2-interferon in Chinese patients with chronic hepatitis B infection. *Lancet* 1988;**2**:298–302.

18 Porres JC, Carreño V, Mora I *et al.* Different doses of recombinant alpha interferon in the treatment of chronic hepatitis B patients without antibodies against the human immunodeficiency virus. *Hepatogastroenterology* 1988;**6**:300–3.

19 Pastore G, Santantonio T, Monno L, Milella M, Luchena N, Angarano G. Permanent inhibition of viral replication induced by low dosage of human leukocyte interferon in patients with chronic hepatitis B. *Hepatogastroenterology* 1988;**35**:57–61.

20 Brook MG, McDonald JA, Karayiannis P *et al.* Randomised controlled trial of interferon alpha 2A (Roferon-A) for the treatment of chronic hepatitis B virus (HBV) infection: factors that influence response. *Gut* 1989;**30**:1116–22.

21 Brook MG, Chan G, Yap I *et al.* Randomised controlled trial of lymphoblastoid IFN alpha in Europid men with chronic hepatitis B virus infection. *BMJ* 1989;**299**:652–6.

22 Saracco G, Mazzella G, Rosina F *et al.* A controlled trial of human lymphoblastoid interferon in chronic hepatitis B in Italy. *Hepatology* 1989;**10**:336–41.

23 Fattovich G, Brollo L, Boscaro S *et al.* Long-term effect of low dose recombinant interferon therapy in patients with chronic hepatitis B. *J Hepatol* 1989;**3**:331–7.

24 Müller R, Baumgarten R, Markus R *et al.* Treatment of chronic hepatitis B with interferon alpha-2b. *J Hepatol* 1990;**11**:S137–40.

25 Perrillo RP, Schiff ER, Davis GL *et al.* A randomized, controlled trial of interferon alpha-2b alone and after prednisone withdrawal for the treatment of chronic hepatitis B. The Hepatitis Interventional Therapy Group. *N Engl J Med* 1990;**323**:295–301.

26 Williams SJ, Craig PI, Cooksley WG *et al.* Randomised controlled trial of recombinant human interferon-alpha A for chronic active hepatitis B. *Aust NZ J Med* 1990;**20**:9–19.

27 Waked I, Amin M, Abd el Fattah S, Osman LM, Sabbour MS. Experience with interferon in chronic hepatitis B in Egypt. *J Chemother* 1990;**2**:310–18.

28 Realdi G, Fattovich G, Pastore G *et al.* Problems in the management of chronic hepatitis B with interferon: experience in a randomized, multicentre study. *J Hepatol* 1990;**11**:S129–32.

29 Lok AS, Wu PC, Lai CL *et al.* A controlled trial of interferon with or without prednisone priming for chronic hepatitis B. *Gastroenterology* 1992;**102**:2091–7.

30 Di Bisceglie AM, Fong TL, Fried MW *et al.* A randomized, controlled trial of recombinant alpha-interferon therapy for chronic hepatitis B. *Am J Gastroenterol* 1993;**88**:1887–92.

31 Bayraktar Y, Uzunalimoglu B, Arslan S, Koseoglu T, Kayhan B, Telatar H. Effects of recombinant alpha interferon on chronic active hepatitis B: preliminary results. *Gut* 1993; **34**:S101.

32 Müller R, Baumgarten R, Markus R *et al.* Low dose alpha interferon treatment in chronic hepatitis B virus infection. *Gut* 1993;**34**:S97–8.

33 Wong DK, Yim C, Naylor CD, Chen E *et al.* Interferon alpha treatment of chronic hepatitis B: randomized trial in a predominantly homosexual male population. *Gastroenterology* 1995;**108**:165–71.

34 Sarin SK, Guptan RC, Thakur V *et al.* Efficacy of low-dose alpha interferon therapy in HBV-related chronic liver disease in Asian Indians: a randomized controlled trial. *J Hepatol* 1996;**24**:391–6.

35 Janssen HL, Gerken G, Carreno V *et al.* Interferon alpha for chronic hepatitis B infection: increased efficacy of prolonged treatment. The European Concerted Action on Viral Hepatitis (EUROHEP). *Hepatology* 1999;**30**:238–43.

36 Krogsgaard K, Bindslev N, Christensen E *et al.* and EUROHEP, The treatment effect of alpha interferon in chronic hepatitis B is independent of pre-treatment variables. Results based on individual patient data from 10 clinical controlled trials. *J Hepatol* 1994;**21**:646–55.

37 Krogsgaard K, Christensen E, Bindslev N *et al.* Relation between treatment efficacy and cumulative dose of alpha interferon in chronic hepatitis B. *J Hepatology* 1996;**25**: 795–802.

38 Thomas HC, Karayiannis P, Brook G. Treatment of hepatitis B virus infection with interferon. Factors predicting response to interferon. *J Hepatol* 1991;**13**(Suppl 1):S4–S7.

39 Carreño V, Castillo I, Molina J, Porres JC, Bartolomé J. Long-term follow-up of hepatitis B chronic carriers who responded to interferon therapy. *J Hepatol* 1992;**15**:102–6.

40 Krogsgaard K. Does corticosteroid pretreatment enhance the effect of alpha interferon treatment in chronic hepatitis B. *J Hepatol* 1994;**20**:159–62.

41 Krogsgaard K, Marcellin P, Trepo C *et al.* Prednisolone withdrawal therapy enhances the effect of human lymphoblastoid interferon in chronic hepatitis B. *J Hepatol* 1996;**25**:803–13.

42 Cohard M, Poynard T, Mathurin P *et al.* Prednisone-interferon combination in the treatment of chronic hepatitis B: direct and indirect metanalysis. *Hepatology* 1994;**20**: 1390–8.

43 Perrillo R, Tamburro C, Regenstein F *et al.* Low-dose, titratable interferon alpha in decompensated liver disease caused by chronic infection with hepatitis B virus. *Gastroenterology* 1995;**109**:908–16.

44 Perrillo RP. Chronic hepatitis B: problem patients (including patients with decompensated disease). *J Hepatol* 1995;**22**: 45–8.

45 Pastore G, Santantonio T, Milella M *et al.* Anti-HBe-positive chronic hepatitis B with HBV-DNA in the serum response to a 6-month course of lymphoblastoid interferon. *J Hepatol* 1992;**14**:221–5.

46 Hadziyannis S, Bramou T, Makris A *et al.* Interferon alpha-2b treatment of HBeAg negative/serum HBV DNA positive chronic active hepatitis type B. *J Hepatol* 1990;**11**: S133–36.

47 Fattovich G, Farci P, Rugge M *et al.* A randomized controlled trial of lymphoblastoid interferon-a in patients with chronic hepatitis B lacking HBeAg. *Hepatology* 1992;**15**:584–9.

48 Brunetto MR, Giarin M, Saracco G *et al.* Hepatitis B virus unable to secrete e antigen and response to interferon in chronic hepatitis B. *Gastroenterology* 1993;**105**:845–50.

49 Lampertico P, Del Ninno E, Manzin A *et al.* A randomized, controlled trial of a 24-month course of interferon alpha 2b in patients with chronic hepatitis B who had hepatitis B virus DNA without hepatitis B e antigen in serum. *Hepatology* 1997;**26**:1621–5.

50 Oliveri F, Santantonio T, Bellati G, *et al.* Long term response to therapy of chronic anti-HBe-positive hepatitis B is poor independent of type and schedule of interferon. *Am J Gastroenterol* 1999;**94**:1366–72.

51 Lopez-Alchorocho JM, Bartolome J, Cotonat T, Carreno V. Efficacy of prolonged interferon-alpha treatment in chronic hepatitis B patients with HbeAb: comparison between 6 and 12 months of therapy. *J Viral Hepat* 1997;**4**:27–32.

52 Niederau C, Heintges T, Lange S *et al.* Long-term follow-up of HBeAg-positive patients treated with interferon alpha for chronic hepatitis B. *N Engl J Med* 1996;**334**:1422–7.

53 Lin SM, Sheen IS, Chien RN, Chu CM, Liaw YF. Long-term beneficial effect of interferon therapy in patients with chronic hepatitis B virus infection. *Hepatology* 1999;**29**:971–5.

54 Fattovich G, Giustina G, Realdi G, Corrocher R, Schalm SW. Long-term outcome of hepatitis B e antigen-positive patients with compensated cirrhosis treated with interferon alpha. European Concerted Action on Viral Hepatitis (EUROHEP). *Hepatology* 1997;**26**:1338–42.

55 Di Marco V, Lo Iacono O, Camma C *et al.* The long-term course of chronic hepatitis B. *Hepatology* 1999;**30**:257–64.

56 Yuen MF, Hui CK, Cheng CC, Wu CH, Lai YP, Lai CL. Long-term follow-up of interferon alpha treatment in Chinese patients with chronic hepatitis B infection: the effect on hepatitis B e antigen seroconversion and the development of cirrhosis-related complications. *Hepatology* 2001;**34**: 139–45.

57 Chen DK, Yim C, O'Rourke K, Krajden M, Wong DK, Heathcote EJ. Long-term follow-up of a randomized trial of interferon therapy for chronic hepatitis B in a predominantly homosexual male population. *J Hepatol* 1999;**30**:557–63.

58 Evans AA, Fine M, London WT. Spontaneous seroconversion in hepatitis B e antigen-positive chronic hepatitis B: implications for interferon therapy. *J Infect Dis* 1997;**176**:845–50.

59 Korenman J, Baker B, Waggoner J, Everhart JE, Di Bisceglie AM, Hoofnagle JH. Long-term remission of chronic hepatitis B after alpha-interferon therapy. *Ann Intern Med.* 1991;**114**: 629–34.

60 Lok AS, Chung HT, Liu VW, Ma OC. Long-term follow-up of chronic hepatitis B patients treated with interferon alpha. *Gastroenterology* 1993;**105**:1833–8.

61 Lau DT, Everhart J, Kleiner DE *et al.* Long-term follow-up of patients with chronic hepatitis B treated with interferon alpha. *Gastroenterology* 1997;**113**:1660–7.

62 Fattovich G, Giustina G, Christensen E *et al.* Influence of hepatitis delta virus infection on morbidity and mortality in compensated cirrhosis type B. The European Concerted Action on Viral Hepatitis (Eurohep). Gut 2000;**46**:420–6.

63 Hsu YS, Chien RN, Yeh CT *et al.* Long-term outcome after spontaneous HBeAg seroconversion in patients with chronic hepatitis B. *Hepatology* 2002;**35**:1522–7.

64 Benvegnù L, Chemello L, Noventa F, Fattovich G, Pontisso P, Alberti A. Retrospective analysis of the effect of interferon therapy on the clinical outcome of patients with viral cirrhosis. *Cancer* 1998;**83**:901–9.

65 Papatheodoridis GV, Manesis E, Hadziyannis SJ. Long term outcome of interferon-alpha treated and untreated patients with HBeAg negative chronic hepatitis B. *J Hepatol* 2000;**34**:306–13.

66 Manesis E, Hadziyannis S. Interferon alpha treatment and retreatment of hepatitis B e antigen-negative chronic hepatitis B. *Gastroenterology* 2001;**121**:101–9.

67 Brunetto MR, Oliveri F, Coco B *et al.* Outcome of anti-HBe positive chronic hepatitis B in alpha-interferon treated and untreated patients: a long term cohort study. *J Hepatol* 2002;**36**:263–70.

68 Zoulim F, Trépo C. Drug therapy for chronic hepatitis B: antiviral efficacy and influence of hepatitis B virus polymerase mutations on the outcome of therapy. *J Hepatol* 1998;**29**:151–68.

69 Atkins M, Gray DF. Lamivudine resistance in chronic hepatitis B. *J Hepatol* 1998;**28**:169.

70 Allen MI, Deslauriers M, Andrews CW *et al.* Clinical Investigation Group: identification and characterization of mutations in hepatitis B virus resistant to lamivudine. *Hepatology* 1998;**27**:1670–7.

71 Chayama K, Suzuki Y, Kobayashi M *et al.* Emergence and takeover of YMDD motif mutant hepatitis B virus during long-term lamivudine therapy and re-takeover by wild type after cessation of therapy. *Hepatology* 1998;**27**:1711–16.

72 Pichoud C, Seignéres B, Wang ZR *et al.* Transient selection of a hepatitis B virus polymerase gene mutant associated with a decreased replication capacity and famciclovir resistance. *Hepatology* 1999;**29**:230–7.

73 Benhamou Y, Dohin E, Lunel-Fabiani F *et al.* Efficacy of lamivudine on replication of hepatitis B virus in HIV-infected patients. *Lancet* 1995;**345**:396–7.

74 Benhamou Y, Katlama C, Lunel F *et al.* Effects of lamivudine on replication of hepatitis B virus in HIV-infected men. *Ann Intern Med* 1996;**125**:705–12.

75 Schnittman SM, Pierce PF. Potential role of lamivudine (3TC) in the clearance of chronic hepatitis B virus infection in a patient coinfected with human immunodeficiency virus type 1. *Clin Infect Dis* 1996;**23**:638–9.

76 Altfeld M, Rockstroh JK, Addo M *et al.* Reactivation of hepatitis B in a long-term anti-HBs-positive patient with AIDS following lamivudine withdrawal. *J Hepatol* 1998;**29**:306–9.

77 Bain VG, Kneteman NM, Ma MM *et al.* Efficacy of lamivudine in chronic hepatitis B patients with active viral replication and decompensated cirrhosis undergoing liver transplantation. *Transplantation* 1996;**62**:1456–62.

78 Grellier L, Mutimer D, Ahmed M *et al.* Lamivudine prophylaxis against reinfection in liver transplantation for hepatitis B cirrhosis. *Lancet* 1996;**348**:1212–15.

79 Ling R, Mutimer D, Ahmed N *et al.* Selection of mutations in the hepatitis B virus polymerase during therapy of transplant recipients with lamivudine. *Hepatology* 1996;**24**:711–13.

80 Al Faraidy K, Yoshida EM, Davis JE *et al.* Alteration of the dismal natural history of fibrosing cholestatic hepatitis secondary to hepatitis B virus with the use of lamivudine. *Transplantation* 1997;**64**:926–8.

81 Ben-Ari Z, Shmueli D, Mor E *et al.* Beneficial effect of lamivudine in recurrent hepatitis B after liver transplantation. *Transplantation* 1997;**63**:393–6.

82 Ben-Ari Z, Shmueli D, Mor E *et al.* Beneficial effect of lamivudine pre- and post-liver transplantation for hepatitis B infection. *Transplant Proc* 1997;**29**:2687–8.

83 Rostaing L, Henry S, Cisterne JM *et al.* Efficacy and safety of lamivudine on replication of recurrent hepatitis B after cadaveric renal transplantation. *Transplantation* 1997;**64**:1624–7.

84 Andreone P, Caraceni P, Grazi GL *et al.* Lamivudine treatment for acute hepatitis B after liver transplantation. *J Hepatol* 1998;**29**:985–9.

85 De Man RA, Bartholomeusz AI, Niesters HGM *et al.* The sequential occurrence of viral mutations in a liver transplant recipient re-infected with hepatitis B: hepatitis B immune globulin escape, famciclovir non-response, followed by lamivudine resistance resulting in graft loss. *J Hepatol* 1998;**29**:669–75.

86 Goffin E, Horsmans Y, Cornu C *et al.* Lamivudine inhibits hepatitis B virus replication in kidney graft recipients. *Transplantation* 1998;**66**:407–9.

87 Herrero JI, Quiroga J, Sangro B *et al.* Effectiveness of lamivudine in treatment of acute recurrent hepatitis B after liver transplantation. *Dig Dis Sci* 1998;**43**:1186–9.

88 Jung YO, Lee YS, Yang WS *et al.* Treatment of chronic hepatitis B with lamivudine in renal transplant recipients. *Transplantation* 1998;**66**:733–7.

89 Markowitz JS, Martin P, Conrad AJ *et al.* Prophylaxis against hepatitis B recurrence following liver transplantation using combination lamivudine and hepatitis B immune globulin. *Hepatology* 1998;**28**:585–9.

90 Marzano A, Debernardi-Venon W, Condreay L *et al.* Efficacy of lamivudine re-treatment in a patient with hepatitis B virus (HBV) recurrence after liver transplantation and HBV-DNA breakthrough during the first treatment. *Transplantation* 1998;**65**:1499–500.

91 Nery JR, Weppler D, Rodriguez M *et al.* Efficacy of lamivudine in controlling hepatitis B virus recurrence after liver transplantation. *Transplantation* 1998;**65**:1615–21.

92 Picardi M, Selleri C, De Rosa G *et al.* Lamivudine treatment for chronic replicative hepatitis B virus infection after allogeneic bone marrow transplantation. *Bone Marrow Transplant* 1998;**21**:1267–9.

93 Liao CA, Lee CM, Wu HC, Wang MC, Lu SN, Eng HL. Lamivudine for the treatment of hepatitis B virus reactivation following chemotherapy for non-Hodgkin's lymphoma. *Br J Haematol* 2002;**116**:166–9.

94 Ahmed A, Keeffe EB. Lamivudine therapy for chemotherapy-induced reactivation of hepatitis B virus infection. *Am J Gastroenterol* 1999;**94**:249–51.

95 Persico M, De Marino F, Russo GD *et al.* Efficacy of lamivudine to prevent hepatitis reactivation in hepatitis B virus-infected patients treated for non-Hodgkin lymphoma. *Blood* 2002 15;**99**:724–5.

96 Stroffolini T, Andriani A, Bibas M, Barlattani A. Successful treatment with lamivudine for reactivated hepatitis B infection following chemotherapy for non-Hodgkin's lymphoma. *Ann Hematol* 2002;**81**:48–9.

97 Silvestri F, Ermacora A, Sperotto A *et al.* Lamivudine allows completion of chemotherapy in lymphoma patients with hepatitis B reactivation. *Br J Haematol* 2000;**108**:394–6.

98 Saif MW, Little RF, Hamilton JM, Allegra CJ, Wilson WH. Reactivation of chronic hepatitis B infection following intensive chemotherapy and successful treatment with lamivudine: a case report and review of the literature. *Ann Oncol* 2001;**12**:123–9.

99 Al-Taie OH, Mork H, Gassel AM, Wilhelm M, Weissbrich B, Scheurlen M. Prevention of hepatitis B flare-up during chemotherapy using lamivudine: case report and review of the literature. *Ann Hematol* 1999;**78**:247–9.

100 Nakagawa M, Simizu Y, Suemura M, Sato B. Successful long-term control with lamivudine against reactivated hepatitis B infection following intensive chemotherapy and autologous peripheral blood stem cell transplantation in non-Hodgkin's lymphoma: experience of 2 cases. *Am J Hematol* 2002;**70**:60–3.

101 Maguire CM, Crawford DH, Hourigan LF, Clouston AD, Walpole ET, Powell EE. Case report: lamivudine therapy for submassive hepatic necrosis due to reactivation of hepatitis B following chemotherapy. *J Gastroenterol Hepatol* 1999;**14**:801–3.

102 Yeo W, Steinberg JL, Tam JS *et al.* Lamivudine in the treatment of hepatitis B virus reactivation during cytotoxic chemotherapy. *J Med Virol* 1999;**59**:263–9.

103 Kawai Y, Ikegaya S, Hata M *et al.* Successful lamivudine therapy for post-chemotherapeutic fulminant hepatitis B in a hepatitis B virus carrier with non-Hodgkin's lymphoma: case report and review of the literature. *Ann Hematol* 2001;**80**:482–4.

104 Rossi G, Pelizzari A, Motta M, Puoti M. Primary prophylaxis with lamivudine of hepatitis B virus reactivation in chronic HBsAg carriers with lymphoid malignancies treated with chemotherapy. *Br J Haematol* 2001;**115**:58–62.

105 Ter Borg F, Smorenburg S, De Man RA *et al.* Recovery from life-threatening, corticosteroid-unresponsive, chemotherapy-related reactivation of hepatitis B associated with lamivudine therapy. *Dig Dis Sci* 1998;**43**:2267–70.

106 Dienstag JL, Perrillo RP, Schiff ER *et al.* A preliminary trial of lamivudine for chronic hepatitis B infection. *N Engl J Med* 1995;**333**:1657–61.

107 Honkoop P, De Man RA, Heijtink RA *et al.* Hepatitis B reactivation after lamivudine. *Lancet* 1995;**346**:1156–7.

108 Nowak MA, Bonhoeffer S, Hill AM *et al.* H. Viral dynamics in hepatitis B virus infection. *Proc Natl Acad Sci USA* 1996;**93**:4398–402.

109 Tipples GA, Ma MM, Fischer KP *et al.* Mutation in HBV RNA-dependent DNA polymerase confers resistance to lamivudine *in vivo*. *Hepatology* 1996;**24**:714–17.

110 Heijtink RA, Kruining J, Honkoop P *et al.* Serum HBeAg quantitation during antiviral therapy for chronic hepatitis B. *J Med Virol* 1997;**53**:282–7.

111 Honkoop P, De Man RA, Scholte HR *et al.* Effect of lamivudine on morphology and function of mitochondria in patients with chronic hepatitis B. *Hepatology* 1997;**26**:211–15.

112 Honkoop P, Niesters HGM, De Man RAM *et al.* Lamivudine resistance in immunocompetent chronic hepatitis B – incidence and patterns. *J Hepatol* 1997;**26**:1393–5.

113 Jaeckel E, Manns MP. Experience with lamivudine against hepatitis B virus. *Intervirology* 1997;**40**:322–36.

114 Lai CL, Ching CK, Tung AKM *et al.* Lamivudine is effective in suppressing hepatitis B virus DNA in Chinese hepatitis B surface antigen carriers: a placebo-controlled trial. *Hepatology* 1997;**25**:241–4.

115 Nevens F, Main J, Honkoop P *et al.* Lamivudine therapy for chronic hepatitis B: a six-month randomized dose-ranging study. *Gastroenterology* 1997;**113**:1258–63.

116 Schalm SW. Clinical implications of lamivudine resistance by HBV. *Lancet* 1997;**349**:3–4.

117 Schiano TD, Lissoos TW, Ahmed A *et al.* Lamivudine-stavudine-induced liver failure in hepatitis B cirrhosis. *Am J Gastroenterol* 1997;**92**:1563–4.

118 Zeuzem S, De Man RA, Honkoop P *et al.* Dynamics of hepatitis B virus infection *in vivo*. *J Hepatol* 1997;**27**:431–6.

119 Allen MI, Deslauriers M, Andrews CW *et al.* and Lamivudine Clinical Investigation Group. Identification and characterization of mutations in hepatitis B virus resistant to lamivudine. *Hepatology* 1998;**27**:1670–7.

120 Atkins M, Gray DF. Lamivudine resistance in chronic hepatitis B. *J Hepatol* 1998;**28**:169.

121 Bernasconi E, Battegay M. Lamivudine for chronic hepatitis B. *N Engl J Med* 1998;**339**:1786.

122 Boni C, Bertoletti A, Penna A *et al.* Lamivudine treatment can restore T cell responsiveness in chronic hepatitis B. *J Clin Invest* 1998;**102**:968–75.

123 Buti M, Jardi R, Cotrina M *et al.* Transient emergence of hepatitis B variants in a patient with chronic hepatitis B resistant to lamivudine. *J Hepatol* 1998;**28**:510–13.

124 Chayama K, Suzuki Y, Kobayashi M *et al.* Emergence and takeover of YMDD motif mutant hepatitis B virus during long-term lamivudine therapy and re-takeover by wild type after cessation of therapy. *Hepatology* 1998;**27**:1711–16.

125 Honkoop P, De Man RA, Niesters HGM. Quantitative assessment of hepatitis B virus DNA during a 24-week course of lamivudine therapy. *Ann Intern Med* 1998;**128**:697.

126 Honkoop P, De Man RA, Niesters HGM *et al.* Clinical impact of lamivudine resistance in chronic hepatitis B. *J Hepatol* 1998;**29**:510–11.

127 Lai CL, Chien RN, Leung NWY *et al.* and Asia Hepatitis Lamivudine Study Group. A one-year trial of lamivudine for chronic hepatitis B. *N Engl J Med* 1998;**339**:61–8.

128 Niesters HGM, Honkoop P, Haagsma EB *et al.* Identification of more than one mutation in the hepatitis B virus polymerase gene arising during prolonged lamivudine treatment. *J Infect Dis* 1998;**177**:1382–5.

129 Song BC, Suh DJ, Lee HC, Chung YH, Lee YS. Hepatitis B e antigen seroconversion after lamivudine therapy is not durable in patients with chronic hepatitis B in Korea. *Hepatology.* 2000;**32**:803–6.

130 Leung NW, Lai CL, Chang TT *et al.* Extended lamivudine treatment in patients with chronic hepatitis B enhances hepatitis B e antigen seroconversion rates: results after 3 years of therapy. *Hepatology* 2001;**33**:1527–32.

131 Hadziyannis SJ, Papatheodoridis GV, Dimou E, Laras A, Papaioannou C. Efficacy of long-term lamivudine monotherapy in patients with hepatitis B e antigen-negative chronic hepatitis B. *Hepatology* 2000;**32**:847–51.

132 Santantonio T, Mazzola M, Lacovazzi T, Miglietta A, Guastadisegni A, Pastore G. Long-term follow-up of patients with anti-HBe/HBV DNA-positive chronic hepatitis B treated for 12 months with lamivudine. *J Hepatol* 2000;**32**:300–6.

133 Buti M, Cotrina M, Jardi R *et al.* Two years of lamivudine therapy in anti-HBe-positive patients with chronic hepatitis B. *J Viral Hepatitis* 2001;**8**:270–5.

134 Dienstag JL, Schiff ER, Wright TL *et al.* Lamivudine as initial treatment for chronic hepatitis B in the United States. *N Engl J Med* 1999 21;**341**:1256–63.

135 Schalm SW, Heathcote J, Cianciara J *et al.* Lamivudine and alpha interferon combination treatment of patients with chronic hepatitis B infection: a randomised trial. *Gut* 2000;**46**:562–8.

136 Tassopoulos NC, Volpes R, Pastore G *et al.* Efficacy of lamivudine in patients with hepatitis B eantigen-negative/hepatitis B virus DNA-positive (precore mutant) chronic hepatitis B. Lamivudine Precore Mutant Study Group. *Hepatology* 1999;**29**:889–96.

137 Van Nunen AB, Hansen BE, Suh DJ *et al.* Durability of HBeAg seroconversion following antiviral therapy for chronic hepatitis B: relation to type of therapy and pretreatment serum hepatitis B virus DNA and alanine aminotransferase. *Gut* 2003;**52**:420–4.

138 Lee KM, Cho SW, Kim SW, Kim HJ, Hahm KB, Kim JH. Effect of virological response on post-treatment durability of lamivudine-induced HBeAg seroconversion. *J Viral Hepat* 2002;**9**:208–12.

139 Song BC, Suh DJ, Lee HC, Chung YH, Lee YS. Hepatitis B e antigen seroconversion after lamivudine therapy is not durable in patients with chronic hepatitis B in Korea. *Hepatology* 2000;**32**:803–6.

140 Dienstag JL, Cianciara J, Karayalcin S *et al.* Durability of serologic response after lamivudine treatment of chronic hepatitis B. *Hepatology* 2003;**37**:748–55.

141 Papatheodoridis GV, Dimou E, Laras A, Papadimitropoulos V, Hadziyannis SJ. Course of virologic breakthroughs under long-term lamivudine in HBeAg-negative precore mutant HBV liver disease. *Hepatology* 2002;**36**:219–26.

142 Schalm SW, Heathcote J, Cianciara J *et al.* Lamivudine and alpha interferon combination treatment of patients with chronic hepatitis B infection: a randomised trial. *Gut* 2000;**46**:562–8.

143 Barbaro G, Zechini F, Pellicelli AM *et al.* Long-term efficacy of interferon alpha-2b and lamivudine in combination compared to lamivudine monotherapy in patients with chronic hepatitis B. An Italian multicenter, randomized trial. *J Hepatol* 2001;**35**:406–11.

144 Tatulli I, Francavilla R, Rizzo GL *et al.* Lamivudine and alpha-interferon in combination long term for precore mutant chronic hepatitis B. *J Hepatol* 2001;**35**:805–10.

145 Xiong XF, Flores C, Yang H *et al.* Mutations in hepatitis B DNA polymerase associated with resistance to lamivudine do not confer resistance to adefovir *in vitro. Hepatology* 1998;**28**:1669–73.

146 Marques AR, Lau DTY, McKenzie R *et al.* Combination therapy with famciclovir and interferon-a for the treatment of chronic hepatitis B. *J Infect Dis* 1998;**178**:1483–7.

147 Marcellin P, Chang TT, Lim SG *et al.* Adefovir dipivoxyl for the treatment of hepatitis B e antigen-positive chronic hepatitis B. *N Engl J Med* 2003 27;**348**:808–16.

148 Hadziyannis SJ, Tassopoulos NC, Heathcote EJ *et al.* Adefovir dipivoxyl for the treatment of hepatitis B e antigen-negative chronic hepatitis B. *N Engl J Med.* 2003;**348**:800–7.

149 EASL Consensus Conference on Hepatitis B. *J Hepatol* 2003;**39**(suppl):51–5236.

25 Alcoholic liver disease

Philippe Mathurin, Thierry Poynard

Screening

In heavy drinkers, liver-related mortality is mainly attributed to cirrhosis and hepatocellular carcinoma (HCC). Therefore, the main objectives of the screening are: (i) to identify patients with significant liver injury, (ii) to characterize the main risk factors for HCC and (iii) to make an early diagnosis of HCC.

In the present chapter, we focus on the non-invasive screening of cirrhosis and on screening of HCC.

Non-invasive screening of cirrhosis

Assessment of the stage and severity of liver injury requires liver biopsy, an invasive procedure associated with severe complications leading to death in 0·02% of patients.[1] Less than 30% of heavy drinkers have some features of significant liver injury such as extensive fibrosis, alcoholic hepatitis or cirrhosis.[2] Routine liver biopsy is non-essential in 70% of heavy drinkers. Indirect diagnostic tests for cirrhosis are clearly necessary to avoid screening with routine liver biopsy.

Several serum proteins have been widely evaluated for their use as a non-invasive test for liver fibrosis: (i) extracellular matrix proteins (procollagen I, procollagen III propeptide (PIIIP), laminin, transforming growth factor (TGF)-β1, hyaluronate); (ii) prothrombin time; (iii) apolipoprotein A-I (ApoA-I); and (iv) α-2 macroglobulin. The number of studies evaluating the diagnostic accuracy of procollagen I, laminin and TGF-β1 is clearly insufficient for reaching a conclusion. For PIIIP and hyaluronate, previous studies yield interesting results even though some data are still controversial.

Serum PIIIP did not provide any significant improvement in assessing the degree of fibrosis in two studies whereas one study observed that PIIIP could be useful in detecting patients with underlying cirrhosis.[3-5] Recently, two studies observed the ability of PIIIP to correctly identify patients with fibrosis or cirrhosis.[6,7] In Teare *et al.*'s study, with the receiver operating curve it was observed that at a cut-off of 0·7 U/ml, the sensitivity was 94% and the specificity 81% (positive predictive value 85%, negative predictive value 92%). A major problem, beside the wide heterogeneity of the assays used in the studies, is that even with the same assay the PIIIP screening cut-off is still unknown.

Hyaluronate, an unbranched polysaccharide, is a component of extracellular matrix. In one study it was observed that hyaluronate may be useful for the diagnosis of cirrhosis.[8] Serum hyaluronate concentrations were significantly higher in alcoholic patients with cirrhosis (467 micrograms/l, range 205–800 micrograms/l) than in alcoholic patients without cirrhosis (53 micrograms/l, range 14–78 micrograms/l). The diagnostic accuracy of serum hyaluronate for the evaluation of cirrhosis was confirmed in patients with primary biliary cirrhosis.[9,10] For routine practice, a unit analyzed the screening cut-off for the diagnosis of cirrhosis.[6] Hyaluronate concentration of ≥ 60 micrograms/l had a sensitivity of 97% and a specificity of 73% for the diagnosis of cirrhosis. In terms of applicability, the diagnostic accuracy of this cut-off should be confirmed in another population by another group.

Prothrombin time was initially designed to assess hepatocellular dysfunction. However, improvement in the measurement of this index leads to additional properties. Indeed, prothrombin time seemed to predict liver fibrosis and to be inversely correlated with the area of fibrosis measured by image analysis.[6,11,12] A recent study evaluated the predictive value of the prothrombin index for liver fibrosis in an initial group of patients with chronic liver disease, and the results were subsequently validated in another group of patients.[13] The reproducibility of measurement of the prothrombin index was compared in different laboratories. Prothrombin index ≤ 80% or ≤ 70% diagnosed severe fibrosis or cirrhosis, respectively, and prothrombin index ≥ 105% or ≥ 100% excluded a diagnosis of severe fibrosis or cirrhosis, respectively, at the 95% probability level. The prothrombin indices measured in different laboratories were similar (78 ± 18% *v* 78 ± 14%) and well correlated (r = 0·91). The authors concluded that prothrombin index had a high diagnostic accuracy for severe fibrosis or cirrhosis especially due to alcohol. Moreover, the prothrombin index was highly reproducible.[13]

Table 25.1   PGA index: the scores range from 0 to 12[a]

Score	Prothrombin time % of normal (seconds over control) (P)	GGT (IU/l) (G)	Apolipoprotein AI (mg/dl) (A)
0	≥ 80% (< 1)	< 20	≥ 200
1	70–79% (1–2)	20–49	175–199
2	60–69% (2–3)	50–99	150–174
3	50–59% (3–4)	100–199	125–149
4	< 50% (≥ 4)	≥ 200	< 125

[a]Each item of the score (prothombin, GGT and apolipoprotein A1) is scored from 0 to 4. The final score combines the three scores of each item and ranges from 0 to 12.

GGT, γ-glutmyl transpeptidase

ApoA-I, the major component of high density lipoprotein cholesterol, was significantly correlated with liver injury.[14] In a study of 581 alcoholic patients, ApoA-I had an independent and discriminate value for the diagnosis of fibrosis versus steatosis ($P < 0.001$) and for the diagnosis of cirrhosis versus non-cirrhotic fibrosis ($P < 0.001$) or versus alcoholic hepatitis without alcoholic cirrhosis ($P < 0.001$).[15] Conversely, serum ApoB was not correlated with hepatic fibrosis. We analyzed the mechanisms involved in the decrease of serum ApoA-I in heavy drinkers with fibrosis.[16–19] Those studies observed that: (i) an increase of ApoA-I mRNA may explain, at least in part, the increase of serum ApoA-I in heavy drinkers with steatosis; (ii) fibrosis is associated with decreased serum ApoA-I, probably due to post-transcriptional mechanisms; and (iii) severe alcoholic cirrhosis is associated with a non-specific decrease in ApoA-I mRNA. However, with regard to the wide overlap of serum ApoA-I in patients with different stages of liver fibrosis, the diagnostic accuracy of ApoA-I for the evaluation of cirrhosis was insufficient. Therefore we analyzed the diagnostic accuracy of a simple index called PGA that combines prothrombin index (P), γ-glutamyl transpeptidase (GGT) concentration (G) and apolipoprotein A-I (A).[12] The PGA value ranged from 0 to 12 (Table 25.1). When the PGA was < 2, the probability of cirrhosis was 0% and the probability of normal liver was 83%. Conversely, when the PGA was > 9, the probability of cirrhosis was 86%. A study observed that the combination of PGA and PIIIP concentration may be useful to reduce the need of liver biopsy.[7]

Serum α-2 macroglobulin, a proteinase inhibitor, has been evaluated as a marker of cirrhosis. Serum level was higher in patients with cirrhosis than in patients without cirrhosis.[20,21] Based on those results, we assessed whether serum α-2 macroglobulin could improve the diagnostic accuracy of PGA.[22] We showed that addition of α-2-macroglobulin to the PGA index (PGAA index) could be useful in the detection of cirrhosis.

The diagnostic accuracy of non-invasive serum markers (PIIIP, hyaluronate, laminin, TGF-β1, prothrombin time, α-2 macroglobulin, PGA and PGAA) were compared.[6] The authors observed that hyaluronate concentration and prothrombin index were the most sensitive variables for screening.

Recently, a score named Fibrotest was developed to predict the extent of liver fibrosis in patients with chronic hepatitis C. Fibrotest combined necroinflammatory factors and serum markers including total bilirubin, GGT activity, α-2 macroglobulin, γ globulin, haptoglobin and ApoA-1. A high negative predictive value (100% certainty of absence of F2 (portal fibrosis with few septa), F3 (portal fibrosis with many septa), or F4 (cirrhosis) was obtained for scores ranging from zero to 0.10 (12% of all patients), and a high positive predictive value (> 90% certainty of presence of F2, F3, or F4) for scores ranging from 0.60 to 1.00 (34% of all patients) was observed.[23] This test could be used to reduce substantially the number of liver biopsies done in patients with chronic HCV infection. Studies evaluating the diagnosis accuracy of Fibrotest in patients with alcoholic liver disease are ongoing in French centers.

In summary, controversies surrounding extracellular matrix serum markers persist. The methods for their quantification and the units of quantification varied widely. The discrepancies between assays contributed to the wide heterogeneity of cut-off levels reported in various studies. Therefore, in routine practice, additional studies are required to determine the screening cut-off of PIIIP and hyaluronate. Conversely, prothrombin index, PGA and PGAA scores, PIIIP and serum hyaluronate may be used in the screening for cirrhosis in heavy drinkers. Further studies are required to evaluate the predictive value of recently available tests such as Fibrotest in patients with alcoholic liver disease. In the near future, for the diagnosis of extensive liver fibrosis in heavy drinkers, the use of serum markers will reduce the need for liver biopsy.

Screening for hepatocellular carcinoma

In cirrhotic patients, the probability of developing HCC at 5 years is approximately 20%, with a yearly incidence rate of 3%. The identification of the subgroup of patients with higher risk for HCC, and its early detection constitute two of the main challenges for hepatologists in the near future. In heavy drinkers, presence of cirrhosis, age > 50 years, male sex, serum alpha fetoprotein (AFP) ≥ 15 ng/ml, HBsAg and anti-HCV antibodies were independently associated with the occurrence of HCC.[24–26] A center developed a clinicobiological score which identified two groups at low (3-year cumulative incidence, 0%) and high risk of HCC (3-year cumulative incidence, 24%).[27] Beside these factors, the preneoplastic role of liver large cell dysplasia has been suggested.[28] In a study the estimated cumulative incidence of HCC at 3 years was 38% and 10% in patients with and without large cell dysplasia, respectively.[27] Another group confirmed that large cell dysplasia, detected in 24% of patients, was a major risk factor for HCC.[29] Based on those results, liver biopsy would be necessary for the identification of patients with a higher risk for HCC.

Screening for HCC is usually done with ultrasonography and the determination of serum AFP. However, contrasting data have been reported on the effectiveness of ultrasonography for early detection of HCC. A French center observed that an initial diagnosis of tumor less than 3 cm was made in only 21% of cases.[30] Conversely, in two studies, ultrasonography allowed the detection of small HCC in 76% of cases.[31,32] Regardless of these contrasting data, most liver units recommend regular ultrasonography in the screening for HCC.

In conclusion, for heavy drinkers in routine practice the following strategy for screening for HCC is recommended. Screening for cirrhosis can be done using serum markers such as PGA, PIIIP or serum hyaluronate. Liver biopsy will be necessary in patients with a PGA score $P < \geq 9$, a PIIIP ≥ 0·7 U/ml or serum hyaluronate ≥ 60 micrograms/l to confirm the diagnosis of cirrhosis and to detect the presence of large cell dysplasia. However, further studies are required to validate this strategy. Among the subgroup of patients at high risk for HCC, further studies will be needed to test the usefulness of intensive screening and preventive measures.

Treatment

In heavy drinkers, pharmacological treatments and liver transplantation have been tested to improve survival of heavy drinkers with severe liver injury such as alcoholic hepatitis or cirrhosis. However, the usefulness of pharmacological treatments for controlling the alcohol-induced liver injury is still unsettled, and controversies persist with regard to the selection of patients for liver transplantation.[33,34]

Pharmacological treatments

To identify the pharmacological treatments associated with efficacy we have used literature-based meta-analysis, a useful technique for evaluation of treatment effect.[35] Meta-analysis was performed when an intervention was evaluated in two or more randomized controlled trials (RCTs) published as complete articles using the same endpoint of survival (short-term or long-term).

Colchicine

In the first RCT evaluating effect of colchicine on the long-term survival of patients with alcoholic cirrhosis, 5- and 10-year survival rates were significantly higher in the colchicine group (75 and 56%, respectively) than in the placebo group (34% and 20%, $P < 0.001$).[36] However in patients with alcoholic hepatitis, two other studies did not observe any effect of colchicine on short-term survival.[37,38] Ald

In a recent randomized placebo-controlled multicenter Veterans Affairs (VA) trial (CSP 352)[39] patients were randomized to receive colchicine 0·6 mg twice daily ($n = 274$) or placebo ($n = 275$) for at least 24 months. The mortality rates in the colchicine and placebo groups were similar: 49% versus 45%. In addition the liver-related deaths were not significantly different: 32% versus 28%. In summary, this trial does not support the conclusion from Kershenobich *et al.*'s[36] study. Ald

Propylthiouracil

In two RCTs there was no observed effect of propylthiouracil on short-term survival.[40,41] Meta-analysis of these RCTs confirms the lack of benefit on short-term survival, with a mean difference of 1% (CI − 7 to 9%) between propylthiouracil-treated and control patients. Alc

The effect of propylthiouracil on long-term survival was analyzed in an RCT with 310 alcoholic patients who received propylthiouracil ($n = 157$) or a placebo ($n = 153$) for 2 years.[42] The two-year mortality rate was lower in the propylthiouracil group than in the placebo group: 13% versus 26%, $P < 0.05$. Propylthiouracil treatment, prothrombin time, hemoglobin levels and mean daily urinary alcohol levels were independent prognostic factors. However, this study has two main limitations: (i) the statistical analysis was carried out using "per protocol analysis" and (ii) the cumulative dropout rates in both groups were approximately 60%. The authors stated that per protocol analysis was appropriate, since compliance was accurately quantified using elaborate monitoring with a fluorescent compound detectable in urine.[43] However, in RCTs the "intention to treat analysis" is usually preferred and the observed high rates of dropouts have to be taken into account. Alc

A recent systematic review of six randomized controlled trials including 710 patients demonstrated no significant benefit of propylthiouracil compared with placebo on mortality (odds ratio 0·91, 95% CI 0·59 to 1·4).[44] Ald In addition propylthiouracil was associated with a non-significant trend towards an increased risk of non-serious events and the infrequent occurrence of serious adverse events (leukopenia).[44] Taking into account this systematic review and the adverse effect profile of propylthiouracil, additional RCTs evaluating propylthiouracil would be difficult to justify.

Other drugs

D-penicillamine, vitamin E, (+)-cyanidanol-3, thioctic acid, malotilate and the calcium antagonist amlodipine have been evaluated in randomized trials, but none has been shown to decrease mortality.[45–51] Ald

Silymarin The first RCT suggested that silymarin would improve long-term survival of patients with cirrhosis.[52] However, another RCT did not confirm any effect of silymarin on survival.[53] Ald

Insulin and glucagon association The infusion of insulin–glucagon was tested in five RCTs (three published in article form and two as abstracts) in patients with alcoholic hepatitis.[54–58] Only one study reported a significant effect on short-term survival.[53] Meta-analysis of these RCTs did not show any significant survival effect of insulin–glucagon infusion on short-term survival, with a mean difference of 95% (CI −11 to 23%). Alc

Anabolic-androgenic steroids Five RCTs evaluating anabolic steroids reported negative results.[59–63] In one study, a sensitivity analysis suggested that anabolic steroids were effective in the subgroup of patients with moderate malnutrition.[62] A recent systematic review confirmed that for alcoholic patients anabolic-androgenic steroids did not have any significant benefit on mortality (relative risk (RR) 0·83, 95% CI 0·6 to 1·15).[64] Moreover, anabolic-androgenic steroids were associated with the infrequent occurrence of serious adverse events (RR 4·54).[64] Based on these results, anabolic steroids are not indicated in patients with alcoholic liver disease. Furthermore, the use of anabolic-androgenic drugs is questionable when considering the potential risk of development of HCC associated with these drugs.

Corticosteroids

Thirteen RCTs tested corticosteroids in patients with alcoholic hepatitis.[61,65–76] Only four trials observed a survival benefit in treated patients.[65–68] The wide variability of disease severity between the studies, the lack of histological analysis before enrollment of patients, the small sample size, and confounding factors prior to randomization such as renal insufficiency or gastrointestinal bleeding explained, at least in part, these contradictory results.[77,78]

The Maddrey criterion is now used for identifying a subgroup of patients with a high risk of mortality.[72] In the most recent RCT, we confirmed Carithers' original observation that corticosteroid therapy significantly decreased short-term mortality in patients with severe alcoholic hepatitis (spontaneous encephalopathy or a Maddrey function

≥ 32): 94% versus 65% at 28 days in Carithers *et al.*'s study (NNT = 3, *P* = 0·006) and 88% versus 45% at 66 days in Ramond *et al.*'s study (NNT = 2, *P* = 0·001).[65,66] Ald

The meta-analysis of the 13 RCTs showed a significant short-term survival benefit of corticosteroids, with a mean difference of 15% (CI 6 to 24%, *P* < 0·01). The effect of corticosteroids on short-term survival was higher in the subgroup of patients with encephalopathy, with a mean difference of 27% (CI 11 to 44%, *P* < 0·0001).[80] Ald

In a study of 122 alcoholic patients with severe biopsy proven alcoholic hepatitis we showed that: (i) corticosteroids are associated with short-term survival benefit; (ii) young patients obtained much greater benefit from corticosteroid treatment; and (iii) survival benefit due to corticosteroid treatment persisted for at least 1 year and disappeared at 2 years.[79] B4

Three meta-analyses provided evidence that corticosteroids improved short-term survival of patients with a severe form of alcoholic hepatitis.[64,78,81] However, two meta-analyses which attempted to adjust for prognostic factors, questioned the efficacy of corticosteroids in alcoholic hepatitis.[64,81] These meta-analyses used a different weighting method than previous meta-analyses that may give too much weight to the results of Mendenhall *et al.*'s[61] RCT. The authors encouraged Mendenhall *et al.* (the authors of the largest trial[61]) to make their data available for analysis of individual patient data, as this study preceded the use of Maddrey's criteria for assessment of disease severity and based severity only on the serum bilirubin level.[82] Therefore, the three investigators of the three RCTs (Mendenhall, Carithers, Ramond) used the more accurate approach in the analysis of the individual data for patients with discriminant function of Maddrey (DF) ≥ 32.[83] Data of 102 placebo and 113 corticosteroid patients with DF ≥ 32 were analyzed. At 28 days, corticosteroid-treated patients had a significantly better survival: 84·6 ± 3·4% versus 65·1 ± 4·8%, *P* = 0·001. Ald In multivariate analysis, age (*P* = 0·003), serum creatinine (*P* = 0·006) and corticosteroid treatment (*P* = 0·01) were independent prognostic variables. The NNT, the number of patients needed to treat with corticosteroids in order to prevent 1 death was 5.[83] Recently, representatives of the American College of Gastroenterology recommended the use of glucocorticosteroids for patients with severe alcoholic hepatitis as defined by the Maddrey criteria.[84] More recently, a randomized trial of total enteral nutrition versus steroids showed similar early mortality with reduced later mortality in patients who received enteral nutrition: at 1 year mortality was 61% (steroid treatment) and 38% (enteral nutrition) (*P* = 0·026). The study is ongoing.[85] Ald

Newer drugs

These include pentoxifylline, anti-tumor necrosis factor (TNF)-α antibodies, phosphatidylcholine and *S*-adenosylmethionine.

In a recent RCT evaluating pentoxifylline in patients with severe alcoholic hepatitis a significant difference in survival was observed between pentoxifylline and placebo groups – 24·5% of patients who received pentoxifylline and 46% of patients who received placebo died.[86] Hepatorenal syndrome was the cause of death in 50% of pentoxifylline patients and 92% of placebo patients. Pentoxifylline treatment, age and creatinine were independently associated with survival. Ald Further trials evaluating pentoxifylline versus corticosteroids are required.

In animal models administration of anti-TNF-α antibody attenuated inflammation and necrosis. A double blind, randomized controlled trial evaluated the safety and tolerance of anti-TNFα antibody (infliximab) combined with steroids in patients with severe alcoholic hepatitis.[87] The authors observed that improvement of Maddrey function (39 to 12) was more pronounced in patients treated with infliximab and steroids. They concluded that the study lacked the power to allow comparison between groups, but that the promising results should encourage a larger trial. In an uncontrolled pilot study of 12 patients treated with a single infusion of infliximab, there was a significant modification in biochemical endpoints between baseline and follow up.[88] In October 2002, a multicenter randomized trial of infliximab in severe alcoholic hepatitis was stopped by the French drug agency (AFSSAPS).[89] There was a two-fold increase in deaths in the infliximab group versus the corticosteroid group. In both groups the main cause of death was infection.[89] The detailed analysis is still ongoing. Ald

The results of a multicenter randomized placebo-controlled trial (CSP 391) evaluating phosphatidylcholine have been recently presented. There was no significant effect of phosphatidylcholine on survival.[90] Ald

An RCT reported that adenosylmethionine might improve survival of patients with alcoholic cirrhosis.[91] Overall survival in the adenosylmethionine group (90%) was significantly better than in the placebo group (73%), $P = 0.04$. The authors observed that adenosylmethionine effect is restricted to the subgroup of patients with moderate liver disease (Child–Pugh A or B). This promising result will have to be confirmed in further RCTs. Ald

Four randomized studies have evaluated a variety of anti-oxidants, but no survival benefit or histological improvement was shown[92–95] with vitamin E.

In summary, only corticosteroids have been shown to be associated with a benefit on short-term survival in patients with severe alcoholic hepatitis (Maddrey discriminant function ≥ 32). The NNT, number of patients needed to treat with corticosteroids in order to prevent 1 death is 5. Ala Future studies evaluating the effect of colchicine and propylthiouracil on long-term survival are not recommended. Recent studies report interesting data concerning new drugs such as pentoxifylline, anti-TNF-α antibody and *S*-adenosylmethionine. Randomized controlled trials are ongoing for some of these drugs.

Liver transplantation

Liver transplantation is a highly effective therapeutic option for endstage liver disease. In patients with alcoholic cirrhosis, liver transplantation leads to survival rates similar to those in patients with non-alcoholic cirrhosis.[96–98] Due to the scarcity of donor organs, controversies surrounding liver transplantation in alcoholic patients have been focused on the identification of the subgroup with survival benefit, the validity of the abstinence criterion for patient selection and the societal issue of using an expensive intervention for the treatment of a self-inflicted illness.

To assess the efficacy of liver transplantation in patients with alcoholic cirrhosis, we compared 2-year survival of 169 transplant patients with matched control patients and simulated control patients.[99] The simulated control group survival was derived from a prognostic model (Beclere model) using the natural history of alcoholic cirrhosis. The final Beclere model combined four variables to obtain a risk score (R) for each patient in the following equation: $R = (0.0484 \times (\text{age in years}) + 0.469 \times (\text{encephalopathy}) + 0.537 \times \text{Log}_e (\text{bilirubin in } \mu\text{mol/l}) - 0.052 \times (\text{albumin in g/l})$. Encephalopathy was rated 0 if absent and 1 if asterixis, confusion or coma was present. Survival function for the Beclere model was S_1 at 1 year and S_2 at 2 years: $S_1 = 0.7334^{\exp. (R-3.058)}$ and $S_2 = 0.643^{\exp. (R-3.058)^2}$. Two-year survival of transplant patients (73%, 67–79%) was similar to matched patients (67%, 63–71%) and simulated patients (67%, 63–70%). In a sensitivity analysis of patients with severe liver disease, 2-year survival of transplant patients was significantly higher (64%, (42–86%) than matched patients (41%, 23–59%) and simulated patients (23%, 19–27%). B2 We concluded that: (i) efficacy of liver transplantation is limited to the subgroup of patients with severe liver disease and (ii) the Beclere model may be useful in the selection of alcoholic patients. However, it was observed in another study that this model may overestimate the risk of death for patients specifically referred for transplantation.[100]

A study evaluated 14 transplant centers with regard to their selection practices.[100] Eight of the centers reported that they would accept candidates with less than 1 year of alcoholic abstinence, four with less than 6 months of abstinence and one program would accept candidates who currently continued to drink alcohol. Most programs reported recommending a 6-month abstinence criterion for listing patients with alcoholic liver disease. However, the validity of the 6-month criterion has been recently called into question. Yates *et al.* observed that the use of the 6-month abstinence criterion forces a significant number of patients with a low risk of relapse to wait for transplant listing.[102] In a study of 84 transplant patients, the receiver operating curve showed that despite the 6-month criterion being the best cut-off in predicting subsequent abstinence, this cut-off was a poor predictor of post-transplantation abstinence (sensitivity 72%, specificity 66%).[103] Five variables were independently associated with post-transplant abstinence: the psycho-social inclusion criteria, absence of previous illicit drug use, presence of a personal life insurance policy, number of alcoholic sisters and the length of pre-transplant abstinence. The pooling of the previous studies observed that the sensitivity of the 6-month abstinence criterion in predicting post-transplant abstinence ranged from 28% to 100% and the specificity from 76% to 92%.[103–106]

A major objection to liver transplantation in alcoholic patients was the concern about the risk of alcoholism recidivism. In previous studies, the risk of recidivism ranged from 10% to 30%.[103,107–109] However, the authors did not observe any difference between abstinent and non-abstinent patients for survival and for compliance with immunosuppressive regimen. Therefore, the reluctance to accept alcoholic patients because of the risk of recidivism is no longer relevant.

In conclusion, patients with severe alcoholic cirrhosis benefit from liver transplantation. Most of the centers recommend a 6-month abstinence for listing the patients. However, this sole criterion is insufficient to predict the abstinence after transplantation. Moreover, after transplantation, the recidivism of alcoholism seems to have no effect on patient outcome.

References

1 Piccinino F, Sagnelli E, Pasquale G, Guisti G. Complications following liver biopsy: a multicentre retrospective study on 68276 biopsies. *J Hepatol* 1986;**2**:165–73.

2 Bedossa P, Poynard T, Naveau S, Martin ED, Agostini H, Chaput JC. Observer variation in assessment of liver biopsies of alcoholic patients. *Alcohol Clin Exp Res* 1988;**12**:173–8.

3 Torres-Salinas M, Pares A, Caballeria J *et al.* Serum procollagen type III peptide as a marker of hepatic fibrogenesis in alcoholic patients. *Gastroenterology* 1986;**90**: 1241–6.

4 Niemelä O, Ristelli L, Sotaniemi EA, Risteli J. Aminoterminal propeptide of type III procollagen in serum in alcoholic liver disease. *Gastroenterology* 1983;**85**:254–9.

5 Annoni G, Colombo M, Cantaluppi MC, Bourtos Khlat, Lambertico P, Rojkind M. Serum type III procollagen and Laminin (Lam-P1) detect alcoholic hepatitis in chronic alcohol abusers. *Hepatology* 1989;**9**:693–7.

6 Oberti F, Valsesia E, Pilette C *et al.* Noninvasive diagnosis of hepatic fibrosis or cirrhosis. *Gastroenterology* 1997;**113**: 1609–16.

7 Teare JP, Sherman D, Greenfield SM *et al.* Comparison of serum procollagen III peptide concentrations and PGA index for assessment of hepatic fibrosis. *Lancet* 1993;**342**:895–8.

8 Engström-Laurent A, Loöf L, Nyberg A, Schroder T. Increased serum levels of hyaluronate in liver disease. *Hepatology* 1985; **5**:638–42.

9 Nyberg A, Engström-Laurent A, Loöf L. Serum hyaluronate in primary biliary cirrhosis-a biochemical marker for progressive liver damage. *Hepatology* 1988;**8**:142–6.

10 Plebani M, Giacomini A, Floreani A *et al.* Biochemical markers of hepatic fibrosis in primary biliary cirrhosis. *Ric Clin Lab* 1990;**20**:269–74.

11 Pilette C, Rousselet MC, Bedossa P *et al.* Histopathological evaluation of liver fibrosis: quantitative image analysis vs semi-quantitative scores. *J Hepatol* 1998;**28**:439–46.

12 Poynard T, Aubert A, Bedossa P *et al.* A simple biological index for detection of alcoholic liver disease in drinkers. *Gastroenterology* 1991;**100**:1397–402.

13 Croquet V, Vuillemin E, Ternisien C *et al.* Prothrombin index is an indirect marker of severe liver fibrosis. *Eur J Gastroenterol Hepatol* 2002;**14**:1133–41.

14 Duhamel G, Nalpas B, Goldstein S, Laplaud PM, Berthelot P, Chapman MJ. Plama lipoprotein and apolipoprotein profile in alcoholic patients with and without liver disease: on the relative roles of alcohol and liver injury. *Hepatology* 1984;**4**:577–85.

15 Poynard T, Abella A, Pignon JP, Naveau S, Leluc R, Chaput JC. Apolipoprotein AI and alcoholic liver disease. *Hepatology* 1986;**6**:1391–5.

16 Bedossa P, Poynard T, Abella A *et al.* Apolipoprotein AI is a serum and tissue marker of liver fibrosis in alcoholic patients. *Alcohol Clin Exp Res* 1989;**13**:829–33.

17 Paradis V, Laurent A, Mathurin P, Poynard T, Vidaud D, Vidaud M, Bedossa P. Role of liver extracellular matrix in transcriptional and post-transcriptional regulation of apolipoprotein A-I by hepatocytes. *Cell Mol Biol* (Noisy-le-grand) 1996;**42**:525–34.

18 Paradis V, Mathurin P, Ratziu V, Poynard T, Bedossa P. Binding of apolipoprotein A-I and acetaldehyde-modified apolipoprotein A-I to liver matrix. *Hepatology* 1996;**23**:1232–8.

19 Mathurin P, Vidaud D, Vidaud M *et al.* Quantification of apolipoprotein A-I and B messenger RNA in heavy drinkers according to liver disease. *Hepatology* 1996;**23**:44–51.

20 Nalpas B, Boigne JM, Zafrani ES, Zimmermann R, Berthelot P. Perturbations de dix proteines plasmatiques au cours des hépatopathies alcooliques. *Gastroenterol Clin Biol* 1980;**4**: 646–54.

21 Murrray-Lyon IM, Michin Clarke HG, McPherson K, Williams R. Quantitative immunoelectrophoresis of serum proteins in cryptogenic cirrhosis, alcoholic cirrhosis and active chronic hepatitis. *Clin Chim Acta* 1972;**39**:215–20.

22 Naveau S, Poynard T, Benattar C, Bedossa P, Chaput JC. Alpha-2-Macroglobulin and hepatic fibrosis. *Dig Dis Sci* 1994;**39**:2426–32.

23 Imbert-Bismut F, Ratziu V, Pieroni L, Charlotte F, Benhamou Y, Poynard T. Biochemical markers of liver fibrosis in patients with hepatitis C virus infection: a prospective study. *Lancet* 2001;**357**:1069–75.

24 Bruix J, Barrera JM, Calvet X *et al.* Prevalence of antibodies to hepatitis C virus in Spanish patients with hepatocellular carcinoma and hepatic cirrhosis. *Lancet* 1989;**2**:1004–6.

25 Di Bisceglie AM, Rustgi VK, Hoofnagle JH, Dusheiko GM, Lotze MT. Hepatocellular carcinoma. *Ann Intern Med* 1988; **108**:390–401.

26 Poynard T, Aubert A, Lazizi Y *et al.* Independent risk factors for hepatocellular carcinoma in French drinkers. *Hepatology* 1991;**13**:896–901.

27 Ganne-Carrie N, Chastang C, Chapel F *et al.* Predictive score for the development of hepatocellular carcinoma and additional value of liver large cell dysplasia in western patients with cirrhosis. *Hepatology* 1996;**23**:1112–18.

28 Anthony PP, Vogel CL, Barker LF. Liver cell dysplasia: a premalignant condition. *J Clin Pathol* 1973;**26**:217–23.

29 Borzio M, Bruno S, Roncalli M *et al.* Liver cell dysplasia is a major risk factor for hepatocellular carcinoma in cirrhosis: a prospective study. *Gastroenterology* 1996;**108**:812–17.

30 Pateron D, Ganne N, Trinchet JC *et al.* Prospective study of screening for hepatocellular carcinoma in Caucasian patients with cirrhosis. *J Hepatol* 1994;**20**:65–71.

31 Zoli M, Magalotti D, Bianchi G, Gueli C, Marchesini G, Pisi E. Efficacy of a surveillance program for early detection of hepatocellular carcinoma. *Cancer* 1996;**78**:977–85.

32 Cottone M, Turri M, Caltagirone M *et al.* Screening for hepatocellular carcinoma in patients with Child's A cirrhosis: an 8-year prospective study by ultrasound and alphafetoprotein. *J Hepatol* 1994;**21**:1029–34.

33 Mezey E. Treatment of alcoholic liver disease. *Semin Liver Dis* 1993;**13**:210–16.

34 Maddrey WC. Alcoholic hepatitis: clinicopathologic features and therapy. *Semin Liver Dis* 1988;**8**:91–102.

35 Sacks HS, Berrier J, Reitman D, Angoma-Berk VA, Chalmers TC. Meta-analysis of randomized controlled trials. *N Engl J Med* 1987;**19**:450–5.

36 Kershenobich D, Vargas F, Garcia-Tsao G, Perez-Tamayo R, Gent M, Rojkind M. Colchicine in the treatment of cirrhosis of the liver. *N Engl J Med* 1988;**318**:1709–13.

37 Trinchet JC, Beaugrand M, Callard P *et al.* Treatment of alcoholic hepatitis with colchicine. Results of a randomized double blind trial. *Gastroenterol Clin Biol* 1989;**13**:551–5.

38 Akriviadis EA, Steindel H, Pinto PC, Fong TL, Kanel G, Reynolds TB, Gupta S. Failure of colchicine to improve short-term survival in patients with alcoholic hepatitis. *Gastroenterology* 1990;**99**:811–18.

39 Morgan TR, Nemchausky B, Schiff E *et al.* Colchicine does not prolong life in patients with advanced alcoholic cirrhosis: results of a prospective, randomized, placebo-controlled, multicenter VA trial (Csp 352). *Gastroenterology* 2002;**122**:Abstract 342.

40 Halle P, Pare P, Kaptein K, Kanel G, Redeker AG, Reynolds TB. Double-blind controlled trial of propylthiouracyl in patients with severe acute alcoholic hepatitis. *Gastroenterology* 1982;**82**:925–31.

41 Orrego H, Kalant H, Israel Y *et al.* Effect of short-term therapy with propylthiouracil in patients with alcoholic liver disease. *Gastroenterology* 1978;**76**:105–15.

42 Orrego H, Blake JE, Blendis LM, Compton KV, Israel Y. Long-term treatment of alcoholic liver disease with propylthiouracil. *N Engl J Med* 1987;**317**:1421–7.

43 Orrego *et al. J Hepatol* 1994;**20**:343–9.

44 Rambaldi A, Gludd C. Propylthiouracil for alcoholic liver disease. *Cochrane Data Base Syst Rev* 2002;**2**; CD002800.

45 Bird GL, Prach AT, McMahon AD, Forrest JA, Mills PR, Danesh BJ. Randomised controlled double-blind trial of the calcium channel antagonist amlodipine in the treatment of acute alcoholic hepatitis. *J Hepatol* 1998;**28**;194–8.

46 Resnick RH, Boinott J, Iber IL, Makopour H, Cerda JJ. Preliminary observations of d-penicillamine therapy in acute alcoholic liver disease. *Digestion* 1974:**11**;257–65.

47 Pia de la Maza M, Petermann M, Bunout D, Hirsh S. Effects of long-term vitamine E supplementation in alcoholic cirrhosis. *J Am Coll Nutr* 1995:**2**;192–6.

48 Colman JC, Morgan MY, Sheuer PJ, Sherlock S. Treatment of alcohol-related liver disease with (+)-cyanidanol-3: a randomised double-blind trial. *Gut* 1980:**21**;965–9.

49 Marshall AW, Graul RS, Morgan MY, Sherlock S. Treatment of alcohol-related liver disease with thioctic acid: a six month randomised double-blind trial. *Gut* 1982:**23**;1088–93.

50 Multimer D, Brunner H, Berthelot P, Portmann B, James O. Malotilate in alcoholic hepatitis: lessons from 3 European controlled trials [Abstract]. *Hepatology* 1988:**8**;1411.

51 Keiding S, Badsberg JH, Becker U *et al.* The prognosis of patients with alcoholic liver disease. An international randomized, placebo-controlled trial on the effect of malotilate on survival. *J Hepatol* 1994;**20**:454–60.

52 Ferenci P, Dragsics B, Dittrich H *et al.* Randomized controlled trial of silymarin treatment in patients with cirrhosis of the liver. *J Hepatol* 1989;**9**:105–13.

53 Pares A, Planas R, Torres M *et al.* Effects of silymarin in alcoholic patients with cirrhosis of the liver: results of a controlled, double-blind, randomized and multicenter trial. *J Hepatol* 1998;**28**:615–21.

54 Feher J, Cornides A, Romany A, Karteszi M, Szalay L, Gogl, Picazo J. A prospective multicenter study of insulin and glucagon infusion therapy in acute alcoholic hepatits. *J Hepatol* 1987;**5**:224–31.

55 Bird G, Lau JYN, Koskinas J, Wicks C, Williams R. Insulin and glucagon infusion in acute alcoholic hepatits: a randomized controlled trial. *Hepatology* 1991;**14**:1097–101.

56 Mirouze, Redeker AG, Reynolds TB, Michel H. Traitement de l'hépatite alcoolique aiguë grave par insulin et glucagon: étude controlée sur 26 malades [Abstract]. *Gastroenterol Clin Biol* 1981;**5**:1187A–1188A.

57 Radvan G, Kanel G, Redeker A. Insulin and glucagon infusion in acute acoholic hepatitis [Abstract]. *Gastroenterology* 1982;**82**:1154.

58 Trinchet JC, Balkau B, Poupon RE *et al.* Treatment of severe alcoholic hepatitis by infusion of insulin and glucagon: a multicenter sequential trial. *Hepatology* 1992;**15**:76–81.

59 Islam N, Islam A. Testosterone propionate in cirrhosis of the liver. A controlled trial. *Br J Clin Pract* 1973;**27**:125–8.

60 Gluud C, Copenhagen Study Group For Liver diseases. Testosterone treatment of men with alcoholic cirrhosis: a double-blind study. *Hepatology* 1986;**6**:807–13.

61 Mendenhall CL, Anderson S, Garcia-Pont P *et al.* Short-term and long-term survival in patients with alcoholic hepatitis treated with oxandrolone and prednisolone. *N Engl J Med* 1984;**311**:1464–70.

62 Mendenhall CL, Moritz TE, Roselle GA *et al.* A study of oral nutritional support with oxandrolone in malnourished

patients with alcoholic hepatitis: results of a department of veterans affairs cooperative study. *Hepatology* 1993;**17**: 564–76.

63 Wells R. Prednisolone and testosterone propionate in cirrhosis of the liver. A controlled trial. *Lancet* 1960;**2**: 1416–19.

64 Rambaldi A, Iaquinto G, Gluud C. Anabolic-androgenic steroids for alcoholic liver disease: a Cochrane review. *Am J Gastroenterol* 2002;**97**:1674–81.

65 Ramond MJ, Poynard T, Rueff B *et al.* A randomized trial of prednisolone in patients with severe alcoholic hepatitis. *N Engl J Med* 1992;**326**:507–12.

66 Carithers RL Jr, Herlong HF, Diehl AM *et al.* Methylprednisolone therapy in patients with severe alcoholic hepatitis: a randomized multicenter trial. *Ann Intern Med* 1989;**110**:685–90.

67 Lesesne HR, Bozymski EM, Fallon HJ. Treatment of alcoholic hepatitis with encephalopathy. Comparison of prednisolone with caloric supplements. *Gastroenterology* 1978;**74**:169–73.

68 Helman RA, Temko MH, Nye SW, Fallon HJ. Natural history and evaluation of prednisolone therapy. *Ann Intern Med* 1971;**74**:311–21.

69 Blitzer BL, Mutchnick MG, Joshi PH, Phillips MM, Fessel JM, Conn HO. Adrenocorticosteroid therapy in alcoholic hepatitis: A prospective, double-blind randomized study. *Am J Dig Dis* 1977;**22**:477–84.

70 Bories P, Guedj JY, Mirouze D, Yousfi A, Michel H. Traitement de l'hépatite alcoolique aiguë par la prednisolone. *Presse Med* 1987;**16**:769–72.

71 Campra JL, Hamlin EM, Kirshbaum RJ, Olivier M, Redeker AG, Reynolds TB. Prednisone therapy of acute alcoholic hepatitis. *Ann Intern Med* 1973;**79**:625–31.

72 Depew W, Boyer T, Omata M, Redeker A, Reynolds T. Double-blind controlled trial of prednisolone therapy in patients with severe acute alcoholic hepatitis and spontaneous encephalopathy. *Gastroenterology* 1980;**78**:524–9.

73 Maddrey WC, Boitnott JK, Bedine MS, Weber FL, Mezey E, White RI. Corticosteroid therapy of alcoholic hepatitis. *Gastroenterology* 1978;**75**:193–9.

74 Shumaker JB, Resnick RH, Galambos JT, Makopour H, Iber FL. A controlled trial of 6-methylprednisolone in acute alcoholic hepatitis. *Am J Gastroenterol* 1978;**69**: 443–49.

75 Porter HP, Simon FR, Pope CE, Volwiler W, Fenster F. Corticosteroid therapy in severe alcoholic hepatitis. *N Engl J Med* 1971;**284**:1350–5.

76 Theodossi A, Eddleston ALWF, Williams R. Controlled trial of methylprednisolone therapy in severe acute alcoholic hepatitis. *Gut* 1982;**23**:75–9.

77 Mathurin P, Bernard B, Quichon JP, Opolon P, Poynard T. L'hémorragie digestive et l'insuffisance rénale: deux facteurs de confusion dans l'analyse de l'efficacité des corticoïdes dans l'hépatite alcoolique aiguë [Abstract]. *Gastroenterol Clin Biol* 1995;**19**:A162.

78 Imperiale TF, McCullough AJ. Do corticosteroids reduce mortality from alcoholic hepatitis? *Ann Intern Med* 1990;**113**:299–307.

79 Mathurin P, Duchatelle V, Ramond MJ *et al.* Survival and prognostic factors in patients with severe biopsy-proven alcoholic hepatitis treated by prednisolone: randomized trial, new cohort, and simulation. *Gastroenterology* 1996; **110**:1847–53.

80 Imperiale TF, O'Connor J, McCullough AJ. Corticosteroids are effective in patients with severe alcoholic patients. *Am J Gastroenterol* 1999;**94**:3066–7.

81 Christensen E, Gludd C. Glucocorticosteroids are ineffective in alcoholic hepatitis: a meta-analysis adjusting for confounding variables. *Gut* 1995;**37**:113–18.

82 Christensen E, Gluud C. Glucocorticosteroids are not effective in alcoholic patients. *Am J Gastroenterol* 1999;**94**:3065–6.

83 Mathurin P, Mendenhall C, Carithers RL Jr *et al.* Corticosteroids improve short term survival in patients with severe alcoholic hepatitis (AH): individual data analysis of the last three randomized placebo controlled double blind trials. *J Hepatol* 2002;**36**:480–7.

84 Mc Cullough AJ, O'Connor JFB. Alcoholic liver disease: proposed recommendations for the American College of Gastroenterology. *Am J Gastroenterol* 1998;**93**:2022–36.

85 Cabre E, Rodriguez-Iglesias P, Caballeria J, Quer J, Sanchez-Lombrana JL, Pares A *et al.* Short and long term outcome of severe alcohol induced hepatitis treated with steroids or enteral nutrition: A multicentre randomized trial. *Hepatology* 2000;**32**:36–42

86 Akriviadis E, Botla R, Briggs W, Han S, Reynolds T, Shakil O. Pentoxifylline improves short-term survival in severe acute alcoholic hepatitis: a double-blind, placebo-controlled trial. *Gastroenterology* 2000;**119**:1637–48.

87 Spahr L, Rubbia-Brandt L, Frossard JL *et al.* Combination of steroids with infliximab or placebo in severe alcoholic hepatitis: a randomized pilot study. *J Hepatol* 2002;**37**: 448–55.

88 Tilg H, Jalan R, Kaser A *et al.* Anti-tumor necrosis factor-alpha monoclonal antibody therapy in severe alcoholic hepatitis. *J Hepatol* 2003 (in press).

89 Poynard T, Thabut D, Chryssostalis A, Taieb J, Ratziu V. Anti-tumor necrosis factor-alpha therapy in severe alcoholic hepatitis: are large randomized trials still possible? *J Hepatol* 2003 (in press).

90 Lieber CS, Weiss DG, Groszmann R *et al.* Effect of moderation of ethanol consumption combined with PPC administration on liver injury in alcoholics: prospective, randomized, placebo-controlled multi-center VA trial (CSP 391). *Hepatology* 2002;**36**:381A.

91 Mato JM, Camara J, Fernandez de Paz J *et al.* S-adenosylmethionine in alcoholic liver cirrhosis: a randomized, placebo-controlled, double-blind, multicenter clinical trial. *J Hepatol* 1999;**30**:1081–9.

92 Wenzel G, Kuklinski B, Ruhlmann C, Ehrhardt D. Alcohol induced toxic hepatitis – a 'free' radical associated disease. Lowering fatality by adjuvent anti-oxidant therapy. *Z die Gesamte Innere Med Ihre Grenzgeb* 1993;**48**:490–96.

93 Phillips M, Curtis H, Portmann B, Donaldson N, Bomford A, O'Grady J. Antioxidants versus corticoteroids in the treatment of severe alcoholic hepatitis: a randomized trial. *Hepatology* 2001;**34**:250A.

94 Stewart SF, Prince M, Bassendine M, Hudson M, James O, Jones D *et al.* A trial of antioxidant therapy alone or with corticosteroids in acute alcoholic hepatitis. *J Hepatol* 2002; **36**:16.

95 Mezey E, Potter JJ, Rennie-Tankersley L, Caballeria J, Pares A. A randomized placebo controlled trial of vitamin E for alcoholic hepatitis. *J Hepatol* 2004;**40**:40–6.

96 Stefanini GF, Biselli M, Grazi GL *et al.* Orthotopic liver transplantation for alcoholic liver disease: rates of survival, complications and relapse. *Hepatogastroenterology* 1997;**44**:1356–9.

97 Starzl TE, Van Thiel D, Tzakis AG *et al.* Orthotopic liver transplantation for alcoholic cirrhosis. *JAMA* 1988;**260**: 2542–4.

98 Lucey MR, Merion MR, Henley KS *et al.* Selection for and outcome of liver transplantation in alcoholic liver disease. *Gastroenterology* 1992;**102**:1736–41.

99 Poynard T, Barthelemy P, Fratte S *et al.* Evaluation of liver transplantation in alcoholic cirrhosis by a case–control study and simulated controls. *Lancet* 1994;**344**:502–7.

100 Anand AC, Ferraz-Neto BH, Nightingale P *et al.* Liver transplantation for alcoholic liver disease: evaluation of a selection protocol. *Hepatology* 1997;**25**:1478–84.

101 Snyder SL, Drooker M, Strain JJ. A survey estimate of academic liver transplant teams' selection practices for alcohol-dependent applicants. *Psychosomatics* 1996;**37**: 432–7.

102 Yates WR, Martin M, LaBrecque D, Hillebrand D, Voigt M, Pfab D. A model to examine the validity of the 6-month abstinence criterion for liver transplantation. *Alcohol Clin Exp Res* 1998;**22**:513–17.

103 Foster PF, Fabrega F, Karademir S, Sankary HN, Mital D, WIlliams JW. Prediction of abstinence from ethanol in alcoholic recipients following liver transplantation. *Hepatology* 1997;**25**:1469–77.

104 Bird JLA, O'Grady JG, Harvey FAH, Calne RY, Williams R. Liver transplantation in patients with alcoholic cirrhosis: selection criteria and rates of survival and relapse. *BMJ* 1990;**301**:15–17.

105 Kumar S, Strauber RE, Gavaler JS *et al.* Orthotopic liver transplantation for alcoholic liver disease. *Hepatology* 1990; **11**:159–64.

106 Osorio RW, Ascher NL, Avery M, Bachetti P, Roberts JP, Lake JR. Predicting recidivism after orthotopic liver transplantation for alcoholic liver disease. *Hepatology* 1994; **20**:105–10.

107 Lucey MR, Carr K, Beresford TP *et al.* Alcohol use after liver transplantation in alcoholics: a clinical cohort follow-up study. *Hepatology* 1997;**25**:1223–7.

108 Shelton W, Balint JA. Fair treatment of alcoholic patients in the context of liver transplantation. *Alcohol Clin Exp Res* 1997;**21**:93–100.

109 Berlakovich GA, Steininger R, Herbst F, Barlan M, Mittlböck M, Mühlbacher F. Efficacy of liver transplantation for alcoholic cirrhosis with respect to recidivism and compliance. Transplantation 1994;**58**:560–5.

26 Non-alcoholic fatty liver disease

Chris P Day

Introduction

In the past few years an increasing amount of research effort has been expended on various aspects of non-alcoholic fatty liver disease (NAFLD) for at least two main reasons. First is the recognition that NAFLD is extremely common, and second the accumulating body of evidence that a proportion of patients with NAFLD can progress to cirrhosis, liver failure and hepatocellular carcinoma. With respect to prevalence, although some high profile reviews have suggested that up to 24% of the general population suffer from NAFLD in various countries,[1] a more evidence-based estimate has come from two analyses of data from the third National Health and Nutrition Examination Survey (NHANES III) carried out between 1988 and 1994 in the USA. These reports have suggested that between 3–6% of the US population have some degree of NAFLD with the diagnosis based on raised aminotransferases in the absence of any alternative etiologies.[2,3] Evidence that this diagnostic label is reasonable has come from a large histological survey of 354 consecutive patients presenting with abnormal liver function tests of unknown etiology. "Abnormal" was defined as either an alanine transaminase (ALT), a γ-glutamyl transferase or an alkaline phosphatase more than twice the upper limit of normal for at least 6 months. Two-thirds of the patients had NAFLD, one-third with simple steatosis and one-third with more advanced disease – non-alcoholic steatohepatitis (NASH) either with or without fibrosis.[4]

Natural history of non-alcoholic fatty liver disease

In marked contrast to patients with alcoholic steatohepatitis, the short-term prognosis of patients with NAFLD is largely excellent. There has been a recent case report of three patients presenting with subacute liver failure[5] and isolated reports of patients developing hepatic failure following obesity surgery.[6,7] However, given the prevalence of fatty liver, these cases appear to be rare exceptions. Although information from a large scale, prospective study examining the natural history of NAFLD in an inception cohort of patients is currently lacking, the available data suggest that the long-term prognosis of patients with NAFLD depends critically on the histological stage of disease at presentation (Figure 26.1). With respect to clinical follow up studies, the largest retrospective study thus far reported on 132 patients with NAFLD of a variety of stages followed up for a median of almost 9 years. While 25% of patients with NASH (± fibrosis) on their index biopsy developed "clinical" evidence of cirrhosis and 11% died a "liver" death, only 3·4% (2/59) with simple fatty liver developed clinical cirrhosis, one of whom (1·7%) died from a liver-related cause.[8] In another study of patients with simple non-alcoholic fatty liver followed for a median 11·5 years, none had clinical evidence of disease progression.[9] With respect to histological follow up studies, to date six paired liver biopsy studies have been reported.[9–14] In most of the included cases the second biopsy was done for normal "clinical" indications, rather than as part of a study protocol and therefore the reported progression rates are almost certainly an overestimate. However, with this proviso the evidence is similar to that in the clinical studies, i.e. the risk of progression differs markedly between patients with simple steatosis and those with NASH ± fibrosis. Of the 14 patients with simple steatosis,[9,14] 3 (21%) developed grade 1 (out of 4) fibrosis (follow up 4.5–15·6 years), while 38% of the 50 patients with NASH[10–14] had an increase in their fibrosis score with 16% progressing to grade 3 (bridging) or 4 (cirrhosis) fibrosis (follow up 1·0–15·7 years).

Further evidence that some patients with NAFLD can progress to cirrhosis has been provided by a study of patients with apparently "cryptogenic" (of no known cause) cirrhosis.[15] The prevalence of the most established risk factors for NAFLD, obesity and diabetes, was over 70% in these patients, which was identical to that seen in the patients with NASH. The cryptogenic patients were, on average, 13 years older than the NASH patients, providing indirect evidence that at least some cases of cryptogenic cirrhosis result from longstanding NASH. These results were confirmed by a subsequent study using a similar strategy to look for NAFLD risk factors in patients with cirrhosis of different aetiologies awaiting liver transplantation.[16] More recently, Ratziu and

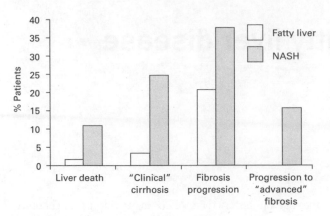

Figure 26.1 Natural history of non-alcoholic fatty liver and non-alcoholic steatohepatitis (NASH).[8–14] Follow up ranged from 1 to 15 years in the different studies. Advanced fibrosis: bridging fibrosis or cirrhosis

colleagues have reported on the natural history of patients with obesity-related cryptogenic cirrhosis.[17] They compared the natural history of 27 patients with obesity-related cirrhosis with that of 85 patients with chronic hepatitis C-related cirrhosis matched for age and sex at the time of diagnosis. Over a median 2·2-year follow up 33% of patients with cryptogenic cirrhosis died a "liver" death compared with only 24% of the hepatitis C cases, with mean time to death in the cryptogenic patients only 9 months compared with over 2 years in the hepatitis C patients. Moreover, the risk of hepatocellular carcinoma (HCC) – 25% – was similar in the two groups of patients. This observation is consistent with several other case reports and series over the past 2 years,[18–20] which, taken together, provide strong evidence that the NAFLD-related cirrhosis is associated with a risk of developing HCC that appears to be of a similar magnitude to the risk associated with alcohol and HCV-related cirrhosis, intermediate between the risks associated with cirrhosis due to autoimmune diseases and chronic hepatitis B infection.[20] This offers at least one plausible explanation for the recently reported linear association between the risk of liver cancer and body mass index (BMI).[21] The difference between the prognosis of patients with simple steatosis compared with those with NASH ± fibrosis has clear implications for both the investigation and subsequent management of patients with suspected NAFLD.

Investigation of patients with suspected non-alcoholic fatty liver disease

The most important issue to consider when devising a protocol for the investigation of patients with suspected NAFLD is to consider which (if any) patients warrant a liver biopsy. This question is best answered by considering the arguments for and against taking a liver biopsy in the investigation of patients with suspected liver disease in general. The first potential justification is that it helps to establish a diagnosis. In a patient presenting with abnormal liver function tests (LFTs) in association with the classic risk factors for NAFLD – obesity, type 2 diabetes mellitus (DM), hypertension and/or dyslipidemia – and an ultrasound showing steatosis, the diagnosis of NAFLD can almost certainly be made with relative confidence without a liver biopsy after the other common causes of abnormal LFTs have been excluded by careful history taking (for alcohol intake and hepatotoxic drugs) and a standard liver "screen" including serological markers for hepatitis B and C infection, autoantibodies, serum ferritin, ceruloplasmin and α-1 anti-trypsin phenotype. As discussed above, several studies have reported that up to two-thirds of patients presenting with unexplained abnormal liver blood tests will have NAFLD[4,22,23] and it seems likely that this proportion will be even higher in patients with established risk factors for NAFLD. Much has been written about how much alcohol intake is "allowed" for a diagnosis of NAFLD. The only study to have examined this issue has reported that "light" to "moderate" alcohol intake reduces the risk of steatosis and NASH in morbidly obese patients undergoing obesity surgery,[24] possibly by reducing insulin resistance and the risk of type 2 DM.[25] In the absence of strong evidence to the contrary, it therefore appears reasonable to suggest that a weekly alcohol intake at or below currently recommended "sensible" limits (21 units for men, 14 units for women) is compatible with a diagnosis of NAFLD.

The second justification for a liver biopsy in patients with suspected liver disease is that the histology will provide prognostic information. As discussed above, this is certainly the case for patients with suspected NAFLD given the different prognoses of simple steatosis and more advanced forms of the disease. Although a number of clinical and biochemical parameters are undoubtedly associated with an increased risk of advanced disease, as yet no factor or combination of factors has been identified that has sufficient sensitivity and specificity to replace biopsy for reliable disease staging. With respect to the various imaging modalities, a recent study comparing ultrasonography, magnetic resonance imaging (MRI) and computed tomography (CT) in patients with biopsy-proven NAFLD has shown that all three modalities are excellent at quantifying the severity of steatosis, but none can accurately distinguish between steatosis and NASH ± fibrosis.[26]

The third reason is that it changes management strategy. For patients with suspected NAFLD, the observations indicating different prognoses for the different stages clearly suggest that different management strategies are appropriate. For patients with simple steatosis, the commonly associated

Table 26.1   Factors predicting advanced fibrosis (bridging or cirrhosis) in biopsy series of patients with or at risk of non-alcoholic fatty liver disease

Factor	Predictive cut-off	Reference
Age	≥ 45 years	29
	≥ 50 years	13
Type 2 diabetes	Presence	29
Hypertension	$\geq 140/90$ mmHg or on treatment	24
Body mass index	≥ 28 kg/m^2	13
	$> 31 \cdot 1$ kg/m^2 (men) $32 \cdot 3$ kg/m^2 (women)	29
ALT	$\geq \times 2$ upper limit of normal	13
	$>$ upper limit of normal	24
AST/ALT ratio	> 1	29
Triglycerides	$\geq 1 \cdot 7$ mmol/l	13
C-peptide	$>$ upper limit of normal	24
Metabolic syndrome	Presence of $\geq$ three features (see Table 26.3)	28

ALT, alanine transaminase; AST, aspartate transaminase

conditions should be sought and treated appropriately. In view of their benign prognosis, these patients should probably be discharged back to their primary care physicians. In contrast, patients with NASH ± fibrosis, with their increased propensity for disease progression, require long-term follow up. Advanced cases (bridging fibrosis or cirrhosis) should be entered into appropriate screening programs for esophageal varices and HCC. C5 In a recent case series of patients with HCC it was reported that patients with NAFLD related cirrhosis were less likely to have undergone HCC surveillance and had larger tumors at diagnosis compared with patients whose cirrhosis was attributable to other aetiologies.[27] Finally, in the next few years when evidence supporting the use of newer therapies may be provided by currently ongoing randomized clinical trials (RCTs), liver biopsy may be required to determine which patients are suitable candidates for these "second-line" therapies which will be primarily indicated for patients with potentially progressive forms of NAFLD.

Risk factors for advanced non-alcoholic fatty liver disease

If we accept that determining disease severity is critical to the future management of a patient with probable NAFLD, and given the large number of such patients currently presenting to liver outpatient departments, it is important to consider the clinical and biochemical factors that have been associated with an increased risk of advanced disease. While not a replacement for liver biopsy, these factors can help to identify those patients most likely to have advanced NAFLD in whom liver biopsy is probably justified. Several studies in

different groups of patients have identified a number of independent clinical and laboratory predictors of advanced fibrosis that can be used to aid the decision of whether or not to biopsy a patient with suspected NAFLD (Table 26.1).[13,24,28,29] Other than the ALT and the aspartate transaminase (AST), almost all of the predictive factors can essentially be considered to be part of the metabolic syndrome, with the presence of the syndrome *per se* associated with an odds ratio of 3·5 (CI 1·1 to 11·2) for advanced fibrosis in the most recent study of 163 patients with biopsy-proven NAFLD.[28] Age (greater than 45 or 50 years) has been identified as risk factor for advanced fibrosis in some,[13,29] but not all,[24] studies. This may also be explained, at least in part, by the increased risk of the metabolic syndrome with increasing age.[28] On the basis of these data, it is reasonable to restrict liver biopsy to patients with at least some, if not all, of these risk factors. It has been suggested that biopsy should be reserved for patients whose abnormal LFTs persist after correction of some of the predictive factors. However, at present there is no evidence that patients whose LFTs respond to these maneuvers are less likely to have advanced disease than patients whose LFTs fail to improve.

General management strategies

There are no published large RCTs of therapies for NAFLD on which to base definitive treatment recommendations. Encouraging results from pilot studies of several treatment modalities have been reported over the past few years and many are currently being tested in large RCTs with histological improvement as their appropriate primary

Table 26.2 Therapeutic strategies for NAFLD/NASH with evidence of benefit from human studies

Strategy	Specific treatment
Weight loss	Calorific restriction
	Calorific restriction and exercise
	Weight-reducing surgery
Insulin sensitization	Troglitazone
	Pioglitazone (+ vitamin E)
	Rosiglitazone
	Metformin
	Iron depletion[a]
Lipid lowering	Gemfibrozil
	Probucol[a]
Antioxidant	Betaine[a]
	Probucol[a]
	Iron depletion[a]
Hepatoprotection	Betaine[a]

[a]Treatments with more than one potential beneficial effect.
NAFLD, non-alcoholic fatty liver disease; NASH, non-alcoholic steatohepatitis

endpoint (Table 26.2). Until results from these trials become available, it seems sensible to direct management strategies for patients with NAFLD at the commonly associated conditions, obesity, type 2 DM, dyslipidemia and hypertension, now considered to be the main features of the metabolic syndrome.[30] C5 These strategies will undoubtedly reduce the risk of patients dying from a cardiovascular cause and may also improve the underlying liver disease. In addition to managing the metabolic syndrome, since several drugs have been recognized as causes of NAFLD (for example amiodarone, tamoxifen),[31] these agents should be stopped if possible, since their withdrawal usually leads to resolution of the hepatic pathology.[31] With respect to alcohol intake, for reasons outlined above,[24] it is reasonable to advise patients to drink alcohol within currently recommended "sensible" limits.

Management of the metabolic syndrome

Over the past 4 years several studies have reported that the majority of patients with NAFLD will have some, if not all, features of the recently characterized metabolic syndrome.[32–35] The Third Report of the National Cholesterol Education Expert Panel on Detection, Evaluation and Treatment of High Blood Cholesterol in Adults (Adult Treatment Panel III (ATPIII)) has recently provided a working definition of the syndrome based on a combination of five factors – central obesity, hypertension, abnormal glucose tolerance, hypertriglyceridemia and low high-density lipoprotein (HDL) cholesterol (see Table 26.3 for

definitions).[36] Subjects with three or more of these factors are considered to have the metabolic syndrome. Since patients with this syndrome have a 30% increased risk of cardiovascular death in the absence of type 2 DM, and a 40–70% increased risk of cardiovascular death in the presence of type 2 DM,[37] patients with the metabolic syndrome require treatment of the syndrome regardless of the severity of any associated NAFLD. First-line management of patients with the metabolic syndrome consists of lifestyle interventions with weight loss, increased exercise and smoking cessation as the primary goals. A large randomized placebo-controlled trial in over 3000 overweight non-diabetic individuals showed that intensive dietary and lifestyle modification directed at achieving modest weight loss (7%) and including exercise (150 minutes per week) reduced the incidence of type 2 DM by 58% (95% CI 48% to 66%) over a mean 2·8 year follow up.[38] The incidence of type 2 DM over 100 patient-years was: control 11, lifestyle intervention 4·8 and the NNT (the number of patients needed to be treated with intensive lifestyle intervention rather than a placebo for three years to prevent one case of type 2 DM) was 7. A1d If the individual components of the syndrome persist despite these lifestyle modifications they should be treated according to conventional guidelines, since the treatment of type 2 DM, hypertension and dyslipidemia occurring either in isolation[39–41] or in combination[42–44] has been shown in large RCTs to result in significant reductions in mortality. Recently evidence has been provided by the Heart Protection Study Collaborative Group that statin therapy reduces the risk of major vascular events (major coronary event, stroke or revascularization) in patients with diabetes irrespective of their initial cholesterol concentration.[44] Patients who have history of cardiovascular disease or adequately treated hypertension *and* are aged 50 years or more, have type 2 DM or a 10-year coronary heart disease risk of ≥ 5% estimated by the Joint British Societies Risk Prediction Chart/Programme and no contraindication, should take aspirin 75 mg daily.[45] Although direct evidence from RCTs is currently lacking, there are good theoretical reasons to believe that treatment strategies directed at components of the metabolic syndrome may have beneficial effects on the livers of patients with NAFLD. C5 As our understanding of the pathogenesis of NAFLD increases it is likely that the choice of therapy for hypertension, type 2 DM and dyslipidemia will be influenced by their perceived or established beneficial hepatic effects.

Treatment directed at achieving weight reduction

There is a sound theoretical basis for believing that strategies aimed at achieving and maintaining weight reduction in patients with NAFLD will improve hepatic histology. Excessive adipose tissue and the associated insulin

**Table 26.3 Components of the metabolic syndrome[a]
(ATP III recommendations)[36]**

Component	Defining level
Glucose intolerance	Fasting glucose ≥ 6·1 mmol/l or known type 2 diabetes mellitus
Central obesity	Waist circumference > 102 cm (men); > 88 cm (women)
Hypertension	≥ 130/85 mm Hg or on treatment
Hypertriglyceridemia	Fasting triglyceride > 1·7 mmol/l or current use of fibrates
Low HDL-cholesterol	< 1·0 mmol/l (men); < 1·3 mmol/l (women)

[a]Metabolic syndrome is defined by the presence of three or more of these features.
HDL, high density lipoprotein; ATP, Adult Treatment Panel

resistance is the primary source of free fatty acids (FFA) coming into the liver. The combination of an increased hepatic supply of FFA and hyperinsulinemia leads to the accumulation of triglyceride and the development of steatosis – the so-called "first-hit" in NAFLD.[46] The increased hepatic FFA oxidation coupled with the adverse mitochondrial effects of the cytokine tumor necrosis factor (TNF)-α, also secreted by adipose tissue, results in oxidative stress – the most likely "second hit" required for steatosis-related hepatocyte injury and associated inflammation.[46] The hyperinsulinemia associated with obesity along with several other "adipocytokines" secreted by adipose tissue including leptin, angiotensinogen and norepinephrine may also contribute to obesity-related hepatic fibrosis via their effects on hepatic stellate cells.[47]

Unfortunately, despite the sound rationale, at present the evidence that weight loss in patients with NAFLD leads to improved liver histology, rather than biochemistry, is largely anecdotal[48,49] and, with one exception,[50] restricted to uncontrolled case series. Importantly, several of these series have demonstrated that too rapid weight loss (usually following surgery) can lead to an increase in hepatic necroinflammation and/or portal fibrosis despite a reduction in steatosis and an improvement in liver blood tests.[51,52] The majority of studies using diet to achieve weight loss relied on simple calorie restriction with no studies examining the value of specific diets. This may be an area for future study since both the saturated fat content of the diet and the fiber intake are known to influence insulin resistance,[53] and a diet high in saturated fat appears to be a risk factor for NASH in obese individuals.[54] The value of exercise in achieving and maintaining weight loss is now well established and the only controlled study of weight loss that has achieved an improvement in histology in treated patients (only steatosis was significant) combined 3 months of increased exercise with moderate calorie restriction.[50] The addition of exercise to calorie restriction makes physiological sense, since exercise

reduces the FFA and triglyceride content of skeletal muscle cells resulting in a reduction in insulin resistance.

As regards "non-lifestyle" interventions for obesity, there are currently three drugs available as adjuncts to dietary therapy in weight reduction: phentermine, sibutramine and orlistat.[53] The National Heart, Lung, and Blood Institutes (NHLBI) and National Institute of Diabetes and Digestive and Kidney Diseases (NIDDK) guidelines for the management of obesity currently recommend that pharmacotherapy be added to lifestyle modification for patients with a BMI ≥ 30 kg/m[2] and no comorbidity, and ≥ 27 kg/m[2] for patients with obesity-related comorbidity. As yet there is no evidence from RCTs that any of these agents are beneficial in the management of NAFLD. However, a recent observational study of 6 months of orlistat therapy in patients with NASH has shown improvement in both steatosis and fibrosis,[55] and large RCTs are currently ongoing. C5 In addition patients with morbid obesity (BMI ≥ 35 kg/m[2]) may be candidates for weight-reducing surgery; either proximal gastric bypass or laparoscopically placed adjustable gastric banding. Jejuno-ilieal bypass has been abandoned, mainly due to the high frequency of severe NASH and subsequent liver failure. As discussed previously, liver failure[6,7] and a deterioration in histology[51,52] has been reported to occur in association with the rapid weight loss that follows gastric bypass surgery and patients therefore require careful assessment and monitoring prior to and following this procedure.

In the absence of data from RCTs, at present it seems appropriate to advise obese patients with NASH to lose weight by combining moderate calorie restriction with increased exercise. Based on the NHLBI-NIDDK guidelines they should aim to lose 10% of their baseline weight at a rate of 500 g–1 kg/week. Patients should be advised against more rapid weight loss in view of the risks of exacerbating liver damage. Diet should be based on a normal "heart-healthy" diet or a standard diabetic diet where indicated.[53] The use of adjunctive pharmacotherapies should be considered for markedly obese patients (BMI ≥ 30 kg/m[2]) who fail to lose weight despite these measures. For less obese patients with NASH they should only be used in the context of a clinical trial. Morbidly obese patients may be considered for surgery and require careful monitoring in view of the potential risk of precipitating liver failure.

Treatment directed at associated diabetes mellitus/insulin resistance

In overweight patients with NAFLD and type 2 DM, tight glycemic control with metformin is recommended since this has been shown to reduce the risk of diabetes-related microvascular complications, diabetes-related death and all-cause mortality.[39] This beneficial effect is greater than that obtained with either insulin or sulfonylureas.[39] There is, however, currently no evidence that improving glycemic control with metformin or any other agent leads to an improvement in hepatic histology in diabetic patients with NASH. Despite this, recent reports that insulin resistance is a universal finding in patients with NASH,[32,35,56] along with increasing evidence that insulin resistance and the associated hyperinsulinemia may play a role in the pathogenesis of advanced NAFLD[47] has led to pilot studies of metformin and other insulin-sensitizing agents in NAFLD patients with and without diabetes. A further attraction of these drugs in NAFLD is that they appear to exert their insulin-sensitizing effect by reducing hepatic and muscle steatosis.[57,58] C5 Whilst there is, as yet, no direct evidence that the use of insulin or sulfonylureas has any adverse effect on the liver of diabetic patients, the putative role of insulin in the pathogenesis of steatosis and fibrosis in NAFLD suggests that these agents should be avoided if glycemic control can be achieved with other treatment modalities. C5

Metformin

Metformin is a member of the biguanide class of drugs. It appears to improve insulin resistance by reducing the fat content of liver and muscle through activation of the enzyme adenine monophosphate (AMP)-dependent protein kinase that results in increased mitochondrial FFA oxidation and decreased FFA and very-low-density lipoprotein (VLDL) synthesis.[57] In the *ob/ob* mouse, an animal model of fatty liver, metformin reverses hepatomegaly and steatosis and improves liver biochemistry.[59] Intrahepatic expression of TNF-α and several TNF-α inducible factors are also reduced by metformin in this model. In two recent pilot studies, metformin given for 3–6 months to non-diabetic patients with NASH was associated with a significant improvement in ALT, glucose disposal, BMI, and hepatomegaly (assessed by CT) compared with non-compliant patients.[60,61] B4 Large RCTs of metformin are currently ongoing in Europe and North America.

Thiazolidinediones

Thiazolidinediones are a new class of anti-diabetic drug that act as agonists for peroxisome proliferator activated receptor γ (PPARγ) and improve insulin sensitivity at least in part via anti-steatotic effects in liver and muscle.[58] They also exert anti-inflammatory effects *in vitro*[62] and antifibrotic effects *in vitro* and *in vivo*.[63] Pilot studies have been carried out with three members of this class of drug in patients with NAFLD. In the first, troglitazone was given to 10 patients with NASH for 3–6 months[64]; one patient had type 2 DM and three had cirrhosis. ALT levels improved in nine patients and, although features of NASH remained in the post-treatment liver biopsies, the grade of necroinflammation improved in

five patients and deteriorated in only one patient. Troglitazone has, however, been associated with rare cases of severe hepatotoxicity and has now been withdrawn from the market. The second thiazolidinedione, rosiglitazone, does not appear to be associated with hepatotoxicity. In a recent uncontrolled pilot study in 22 patients with NASH including 7 with type 2 DM, 48 weeks of therapy led to improved insulin sensitivity and ALT levels, with the histological fibrosis score improving in 8 patients, deteriorating in 3 and remaining unchanged in 11.[65] B4 Of some concern was the observation that 67% of patients gained weight with a mean increase of 7·3%. Pioglitazone, the third member of this class of drug, has also been shown to improve steatosis and liver cell injury (ballooning and Mallory's hyaline) in non-diabetic patients with NASH when given for 6 months in combination with vitamin E.[66] A1c In this randomized study no significant changes were observed with vitamin E alone. In a further pilot study of 18 non-diabetic NASH patients, pioglitazone, given for 48 weeks improved histology on two-thirds of patients.[67] Importantly one patient in two of these studies had therapy withdrawn as a result of a rising ALT. Therefore concern over the safety of these drugs remains a significant issue that can only be addressed by currently ongoing large RCTs.

IκB kinase inhibitors

Recent evidence from animal models demonstrating a role for IκB kinase (IKK) in insulin resistance and an improvement in fat-induced skeletal muscle insulin resistance with salicylate,[68] an IKK inhibitor, suggests that selective IKK inhibition may be the next therapeutic strategy directed at improving insulin sensitivity. Since IKK inhibition will also reduce the expression of several NFκ-B-dependent proinflammatory cytokines and adhesion molecules, once developed, these inhibitors may be particularly useful for the treatment of NASH.

At present there is not enough evidence to support the routine use of antidiabetic agents in non-diabetic patients with NASH, although such evidence may be forthcoming from ongoing RCTs. At present, for patients with NASH and type 2 DM, it would seem reasonable to suggest that, where treatment with oral hypoglycemic agents is indicated for "conventional" reasons, insulin sensitizers such as metformin are the preferred drugs, particularly in obese patients.

Treatment directed at associated lipid abnormalities

Dyslipidemia, particularly hypertriglyceridemia is present in between 20% and 80% of patients with NAFLD. As with weight loss and insulin sensitizers, there is good scientific rationale supporting the use of fibrates – the conventional triglyceride-lowering agents – in patients with NAFLD. C5 Fibrates are agonists for PPAR-α receptors, transcription factors that upregulate the transcription of genes encoding a variety of FFA oxidizing enzymes in mitochondria, peroxisomes and endoplasmic reticulum.[69] The use of potent PPAR-α agonists ameliorates liver injury in the methionine-choline deficient (MCD) animal model of NASH and PPAR-α "knockout" mice develop more severe disease.[70] Several observational studies have examined the effect of lipid-lowering agents on parameters of liver function in patients with NAFLD. However, in the only small observational study in which there was histological follow up, 1 year of clofibrate therapy had no effect on liver biochemistry or histology.[71] Combined PPAR-α/PPAR-γ agonists have recently been developed and have been shown to improve insulin sensitivity and reduce hepatic steatosis in fat-fed rats.[72] These agents have great potential for the treatment of NAFLD and the results of clinical trials are awaited with interest. There is no rationale for the use of HMG CoA reductase inhibitors ("statins") in the treatment of NAFLD. However, they should be prescribed for the "conventional" indications including type 2 DM regardless of cholesterol concentration.[44] Importantly there is no evidence that patients with NAFLD are more likely to suffer from statin-induced idiosyncratic hepatotoxicity.

Antihypertensive therapy

Hypertension should be sought and treated appropriately in patients with NAFLD, particularly those with type 2 DM in whom tight blood pressure control (< 140/80 mmHg) with an angiotensin converting enzyme (ACE) inhibitor or a β-blocker significantly reduces the risk of cardiovascular morbidity, sudden death, stroke and peripheral vascular disease.[42,43] No studies have specifically examined the effect of different antihypertensive agents on the livers of hypertensive patients with NAFLD. However, recent evidence that angiotensin 2 receptor antagonists and ACE inhibitors are antifibrotic in animal models of hepatic fibrosis,[73] suggests that these agents are worth examining in clinical trials. In the meantime, in the absence of contraindications, these drugs may be considered as the drugs of choice for hypertensive patients with NAFLD. C5

Liver-specific therapies

In view of the difficulties in achieving weight loss in patients with NASH, the concern over the potential toxicity of insulin-sensitizing agents, and the apparent lack of efficacy of hypolipidemic drugs, it is not surprising that investigators have begun to examine the effects of alternative forms of therapy for patients with NASH. The rationale for these studies, most of which are at the animal model or "pilot" stage, has been based either on reducing the severity of the putative second hits – oxidative stress and endotoxin-mediated cytokine release[44] – or on the use of general hepatoprotective agents.

Antioxidants

The accumulating body of evidence supporting a role for oxidant stress in the pathogenesis of NASH[44] has lead to trials of several agents, whose potential beneficial effects might be attributed, at least in part, to their antioxidant effects. In a recent placebo-controlled RCT, probucol, a lipid-lowering agent with antioxidant properties, led to a significant reduction in ALT and AST in 30 patients with biopsy-proven NASH.[74] A1c No histological follow up was done. Betaine is required for the hepatic synthesis of S-adenosylmethionine, which, in addition to being an important donor of methyl groups, is a precursor of glutathione (GSH), an important intracellular antioxidant. Betaine given to seven patients with NASH for 1 year led to a significant improvement or normalization of serum ALT levels and to improved or unchanged histological parameters (steatosis, necroinflammation and fibrosis).[75] B4 Vitamin E, (α-tocopherol), is a lipid-soluble antioxidant particularly effective against oxidative attack on membrane phospholipids. Vitamin E (400–1200 IU/day) given to 11 children with NAFLD for 4–10 months, led to a significant improvement in liver biochemistry. B4 However, in this study there was no pre or post-treatment histological assessment.[76] In adults, two small pilot studies of oral vitamin E have reported non-significant improvements in histology after 6[66] and 12[77] months. B4 However, a recent small RCT of vitamin E combined with vitamin C found no difference in the proportion of patients with improvement in their fibrosis score between the drug and placebo groups, although this study may have lacked power to show a benefit from this intervention, should it exist.[78] Finally, the recently reported improvement in liver biochemistry in non-iron overloaded patients with clinical evidence of NASH following phlebotomy to near iron depletion has been attributed to a reduction in iron-mediated oxidative stress as well as to improved insulin sensitivity.[79]

Anti-endotoxin/cytokine therapy

At present, studies examining therapies for NASH based on reducing levels of gut-derived endotoxin or on the resulting release of TNF-α from Kupffer cells have been restricted to the *ob/ob* leptin-deficient, murine model of NASH.[80] Studies with probiotics and anti-TNF antibodies have, however, been encouraging and pilot studies with the anti-TNF-α agent pentoxifylline are ongoing.

Ursodeoxycholic acid

Ursodeoxycholic acid (UCDA) is the epimer of chenodeoxycholic acid and appears to replace endogenous, hepatotoxic bile acids. UDCA has membrane stabilizing or cytoprotective, immunological and anti-apoptotic effects. Initial observational studies evaluating the therapeutic benefit of UDCA (10–15 mg/kg per day) in patients with NASH reported a significant improvement or normalization of liver test results and a reduction in the degree of steatosis in the only study with post-treatment histology.[71,81] However, a recent large placebo-controlled randomized trial in 166 patients with NASH has shown no benefit of 2 year long therapy with UDCA (13–15 mg/kg per day).[82] Weight was stable in both groups. In 107 paired biopsies, changes in the degree of steatosis, necroinflammation and fibrosis were not different between UDCA and placebo. Ala

Liver transplantation for patients with non-alcoholic fatty liver disease

Patients with NAFLD that progress to decompensated cirrhosis or who develop HCC are candidates for liver transplantation. Unsurprisingly, steatosis recurs in the majority of patients by 4 years, with 50% developing recurrent NASH and fibrosis, and cases of recurrent cirrhosis are also reported.[83,84] Risk factors for recurrence are the presence of insulin resistance/type 2 DM pre and post-transplantation, weight gain post-transplantation and cumulative steroid

Table 26.4   Minimum requirements for clinical trials of NASH therapy

Study parameter	Requirement
Basic design	Double-blind, randomized, controlled
Entry criteria	Recent biopsy evidence of NASH
	Drinking within "sensible" alcohol limits
	Secondary causes of NASH and other primary liver diseases excluded
Patient numbers	Sufficient for adequate statistical power
Study duration	At least a year, preferably 2 years
Stratification	For presence of type 2 diabetes mellitus
Primary study endpoints	Improvement in fibrosis stage
	Improvement in necroinflammation grade
Secondary endpoints	Quality of life
	Cost benefit

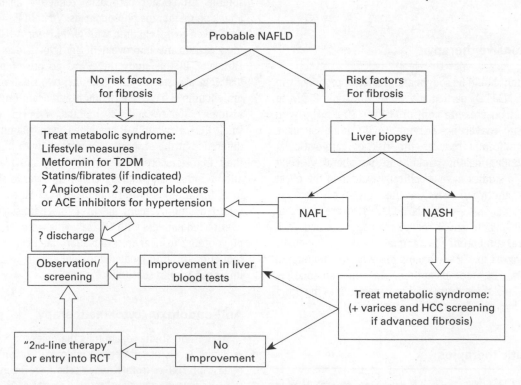

Figure 26.2   Management strategy for patient presenting with suspected non-alcoholic fatty liver disease. It is assumed that these patients have had other causes of abnormal liver blood tests excluded by history (for alcohol excess and hepatotoxic drugs) and serology (for autoimmune disease and viral hepatitis) and have steatosis detected on abdominal ultrasound. ACE, angiotensin converting enzyme; HCC, hepatocellular carcinoma; RCT, randomized controlled trials; T2DM, type 2 diabetes mellitus; NAFLD, non-alcoholic fatty liver disease; NASH, non-alcoholic steatohepatitis; HCC, hepatocellular carcinoma

dose.[84] These factors clearly suggest several strategies aimed at reducing the frequency of disease recurrence in a group of patients that seem likely to contribute increasing numbers to transplant programs in the future.

Conclusions

At present there is no established therapy for NAFLD based on evidence from large, RCTs. Treatment for all patients, whatever the severity of their disease, should therefore be directed at the associated risk factors: obesity, type 2 DM, hyperlipidemia and hypertension. This strategy will reduce morbidity and mortality and may also be beneficial to the liver. Patients with one or more risk factors for advanced NAFLD should probably undergo liver biopsy to determine their disease stage. Patients with advanced fibrotic disease should be followed up and enter surveillance programs for varices and HCC. For the future, studies in animal models of NAFLD and pilot studies in humans have reported encouraging data for a variety of novel treatment strategies based on our increasing understanding of disease pathogenesis. It is hoped that within the next few years results from currently ongoing large clinical trials of these strategies (Table 26.4) will provide a firm evidence base for the use of safe, well-tolerated lifestyle modifications and/or pharmaceutical agents with beneficial effects on liver histology, currently the best available surrogate marker for long-term prognosis.[77] An overall management strategy for patients presenting with suspected NAFLD is suggested in Figure 26.2.

References

1 Angulo P. Nonalcoholic fatty liver disease. *N Engl J Med* 2002;**346**:1221–31.
2 Clark JM, Brancati FL, Diehl AM. The prevalence and etiology of elevated aminotransferase levels in the United States. *Am J Gastroenterol* 2003;**98**:960–7.
3 Ruhl CE, Everhart JE. Determinants of the association of overweight with elevated serum alanine aminotransferase activity in the United States. *Gastroenterology* 2003;**124**:71–9.
4 Skelly MM, James PD, Ryder SD. Findings on liver biopsy to investigate abnormal liver function tests in the absence of diagnostic serology. *J Hepatol* 2001;**35**:195–9.
5 Caldwell SH, Hespenheide EE. Subacute liver failure in obese women. *Am J Gastroenterol* 2002;**97**:2058–62.
6 Cairns SR, Kark AE, Peters TJ. Raised hepatic free fatty acids in a patient with acute liver failure after gastric surgery for morbid obesity. *J Clin Pathol* 1986;**39**:647–9.
7 Grimm IS, Schindler W, Haluszka O. Steatohepatitis and fatal hepatic failure after biliopancreatic diversion. *Am J Gastroenterol* 1992;**87**:775–9.
8 Matteoni CA, Younossi ZM, Gramlich T *et al.* Non-alcoholic fatty liver disease: a spectrum of clinical and pathological severity. *Gastroenterology* 1999;**116**:1413–19.
9 Teli MR, James OFW, Burt AD *et al.* The natural history of non-alcoholic fatty liver: a follow up study. *Hepatology* 1995;**22**:1714–19.
10 Lee RG. Nonalcoholic steatohepatitis: a study of 49 patients. *Hum Pathol* 1989;**20**:594–8.
11 Powell EE, Cooksley WG, Hanson R *et al.* The natural history of non-alcoholic steatohepatitis: a follow up study of forty-two patients for up to 21 years. *Hepatology* 1990;**11**:74–80.
12 Bacon BR, Farahvash MJ, Janney CG *et al.* Nonalcoholic steatohepatitis: an expanded clinical entity. *Gastroenterology* 1994;**107**:1103–9.
13 Ratziu V, Giral P, Charlotte F *et al.* Liver fibrosis in overweight patients. *Gastroenterology* 2000;**118**:1117–23.
14 Harrison SA, Torgerson S, Hayashi PH. The natural history of non-alcoholic fatty liver disease: a clinical histopathologic study. *Am J Gastroenterol* 2003;**98**:2042–7.
15 Caldwell SH, Oelsner DH, Lezzoni JC *et al.* Cryptogenic cirrhosis: clinical characterization and risk factors for underlying disease. *Hepatology* 1999;**29**:664–70.
16 Poonwala A, Nair S, Thuluvath PJ. Prevalence of obesity and diabetes in patients with cryptogenic cirrhosis: a case–control study. *Hepatology* 2000;**32**:689–92.
17 Ratziu V, Bonyhay L, Di Martino V, *et al.* Survival, liver failure, and hepatocellular carcinoma in obesity-related cryptogenic cirrhosis. *Hepatology* 2002;**35**:1485–93.
18 Shimada M, Hashimoto E, Taniai K *et al.* Hepatocellular carcinoma in patients with non-alcoholic steatohepatitis. *J Hepatol* 2002;**37**:154–60.
19 Bugianesi E, Leone N, Vanni E *et al.* Expanding the natural history of nonalcoholic steatohepatitis: from cryptogenic cirrhosis to hepatocellular carcinoma. *Gastroenterology* 2002;**123**:134–40.
20 Nair S, Mason A, Eason J *et al.* Is obesity an independent risk factor for hepatocellular carcinoma in cirrhosis? *Hepatology* 2002;**36**:150–5.
21 Calle EE, Rodriguez C, Walker-Thurmond K, Thun MJ. Overweight, obesity and mortality from cancer in a prospectively studied cohort of US adults. *N Engl J Med* 2003;**348**:1625–38.
22 Hultcrantz R, Glaumann H, Lindberg G, Nilsson LH. Liver investigation in 149 asymptomatic patients with moderately elevated activities of serum aminotransferases. *Scand J Gastroenterol* 1986;**21**:109–13.
23 Daniel S, Ben-Menachem T, Vasudevan G, Ma CK, Blumenkehl M. Prospective evaluation of unexplained chronic liver transaminase abnormalities in asymptomatic and symptomatic patients. *Am J Gastroenterol* 1999;**94**:3010–14.
24 Dixon JB, Bhathal PS, O'Brian PE. Non-alcoholic fatty liver disease: predictors of non-alcoholic steatohepatitis and liver fibrosis in the severely obese. *Gastroenterology* 2001;**121**:91–100.
25 Rimm EB, Chan J, Stampfer MJ, Colditz GA, Willett WC. Prospective study of cigarette smoking, alcohol use, and the risk of diabetes in men. *BMJ* 1995;**310**:555–9.

26 Saadeh S, Younossi ZM, Remer EM *et al.* The utility of radiological imaging in nonalcoholic fatty liver disease. *Gastroenterology* 2002;**123**:745–50.

27 Marrero JA, Fontana RJ, Su GL, Conjeevaram HS, Emick DM, Lok AS. NAFLD may be a common underlying liver disease in patients with hepatocellular carcinoma in the United States. *Hepatology* 2002;**36**:1349–54.

28 Marchesini G, Bugianesi E, Forlani G *et al.* Nonalcoholic fatty liver, steatohepatitis and the metabolic syndrome. *Hepatology* 2003;**37**:917–23.

29 Angulo P, Keach JC, Batts KP *et al.* Independent predictors of liver fibrosis in patients with non-alcoholic steatohepatitis. *Hepatology* 1999;**30**:1356–62.

30 Alberti KGMM, Zimmet PZ. Definition, diagnosis and classification of diabetes mellitus and its complications. Part 1: diagnosis and classification of diabetes mellitus. Provisional report of a WHO consultation. *Diabet Med* 1998;**15**:539–53.

31 Farrell GC. Steatohepatitis. In: Farrell GC (ed). *Drug Induced Liver Disease.* Edinburgh: Churchill Livingstone, 1994.

32 Marchesini G, Brizi M, Morselli-Labate AM *et al.* Association of non-alcoholic fatty liver disease with insulin resistance. *Am J Med* 1999;**107**:450–5.

33 Cortez-Pinto H, Camilo ME, Baptista A, De Oliveira AG, De Moura MC. Non-alcoholic fatty liver: another feature of the metabolic syndrome? *Clin Nutr* 1999;**18**:353–8.

34 Marchesini G, Brizi M, Bianchi G *et al.* Nonalcoholic fatty liver disease: a feature of the metabolic syndrome. *Diabetes* 2001;**50**:1844–50.

35 Sanyal AJ, Campbell-Sargent C, Mirshahi F *et al.* Non-alcoholic steatohepatitis: association of insulin resistance and mitochondrial abnormalities. *Gastroenterology* 2001; **120**:1183–92.

36 Expert Panel on Detection Evaluation and Treatment of High Blood Cholesterol in Adults. Executive summary of the third report of the National Cholesterol Education Program (NCEP) expert panel on detection, evaluation and treatment of high blood cholesterol in adults (Adult Treatment Panel III). *JAMA* 2001;**285**:2486–97.

37 Isomaa B, Almgren P, Tuomi T *et al.* Cardiovascular morbidity and mortality associated with the metabolic syndrome. *Diabetes Care* 2001;**24**:683–9.

38 Diabetes Prevention Program Research Group. Reduction in the incidence of type 2 diabetes with lifestyle intervention or metformin. *N Engl J Med* 2002;**346**:393–403.

39 UK Prospective Diabetes Study Group. Effect of intensive blood-glucose control with metformin on complications in overweight patients with type 2 diabetes. (UKPDS 34). *Lancet* 1998;**352**:854–65.

40 Peto R, Collins R. Antihypertensive drug therapy: effects on stroke and coronary heart disease. In: Swales JD (ed). *Textbook of Hypertension.* Oxford: Blackwell, 1994.

41 Heart Protection Study Collaborative Group. MRC/BHF Heart Protection Study of cholesterol lowering with simvastatin in 20 536 high-risk individuals: a randomised placebo-controlled trial. *Lancet* 2002;**360**:7–22.

42 UK Prospective Diabetes Study Group. Tight blood pressure control and risk of macrovascular and microvascular complications in type 2 diabetes (UKPDS 38). *BMJ* 1998;**317**:703–13.

43 The Heart Outcomes Prevention Evaluation Study Investigators. Effects of angiotensin-converting-enzyme inhibitor, ramipril, on cardiovascular events in high-risk patients. *N Engl J Med* 2000;**342**:145–53.

44 Heart Protection Study Collaborative Group. MRC/BHF Heart Protection Study of cholesterol-lowering with simvastatin in 5963 people with diabetes: a randomised placebo-controlled trial. *Lancet* 2003;**361**:2005–16.

45 Joint British recommendations on prevention of coronary heart disease in clinical practice. *Heart* 1998;**80(Suppl 2)**: S1–S29.

46 Day CP, James OFW. Steatohepatitis: a tale of two "hits"? *Gastroenterology* 1998;**114**:842–5.

47 Day CP. Pathogenesis of steatohepatitis. *Best Pract Res Clin Gastroenterology* 2002;**16**:663–78.

48 Eriksson S, Eriksson KF, Bondesson L. Nonalcoholic steatohepatitis in obesity: a reversible condition. *Acta Med Scand* 1986;**20**:83–8.

49 Rozental P, Biava C, Spencer H, Zimmerman H. Liver morphology and function tests in obesity and during total starvation. *Am J Dig Dis* 1967;**12**:198–208.

50 Ueno T, Sugawara H, Sujaku K *et al.* Therapeutic effects of restricted diet and exercise in obese patients with fatty liver. *J Hepatol* 1997;**27**:103–7.

51 Anderson T, Gluud C, Franzmann M, Christoffersen P. Hepatic effects of dietary weight loss in morbidly obese patients. *J Hepatol* 1991;**12**:224–9.

52 Luyckx FH, Desaive C, Thiry A *et al.* Liver abnormalities in severely obese subjects: effect of drastic weight loss after gastroplasty. *Int J Obes* 1998;**22**:222–6.

53 American Gastroenterological Association. AGA technical review on nonalcoholic fatty liver disease. *Gastroenterology* 2002;**123**:1705–25.

54 Musso G, Gambino R, De Michieli F *et al.* Dietary habits and their relations to insulin resistance and postprandial lipemia in nonalcoholic steatohepatitis. *Hepatology* 2003;**37**:909–16.

55 Harrison SA, Fincke C, Helinski D, Torgerson S. Orlistat treatment in obese, non-alcoholic steatohepatitis patients: a pilot study [Abstract]. *Hepatology* 2002;**36**:406A.

56 Pagano G, Pacinin G, Musso G *et al.* Nonalcoholic steatohepatitis, insulin resistance, metabolic syndrome: further evidence for an etiologic association. *Hepatology* 2002;**35**:367–72.

57 Zhou G, Myers R, Li Y *et al.* Role of AMP-activated protein kinase in mechanism of metformin action. *J Clin Invest* 2001;**108**:1167–74.

58 Mayerson AB, Hundal RS, Dufour S *et al.* The effects of rosiglitazone on insulin sensitivity, lipolysis, and hepatic and skeletal muscle triglyceride content in patients with type 2 diabetes. *Diabetes* 2002;**51**:797–802.

59 Lin HZ, Yang SQ, Chuckaree C, Kuhajda F, Ronnet G, Diehl AM. Metformin reverses fatty liver disease in obese, leptin deficient mice. *Nat Med* 2000;**6**:998–1003.

60 Marchesini G, Brizi M, Bianchi G, Tomassetti S, Zoli M, Melchionda N. Metformin in non-alcoholic steatohepatitis. *Lancet* 2001;**358**:893–4.

61 Nair S, Diehl AM, Perrillo R. Metformin in non-alcoholic steatohepatitis (NASH): efficacy and safety. A preliminary report [Abstract]. *Gastroenterology* 2002;**122**:A621–A622.

62 Jiang C, Ting AT, Seed B. PPAR-gamma agonists inhibit production of monocyte inflammatory cytokines. *Nature* 1998;**391**:82–6.

63 Galli A, Crabb DW, Ceni E *et al.* Antidiabetic thiazolidinediones inhibit collagen synthesis and hepatic stellate cell activation *in vivo* and *in vitro*. *Gastroenterology* 2002;**122**:1924–40.

64 Caldwell SH, Hespenheide EE, Redick JA, Iezzoni JC, Battle EH, Sheppard BL. A pilot study of a thiazolidinedione, troglitazone, in nonalcoholic steatohepatitis. *Am J Gastroenterol* 2001;**96**:519–25.

65 Neuschwander-Tetri BA, Brunt EM, Wehmeier KR, Oliver D, Bacon BR. Improved non-alcoholic steatohepatitis after 48 weeks of treatment with the PPAR-γ ligand rosiglitazone. *Hepatology* 2003;**38**:1008–17.

66 Sanyal AJ, Contos MJ, Sargeant C *et al.* A randomized controlled pilot study of pioglitazone and vitamin E versus vitamin E for nonalcoholic steatohepatitis [Abstract]. *Hepatology* 2002;**36**:382A.

67 Promrat K, Lutchman G, Uwaito G *et al.* A pilot study of pioglitazone treatment for non-alcoholic steatohepatitis. *Hepatology* 2004;**39**:188–96.

68 Yuan M, Konstantopoulos N, Lee J *et al.* Reversal of obesity- and diet-induced insulin resistance with salicylates or targeted disruption of IKKβ. *Science* 2001;**293**:1673–7.

69 Berger J, Moller DE. The mechanism of action of PPARs. *Annu Rev Med* 2002;**53**:409–35.

70 Ip E, Farrell GC, Robertson G, Hall P, Kirsch R, Leclercq I. Central role of PPARα-dependent hepatic lipid turnover in dietary steatohepatitis in mice. *Hepatology* 2003;**38**:123–32.

71 Laurin J, Lindor KD, Crippin JS *et al.* Ursodeoxycholic acid or clofibrate in the treatment of non-alcoholic-induced steatohepatitis: a pilot study. *Hepatology* 1996;**23**:1464–7.

72 Ye J-M, Iglesias MA, Watson DG *et al.* PPARα/γ ragaglitizar eliminates fatty liver and enhances insulin action in fat-fed rats in the absence of hepatomegaly. *Am J Physiol Endocrinol Metab* 2003;**284**:E531–E540.

73 Yoshiji H, Kuriyama, Yoshii J *et al.* Angiotensin II type 1 receptor interaction is a major regulator for liver fibrosis in rats. *Hepatology* 2001;**34**:745–50.

74 Merat S, Malekzadeh R, Sohrabi MR *et al.* Probucol in the treatment of non-alcoholic steatohepatitis: a double-blind randomized controlled study. *J Hepatolatol* 2003;**38**:414–18.

75 Abdelmalek MF, Angulo P, Jorgensen RA *et al.* Betaine, a promising new agent for patients with non-alcoholic steatohepatitis: Results of a pilot study. *Am J Gastroenterol* 2001;**96**:2711–17.

76 Lavine JE. Vitamin E treatment of non-alcoholic steatohepatitis in children: a pilot study. *J Pediatr* 2000;**136**:734–8.

77 Hasegawa T, Yonada M, Nakamura K *et al.* Plasma transforming growth factor-β1 level and efficacy of α-tocopherol in patients with non-alcoholic steatohepatitis: a pilot study. *Alim Pharm Ther* 2001;**15**:1667–72.

78 Harrison SA, Torgerson S, Hayashi P, Ward J, Schenker S. Vitamin E and Vitamin C treatment improves fibrosis in patients with non-alcoholic steatohepatitis. *Am J Gastroenterol* 2003;**98**:2485–90.

79 Facchini FS, Hua NW, Stoohs RA. Effect of iron depletion in carbohydrate-intolerant patients with clinical evidence of nonalcoholic fatty liver disease. *Gastroenterology* 2002;**122**:931–9.

80 Li Z, Yang S, Lin H *et al.* Probiotics and antibodies to TNF inhibit inflammatory activity and improve non-alcoholic fatty liver disease. *Hepatology* 2003;**37**:343–50.

81 Angulo P, Lindor KD. Treatment of non-alcoholic fatty liver: present and emerging therapies. *Semin Liver Dis* 2001;**21**:81–8.

82 Lindor KD, Kowdley KV, Heathcote CJ *et al.* Ursodeoxycholic acid for treatment of non-alcoholic steatohepatitis: results of a randomised, placebo-controlled trial. *Hepatology* 2004;**39**:770–8.

83 Contos MJ, Cales W, Sterling RK *et al.* Development of nonalcoholic fatty liver disease after orthotopic liver transplantation for cryptogenic cirrhosis. *Liver Transpl* 2001;**7**:363–73.

84 Ong J, Younossi ZM, Reddy V *et al.* Cryptogenic cirrhosis and posttransplantation nonalcoholic fatty liver disease. *Liver Transpl* 2001;**7**:797–801.

27 Hemochromatosis and Wilson disease

Gary Jeffrey, Paul C Adams

Introduction

Hemochromatosis is the most common genetic disease in populations of European ancestry. Despite estimates in different countries ranging from 1 in 100 to 1 in 300, hemochromatosis is still considered by many physicians to be a rare disease. The diagnosis can be difficult because of the non-specific nature of the symptoms. The discovery of the hemochromatosis gene in 1996,[1] has led to new insights into the pathogenesis of the disease and new diagnostic strategies.[2]

Pathogenesis of hemochromatosis

There is increasing evidence that the HFE protein produced by the hemochromatosis gene interacts with the transferrin receptor on the cell membrane to control intracellular iron concentration. The typical C282Y mutation of the *HFE* gene seen in hemochromatosis results in a conformational change in the HFE protein and intracellular iron decreases. As the iron-depleted cells in the intestinal crypts migrate to the tips of the villi of the duodenum, another gene is activated, DMT1, which facilitates increased iron absorption. A new iron transporter gene, ferroportin 1, which exports iron out of the cells into the circulation has also been implicated in the pathogenesis of iron overload. Hepcidin is a regulatory hormone produced in the liver which may be abnormally regulated in hemochromatosis.[3] Experiments in knockout mice models for a variety of iron-related genes have demonstrated the importance of multiple genes and proteins in the phenotypic expression of iron overload.[4] Therefore it is likely that the control of iron absorption is a cascade of events similar conceptually to blood coagulation or complement activation.[5,6]

Diagnosis of hemochromatosis

A paradox of genetic hemochromatosis is the observation that the disease is underdiagnosed in the general population with hemochromatosis, and overdiagnosed in patients with secondary iron overload.

Underdiagnosis of hemochromatosis

Population studies using genetic testing in patients of northern European ancestry have demonstrated a prevalence of C282Y homozygotes of approximately 1 in 200. The fact that many physicians consider hemochromatosis to be rare implies either a lack of penetrance of the gene (non-expressing homozygote) or a large number of patients that remain undiagnosed in the community.

A major problem in the diagnosis of hemochromatosis is the lack of symptoms and the non-specific nature of the symptoms. An elderly patient who presents with joint symptoms and diabetes is not often considered to have genetic hemochromatosis. The presenting features vary depending on age and sex but fatigue is the most common complaint. Women are more likely to have fatigue, arthralgia and pigmentation rather than liver disease.[7]

Diagnostic tests for hemochromatosis

Serum iron

An elevated serum iron is found in most but not all cases. Serum iron can vary throughout the day and it has been estimated that approximately 5–10% of homozygotes have a normal serum iron.[8]

Transferrin saturation

The transferrin saturation is the serum iron/total iron binding capacity. The transferrin saturation has a sensitivity of greater than 90% for hemochromatosis in referral studies of iron loaded patiients, however, in population studies the sensitivity may be as low as 50%.[9,10] A fasting value has even greater predictive value but may not always be practical. The transferrin saturation is often elevated even in children or young adults with hemochromatosis before the development of iron overload and a rising ferritin. The threshold to pursue further diagnostic studies has varied from 45% to 62% in previous studies. A lower threshold picks up more patients with hemochromatosis but also leads to more investigations in patients without hemochromatosis. A higher threshold leads to fewer investigations overall with a greater possibility of missing some patients. These concepts are most relevant when considering population screening.[11]

Serum ferritin

The relationship between serum ferritin and total body iron stores has been clearly established by strong correlations with hepatic iron concentration and amount of iron removed by venesection.[12] However, ferritin can be elevated secondary to chronic inflammation and histiocytic neoplasms. A major diagnostic dilemma in the past was whether the serum ferritin was related to hemochromatosis or another underlying liver disease such as alcoholic liver disease, chronic viral hepatitis or non-alcoholic steatohepatitis. It is likely that many of these difficult cases will now be resolved by genetic testing. Large population studies have demonstrated that a mild elevation in ferritin (300–1000 micrograms/l) is very common, and may be related to obesity with steatohepatitis, regular alcohol consumption or inflammation.

Iron removed by venesection

Since hemochromatosis has usually been diagnosed when symptoms developed in the fifth or sixth decade, patients had significant iron overload at the time of diagnosis. The removal of 500 ml of blood weekly (0·25 g iron) was well tolerated often for years without the development of significant anemia. If a patient became anemic (hemoglobin < 100 g/l) after only six venesections, it suggested mild iron overload incompatible with the diagnosis of hereditary hemochromatosis. These guidelines may no longer apply as population and pedigree studies uncover patients in the second and third decade.[13] At our center, only 71% of homozygotes would have met the arbitrary criterion that more than 5 g of iron (20 venesections) were removed without anemia.[14] This is a historical diagnostic criterion for hemochromatosis which is no longer relevant in the era of genetic testing.

Liver biopsy

Liver biopsy has been the "gold standard" diagnostic test for hemochromatosis and has shifted from a diagnostic tool to a prognostic guide. The need for liver biopsy seems less apparent in the young asymptomatic patient with a low clinical suspicion of cirrhosis based on history, physical examination and iron studies. Clinical guidelines have been suggested, such as a serum ferritin < 1000 micrograms/l or age < 40 years to reduce the need for liver biopsy.[15] Clinical judgment and assessment of concomitant risk factors (alcohol, viral hepatitis) would be a better guide for the need for liver biopsy rather than an arbitrary threshold. Most non-cirrhotic patients with hemochromatosis have serum ferritin < 1000 micrograms/l *and* a normal aspartate transaminase (AST).[16] Cirrhosis can be predicted non-invasively in C282Y homozygotes if the serum ferritin is > 1000 micrograms/l, the platelet count is less than 200×10^6/l and the AST is > 40 U/l.[17]

Patients with cirrhosis have a 5·5-fold relative risk of death compared with non-cirrhotic hemochromatosis patients.[18,19] Cirrhotic patients are also at risk of hepatocellular carcinoma. The mean age of cirrhotic patients with hepatocellular carcinoma was 68 years in a Canadian series but was lower in Italian patients with concomitant viral hepatitis.[20] Although early detection has been clearly demonstrated by serial ultrasound and α-fetoprotein determination, curative treatment options remain limited. An elderly cirrhotic patient may not withstand a major resection and the residual cirrhotic liver remains a fertile ground for new tumor development. Organ shortages often preclude the possibility of immediate liver transplantation although living related adult liver transplantation may improve this situation in the future.

Hepatic iron concentration and hepatic iron index

The traditional method of assessing iron status by liver biopsy uses the semi-quantitative staining method of Perls. However, when moderate iron overload is present, the degree of iron overload can be difficult to interpret. Iron concentration can be measured using atomic absorption spectrophotometry. This can be done on a piece of paraffin embedded tissue so special preparation is not required at the time of the biopsy. An advantage of cutting the tissue from the block is that one can be more certain that the tissue assayed is the same as the tissue examined microscopically. The normal reference range for hepatic iron concentration is 0–35 μmol/g dry weight (< 2000 micrograms/g). The hepatic iron concentration (μmol/g) divided by age (years) is the hepatic iron index. Before genetic testing became available, this was demonstrated by Bassett *et al.* to be a useful test in differentiating the patient with genetic hemochromatosis from the patient with alcoholic siderosis.[21] The index remains a useful test in this clinical setting but has been extrapolated to be a diagnostic criterion for hemochromatosis. A threshold of 1·9 for the hepatic iron index had a 91% sensitivity for hemochromatosis and area under the receiver operating characteristic curve was 0·94 (95% CI 0·9 to 0·99).[22] Early diagnosis in population screening and pedigree studies have led to the recognition of many homozygotes with a hepatic iron index > 1·9.[23] Increasing awareness of the concept of

Table 27.1   Prevalence of C282Y homozygotes in hemochromatosis studies

Source	Population	Country	C282Y Homozygotes n/N (%)
Adams and Chakrabarti[14]	Suspected clinical diagnosis[a]	Canada	122/128 (95)
Feder *et al.*[1]	Suspected clinical diagnosis	USA	148/178 (83)
Beutler *et al.*[30]	Suspected clinical diagnosis	USA	121/147 (82)
Jouanelle *et al.*[26]	Suspected clinical diagnosis	France	59/65 (93)
Carella *et al.*[29]	Suspected clinical diagnosis	Italy	48/75 (64)
UK Haemochromatosis Consortium[28]	Suspected clinical diagnosis	UK	105/115 (91)
Jazwinzka *et al.*[31]	Family studies	Australia	112/112 (100)

[a]Suspected clinical diagnosis includes isolated iron loaded probands and probands with discovered relatives.

moderate iron overload in cirrhosis of any etiology has demonstrated many patients without hemochromatosis who have a hepatic iron index > 1·9.[24] The hepatic iron index has therefore become less useful with the advent of genetic testing. The commentary on liver biopsy reports that the hepatic iron index is > 1·9, confirming a diagnosis of genetic hemochromatosis should be strongly discouraged.

Imaging studies of the liver

Magnetic resonance imaging (MRI) can demonstrate moderate to severe iron overload of the liver. The technology is advancing and it is possible that eventually it may become as precise as hepatic iron determination.[25] Proponents of MRI have emphasized the non-invasive nature of the test for the diagnosis and alleviated need for liver biopsy. As previously discussed, the role of liver biopsy has now shifted from a diagnostic tool to a prognostic tool. It is likely that the presence of an elevated ferritin with a positive genetic test will satisfy the non-invasive clinician more than an MRI study. MRI can also demonstrate the clinical features of cirrhosis such as nodularity of the liver, ascites, portal hypertension and splenomegaly as well as hepatocellular carcinoma. These features can be more readily assessed by abdominal ultrasound at a lower cost.

Genetic testing for hemochromatosis

A major advance which stems from the discovery of the hemochromatosis gene, is the diagnostic genetic test. The original publication reported that 83% of a group of patients with suspected hemochromatosis had the characteristic C282Y mutation of the *HFE* gene. In this report, the gene was called HLA-H but this name was later changed to *HFE*.[1] The C282Y mutation is also reported as 845A in some laboratories reflecting the base pair change rather than the amino acid change. Subsequent studies in well defined hemochromatosis pedigrees reported that 90–100% of typical hemochromatosis patients had the C282Y mutation.[14,22,26–28] (Table 27.1). The presence of a single mutation in most patients was in marked contrast to other genetic diseases in which multiple mutations have been discovered (cystic fibrosis, Wilson disease,

α-1-antitrypsin deficiency). A second minor mutation, H63D, was also described in the original report.[1] This mutation does not cause the same intracellular trafficking defect of the HFE protein and many homozygotes for H63D have been found without iron overload in the general population. Compound heterozygotes (C282Y/H63D) may resemble homozygotes with mild to moderate iron overload.[32,33]

The interpretation of the genetic test in several settings is shown in Box 27.1. The test may also be performed on DNA extracted from paraffin embedded tissue such as liver explants. Studies of explanted livers have demonstrated that many liver transplant patients classified as hemochromatosis patients are negative for the C282Y mutation.[34] This suggests that those patients may have had iron overload secondary to chronic liver disease rather than hemochromatosis. Therefore any interpretation of iron reaccumulation post liver transplant for hemochromatosis must be done with caution.

Genetic discrimination is a concern with the widespread use of genetic testing. A positive genetic test even without iron overload could disqualify a patient for health or life insurance. In the case of hemochromatosis, the advantages of early diagnosis of a treatable disease outweigh the disadvantages of genetic discrimination.

Genotypic–phenotypic correlation in hemochromatosis   If we define the presence of homozygosity for the C282Y mutation as the new gold standard for hemochromatosis, it provides for the first time a benchmark for the assessment of the phenotypic diagnostic tools that have been used for decades. In one study transferrin saturation, ferritin, hepatic iron index and iron removed by venesection were evaluated in putative homozygotes. Ninety-five percent (122/128) patients were homozygous for the C282Y mutation. The hepatic iron index was > 1·9 in 91·3% of these cases, transferrin saturation > 55% in 90%, serum ferritin > 300 micrograms/l in 96% of men and > 200 micrograms/l in 97% of women, and iron removed > 5 g in 70% of men and 73% of women. Four homozygotes for C282Y had no biochemical evidence of iron overload. The sensitivity of the phenotypic tests in decreasing order was: serum ferritin, hepatic iron index, transferrin saturation and iron removed by venesection. Although the

---

Box 27.1   Interpretation of C282Y genetic testing for hemochromatosis

C282Y homozygote: This is the classic genetic pattern that is seen in >90% of typical cases. Expression of disease ranges from no evidence of iron overload to massive iron overload with organ dysfunction. Siblings have a 1 in 4 chance of being affected and should have genetic testing. For children to be affected the other parent must be at least a heterozygote. If iron studies are normal, false positive genetic testing or a non-expressing homozygote should be considered

C282Y/H63D (compound heterozygote): This patient carries one copy of the major mutation and one copy of the minor mutation. Most patients with this genetic pattern have normal iron studies. A small percentage of compound heterozygotes have been found to have mild to moderate iron overload. Severe iron overload is usually seen in the setting of another concomitant risk factor (alcoholism, viral hepatitis)

C282Y heterozygote: This patient carries one copy of the major mutation. This pattern is seen in about 10% of the Caucasian population and is usually associated with normal or mildly increased iron studies. In rare cases the iron studies are high in the range expected in a homozygote rather than a heterozygote. These cases may carry an unknown hemochromatosis mutation and liver biopsy is helpful to determine the need for venesection therapy

H63D homozyote: This patient carries two copies of the minor mutation. Most patients with this genetic pattern have normal iron studies. A small percentage of these cases have been found to have mild to moderate iron overload. Severe iron overload is usually seen in the setting of another concomitant risk factor (alcoholism, viral hepatitis)

H63D heterozygote: This patient carries one copy of the minor mutation. This pattern is seen in about 20% of the Caucasian population and is usually associated with normal iron studies. This pattern is so common in the general population that the presence of iron overload may be related to another risk factor. Liver biopsy may be required to determine the cause of the iron overload and the need for treatment in these cases

No *HFE* mutations: There are currently some new mutations associated with iron overload that are being studied in research laboratories (ferroportin, transferrin receptor 2). There will likely be other hemochromatosis mutations discovered in the future. If iron overload is present without any *HFE* mutations, a careful history for other risk factors must be reviewed and liver biopsy may be useful to determine the cause of the iron overload and the need for treatment. Many of these cases are isolated, non-familial cases

---

genetic test is useful in the diagnostic algorithm (Figure 27.1), this study demonstrated both iron loaded patients without the mutation and homozygous patients without iron overload.[14]

Non-expressing homozygotes   As genetic testing becomes more widespread an increasing number of persons have been found with the hemochromatosis gene without iron overload.[35] Large scale population studies in North America and northern Europe have demonstrated that approximately 50% of C282Y homozygous women and 86% of homozygous men will have an elevated ferritin. It is apparent that the prevalence of *HFE* mutations far exceeds the prevalence of biochemical iron overload and clinical symptoms attributable to hemochromatosis. Patients who are homozygous for the C282Y mutation should be considered at risk of developing iron overload but if there are no abnormalities in transferrin saturation or ferritin in adulthood, it seems more likely that they are non-expressing homozygotes rather than patients who will develop iron overload later in life.[36]

Family studies in hemochromatosis   Once the proband case is identified and confirmed with genetic testing for the C282Y mutation, family testing is imperative. Siblings have a one in four chance of carrying the gene and should be screened with the genetic test and serum ferritin. The risk to a child is dependent on the prevalence of heterozygotes in the community and is probably greater than 1 in 20 and much lower if the spouse is non-Caucasian. A cost effective strategy now possible with the genetic test is to test the spouse for the C282Y mutation to assess the risk in the children. If the spouse is not a heterozygote or homozygote, the children will be obligate heterozygotes. This assumes paternity and no other gene or mutation causing hemochromatosis. This strategy is particularly advantageous where the children are geographically separated or may be under a different physician or healthcare system.[37] Genetic testing in general raises many perplexing questions such as premarital testing, *in utero* testing, and paternity issues which have not yet been tested in hemochromatosis.

If an isolated heterozygote is detected by genetic testing, it is recommended to test siblings. Extended family studies are less revealing than a family study with a homozygote but more likely to uncover a homozygote than random population screening.

It is important to remember that there will be patients with a clinical picture indistinguishable from genetic hemochromatosis who will be negative for the C282Y mutation. Most of these patients will be isolated cases although a few cases of familial iron overload (ferroportin and transferrin receptor 2 mutations) have been reported with negative C282Y testing.[29] A negative C282Y test should alert the physician to question the diagnosis of genetic hemochromatosis and reconsider secondary iron overload related to cirrhosis, alcohol, viral hepatitis or iron loading

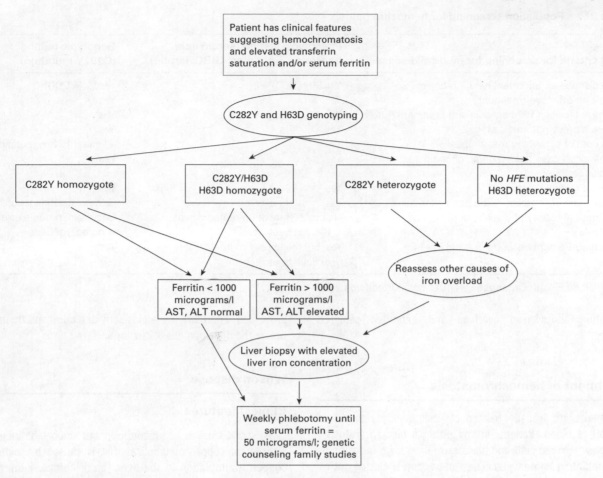

Figure 27.1 Diagnostic algorithm for a patient suspected of having hemochromatosis. AST, aspartate transaminase; AlT, alanine transaminase

anemias. If no other risk factors are found, the patient should begin venesection treatment similar to any other hemochromatosis patient.

Population screening

Soon after the development of the genetic test for hemochromatosis, it seemed that hemochromatosis would be an ideal disease for population screening. It seemed to have a high prevalence, could be detected with low cost iron tests, confirmed by a specific genetic test and easily be treated.[38] Hemochromatosis meets many of the guidelines established by the World Health Organization for screening (Table 27.2). Large population screening studies have been done in North America, Europe and Australia using a variety of approaches and patient populations. Several population studies have included large control populations with no *HFE* mutations (wild type). In one study of 41 038 patients attending a health appraisal clinic in San Diego there were no apparent differences in the symptoms of arthritis, fatigue, diabetes, pigmentation or impotence between C282Y homozygotes and the control participants. Liver disease appeared to be slightly more prevalent in the C282Y homozygotes.[39,40] In another large screening study with control wild type participants, liver disease was more common in male C282Y homozygotes and arthralgia and infertility in female C282Y homozygotes.[41] The screening of 65 238 patients in Norway led to 147 liver biopsies and found only four men and no women with cirrhosis.[9,42] A consistent finding has been a significant percentage of non-expressing C282Y homozygotes. Iron overload in non-Caucasian populations is under investigation in the Hemochromatosis and Iron Overload Screening (HEIRS) study which will screen 100 000 primary care patients in North America. Preliminary results have confirmed the rarity of the C282Y mutation in African-Americans, Asians and Hispanics, and Pacific Islanders. Hyperferritinemia is common in Asian men.[43] Universal screening is unlikely to be widely implemented but selective screening in high risk populations such as men of northern European ancestry may be a preferred strategy. Other strategies include more intense physician and patient

Table 27.2   Population screening for hemochromatosis

WHO criteria for screening for medical disease	Phenotypic testing (serum iron, transferrin saturation, UIBC, ferritin)	Genotypic testing (C282Y mutation)
Is the disease an important health problem?	Yes (1 in 300)	Yes (1 in 200)
Is there an effective treatment?	Yes	Yes
Are there facilities for diagnosis and treatment?	Yes	Yes
Is there a presymptomatic stage?	Yes	Yes
Is the cost of screening reasonable?	Yes	If limited to few mutations
Is continuous case finding on an ongoing basis feasible?	Yes	Yes
Is there a suitable test?	Yes	Yes
Is the testing acceptable to the population?	Yes	Genetic discrimination?
Is the natural history of disease understood?	Natural history of untreated disease has not been studied	Uncertain in non-expressing homozygotes
Is there agreement on whom to treat?	Yes, but the impact of treatment is difficult to assess	Yes

WHO, World Health Organization; UIBC, unsaturated iron binding capacity

education about iron overload and extended pedigree studies.[44]

Treatment of hemochromatosis

Patients are initially treated by the weekly removal of 500 ml of blood. Patients attend either a blood transfusion service where red cells and plasma are used for transfusion or an ambulatory care facility. The venesection is carried out by a nurse using a kit containing a 16-gauge straight needle and collection bag (Blood Pack MR6102). Blood is removed with the patient in the reclining position over 15–30 minutes. A hemoglobin is done at the time of each venesection. If the hemoglobin decreases to less than 100 g/l the venesection schedule is modified to 500 ml every other week. Serum ferritin is measured periodically (every 3 months in severe iron overload, monthly in mild iron overload) and weekly venesections are continued until the serum ferritin is approximately 50 micrograms/l. Transferrin saturation often remains elevated despite therapy. Patients may then begin maintenance venesections three to four times per year.[45] Iron reaccumulation is an inconsistent observation and many patients will go for years without treatment and without a rise in serum ferritin.[46] Chelation therapy is not used for the treatment of hereditary hemochromatosis.

There are no randomized trials comparing venesection therapy to no treatment. Iron depletion before the development of cirrhosis can prevent cirrhosis and the development of hepatocellular carcinoma. Patients with cirrhosis had a 5·5 fold relative risk of death and non-cirrhotic treated patients had a survival similar to an age and sex matched control group.[18,19] B4 Other disabling diseases such as arthritis, diabetes and impotence will likely be prevented. Therefore the goal is early detection and treatment before the development of cirrhosis. C

Wilson disease

Clinical features

Wilson disease is an uncommon but important inherited disorder of copper metabolism that is caused by increased copper accumulation in the liver, brain, cornea, kidney and other tissues. It occurs worldwide with a prevalence of 1 in 30 000 and is inherited as an autonomic recessive disorder. If left untreated the natural history is progressive with 42% of patients presenting with acute or chronic liver disease, the majority during childhood or early adolescence, although rarely patients may present as late as 58 years. As many as 15% of patients also present with hemolysis in this same young age group. Severe debilitating neurological and psychiatric symptoms are the presenting feature in 44% of patients and these symptoms present somewhat later in adolescence or early adulthood. Prior to the availability of liver transplantation death commonly resulted from the complications of liver failure, although others died from progressive neurological dysfunction or hemolysis. Early recognition of Wilson disease allows initiation of treatment that results in the reversal of symptoms and prevents complications and death.

Genetic analysis

The recent cloning of the Wilson disease gene and the identification of mutations responsible for this disorder has resulted in exciting advances in our understanding of the pathophysiology of this disease.[47,48] The gene encodes for a

Table 27.3 Predictive value of diagnostic criteria of Wilson disease

Criterion	Abnormality	Advantage	Disadvantage
Kayser–Fleischer corneal rings	Found on slit lamp examination	Easily assessed physical finding	Normal in 10–45% of patients, mainly the young
Serum ceruloplasmin	Less than 20 mg/l	Decreased in 73–95% of patients	Maybe normal, mainly with liver disease
24-hour copper excretion	More than 100 micrograms/ 24 hours	Increased in 85% of patients; useful in acute liver failure	Copper contamination and incomplete sample
Non-ceruloplasmin bound copper	More than 12 micrograms/dl	Increased when ceruloplasmin levels are normal	Not routinely reported
Liver copper quantitation	More than 250 micrograms/g dry weight	Increased in 90% or more of patients	Elevated in chronic cholestasis Sampling errors
Radiocopper scan	Lack of copper binding by ceruloplasmin	Differentiates homozygotes and heterozygotes	Blood samples over 48 hours

cation-transporting P-type ATPase that is expressed in the liver and brain. Within the hepatocyte the protein is found diffusely throughout the cytoplasm but is also localized to the Golgi.[49] Mutations in the gene result in defective biliary excretion of copper and increased tissue copper levels. A number of additional proteins are now being recognized as important in copper transport. Atox 1 is a copper chaperone that binds with the Wilson disease ATPase and is required for copper excretion from cells.[50] The identification of the Wilson disease gene also has implications for the genetic diagnosis of this disorder. Genotype analysis of the Wilson disease gene has found that no single mutation is responsible for all or even the majority of patients with the disorder and more than 200 different mutations have now been reported. The most common mutation is a His1069Gln substitution, which occurs in between 20% and 60% of patients depending on the population studied. Some studies suggest an association between the His1069Gln mutation and late onset disease and neurological symptoms, however this has not been confirmed by others.[51,52]

Diagnosis

The diagnosis of Wilson disease is made on the basis of clinical and biochemical features with the addition of haplotype or genotype analysis in family studies (Table 27.3). The diagnostic utility of individual biochemical abnormalities depends on the manner in which a patient presents. In most patients the presence of a serum ceruloplasmin level less than 20 mg/dl and the finding of Kayser–Fleischer rings by slit lamp examination are diagnostic. In those patients with only one of these abnormalities an elevated liver copper level greater than 250 micrograms/g dry weight on liver biopsy will confirm the diagnosis. If liver biopsy is contraindicated then an elevated 24-hour urinary copper excretion greater than 100 micrograms/24 hours, an abnormal radiocopper scan or increased non-ceruloplasmin bound serum copper levels greater than 12 micrograms/dl may be confirmatory.

Screening

Screening the general population for Wilson disease is not presently cost effective given the low prevalence of disease and the lack of a single accurate diagnostic test (Table 27.3). Screening should be performed in siblings of patients with Wilson disease, as one in four of this group will have homozygous disease. A recent series found that 18% of patients were diagnosed on the basis of family screening and that only one (10%) of these patients was symptomatic at the time of diagnosis.[53] It has been recommended that all psychiatric patients with signs of liver or neurological disease, or who are refractory to therapy should be screened for Wilson disease. The cost effectiveness of this strategy has not yet been analyzed. Screening all patients with liver disease with a serum ceruloplasmin estimation found that the positive predictive value of this test was only 5·9%.[54] Screening unselected patients with liver disease was therefore not cost effective and it was recommended that screening should be restricted to those patients with liver disease of unknown etiology. The cost effectiveness of this recommendation needs to be further analyzed.

Management

The key to effective drug therapy for Wilson disease is the early detection of disease before the onset of structural neurological abnormalities or cirrhosis. The mainstay of drug treatment for Wilson disease for the past 40 years has been penicillamine.[55] This drug given at a dose of 1·5–2·0 g/day has proved to be an effective copper chelating agent and will reverse or improve the symptoms and signs of Wilson disease. C3 It also prevents the onset of symptoms in asymptomatic patients. Side effects occur in 20% of patients within the first month but most are due to hypersensitivity and respond to cessation of the drug and reintroduction of penicillamine in small doses (250 mg/day) with gradual increases and short-term prednisolone. Long term penicillamine needs to be stopped in only 5% of patients. Pyridoxine deficiency may rarely be induced by penicillamine and 25 mg daily supplements are recommended. Unfortunately penicillamine causes significant symptomatic deterioration in 20% of those patients presenting with neurological symptoms and alternative drugs may be required in this situation. C3

A small number of alternative agents have been shown to be effective in the treatment of Wilson disease. Trientine at a dose of 1–2 g/day is an effective copper chelating agent and may be used in those patients who suffer severe reactions to penicillamine or develop deteriorating neurological symptoms with this drug. C3 Zinc therapy of 75–150 mg/day has been shown to maintain low copper levels in those patients already on maintenance therapy by increasing gastrointestinal copper excretion.[56] It may be useful in those patients unable to tolerate either penicillamine or trientine. C3 Most recently ammonium thiomolybdate at 60–100 mg/day was shown to effectively bind copper and block intestinal copper absorption and was able to decrease hepatic copper levels in a limited number of patients.[57] C3 Only two of 55 patients with neurological symptoms who were initially treated with this drug showed neurological deterioration. Trials are presently examining the effectiveness of combination therapy of trientine and zinc or thiomolybdate and zinc. Acceptable patient and newborn outcomes have been achieved with long-term penicillamine, trientine or zinc therapy during pregnancy.[58,59]

Liver transplantation is required in those patients with acute liver failure or those suffering from complications of cirrhosis. The procedure cures the hepatic copper excretory abnormality, and survival post-transplantation is similar to patients with other causes of liver disease undergoing this procedure.[60] C3 This procedure is not recommended for those patients with only extrahepatic manifestations of Wilson disease.

Reference list

1 Feder JN, Gnirke A, Thomas W *et al.* A novel MHC class I-like gene is mutated in patients with hereditary hemochromatosis. *Nat Genet* 1996;**13**:399–408.

2 Bacon BR, Powell L, Adams PC, Kresina T, Hoofnagle J. Molecular medicine and hemochromatosis: at the crossroads. *Gastroenterology* 1999;**116**:193–207.

3 Bridle K, Frazer D, Wilkins S *et al.* Disrupted hepcidin regulation in HFE-associated haemochromatosis and the liver as a regulator of body iron homeostasis. *Lancet* 2003;**361**: 661–73.

4 Muckenthaler M, Roy C, Custodio A *et al.* Regulatory defects in liver and intestine implicate abnormal hepcidin and Cybrd1 in mouse hemochromatosis. *Nat Genet* 2003;**34**:102–6.

5 Philpott C. Molecular aspects of iron absorption: insights into the role of HFE in hemochromatosis. *Hepatology* 2002;**35**: 993–1001.

6 Parkkila S, Niemela O, Britton R *et al.* Molecular aspects of iron absorption and HFE expression. *Gastroenterology* 2001;**121**:1489–96.

7 Moirand R, Adams PC, Bicheler V, Brissot P, Deugnier Y. Clinical features of genetic hemochromatosis in women compared to men. *Ann Intern Med* 1997;**127**:105–10.

8 Adams PC, Valberg LS. Evolving expression of hereditary hemochromatosis. *Semin Liver Dis* 1996;**16**:47–54.

9 Asberg A, Hveem K, Thorstensen K *et al.* Screening for hemochromatosis – high prevalence and low morbidity in an unselected population of 65 238 persons. *Scand J Gastroenterol* 2001;**36**:1108–15.

10 Beutler E, Felitti V, Gelbart T, Ho N. The effect of HFE genotypes on measurement of iron overload in patients attending a health appraisal clinic. *Ann Intern Med* 2000; **133**:329–37.

11 Adams PC. Population screening for hemochromatosis. *Hepatology* 1999;**29**:1324–7.

12 Brissot P, Bourel M, Herry D *et al.* Assessment of liver iron content in 271 patients: a reevaluation of direct and indirect methods. *Gastroenterology* 1981;**80**:557–65.

13 Adams PC, Kertesz AE, Valberg LS. Clinical presentation of hemochromatosis: a changing scene. *Am J Med* 1991;**90**: 445–9.

14 Adams PC, Chakrabarti S. Genotypic/phenotypic correlations in genetic hemochromatosis: evolution of diagnostic criteria. *Gastroenterology* 1998;**114**:319–23.

15 Tavill AS. Diagnosis and management of hemochromatosis. *Hepatology* 2001;**33**:1321–1328.

16 Guyader D, Jacquelinet C, Moirand R, Turlin B, Mendler M, Chaperon J *et al.* Non-invasive prediction of fibrosis in C282Y homozygous hemochromatosis. *Gastroenterology* 1998; **115**:929–936.

17 Beaton M, Guyader D, Deugnier Y, Moirand R, Chakrabarti S, Adams P. Non-invasive prediction of cirrhosis in C282Y-linked hemochromatosis. *Hepatology* 2002;**36**:673–8.

18 Adams PC, Speechley M, Kertesz AE. Long-term survival analysis in hereditary hemochromatosis. *Gastroenterology* 1991;**101**:368–72.

19 Niederau C, Fischer R, Purschel A, Stremmel W, Haussinger D, Strohmeyer G. Long-term survival in patients with hereditary hemochromatosis. *Gastroenterology* 1996;**110**: 1107–19.

20 Fargion S, Mandelli C, Piperno A *et al.* Survival and prognostic factors in 212 Italian patients with genetic hemochromatosis. *Hepatology* 1992;**15**:655–9.

21 Bassett ML, Halliday JW, Powell LW. Value of hepatic iron measurements in early hemochromatosis and determination of the critical iron level associated with fibrosis. *Hepatology* 1986;**6**:24–9.

22 Adams PC, Bradley C, Henderson AR. Evaluation of the hepatic iron index as a diagnostic criterion in hereditary hemochromatosis. *J Lab Clin Med* 1997;**130**:509–14.

23 Adams PC, Deugnier Y, Moirand R, Brissot P. The relationship between iron overload, clinical symptoms and age in 410 patients with genetic hemochromatosis. *Hepatology* 1997; **25**:162–6.

24 Ludwig J, Hashimoto E, Porayko M, Moyer T, Baldus W. Hemosiderosis in cirrhosis: a study of 447 native livers. *Gastroenterology* 1997;**112**:882–8.

25 Gandon Y, Olivie D, Guyader D *et al.* Non-invasive assessment of hepatic iron stores by MRI. *Lancet* 2004 **363**:357–62.

26 Jouanolle A-M, Gandon G, Jezequel P *et al.* Haemochromatosis and HLA-H. *Nat Genet* 1996;**14**:251–2.

27 Burke W, Thomson E, Khoury M *et al.* Hereditary hemochromatosis: gene discovery and its implications for population-based screening. *JAMA* 1998;**280**:172–8.

28 The UK Haemochromatosis Consortium. A simple genetic test identifies 90% of UK patients with haemochromatosis. *Gut* 1997;**41**:841–5.

29 Carella M, D'Ambrosio L, Totaro A *et al.* Mutation analysis of the HLA-H gene in Italian hemochromatosis patients. *Am J Hum Genet* 1997;**60**:828–32.

30 Beutler E, Gelbart T, West C *et al.* Mutation analysis in hereditary hemochromatosis. *Blood Cells Mol Dis* 1996;**22**: 187–94.

31 Jazwinska EC, Cullen LM, Busfield F *et al.* Haemochromatosis and HLA-H. *Nat Genet* 1996;**4**:249–51.

32 Bacon BR, Schratz C, Britton RS, Wolff RK. Presence of the hemochromatosis genotype in patients with liver disease. *Gastroenterology* 1997;**112**:A1218.

33 Moirand R, Jouanolle A-M, Brissot P, Le Gall J-Y, David V, Deugnier Y. Phenotypic expression of HFE mutations: a French study of 1110 unrelated iron-overloaded patients and relatives. *Gastroenterology* 1999;**116**:372–7.

34 Minguillan J, Lee R, Britton R *et al.* Genetic markers for hemochromatosis in patients with cirrhosis and iron overload. *Hepatology* 1997;**26**:158A.

35 Adams PC. Non-expressing C282Y homozygotes for hemochromatosis: minority or majority of cases? *Mol Genet Metab* 2000;**71**:81–6.

36 Yamashita C, Adams PC. Natural history of the C282Y homozygote of the hemochromatosis gene *(HFE)* with a normal serum ferritin. *Clin Gastroenterol Hepatol* 2003; **1**:388–91.

37 Adams PC. Implications of genotyping of spouses to limit investigation of children in genetic hemochromatosis. *Clin Genet* 1998;**53**:176–8.

38 Adams PC. Population screening for haemochromatosis. *Gut* 2000;**46**:301–3.

39 Beutler E, Felitti V, Koziol J, Ho N, Gelbart T. Penetrance of the 845G to A (C282Y) HFE hereditary hemochromatosis mutation. *Lancet* 2002;**359**:211–18.

40 Waalen J, Felitti V, Gelbart T, Ho N, Beutler E. Prevalence of hemochromatosis-related symptoms among individuals with mutations in the *HFE* gene. *Mayo Clin Proc* 2002;**77**: 522–30.

41 Asberg A, Hveem K, Kruger O, Bjerve K. Persons with screening-detected haemochromatosis: as healthy as the general population? *Scand J Gastroenterol* 2002;**37**: 719–24.

42 McLaren G, Barton J, Gordeuk V *et al.* High *HFE* C282Y homozygote frequency in Caucasians but not in Hispanics, African Americans, or Asians: an analysis of 50 290 primary care patients in the hemochromatosis and iron overload screening study (HEIRS). *Blood* 2002;**100**:447a.

43 Khoury M, McCabe L, McCabe E. Population screening in the era of genomic medicine. *N Eng J Med* 2003;**348**:50–8.

44 Adams PC. Factors affecting rate of iron mobilization during venesection therapy for hereditary hemochromatosis. *Am J Hematol* 1998;**58**:16–19.

45 Adams PC, Kertesz AE, Valberg LS. Rate of iron reaccumulation following iron depletion in hereditary hemochromatosis. Implications for venesection therapy. *J Clin Gastroenterol* 1993;**16**:207–10.

46 Bull PC, Thomas GR, Rommens JM, Forbes JR, Cox DW. The Wilson disease gene is a putative copper transporting P-type ATPase similar to the Menkes gene. *Nat Genet* 1993;**5**: 327–37.

47 Tanzi RE, Petrukhin K, Chernov I *et al.* The Wilson disease gene is a copper transporting ATPase with homology to the Menkes disease gene. *Nat Genet* 1993;**5**:344–50.

48 Hung I, Suzuki M, Yamaguchi Y, Yuan D, Klausner R, Gitlin J. Biochemical characterization of the Wilson disease protein and functional expression in the yeast *Saccharomyces cerevisiae. J Biol Chem* 1997;**272**: 21461–6.

49 Hazma I, Faisst A, Prohaska J, Chen J, Gruss P, Gitlin JD. The metallochaperone Atox1 plays a critical role in perinatal copper homeostasis. *Proc Natl Acad Sci USA* 2001;**98**: 6848–52.

50 Shah A, Chernov I, Zhang H *et al.* Identification and analysis of mutations in the Wilson disease gene (ATP7B): population frequencies, genotype-phenotype correlation, and functional analysis. *Am J Hum Genet* 1997;**61**:317–28.

51 Thomas G, Forbes J, Roberts E, Walshe J, Cox D. The Wilson disease gene: spectrum of mutations and their consequences. *Nat Genet* 1995;**9**:210–7.

52 Steindl P, Ferenci P, Dienes H *et al.* Wilson's disease in patients presenting with liver disease: a diagnostic challenge. *Gastroenterology* 1997;**113**:212–18.

53 Cauza E, Dobersberger T, Polli C, Kaserer K, Kramer L, Ferenci P. Screening for Wilson's disease in patients with liver disease by serum ceruloplasmin. *J Hepatol* 1997;**27**:358–62.

54 Walshe JM. Penicillamine, a new oral therapy for Wilson's disease. *Am J Med* 1956;**21**:487–95.

55 Hoogenrad T. Zinc treatment of Wilson's disease. *J Lab Clin Med* 1998;**132**:240–1.

56 Brewer G, Hedera P, Kluin K *et al.*Treatment of Wilson's disease with ammonium tetrathiomolybdate. II. Initial therapy in 33 neurologically affected patients and follow up with zinc therapy. *Arch Neurol* 1996;**53**:1017–25.

57 Sternlieb I. Wilson's disease and pregnancy. *Hepatology* 2000;**31**:531–32.

58 Brewer GJ, Johnson VD, Dick RD, Hedera P, Fink JK, Kluin KJ. Treatment of Wilson's disease with zinc. XVII: Treatment during pregnancy. *Hepatology* 2000;**31**:364–70.

59 Schilsky ML, Scheinberg I, Sternlieb I. Liver transplantation for Wilson's disease: indications and outcome. *Hepatology* 1994;**19**:583–7.

28 Primary biliary cirrhosis

Jenny Heathcote

Introduction

Primary biliary cirrhosis (PBC) is an inflammatory disease of the interlobular and septal bile ducts within the liver and is thought to be immune mediated.[1] Granulomatous destruction of these bile ducts leads to ductopenia and hence persistent cholestasis. Progressive fibrosis and eventually cirrhosis develop and liver failure is a terminal event unless intervention occurs with a liver transplant.

This disease predominantly affects middle aged women from all racial groups,[2] but there is considerable geographic variation in its prevalence.[3] It appears to be most common in women of European ancestry, but by no means is this disease confined to Caucasians.

Diagnosis

When PBC was first described, patients were noted to be jaundiced and to have tuberous xanthoma.[4] It was recognized as a primary disease of the liver in 1950.[5] Once routine biochemical screening at annual check-ups became common practice, patients were diagnosed with PBC in the absence of jaundice. In the 1960s, serological tests using immuno-fluorescence techniques indicated that non-organ and non-species-specific mitochondrial antibodies were very specific for patients with PBC.[6] At much the same time, the histological characteristics of this disease were first described and "staging" was introduced.[7,8] These studies indicated that the early bile duct destruction was often secondary to granulomatous infiltration of the ducts, not dissimilar to that seen in sarcoidosis. In fact, PBC and sarcoidosis have frequently been described as being present at the same time in the same patient.[9] In the 1970s, descriptions of the many autoimmune disorders frequently seen in association with patients with PBC were reported.[10,11]

In the late 1980s, it was recognized that the substrates for anti-mitochondrial antibodies (AMA) were the family of 2-oxo acid dehydrogenase enzymes located on the inner membrane of mitochondria.[12] The isolation of these substrates led to the development of more specific and sensitive testing for AMA using enzyme-linked immunosorbent assay (ELISA) or immunoblotting, which showed that the AMA test is positive in 95% of patients with PBC. It is extremely rare to find AMA in any other clinical situation apart from otherwise clear-cut autoimmune hepatitis, in which this is still very uncommon.[13] AMA are not associated with any other acute or chronic cholestatic condition.

It has now become recognized that sampling error of liver tissue using needle biopsies is common in PBC.[14] It is not unusual to see what are described as early stage I or II lesions in the same sample which, in another area, shows fibrosis and even cirrhosis. It has recently been suggested that in order to accurately diagnose ductopenia in a needle biopsy, 20 portal tracts need to be present for analysis.[15] It is rare for 20 portal tracts to be present in one needle biopsy!

Although asymptomatic individuals with PBC were reported by Sherlock in 1959[16] the natural history of such patients was more fully described by Long *et al.* in 1977.[17] Later it became evident that AMA positive subjects with normal liver biochemistry, undergoing serological tests because of the presence of another autoimmune disease, may also have the histological lesions of PBC on biopsy.[18] A 10-year follow up of these individuals has shown that the majority develop biochemical cholestasis and many have developed symptomatic disease.[19]

The many presentations of primary biliary cirrhosis

PBC may be diagnosed in several situations. The classic description of the patient with jaundice, xanthoma, pruritus, cholestatic liver tests, AMA positive serology, with a diagnostic or confirmatory liver biopsy may still present *de novo* on rare occasions. More commonly (60% of the time), PBC is diagnosed in an individual without symptoms but with abnormal biochemical tests characteristic of anicteric cholestasis, with a positive serological test for AMA, and with a diagnostic or confirmatory histological pattern on liver biopsy. It has become apparent that some patients may have the clinical, biochemical, and histological features of PBC and also have the same associated autoimmune diseases, but test negative for serum AMA[20–24] (even when highly sophisticated tests are employed to test for AMA[25]). These latter patients tend to test seropositive for antinuclear antibodies (ANA) or smooth muscle antibodies (SMA), often with high titers. The typical histological findings of PBC described in a retrospective study of histological tissue and chart review of 200 patients indicated that 12% had no positive serological tests.[26] Thus the diagnosis of PBC has become much more diverse. It is unclear whether the same disease process causes the classic histological lesions of PBC or whether there are multiple etiological factors which all cause the same histological response.

Natural history

As the diagnosis of PBC is made at earlier and earlier stages of the disease, so we learn more about its natural history. It now seems likely that there is a long preclinical course when AMA alone are present in the serum. However, the study that described such patients[19] included mostly patients who were well past middle age, i.e. more than 60 years old. The diagnosis of asymptomatic PBC tends to be made in patients who are 2–10 years older than patients with symptomatic disease.[2] This relationship suggests that asymptomatic disease is not necessarily a precursor of symptomatic disease, and could a be a *form fruste* of symptomatic disease. However, the natural history of the progression of the disease in older patients seems to be somewhat more rapid than that seen in younger patients.[27]

The initial 10-year follow up report of asymptomatic disease suggested that 50% of asymptomatic patients became symptomatic over this period of time.[17] More recent studies with longer follow ups indicate that although asymptomatic disease tends to progress at a much slower rate than symptomatic disease, survival of both symptomatic and asymptomatic patients with PBC is significantly less than that of the general population.[28,29] Mean survival for patients with symptomatic PBC is 8 years whereas that for asymptomatic disease is closer to 16 years.[30]

Information from the many randomized controlled trials (RCTs) of therapy in patients with PBC conducted over the past 20 years also indicates that the course of PBC is not the same for all patients. About one-third of asymptomatic patients develop symptomatic disease within 5 years. The other two-thirds may not develop symptomatic disease for much longer. A large study from Newcastle in the north of England has reported that 54% of patients with asymptomatic PBC do not die of their liver disease.[31] It is crucial that we identify markers to accurately predict which asymptomatic subjects will and will not develop progressive disease. Once a patient develops biochemical hyperbilirubinemia, the natural history of this disease is much more predictable.

Surrogate markers of outcome

Symptoms typical of PBC, such as fatigue, do not correlate with the severity of disease as judged by the height of the serum bilirubin or the Mayo risk score.[32] Similarly, pruritus, the next most common symptom in patients with PBC is not a marker of disease severity; in fact pruritus frequently lessens as decompensated disease develops, just as skin xanthomata diminish with disease progression. Unlike other chronic liver diseases, variceal hemorrhage is not necessarily a sign of advanced liver disease, as the portal hypertension may initially be due to presinusoidal causes,[33] that is nodular regenerative hyperplasia, cirrhosis being absent. In this situation, variceal hemorrhage, as long as liver ischemia is avoided, does not necessarily indicate a poor outcome. As PBC is primarily a disease of the biliary system, when signs of failure of hepatocyte function develops, such as uncorrectable coagulopathy, these indicate terminal disease. There are no symptoms present in patients with purely compensated disease which correlate with outcome. Some have suggested that the presence of associated autoimmune diseases is associated with a worse prognosis, but the data on which this suggestion was based have been refuted.[29,34]

The degree of hyperbilirubinemia has been shown to correlate extremely well with survival.[35] This was first shown prior to the introduction of liver transplantation for liver failure in PBC and the study indicated that the height of the bilirubin was a valid marker of final outcome, i.e. death. Standard liver biochemical tests, namely serum levels of alkaline phosphatase and the aminotransferases, have never been shown to correlate with prognosis in patients with PBC. More sophisticated risk scores designed to predict prognosis in patients with PBC have been developed by several different authors.[36–38] It is noteworthy that serum bilirubin features in each of the scores described. The most widely used composite score, the Mayo risk score,[36] is popular because it does not require any invasive procedures, i.e. liver biopsy, so is very convenient for everyday use. The components of the Mayo risk score, age, serum albumin, coagulation time, and the presence of fluid retention and/or use of diuretics, seem to be sufficient to accurately predict outcome in PBC. However, an earlier study (on a relatively small number of patients) did indicate that patients who have liver fibrosis or cirrhosis on biopsy had a worse survival than those without fibrosis or cirrhosis.[39] On its own, presence or absence of cirrhosis is not a highly predictive surrogate marker for final outcome, i.e. death, presumably because there are other features which factor into progression of disease. A recent detailed review of liver histology in PBC suggests that the presence of a lymphoplasmacytic interface hepatitis is a marker of more rapidly progressive disease[40] and in another report of four cases, rapidly progressive bile duct loss, even in the absence of cirrhosis led to liver failure.[41]

The recent introduction of ursodeoxycholic acid (UDCA) therapy, which markedly reduces the serum bilirubin concentration, has been shown not to invalidate either the serum bilirubin or the Mayo risk score as a prognostic marker, at least within the first 6 months of therapy.[42] However, it is still unknown whether the serum bilirubin in patients treated with UDCA remains a valid marker of survival in those with endstage disease. The Mayo risk score was first developed and validated for patients who were not treated with a liver transplant for endstage disease. Since liver transplantation has become the alternative endpoint, the Mayo risk score has been re-evaluated along with other factors thought to predict post-transplant survival.[43]

Only in the context of clinical trials when large numbers of liver biopsy specimens are available can the effect of sampling error be minimized, although it is likely that sampling error will only truly be reduced to an insignificant degree if many hundreds of paired biopsy samples are evaluated. Whereas in the past a composite score for inflammation and fibrosis was developed to stage PBC,[8] it may be more appropriate for the degree of inflammation to be graded separately from the degree of fibrosis, very much like the score that has been developed for the assessment of chronic viral hepatitis. As previously mentioned, the degree of ductopenia can only be adequately assessed in liver tissue specimens with a sufficient number of portal tracts present. Similarly, the degree and pattern of inflammation and fibrosis can only be adequately assessed when the tissue specimens are more than a minimum size – generally considered to be > 1 cm in length.

There is no evidence that the AMA titer in any way correlates with the course of PBC.[44] The only biochemical marker with prognostic value is the serum bilirubin concentration. Other factors important in determining outcome have not as yet been validated. These include lymphoplasmacytic interface hepatitis,[40] vascular supply to the liver,[45] and the presence of various inflammatory mediators and markers of tissue fibrosis.[46]

It has now become very difficult to use death as an endpoint, since most patients with decompensated PBC, if they have no contraindication, are referred for liver transplantation. The identification of valid surrogate markers of outcome is extremely important in evaluating specific therapies in PBC, particularly as the mean survival time of this disease, in both symptomatic and asymptomatic patients, is long (8 and 12 years, respectively). As more and more asymptomatic patients, (whose survival may be influenced by factors external to the liver) are included in drug trials, these trials will need to be very large in size and of long duration to effectively evaluate the effect of therapy on survival. Hence the urgent need to establish which asymptomatic patients are at risk of dying from liver failure. Large trials are unwieldy, expensive and intolerable for patients.

Timing for liver transplantation

As liver transplantation has become available for patients with PBC in liver failure, the need for this procedure has been used as a final measure of outcome in many therapeutic trials. However, the validity of this outcome can be questioned, since liver transplantation is sometimes done for intolerable symptoms such as uncontrollable pruritus or severe osteoporosis rather than for liver failure. Even in patients who undergo liver transplantation for decompensated liver disease, timing of the transplantion will vary considerably between patients simply because of their blood type. Variations will also depend on external forces such as availability of donated organs, limitations of health insurance, distance from a major healthcare center, and more recently, whether or not there is a living donor. Hence, there are many reasons why time to liver transplantation is a rather variable endpoint and not necessarily as valid as may appear on the surface.

Therapeutic trial design: assessment of credibility

RCTs of therapy in PBC have been published for the past 25 years. During this time, many refinements have been made in trial design to enhance accuracy. For example, the first trial was not double blind[47] and thus several biases which might have been minimized by blinding were present. In addition, the sample size needed to ensure that the study has adequate power was not calculated, and no "stopping rules" were described.

The more asymptomatic patients recruited the less likely any of the usual "endpoints" in the control group will be observed over the 3–5-year funding period for most trials. Thus the probability of observing an effect of therapy on endpoints such as death or need for liver transplant is low. The sample size required in the trials of mainly asymptomatic patients with early disease is so large that trials would became impossible to conduct and too expensive to fund. The compromise has been to conduct meta-analyses of data from several published series. This generally requires many assumptions to be made and it is probably preferable to combine all the raw data for analysis when these are available.

To determine the appropriate sample size for a clinical trial requires not only a large sample of historical data to establish the natural history of the disease in a particular population (event rate in the control group) but also pilot study data, from which an estimate of the expected therapeutic benefit can be made. These two conditions have rarely been met in the many trials of therapy reported in PBC.

It is important that a valid primary measure of outcome be established prior to starting a study. This outcome measure needs to be reliable and easy to quantify and should ideally have been validated in both the historical sample and pilot study used to calculate the sample size. The primary measure of outcome in PBC cannot feasibly be death or even need for liver transplantation, in view of the sample size that would be necessary (> 700 patients).[48] Hence, surrogate markers for outcome are often employed. Unfortunately, some trials have employed surrogate endpoints which have not been shown to correlate with outcome, for example serum alkaline phosphatase concentration. Others have failed to address the issue of sampling error with liver histology.[14] Recently, "composite failure to respond to treatment" scores have been introduced, but these have not been validated as measures of outcome.

The intention to treat principle is vital when carrying out statistical analysis of outcome to avoid as much bias as possible when interpreting the data. This means that all patients who are randomized need to be included in the final analysis, even though they may have been censored at a very early point in the trial because of untimely death, need to withdraw from the study, non-compliance, etc. Using the intention to treat principle allows for only a very conservative analysis of the effectiveness of therapy, but it permits assessment of the "real life" situations, i.e. the generalizability of the study.

Just as the sample size needs to be adequate to demonstrate an effect of therapy, it also should be adequate to assess the frequency of adverse events. Whereas this may be obvious with a drug that has a profound systemic effect, that is chlorambucil,[49] it may be less obvious with drugs which have fewer adverse effects. As patients with PBC, particularly if they have asymptomatic disease at trial entry, have a quite long natural survival without any therapeutic intervention, it is obviously vital to establish whether adverse effects cause greater morbidity and mortality than if the disease were left untreated! In addition, the effect of any therapy on enhancing the rate of progress of various conditions complicating PBC, such as the effect of prednisolone on osteoporosis, may need to be monitored.[50]

In determining the thoroughness and hence accuracy of any trial report, as much can be learned from what is not written in the methods section as can be gained from the results. The discussion is generally the opinion of the author. For an independent analysis of the validity of the data, a combination of excellent clinical judgment and understanding of the rationale for the intervention, as well as the basic concepts of trial design, need to be considered. Only then can a decision be made whether or not the benefit of an evaluated intervention is generalizable to a specific individual with PBC.

Randomized controlled trials of treatment for primary biliary cirrhosis

Immunosuppressives

Once it was recognized that PBC was an autoimmune disease, the logical approach to therapy was to employ an immunosuppressive. Because the majority of patients with PBC are women and osteoporosis complicates PBC (mostly in those with advanced liver disease)[50] regardless of menopausal status,[51] corticosteroid therapy has for the most part been avoided. RCTs of immunosuppressive therapy in PBC have employed azathioprine, cyclosporin, methotrexate, prednisolone, chlorambucil, thalidomide and more recently, budesonide.[52-62] Neither of the two trials of azathioprine showed a beneficial effect of this drug on survival. The first trial had an inadequate sample size,[47] lacked a placebo control group and predetermined stopping rules, and the results were not analyzed according to intention to treat. The second trial of azathioprine[53] although much larger (248 patients), did not include a sample size calculation to assure that it had adequate power, and the withdrawal rate was greater than 20% in both the azathioprine and placebo groups. Despite randomization, the two groups were not stratified for factors known to influence survival and were not comparable at baseline. Only after employment of the Cox multiple regression analysis to adjust for these baseline differences was a benefit of treatment on survival observed. This difference in survival between the treatment groups could only be measured in months, which may not be clinically important. Patients were followed for up to 10 years, but the number of patients still being followed at that period was only nine in the azathioprine and none in the placebo group. It appears that the intention to treat principle was not used in the analysis, since 32 patients were excluded from the analysis because of incomplete data. Thus the validity of the small benefit in survival can be further questioned. Ald

Several small trials[54-55] and one large trial (349 patients) of cyclosporin therapy have been published.[56] This trial ran into the same problems as had been encountered with the large azathioprine trial, i.e. lack of comparability of the two treatment groups at baseline. Even though there was a similar number of deaths, 30 in the cyclosporin group and 31 in the placebo group, the authors concluded that survival was improved in the cyclosporin-treated patients. Renal impairment was observed in 9% and systemic hypertension in 11% of the cyclosporin-treated patients (1·7% and 1% in placebo-treated, respectively). These two serious adverse effects in patients whose disease is relatively slowly progressive precludes the use of this drug in the long-term treatment of PBC.

Methotrexate has been claimed to be of value in pilot studies,[57] but only one RCT of therapy has been published.[58]

Sixty patients were recruited, 30 randomized to low dose therapy (2·5 mg three times per week). At the end of 6 years, the serum bilirubin and Mayo risk score were higher in those receiving methotrexate, suggesting that the drug may be toxic in patients with PBC. Ald A large multicenter trial in the USA comparing UDCA alone with the same intervention combined with methotrexate has just been completed and the results reported only in abstract form indicate no benefit of methotrexate.[63] Ald

A small, 3-year RCT of prednisolone has been done.[52] A significant reduction in the serum bilirubin level (a valid surrogate outcome measure) was observed in treated patients, but osteoporosis in those who received corticosteroids worsened. Ald However, a trial with a very small sample size of bisphosphonates in patients with PBC treated with corticosteroids indicates that etidronate significantly stabilizes bone mineral density in vertebrae of patients with PBC receiving corticosteroids.[60] Hence, it may be appropriate that corticosteroids be re-evaluated in the therapy of PBC now that patients can be given preventive therapies to reduce the complication of osteoporosis.

Budesonide is an oral corticosteroid which is eliminated on first pass through the liver. Thus it was hoped that this agent could benefit patients with PBC without having a deleterious effect on bone mineral density. In the first small RCT by Leuschner *et al.*,[61] improvement in liver biochemistry, IgM values and liver histology was observed in the few patients studied, most of whom had very early disease. In a second study by Angulo *et al.*,[62] no benefit was observed and the Mayo risk score increased significantly in those randomized to budesonide for a year and bone mineral density measurements deteriorated in the lumbar spine ($P < 0.01$) – it is likely that many of these patients had advanced PBC so that the benefit of the first pass effect was lost. Ala Wolfhagen *et al.* in another small RCT involving 50 patients with PBC with suboptimal response to UDCA, treated patients with additional prednisone (30 mg/day tapered to 10 mg/day) and azathioprine (50 mg/day). There was no improvement in bilirubin. The trial was too small and of too short a duration to examine the effect on survival.[64] Ald

A small study of 13 patients randomized to 0·5–4 mg daily of chlorambucil (mean 2 mg daily) compared with placebo has been reported.[49] All treated patients developed some degree of bone marrow suppression and discontinuation of therapy was required in four. A 30% withdrawal rate due to drug toxicity indicates that this drug should not undergo further evaluation in patients with PBC. Ald

A very small and short (6-month) RCT of 18 PBC patients taking thalidomide has been reported, showing little benefit of this treatment. However, this study lacked adequate power to evaluate this form of therapy in any meaningful way. No benefit on serum bilirubin was observed during the 6 months of treatment.[59] Ald

An alternative approach has been to use drugs that may not interfere with the primary cause, i.e. immune-mediated bile duct destruction, but interfere with the progression of the disease, either by reducing fibrogenesis or by reducing cholestasis.

Two antifibrotic drugs have been assessed: colchicine in three small RCTs and D-penicillamine in many more. The studies of colchicine therapy are interesting, but unfortunately, all three trials recruited fewer than 100 patients each.[65–67] They all used approximately the same dose of colchicine and a meta-analysis of these three studies may prove to be worthwhile in the future. The first study introduced the concept of a multiple criteria "treatment failure" composite index as a measure of outcome. There was no evidence of the validation of this composite index, but similar treatment failure composite indices have been employed in several other clinical trials in PBC. Frequently these indices have included factors not known to be relevant to PBC survival. The observation in two of the colchicine studies – that colchicine had a beneficial effect on liver function, i.e. serum albumin and bilirubin – was encouraging. None of these three studies suggested a benefit on symptoms or histology. One study suggested that there was a survival advantage to receiving colchicine, even though only 64 patients were recruited and 10 patients withdrew, 8 of whom were randomized to colchicine. The third study also had a high dropout rate (32%) among those randomized to colchicine. A long term, i.e. 8-year follow up of this latter study indicated that there was no survival advantage in treated patients, although the original sample size was small.[68] Ald

While there are eight RCTs of D-penicillamine, the results are disappointing.[48] Unlike patients with Wilson disease, adverse effects of therapy were common, resulting in a high withdrawal rate, similar to the experience with rheumatoid arthritis. This drug is no longer recommended for the treatment of PBC. Ald

Reduction of cholestasis

Hydrophilic bile acids

Leuschner, in the early 1980s, reported that administration of UDCA in patients with gallstones, who coincidentally also had chronic hepatitis, led to an improvement of liver biochemistry.[69] A 2-year pilot study in 15 patients with PBC conducted by Poupon *et al.*[70] indicated that treatment with UDCA in a dose of 13–15 mg/kg daily reduced serum bilirubin concentration in patients who had elevated levels prior to the start of therapy. B4 Many RCTs of UDCA therapy have been conducted subsequently. The mechanisms of action of UDCA are slowly being identified. The original premise that the introduction of the less toxic hydrophilic dihydroxy bile acid UDCA would reduce the exposure of hepatocyte membranes to the toxic effects of the retained hydrophobic endogenous bile acids has now been proved to be the case.[71] In addition, UDCA inhibits the uptake of endogenous bile acids at the terminal ileum,[72] although most is absorbed passively throughout the small bowel in its unconjugated state. The marked benefit on serum bilirubin levels may be due in part to upregulation of the canalicular transporter Mrp2[73] by UDCA. *In vitro* studies of hepatocytes in culture indicate that the apoptotic effect of hydrophobic bile acids can be abrogated by the addition of UDCA (in physiological doses) to the culture medium[74] – whether UDCA has a similar effect on biliary epithelial cells is unknown.

There have now been two meta-analyses of up to 16 studies of UDCA in PBC.[75,76] The more recent was published in the *Cochrane Library* in 2003.[76] Both Goulis *et al.*[75] and Gluud and Christensen[76] did a detailed analysis of these rather heterogeneous studies in which treatment periods ranged from as little as 6 months up to 4 years, the daily dose of UDCA ranged from 7·7 mg/kg to 15 mg/kg, and there was a wide range of disease severity. In addition, the Jadad scores for methodological quality were only ≥ 4 in five of the 16 trials. Sensitivity analyses for dose, length of study, and quality did not show differences in the first meta-analysis.[75] The authors of the more recent review[76] also attempted to take these variations into consideration and concluded that whereas at 2 years there was no survival advantage, in those studies where patients had received up to 4 years of UDCA the need for liver transplantation was marginally but statistically significantly reduced ($P < 0·04$) (Figure 28.1). The absolute risk reduction (ARR) was 3% (NNT, the number of patients needed to be treated with UDCA for 4 years to avoid or delay one transplant was 33). Survival without transplant was not significantly influenced by UDCA therapy. Ala Since not all placebo or non-intervention patients were eventually given UDCA, the evaluation of the non-randomized phases of these trials has intrinsic biases and lacks the appropriate basis for an intention to treat analysis. Why patients who were given UDCA 2 years after randomization worsened progressively compared with those given UDCA from the start of the study is unclear.[77] Some benefit might have been expected. It could be argued that the only reason liver transplantation was delayed in those receiving UDCA was because patients had lower serum bilirubin levels that those on placebo – serum bilirubin has been shown to be a valid prognostic marker in PBC – both on its own and when incorporated into the many risk scores. However, serum bilirubin levels remain valid prognostic markers in patients on UDCA.[42] Simply delaying liver transplantation by treating with UDCA could potentially lead to a worse outcome once transplantation becomes necessary as patients are likely to be older; however, the outcome following liver transplantation was found to be no different despite the older age of the UDCA-treated patients.[78] B4

In all studies, the administration of UDCA was associated with an improvement of liver biochemistry. The more recent meta-analysis[76] also indicated that overt ascites and obvious jaundice were less frequent in patients randomized to UDCA (ARR 5%, NNT 20, $P < 0·02$ and ARR 10%, NNT 10, $P < 0·001$, respectively, Figure 28.2), but there was no difference in the number of patients with bleeding varices or hepatic encephalopathy. Ala These data suggest that prolonged treatment with UDCA may be required to exert a beneficial effect on the natural history of PBC. Although clinical benefit appears to be modest, systematic review has not shown an association of this therapy with adverse events.[76]

One report suggests that in those individuals with endstage disease, treatment with UDCA may cause a sudden rise in bilirubin and hence it is advised that when UDCA is prescribed to patients with decompensated PBC, they should be followed very closely.[79]

Three of the four larger double blind randomized trials[80–82] used the same dose of UDCA (13–15 mg/kg per day), and the results were analyzed according to the intention to treat principle. In two of these a composite "treatment failure" outcome measure was used, and in the third the percentage change in total serum bilirubin over 2 years was used as the primary outcome measure. Detailed sample size calculations and clear-cut predetermined definition of study duration were only described for this latter study. Few adverse effects of UDCA were reported and the withdrawal rate was less than 20% in all three studies. A combined analysis of the raw data from these three studies, continued beyond the initial 2 years, has been published.[83] In two of the three trials, some patients initially randomized to placebo were switched to open label UDCA after the first 24 months. However, the results were analyzed according to intention to treat, so that those patients initially randomized to receive placebo and subsequently switched to receive UDCA remained in the placebo group for the purposes of analysis. Intuitively, it seems likely that this procedure would reduce the probability of demonstrating benefit with UDCA in the analysis of the longer-term data, should a true benefit exist. Despite this consideration, the combined analysis of survival data from the three trials suggested that UDCA therapy for up to 4 years led to an increase in time free of liver transplantation in treated patients. Alc

Subgroup analyses did not show any benefit in patients who, at baseline, had a total serum bilirubin of less than 1·4 mg/dl and/or stage I/II liver histology. These subgroup analyses do not prove that UDCA is ineffective in patients with asymptomatic and/or early disease, but they do suggest that clinical trials in such patients would require very large numbers of patients and would be required to be of such long duration to show any benefit of the treatment that they would not be feasible.

The fourth large trial (151 patients) employed a smaller dose (10–12 mg/kg bodyweight daily) and a different

Review: Ursodeoxy cholic acid for primary biliary cirrhosis
Comparison: 04 UDCA-UDCA versus placebo/no intervention-UDCA
Outcome: 02 Liver transplantation

Study	UDCA n/N	Control n/N	Risk difference (Fixed) 95% CI	Weight %	Risk difference (Fixed) 95% CI
01 Jadad score = 4 or 5					
BARCELONA	7/99	7/93		13·8	0·00 (−0·08 to 0·07)
FRANKFURT	0/10	0/10		1·4	0·00 (−0·17 to 0·17)
GÖTEBORG	2/60	3/56		8·3	−0·02 (−0·09 to 0·05)
HELSINKI	0/30	3/31		4·4	−0·10 (−0·21 to 0·02)
MAYO-I	7/89	7/91		12·9	0·00 (−0·08 to 0·08)
MILAN	0/44	0/44		6·3	0·00 (−0·04 to 0·04)
TORONTO	15/111	22/111		16·0	−0·06 (−0·16 to 0·03)
Subtotal (95% CI)	31/443	42/436		63·2	−0·03 (−0·06 to 0·01)

Test for heterogeneity $\chi^2 = 4·26$ df = 6 $P = 0·6419$
Test for overall effect = 1·40 $P = 0·1602$

02 Jadad score = 1, 2 or 3					
ATHENS	4/43	3/43		6·2	0·02 (−0·09 to 0·14)
DALLAS	16/77	20/74		10·9	−0·06 (−0·20 to 0·07)
NEWARK-II	0/9	0/10		1·4	0·00 (−0·18 to 0·18)
NEWCASTLE	2/22	1/24		3·3	0·05 (−0·10 to 0·19)
TAIPEI	0/6	0/6		0·9	0·00 (−0·27 to 0·27)
TOKYO	0/26	0/26		3·7	0·00 (−0·07 to 0·07)
VILLEJUIF	4/73	12/73		10·5	−0·11 (−0·21 to −0·01)
Subtotal (95% CI)	26/256	36/256		36·8	−0·04 (−0·10 to 0·01)

Test for heterogeneity chi−square = 6·16 df = 6 $P = 0·405$
Test for overall effect = −1·45 $P = 0·15$

Total (95% CI)	57/699	78/692		100·0	−0·03 (−0·06 to 0·00)

Test for heterogeneity $\chi^2 = 10·60$ df = 13 $P = 0·6441$
Test for overall effect = −2·01 $P = 0·04$

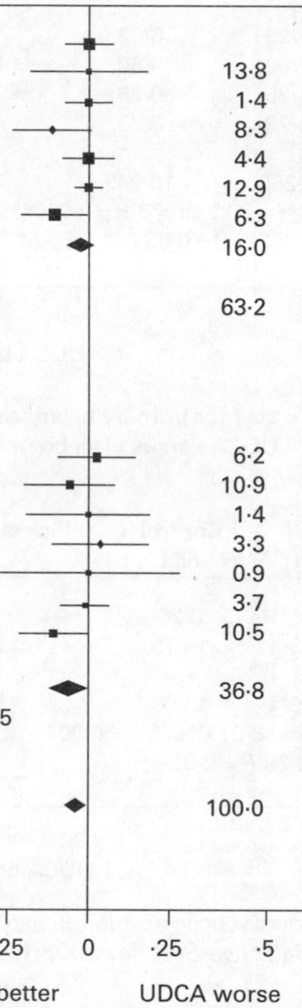

```
        −·5    −·25     0     ·25    ·5
            UDCA better      UDCA worse
```

Figure 28.1 Meta-analysis of ursodeoxycholic acid for primary biliary cirrhosis: outcome liver transplantation (Source: Gluud C, Christensen E. *Cochrane Database Syst Rev* 2003;**1**:CD000551[76])

preparation of UDCA. After 2 years of treatment no difference in survival was seen, there being eight deaths in those randomized to UDCA and 12 in those randomized to placebo.[82] Alc

It should be pointed out that the pooled analysis of the three trials is not a systematic review or meta-analysis, but rather was done by pooling of results from three trials which were of similar design but which had rather dissimilar results. This procedure differs from a systematic review or formal meta-analysis, which attempts to minimize bias by the consideration and inclusion of all relevant trials, justifies the exclusion of trials from the analysis, and explores heterogeneity between trials and the reasons for variation in results. A formal meta-analysis which demonstrates benefit from an intervention may also include a sensitivity analysis to indicate the number of unpublished or excluded trials of specified size

with negative results which would be required to negate the results of the meta-analysis. Meta-analyses may suffer from the opposite weakness cited for the combined analysis of similar trials, that is, they may involve pooled analysis of trials which differ sufficiently in their design that they are not truly comparable. Accordingly, caution should be exercised in interpreting both the combined analysis of selected trials[83] on one hand as proof of a beneficial effect of UDCA on mortality in PBC, and the most recent meta-analysis on the other, as evidence that no such effect *on mortality* exists.[76]

Osteoporosis

No effect of UDCA on bone mineral density was demonstrated in the RCT of UDCA in PBC published by

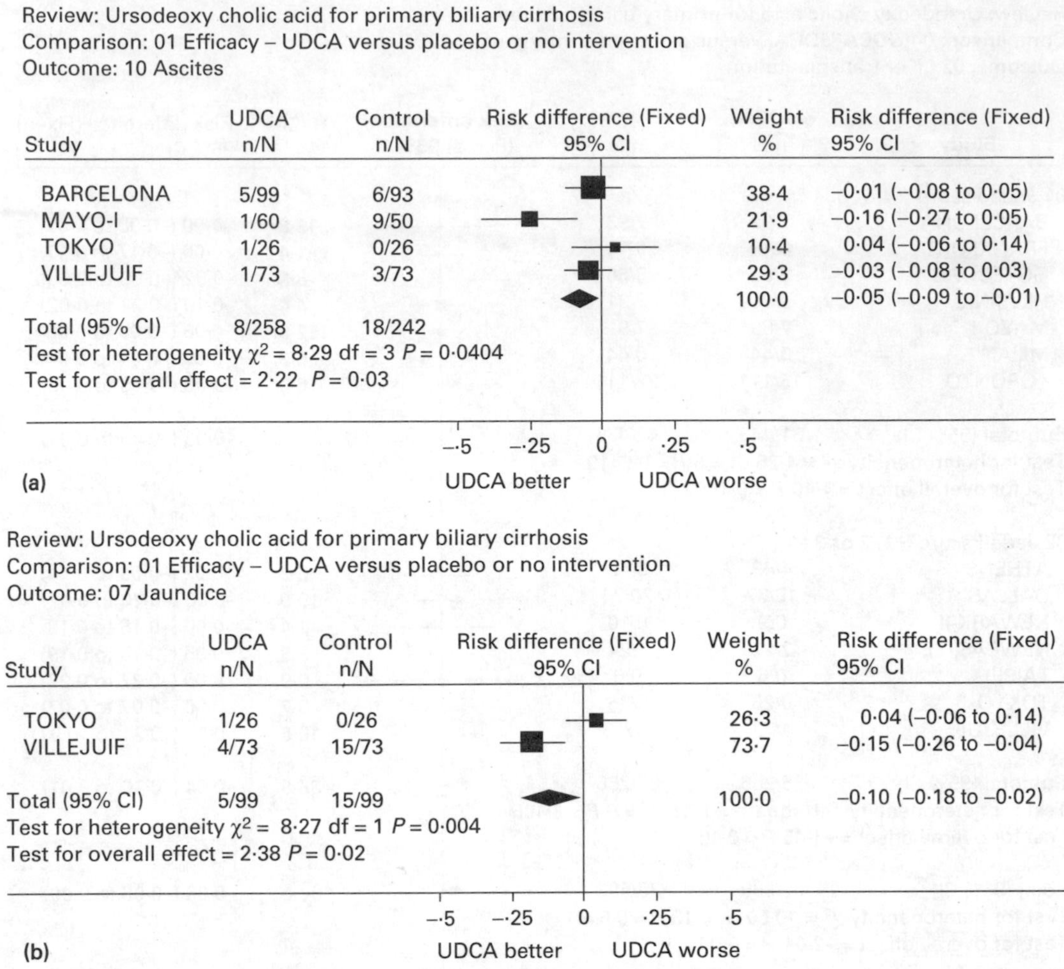

Review: Ursodeoxy cholic acid for primary biliary cirrhosis
Comparison: 01 Efficacy – UDCA versus placebo or no intervention
Outcome: 10 Ascites

Study	UDCA n/N	Control n/N	Risk difference (Fixed) 95% CI	Weight %	Risk difference (Fixed) 95% CI
BARCELONA	5/99	6/93		38·4	−0·01 (−0·08 to 0·05)
MAYO-I	1/60	9/50		21·9	−0·16 (−0·27 to 0·05)
TOKYO	1/26	0/26		10·4	0·04 (−0·06 to 0·14)
VILLEJUIF	1/73	3/73		29·3	−0·03 (−0·08 to 0·03)
				100·0	−0·05 (−0·09 to −0·01)

Total (95% CI) 8/258 18/242
Test for heterogeneity $\chi^2 = 8\cdot29$ df = 3 $P = 0\cdot0404$
Test for overall effect = 2·22 $P = 0\cdot03$

$$-\cdot5 \quad -\cdot25 \quad 0 \quad \cdot25 \quad \cdot5$$
UDCA better   UDCA worse

(a)

Review: Ursodeoxy cholic acid for primary biliary cirrhosis
Comparison: 01 Efficacy – UDCA versus placebo or no intervention
Outcome: 07 Jaundice

Study	UDCA n/N	Control n/N	Risk difference (Fixed) 95% CI	Weight %	Risk difference (Fixed) 95% CI
TOKYO	1/26	0/26		26·3	0·04 (−0·06 to 0·14)
VILLEJUIF	4/73	15/73		73·7	−0·15 (−0·26 to −0·04)

Total (95% CI) 5/99 15/99   100·0   −0·10 (−0·18 to −0·02)
Test for heterogeneity $\chi^2 = 8\cdot27$ df = 1 $P = 0\cdot004$
Test for overall effect = 2·38 $P = 0\cdot02$

$$-\cdot5 \quad -\cdot25 \quad 0 \quad \cdot25 \quad \cdot5$$
UDCA better   UDCA worse

(b)

Figure 28.2 Meta-analysis of ursodeoxycholic acid for primary biliary cirrhosis: outcome (a) acites and (b) jaundice (Source: Gluud C, Christensen E. *Cochrane Database Syst Rev* 2003;**1**:CD000551[76])

Lindor *et al*,[84] although the study may have lacked power. Ald A small study assessing bone mineral density and vertebral fractures in PBC patients randomized to cyclosporin A or placebo suggested that cyclosporin-treated patients have less bone loss and better biochemical parameters of bone remodelling.[85] Ald

Fatigue and pruritus

Although there are now some very sophisticated methods to measure these symptoms, none of the RCTs of therapy for PBC employed such instruments to monitor the effect of therapy. There are many anecdotal case reports of marked improvement and marked worsening of both fatigue and pruritus in patients receiving UDCA. Pilot studies of methotrexate have reported dramatic improvement in both fatigue and pruritus, but these uncontrolled studies provide only weak evidence for benefit. B4

Histology

Assessment of the effect of UDCA in liver histology after 2 years of therapy have been conflicting[80–82] and thus inconclusive. However in the study by Pares *et al*.[77] the apparent benefit of 5 years of UDCA therapy on liver histology in terms of stage of disease, progression of bile duct destruction and interface hepatitis was significantly greater than that observed in those randomized to placebo. Ald The majority of patients included in this trial had early asymptomatic disease. Assessment of liver histology from the French multicenter study using the Markov model indicated that regression of cirrhosis was never seen but that the progression to cirrhosis was markedly delayed in those who received UDCA.[86] It must be emphasized that follow up liver histology was not available in all randomized patients, some refused to have a second biopsy, and more importantly, no second biopsy was obtained from those patients who died or required a liver transplant, i.e. those whose liver disease clearly had progressed. Only 44% of patients had second biopsies available for evaluation. This factor introduces the potential for significant bias into observations concerning effect of both UDCA and placebo on histology.

These histological data suggest that if UDCA exerts a long-term benefit in PBC it may be more likely to do so in individuals with early asymptomatic disease. However, recent data indicate that less than 50% of individuals with asymptomatic PBC die of their liver disease.[31] For therapy to be cost effective, it is important to be able to identify which asymptomatic patients are most likely to develop progressive disease. Corpechot *et al.*[40] have suggested that surrogate markers for disease progression include lymphoplasmacytic interface hepatitis (as well as serum bilirubin and albumin values). So, whereas a liver biopsy may not be necessary for diagnostic purposes, it may be necessary to assess the likelihood of disease progression in patients with asymptomatic disease. Other prognostic markers in patients with early disease (i.e. where the Mayo risk score is not applicable) may be genetic markers not currently available for widespread use, for example human leukocyte anti-gen (HLA).[87]

Assessment of adverse effects in therapeutic trials of primary biliary cirrhosis

No clear-cut hepatotoxic effect of any of the drugs described above has been described, although other toxic effects, for example bone marrow suppression with chlorambucil or pulmonary toxicity with methotrexate have been well described. Other drug-related adverse events include the effect of cyclosporin on renal function and systemic blood pressure and a neuropathy thought to be induced by colchicine seen in the two RCTs of this agent. Certainly the safest and apparently most effective drug to date remains UDCA.

The future for primary biliary cirrhosis

Treatment with UDCA is not curative. It may delay the progression of disease in some patients, but the evidence for this benefit is not clear-cut. Several small trials of UDCA in combination with methotrexate,[88–90] colchicine,[91–94] and prednisolone[95,96] have been conducted, but no study has been large enough to adequately assess effectiveness. There have been small pilot studies employing different classes of drug, for example silymarin and bezafibrate.[97,98] As UDCA is the current standard of care[98] it is very hard for any new agent to show a benefit using a valid surrogate marker, for example serum bilirubin, as UDCA has such a profound effect on bilirubin level. However, these studies are necessary if only to examine possible agents for larger RCT. One such agent currently being assessed is the immunosuppressive mycophenolate motefil.[100] It will take many years before we know the answer. Meanwhile, liver transplantation remains

the last resort when other treatments have failed. Clearly, no RCT of liver transplantation is feasible. However, when the assessment of survival following transplantation is compared with the predicted survival using the Mayo risk score at the time transplantation is done the evidence is that liver transplantation leads to a marked survival benefit in patients with PBC and currently it remains the only curative therapy for this disease.[101,102] B4

References

1 Gershwin ME, Mackay IR. Primary biliary cirrhosis: paradigm or paradox for autoimmunity. *Gastroenterology* 1990;**99**: 822–33.

2 Witt-Sullivan H, Heathcote J, Cauch K *et al.* The demography of primary biliary cirrhosis in Ontario, Canada. *Hepatology* 1990;**12**:98–105.

3 Watson RG, Angus PW, Dewar M *et al.* and the Melbourne Liver Group. Low prevalence of primary biliary cirrhosis in Victoria, Australia. *Gut* 1995;**36**:927–30.

4 Addison T, Gull W. On a certain affection of the skin, vitiligo idea – plana, tuberosa. *Guy's Hosp Rep* 1851;**7**:265–76.

5 Ahrens EH, Rayne MA, Kunkle HG *et al.* Primary biliary cirrhosis. *Medicine* 1950;**29**:299–364.

6 Doniach D, Roitt IM, Walker JG *et al.* Tissue antibodies in primary biliary cirrhosis, active chronic (lupoid) hepatitis, cryptogenic cirrhosis and other liver diseases and their clinical implications. *Clin Exp Immunol* 1966;**1**:237–62.

7 Scheuer PJ. Primary biliary cirrhosis. *Proc R Soc Med* 1967; **60**:1257–60.

8 Ludwig J, Dickson ER, Mcdonald GSA. Staging of chronic nonsuppurative destructive cholangitis (syndrome of primary biliary cirrhosis). *Virchows Arch (A)* 1978;**379**:103–12.

9 Keeffe EB. Sarcoidosis and primary biliary cirrhosis. Literature review and illustrative case. *Am J Med* 1987;**83**: 977–80.

10 Golding PL, Smith M, Williams R. Multisystem involvement in chronic liver disease. *Am J Med* 1973;**55**:772–82.

11 Culp KS, Fleming CR, Duffy J *et al.* Autoimmune associations in primary biliary cirrhosis. *Mayo Clin Proc* 1982;**57**:365–70.

12 Fussey S, Guest JR, James O *et al.* Identification and analysis of the major M2 autoantigens in primary biliary cirrhosis. *Proc Natl Acad Sci USA* 1988;**85**:8654–8.

13 Czaja AJ, Carpenter HA, Manns MP. Antibodies to soluble liver antigen, P455011D6, and mitochondrial complexes in chronic hepatitis. *Gastroenterology* 1993;**105**:1522–8.

14 Garrido MC, Hubscher SG. Accuracy of staging in primary biliary cirrhosis. *J Clin Pathol* 1996;**49**:556–9.

15 Tadrou PJ, Goldin RD. How many portal tracts are necessary to make a diagnosis of significant bile duct loss (SBDL)? *J Pathol* 1997;**181**:11A.

16 Sherlock, S. Primary biliary cirrhosis (chronic intrahepatic obstructive jaundice). *Gastroenterology* 1959;**37**:574–86.

17 Long RG, Scheuer PJ, Sherlock S. Presentation and course of asymptomatic primary biliary cirrhosis. *Gastroenterology* 1977;**72**:1204–7.

18 Mitchison HC, Bassendine MF, Hendrick A *et al.* Positive anti-mitochondrial antibody but normal alkaline phosphatase: is this primary biliary cirrhosis? *Hepatology* 1986;**6**:1279–84.

19 Metcalf JV, Mitchison HC, Palmer JM *et al.* Natural history of early primary biliary cirrhosis. *Lancet* 1996;**348**:1399–402.

20 Brunner G, Klinge O. Ein der chronisch-destruierenden nicht-eitrigen Cholangitis ähnliches Krankheitsbild mit anti-nukleären Antikörpern (Immunocholangitis). *Dtsch Med Wochenschr* 1987;**112**:1454–8.

21 Ben-Ari Z, Dhillon AP, Sherlock S. Autoimmune cholangiopathy: part of the spectrum of autoimmune chronic active hepatitis. *Hepatology* 1993;**18**:10–15.

22 Michieletti P, Wanless IR, Katz A *et al.* Antimitochondrial antibody negative primary biliary cirrhosis: a distinct syndrome of autoimmune cholangitis. *Gut* 1994;**35**:260–5.

23 Taylor SL, Dean PJ, Riely CA. Primary autoimmune cholangitis. An alternative to antimitochondrial antibody-negative primary biliary cirrhosis. *Am J Surg Pathol* 1994;**18**:91–9.

24 Lacerda MA, Ludwig J, Dickson ER *et al.* Antimitochondrial antibody-negative primary biliary cirrhosis. *Am J Gastroenterol* 1995;**90**:247–9.

25 Miyakawa H, Tanaka A, Kikuchi K, Matsushita M, Kitazawa E, Kawaguchi N *et al.* Detection of anti-mitochondrial autoantibodies in immunofluorescent AMA-negative patients with primary biliary cirrhosis using recombinant autoantigens. *Hepatology* 2001;**34**:243–8.

26 Goodman ZD, McNally PR, Davis DR *et al.* Autoimmune cholangitis: a variant of primary biliary cirrhosis. Clinicopathologic and serologic correlations in 200 cases. *Dig Dis Sci* 1995;**40**:1232–42.

27• Newton JL, Jones DE, Metcalf JV *et al.* Presentation and mortality of primary biliary cirrhosis in older patients. *Age Aging* 2000;**29**:305–9.

28 Balasubramaniam K, Grambsch PM, Wiesner RH *et al.* Diminished survival in asymptomatic primary biliary cirrhosis: a prospective study. *Gastroenterology* 1990;**98**:1567–71.

29 Springer J, Cauch-Dudek K, O'Rourke K *et al.* Asymptomatic primary biliary cirrhosis: a study of its natural history and progression. *Am J Gastroenterol* 1999;**94**:47–53.

30 Mahl T, Shockcor W, Boyer JL. Primary biliary cirrhosis: survival of a large cohort of symptomatic and asymptomatic patients followed for 24 years. *J Hepatol* 1994;**20**:707–13.

31 Prince M, Chetwynd A, Newman W, Metcalf JV, James OFW. Survival and symptom progression in a geographically based cohort of patients with primary biliary cirrhosis: follow up for up to 28 years. *Gastroenterology* 2002;**133**:1044–51.

32 Cauch-Dudek K, Abbey S, Stewart DE *et al.* Fatigue in primary biliary cirrhosis. *Gut* 1998;**43**:705–10.

33 Colina F, Pinedo F, Solis JA *et al.* Nodular regenerative hyperplasia of the liver in early histological stages of primary biliary cirrhosis. *Gastroenterology* 1992;**102**:1319–24.

34 Mitchison HC, Lucey MR, Kelly PJ *et al.* Symptom development and prognosis in primary biliary cirrhosis: a study in two centers. *Gastroenterology* 1990;**99**:778–84.

35 Shapiro JM, Smith H, Schaffner F. Serum bilirubin: a prognostic factor in primary biliary cirrhosis. *Gut* 1979;**20**:137–40.

36 Dickson E, Grambsch PM, Fleming TR *et al.* Prognosis in primary biliary cirrhosis: model for decision making. *Hepatology* 1989;**10**:1–7.

37 Bonsel GJ, Klompmaker IJ, Van 'T Veer F *et al.* Use of prognostic models for assessment of value of liver transplantation in primary biliary cirrhosis. *Lancet* 1990;**335**:493–7.

38 Hughes MD, Raskino CL, Pocock SJ *et al.* Prediction of short-term survival with an application in primary biliary cirrhosis. *Stat Med* 1992;**11**:1731–45

39 Roll J, Boyer JL, Barry D *et al.* The prognostic importance of clinical and histological features in asymptomatic and symptomatic primary biliary cirrhosis. *N Engl J Med* 1983;**308**:1–7.

40 Corpechot C, Carrat F, Poupon R, Poupon RE. Primary biliary cirrhosis: incidence and predictive factors of cirrhosis development in ursodiol-treated patients. *Gastroenterology* 2002;**122**:652–8.

41 Vleggaar FP, van Buuren HR, Zondervan PE, ten Kate FJW, Hop WCJ, and the Dutch multicenter PBC study group. Jaundice in non-cirrhotic primary biliary cirrhosis: the premature ductopenic variant. *Gut* 2001;**49**:276–81.

42 Kilmurry M, Heathcote EJ, Cauch-Dudek K *et al.* Is the Mayo model for predicting survival useful after the introduction of ursodeoxycholic acid treatment for primary biliary cirrhosis? *Hepatology* 1996;**23**:1148–53.

43 Ricci P, Therneau TM, Malinchoc M *et al.* A prognostic model for the outcome of liver transplantation in patients with cholestatic liver disease. *Hepatology* 1997;**25**:672–7.

44 Van Norstrand MD, Malinchoc M, Lindor KD *et al.* Quantitative measurement of autoantibodies to recombinant mitochondrial antigens in patients with primary biliary cirrhosis: relationship of levels of autoantibodies to disease progression. *Hepatology* 1997;**25**:6–11.

45 Wanless IR, Wong F, Blendis LM *et al.* Hepatic and portal vein thrombosis in cirrhosis: possible role in development of parenchymal extinction and portal hypertension. *Hepatology* 1995;**21**:1238–47.

46 Poupon RE, Balkau B, Guechot J *et al.* Predictive factors in ursodeoxycholic acid-treated patients with primary biliary cirrhosis: role of serum markers of connective tissue. *Hepatology* 1994;**19**:635–40.

47 Heathcote J, Ross A, Sherlock S. A prospective controlled trial of azathioprine in primary biliary cirrhosis. *Gastroenterology* 1976;**70**:656–9.

48 James OFW. D-penicillamine for primary biliary cirrhosis. *Gut* 1985;**26**:109–13.

49 Hoofnagle JH, Davis GL, Schafer DF *et al.* Randomized trial of chlorambucil for primary biliary cirrhosis. *Gastroenterology* 1986;**91**:1327–34.

50 Menon KVN, Angulo P, Weston S, Dickson ER, Lindor KD. Bone disease in primary biliary cirrhosis: independent indicators and rate of progression. *J Hepatol* 2001;**35**:316–23.

51 Pares A, Guanabens N, Alvarez L *et al.* Collagen Type Iα1 and vitamin D receptor gene polymorphisms and bone mass in primary biliary cirrhosis. *Hepatology* 2001;**33**:554–60.

52 Mitchison HC, Palmer JM, Bassendine MF *et al.* A controlled trial of prednisolone treatment in primary biliary cirrhosis. Three-year results. *J Hepatol* 1992;**15**:336–44.

53 Christensen E, Neuberger J, Crowe J *et al.* Beneficial effect of azathioprine and prediction of prognosis in primary biliary cirrhosis: final results of an international trial. *Gastroenterology* 1985;**89**:1084–91.

54 Minuk G, Bohme C, Gurgess E *et al.* Pilot study of cyclosporin A in patients with symptomatic primary biliary cirrhosis. *Gastroenterology* 1988;**95**:1356–63.

55 Wiesner RH, Ludwig J, Lindor K *et al.* A controlled trial of cyclosporine in the treatment of primary biliary cirrhosis. *N Engl J Med* 1990;**322**:1419–24.

56 Lombard M, Portmann B, Neuberger J. Cyclosporin A treatment in primary biliary cirrhosis: results of a long-term placebo controlled trial. *Gastroenterology* 1993;**104**:519–26.

57 Kaplan MM, Knox TA. Treatment of primary biliary cirrhosis with low-dose weekly ethotrexate. *Gastroenterology* 1991;**101**:1332–8.

58 Hendrickse M, Rigney E, Giaffer MH *et al.* Low-dose methotrexate in primary biliary cirrhosis: long-term results of a placebo-controlled trial. *Gastroenterology* 1999;**117**:400–7.

59 McCormick PA, Scott F, Epstein O *et al.* Thalidomide as therapy for primary biliary cirrhosis: a double-blind placebo controlled pilot study. *J Hepatol* 1994;**21**:496–9.

60 Wolfhagen FHJ, van Buren HR, denOuden JW *et al.* Cyclical etidronate in the prevention of bone loss in corticosteroid-treated primary biliary cirrhosis. A prospective, controlled pilot study. *J Hepatol* 1997;**26**:325–30.

61 Leuschner M, Maier KP, Schlichting J *et al.* Oral budesonide and ursodeoxycholic acid for treatment of primary biliary cirrhosis: results of a prospective double-blind trial. *Gastroenterology* 1999;**117**:918–25.

62 Angulo P, Jorgensen RA, Keach JC, Dickson ER, Smith C, Lindor K. Oral budesonide in the treatment of patients with primary biliary cirrhosis with a suboptional response to ursodeoxycholic acid. *Hepatology* 2000;**31**:318–23.

63 Combes B, Emerson SS, Flye NL. The primary biliary cirrhosis (PBC) ursodiol (UDCA) plus methotrexate (MTX) or its placebo study (PUMPS) – a multicentre randomized trial. *Hepatology* 2003;**38**:112A.

64 Wolfhagen FHJ, van Hoogstraten HJF, van Buuren HR *et al.* Triple therapy with ursodeoxycholic acid, prednisone and azathioprine in primary biliary cirrhosis: a 1-year randomized, placebo-controlled study. *J Hepatol* 1998;**29**:736–42.

65 Kaplan MM, Alling DW, Zimmerman HJ *et al.* A prospective trial of colchicine for primary biliary cirrhosis. *N Engl J Med* 1986;**315**:1448–54.

66 Warnes TW, Smith A, Lee F *et al.* A controlled trial of colchicine in primary biliary cirrhosis. *Hepatology* 1987;**5**:1–7.

67 Bodenheimer H, Schaffner F, Pessullo J. Evaluation of colchicine therapy in primary biliary cirrhosis. *Gastroenterology* 1988;**95**:124–9.

68 Zifroni A, Schaffner F. Long-term follow up of patients with primary biliary cirrhosis on colchicine therapy. *Hepatology* 1991;**14**:990–3.

69 Leuschner U, Leuschner M, Sieratzki J *et al.* Gallstone dissolution with ursodeoxycholic acid in patients with

70 Poupon R, Poupon RE, Calmus Y *et al.* Is ursodeoxycholic acid an effective treatment for primary biliary cirrhosis? *Lancet* 1987;**i**:834–6.

71 Setchell KDR, Rodrigues CMP, Clerici C *et al.* Bile acid, concentrations in human and rat liver tissue and in hepatocyte nuclei. *Gastroenterology* 1997;**112**:226–35.

72 Stiehl A, Raedsch R, Rudolph G. Acute effects of ursodeoxycholic and chenodeoxycholic acid on the small intestinal absorption of bile acids. *Gastroenterology* 1990;**98**:424–8.

73 Beuers U, Bilzer M, Chittattu A *et al.* Tauroursodeoxycholic acid inserts the apical conjugate export pump, Mrp2, into canalicular membranes and stimulates organic anion secretion by protein kinase C-dependent mechanisms in cholestatic rat liver. *Hepatology* 2001;**33**:1206–16.

74 Rodrigues CM, Fan G, Ma X, Kren BT, Steer CJ. A novel role for ursodeoxycholic acid in inhibiting apoptosis by modulating mitochondrial membrane perturbation. *J Clin Invest* 1998;**101**:2790–9.

75 Goulis J, Leandro G, Burroughs AK. Randomised controlled trials of ursodeoxycholic acid therapy for primary biliary cirrhosis: a meta-analysis. *Lancet* 1999;**354**:1053–60.

76 Gluud C, Christensen E. Ursodeoxycholic acid for primary biliary cirrhosis (Cochrane Review). *Cochrane Database Syst Rev* 2003;**(1)**:CD000551.

77 Pares A, Caballeria L, Rodes J *et al.* Long-term effects of ursodeoxycholic acid in primary biliary cirrhosis results of a double blind controlled multicentric trial. *J Hepatol* 2000;**32**:561–6.

78 Heathcote EJ, Stone J, Cauch-Dudek K *et al.* Effect of pretransplantation ursodeoxycholic acid therapy on the outcome of liver transplantation in patients with primary biliary cirrhosis. *Liver Transplant Surg* 1999;**5**:269–74.

79 Poupon R, Poupon RE. Deterioration in primary biliary cirrhosis in a patient on ursodeoxycholic acid. *Lancet* 1988;**ii**:166.

80 Poupon RE, Balkau B, Eschwege E *et al.* A multicentre controlled trial of ursodiol for the treatment of primary biliary cirrhosis. *N Engl J Med* 1991;**324**:1548–554.

81 Lindor KD, Dickson ER, Baldus WP *et al.* Ursodeoxycholic acid in the treatment of primary biliary cirrhosis. *Gastroenterology* 1994;**106**:1284–90.

82 Heathcote EJ, Cauch-Dudek, Walker V *et al.* The Canadian Multicentre double-blind randomized controlled trial of ursodeoxycholic acid in primary biliary cirrhosis. *Hepatology* 1994;**19**:1149–56.

83 Poupon RE, Lindor KD, Cauch-Dudek K *et al.* Combined analysis of randomized controlled trials of ursodeoxycholic acid in primary biliary cirrhosis. *Gastroenterology* 1997;**113**:884–90.

84 Lindor KD, Janes CH, Crippen JS *et al.* Bone disease in primary biliary cirrhosis: does ursodeoxycholic acid make a difference? *Hepatology* 1995;**21**:389–92.

85 Guanabens N, Pares A, Navasa M *et al.* Cyclosporin A increases the biochemical markers of bone remodeling in primary biliary cirrhosis. *J Hepatol* 1994;**21**:24–8.

86 Corpechot C, Carrat F, Bonnand AM, Poupon RE, Poupon R. The effect of ursodeoxycholic acid therapy on liver fibrosis progression in primary biliary cirrhosis. *Hepatology* 2000;**32**:1196–9.

87 Donaldson P, Agarwal K, Craggs A, Craig W, James O, Jones D. HLA and interleukin 1 gene polymorphisms in primary biliary cirrhosis: associations with disease progression and disease susceptibility. *Gut* 2001;**48**:397–402.

88 Lindor KD, Dickson ER, Jorgenson RA *et al*. The combination of ursodeoxycholic acid and methotrexate for patients with primary biliary cirrhosis: the results of a pilot study. *Hepatology* 1995;**22**:1158–62.

89 Gonzalez-Koch A, Brahm J, Antezana C *et al*. The combination of ursodeoxycholic acid and methotrexate for primary biliary cirrhosis is not better than ursodeoxycholic acid alone. *J Hepatol* 1997;**27**:143–9.

90 Buscher HP, Zietzschmann Y, Gerok W. Positive responses to methotrexate and ursodeoxycholic acid in patients with primary biliary cirrhosis responding insufficiently to ursodeoxycholic acid alone. *J Hepatol* 1993;**18**:9–14.

91 Vuoristo M, Farkkila M, Karvonen A-L *et al*. A placebo-controlled trial of primary biliary cirrhosis treatment with colchicines and ursodeoxycholic acid. *Gastroenterology* 1995;**108**:1470–8.

92 Shibata J, Fujiyama S, Honda Y *et al*. Combination therapy with ursodeoxycholic acid and colchicines for primary biliary cirrhosis. *J Gastroenterol Hepatol* 1992;**7**:277–82.

93 Ikeda T, Tozuka S, Noguchi O *et al*. Effects of additional administration of colchicines in ursodeoxycholic acid-treated patients with primary biliary cirrhosis: a prospective randomized study. *J Hepatol* 1996;**24**:88–94.

94 Poupon RE, Huet PM, Poupon R *et al*. A randomized trial comparing colchicines and ursodeoxycholic acid combination to ursodeoxycholic acid in primary biliary cirrhosis. *Hepatology* 1996;**4**:1098–103.

95 Leuschner M, Guldutuna S, You T *et al*. Ursodeoxycholic acid and prednisolone versus ursodeoxycholic acid and placebo in the treatment of early stages of primary biliary cirrhosis. *J Hepatol* 1996;**25**:49–57.

96 Wolfhagen FH, van Buren HR, Schalm SW. Combined treatment with ursodeoxycholic acid and prednisone in primary biliary cirrhosis. *Neth J Med* 1994;**44**:84–90.

97 Angulo P, Patel T, Jorgensen RA, Therneau TM, Lindor K. Silymarin in the treatment of patients with primary biliary cirrhosis with a suboptional response to ursodeoxycholic acid. *Hepatology* 2000;**32**:897–900.

98 Kurihara T, Sibuya-ku S. Bezafibrate in the treatment of primary biliary cirrhosis: comparison with ursodeoxycholic acid. *Am J Gastroenterol* 2000;**95**:2990–2.

99 Heathcote EJ. Management of primary biliary cirrhosis. *Hepatology* 2000;**31**:1005–13.

100 Jones EA. Rationale for trials of long-term mycophenolate mofetil therapy for primary biliary cirrhosis. *Hepatology* 2002;**35**:258–62.

101 Markus BH, Dickson E, Grambsch P *et al*. Efficiency of liver transplantation in patients with primary biliary cirrhosis. *N Engl J Med* 1989;**320**:1709–13.

102 Tinmouth J, Tomlinson G, Heathcote J, Lilly L. Benefit of transplantation in primary biliary cirrhosis. *Transplantation* 2002;**73**:224–7.

29 Autoimmune hepatitis

Michael Peter Manns, Andreas Schüler

Introduction

Autoimmune hepatitis is a self-perpetuating necroinflammatory disease of unknown etiology, which is characterized by a loss of tolerance towards the patient's own liver tissue. If left untreated the disease leads to cirrhosis and liver failure. Since the recognition of immunologically based liver disease in the 1950s, efforts have been directed toward the development of tools for diagnosis, classification according to serological markers and clinical course, and distinguishing autoimmune hepatitis from other liver diseases.

In the early years diagnosis of autoimmune hepatitis was hampered by the lack of knowledge about the etiology of most acute and chronic liver diseases. The detection of hepatitis viruses and a better understanding of the etiology of other forms of liver disease allowed for the exclusion of patients with these disorders from studies of autoimmune hepatitis and more accurate determination of prognosis and effects of immunosuppressive drugs. The characterization of distinctive autoantibodies and the identification of autoantigens led to a more specific diagnosis of the disease and to the ability to characterize distinct subclasses according to prognosis, treatment response and outcome.

Features of autoimmune hepatitis

Autoimmune hepatitis is a syndrome which is characterized by a typical constellation of epidemiological, laboratory and clinical features: female predominance (female:male ratio 4:1), overrepresentation of the human leukocyte antigen (HLA) alleles DR3 and DR4, hypergammaglobulinemia, circulating autoantibodies, response to immunosuppressive therapy and coexistence of extrahepatic autoimmune diseases.

Epidemiology and genetic predisposition

The incidence of autoimmune hepatitis in western Europe and ethnically comparable populations is 0·7 cases per 100 000 inhabitants per year.[1] Autoimmune hepatitis is recognized more frequently in geographic areas where the prevalence of viral hepatitis is low.

It is generally accepted that occurrence and probably the severity of autoimmune hepatitis is based on an immunogenetic background. Autoimmune hepatitis is strongly associated with the HLA haplotype A1, B8, DR3 or DR4.[2–5] In Caucasian patients autoimmune hepatitis type 1 is strongly associated with the HLA-B8-DR3 haplotype. HLA-B8 is in strong linkage dysequilibrium with HLA-DR3 (94% co-occurrence), which results in a close association between autoimmune hepatitis (AIH) type 1 and B8.[2,5]

HLA-B8 is found in 47%, HLA-A1-B8-DR3 in 37%, HLA-DR3 in 52%, and HLA-DR4 in 42% of patients.[6] Patients with HLA-DR3 have an early onset and a more severe course of the disease. Patients with the HLA-DR4 allele are older, have a more benign disease course, but have extrahepatic autoimmune diseases more frequently. HLA and HLA-B54 are common in Japan where AIH type 1 is rare.[7]

It is unlikely that a single gene determines susceptibility for autoimmune hepatitis, since HLA-DR3 and DR4 are independent risk factors for the disease and are associated with distinct clinical syndromes.[3,8]

Prognosis

The mortality in untreated autoimmune hepatitis in the placebo control groups of early clinical trials was greater than 50% within 3–5 years of diagnosis.[9–12] However, only cases with severe inflammatory activity or fibrosis were included in these early trials. Although the etiology of the chronic hepatitis was not certain, due to the lack of viral markers, the majority of patients in these trials appear to have been suffering from autoimmune hepatitis. However, it was impossible to exclude hepatitis C infection until the early 1990s.

Verification of these data on naive patients in whom the diagnosis of hepatitis C has been excluded is not possible, since studies including untreated control groups or cohort studies of untreated patients can no longer be justified ethically.

The poor survival observed in the control group in early studies may have been influenced also by the late diagnosis of autoimmune hepatitis, and an overrepresentation of patients with advanced liver disease. Conversely, the response to newer therapies may also appear to be better today, since more patients are diagnosed at early disease stages without cirrhosis. Nevertheless, it can be concluded that untreated autoimmune hepatitis is associated with a high risk for the development of endstage cirrhosis.

Outcome in untreated autoimmune hepatitis depends on the degree of inflammatory activity and on the stage of fibrosis. In untreated patients more than 10-fold elevation of aspartate aminotransferase (AST), or more than five-fold elevation of AST together with more than two-fold elevation of γ-globulins, are associated with average 50% 3-year and 90% 10-year mortality. In contrast, AST elevation less than five-fold together with γ-globulin elevation less than two-fold are associated with only an average of 10% 10-year mortality.[13]

Periportal hepatitis without fibrosis is associated with a 17% incidence of cirrhosis at 5 years, but a normal 5-year survival.[14,15] The presence of bridging necrosis or multilobular necrosis is associated with an incidence of cirrhosis at 5 years as high as 82% and with a 5-year survival of only 55%.[15] Patients with cirrhosis at presentation have 58% 5-year mortality.

Patients in whom remission is achieved have a 10-year life expectancy of 90% which does not differ from that of patients with cirrhosis at the beginning of treatment (89%).[13,16] Thus the presence of cirrhosis before or after therapy does not influence survival.[13,17]

Clinical features

Although autoimmune hepatitis occurs mainly in young women, the disease may develop at any age and in either sex.[17] There appears to be a bimodal distribution to the peak incidence of the disease, with the first peak occurring between the ages of 10 and 30 years and the second over 40 years.[17] Data regarding the distribution of cirrhosis at presentation in these two age groups are not available but differences were not seen when comparing patients with HLA-DR3, which predominates in young patients and DR4.[18] Forty percent of patients present with acute hepatitis.[19] Fulminant liver failure may occur but is rare. In the majority of patients the disease progresses without major symptoms, and the diagnosis is not made until symptoms of severe liver disease are present. Jaundice is present in a large proportion of patients at diagnosis. Patients' complaints include fatigue, anorexia, abdominal pain (10–20%) and fever (20%). Amenorrhea occurs in women with severe hepatic inflammation. Hepatomegaly is common and an enlarged spleen is palpable in 50% of patients. Liver cirrhosis is a presenting feature in 30–80% of patients and 10–20% exhibit signs of decompensated liver disease.

Table 29.1 Extrahepatic autoimmune syndromes in autoimmune hepatitis

Frequent symptoms	Rare symptoms
Arthritis	Mixed connective tissue disease
Vitiligo	Lichen planus
Autoimmune thyroid disease	Ulcerative colitis
Insulin dependent diabetes	
Hirsutism, cushingoid features	

Extrahepatic manifestations

Coexisting extrahepatic autoimmune diseases are frequently found in patients with autoimmune hepatitis. Whereas arthropathies and periarticular swelling of both large and small joints occurs in 6–36% of patients, arthritis with joint erosions is rarely seen. Additional clinical features are listed in Table 29.1.

Diagnosis

Since autoimmune hepatitis is a syndrome of unknown etiology, diagnosis requires the assessment of typical clinical and laboratory features. Histology confirms disease activity and stage but by itself is not sufficient for diagnosis.

Advances in the characterization of autoantibodies and their antigens and the exclusion of etiologically distinct liver diseases facilitate early diagnosis in autoimmune hepatitis. Since treatment of autoimmune hepatitis in advanced stages is less effective and is associated with a higher risk of relapse, early treatment improves outcome.

Definitive diagnosis of autoimmune hepatitis requires the presence of circulating autoantibodies at titers of at least 1:80 (in children 1:20) for most autoantibodies associated with autoimmune hepatitis, hypergammaglobulinemia 1–1·5 times the upper limit of normal, and periportal or lobular hepatitis on liver biopsy. Other chronic liver diseases must be excluded by a search for the presence of viral markers, the history of parenteral blood exposure, alcoholic liver disease, drug-induced liver disease, other forms of autoimmune liver disease including primary biliary cirrhosis, and primary sclerosing cholangitis, and genetically determined diseases such as Wilson's disease or hemochromatosis.

The International Autoimmune Hepatitis Group has proposed a scoring system which may help to verify the diagnosis of autoimmune hepatitis and to distinguish it as much as possible from other forms of chronic hepatitis.[20,21] The system documents clinical, laboratory and histological

Table 29.2 Scoring system for diagnosis of autoimmune hepatitis[21]

Parameter	Score
Sex	
Female	+2
Male	0
Serum biochemistry	
Alkaline phosphatase-to-AST levels (ratio of elevations above normal)	
>3·0	−2
1·5–2·0	0
<3·0	+2
Total serum globulin, γ-globulin, or IgG (times upper normal limit)	
>2·0	+3
1·5–2·0	+2
1·0–1·5	+1
<1·0	0
Autoantibodies (titers by immunofluorescence on rodent tissues)	
Adults	
ANA, SMA or LKM-1	
>1:80	+3
1:80	+2
1:40	+1
<1:40	0
Children	
ANA or LKM-1	
>1:20	+3
1:10 or 1:20	+2
<1:20	0
SMA	
>1:20	+3
1:20	+2
<1:20	0
Antimitochondrial antibody	
Positive	−4
Negative	0
Seropositivity for other defined autoantibodies	+2
Hepatitis viral markers	
Negative	+3
Positive	−3
Other etiological factors	
History of recent hepatotoxic drug usage or parenteral exposure to blood products	
Yes	−4
No	+1
Alcohol (average consumption)	
<25 g/day	+2
>60 g/day	−2
Genetic factors	
HLA-DR3 or DR4	+1
Other autoimmune diseases in patient or first degree relatives	+2

(Continued)

Table 29.2 (Continued)

Parameter	Score
Liver histology	
Lobular hepatitis and bridging necrosis	+3
Predominant lymphoplasmocytic infiltrate	+1
Rosetting of liver cells	+1
None of above	−5
Bile duct lesions	−3
Other changes indicating different etiology	−3
Response to therapy	
Complete	+2
Relapse	+3
Diagnostic aggregate scores	
Pretreatment	
Definite	>15
Probable	10–15
Post-treatment	
Definite	>17
Probable	12–17

ANA, antinuclear antibodies; SMA, smooth muscle antibodies; LKM-1, liver kidney microsomal antibodies; AST, aspartate aminotransferase

findings at presentation as well as response to corticosteroid therapy. The latter response may help to clarify the diagnosis even in patients who lack other typical features (Table 29.2). This scoring system has not yet been validated prospectively, but retrospective validation suggests that it is valuable.[22]

Serologically defined subtypes

Three groups of autoimmune hepatitis can be divided serologically according to the presence of distinct autoantibodies. Although this division into three subgroups is regarded as preliminary and is not conclusively validated, it reflects differences with regard to onset, clinical course, treatment response, and outcome.[23]

AIH type 1

Type 1 is characterized by the presence of antinuclear antibodies (ANA) and/or smooth muscle antibodies (SMA). Autoantibody titers do not correlate with disease course, prognosis, progression or disease activity. In pediatric patients SMA may be the only marker of AIH type 1. This group accounts for 80% of patients with autoimmune hepatitis. Although most patients are young at presentation, the disease may also become manifest in older patients. There is a good response to immunosuppressive therapy in up to 80% of patients.[24] ANA, and especially the presence of SMA with anti-actin specificity, are of high diagnostic specificity.[25,26]

Seventy percent of patients are women younger than 40 years of age.[24,27] In 17% of patients concurrent autoimmune disease, including immune thyroiditis, Graves' disease, rheumatoid arthritis or ulcerative colitis, are present.[6,27–29] Twenty-five percent of patients with AIH type 1 are found to have cirrhosis at presentation. Thus the disease may progress without major symptoms, and some patients who present with acute onset may have exacerbation of a long-lasting subclinical disease.[16,27,30]

AIH type 2

Type 2 is characterized by anti-liver kidney microsomal (anti-LKM–1) autoantibodies which are targeted against cytochrome P450 2D6, and is predominantly seen in children.[31,32] In 10%, anti-LKM–3 autoantibodies against uridine diphosphate glucuronyltransferases are also present.[33] Anti-LC–1, directed against formiminotransferase cyclodeaminase, is another marker of autoimmune hepatitis type 2 and appears to correlate with disease activity.[34,35] Autoimmune hepatitis type 2 is characterized by a more rapid progression to cirrhosis, a higher relapse rate, and a comparatively poorer response to corticosteroid therapy. The presence of ANA and/or SMA is detected in only 4% of patients in this group.[36] AIH type 2 is a rare disease that affects up to 20% of patients with autoimmune hepatitis in Europe but only 4% in the USA.[36] At the time of diagnosis liver cirrhosis is frequently present. Especially in Europe AIH type 2 may also be observed in adults.

AIH type 3

Type 3 is characterized by autoantibodies against soluble liver antigen (anti-SLA), which is targeted against a previously identified amino acid sequence, which presumably encodes a UGA-suppressor tRNA-associated protein.[37,38] As anti-SLA and anti-liver-pancreas (LP) have been demonstrated to be identical, the designation anti-SLP/LP has replaced anti-SLA and anti-LP.[37,39] The designation of this as a distinct subtype may be premature since clinical course and response to corticosteroid therapy do not differ significantly from AIH type 1. Anti-SLA/LP may indeed be the only markers of autoimmune hepatitis in patients who are negative for ANA, SMA, and anti-LKM–1 autoantibodies.[40] About 13% of patients with autoimmune hepatitis lack classic autoantibodies but present with typical laboratory and clinical features.

Overlap syndromes

Overlap syndromes between different autoimmune liver diseases are not uncommon and are present in about 18% of patients.[41] About 5% of patients with primary diagnosis of autoimmune hepatitis also present with symptoms and laboratory and histological features of primary biliary cirrhosis

(PBC), whereas 19% of PBC patients also have signs of autoimmune hepatitis.[41] The autoimmune hepatitis scoring system helps to define the strength of the diagnosis and to identify patients with possible overlap syndrome. A switch from PBC to autoimmune hepatitis may occur and require another treatment regimen.

Liver histology

Autoimmune hepatitis cannot be diagnosed by liver histology alone, since there are no pathognomonic histological features. Histology can only support the diagnosis and is used to classify disease activity (grading) and the degree of fibrosis (staging). There is a general agreement that bridging necrosis and multilobular necrosis should be regarded as factors associated with a poor prognosis.[14,42]

Treatment

Corticosteroids should be administered until remission, incomplete response, treatment failure or unacceptable adverse effects occur. Remission is defined by the absence of symptoms, resolution of hepatic inflammation by liver histology, and a normalization of liver enzymes with the exception of AST which may remain up to twice normal.[19]

Conventional corticosteroids

Three controlled trials[10–12] provided evidence that corticosteroid therapy reduces mortality in autoimmune hepatitis (Table 29.3), and this benefit was further substantiated by longer follow up of the patients in one of these studies[9] (Table 29.4). Ald In these studies steroids also relieved symptoms, improved biochemical abnormalities including transaminases, bilirubin levels and hypoalbuminemia, and improved liver histology. Each of these early trials enrolled only small numbers of patients. There were also some design flaws, such as lack of blinding, repeated analyses, and the exclusion from analysis of patients who were withdrawn after randomization because of changes in diagnoses. In one of the trials[10] there were five such examples out of 54 patients who were randomized, and four of these were in the group receiving steroid treatment. However, clinical and biochemical responses to steroid treatment (Figures 29.1–29.3) were sufficiently large, when compared with placebo or azathioprine, that there is a high level of confidence that a significant treatment effect exists. The magnitude of the reduction of mortality produced by steroids can be estimated from the original analysis of the study of Cook *et al.*[10] (control 55%, steroid 14%, absolute risk reduction (ARR) 42%, numbers needed to treat (NNT) = 3) Ald and

Table 29.3 Effect of prednisone on mortality in randomized controlled trials of chronic autoimmune hepatitis (CAH)

Study	Patients	Steroid regimen	Control intervention	Mortality Control	Steroid	P
Cook *et al.* (1971)[10]	49 patients with CAH, 35 with cirrhosis; no previous steroids; 5 patients (4 in steroid group) excluded from analysis because of change in diagnosis	Prednisone 15 mg (3–72 months) attempts to withdraw after 1 month	"No specific treatment"	3/22	15/27	<0·01
Soloway *et al.* (1972)[11]	35[a] patients with chronic liver disease biochemically and histologically, 16 with cirrhosis	Prednisone 20 mg after 4 weeks tapering course from 60 mg (3 months to 3·5 years)	Placebo	1/18	7/17	<0·05
Murray-Lyon *et al.* (1973)[12]	47 patients with chronic aggressive hepatitis, 33 with cirrhosis; approximately half had previous steroid or azathioprine	15 mg daily (up to 2 years); discontinued in 1 month if no improvement in liver function	Azathioprine 75 mg	1/22	6/25	N/A[b]

[a]Additional patients were randomized to receive prednisone 10 mg plus azathioprine 50 mg (14 patients), or azathioprine 100 mg (14 patients); see text.
[b]N/A, not available. Estimated probability of survival at 2 years: steroid 95%, azathioprine 72%.

from the analysis conducted after 10 years follow up of the same patient groups (control 73%, steroid 37%, ARR 36%, NNT = 3).[9]

Corticosteroids are now regarded as standard therapy for patients with moderate to severe autoimmune hepatitis. Data from the randomized trials and from uncontrolled studies suggest that the remission rate is approximately 80% with initial therapy within a time frame of 2–4 years.[43] Usually a significant decrease in transaminases is seen within a few months. In the Mayo study of 111 patients treated with daily prednisone alone or prednisone plus azathioprine, 82 (74%) entered remission, 16 (14%) were treatment failures, and 13 patients (12%) neither relapsed nor experienced treatment failure. B4 It is important to note that histological remission may lag behind improvement of symptoms and biochemical parameters. In the patients treated in the Mayo study symptoms improved first (87% by 6 months), followed by biochemical resolution (68% by 6 months), while histological resolution was seen in only 8% at 6 months and 29% at 12 months.[44] Complete remission, including histologic resolution, was accomplished by 2 years in 61 (74%) of the 82 patients who entered remission, by 3 years in 73 (89%), and by 4 years in 78 (95%).[43] About 10% of patients showed progressive disease in spite of corticosteroid therapy, 13% had an incomplete response after at least 3 years of treatment, and 13% of patients developed severe adverse effects of therapy. Furthermore, the risk of relapse is more than 50% within 6 months and 70% within 3 years after induction therapy or after treatment cessation.[19,45,46] Patients who do not enter

Table 29.4 Long-term outcome of patients with treated and untreated autoimmune hepatitis[a]

	Control	Prednisolone
Patients treated	22	22
Cirrhosis	15/22	15/21
Alive at 10 years	6	13
Dead at 10 years	16[a]	8
Deaths 0–5 years	14	4
Deaths 6–10 years	2	4
Lost to follow up	1	

[a]Two not related to liver disease.

remission have a 40% risk of developing cirrhosis within 10 years.[16] B4

The benefits of corticosteroid therapy have been shown only in a subgroup of patients with severe liver disease, symptoms, and markedly elevated transaminases and γ-globulin levels.[11,44,47,48] A1d, B4 For example, the Mayo Clinic studies included patients according to pre-set criteria,[11,48] which included hepatitis lasting for at least 10 weeks and AST greater than 10 times normal (or AST greater than five times normal together with two-fold elevated γ-globulins). Disease was verified by liver biopsy in all patients and those with hepatic encephalopathy, malignancy or massive alcohol intake were excluded.

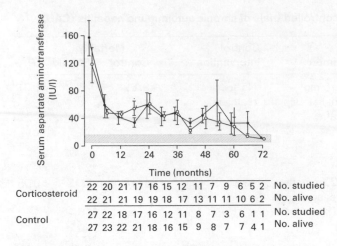

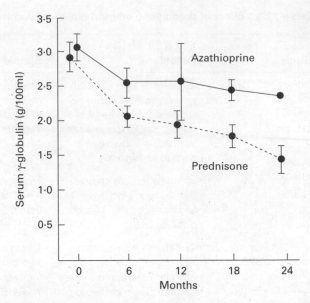

Figure 29.1 Serum aspartate aminotransferase levels following treatment with steroids in active chronic hepatitis. (Reproduced with permission from Cook GC *et al. QJM* 1971;**40**:159–85[10])

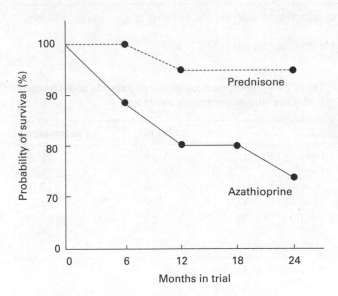

Figure 29.2 The calculated probability of survival in the prednisone and azathioprine groups over the 2 years of treatment. (Reproduced with permission from Murray-Lyon IM *et al. Lancet* 1973;**i**:735–7[12])

Figure 29.3 Mean values (± SEM) of serum γ-globulin in the prednisone and azathioprine groups at 6-month intervals. (Reproduced with permission from Murray-Lyon IM *et al. Lancet* 1973;**i**:735–7[12])

Controlled trials have not been done in patients with mild asymptomatic autoimmune hepatitis. In these patients, who numerically far outnumber patients with severe liver disease, the role for steroid therapy remains unclear.[47]

Since the average duration of treatment until remission is achieved is 22 months (range 6 months to 4 years), treatment withdrawal should not be attempted less than 2 years from the start of therapy to prevent early relapse. Drug withdrawal should be preceded by liver biopsy. The rate of relapse depends on the degree of continuing inflammation and increases from 20% with complete resolution of hepatic inflammation to 50% with ongoing portal inflammation, and 100% with progression to cirrhosis or persisting periportal hepatitis.[47] The rate of relapse after treatment withdrawal is as high as 80%. The remaining 20% patients have to be regularly assessed by clinical parameters and liver biopsy as the risk of relapse cannot be predicted reliably. Ongoing inflammation may exist without significantly elevated transaminases. Normal liver histology after 2 years of steroid therapy does not exclude relapse following treatment withdrawal.

The proportion of patients who continue without inflammatory activity after treatment withdrawal is low. In some of those patients the initial diagnosis may have been incorrect. Valid data on the long-term outcome of this patient group are not available.

Budesonide, a short half-life corticosteroid with 90% hepatic first pass elimination, was shown to improve liver inflammation in an uncontrolled study of patients with acute autoimmune hepatitis.[49] B4 Plasma cortisol levels were suppressed significantly only in cirrhotic patients, possibly due to a reduced capacity of the cirrhotic liver to metabolize steroids. Budesonide was not useful in a small number of patients with treatment failure.[50]

Azathioprine

In one of the trials[11] of prednisone therapy patients were randomized to receive prednisone, azathioprine, a combination of azathioprine and prednisone, or a placebo. No differences in outcomes were observed between the azathioprine and placebo groups, while patients in the combined therapy group appeared to respond in a fashion similar to the prednisone-treated patients. In a second study,[12] a direct comparison of steroids and azathioprine was made, and steroids were clearly more effective. A1d

There is no evidence that azathioprine is more effective than placebo for induction of remission, but in uncontrolled studies it was reported to maintain remission induced by combined therapy with azathioprine and corticosteroids for periods of 1–10 years in as many as 83% of patients.[51,52]

Other immunosuppressive drugs

Cyclosporin A has been used successfully in children[53] and adults,[54] but has not been compared with conventional treatment regimen in a randomized fashion. B4 The impact of other novel immunosuppressive drugs such as tacrolimus, rapamycin or mycophenolate in the treatment of autoimmune hepatitis has not yet been established and they cannot be recommended for general use in patients with intractable disease.

Liver transplantation

Liver transplantation has resulted in excellent long-term survival rates that exceed 90% after 5 years.[43] B4 Patients who fail to enter remission after 4 years of conventional treatment are regarded as potential candidates for liver transplantation. Autoantibodies and hypergammaglobulinemia disappear within 2 years after transplantation. However, recurrence in the graft occurs in 17% patients after 5 ± 1 years and mostly responds to adjustments in the immunosuppression regimen.[55] B4 Development of *de novo* autoimmune hepatitis in patients who undergo transplantation for non-autoimmune liver disease is rare (2·5–3·4% of allografts) and predominantly occurs in children.[56,57] Treatment with prednisolone and azathioprine is effective in those patients.[58] B4

References

1 Hodges JR, Millward-Sadler GH, Wright R. Chronic active hepatitis: the spectrum of disease. *Lancet* 1982;**1**:550–2.

2 Mackay IR, Tait BD. HLA associations with autoimmune-type chronic active hepatitis: identification of B8-DRw3 haplotype by family studies. *Gastroenterology* 1980;**79**:95–8.

3 Donaldson PT, Doherty DG, Hayllar KM *et al.* Susceptibility to autoimmune chronic active hepatitis: human leukocyte antigens DR4 and 4 A1-B8-DR3 are independent risk factors. *Hepatology* 1990;**13**:701–6.

4 Czaja AJ, Carpenter HA, Santrach PJ *et al.* Significance of HLA DR4 in type 1 autoimmune hepatitis. *Gastroenterology* 1993;**105**:1502–7.

5 Mackay IR, Morris PJ. Association of autoimmune active chronic hepatitis with HLA-A1,8. *Lancet* 1972;**ii**:793–5.

6 Czaja AJ, Carpenter HA, Santrach PJ *et al.* Genetic predispositions for the immunological features of chronic active hepatitis. *Hepatology* 1993;**18**:816–22.

7 Seki T, Kiyosawa K, Inoko H *et al.* Association of autoimmune hepatitis with HLA-Bw54 and DR4 in Japanese patients. *Hepatology* 1990;**12**:1300–4.

8 Doherty DG, Donaldson PT, Underhill JA *et al.* Allelic sequence variation in the HLA class 11 genes and proteins in patients with autoimmune hepatitis. *Hepatology* 1994;**19**:609–15.

9 Kirk AP, Jain S, Pocock S *et al.* Late results of the Royal Free Hospital prospective controlled trial of prednisolone therapy in hepatitis B surface antigen negative chronic active hepatitis. *Gut* 1980;**21**:78–83.

10 Cook GC, Mulligan R, Sherlock S. Controlled prospective trial of corticosteroid therapy in active chronic hepatitis. *QJM* 1971;**40**:159–85.

11 Soloway RD, Summerskill WHJ, Baggenstoss AH *et al.* Clinical, biochemical and histological remission of severe chronic active liver disease: a controlled study of treatments and early prognosis. *Gastroenterology* 1972;**63**:820–33.

12 Murray-Lyon IM, Stern RB, Williams R. Controlled trial of prednisone and azathioprine in active chronic hepatitis. *Lancet* 1973;**i**:735–7.

13 Roberts SK, Therneau T, Czaja AJ. Prognosis of histologic cirrhosis in type 1 autoimmune hepatitis. *Gastroenterology* 1996;**110**:848–57.

14 Cooksley WGE, Bradbear RA Robinson W *et al.* The prognosis of chronic active hepatitis without cirrhosis in relation to bridging necrosis. *Hepatology* 1986;**6**:345–8.

15 Schalm SW, Korman MG, Summerskill WHJ *et al.* Severe chronic active liver disease: prognostic significance of initial morphologic patterns. *Am J Dig Dis* 1977;**22**:973–80.

16 Davis GL, Czaja AJ, Ludwig J. Development and prognosis of histologic cirrhosis in corticosteroid-treated hepatitis B surface antigen-negative chronic active hepatitis. *Gastroenterology* 1984;**87**:1222–7.

17 Meyer zum Büschenfelde KH, Hoofnagle J, Manns M. *Immunology and liver*. Dordrecht: Kluwer Academic, 1993.

18 Czaja AJ, Carpenter HA, Santrach PJ *et al.* Significance of HLA DR4 in Type 1 autoimmune hepatitis. *Gastroenterology* 1993;**105**:1502–7.

19 Czaja AJ. Diagnosis, prognosis, and treatment of classical autoimmune chronic active hepatitis. In: Krawitt EL, Wiesner RH (eds). *Autoimmune liver diseases*. New York: Raven Press, 1991.

20 Johnson PJ, McFarlane IG, Alvarez F *et al.* Meeting Report. International Autoimmune Hepatitis Group. *Hepatology* 1993;**18**:998–1005.

21 Alvarez F, Berg PA, Bianchi FB *et al.* International Autoimmune Hepatitis Group report: review of criteria for diagnosis of autoimmune hepatitis. *J Hepatol* 1999;**31**:929–38.

22 Czaja AJ, Carpenter HA. Validation of scoring system for diagnosis of autoimmune hepatitis. *Dig Dis Sci* year;**41**:305–14.

23 Maddrey WC. Subdivisions of idiopathic autoimmune chronic active hepatitis. *Hepatology* 1987;**7**:1372–5.

24 Czaja AJ. Natural history, clinical features, and treatment of autoimmune hepatitis. *Semin Liver Dis* 1984;**4**:1–12.

25 Lidman K, Biberfield G, Fagraeus A *et al.* Anti-actin specificity of human smooth muscle antibodies in chronic active hepatitis. *Clin Exp Immunol* 1976;**24**:266–72.

26 Toh B-H. Smooth muscle autoantibody and autoantigens. *Clin Exp Immunol* 1979;**38**:621–8.

27 Czaja AJ, Davis GL, Ludwig J *et al.* Autoimmune features as determinants of prognosis in steroid-treated chronic active hepatitis of uncertain etiology. *Gastroenterology* 1983;**85**: 713–17.

28 Perdigoto R, Carpenter HA, Czaja AJ. Frequency and significance of chronic ulcerative colitis in severe corticosteroid-treated autoimmune hepatitis. *J Hepatol* 1992;**14**:325–31.

29 Czaja AJ, Carpenter HA, Santrach PJ *et al.* Evidence against hepatitis viruses as important causes of severe autoimmune hepatitis in the United States. *J Hepatol* 1993;**18**:342–52.

30 Nikias GA, Batts KP, Czaja AJ. The nature and prognostic implications of autoimmune hepatitis with an acute presentation. *J Hepatol* 1994;**21**:866–71.

31 Rizzetto M, Swana G, Doniach D. Microsomal antibodies in active chronic hepatitis and other disorders. *Clin Exp Immunol* 1973;**15**:331–44.

32 Homberg JC, Abuaf N, Bernard O *et al.* Chronic active hepatitis associated with anti-liver/kidney microsome antibody type I: a second type of "autoimmune hepatitis". *Hepatology* 1987;**197**:1333–9.

33 Strassburg C, Obermayer-Straub P, Alex B *et al.* Autoantibodies against glucuronosyltransferases differ between viral hepatitis and autoimmune hepatitis. *Gastroenterology* 1996;**11**:1582–92.

34 Martini E, Abuaf N, Caalli F *et al.* Antibody to liver cytosol (anti-LC1) in patients with autoimmune chronic active hepatitis type 2. *Hepatology* 1988;**8**:1662–6.

35 Lapierre P, Hajoui O, Homberg J-C *et al.* Formiminotransferase cyclodeaminase is an organ specific autoantigen recognized by sera of patients with autoimmune hepatitis. *Gastroenterology* 1999;**116**:643–649.

36 Czaja AJ, Manns MP, Homburger HA. Frequency and significance of antibodies to liver/kidney microsome type 1 in adults with chronic active hepatitis. *Gastroenterology* 1992;**103**:1290–5.

37 Wies I, Brunner S, Henninger J *et al.* Identification of target antigen for SLA/LP autoantibodies in autoimmune hepatitis type 3. *Lancet* 2000;**355**:1510–15.

38 Volkmann M, Martin L, Bäurle A *et al.* Soluble liver antigen: isolation of a 35 kD recombinant protein (SLA-P35) specifically recognizing sera from patients with autoimmune hepatitis type 3. *Hepatology* 2001;**33**:591–6.

39 Stechemesser E, Klein R, Berg PA. Characterisation and clinical relevance of liver-pancreas antibodies in autoimmune hepatitis. *Hepatology* 1993;**18**:1–9.

40 Czaja AJ, Manns MP. The validity and importance of subtypes in autoimmune hepatitis: a point of view. *Am J Gastroenterol* 1995;**90**:1206–11.

41 Czaja AJ. Frequency and nature of the variant syndromes of autoimmune liver disease. *Hepatology* 1998;**28**:360–5.

42 Combes B. The initial morphologic lesion in chronic hepatitis. Important or unimportant? *Hepatology* 1986;**6**: 518–22.

43 Sanchez-Urdazpal LS, Czaja AJ, van Hoek B *et al.* Prognostic features and role of liver transplantation in severe corticosteroid-treated autoimmune chronic active hepatitis. *Hepatology* 1992;**15**:215–21.

44 Davis GL, Czaja AJ. Immediate and long-term results of corticosteroid therapy for severe idiopathic chronic active hepatitis. In: Czaja AJ, Dickson ER (eds). *Chronic active hepatitis: the Mayo Clinic experience.* New York: Marcel Dekker, 1986.

45 Hegarty JE, Nouri Aria KT, Portmann B *et al.* Relapse following treatment withdrawal in patients with autoimmune chronic active hepatitis. *Hepatology* 1993;**3**:685–9.

46 Czaja AJ, Ammon HV, Summerskill WHJ. Clinical features and prognosis of severe chronic active liver disease (CALD) after corticosteroid-induced remission. *Gastroenterology* 1980;**78**:518–23.

47 Koretz RL, Lewin KJ, Fagen ND *et al.* Chronic active hepatitis. Who meets treatment criteria? *Dig Dis Sci* 1980;**25**:695–9.

48 Ammon HV. Assessment of treatment regimens. In: Czaja AF, Dickson ER (eds). *Chronic active hepatitis: the Mayo Clinic experience.* New York: Marcel Dekker, 1986.

49 Danielsson Ü, Prytz H. Oral budesonide for treatment of autoimmune chronic active hepatitis. *Aliment Pharmacol Ther* 1994;**8**:585–90.

50 Failure of budesonide in a pilot study of treatment-dependent autoimmune hepatitis. *Gastroenterology* 2001;**119**:1312–16.

51 Stellon AJ, Keating JJ, Johnson PH *et al.* Maintenance of remission in autoimmune chronic active hepatitis with azathioprine after corticosteroid withdrawal. *Hepatology* 1988;**8**:781–4.

52 Johnson PJ, McFarlane IG, Williams R. Azathioprine for long-term maintenance of remission in autoimmune hepatitis. *N Engl J Med* 1995;**333**:958–63.

53 Alvarez F, Ciocca M, Canero-Velasco C *et al.* Short term cyclosporine induces a remission of autoimmune hepatitis in children. *J Hepatol* 1999;**30**:222–7.

54 Malekzadeh R, Nasser-Moghaddam S, Kaviani M-J *et al.* Cyclosporine A is a promising alternative to corticosteroids in autoimmune hepatitis. *Dig Dis Sci* 2001;**46**:1321–7.

55 Gonzázez-Koch A, Czaja AJ, Carpenter HA *et al.* Recurrent autoimmune hepatitis after orthotopic liver transplantation. *Liver Transpl* 2001;**4**:302–10.

56 Kerkar N, Hadzic N, Davies ET *et al.* De-novo autoimmune hepatitis after liver transplantation. *Lancet* 1998;**353**:409–13.

57 Heneghan MA, Portmann BC, Norris SM *et al.* Graft dysfunction mimicking autoimmune hepatitis following liver transplantation in adults. *Hepatology* 2001;**34**:464–70.

58 Salcedo M, Vaquero J, Banares R *et al.* Response to steroids in *de novo* autoimmune hepatitis after liver transplantation. *Hepatology* 2002;**35**:349–56.

30 Primary sclerosing cholangitis

Roger Chapman, Sue Cullen

Introduction

Primary sclerosing cholangitis (PSC) is a chronic cholestatic liver disease in which a progressive obliterating fibrosis of the intrahepatic and extrahepatic bile ducts leads to biliary cirrhosis, portal hypertension and eventually hepatic failure, and in addition 10–30% of patients will develop a cholangiocarcinoma. In comparison with some of the conditions discussed in this book, PSC is a rare disease. But the absence of large randomized clinical trials and meta-analyses in PSC does not prevent us from gathering the best evidence with which to attempt to answer the many questions posed by patients and clinicians about the etiology, diagnosis, prognosis and management of this disease. Inevitably, where good external evidence is lacking, personal clinical expertise may play a greater role in the decision making process. This integration of clinical expertise and best available clinical evidence from systematic research constitutes the practice of "evidence-based gastroenterology".

Etiology

A number of causative agents have been implicated in the pathogenesis of PSC but no single hypothesis has provided a unifying explanation for all the clinical and pathological features of this disease. PSC is closely associated with inflammatory bowel disease (IBD), the majority (65–86%) of patients with PSC have coexistent ulcerative colitis and the prevalence of PSC in ulcerative colitis populations is between 2% and 6%.[1-3] In a patient with ulcerative colitis, abnormal liver function tests, particularly an elevated serum alkaline phosphatase, may be the first indication of this insidious condition. Endoscopic retrograde cholangiopancreatography (ERCP) remains the "gold standard" for diagnosis, although magnetic resonance cholangiography (MRC) a less invasive technique will probably become the preferred choice in the next 5 years. The precise etiology and pathogenesis of PSC is still not completely understood. This chapter sets out the evidence that immune mechanisms play a key role in the development of the disease.

Autoimmunity

The 2:1 male to female ratio of patients with PSC and the relatively poor response of the disease to immunosuppression suggest that PSC is not a classic autoimmune disease. PSC patients do have an increased frequency of the HLA B8 DR3 DQ2 haplotype, however, in common with a number of organ-specific autoimmune diseases such as lupoid chronic active hepatitis, type 1 diabetes mellitus, myasthenia gravis and thyrotoxicosis.[1-3] PSC is also independently associated with a range of autoimmune diseases, diabetes mellitus and Graves' disease being the most common. Saarinen *et al.* found that 25% of patients with PSC had one or more autoimmune disease, compared with 9% of patients with IBD alone.[4]

Autoantibodies

A wide range of autoantibodies can be detected in the serum of patients with PSC clearly indicating an altered state of immune responsiveness or immune regulation. Although a few studies have demonstrated some correlation between particular clinical parameters and the presence of autoantibodies, there is presently insufficient evidence to make use of any of them in determining prognosis. Most are present at low prevalence rates and at relatively low titers (Table 30.1).

Anti-neutrophil specific antibodies are a fairly consistent feature of PSC, occurring in up to 88% of patients. The anti-neutrophil cytoplasmic antibodies (ANCA) associated with PSC are distinct from cANCA and classic pANCA that are commonly used as diagnostic and therapeutic seromarkers for Wegener's granulomatosis and microscopic polyangiitis respectively. PSC, ulcerative colitis and autoimmune hepatitis (AIH) are associated with "atypical pANCA" which has a distinct staining pattern on indirect immunofluorescence microscopy. The prevalence of atypical pANCA in PSC, ulcerative colitis and AIH is 33–88%, 40–87% and 50–96%, respectively.[5] Work by Terjung and Worman has demonstrated that the target antigen for atypical pANCA appears to be localized to the nuclear periphery, and it has been suggested that the anti-neutrophil antibody in PSC therefore be renamed pANNA (anti-neutrophil nuclear antibody).[6] The specific target antigen of this antibody remains to be clarified, but Terjung's group has demonstrated that about 90% of

Table 30.1 Serum autoantibodies in primary sclerosing cholangitis

Antibody[a]	Prevalence
Anti-nuclear antibody	7–77%
Anti-smooth muscle antibody	13–20%
Anti-endothelial cell antibody	35%
Anti-cardiolipin antibody	4–66%
Thyroperoxidase	7–16%
Thyroglobulin	4%
Rheumatoid factor	15%

[a]Antimitochondrial antibody is only rarely detected in PSC (< 10%). This is useful in differentiating primary sclerosing cholangitis from primary biliary cirrhosis.

Table 30.2 Key HLA haplotypes associated with primary sclerosing cholangitis (PSC)

Haplotype	Significance in PSC
B8-TNF*2-DRB3*0101-DRB1* 0301-DQA1*0501-DQB1*0201	Strong association with disease susceptibility
DRB3*0101-DRB1*1301- DQA1*0103-DQB1*0603	Strong association with disease susceptibility
DRB5*0101-DRB1*1501- DQA1*0102-DQB1*0602	Weak association with disease susceptibility
DRB4*0103-DRB1*0401- DQA1*03-DQB1*0302	Strong association with protection against disease
MICA*008	Strong association with disease susceptibility

pANNA from individuals with PSC reacted with a neutrophil-specific nuclear envelope protein with a molecular mass of approximately 50 kDa. However, the molecular identity of this nuclear envelope protein remains unknown.

The importance of autoantibodies in the development of PSC remains unclear. To date there is no convincing model of the pathogenesis of PSC, ulcerative colitis or AIH that implicates anti-neutrophil antibodies, and it may be that these antibodies are simply a marker for an as yet undetermined immune dysregulation. There is, however, some evidence that a monoclonal antibody to a colonic epithelial protein in patients with ulcerative colitis cross-reacts with epithelial cells lining the extrahepatic bile ducts of PSC patients with ulcerative colitis, suggesting that the pathogenesis of these two conditions might be associated with a common antigen.[7]

An interesting paper by Xu *et al.* has demonstrated the presence of autoantibodies to surface antigens expressed on biliary epithelial cells in PSC. This study also showed that these autoantibodies induced increased expression of CD44 on the biliary epithelial cell, demonstrating that the biliary epithelial cell may be the candidate epithelial cell in PSC.[8] More work is needed in this area to clarify if this might be mechanism of action of autoantibodies in the development of the clinical disease. It is not yet clear whether there is a single primary susceptibility allele on each of these haplotypes, although *MICA*008* (mapping to the human leukocyte antigen (HLA) class I/class III boundary between B8 and *TNFA*) occurs on two of the key haplotypes and is therefore a candidate epithelial cell and production of interleukin (IL)-6 by biliary epithelial cells.[9] More work is needed in this area to clarify if this might be mechanism of action of autoantibodies in the development of the clinical disease.

Immunogenetics

Studies of genes encoding the key proteins in the immune system have contributed towards our understanding of the influence of the immune system on the development and progression of PSC.

PSC appears to be a "complex" disease in that it is not attributable to a single gene locus. Susceptibility to PSC is probably acquired through inheriting one of a number of patterns of genetic polymorphisms which together cause a predisposition to development of the disease.

MHC genes

The major histocompatibility complex on the short arm of chromosome 6 encodes the HLA molecules which have a central role in T cell response and are highly polymorphic. The major histocompatibility complex (MHC) class I and class II regions encode the classical transplantation antigens of the HLA A, B, Cw, and DR, DQ and DP families. The class III region encodes a range of immune response genes, including those encoding tumor necrosis factor-α and β (TNFα and β), the heat shock protein family (HSP-70), complement proteins C2, C4A, C4B, Bf, and the genes encoding the MHC class I chain-related proteins, MICα and β (*MICA* and *MICB*).

Early studies based on HLA serotyping found an increased frequency of the HLA B8 DR3 haplotype in PSC patients compared with controls. More recently serotyping has been replaced by the more detailed technique (Table 30.2).[10] The technique of molecular genotyping has elucidated five key HLA haplotypes associated with PSC.[9] It is not yet clear whether there is a single primary susceptibility allele on each of these haplotypes, although *MICA*008* (mapping to the HLA Class I/Class III boundary between B8 and *TNFA*) occurs on two of the key haplotypes.

Non-MHC immunoregulatory genes

A range of non-MHC immunoregulatory genes has been studied in relation to PSC. Cytotoxic lymphocyte antigen-4 (CTLA-4, CD152) is one of the differentiation antigens exclusively expressed on activated CD4+ and CD8+ T cells. It acts by binding to B7, the same ligand as CD28, thereby disrupting the crucial CD28-B7 interaction, one of the key co-stimulatory events in the initiation and progression of the T cell immune response. An amino acid changing single nucleotide polymorphism (SNP) in codon 17 of the leader peptide of CTLA-4 has been associated with susceptibility to autoimmune thyroid disease, insulin-dependent diabetes mellitus, AIH and PBC. The role of this polymorphism in PSC, however, is controversial and to date results have been conflicting.

After antigen presentation, the next step in the adaptive immune response is the release of cytokines and chemokines at the site of inflammation. One polymorphism in TNF-α, as discussed above, is associated with PSC but this appears to be related to the extended HLA B8, DR3 DQ2 haplotype rather than being an independent effect.[11,12] Polymorphisms have also been studied in IL-1 and IL-10, and chemokine CCR-5 to assess a relationship to PSC.[13] So far these studies have been negative or controversial and no clear association has emerged.

The end result of inflammation in PSC is periductal fibrosis. Genes involved in the regulation of the production and destruction of extracellular matrix are therefore also good candidate genes for study. One such family of genes is that comprising the matrix metalloproteinases (MMPs). A functional polymorphism of MMP-3 (stromelysin) has been shown to be associated with both susceptibility to PSC and progression to portal hypertension.[14]

Cellular immune abnormalities

The initiation and maintenance of the immune cascade is determined not only by MHC recognition but also by the presence of accessory cells and molecules to provide co-stimulatory signals and the production of cytokines to amplify or modify the immune response.

Studies of circulating lymphocyte subsets in PSC have produced rather conflicting results, although there does seem to be some consensus on the finding that there is a fall in CD8+ T cells as the disease progresses.[15] The fact that this change occurs only in advanced disease however, means that it is unlikely to be significant in the pathogenesis of the disease. The cellular infiltrate at the site of tissue injury is probably more relevant than the circulating population. Although it is clear that there is a T cell predominant portal tract infiltrate in PSC, there is still some uncertainty regarding the relative importance of CD4+ and CD8+ cells in this infiltrate (Figure 30.1). The hypothesis that these T lymphocytes are involved in the pathogenesis of the disease (rather than simply being markers for its presence) is supported by evidence that these cells are functional. This evidence comes from studies of surface markers expressed on activated and memory T cells.

T cell receptor

Most T cells carry a T cell receptor (TCR) consisting of two disulphide-linked polypeptides, termed α and β. A group of T cells carrying an alternative receptor, termed $\gamma\delta$, has been identified over the past 13 years. These cells appear to be involved in autoimmunity, although their exact function is not clear.[16] An increase in the number of $\gamma\delta$ T cells has been found in the peripheral blood and portal infiltrates of patients with both PSC and AIH compared with controls.[17] There was no concentration of the $\gamma\delta$ cells in the areas of bile ducts or interface hepatitis however, and the predominant cell type was still $\alpha\beta$. The significance of $\gamma\delta$ cells in the pathogenesis of PSC is therefore not clear although they might function by modulating $\alpha\beta$ T cell activation or regulating antibody or autoantibody production from B cells.

Although T cell receptor gene rearrangements serve to generate genetic diversity, a particular V$\alpha\beta$ gene segment can play a dominant role in recognition of certain peptide-MHC complexes. Expanded T cell populations using restricted sets of T cell receptor V gene segments have been identified in areas of inflammation in diseases such as rheumatoid arthritis and Sjögren's disease. This suggests the presence of a specific antigen with the capacity of driving the production of T cells with this restricted V$\alpha\beta$ segment product.[18,19] Studies from Broome *et al.* indicated that the hepatic, but not peripheral, T cells in PSC preferentially have Vβ3 T cell repertoires.[20] An oligoclonal expansion was not demonstrated in this study, but oligoclonal T cells receptors which proliferate in culture with enterocytes and are cytotoxic to enterocyte cell lines *in vitro* have also been reported in PSC.[21]

Cytokines

Most studies in the context of PSC have looked at cytokine secretion from peripheral rather than liver-derived lymphocytes. This work has not been conclusive. There are some preliminary data (published only in abstract form to date) that show an increased expression of both T helper (Th)1 and Th2 cytokines within the liver of PSC patients compared with healthy controls.[22] Downregulation of IL-10 mRNA expression in PSC and PBC was also demonstrated. These changes were reversed after treatment with ursodeoxycholic acid (UDCA).[23]

An abnormal cytokine repertoire and the high expression of cytokine mRNA in the early stages of PSC suggest that Th1 and Th2 cytokines may play a role in the pathogenesis of the disease. Cytokines could have an influence on many aspects of the progression of PSC including the cytotoxic T cell development, aberrant expression of class II MHC molecules on biliary epithelial cells, and MMP gene expression in fibroblasts.[24] Their true role in the development and progression of PSC has yet to be clearly defined.

Biliary epithelial cells

The biliary epithelial cell is the target of immune attack in PSC, while at the same time appearing to be an active

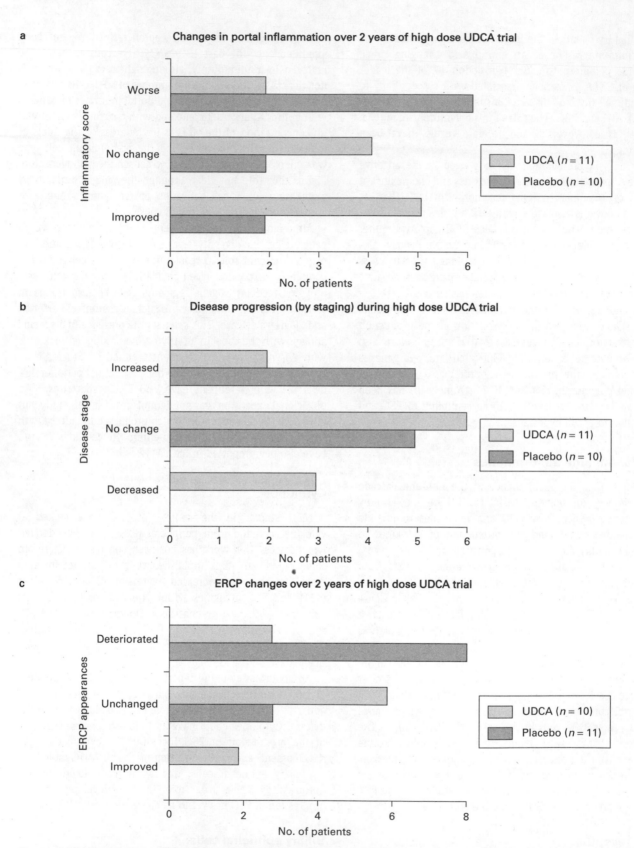

Figure 30.1 Comparison of (a) changes in portal inflammatory score, (b) disease progression by staging, and (c) cholangiographic assessment in patients treated with high dose ursodeoxycholic acid (UDCA) versus placebo over the 2-year trial. (Reproduced from Mitchell *et al. Gastroenterology* 2001;**121**:900–7[100])

participant in the immune response. Aberrant expression of HLA molecules on target cells is important in the pathogenesis of autoimmune diseases. Normal biliary epithelial cells express only HLA class I and not class II antigens. However, the HLA class II antigens HLA-DR, DQ and DP have all been found to be expressed by the biliary epithelial cells of patients with PSC.[25,26] These antigens have the potential to initiate an immune response by binding autoantigens or exogenous antigens and presenting the peptides to class II restricted T lymphocytes.

"Professional" antigen-presenting cells (APC) also express cell surface co-stimulatory molecules such as CD54 (intercellular adhesion molecule-1 (ICAM-1)) and members of the B7 family (CD80 and CD84) which are required for T cell activation. These co-stimulatory molecules appear to be lacking on the biliary epithelial cells in PSC, and this observation has cast doubt upon the theory that biliary epithelial cells act as APCs.[27] Aberrant expression of CD54 (ICAM-1), however, has recently been demonstrated as occurring in patients with endstage PSC. This finding could not be replicated in patients with earlier stage disease.[28,29] Recently, Cruickshank *et al.* has also demonstrated that CD44, the lymphocyte homing receptor, is highly expressed on biliary epithelial cells in a range of inflammatory liver diseases including PSC.[30] This phenomenon may occur as a function of biliary cell response to stress or damage and, through the ability of CD44 to bind chemokines and growth factors, might mediate local inflammatory responses. Biliary epithelial cells therefore, may act as APCs although they seem to be less active in this role than dendritic cells or macrophages.

Role of bacteria in the etiopathogenesis of primary sclerosing cholangitis

The coexistence of inflammatory colitis in around 75% of northern European patients with PSC has led to the hypothesis that the initiating step in this disease is the access of intestinal bacteria through an inflamed and leaky bowel wall, to the portal circulation. An abnormal immune response to bacterial antigens (possibly acting as molecular mimics for autoantigens) in an immunogenetically susceptible host might be sufficient to precipitate the cascade of immune reactions detailed above.

Investigation of bacterial growth from human tissue is confounded by the bacterial contamination caused by intubation of the bile duct at ERCP. Several animal models however, have been used to investigate this proposal. Wistar and Sprague-Dawley rats develop a pattern of hepatic injury somewhat similar to human PSC after artificially induced small bowel bacterial overgrowth.[31] Rat models have also demonstrated that bacterial peptides instilled into the rectum of rats with a chemically induced colitis appear very quickly in the bile and will initiate a small duct cholangitis, although no extrahepatic strictures are produced.[32]

Hypotheses for the etiopathogenesis of PSC

A plausible unifying hypothesis for the etiopathogenesis of PSC has been put forward by Vierling.[33] This suggests that the initial insult is the reaction of an immunogenetically susceptible host to bacterial cell wall products entering the portal circulation through a permeable gut wall either due to colitis or possibly during episodes of intestinal infection. The resulting Kupffer cell (hepatic macrophage) activation would result in peribiliary cytokine and chemokine secretion attracting activated neutrophils, monocyte/macrophages, lymphocytes and fibroblasts to the site of infection. The resultant concentric fibrosis around the bile ducts could then lead to ischemia and then atrophy of the biliary epithelial cell. The bile duct loss would then lead to progressive cholestasis, fibrosis and secondary biliary cirrhosis. This hypothesis does not explain why there is a relative paucity of patients with PSC and underlying Crohn's colitis, nor the association of PSC with stricturing of the pancreatic duct.

More recently, Grant *et al.* have proposed the existence of an enterohepatic circulation of lymphocytes, whereby some mucosal lymphocytes produced in the gut during active inflammation persist as memory cells capable of recirculation through the liver.[34] Under certain circumstances these gut-derived lymphocytes might become activated resulting in hepatic inflammation. This hypothesis is supported by the finding that some lymphocyte homing receptors are shared by the liver and gut. This concept of dual homing lymphocytes helps to explain the observation that PSC runs a course independent of inflammation in the bowel and indeed can develop even after proctocolectomy.

In conclusion, current evidence suggests that PSC is an immune-mediated rather than a classic autoimmune disease. The association with inflammatory colitis suggests that an abnormal immune response may be initiated in an immunogenetically susceptible host by the access of bacterial antigen, through a permeable gut wall, to the portal circulation. This bacterial antigen might then act as a molecular mimic of an autoantigen precipitating an immune cascade which results in stricturing and scarring of the intrahepatic and extrahepatic bile ducts, peribiliary fibrosis and ultimately, cirrhosis. There are difficulties in determining which of the wide range of immune abnormalities identified in these patients, are causal and which are the consequences of tissue injury.

Diagnosis

Although ERCP remains the gold standard for the diagnosis of PSC, it is an invasive technique that carries a small but significant risk of morbidity and mortality. A non-invasive and inexpensive test could not only be used for diagnosis but also for screening an asymptomatic patient population in order to detect early stage disease. The operating characteristics of such a diagnostic test should be compared with the gold standard and the test should be applied to patients with and without PSC as diagnosed by the gold standard test (ERCP).

MRC is a new non-invasive technique and increasing data exists on its performance relative to ERCP. In one recent study[35] the ERCP and MRC of patients with a suspected diagnosis of PSC were independently evaluated, and MRC was as sensitive and specific as either ERCP or percutaneous hepatic cholangiography. Current evidence suggests that MRC can be used in place of ERCP to exclude the diagnosis of PSC.

Prognosis

The clinical course of PSC is quite variable; the disease is indolent in some patients and more rapidly progressive in others. The natural history of PSC is described in a number of retrospective studies with the median survival time from diagnosis to death or orthotopic liver transplantation (OLT) reported between 12 and 21 years.[36–39] Differences in survival estimations may reflect the variation in the definition of onset and outcome. As there is no reliable marker of early disease in PSC the onset is difficult to identify clearly. Whether the onset is defined as the occurrence of the first symptoms consistent with PSC, as the time of the first abnormal liver function test, or as the time of diagnosis by ERCP will result in differences in survival estimates. In retrospective studies details of distant events may be sparse and there is likely to be failure to recognize early signs and symptoms. Patients with late stage disease may predominate, while patients who die from rapidly progressive disease may be missed.

The ideal study of prognosis is prospective and follows patients from a defined point in the disease process, usually diagnosis. There have been no studies using such an inception cohort in PSC because the disease is rare and its slow progression makes a prospective study impractical. A large retrospective study published by Broome *et al.*[36] did include a high proportion (46%) of patients with early (stage I and II) disease. Forty-four percent of patients were asymptomatic at diagnosis, and these patients exhibited longer survival than symptomatic patients. The estimated median survival for the whole PSC group was 144 months. For patients with symptoms at the time of diagnosis the estimated median survival was significantly less, at 112 months. Over one-fifth of the asymptomatic patients became symptomatic during the median follow up period of 63 months. From these studies a number of prognostic models have been developed, mainly using parameters defined at diagnosis (Tables 30.3 and 30.4). Perhaps the most controversial prognostic factor is HLA DR4. Studies from Oxford[41] and the Mayo Clinic[43] suggest that HLA DR4 is associated with poor prognosis, whilst studies from London[44] and Sweden[17] were unable to confirm this association. Although these models successfully predict the natural history of the disease in a cohort of PSC patients, they

are less successful when applied to individual patients. The confounding factor is the development of hepatobiliary or colonic cancer.

Cholangiocarcinoma is difficult to diagnose,[45] is associated with poor prognosis,[46] and precludes OLT.[47] In Broome *et al.*'s study cholangiocarcinoma was found in 8% of patients with PSC but occurred in 30% of the 79 patients who died or underwent OLT.[36] In this and other studies none of the investigated clinical or laboratory parameters could identify those patients who would subsequently develop cholangio-carcinoma, although PSC patients with coexistent ulcerative colitis have a three to four-fold higher risk of developing cholangiocarcinoma. A recent case–control study has suggested that long duration of ulcerative colitis and smoking are independent risk factors associated with the development of hepatobiliary malignancy in PSC.[48]

Two studies have shown that biliary dysplasia seen on liver biopsy can antedate the development of cholangiocarcinoma by at least 2 years, and may be an indication for early liver transplantation. Patients with ulcerative colitis and PSC are also considered to be at higher risk of developing colonic dysplasia and carcinoma.[49] Early studies[54,51] investigating this risk gave conflicting results due to the different methodologies employed, small numbers, design flaws, and different endpoints.[52] However, a recent study of a retrospectively defined inception cohort[53] has shown that the risk of developing colonic dysplasia or cancer is significantly increased in ulcerative colitis patients with PSC compared with patients with ulcerative colitis alone. A high proportion of right-sided cancers was noted in the PSC patients, consistent with the hypothesis that these cancers arise due to exposure to carcinogenic bile acids.[54] Consensus has emerged that PSC definitely predisposes to colonic dysplasia and cancer. Recent studies have shown that patients treated with UDCA have a 30% reduction in the incidence of colonic dysplasia or carcinoma.[55] PSC patients with ulcerative colitis remain at risk of developing colon cancer or dysplasia even after they have undergone OLT.[56]

The evidence is that physicians can only provide their PSC patients with a tentative survival estimate using the variables derived from prognostic models. The development of cholangiocarcinoma is often insidious and unpredictable. Although a significant impact of screening on mortality is unproved, we recommend that PSC patients with ulcerative colitis should immediately enter a yearly colonoscopic surveillance program, in contrast to the 2-yearly surveillance program after 8 years of colitis that is recommended for ulcerative colitis patients without PSC.

Management of complications

As PSC slowly progresses to biliary cirrhosis and portal hypertension, complications may arise from chronic cholestasis or chronic liver failure (as in PBC and other liver

Table 30.3 Studies of prognosis in primary sclerosing cholangitis: multivariate analysis

Study	No. of patients	% Asymptomatic	Median survival (years)	Independent prognostic factors
Helzberg *et al.* (1987)[39]	53	25	a	Hepatomegaly Serum bilirubin > 1·5 mg/dl at onset of disease
Wiesner *et al.* (1989)[37]	174	21	11·9	Age Serum bilirubin Blood hemoglobin concentration Presence of IBD Histological stage
Farrant *et al.* (1991)[38]	126	16	12·0	Hepatomegaly Splenomegaly Serum alkaline phosphatase Histological stage Age Presence of symptoms not a significant prognostic factor
Broome *et al.* (1996)[36]	305	44	12·0	Age Serum bilirubin Histological stage

[a]5% survival = 9 years.
IBD, inflammatory bowel disease

Table 30.4 Studies of prognosis in primary sclerosing cholangitis (PSC): univariate analysis

Study	No. of patients	Prognostic indicator	Comments
Craig *et al.* (1991)[40]	129	Disease assessment by cholangiography	Intrahepatic disease worse than extrahepatic
Mehal *et al.* (1994)[41]	83	HLA DR4	HLA DR4 associated with poor prognosis
Olsson and Asztely (1995)[42]	94	Disease assessment by cholangiography	High grade intrahepatic strictures indicate early jaundice and short survival
Maloney *et al.* (1996)[44]	120	HLA DR4	HLA DR4 not associated with poor prognosis but confers resistance to developing PSC

diseases) or complications specific to PSC such as biliary strictures and the development of cholangiocarcinoma. The general management of the complications of cholestasis is discussed elsewhere in this book.

Management of the complications of chronic liver disease

The complications of endstage chronic liver disease, namely esophageal varices, ascites and portosystemic encephalopathy are equally observed in the later stages of PSC. The management of these complications is common to all advanced liver disease and warrants no further discussion here. Special mention should be made of the problem of bleeding from peristomal varices which occur as a consequence of portal hypertension in PSC patients who have undergone procto-colectomy for underlying IBD and have an ileal stoma. Peristomal variceal bleeding can be severe and difficult to treat. Local measures such as injection of sclerosant, venous ligation and ileostomy revision are usually unsuccessful and associated with recurrent bleeding. Portosystemic shunts, i.e. transjugular intrahepatic portosystemic shunt (TIPS), can control severe bleeding episodes but such patients may ultimately require hepatic transplantation. B4

Ideally patients with PSC who require a proctocolectomy for control of their ulcerative colitis should have ileal pouch–anal anastomosis so as to avoid the formation of an ileal stoma and the problem of peristomal varices. With the recognition that PSC patients with ulcerative colitis have a greater risk of developing colonic dysplasia or DNA aneuploidy compared with patients with ulcerative colitis alone[57] surveillance of the anastomosis is required. Although there is no direct evidence, there is consensus that patients with ulcerative colitis with an intact colon should undergo annual surveillance colonoscopy with multiple biopsies. C5 The incidence of pouchitis is also increased in patients with an ileal pouch–anal anastomosis and coexistent PSC.[58]

Management of complications specific to primary sclerosing cholangitis

PSC is characterized by multiple small annular strictures in the biliary tree seen at ERCP. Tight biliary strictures, particularly in the extrahepatic biliary tree, may interrupt the indolent course of disease and cause deterioration of liver function with more rapid progression to biliary cirrhosis. Such benign dominant biliary strictures cannot be reliably differentiated from cholangiocarcinoma by cholangiographic appearance. In one study of patients awaiting OLT ultrasound-guided biopsy of a dominant biliary stricture accurately demonstrated cholangiocarcinoma complicating PSC in 75% of cases.[59] Exfoliative brush cytology of strictures at ERCP has a high specificity and positive predictive value for the diagnosis of cholangiocarcinoma but low sensitivity and negative predictive value.[60] Despite the relatively low sensitivity endoscopic bile duct brush cytology may be diagnostic for malignancy or reveal high grade dysplasia.[61] No single serum marker accurately predicts the development of cholangiocarcinoma but an index combining two serum markers, CA19–9 and carcinoembryonic antigen (CEA), may be useful to identify PSC patients with occult tumours.[62] This finding has not been confirmed by other investigators.[63]

Dominant strictures may be treated endoscopically or surgically. Endoscopic treatment involves balloon dilatation of the stricture and/or placement of a biliary stent. Surgical procedures aim to bypass the obstruction and drain the biliary system into the gut. Unfortunately there are no controlled trials which examine the validity of either approach and guide future management. Since biliary manipulation increases the risk of stricturing and bacterial cholangitis and may jeopardize future OLT, endoscopic and surgical intervention in PSC is as a rule best avoided for as long as possible.

Selected non-cirrhotic PSC patients with dominant extrahepatic strictures may benefit from a bilioenteric bypass.[64] A non-randomized retrospective study of endoscopic intervention including dilatation or stenting of strictures,

placement of nasobiliary drainage and extraction of stones in PSC suggested that 77% of the patients showed improvements of their clinical symptoms, liver function tests or cholangiograms.[65] C4 A report from Amsterdam described 32 patients with dominant strictures treated with short-term endoscopic stenting for a mean of 11 days. Primary endpoints were improvements in symptoms and cholestasis which were seen in all patients, and which were maintained for several years. Seven transient procedure-related complications occurred in 45 therapeutic procedures.[66] Where OLT is precluded, as in biliary obstruction due to cholangiocarcinoma, endoscopic stenting is undoubtedly the best option for more distal lesions. C4

Medical therapy – the prevention of disease progression

In both PBC and PSC the primary site of inflammation and damage is the biliary epithelium. When severely damaged or destroyed the bile ducts do not have the capacity to regenerate like hepatocytes which are the primary target for injury in various parenchymal liver diseases. Given the finite number of bile ducts in the liver the natural history of PSC, like PBC, is that of progressive loss of functioning intrahepatic bile ducts (ductopenia). This ductopenia leads to a progressive and irreversible failure of hepatic biliary excretion. To delay and reverse this process physicians have tried a variety of agents but in PSC, in contrast to PBC, few randomized controlled trials have been done.

D-Penicillamine

Increased hepatic copper levels are detected in all patients with prolonged cholestasis including those with PSC. This observation provided the rationale for the controlled trial of the cupruretic, D-pencillamine, performed by the Mayo Clinic.[67] Seventy patients were randomized to either D-pencillamine or placebo for 36 months. No improvement was observed on disease progression or overall survival in the treatment group. Major adverse effects including pancytopenia and proteinuria led to the permanent discontinuation of penicillamine in 21% of the treated patients. A1c

Corticosteroids

It is surprising that there have been no long-term studies of the effect of corticosteroid therapy on histological progression and survival in PSC, especially as the disease may be immune mediated. This may reflect concerns about the long-term adverse effect profile of corticosteroids. Systemic and topical corticosteroid therapy has been evaluated in a number of small often uncontrolled trials.[68,69] In one such study 10 patients diagnosed by ERCP and liver biopsy with early PSC (elevated serum alkaline phosphatase, but none with biliary cirrhosis) were treated with prednisone without a significant response.[68] B4 In another uncontrolled pilot study 10 patients with PSC, selected because they had elevated aminotransferases, were given prednisolone, and the majority responded with improvement in their biochemistry.[69] In a subsequent study Lindor et al.[70] were unable to confirm these optimistic results. They treated 12 patients with a combination of low dose prednisone (10 mg daily) and colchicine (0·6 mg twice daily). The clinical course of the treated patients was compared with a control group, but the study was not randomized. After 2 years no significant differences in the biochemistry and liver histology were detected between the two groups. In this study treatment did not alter the rate of disease progression or improve survival. B4 The absence of a beneficial response, and the suspicion that corticosteroid therapy enhanced cortical bone loss and hence the risk of developing compression fractures of the spine even in young male patients, led the authors to advise against empirical corticosteroid therapy in these patients. This conclusion was strengthened by the observation that spontaneous fractures in patients who have undergone liver transplantation occur almost exclusively in PSC patients who are already osteopenic at the time of transplantation.[71]

Topical corticosteroids are usually administered through a nasobiliary drain left *in situ* following ERCP. Three anecdotal studies,[72–74] have reported benefit. The only controlled trial of nasobiliary lavage with corticosteroids from the Royal Free Hospital[75] showed no benefit when compared with a placebo group. Ald Although the numbers were small, the bile of all the treated patients became rapidly colonized with enteric bacteria and a higher incidence of bacterial cholangitis was recorded in the treatment group.

More recent clinical trials have studied the possible benefit of budesonide, a second-generation corticosteroid with a high first-pass metabolism and minimal systemic availability. Unfortunately preliminary results both alone[76] and in combination with UDCA[77] have been disappointing. Ald

There is no direct evidence to suggest that either oral or topical corticosteroids are beneficial in PSC. Indeed when PSC patients with coexistent ulcerative colitis are given courses of corticosteroids to treat their ulcerative colitis this treatment appears to have little influence on the behavior of their liver disease. It may be difficult to justify a trial using corticosteroids as monotherapy but a large controlled trial could clarify their role in combination with a choleretic agent. Potentially serious adverse effects may be reduced by new agents such as bisphosphonates which prevent cortical bone loss.

Methotrexate

After demonstrating a promising response to low dose oral pulse methotrexate in an open study[78] involving 10 PSC patients without evidence of portal hypertension, Knox and Kaplan[79] carried out a double blind, randomized placebo-controlled trial of oral pulse methotrexate at a dose of 15 mg per week. Twelve patients with PSC were entered into each group. Although each patient was monitored with both liver biopsy and ERCP (at baseline and yearly) and biochemical tests, the only significant change was a fall in the serum alkaline phosphatase by 31% in those receiving methotrexate. Ald

There were no significant improvements in liver histology, treatment failure or mortality rates. The only toxicity attributed to methotrexate during the study was a transient decrease in the white cell count related to a bout of bacterial cholangitis and *Campylobacter* enterocolitis in a single patient.

The study was too small in terms of numbers of patients and of too short duration to have adequate power to detect a significant benefit in patients with early disease, should such a benefit exist. Nevertheless, with the negative results of this controlled trial and more recent reports of the toxicity of pulse methotrexate in patients with PBC (interstitial pneumonitis, severe lung damage, hepatotoxicity) it would be difficult to justify a larger controlled trial of methotrexate therapy at present. In a pilot study Lindor et al.[80] found that methotrexate given in combination with UDCA to 19 PSC patients was associated with toxicity (alopecia, pulmonary complications) but showed no additional improvement in liver biochemistry compared with a control group of nine patients treated with UDCA alone. Ald

Other immunosuppressants

Despite the evidence that PSC may be an immune-mediated disease, there have been few randomized controlled trials of immunosuppressive agents containing sufficient numbers of patients with early disease. Immunosuppression is unlikely to be effective in patients with advanced liver disease and irreversible bile duct loss, and this may account for the disappointing results so far seen in PSC with these agents. No controlled trials of azathioprine in PSC have been reported. In one case report[81] two patients improved clinically on azathioprine but in another[82] the patient deteriorated. The use of cyclosporine in PSC has been evaluated in a randomized controlled trial from the Mayo Clinic[85] involving 34 patients with PSC and, in the majority, coexistent ulcerative colitis. Treatment with cyclosporine reduced the symptoms of ulcerative colitis[84] but had no effect on the course or prognosis of PSC. Follow up liver histology after 2 years of treatment revealed progression in 9/10 of the placebo group but only 11/20 of the cyclosporine-treated group. Ald

This was not reflected by any beneficial effect on the biochemical tests. The prevalence of adverse effects was low; serious renal complications were not reported. A combination of cyclosporine and prednisolone elicited a beneficial response in a 65-year-old man with PSC accompanied by pancreatic duct abnormalities.[85]

Tacrolimus (FK 506) an immunosuppressive macrolide antibiotic, has been used to treat 10 patients with PSC in an open study.[86] After 1 year of treatment with a twice daily oral regimen all patients experienced an improvement in their liver biochemical tests. Ald For example the median serum bilirubin level was reduced by 75% and the serum alkaline phosphatase was reduced by 70%. No major adverse events were reported in this initial study in PSC. A randomized controlled trial is required to confirm these encouraging preliminary results.

Cladribine, a nucleoside analog with specific antilymphocyte properties, has been used to treat a variety of autoimmune disorders. In a recent pilot study in PSC six patients with early disease were treated for 6 months and followed for 2 years. Whilst significant decreases were seen in peripheral and hepatic lymphocyte counts no significant changes were observed in symptom scores, liver function tests or cholangiograms.[87] C4

The hepatobiliary injury which occurs in rats with experimental bacterial overgrowth is said to result from peptidoglycan-polysaccharide-mediated activation of Kupffer cells, which in turn release cytokines such as TNF-α. In rats the liver injury can be prevented by pentoxifylline. In an open pilot study, 20 patients with PSC were treated with pentoxifylline 400 mg four times daily for 1 year. In this dose pentoxifylline did not improve symptoms or liver tests.[88] C4

Antifibrogenic agents

In the light of initial reports which suggested a positive trend of the antifibrogenic agent colchicine on survival in PBC and other types of cirrhosis, a randomized trial from Sweden[89] compared colchicine in a dose of 1 mg daily by mouth in 44 patients with PSC with a matched placebo group of 40 patients. At 3-year follow up there were no differences in clinical symptoms, serum biochemistry, liver histology or survival between the two groups. Ald The only recorded adverse effect attributable to colchicine was diarrhea in a single patient. The absence in this study of any proved effect of colchicine on disease progression, outcome or survival is in keeping with more recent long-term studies of colchicine in PBC and other chronic liver diseases which have failed to confirm the initial reported survival benefits.

Ursodeoxycholic acid

This hydrophilic bile acid has become widely used in the treatment of cholestatic liver of all causes. UDCA appears to exert a number of effects all of which may be beneficial in chronic cholestasis: a choleretic effect by increasing bile flow; a direct cytoprotective effect; an indirect cytoprotective effect by displacement of the more hepatotoxic endogenous hydrophobic bile acids from the bile acid pool; an immunomodulatory effect; and finally an inhibitory effect on apoptosis.

Using a labeled bile acid analog Jazrawi *et al.*[90] demonstrated a defect in hepatic bile acid excretion but not in uptake in patients with PBC and PSC, resulting in bile acid retention. They observed an improvement of hepatic excretory function with UDCA in patients with PBC but only a trend towards improvement in the small number of patients with PSC. Not only is hepatic bile acid excretion affected by UDCA but so is ileal reabsorption of endogenous bile acids. The net result is enrichment of the bile acid pool with UDCA. Hydrophobic bile acids are more toxic than UDCA which can protect and stabilize membranes.

Studies have demonstrated that long-term treatment with UDCA decreases aberrant expression of HLA class I on hepatocytes and reduces levels of soluble cell adhesion molecules (sICAM) in PBC patients. *In vitro* studies have shown that UDCA may alter cytokine production by human peripheral mononuclear cells. In PSC one study has shown that UDCA has been shown to decrease aberrant HLA DR expression on bile ducts.[91] However, a more recent study could not demonstrate any alteration in expression of either HLA class I and II or ICAM-1 on either biliary epithelial cells or hepatocytes.[92] The body of evidence suggests that UDCA does have some modulatory effects on immune function, but how important these are remains unclear.

Numerous studies have attempted to address the clinical efficacy of UDCA treatment in PSC. The majority have been uncontrolled studies in small numbers of patients. In a pilot study O'Brien *et al.*[93] treated 12 patients with UDCA on an open basis over 30 months. They documented improvement in fatigue, pruritus and diarrhea and significant improvement of all liver biochemical tests, particularly alkaline phosphatase during the two UDCA treatment periods. Symptoms and liver biochemistry relapsed during a 6-month withdrawal period between treatment phases. During UDCA treatment the amount of cholic acid declined slightly but the levels of other relatively hydrophobic bile acids did not change significantly.

In the first randomized double blind controlled trial of UDCA in PSC Beuers *et al.*[94] compared over a 12-month period six patients who received UDCA 13–15 mg/kg bodyweight with eight patients who received placebo. The majority of patients had early disease (Ludwig classification stages I and II). After 6 months a significant reduction in alkaline phosphatase and aminotransferases was achieved in the treatment group. A significant fall in bilirubin was only noted after 12 months. Using a multiparametric score the UDCA-treated group showed significant improvement in their liver histology, mainly attributed to decreased portal and parenchymal inflammation. Unfortunately treatment did not ameliorate their symptoms. UDCA-induced diarrhea was the only important side effect requiring a patient to withdraw.

Similar results were obtained by Stiehl *et al.*[95] who randomized 20 patients to either 750 mg daily of UDCA or placebo. However in a larger randomized placebo-controlled trial of UDCA in PSC by Lindor *et al.*[96] no benefit was demonstrated. In this trial 105 patients were randomized to treatment with UDCA in conventional doses (13–15 mg/kg bodyweight daily) or placebo and followed up for up to 6 years (mean 2·9 years). Treatment with UDCA had no effect upon the time until treatment failure defined as death, liver transplantation, the development of cirrhosis, quadrupling of bilirubin, marked relapse of symptoms or the development of signs of chronic liver disease. Furthermore the significant improvement in liver biochemical tests seen in the treated group was not reflected by any beneficial changes in liver histology. On the contrary there was a suggestion that the liver histology of patients on UDCA showed a greater tendency to progress towards fibrosis. However, this could also be explained by sampling variability between serial liver biopsies.[97]

The failure of standard doses of UDCA to provide clinical benefit led our group to consider the use of higher doses. Our rationale is that with increasing cholestasis there is decreasing enrichment of the bile acid pool with UDCA and higher doses are required to achieve the same level of enrichment.[98] Furthermore, the *in vitro* immunomodulatory effects of UDCA are enhanced with increasing UDCA concentrations.[99] In a pilot study we evaluated 26 patients with PSC who were randomized to either high dose (20–25 mg/kg) UDCA or placebo[100] for 2 years. High dose UDCA had no effect on symptoms but as expected there was a significant improvement in liver biochemistry. More importantly we found a significant reduction in cholangiographic appearances and liver fibrosis (Figure 30.1 and Table 30.5). In the treatment group bile acid saturation with UDCA >70% confirmed patient compliance. No significant adverse effects were reported, in particular no worsening of colitis was seen.

Similar encouraging results were obtained in an open study in 30 patients with PSC treated for 1 year.[102] When compared with historical controls a significant improvement in projected survival using the Mayo risk score was observed with high dose but not with the conventional dose (13–15 mg/kg per day) of UDCA. In the light of these promising results a large controlled trial of high dose UDCA is in progress in Scandinavia.

The treatment of PSC with bile acids has been the subject of a recent Cochrane systematic review by Chen and Gluud.[103] They concluded that treatment with UDCA leads to a significant improvement in liver biochemistry but that the evidence is insufficient to either support of refute its clinical effects in patients with PSC (Figure 30.2). They recommend that large scale high quality randomized clinical trials should be performed.

Whilst it is established that hydrophilic bile acid UDCA inhibits injury by hydrophobic bile acids, hepatocyte cell death from bile acid-induced toxicity occurs more frequently from apoptosis than from necrosis. It has been demonstrated that UDCA inhibits deoxycholic acid-induced apoptosis by modulating mitochondrial transmembrane potential and reactive oxygen species production.[104] Moreover, UDCA inhibited *in vitro* deoxycholic acid stimulated growth in several tumor cell lines

including colon cancer.[105] This has led to the suggestion that UDCA may reduce the risk of dysplasia and cancer in the biliary tree and/or the colon. Tung *et al.* studied 59 patients with PSC and ulcerative colitis followed with 3-yearly surveillance colonoscopy.[106] Colonic dysplasia was significantly less common in those patients treated with UDCA. However, these results were not confirmed in a study of 120 patients followed with 2-yearly colonoscopic surveillance.[107] The recent study of Pardi *et al.* has confirmed the chemopreventive effect of UDCA.[55] To date, there is no evidence that the high rate of bile duct cancer is reduced by UDCA therapy.

Miscellaneous treatments

In keeping with ulcerative colitis, there is a strong inverse relationship between PSC and cigarette smoking. This led Angulo *et al.*[108] to test the hypothesis that oral nicotine might have a beneficial effect in PSC. Eight non-smoking patients with PSC were treated with nicotine 6 mg four times daily for up to 1 year. Adverse effects were frequent requiring cessation in three patients and no beneficial effects were seen.

Combined therapy

In an important pilot study, the potential of combination therapy was explored by Schramm *et al.*,[109] who treated 15 patients with PSC. All patients received low dose UDCA (500–750 mg daily), prednisolone 1 mg/kg daily and azathioprine 1–1·5 mg/kg daily. After a median follow up period of 41 months, all patients had a significant improvement in liver function tests. Seven patients had been previously treated with UDCA but liver enzymes improved only after immunosuppressive therapy was added. More importantly, six of 10 with follow up biopsies showed histological improvement and significant radiological deterioration was only seen in one of 10 patients who had had ERCP.

In a 13-year prospective study Stiehl *et al.*[110,111] studied the survival of 106 patients with PSC treated with 750 mg UDCA daily and by endoscopic balloon dilatation of major dominant stenoses whenever necessary. Ten patients had a dominant stricture at entry and over a median follow up of 5 years another 43 developed a dominant stenosis. This was not prevented by low dose UDCA treatment but successfully treated by balloon dilatation in the majority, only five requiring temporary stenting. This combined approach of UDCA and endoscopic intervention significantly improved the survival compared with predicted survival rates. This was an uncontrolled study provides only relatively weak evidence that UDCA and/or endoscopic therapy prolonged survival, although the results are promising.

Orthotopic liver transplantation

For patients with advanced PSC, OLT is the only therapeutic option. A number of centers report a 5-year

Table 30.5 Controlled trials of ursodeoxycholic acid in primary sclerosing cholangitis

Authors	No of patients	Type of study	Dose	Duration	LFTs improved				Symptoms improved	Liver histology improved	Proportion with early disease[a]
					Alk P	GGT	Bili	AT			
Beuers et al. (1992)[94]	14	DBPC	13–15 mg/kg daily	12 months	Yes	Yes	Yes	Yes	No	Yes	57%
Lo et al. (1992)[91]	23	DBPC	10 mg/kg daily	24 months	Trend	Trend	No	Trend	No	No	74%
Stiehl et al. (1994)[95]	20	DBPC, Unc	750 mg daily	Controlled for 3 months, uncontrolled up to 4 years	Yes	Yes	No	Yes	No	Yes	35%
Mitchell et al. (2001)[100]	26	DBPC	20–25 mg/kg daily	12 months	Yes	Yes	No	No	No	Yes	30%
van Hoogstraten et al. (1998)[101]	48	DB	10 mg/kg daily in single (Grp 1) or three (Grp 2) doses	24 months	Yes	Yes	No	Yes	No	NA	NA
Lindor et al. (1997)[96]	105	DBPC	13–15 mg/kg daily	Mean 29 years	Yes	Yes	Yes	Yes	No	No	NA

[a] Proportion with early disease, i.e. stages I and II. Unc, uncontrolled; DB, Double blinded trial; PC, Placebo-controlled trial; Alk P, alkaline phosphatase; GGT, γ-glutamyltranspeptidase; Bili, bilirubin; NA, data not available; LFTs, liver function tests

Review: 97% solids for primary sclerosing cholangitis
Comparison: 01 UDCA versus control (placebo or no treatment)
Outcome: 01 Mortality at the end of treatment

Study	UDCA n/H	Control n/H	Relative risk (fixed) 95% CI	Weight (%)	Relative risk (fixed) 95% CI
Beutre 1997	0/6	1/8		22·5	0·47 (0·07, 0·00)
Linder 1997	4/53	3/62		61·8	1·31 (0·31, 6·60)
x Lo 1992	0/8	0/10		0·0	Not estimable
Michell 2001	0/13	1/13		26·7	0·33 (0·01, 7·60)
x Stiehl 1994	0/10	0/10		0·0	Not estimable
x de bois 1998	0/20	0/20		0·0	Not estimable
Total (95% CI)	4/110	5/113		100·0	0·88 (0·27, 2·73)

Test for heterogeneity chi squared 0·88 df = 2 $P = 0·8442$
Test for overall effect = −0·20 $P = 0·8$

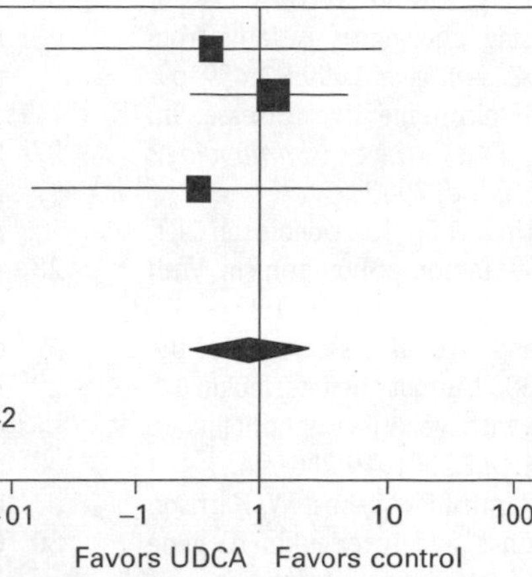

```
       −01    −1     1     10    100
          Favors UDCA  Favors control
```

Figure 30.2   Meta-analysis of five trials of UDCA versus control (placebo or no treatment). Mortality at the end of treatment. (From Chen and Gluud[103], with permission)

survival rate in excess of 75%.[112] Farges *et al.*[113] advocate assessment for OLT earlier in the course of the disease to reduce the operative risk and to prevent the development of hepatobiliary malignancy. Against this approach is the recognition that PSC may recur in the graft[114] and that colon cancer is the most frequent cause of death in PSC patients after OLT.[115] A recent study has shown that PSC recurrence is more common in male IBD patients who have an intact colon. Five-year survival rates are also improved in colectomized patients. In the absence of prognostic models capable of predicting the course of disease or the onset of complications in individual patients, the timing of OLT continues to be controversial.[112] A recent report suggests that prior treatment with UDCA is associated with a better outcome after transplantation.[116]

Conclusion

There is no established effective medical treatment for PSC. Recent studies suggest that high dose UDCA may have a role in at least slowing disease progression, although the results of larger long-term randomized trials are awaited. Randomized controlled trials of immunosuppressive agents in early PSC are needed, possibly in combination with high dose UDCA. With the identification of T cell subsets involved in PSC and the cytokines they produce it may be possible to use particular recombinant cytokines or antibodies to specific cytokines such as anti-TNF antibody (infliximab) to manipulate the immune response in PSC and alter disease progression. Greater insight

into the pathogenetic mechanisms involved in PSC would enable therapy to be targeted more specifically at the area of initial damage, namely, the biliary epithelium.

Liver transplantation remains the mainstay of treatment for patients with endstage disease but the disease will recur in at least 30% of patients.

References

1 Schrumpf E, Fausa O, Forre O, Dobloug JH, Ritland S, Thorsby E. HLA antigens and immunoregulatory T cells in ulcerative colitis associated with hepatobiliary disease. *Scand J Gastroenterol* 1982;**17**:187–91.

2 Shepherd HA, Selby WS, Chapman RW *et al.* Ulcerative colitis and persistent liver dysfunction. *QJM* 1983;**52**:503–13.

3 Chapman RW, Varghese Z, Gaul R, Patel G, Kokinon N, Sherlock S. Association of primary sclerosing cholangitis with HLA-B8. *Gut* 1983;**24**:38–41.

4 Saarinen S, Olerup O, Broome U. Increased frequency of autoimmune diseases in patients with primary sclerosing cholangitis. *Am J Gastroenterol* 2000;**95**:3195–9.

5 Terjung B, Worman HJ. Anti-neutrophil antibodies in primary sclerosing cholangitis. *Best Pract Res Clin Gastroenterol* 2001;**15**:629–42.

6 Terjung B, Spengler U, Sauerbruch T, Worman HJ. "Atypical p-ANCA" in IBD and hepatobiliary disorders react with a 50-kilodalton nuclear envelope protein of neutrophils and myeloid cell lines. *Gastroenterology* 2000;**119**:310–22.

7 Mandal A, Dasgupta A, Jeffers L *et al.* Autoantibodies in sclerosing cholangitis against a shared peptide in biliary and colon epithelium. *Gastroenterology* 1994;**106**:185–92.

8 Xu B, Broome U, Ericzon BG, Sumitran-Holgersson S. High frequency of autoantibodies in patients with primary sclerosing cholangitis that bind biliary epithelial cells and induce expression of CD44 and production of interleukin 6. *Gut* 2002;**51**:120–7.

9 Spurkland A, Saarinen S, Boberg KM *et al.* HLA class II haplotypes in primary sclerosing cholangitis patients from five European populations. *Tissue Antigens* 1999;**53**:459–69.

10 Donaldson PT. Genetics of autoimmune liver disease. In: Gershwin E, Manns MP (eds). *Liver Immunology.* Philadelphia: Hanley and Belfus, Inc, 2003.

11 Bernal W, Moloney M, Underhill J, Donaldson PT. Association of tumor necrosis factor polymorphism with primary sclerosing cholangitis. *J Hepatol* 1999;**30**:237–41.

12 Mitchell SA, Grove J, Spurkland A *et al.* Association of the tumour necrosis factor alpha-308 but not the interleukin 10-627 promoter polymorphism with genetic susceptibility to primary sclerosing cholangitis. *Gut* 2001;**49**:288–94.

13 Donaldson PT, Norris S, Constantini PK, Bernal W, Harrison P, Williams R. The interleukin-1 and interleukin-10 gene polymorphisms in primary sclerosing cholangitis: no associations with disease susceptibility/resistance. *J Hepatol* 2000;**32**:882–6.

14 Satsangi J, Chapman RW, Haldar N *et al.* A functional polymorphism of the stromelysin gene (MMP-3) influences susceptibility to primary sclerosing cholangitis. *Gastroenterology* 2001;**121**:124–30.

15 Lindor KD, Wiesner RH, Katzmann JA, LaRusso NF, Beaver SJ. Lymphocyte subsets in primary sclerosing cholangitis. *Dig Dis Sci* 1987;**32**:720–5.

16 Hayday A, Geng L. Gamma delta cells regulate autoimmunity. *Curr Opin Immunol* 1997;**9**:884–9.

17 Martins EB, Graham AK, Chapman RW, Fleming KA. Elevation of gamma delta T lymphocytes in peripheral blood and livers of patients with primary sclerosing cholangitis and other autoimmune liver diseases. *Hepatology* 1996;**23**:988–93.

18 Sumida T, Yonaha F, Maeda T *et al.* T cell receptor repertoire of infiltrating T cells in lips of Sjogren's syndrome patients. *J Clin Invest* 1992;**89**:681–5.

19 Imberti L, Sottini A, Primi D. T cell repertoire and autoimmune diseases. *Immunol Res* 1993;**12**:149–67.

20 Broome U, Grunewald J, Scheynius A, Olerup O, Hultcrantz R. Preferential V beta3 usage by hepatic T lymphocytes in patients with primary sclerosing cholangitis. *J Hepatol* 1997;**26**:527–34.

21 Probert CS, Christ AD, Saubermann LJ *et al.* Analysis of human common bile duct-associated T cells: evidence for oligoclonality, T cell clonal persistence, and epithelial cell recognition. *J Immunol* 1997;**158**:1941–8.

22 Mitchell SA Chapman R, Fleming KA. Enhanced cytokine mRNA expression in primary sclerosing cholangitis and autoimmune liver disease [Abstract]. *Gastroenterology* 1997;**112**:A757.

23 Mitchell SA Chapman R, Fleming KA. Decreased interleukin-10 mRNA expression in primary sclerosing cholangitis and primary biliary cirrhosis: A role for IL-10 in pathogenesis [Abstract]. *Hepatology* 1997;**26**:442A.

24 Mitchell SA, Chapman RW. Primary sclerosing cholangitis. *Clin Rev Allergy Immunol* 2000;**18**:185–214.

25 Chapman RW, Kelly PM, Heryet A, Jewell DP, Fleming KA. Expression of HLA-DR antigens on bile duct epithelium in primary sclerosing cholangitis. *Gut* 1988;**29**:422–7.

26 Broome U, Glaumann H, Hultcrantz R, Forsum U. Distribution of HLA-DR, HLA-DP, HLA-DQ antigens in liver tissue from patients with primary sclerosing cholangitis. *Scand J Gastroenterol* 1990;**25**:54–8.

27 Leon MP, Bassendine MF, Wilson JL, Ali S, Thick M, Kirby JA. Immunogenicity of biliary epithelium: investigation of antigen presentation to CD4+ T cells. *Hepatology* 1996;**24**:561–7.

28 Adams DH, Mainolfi E, Burra P *et al.* Detection of circulating intercellular adhesion molecule-1 in chronic liver diseases. *Hepatology* 1992;**16**:810–14.

29 Broome U, Hultcrantz R, Scheynius A. Lack of concomitant expression of ICAM-1 and HLA-DR on bile duct cells from patients with primary sclerosing cholangitis and primary biliary cirrhosis. *Scand J Gastroenterol* 1993;**28**:126–30.

30 Cruickshank SM, Southgate J, Wyatt JI, Selby PJ, Trejdosiewicz LK. Expression of CD44 on bile ducts in primary sclerosing cholangitis and primary biliary cirrhosis. *J Clin Pathol* 1999;**52**:730–4.

31 Lichtman SN, Sartor RB, Keku J, Schwab JH. Hepatic inflammation in rats with experimental small intestinal bacterial overgrowth. *Gastroenterology* 1990;**98**:414–23.

32 Yamada S, Ishii M, Liang LS, Yamamoto T, Toyota T. Small duct cholangitis induced by N-formyl L-methionine L-leucine L-tyrosine in rats. *J Gastroenterol* 1994;**29**:631–6.

33 Vierling J. Aetiopathogenesis of primary sclerosing cholangitis. In: Manns PCR, Stieihl A, Wiesner R (eds). *Primary sclerosing cholangitis.* London: Kluwer Academic Publishers, 1998.

34 Grant AJ, Lalor PF, Salmi M, Jalkanen S, Adams DH. Homing of mucosal lymphocytes to the liver in the pathogenesis of hepatic complications of inflammatory bowel disease. *Lancet* 2002;**359**:150–7.

35 Angulo P, Pearce DH, Johnson CD, Henry JS, LaRusso NF, Petersen BT, Lindor KD. Magnetic resonance cholangiography in patients with biliary disease, its role in PSC. *J Hepatol* 2000;**33**:659–60

36 Broome U, Olsson R, Loof L *et al.* Natural history of prognostic factors in 305 Swedish patients with primary sclerosing cholangitis. *Gut* 1996;**38**:610–15.

37 Wiesner RH, Grambsch PM, Dickson ER *et al.* Primary sclerosing cholangitis: natural history, prognostic factors and survival analysis. *Hepatology* 1989;**10**:430–6.

38 Farrant JM, Hayllar KM, Wilkinson ML *et al.* Natural history and prognostic variables in primary sclerosing cholangitis. *Gastroenterology* 1991;**100**:1710–17.

39 Helzberg JH, Petersen JM, Boyer JL. Improved survival with primary sclerosing cholangitis. A review of clinicopathologic features and comparison of symptomatic and asymptomatic patients. *Gastroenterology* 1987;**92**:1869–75.

40 Craig DA, MacCarty RL, Wiesner RH *et al.* Primary sclerosing cholangitis: value of cholangiography in determining the prognosis. *Am J Roentgenol* 1991;**157**:959–64.

41 Mehal WZ, Lo YM, Wordsworth BP, Fleming K, Chapman RW. HLA DR4 is a marker for rapid disease progression in primary sclerosing cholangitis. *Gastroenterology* 1994;**106**:160–7.

42 Olsson RG, Asztely MS. Prognostic value of cholangiography in primary sclerosing cholangitis. *Eur J Gastroenterol Hepatol* 1995;**7**:251–4.

43 Aguilar HI, Nuako K, Krom RA *et al.* Do primary sclerosing cholangitis (PSC) patients who express HLA-DR4 haplotype have a more rapidly progressive disease? *Hepatology* 1994; **20**:154A.

44 Maloney MM, Donaldson PT, Thomson LJ, Williams R. HLA-DR4 and DR4 subtypes confer resistance to primary sclerosing cholangitis and are not associated with a poor prognosis. *Hepatology* 1996;**24**:169A.

45 Miros M, Kerlin P, Walker N *et al.* Predicting cholangiocarcinoma in patients with primary sclerosing cholangitis before transplantation. *Gut* 1991;**32**:1369–73.

46 Kornfield D, Ekbom A, Ihre T. Survival and risk of cholangiocarcinoma in patients with primary sclerosing cholangitis. A population-based study. *Scand J Gastroenterol* 1997;**32**:1042–5.

47 Herbener T, Zajko AB, Koneru B *et al.* Recurrent cholangiocarcinoma in the biliary tree after liver transplantation. *Radiology* 1988;**169**:641–2.

48 Bergquist A, Glaumann H, Persson B *et al.* Risk factors and clinical presentation of hepatobiliary carcinoma in patients with primary sclerosing cholangitis: a case–control study. *Hepatology* 1998;**27**:311–16.

49 D'Haens GR, Lashner BA, Hanauer SB. Pericholangitis and sclerosing cholangitis are risk factors for dysplasia and cancer in ulcerative colitis. *Am J Gastroenterol* 1993;**88**: 1174–8.

50 Brentnall TA, Haggitt RC, Rabinovitch PS *et al.* Risk and natural history of colonic neoplasia in patients with primary sclerosing cholangitis and ulcerative colitis. *Gastroenterology* 1996;**110**:331–8.

51 Loftus EVJ, Sandborn WJ, Tremaine WJ *et al.* Risk of colorectal neoplasia in patients with primary sclerosing cholangitis. *Gastroenterology* 1996;**110**:432–40.

52 Ahnen DJ. Controlled clinical trials: the controls are the key. *Gastroenterology* 1996;**110**:628–30.

53 Lashner BA, Shetty B, Rybicki L. Risk factors for cancer or dysplasia in ulcerative colitis with primary sclerosing cholangitis [Abstract]. *Gastroenterology* 1998;**114**:A1018.

54 Marchesa P, Lashner BA, Lavery IC *et al.* The risk of cancer and dysplasia among ulcerative colitis patients with primary sclerosing cholangitis. *Am J Gastroenterol* 1997;**92**:1285–8.

55 Pardi DS, Loftus EV, Kremers WK, Keach J, Lindor KD. Ursodeoxycholic acid as a chemopreventive agent in patients with ulcerative colitis and primary sclerosing cholangitis. *Gastroenterology* 2003;**124**:889–893.

56 Bleday R, Lee E, Jessuran J *et al.* Increased risk of early colorectal neoplasms after hepatic transplant in patients with inflammatory bowel disease. *Dis Colon Rectum* 1993; **36**:908–12.

57 Broome U, Loberg R, Veress B, Eriksso LS. Primary sclerosing cholangitis and ulcerative colitis. Evidence for increased neoplastic potential. *Hepatology* 1995;**22**:1404–8.

58 Penna C, Dubois R, Tremaine WJ *et al.* Pouchitis after pouchanal anastomosierative colitis occurs with increased frequency in patients with associated primary sclerosing cholangitis. *Gut* 1996;**38**:234–239.

59 Mirza DF, Davies M, Olliff S *et al.* Preoperative diagnosis of cholangiocarcinoma in primary sclerosing cholangitis in potential liver tranplantation candidates [Abstract]. *Hepatology* 1994;**20**:154A.

60 Ferrunior AP, Lichtenstein DR, Slivka A, Chang C, Carr-Locke DL. Brush cytology during ERCP for the diagnosis of biliary and pancreatic malignancies [See comments]. *Gastrointest Endosc* 1994;**40**(2 Pt 1):140–8.

61 Lee JG, Leung JW, Baillie J, Layfield LJ, Cotton PB. Benign, dyplasitic or malignant – making sense of endoscopic bile duct brush cytology: results in 149 consecutive patients. *Am J Gastroenterol* 1995;**90**:722–6.

62 Ramage JK, Donaghy A, Farrant JM, Iorns R, Williams R. Serum tumor markers for the diagnosis of cholangiocarcinoma in primary sclerosing cholangitis. *Gastroenterology* 1995;**108**:865–9.

63 Bjornsson E, Kilander A, Olsson R. CA 19–9 and CEA are unreliable markers for cholangiocarcinoma in patients with primary sclerosing cholangitis. *Liver* 1999;**19**:501–5.

64 Hepburgh JA. Surgical biliary drainage in primary sclerosing cholangitis. The role of the Hepp-Couinaud approach. *Arch Surg* 1994;**129**:1057–62.

65 Lee JG, Schutz SM, England RE, Leung JW, Cotton PB. Endoscopic therapy of sclerosing cholangitis. *Hepatology* 1995;**21**:661–7.

66 Ponsioen CY, Lam K, van Milligan de Wit AW, Huibregtse K, Tytgat GN. Four years experience with short term stenting in primary sclerosing cholangitis. *Am J Gastroenterol* 1999; **94**:2403–7.

67 LaRusso NF, Wiesner RH, Ludwig J *et al.* Prospective trial of penicillamine in primary sclerosing cholangitis. *Gastroenterology* 1988;**95**:1036–42.

68 Sivak M Jr, Farmer RG, Lalli AF. Sclerosing cholangitis: its increasing frequency of recognition and association with inflammatory bowel disease. *J Clin Gastroenterol* 1981;**3**: 261–6.

69 Burgert SL, Brown BP, Kirkpatrick RB, LaBrecque DR. Positive corticosteroid response in early primary sclerosing cholangitis [Abstract]. *Gastroenterology* 1984;**86**:1037.

70 Lindor KD, Wiesner RH, Colwell LJ *et al.* The combination of prednisone and colchicine in patients with primary sclerosing cholangitis. *Am J Gastroenterol* 1991;**86**:57–61.

71 Porayko MK, Wiesner RH, Hay JE *et al.* Bone disease in liver transplant recipients: incidence, timing and risk factors. *Transplant Proc* 1991;**23**:1462–5.

72 Grijm R, Huibregtse K, Bartelsman J *et al.* Therapeutic investigations in primary sclerosing cholangitis. *Dig Dis Sci* 1986;**31**:792–8.

73 Jeffrey GP, Reed WD, Laurence BH, Shilkin KB. Primary sclerosing cholangitis: clinical and immunopathological review of 21 cases. *J Gastroenterol Hepatol* 1990;**5**:135–40.

74 Craig PI, Williams SJ, Hatfield ARW, Ng M, Cotton PB. Endoscopic management of primary sclerosing cholangitis [Abstract]. *Gut* 1990;**31**:1182a.

75 Allison MC, Burroughs AK, Noone P, Summerfield JA. Biliary lavage with corticosteroids in primary sclerosing cholangitis. A clinical, cholangiographic and bacteriological study. *J Hepatol* 1986;**3**:118–22.

76 Angulo P, Batts KP, Jorgensen A, Lindor KD. Budesonide in the treatment of primary sclerosing cholangitis: a pilot study [Abstract]. *Hepatology* 1999;**30**:477A.

77 van Hoogstraten HJF, Vieggar FP, Boland GI *et al.* Budesonide or prednisone in combination with ursodeoxycholic acid in primary sclerosing cholangitis. A randomized double-blind pilot study. *Am J Gastroenterol* 2000;**95**:2015–22.

78 Knox TA, Kaplan MM. Treatment of primary sclerosing cholangitis with oral methotrexate. *Am J Gastroenterol* 1991;**86**:546–52.

79 Knox TA, Kaplan MM. A double-blind controlled trial of oral-pulse methotrexate therapy in the treatment of primary sclerosing cholangitis. *Gastroenterology* 1994;**106**:494–9.

80 Lindor KD, Jorgensen RA, Anderson ML *et al.* Ursdeoxycholic acid and methotrexate for primary sclerosing cholangitis: a pilot study. *Am J Gastroenterol* 1996;**91**:511–15.

81 Javett SL. Azathioprine in primary sclerosing cholangitis. *Lancet* 1971;**i**:810–11.

82 Wagner A. Azathioprine treatment in primary sclerosing cholangitis. *Lancet* 1971;**ii**:663–4.

83 Wiesner RH, Steiner B, LaRusso NF, Lindor KD, Baldus WP. A controlled clinical trial evaluating cyclosporine in the treatment of primary sclerosing cholangitis [Abstract]. *Hepatology* 1991;**14**:63A.

84 Sandborn WJ, Wiesner RH, Tremaine WJ, Larusso NF. Ulcerative colitis disease activity following treatment of associated primary sclerosing cholangitis with cyclosporin. *Gut* 1993;**34**:242–6.

85 Kyokane K, Ichihara T, Horisawa M *et al.* Successful treatment of primary sclerosing cholangitis with cyclosporine and corticosteroid. *Hepatogastroenterology* 1994;**41**:449–52.

86 Van-Thiel DH, Carroll P, Abu-Elmagd K *et al.* Tacrolimus (FK 506), a treatment for primary sclerosing cholangitis: results of an open-label preliminary trial. *Am J Gastroenterol* 1995; **90**:455–9.

87 Duchini A, Younossi ZM, Saven A *et al.* An open-label pilot trial of cladibrine (2-cloolordeoxyadenosine) in patients with primary sclerosing cholangitis. *J Clin Gastroenterol* 2000; **31**:271–3.

88 Bharucha AE, Jorgensen R, Lichtman SN, La Russo NF, Lindor KD. A pilot study of pentoxifylline for the treatment of primary sclerosing cholangitis. *Am J Gastroenterol* 2000; **95**:2238–42.

89 Olsson R, Broome U, Danielsson A *et al.* Colchicine treatment of primary sclerosing cholangitis. *Gastroenterology* 1995;**108**:1199–203.

90 Jazrawi RP, de-Caestecker JS, Goggin PM *et al.* Kinetics of hepatic bile acid handling in cholestatic liver disease: effect of ursodeoxycholic acid. *Gastroenterology* 1994; **106**:134–42.

91 Lo SK, Hermann R, Chapman RW *et al.* Ursodeoxycholic acid in primary sclerosing cholangitis; a double blind controlled trial. *Hepatology* 1992:16.

92 van Milligen de Wit AW, Kuiper H, Camoglio L, van Bracht J, Jones EA, Tytgat GN, van Deventer SJ. Does ursodeoxycholic acid mediate immunomodulatory and anti-inflammatory effects in patients with primary sclerosing cholangitis? *Eur J Gastroenterol Hepatol* 1999; **11**:129–36.

93 O'Brien CB, Senior JR, Arora-Mirchandani R, Batta AK, Salen G. Ursodeoxycholic acid for the treatment of primary sclerosing cholangitis: a 30-month pilot study. *Hepatology* 1991;**14**:838.

94 Beuers U, Spengler U, Kruis W *et al.* Ursodeoxycholic acid for treatment of primary sclerosing cholangitis: a placebo-controlled trial. *Hepatology* 1992;**16**:707–14.

95 Stiehl A, Walker S, Stiehl L *et al.* Effect of ursodeoxycholic acid on liver and bile duct disease in primary sclerosing cholangitis. A 3-year pilot study with a placebo-controlled study period. *J Hepatol* 1994;**20**:57–64.

96 Lindor KD, The Mayo PSC/UDCA Study Group. Ursodiol for primary sclerosing cholangitis. *N Engl J Med* 1997; **336**:691–5.

97 Olsson R, Hagerstrand I, Broome U *et al.* Sampling variability of percutaneous liver biopsy in primary sclerosing cholangitis. *J Clin Pathol* 1995;**48**:933–5.

98 Stiehl A, Rudolph G, Sauer P, Theilmann L. Biliary secretion of bile acids and lipids in primary sclerosing cholangitis. Influence of cholestasis and effect of ursodeoxycholic acid treatment. *J Hepatol* 1995;**23**:283–9.

99 Hirano F, Tanaka H, Makino Y, Okamoto K, Makino I. Effects of ursodeoxycholic acid and chenodeoxycholic acid on major histocompatibility complex class I gene expression. *J Gastroenterol* 1996;**31**:55–60.

100 Mitchell SA, Bansi DS, Hunt N, von Bergmann K, Fleming KA, Chapman RW. A preliminary trial of high dose ursodeoxycholic acid in primary sclerosing cholangitis. *Gastroenterology* 2001;**122**:900–7.

101 van Hoogstraten HJ, Wolfhagen FJ, van de Meeberg PC, van Buren HR, Schaerm S. Ursodeoxycholic acid therapy for primary sclerosing cholangitis; single versus multiple doses. *J Hepatol* 1998;**29**:417–23.

102 Harnois DM, Angulo P, Jorgensen RA, La Russo NF, Lindor KD. High-dose ursodeoxycholic acid as a therapy for patients with primary sclerosing cholangitis. *Am J Gastroenterol* 2001;**96**:1558–66.

103 Chen W, Gluud C. Bile acids for primary sclerosing cholangitis (Cochrane Review). The Cochrane Library, Issue 4, 2003. Chichester, UK.

104 Rodrigues CM, Fan G, WongPY, Kren BT, Steer CJ. Ursodeoxycholic acid may inhibit deoxycholic acid-induced aopotosis bymodulating mitochondrial trans-membrane potential and reactive species production. *Mol Med* 1998;**4**:165–78.

105 Martinez JD, Stratagoules ED, La Rue JM *et al.* Different bile acids exhibit distinct biological effects. *Nutr Cancer* 1998;**31**:111–18.

106 Tung BY, Edmond MJ, Haggitt RC *et al.* Ursodiol use is associated with lower prevalence of colonic neoplasia in patients with ulcerative colitis and primary sclerosing cholangitis. *Ann Intern Med* 2001;**134**:89–95.

107 Wolf JM, Rybicki L,Lashner BA. Ursodeoxycholic acid is not chemoprotective for colorectal cancer in ulcerative colitis patients with primary sclerosing cholangitis [Abstract]. *Gastroenterology* 2001;**121**:2276.

108 Angulo P, Bharucha AE, Jorgensen RA *et al.* Oral nicotine in treatment of primary sclerosing cholangitis: a pilot study. *Dig Dis Sci* 1999;**44**:602–7.

109 Schramm C, Schirmacher P, Helmreich-Becker I *et al.* Combined therapy with azathioprine prednisolone and ursodiol in patients with primary sclerosing cholangitis. A case series. *Ann Intern Med* 1999;**131**:943–6.

110 Stiehl A, Rudolph G, Sauer P, Benz C *et al.* Efficacy of ursodeoxycholic acid treatment and endoscopic dilatation of major duct stenoses in primary sclerosing cholangitis. A 8 years prospective study. *J Hepatol* 1997;**26**:56–61.

111 Stiehl A, Rudolph G, Kloteis-Plodsky P, Samuel P, Walker S. Development of dominant bile duct stenoses in patients treated with ursodeoxycholic acid, outcome after endoscopic treatment. *J Hepatol* 2002;**36**:151–6.

112 Gow PJ, Chapman RW. Liver transplantation for primary sclerosing cholangitis. *Liver* 2000;**20**:97–103.

113 Farges O, Malassagne B, Sebagh M, Bismuth H. Primary sclerosing cholangitis: liver transplantation or biliary surgery. *Surgery* 1995;**117**:146–55.

114 Graziadei IW, Wiesner RH, Batts KP *et al.* Recurrence of primary sclerosing cholangitis following liver transplantation. *Hepatology* 1999;**29**:1050–6.

115 Vera A, Gunson BK, Ussatos V *et al.* Colorectal cancer in patients with inflammatory bowel disease after liver transplantation for primary sclerosing cholangitis. *Transplantation* 2003;**75**:1983–8.

116 Brandseter B, Broome U, Isoniemi H *et al.* Liver transplantation for primary sclerosing cholangitis: outcome after acceptance to the waiting list. *Liver Transpl* 2003;**9**:961–9.

31 Portal hypertensive bleeding

John Goulis, Andrew K Burroughs

Introduction

Portal hypertension is a major complication of chronic liver disease, most frequently cirrhosis, leading to the development of portosystemic collaterals of which the most clinically significant are those that form gastroesophageal varices. Variceal hemorrhage is the most serious complication of portal hypertension and is associated with a high mortality rate.[1]

In the past two decades several new therapeutic approaches have been introduced for the prevention and treatment of variceal bleeding. Currently in addition to sclerotherapy and surgical shunts, the therapeutic armamentarium for portal hypertensive bleeding has been considerably expanded by the introduction of pharmacological therapy with various vasoactive agents, the endoscopic ligation of esophageal varices and the transjugular intrahepatic portosystemic shunt (TIPS).

As a result the number of randomized clinical trials dealing with the treatment of portal hypertension is ever increasing. However, making therapeutic decisions is not easy, as most of the new treatments are inadequately or poorly evaluated in trials using heterogeneous criteria for the definition of their main endpoints and usually lacking adequate statistical power.

We evaluated randomized controlled trials for prevention of first bleeding, treatment of acute bleeding and prevention of recurrent bleeding from esophageal varices, using meta-analysis where applicable. The main endpoints selected for analysis were the following: (i) first bleeding episode (for primary prevention trials), or failure to control bleeding including very early re-bleeding (for trials of acute bleeding) or re-bleeding (for trials for prevention of re-bleeding) (ii) mortality (short term or long term) and (iii) incidence of complications. Pooled estimates of efficacy are presented as pooled odds ratios (POR), obtained by the Mantel–Haenszel method (fixed effect model) as modified by Robbins,[2] with 95% confidence intervals (CI). We used a statistical evaluation of heterogeneity by χ^2 test to assess whether the variation in treatment effect within trials of the same group was greater than might be expected. We considered heterogeneity to be present if $P < 0.05$; if so the calculation of POR was carried out by the DerSimonian and Laird method,[3] which is recommended for meta-analysis of studies with significant heterogeneity.

Natural history: prediction of the risk of bleeding

Development of varices

At the time of diagnosis of cirrhosis, varices are present in about 60% of decompensated and 30% of compensated patients.[1] The minimal portal pressure gradient or its equivalent hepatic venous pressure gradient (HVPG) threshold for the development of varices is 10–12 mmHg.[4] In most patients, esophageal varices enlarge over time, although regression of varices in a minority of patients has also been observed.[5] The presence and size of esophageal varices is associated with the severity of liver disease and continued alcohol abuse.[6] Portal hypertensive gastropathy has a prevalence of 80% in cirrhotic patients, with chronic bleeding in 11% and acute bleeding in 2·5% with mortality of 12·5% related to bleeding.[7]

Risk of first variceal bleeding

The incidence of variceal bleeding in unselected patients who have never previously bled is low (4·4/100 per year).[8] However mortality of the first bleeding episode is high (25–50%).[9] Hence the identification of patients with varices who will bleed before they do so is clearly important in order to offer effective prophylactic therapy to those who need it and avoid it in those who do not, particularly if the therapy is invasive or costly. The risk factors for the first episode of variceal bleeding in cirrhotic patients are the severity of liver dysfunction, large size of varices (increased tension of the variceal wall), and the presence of endoscopic red color signs. The combination of these three factors is the basis of the North Italian Endoscopic Club (NIEC) index for the prediction of the first variceal bleeding.[10] It is important to realize that patients with small varices and grade C severity cirrhosis are more at risk of first bleeding than patients with large varices and grade A severity cirrhosis, emphasizing the importance of liver dysfunction.[11] However, only a third of patients who present with variceal hemorrhage have the above risk factors.[12] Hence there is a need to define new predictive factors that could be combined in the NIEC index to improve its validity. The main interest has been the identification of haemodynamic factors that could more readily reflect the pathophysiological changes that lead to variceal bleeding. It is now well accepted that no bleeding occurs if HVPG falls below 12 mmHg[13] and the height of HVPG has been shown to be an independent risk factor of bleeding.[14] Finally variceal pressure has also been shown, prospectively, to be an independent predictive factor for the first variceal bleeding, and its addition to NIEC index could result in a significant gain in prognostic accuracy.[15]

Randomized controlled trials for prevention of first variceal bleeding

Shunt surgery versus non-active treatment

There have been four prophylactic shunt trials,[16–19] which were the first randomized controlled trials in portal hypertension, including 302 patients. A meta-analysis of these trials has been published.[1] Variceal bleeding was significantly reduced (odds ration (OR) 0·31, 95% CI 0·17 to 0·56) in the treated group but survival was significantly worse (OR 1·6, 95% CI 1·02 to 2·57). Alc In addition the risk of chronic or recurrent encephalopathy was significantly increased (OR 2·0, 95% CI 1·2 to 3·1) in shunted patients. In view of the mortality data and the serious adverse effects, prophylactic shunt surgery has been abandoned worldwide. Moreover the advent of liver transplantation removes any rationale for prophylactic surgery of any kind in cirrhotic patients.

Thus the results of Inokuchi *et al.* from Japan who compared devascularization procedures or selective shunts with non-active treatment,[20] showing a significant reduction in bleeding risk and mortality with prophylactic surgery, are not clinically relevant today. Moreover as the method of randomization is not clear the validity of the data is in question.

Sclerotherapy versus non-active treatment

The success of endoscopic sclerotherapy in the treatment of acute variceal bleeding led to extensive evaluation of sclerotherapy for the prevention of the first variceal bleed. There are 21 trials,[21–41] of which four were published in abstract form,[36–39] including a total of 1922 patients. The main characteristic of these trials was the statistically significant heterogeneity ($P < 0.001$) in the direction and size of the treatment effect on bleeding and death, so that meta-analysis is not justified. The first trials reported promising results with a reduction in bleeding rate, and in some a reduction in overall mortality.[22,28,29] However they were of

poor quality.[42] Subsequent larger trials did not confirm benefit and indeed some trials have suggested that prophylactic sclerotherapy is deleterious.[33,35] Alc In evaluating endoscopic sclerotherapy it must be remembered that it as an expensive and invasive treatment, which is associated with potentially serious complications. Hence prophylactic sclerotherapy would have to be clearly superior to no prophylactic treatment by a considerable margin before it could be recommended for widespread use.

Variceal ligation versus non active treatment

In recent years, endoscopic variceal ligation has replaced endoscopic sclerotherapy as the method of choice for the prevention of re-bleeding. In randomized trials and a meta-analysis, ligation was more effective than sclerotherapy in preventing re-bleeding, in part because it resulted in faster eradication of varices and had fewer complications.[43] Six trials of variceal ligation against no treatment have been carried out in patients with esophageal varices who have never bled. Given the published literature and the consensus on the use of non-selective β-blockers one would have expected that banding ligation would have been compared with β-blockade. Although these studies have been widely considered unethical they are commented on in this chapter as a background to the β-blocker versus banding studies.

The six studies included 612 patients with high risk esophageal varices[44–49] (Table 31.1). Variceal ligation significantly reduced the risk of first variceal bleeding (POR 4·26, 95% CI 2·85 to 3·37) and mortality (POR 2·44, 95% CI 1·70 to 3·51). A1 Although some adverse effects of variceal ligation (retrosternal pain, dysphagia, etc.) were transient, two patients died, one because of esophageal perforation related to the insertion of the overtube[45] and the other after postligation ulcer bleeding complicated by aspiration pneumonia.[46]

β-Blockers versus non-active treatment

The optimal prophylactic treatment should be easy to administer, have relatively few adverse effects, and be reasonably effective. Drug therapy potentially fulfills these criteria best. In addition, drug therapy has the potential to protect against gastric mucosal bleeding, which accounts for a sizeable proportion of first bleeding episodes.[50]

There are nine prophylactic trials using β-receptor blockade in cirrhotic patients with large varices,[31,35,38,51–56] comprising 996 patients; seven trials of propranolol[31,35,38,51,54–56] and two of nadolol[52,53] (Table 31.2). Seven trials were published as peer-reviewed articles[31,35,51–55] and two in only abstract form.[38,56] One of the latter trials[56] was an outlier reporting a very low bleeding rate in non-treated patients. This study caused statistically significant heterogeneity in the evaluation

Table 31.1 Randomized controlled trials of variceal ligation versus non-treatment for the primary prophylaxis of variceal bleeding

Study	Child C (%)	No. of patients	Event rate		ARR (95% CI)
			Variceal ligation	Controls	
Outcome: variceal bleeding					
Sarin et al.[44]	31	68	3/35	13/33	0·31 (0·12 to 0·5)
Lay et al.[45]	38	126	12/62	38/64	0·28 (0·15 to 0·41)
Lo et al.[46]	28	127	8/64	14/63	0·40 (0·25 to 0·56)
Svoboda et al.[48]	NR	102	15/52	27/50	0·1 (−0·03 to 0·23)
Chen and Chang[47]	NR	156	7/80	28/76	0·25 (0·07 to 0·44)
Gameel et al.[49]	NR	33	0/16	3/17	0·18 (0·05 to 0·36)
Total		612	45/309	123/303	0·24 (0·18 to 0·3)
Outcome: death					
Sarin et al.[44]	31	68	4/35	8/33	0·12 (−0·05 to 0·31)
Lay et al.[45]	38	126	17/62	37/64	0·22 (0·08 to 0·36)
Lo et al.[46]	28	127	16/64	23/63	0·30 (0·14 to 0·47)
Svoboda et al.[48]	NR	102	12/52	19/50	0·11 (−0·04 to 0·27)
Chen and Chang[47]	NR	156	15/80	31/76	0·15 (−0·03 to 0·33)
Gameel et al.[49]	NR	33	1/16	0/17	−0·06 (−0·18 to 0·06)
Total		612	65/309	149/303	0·12 (0·06 to 0·18)

NR, not reported; ARR, absolute risk reduction

Table 31.2 Randomized controlled trials of β-blockers versus non-active treatment for the prevention of first variceal bleeding

Study	No. of patients C/T	Child C (%)	Bleeding C/T	Death C/T
Pascal and Cales[51]	111/116	46	30/20	40/25
Ideo[52a]	49/30	–	11/1	9/3
Lebrec[53a]	53/53	–	10/7	10/10
Pasta[54]	89/85	7	31/18	28/37
Andreani et al.[31]	41/43	28	13/2	18/13
Conn et al.[55]	51/51	8	11/2	11/8
PROVA[35]	51/51	8	13/12	14/7
Strauss et al.[38b]	16/20	NR	4/4	7/7
Colman et al.[56b]	25/23	NR	2/8	7/6
POR (95% CI)			0·54 (0·39 to 0·74)	0·75 (0·57 to 1·06)

[a]Nadolol.

[b]Abstract only.

C, control; T, β-blockers; NR, not reported; POR, pooled odds ratio

of first bleeding in a comprehensive analysis evaluating the effect of β-blockade therapy in the prevention of variceal bleeding. The heterogeneity disappeared when this trial[56] was excluded from the analysis. There was a statistically significant bleeding risk reduction with β-blocker treatment when the outlier trial was included (OR 0·54, 95% CI 0·39 to 0·74) or excluded (OR 0·48, 95% CI 0·35 to 0·66).[56] The number of patients needed to be treated (NNT) with β-blockers to prevent one bleeding episode was estimated to be 11. There was no heterogeneity in the evaluation of

mortality in these trials ($P = 0.19$). Mortality reduced with β-blockers but not significantly so (OR 0·75, 95% CI 0·57 to 1·06).

β-Blockers have been shown to be effective independently of cause and severity of cirrhosis, presence of ascites and variceal size in an analysis of individual patient data from four of the above trials.[57] However bleeding may occur after stopping β-blocker therapy, suggesting that therapy should be maintained lifelong.[58] Finally, propranolol has been shown to prevent both acute and chronic bleeding from portal

Table 31.3 Randomized controlled trials of variceal ligation versus propranolol for the primary prophylaxis of variceal bleeding

Study	Child C (%)	No. of patients	Event rate Variceal ligation	Controls	ARR (95% CI)
Outcome: variceal bleeding					
Sarin *et al.*[62]	31	99	4/45	12/44	0·18 (0·03 to 0·34)
De *et al.*[63]	13	30	2/15	1/15	−0·07 (−0·28 to 0·15)
de la Mora *et al.*[64]	NR	24	1/12	1/12	0·00 (−22 to 22)
Jutabha *et al.*[65]	NR	35	0/18	1/17	0·059 (−0·053 to 0·17)
Psilopoulos *et al.*[66]	20	35	1/21	1/14	0·024 (−0·043 to 0·18)
Lui *et al.*[67]	33	100	3/44	9/66	0·07 (−0·04 to 0·18)
Schepke *et al.*[68]	12.5	152	19/75	22/77	0·032 (0·11 to 0·17)
Total		475	30/230	47/245	
Outcome: death					
Sarin *et al.*[62]	31	99	5/45	5/44	0·002 (−0·13 to 0·13)
De *et al.*[63]	13	30	NR	NR	
de la Mora *et al.*[64]	NR	24	1/12	1/12	0·00 (−0·22 to 0·22)
Jutabha *et al.*[65]	NR	35	NR	NR	
Psilopoulos *et al.*[66]	20	35	1/21	0/14	−0·048 (−0·14 to 0·044)
Lui *et al.*[67]	NR	100	11/44	18/66	0·02 (−0·14 to 0·19)
Schepke *et al.*[68]	12.5	152	34/75	32/77	−0·038 (−0·195 to 0·12)
Total		229	52/197	56/213	

NR, not reported; ARR, absolute risk reduction

hypertensive gastropathy in a single blind randomized study.[50] Ald Adverse effects of β-blockers are usually reversible after discontinuation of the drug, and no fatal complications have been reported.

β-Blockers versus nitrates

Evidence has been presented from a randomized trial first published in 1996[59] and completed by a long-term analysis in 2000[60] which showed that that the combination of nadolol and isosorbide dinitrate was more effective than nadolol alone for prevention of variceal bleeding.

In the latter study 146 patients with cirrhosis and known esophageal varices, but no bleeding, were treated for 7 years.[60] Sixteen in the nadolol group and eight in the combination group bled (logrank test, $P = 0.02$). The cumulative bleeding risk was 29% and 12%, respectively (95% CI for the difference 1–23%) Addition of isosorbide-5-mononitrate did not increase the incidence of liver failure, development of ascites or renal insufficiency; five patients requested discontinuation of nitrates due to adverse effects. However, the results of the most recent multicenter and larger randomized controlled trial are conflicting. In this study[61] a total of 349 cirrhotic patients with gastroesophageal varices were randomized to receive propranolol + placebo (n=174) or propranolol + isosorbide mononitrate (ISMN)

($n = 175$). There were no significant differences in the 1 and 2-year actuarial probability of variceal bleeding between the two groups (propranolol + placebo 8·3% and 10·6%, respectively; propranolol + ISMN, 5% and 12·5%, respectively). Survival was also similar. Adverse effects were significantly more frequent in the propranolol + ISMN group mainly due to a greater incidence of headache. The combination was otherwise safe and did not produce any deleterious effects on renal function.

β-blockers effectively prevent variceal bleeding. Adding nitrates does not further decrease the low residual risk of bleeding in patients receiving propranolol. In conclusion current data do not support a recommendation for alternative medication to non-selective β-blockers for primary prophylaxis of variceal bleeding. However the long-term combination drug therapy is generally safe and may be an alternative in clinical conditions associated with a greater risk of bleeding. Ald

Variceal ligation versus β-blockers

Recently, seven randomized trials, involving 475 patients, compared endoscopic band ligation of high risk esophageal varices to propranolol[62–68] (Table 31.3). In the first trial, Sarin *et al.*[62] found that ligation was more effective than propranolol for prevention of bleeding (actuarial survival, propranolol 43%, ligation 15%, $P < 0.05$). However, the rate of bleeding in the propranolol group was higher than has been observed in some other studies. This may be because of the lower mean dose of propranolol used (70 mg/day compared with 123 mg/day in previous studies). Alternatively, the difference in bleeding rates between groups may have occurred because of the relatively small number of patients studied and the resultant rather wide confidence intervals. The rate of bleeding in the propranolol group was the same as that in the non-treated group in a previous trial by the same authors in which the same selection criteria were used.[45] In the other six trials such a marked difference in the incidence of the first episode of variceal bleeding between the two treatment arms was not reproduced.[63-68] In the meta-analysis of the seven studies variceal ligation significantly reduced the risk of first variceal bleeding compared with propranolol (POR 1·61, 95% CI 0·98 to 2·66). However the same meta-analysis did not find any difference in terms of mortality, with a trend in a favor of drug treatment (POR 0·93, 95% CI 0·58 to 1·49). Alc

The conflicting results of these studies and the small number of patients randomized and events observed, as well as the cost of endoscopic variceal ligation, do not provide sufficient evidence for recommending any change in the current practice of prescribing propranolol as the treatment of first choice for the primary prevention of variceal bleeding.

Variceal ligation versus sclerotherapy

Variceal ligation was compared with sclerotherapy for the primary prevention of variceal bleeding in three small studies[69-71] of which one was published only in abstract form.[70] The results were conflicting. One study indicated that sclerotherapy was more effective,[71] the second that ligation was more effective[69] and the third that the two interventions are of similar efficacy.[70] Thus it is not surprising that there is significant heterogeneity in the meta-analysis ($P = 0.045$) for bleeding, and combining the data in a meta-analysis may not be justified. There was no significant difference for mortality (POR 0·84, 95% CI 0·35 to 2·05). Alc

Conclusion

The data from prophylactic trials suggest that screening for moderate and large varices in cirrhotic patients should be part of routine clinical practice, and if these are found, prophylactic treatment to prevent first variceal bleeding should be offered. Shunt surgery prevents bleeding but the increase in mortality and the long-term risk of encephalopathy make this treatment unacceptable. Prophylactic sclerotherapy should not be used as it is relatively ineffective, costly and potentially dangerous. The treatment of choice is prophylactic β-blocker therapy; it is inexpensive, easy to administer, and effective for prevention of the first variceal hemorrhage and of bleeding from gastric mucosa. Ald Primary prophylaxis with variceal ligation

appears to be safe and may be a reasonable alternative for: (i) patients with contraindications to β-blockers, (ii) patients who cannot tolerate or have no hemodynamic response to the drug therapy. However, it is unlikely to be a routine prophylactic treatment as it is much more expensive and less available than β-blockers and it will not prevent gastric mucosal bleeding. The trend towards increased mortality with banding needs further observation, as increased mortality was seen with prophylactic sclerotherapy.

Outcome of acute variceal bleeding

Acute variceal bleeding is a life-threatening complication in patients with cirrhosis and portal hypertension, with mortality that ranges from 30% to 50%.[1] Although overall survival may be improving, because of new therapeutic approaches, mortality is still closely related to failure to control hemorrhage or early re-bleeding, which is a distinct characteristic of portal hypertensive bleeding and occurs in as many as 50% of patients in the first days to six weeks after admission.[72,73] Factors that influence this failure in cirrhotic patients have been little studied. Severity of liver disease has been recognized as a risk factor for both early re-bleeding and short-term mortality after an episode of variceal bleeding.[12,73-75] Active bleeding during emergency endoscopy (for example, oozing or spurting from the ruptured varix) has been found to be a significant indicator of the risk of early re-bleeding.[74,75] Increased portal pressure (HVPG >16 mmHg) has been also proposed as a prognostic factor of early re-bleeding in an elegant study of continuous portal pressure measurement immediately after the bleeding episode,[76] and another study has shown that increased HVPG was related to increased failure to control bleeding and mortality.[77]

There is also a strong association between variceal hemorrhage and bacterial infection. Eight recent studies have shown that antibiotic therapy (with oral non-absorbable antibiotics,[78] and more recently with different quinolones or amoxicillin with clavulanic acid,[79-84] imipenem,[85] cefotaxime[86]) prevent bacterial infection in cirrhotic patients with gastrointestinal bleeding.[65-69] This was confirmed in a meta-analysis of these eight trials (significant beneficial effect on mortality (RR 0·70, 95% CI 0,56,089) and prevention of bacterial infections (RR 0·39, 95% CI 0,32,048).[87] Finally our group has recently shown that bacterial infection, diagnosed on admission, is an independent prognostic factor of failure to control bleeding or early re-bleeding.[74] These data may support a role of bacterial infection in the initiation of variceal bleeding.[88] A recent randomized trial has shown a reduction in early re-bleeding after acute bleeding, following prophylactic antibiotics.[82]

The clinician should be aware that most clinical trials have focused on esophageal varices, with very few designed to evaluate therapy for gastric varices. Gastric varices may lead to more severe bleeding initially, and tend to re-bleed frequently.[89] The following sections refer to esophageal varices unless specified.

Randomized controlled trials for the treatment of acute variceal bleeding

Pharmacologic treatment

Vasoactive drug treatment is the only treatment that does not require sophisticated equipment or the skills of a specialist and is immediately available, even before the patient is admitted to hospital, as has been shown recently.[90] Furthermore, as evidence suggests that those patients with high variceal or portal pressure are likely to continue to bleed or re-bleed early,[13,77] prolonged drug therapy that lowers portal pressure over days may be the optimal treatment. The vasoactive drugs that are currently used in the management of acute variceal bleeding are vasopressin, glypressin, somatostatin, octreotide and vapreotide. Vasopressin, which is a powerful vasoconstrictor lowers portal pressure through the induction of smooth muscle contraction, particularly in splanchnic arterioles. However the drug also causes systemic vasoconstriction which leads to serious side effects such as cardiac arrhythmias, myocardial ischemia, mesenteric ischemia and cerebrovascular episodes, resulting in cessation of therapy in up to 25% of cases.[91,92] Terlipressin is a synthetic analogue of vasopressin (triglycyl lysine vasopressin). It has an intrinsic effect as well as being converted *in vivo* into vasopressin by enzymatic cleavage of the triglycyl residues. This prolongs its biological half-life, so that a continuous intravenous infusion is unnecessary. Somatostatin has been used in the pharmacological treatment of variceal bleeding because of its reported ability to reduce splanchnic blood flow,[93] portal pressure and azygous blood flow[94] in cirrhotic patients although only the findings regarding the reduction in azygous flow are consistent. Bolus injections of somatostatin appear to have greater hemodynamic effects as compared with continuous infusion.[95] Finally octreotide has been reported to cause a reduction in portal pressure[96] and a transient decrease in azygous blood flow,[97] but there are some studies that did not confirm these data, using similar or even greater doses of the drug.[98]

Randomized controlled trials of vasoactive drug treatment of acute variceal bleeding

Drugs versus placebo (Table 31.4)

Vasopressin versus placebo

Vasopressin was compared with non-active treatment or placebo in four randomized controlled trials,[91,99–101] including only 157 patients. In two of these trials the intra-arterial route of administration was used.[91,99] There was a significant heterogeneity in the evaluation of failure to control bleeding. There was a clear trend in favor of vasopressin but the result was not statistically significant by the Der Simonian and Laird method (POR 0·23, 95% CI 0·05 to 1·02). Moreover there was no difference in mortality (POR 0·98, 95% CI 0·47 to 2·1). Alc Complications were reported in up to 64% of patients, which led to discontinuation of treatment in 25% of cases. In order to minimize the systemic complications of vasopressin, nitroglycerin has been added to the regime. This drug is a powerful venous dilator and reduces the portal vascular resistance and improves myocardial performance. Three randomized controlled trials have compared vasopressin alone with vasopressin plus nitroglycerin (transdermally,[92] sublingually,[102] and intravenously[103]), including 176 patients. Failure to control bleeding was significantly less common with vasopressin plus nitroglycerin (POR 0·39, 95% CI 0·21 to 0·72) but there was no difference in mortality (POR 0·94, 95% CI 0·49 to 1·79). Alc In two of the trials,[102,103] adverse effects were significantly reduced with the combination treatment. However nitroglycerin because of portocollateral shunting bypasses the liver, and can cause significant systemic effects. Hence this combination therapy must be monitored very closely and is less applicable as an immediate therapy.

Terlipressin versus placebo

The clinical efficacy of terlipressin has been evaluated in six randomized placebo-controlled studies,[90,104–108] including 388 patients. In two of the studies endoscopic sclerotherapy was employed at the initial diagnostic endoscopy.[90,108] In one of these the drug was given while the patient was transferred to hospital.[90] There was a statistically significant reduction in failure to control bleeding with terlipressin compared with placebo (POR 0·49, 95% CI 0·33 to 0·75) and more importantly the same meta-analysis showed that terlipressin is the only vasoconstrictor that significantly reduces mortality (POR 0·51, 95% CI 0·33 to 0·79). Alc However there is some criticism of these studies. The sample sizes were small, allowing a large type 2 error in the first three trials,[104–106] and the evidence in the early administration trial[90] of the effect of terlipressin, given only as three doses up to 8 hours, does not readily explain the apparent benefit on mortality (only in group C patients) or the control of bleeding.

Somatostatin versus placebo

Three placebo-controlled trials of somatostatin exhibit divergent results.[109–111] The trials by Valenzuela *et al.*[109] and Gotzsche *et al.*[111] suggested that somatostatin was no more effective than placebo. Unfortunately both studies had a very long recruitment period, suggesting marked patient selection. Moreover, Gotzsche *et al.*[111] did not evaluate the endpoint of

Table 31.4   Randomized controlled trials of drugs versus placebo for the treatment of the acute bleeding episode

Study	No. of patients C/T	Child C (%)	Failure to control bleeding (*n*) C/T	Death (*n*) C/T
Vasopressin v *placebo*				
Merigan *et al.* (1962)[99]	24/29	NR	24/13	23/28
Conn *et al.* (1975)[91]	16/17	NR	12/5	10/9
Mallory *et al.* (1980)[100]	20/18	NR	17/10	9/8
Fogel *et al.* (1982)[101]	19/14	NR	12/10	8/7
POR (95% CI)			0·23 (0·05 to 1·02)	0·98 (0·47 to 2·1)
Terlipressin v *placebo*				
Walker *et al.* (1986)[104]	25/25	50	12/5	8/3
Freeman *et al.* (1989)[105]	16/15	29	10/6	4/3
Soderlund *et al.* (1990)[106]	29/31	33	13/5	11/3
Pawels *et al.* (1994)[107]	14/17	NR	6/7	5/6
Levacher *et al.* (1995)[90]	43/41	81	23/12	20/12
Patch *et al.* (1999)[108]	66/66	62	40/37	28/22
POR (95% CI)			0·49 (0·33 to 0·75)	0·51 (0·33 to 0·79)
Somatostatin v *placebo or inactive treatment*				
Flati *et al.* (1986)[113]	16/19	40	9/2	7/4
Testoni *et al.* (1986)[114]	14/15	17	1/1	0/1
Loperfido *et al.* (1987)[112]	25/22	19	21/17	7/6
Valenzuela *et al.* (1989)[109]	36/48	32	9/21	10/15
Burroughs *et al.* (1990)[110]	59/61	41	35/22	7/9
Gotzsche (2003)[111]	44/42	NR	NR	16/16
POR (95% CI)			0·6 (0·21 to 1·65)[a]	1·2 (0·64 to 1·61)
Octreotide v *placebo*				
Burroughs *et al.* (1996)[115a]	139/123	40	85/71	37/35
variceal bleeding only	109/88	40	75/56	32/24
Octreotide v *placebo for early re-bleeding*				
Primignani *et al.* (1995)[116]	32/26		10/9[b]	
D'Amico *et al.* (1998)[117]	131/131	31	37/31[c]	20/26

[a]DerSimonian and Laird method.
[b]Evaluation at 30 days.
[c]Evaluation at 15 days.
POR, pooled odds ratio; C, placebo; T, drug; NR, not reported

failure to control bleeding, while Valenzuela *et al.*[109] reported an extremely high response rate (83%) in the placebo group (the highest ever reported). In contrast, the study by Burroughs *et al.*[110] reported a statistically significant benefit for somatostatin in controlling variceal bleeding over a 5-day treatment period. These differences in the reported results caused statistically significant heterogeneity (*P* = 0·006) in the meta-analysis of the six studies which compare somatostatin with placebo[109–111] or inactive treatment.[112–114] There was a trend in favor of somatostatin but the result was not statistically significant by the Der Simonian and Laird method (POR 0·6, 95% CI 0·21 to 1·65). There was no

difference in mortality between the two treatment groups (POR 1·02, 95% CI 0·64 to 1·61). Alc

Octreotide versus placebo

There is only one double blind randomized trial of octreotide versus placebo, the largest ever carried out to evaluate the efficacy of a vasoactive drug (*n* = 262)[115] in the management of acute variceal bleeding, currently available only in abstract form. In this study a continuous 5-day infusion of 50 micrograms/hour octreotide, started as soon as possible after admission was not more effective than placebo,

Table 31.5 Randomized controlled trials of comparisons between drugs for the treatment of the acute bleeding episode

Study	No. of patients C/T	Child C (%)	Failure to control bleeding (n) C/T	Death (n) C/T	Complications C/T
Vasopressin v vasopressin plus nitroglycerin					
Tsai et al. (1986)[102]	20/19	34	11/15	11/11	
Gimson et al. (1986)[103]	38/34	61	12/19	9/9	
Bosch et al. (1989)[92]	30/35	51	8/16	9/10	
Terlipressin v vasopressin					
Freeman et al. (1989)[124]	11/10	15	10/3	3/2	
Desaint et al. (1987)[125]	6/10	43	1/2	2/3	
Lee et al. (1988)[126]	24/21	27	16/17	8/10	
Chiu et al. (1988)[127]	28/26	60	13/13	10/12	
D'Amico et al. (1994)[128]	55/56	9	13/5	9/14	
POR (95% CI)			0·64 (0·36 to 1·14)	1·48 (0·85 to 2·6)	
Somatostatin v vasopressin					
Kravetz et al. (1984)[129]	31/30	41	13/14	17/16	22/3
Jenkins et al. (1985)[130]	12/10	54	8/3	4/2	2/0
Bagarani et al. (1987)[131]	25/24	69	17/8	10/6	3/1
Cardona et al. (1989)[132]	18/20	26	8/12	3/6	15/6
Hsia et al. (1990)[133]	24/22	65	15/10	15/14	11/4
Saari et al. (1990)[134]	22/32	46	10/11	15/22	11/1
Rodriguez-Moreno (1991)[135]	16/15	30	6/9	3/3	11/0
Somatostatin v terlipressin					
Feu et al. (1996)[136]	80/81	29	16/13	13/13	31/19
Walker et al. (1996)[137]	53/53	12	5/10	11/11	0/3
Octreotide v vasopressin					
Hwang et al. (1992)[138]	24/24	44	13/9	12/11	11/3
Octreotide v terlipressin					
Silvain et al. (1993)[140]	41/46	47	17/10	11/10	31/19

C, control; T, treatment; NR, not reported; POR, pooled odds ratio

whether or not injection sclerotherapy was needed for active bleeding or drug failure. Moreover, two other studies[116,117] using octreotide (100 micrograms 8-hourly, subcutaneously) or placebo after the control of the initial bleeding episode failed to show any difference in early re-bleeding or mortality between the two treatment groups. A1c

Drugs versus balloon tamponade

There have been six trials that compared vasoactive drugs and balloon tamponade. The drugs used were terlipressin in three studies,[118–120] somatostatin in two studies[121,122] and octreotide in one study.[123] Meta-analysis of these six trials showed that the drugs were as effective as balloon tamponade for prevention of failure to control bleeding (POR 1·04, 95% CI 0·63 to 1·72) or death (POR 0·65, 95% CI 0·36 to 1·16). A1c Sensitivity analysis showed that there was no difference according to the type of the drug. However, the sample sizes

were small and the endpoints not very clear, indicating that these results should be interpreted with caution. Tamponade if used properly, provides good control of bleeding. However the balloons should not be inflated for more than 12 hours and preferably less, and bleeding frequently recurs when the balloons are deflated. From the trial reports it is not always clear when efficacy is being assessed, for example during therapy or at the end of an interval of 24 hours after termination of drug therapy or tamponade.

Drugs versus drugs (Table 31.5)

Terlipressin versus vasopressin

Terlipressin was compared with vasopressin in five small, unblinded studies[124–128] involving only 247 patients. In two of these studies, vasopressin was associated with nitroglycerin.[127–128] Failure to control bleeding was less frequent with terlipressin, but the result was not statistically significant (POR 0·64, 95% CI 0·36 to 1·14). There was no difference in mortality between the two treatment arms (POR 1·48, 95% CI 0·85 to 2·57). Alc More importantly the complication rate was significantly lower with terlipressin even when vasopressin was combined with nitroglycerin.

Somatostatin versus vasopressin

Somatostatin was compared with vasopressin in seven trials including 301 patients.[129–135] Although these trials showed a trend in favor of somatostatin, the difference was not statistically significant (POR 0·74, 95% CI 0·47 to 1·16). There was no difference in mortality between the two vasoactive agents (POR 0·93, 95% CI 0·57 to 1·5). However, a statistically significant reduction in complications was observed in the group receiving somatostatin (POR 0·11, 95% CI 0·07 to 0·19) as the mean complication rate was 51% with vasopressin and only 10% with somatostatin. Alc

Somatostatin versus terlipressin

Two studies have compared somatostatin with terlipressin,[136,137] involving 267 patients. Both studies showed that the two drugs were similarly effective in preventing failure to control variceal bleeding and death. Moreover, in the larger of these studies,[136] a significantly lower incidence of complications in the somatostatin group was reported. Alc

Octreotide versus other drugs

The efficacy of octreotide treatment in comparison to other vasoactive drugs, for acute variceal bleeding, has not been adequately evaluated. Octreotide was found to be comparable to vasopressin in two low quality studies ($n = 89$ in total)[138,139] and to terlipressin plus nitroglycerin in another ($n = 87$ patients).[140] However the sample sizes were small and the trials may have lacked power to show differences, and the endpoints are not very clear, indicating that these results should be interpreted with caution. Ald

Recombinant activated factor VII

In a placebo-controlled double blind randomized trial, the recombinant factor VIIa was safe but no clearcut benefit in control of bleeding or mortality was seen.[141]

Randomized controlled trials of emergency sclerotherapy in the management of acute variceal bleeding

Injection sclerotherapy, first introduced in 1939 and "rediscovered" in the late 1970s, has rapidly become the endoscopic treatment of choice for the control of acute variceal bleeding over the past two decades. Paradoxically the best evidence for the value of sclerotherapy in the management of acute variceal bleeding has come from a more recently published study by the Veterans Affairs Cooperative Variceal Sclerotherapy Group.[142] In this study sclerotherapy, compared with sham sclerotherapy, stopped hemorrhage from actively bleeding esophageal varices (91% in sclerotherapy arm compared with 60% in sham sclerotherapy, $P < 0.001$, ARR = 29%, NNT = 3) and significantly increased hospital survival (75% v 51%, $P = 0.04$ ARR = 24%, NNT = 3). Alc

Today it is generally accepted that sclerotherapy should be carried out at the diagnostic endoscopy, which should take place as soon as possible, because there is evidence that this is beneficial compared with delayed injection.[143,144] No more than two injection sessions should be used to arrest variceal bleeding within a 5-day period.[72] Several sclerosing agents have been used for injection, polidocanol 1–3%, ethanolamine oleate 5%, sodium tetradecyl sulfate 1–2% and sodium morrhuate 5%. There is no evidence that any one sclerosant can be considered the optimal sclerosant for acute injection. As it has been shown that a substantial proportion of intravariceal sclerosant ends up in the paravariceal tissue and vice-versa there is no evidence that one technique is better than the other. One of the main shortcomings of sclerotherapy is the risk of local and systemic complications – although this varies greatly between trials and may be related to the experience of the operator.[145]

Sclerotherapy plus drugs/balloon tamponade versus drugs/balloon tamponade

Five trials with this clinical design comprised 413 patients: in three vasopressin was used[146–148] and in two octreotide[149] and somatostatin[150] (Table 31.6). The treatment effect was evaluated within 24 hours and up to 120 hours. Failure to control bleeding was significantly less common with sclerotherapy plus drugs than with drugs alone (POR 2·75, 95% CI 1·68 to 4·50), without significant heterogeneity ($P = 0.24$). The NNT with sclerotherapy to prevent one re-bleeding episode was 6 (95% CI 4 to 12). Alc Publication bias assessment showed that 15 null or negative studies would be needed to render the results of this meta-analysis non-significant. There was a trend toward fewer deaths in the sclerotherapy plus drugs arm than in the group treated with drugs alone but the difference was not significant (POR 1·37, 95% CI 0·85 to 2·20). The incidence of complications, when reported, varied considerably between trials with two of them stating that there were more complications in the sclerotherapy arm and one in the control arm.

Sclerotherapy versus drugs

Fifteen studies are summarized in Table 31.7: vasopressin[151] and terlipressin[152] were each used in one study, somatostatin

Table 31.6 Randomized controlled trials of sclerotherapy plus drugs/balloon tamponade versus drugs/balloon tamponade alone for the treatment of the acute bleeding episode

Study	Compared treatment	No. of patients S + D/D	Child C n (%)	Re-bleeding n (S + D/D)	Death n (S + D/D)	Complications n (S + D/D)
Soderlund and Ihre (1985)[146]	Vasopressin ± tamponade	57/50	70 (65)	3/8	16/18	10/8
Larson et al. (1986)[147]	Vasopressin ± tamponade	44/38	47 (57)	5/14	2/5	25/42[a]
Alexandrino et al. (1990)[148a]	Vasopressin/nitroglycerin ± tamponade	41/42	41 (49)	12/12	16/17	NR
Novella et al. (1996)[149a]	Octreotide	22/19	NR	3/7	3/2	NR
Villanueva et al. (1999)[150]	Somatostatin	50/50	25 (26)	7/21	7/10	11/4
POR (95%CI)				2·75 (1·68 to 4·50)	1·37 (0·85 to 2·20)	

[a]Abstract.
S+ D/D, sclerotherapy + drugs/drugs; NR, not reported; POR, pooled odds ratio

Table 31.7 Randomized controlled trials of sclerotherapy versus drugs for the treatment of the acute bleeding episode

Study	Compared treatment	No. of patients S/D	Child C n (%)	Re-bleeding n (S/D)	Death n (S/D)	Complications n (S/D)
Westaby et al. (1989)[151]	Vasopressin + nitroglycerin	33/31	22 (34)	4/11	9/12	NR
Di Febo et al. (1990)[155a]	Somatostatin	24/23	19 (40)	2/5	5/6	2/1
Shields et al. (1992)[153]	Somatostatin	41/39	42 (52·5)	7/9	8/12	12/5
Sung et al. (1993)[157]	Octreotide	49/49	43 (43)	13/15	20/14	18/5
Planas et al. (1994)[154]	Somatostatin	35/35	24 (34)	6/7	8/10	10/5
Poo[a] et al. (1996)[159a]	Octreotide	21/22	20 (47)	2/1	5/3	1/1
Jenkins et al. (1997)[158]	Octreotide	77/73	80 (53)	14/11	13/22	15/19
El-Jackie et al. (1998)[160a]						
Lopez et al. (1999)[161a]	Octreotide	50/50	NR	3/21	NR	NR
	Octreotide	33/31	NR	4/5	7/6	NR
Escorsell et al. (2000)[152]	Terlipressin	114/105	69 (31)	36/35	19/26	34/21
Bildozola et al. (2000)[162]	Octreotide	25/25	5 (10)	7/10	2/5	8/9
Freitas et al. (2000)[163]						
Sivri et al. (2000)[164]	Octreotide	53/58	39 (35)	12/12	8/13	NR
Yousuf et al. (2000)[165]	Octreotide	36/30	35 (53)	9/8	1/1	5/1
Ramires et al. (2000)[156]	Octreotide	48/48	20 (21)	2/4	5/5	6/8
	Somatostatin	19/21	12 (30)	5/5	6/6	NR
POR (95% CI)				1·55 (1·19 to 2·02)	1·40 (1·05 to 1·86)	0·79 (0·57 to 1·09)[b]

[a]Abstract
[b]Der Simonian and Laird method
S, sclerotherapy; D, drugs; NR, not reported; POR, pooled odds ratio

in four studies[153-156] and octreotide in nine studies,[157-165] involving 1324 patients. The evaluation of the treatment effect was done at the end of the infusion of the drug (from 48 hours to 120 hours). The overall efficacy of sclerotherapy was 85% (range 73–96%) in studies of 12–72 hours drug infusion[151,154-161,163-165] and 74% (68–84%) in studies of 120 hours drug infusion.[152,153,162] There was some heterogeneity [that was not statistically significant ($P = 0.067$)] in the evaluation of failure to control bleeding in these studies, that appeared to be due to differences in observed benefit from sclerotherapy rather than different outcomes in individual studies: only three of the 15 studies[57,158,163] reported a nonsignificant trend in favor of drugs over sclerotherapy. Failure to control bleeding was statistically significantly less frequent in patients randomized to sclerotherapy (Mantel–Haenszel method: POR 1·55, 95% CI 1·19 to 2·02). The NNT with sclerotherapy rather than drugs to avoid one

re-bleeding episode is 15 (95% CI 9 to 40). Alc Publication bias assessment showed that 15 null or negative studies would be needed to render the results of this meta-analysis non-significant. Sensitivity analyses including only (i) peer-reviewed articles[151-154,156-158,162-165] (POR 1·34, 95% CI 1·003 to 1·79), (ii) studies using only somatostatin or octreotide,[153-165] (POR 1·54, 95% CI 1·13 to 2·1), (iii) studies with 120 hours drug treatment[152,153,162] (POR 1·42, 95% CI 0·95 to 2·12) and (iv) studies with cirrhotic patients[151-159,161-165] (POR 1·27, 95% CI 0·96 to 1·69) always showed a strong trend in favor of sclerotherapy.

There was no significant heterogeneity in the evaluation of mortality in these studies: only two studies[156-157,159] reported lower mortality in the drug arm but in neither was this statistically significant. Overall there were statistically significantly fewer deaths in patients randomized to sclerotherapy (POR 1·40, 95% CI 1·05 to 1·86) The NNT to

Table 31.8 Randomized controlled trials of sclerotherapy plus drugs versus sclerotherapy alone for the treatment of the acute bleeding episode

Study	Compared treatment	No. of patients S/S+D	Child C *n* (%)	Re-bleeding *n* (S/S+D)	Death *n* (S/S+D)	Complications *n* (S/S+D)
Besson *et al.* (1995)[167]	Sclerotherapy + octreotide	101/98	73 (37)	25/11	12/12	33/34
Signorelli *et al.* (1996)[169a]	Sclerotherapy + somatostatin	30/33	NR	11/6	NR	NR
Brunati *et al.* (1996)[170a]	Sclerotherapy +octreotide/	27/28	NR	11/7	NR	NR
	Sclerotherapy + terlipressin	27/28	NR	11/6		
Signorelli *et al.* (1997)[171a]	Sclerotherapy + octreotide	42/44	NR	12/7	NR	NR
ABOVE (1997)[168]	Sclerotherapy + somatostatin	75/77	NR	48/31	24/27	37/37
Zuberi and Balock (2000)[172]	Sclerotherapy + octreotide	35/35	0 (0)	13/4	1/1	NR
Freitas *et al.* (2000)[163]	Sclerotherapy + octreotide	42/44	29 (37)	18/9	13/12	NR
Cales *et al.* (2001)[166]	Sclerotherapy + vapreotide	98/98	73 (37)	49/33	7/5	8/6
POR (95% CI)				0·42 (0·3 to 0·6)	1·0 (0·68 to 1·48)	

[a]Abstract.

S, sclerotherapy; S+D, sclerotherapy plus drugs; NR, not reported; POR, pooled odds ratio

avoid one death is 23 (95% CI 12 to 730). Alc Publication bias assessment showed that four null or negative studies would be required to render the results of this meta-analysis non-significant.

Finally the type of complications recorded in 10 studies[152–155,157–159,162,164,165] differed considerably, resulting in a significant heterogeneity ($P = 0.05$). Five studies reported more complications in the sclerotherapy arm[153–155,157,163] while four reported more complications[152,158,165,166] in the drug arm and one found equal numbers in both arms.[159] The meta-analysis showed a trend in favor of drug treatment but the result was not statistically significant (Der Simonian and Laird method: POR 0·79, 95% CI 0·57 to 1·09).

Sclerotherapy plus drugs versus sclerotherapy alone

Eight trials[163,166–172] comprised this group (Table 31.8). Two trials, published as abstracts, assigned patients to three treatment arms[169,170] and each comparison with sclerotherapy was evaluated separately (for Signorelli *et al.*'s trial the results

1 year later[171] were used for the octreotide comparison). Hence nine comparisons of sclerotherapy plus drugs (two somatostatin, five octreotide, one vapreotide and one terlipressin) versus sclerotherapy alone in eight studies[166–173] including 962 patients were analyzed. Five studies were placebo-controlled[166–169,172] while three were not.[163,170,171] In six studies the drug was administered for 120 hours[166–169,172] while in two for 48 hours.[163,170] The efficacy of sclerotherapy was only 58% in the 48 hours studies[163,170] and 60% (range 35–88%) in the 120 hours studies.[166–169,172] Re-bleeding was statistically significantly less frequent in patients randomized to sclerotherapy plus drugs (POR 0·42, 95% CI 0·3 to 0·6). The NNT to avoid one re-bleeding episode was 7 (95% CI 5 to 13). Alc Publication bias assessment showed that 47 null or negative studies would be needed to render the results of this meta-analysis statistically non-significant. However, there were equal number of deaths between the two treatment arms and the result was not statistically significant (POR 1·0, 95% CI 0·68 to 1·48). Although it is common to find no survival rate differences between treatments in trials of acute variceal bleeding, one might have expected a trend for lower

mortality in the combined treatment group, given the strongly significant reduction in bleeding, a very marked biological difference.

Only two studies provided data on complications.[148,149] There were no significant differences between the two treatment arms in these studies.

Sclerotherapy versus variceal ligation

Only four studies have been specifically designed to compare sclerotherapy with variceal ligation for the management of the acute bleeding episode.[173-176] Other data come from 10 studies of long-term sclerotherapy versus variceal ligation[177-186] (Table 31.9). There was no statistical heterogeneity ($P = 0.26$) in the analysis of failure to control bleeding from the 14 studies,[173-186] including a total of 841 patients. Meta-analysis showed that initial failure to control bleeding was significantly less common with variceal ligation than with sclerotherapy (POR 0.51, 95% CI 0.34 to 0.79). The NNT with variceal ligation rather than with sclerotherapy to prevent one episode of failure to control bleeding was 15 (95% CI 9 to 44). Alc Publication bias assessment showed that 14 null or negative studies would be needed to render the results of the meta-analysis statistically non-significant. Short-term mortality was reported only in two studies[173,174]: in both there was a trend in favor of variceal ligation but the result was not statistically significant. Finally, only the two studies specifically designed to compare emergency sclerotherapy with variceal ligation[173,174] reported incidence of complications. Complications were less frequent in the variceal ligation arm in both studies and the result reached statistical significance in one.[174]

Randomized controlled trials of emergency surgery in the management of acute variceal bleeding

Four randomized trials, carried out in the 1980s, compared sclerotherapy to emergency staple transection.[187-190] Failure to control bleeding was reported only in two of these studies, with divergent results. Teres *et al.*[189] reported that efficacy of transection in their study was only 71%, the lowest in the literature, compared with 83% in the sclerotherapy arm. In contrast, in the largest study by Burroughs *et al.*,[190] a 5-day bleeding-free interval was achieved in 90% of the patients who underwent transection (none re-bled from varices) compared with 80% in those who had two emergency injection sessions. There was no difference in mortality between the two treatment modalities. Cello *et al.* showed that emergency portacaval shunt was more effective than emergency sclerotherapy (followed by elective sclerotherapy) in preventing early re-bleeding (19% *v* 50%).[191] Hospital and 30-day mortality were not significantly different. Finally

Orloff *et al.*[192] in a small study, reported that portacaval shunt, carried out in less than 8 hours from admission, was significantly better than medical treatment (vasopressin/balloon tamponade) in the control of acute variceal bleeding. Survival was also better in the patients who had shunts but the difference was not statistically significant. Ald

Randomized controlled trials of novel endoscopic therapies in the management of acute variceal bleeding

Tissue adhesives

Two types of tissue adhesives (*n*-butyl-2-cyanoacrylate, Histoacryl and isobutyl-2-cyanoacrylate, Bucrylate) have been used for the control of variceal bleeding.[193] The adhesives could offer better immediate control of bleeding because they harden within seconds upon contact with blood. However extra care must be taken to ensure that the adhesive does not come into contact with the endoscope and block the channels of the instrument. This can be prevented if the adhesive is mixed with lipiodol to delay hardening. Moreover, the sclerotherapy needle must be carefully placed within the varix prior to injection, to avoid leak of the adhesive.[193] A small randomized trial showed that cyanoacrylate was superior to conventional sclerotherapy with 3% ethanolamine oleate solution for control of bleeding and reduction of hospital mortality in Child–Pugh class C patients.[194] Two randomized controlled trials compared sclerotherapy alone with the combination of sclerotherapy and *n*-butyl-2-cyanoacrylate for the control of active variceal bleeding.[195,196] The combined treatment was more effective than sclerotherapy alone in both studies. Moreover, in two studies *n*-butyl-2-cyanoacrylate was compared with variceal ligation for the control of bleeding from esophageal[197] or esophagogastric varices.[198] The overall success rate for initial hemostasis of both treatment modalities was similar in these studies. However, *n*-butyl-2-cyanoacrylate was superior to variceal ligation for the control of fundal variceal bleeding, but it was less effective for the prevention of re-bleeding (67% *v* 28%). Finally, in a small study,[199] a biological fibrin glue (Tissucol) was more effective than sclerotherapy with polidocanol in the prevention of early re-bleeding and had a significantly lower incidence of complications. More studies are necessary to confirm these data and examine the potential risks of activation of coagulation, systemic embolism and transmission of infections with the human plasma-derived fibrin glue.

An endoscopic detachable snare is another ligation device which has the advantage of allowing an unlimited number of ligations by reloading the nylon minisnare while the endoscope remains in the esophagus. The first prospective randomized trial showed that the minisnare performed

Table 31.9 Randomized controlled trials of sclerotherapy versus variceal ligation for the prevention of re-bleeding

Study	No. of patients (S/L)	Child C (%)	Failure of initial hemostasis	Re-bleeding S/L	Death S/L	Variceal obliteration S/L	Variceal recurrence S/L
Stiegmann et al. (1992)[177]	65/64	19	3:13/2:14	31/23	29/18	22/27	11:22/9:27
Laine et al. (1993)[178]	39/38	23	1:9/1:9	17/10	6/4	27/22	
Gimson et al. (1993)[179]	23/21	26	3/3	26/16	17/21	27/32	
Jensen et al. (1993)[173]	18/14	NR	0/3	9/6	3/2	NR	
Mundo et al. (1993)[260]	11/8	37	NR	3/2	4/2	4/4	
Young et al. (1993)[261]	13/10	78	NR	5/2	4/2	11/9	
Lo et al. (1995)[180]	59/61	48	3:15/1:18	30/20	19/10	37/45	
Hou et al. (1995)[181]	67/67	39	2:16/0:20	28/13	11/14	53/58	
Jensen et al. (1993)[173]	26/24	NR	NR	9/7	9/4	NR	
Jain et al. (1996)[182]	24/22	46[a]	2/3	5/9	NR	24/20	2:24/5:20
Mostafa et al. (1996)[183]	89/69	NR	1:21/1:18	9/6	2/3	82/63	7:82/12:63
Baroncini et al. (1997)[263]	54/57	27	NR	10/9	12/12	50/53	7:50/17:53
Lo et al. (1997)[174]	34/37	60	8/1	10/6	12/7	NR	
Sarin et al. (1997)[184]	48/47	14	1:7/1:5	10/3	3/3	45/44	3:45/10:44
Masci et al. (1997)[264]	50/50	NR	NR	26/16	10/12	41/43	6:37/11:37
Avgerinos et al. (1997)[265]	40/37	8	NR	19/10	8/8	39/35	17:39/11:35
Shiha and Farag (1997)[185]	43/42	NR	4:19/2:17	10/6	2/2	37/37	6:37/11:37
Fakhry et al. (1997)[186]	41/43	NR	1:17/1:18	6/7	NR	40/42	8:41/9:42
de la Pena et al. (1998)[266]	46/42	NR	NR	23/13	10/8	29/31	13:29/19:31
Shafqat et al. (1998)[175]	28/24	NR	6/1	NR	6/3	NR	NR
Salem et al. (1999)[176]	180/180	NR	32/16	NR	NR	NR	
POR (95% CI)			0·51 (0·34 to 0·79)	0·53 (0·42 to 0·67)	0·77 (0·59 to 0·99)	1·23 (0·93 to 1·61)	1·36 (0·96 to 1·92)

S, sclerotherapy; L, variceal ligation; NR, not reported; POR, pooled odds ratio

equally well when compared with a multiple variceal ligator.[200] Ald

Gastric varices

The reported incidence of bleeding from gastric varices varies between 3% and 30%, but in most series it is less than 10%.[201] Patients with gastric variceal hemorrhage bleed more profusely and require more transfusions than patients with esophageal variceal bleeding.[202] Moreover these patients have a higher risk of re-bleeding and a decreased survival rate compared with patients bleeding from esophageal varices.[202] The optimal treatment of gastric variceal bleeding is not known. Limited information is available on the role of vasoactive drugs in the control of gastric fundal bleeding and balloon tamponade has been used with little success. Use of standard sclerosants is associated with unacceptable re-bleeding, particularly from necrotic ulceration, as the gastric mucosa appears much more sensitive to this than the esophagus.

Because of this, alternative sclerosant agents have been evaluated. The tissue adhesives *n*-butyl-2-cyanoacrylate and isobutyl-2-cyanoacrylate, mixed with lipiodol, to delay premature hardening, have been evaluated, and found to be efficacious in observational studies.[195,203] Isobutyl-2-cyanoacrylate has been shown to be superior to ethanolamine, in a non-randomized study,[204] achieving hemostasis in 90% of 23 patients, as opposed to 67% of 24 patients ($P < 0.005$).

In a recent randomized controlled trial of 37 patients with isolated fundic varices (acute and recent bleeding)[205] with follow up of 15 months, cyanoacrylate glue was shown to be more effective than alcohol sclerotherapy for variceal obliteration (100% *v* 44%, $P < 0.005$). There was a trend in favor of cyanoacrylate glue for the control of acute bleeding (89% *v* 62%) and the need of surgical intervention (10% *v* 35%), although both were statistically non-significant. Mortality was similar in the two groups. Ald

However, reports of cerebral embolism, with the tissue adhesives identified in the cerebral circulation at post mortem as well splenic embolisation and development of retrogastric abscesses, are worrying, as well splenic embolization and development of retrogastric abscesses and interest has therefore focused on thrombin. This is much easier to administer, and has been shown to provide good early hemostasis.[206] However, in all of these studies, re-bleeding rates have remained high. Hence in patients with re-bleeding or uncontrolled bleeding from gastric varices devascularization surgery or portosystemic shunting has been proposed.[207] It has been shown that "salvage" TIPS is very effective in this situation, with more than 95% success rate for initial hemostasis and an early re-bleeding rate of less than 20%.[201] TIPS appears to be as effective for gastric varices as for esophageal varices.

Non-actively bleeding patients with fundal varices constitute a discrete population. The efficacy of cyanoacrylate in these patients is controversial and bleeding rates in this group can be relatively high. The Japanese experience with balloon-occluded transvenous obliteration as a prophylactic procedure in this patient population appears promising.[208] TIPS, shunt surgery, and of course, liver transplantation are the only other therapeutic options for recurrent bleeding from gastric varices.

Uncontrolled variceal bleeding

Uncontrolled variceal bleeding despite adequate endoscopic and pharmacologic therapy represents a difficult management problem. A large consensus conference failed to agree on a suitable definition for this condition,[209] and this is further complicated by the different behavior of varices in different locations (esophageal or gastric varices) and the varying therapies that are available.

The definition that is commonly used for uncontrolled esophageal variceal bleeding is continued variceal bleeding despite two sessions of emergency endoscopic interventions and vasoactive therapy during a 7-day period, or bleeding past a Sengstaken-Blakemore tube independent of the number of sclerotherapy sessions. Bleeding from gastric varices is said to be uncontrolled when hemorrhage persists despite vasoconstrictor therapy.[209]

There are no randomized controlled trials evaluating different "salvage" therapies in uncontrolled variceal bleeding. However the advent of TIPS has offered a valuable option in this condition. TIPS is an interventional radiologic procedure which involves the creation of a communication between hepatic vein and an intrahepatic branch of the portal vein, thus decompressing the portal venous system. Hence TIPS functions in a similar way to surgical shunts. However, the morbidity and mortality due to the procedure is much more favorable. It has been shown in uncontrolled studies that emergency TIPS is highly effective as salvage therapy in patients with uncontrolled esophageal or gastric variceal bleeding.[201,210] This treatment is the best option for patients with poor liver function awaiting liver transplantation. B3

Conclusion

The available data suggest that emergency endoscopic treatment with banding ligation or sclerotherapy, at the time of the initial diagnostic endoscopy, should be the gold standard for the management of the acute variceal bleeding episode. Sclerotherapy may be more applicable in some acute situations compared with ligation. A diagnostic endoscopy, with visualization unhindered by the ligation device, should be done first as varices may not be the source of bleeding. If a double intubation is considered (placing the ligation device after diagnosis) then this could increase the risk of complications and does lengthen the procedure.

Sclerotherapy is also significantly better than drug treatment alone and there is no need for further studies directly comparing sclerotherapy or ligation with one of the currently available drugs. However, the combination of sclerotherapy with a drug, given as soon as possible after admission, has shown promising results and should be further tested in randomized controlled trials. The drugs of choice for this combination are terlipressin (as mortality is reduced albeit in small placebo-controlled studies) and somatostatin (which has less side effects and has been successfully tested over 5 days). Further studies are needed to assess the role of tissue adhesives or fibrin glues in patients unresponsive to vasoactive drugs or sclerotherapy.

The role of emergency TIPS as "salvage therapy" for uncontrolled bleeding from esophageal or gastric varices has been justified, although randomized trials to compare it with emergency surgical shunts or other therapies are still required.

Prevention of recurrent variceal bleeding

Patients surviving the first episode of variceal bleeding are at very high risk of recurrent bleeding (70% or more) and death (30–50%). There is a general consensus that all patients who have previously bled from varices should have secondary therapy to prevent further variceal bleeding.[12] There is no role for an observational policy, as all randomized studies have shown active therapy to be better than observation alone. Hence, in clinical practice the risk indicators of long-term re-bleeding are of less clinical value, than those for first variceal bleeding. However severity of liver disease,[8] continued alcohol abuse[6] and variceal size has been associated with variceal re-bleeding. A recent development has been the proposed use of hemodynamic indices to identify patients who are more likely to re-bleed. Two such indices have been reported, using the technique of hepatic wedge pressure measurement as an indicator of portal pressure. From the analysis of the Barcelona-Boston-New Haven Primary Prophylaxis trial, it was concluded that variceal bleeding did not occur with an HVPG < 12 mmHg, in patients with predominantly sinusoidal portal hypertension.[211] However with an HVPG >12 mmHg, the correlation between portal pressure and bleeding risk is inconsistent.

An alternative hemodynamic index has been proposed by Feu *et al.*[212] Patients who had a percentage reduction of HVPG of 20% or more from baseline had a re-bleeding rate of 15% compared with 50% in those who did not achieve this hemodynamic target. Unfortunately, these HVPG targets are achieved in only about a third of patients on β-blockers – hence the introduction of combined pharmacologic therapy. Several studies on secondary prevention have used hemodynamic monitoring during combination pharmacotherapy in their design. In these studies the target values are reached only in 45–60% of patients subjected to therapy with β-blockers and nitrates. Moreover, because most re-bleeding episodes occur within 1 month of the index bleed, early repeat HVPG measurements are needed in order to identify the non-responders. However, the above approach, has not been confirmed in one study[213] and has been questioned regarding its clinical applicability and utility.[214]

The options facing the clinician are numerous, including pharmacologic, endoscopic and surgical/radiological therapies.

Randomized controlled trials for the prevention of variceal re-bleeding

β-blockers versus no treatment

A comprehensive meta-analysis of 12 trials comprising 769 patients[56,214–224] has been published.[225] The mean follow up was 21 ± 5 months. There was significant heterogeneity in the evaluation of re-bleeding ($P < 0.01$). Treatment with β-blockers significantly decreased the risk of re-bleeding (Der Simonian and Laird method: POR 21%, 95% CI 10 to 32%). The NNT with β-blockers to prevent one re-bleeding episode was 5. Survival was also significantly improved in patients treated with β-blockers. (Der Simonian and Laird method: POR 5·4%, 95% CI 0 to 11%) although there was significant heterogeneity in this analysis ($P < 0.01$). The NNT needed to be treated to prevent one death is 14. Adverse events occurred in 17% of patients and were generally mild. No fatal complication has been reported with β-blockers. Ald

The use of the recently proposed hemodynamic targets (for example 20% reduction of HVPG and/or fall < 12 mmHg) to identify patients who are "non-responders" to pharmacological therapy could be a useful tool in the planning of treatment for secondary prevention of variceal bleeding. These patients could then be offered alternative therapy such as variceal ligation, or combination drug therapies, before they have further bleeding. The applicability of hemodynamic monitoring has been questioned.[214] β-blockers in association with oral nitrates have been shown to induce a greater drop in portal pressure than β-blockers alone.[226] Other drugs that may work in combination with β-blockers include angiotensin-converting enzyme (ACE) inhibitors and angiotenin-II receptor antagonists,[227] α-adrenoreceptor antagonists like prazosin[228] and spironolactone,[229] but problems with their adverse effects particularly hypotension, and lack of efficacy preclude their use.

β-blockers plus nitrates versus β-blockers alone

The rationale behind the use of combination therapy is that agents acting through different mechanisms may be additive

Table 31.10 Randomized controlled trials of sclerotherapy versus β-blockers for the prevention of re-bleeding

Study	No. of patients D/S	Child C (%)	Bleeding D/S	Death D/S	Adverse events D/S
Alexandrino et al.[237]	34/31	–	25/17	11/9	24/28
Dollet et al.[238]	27/28	27	11/18	12/15	0/10
Fleig et al.[239]	57/58	NR	26/26	16/20	NR
Westaby et al.[240]	52/56	–	29/28	22/21	4/0
Liu et al.[241]	58/60	NR	33/20	27/17	NR
Martin et al.[242]	34/42	24	18/23	8/13	0/19
Rossi et al.[221]	27/26	38	13/13	7/6	3/8
Andreani et al.[243]	35/40	35	12/17	9/17	ND
Dasarathy et al.[244]	53/51	34	31/19	19/10	5/9
Teres et al.[245]	58/58	14	37/26	23/21	10/23
Villanueva et al.[246]**	43/43		11/23	4/9	
POR (95% CI)			0·88 (0·58 to 1·32)	0·95 (0·72 to 1·25)	

[a]All trials used propranolol except one.
**Nadolol plus isosorbide mononitrate.
D, drug; S, sclerotherapy; NR, not reported; POR, pooled odds ratio

or synergestic in terms of their benefit. In a recent randomized trial the addition of ISMN significantly improved the efficacy of propranolol alone in the prevention of variceal re-bleeding – but only after stratification according to age (i.e. < 50 years of age v > 50 years of age; $P = 0.03$), or after evaluation of prolonged follow up (3 years; $P = 0.05$).[230] However, no significant difference was found in the overall rate of re-bleeding and survival. Moreover, more patients in the combination treatment group had to discontinue therapy due to adverse effects.[230] AId Similarly no additional benefit from the combination of β-blockers and ISMN was reported in an abstract.[231] Of note is that in this study, a higher mortality was observed in the combination-therapy group. Recently, combination therapy and its effectiveness in preventing re-bleeding was assessed by hemodynamic monitoring. Although the number of patients studied was small ($n = 34$) and the β-blocker dose was fixed (160 mg of long acting propranolol) the investigators reported that the addition of ISMN increased the number of responders (HVPG < 12 mmHg or > 20% from baseline value) from 38% to 59%, and these patients experienced less bleeding (10% v 64% for non-responders; $P < 0.05$).

Sclerotherapy versus no treatment

There are 8 trials including 1111 patients.[146,221,232–236] The re-bleeding rate was reduced in all studies except one.[232] Meta-analysis showed that the pooled odds ratio was significantly reduced (POR 0·63, 95% CI 0·49 to 0·79). Mortality was also reduced significantly in the sclerotherapy arm (POR 0·77, 95% CI 0·61 to 0·98). However complications were frequent and did not differ from those of prophylactic or emergency sclerotherapy. AId

Sclerotherapy versus drugs

Eleven trials, involving 971 patients compared sclerotherapy with drugs (propranolol in 10 studies[221,237–245] and nadolol plus ISMN in one study[246]) for the prevention of recurrent bleeding (from any source, for example varices, portal hypertensive bleeding, or sclerotherapy ulcers) (Table 31.10). There was a striking heterogeneity in the evaluation of re-bleeding ($P = 0.004$): in five studies[221,238,242,243,246] re-bleeding was less frequent in patients randomized to drugs and in six in patients randomized to sclerotherapy.[237,239–241,244,245] The POR showed that there was no significant difference between the two treatment modalities (Der Simonian and Laird method: POR 0·88, 95% CI 0·72 to 1·25). There was no significant heterogeneity in the evaluation of survival ($P = 0.15$). More patients randomized to sclerotherapy survived but the result was not statistically significant (POR 0·95, 95% CI 0·58 to 1·32). Moreover, the number of patients free of adverse events was significantly higher in the drug group compared with sclerotherapy group (POR 0·85, 95% CI 0·65 to 1·11). AIc

Sclerotherapy plus drugs versus sclerotherapy

Twelve trials of sclerotherapy and drugs (eight propranolol,[247–254] three nadolol[255–257] and one isosorbide-5-mononitrate[258]) versus sclerotherapy alone, comprising 853 patients are summarized in Table 31.11). Theoretically the drug might prevent re-bleeding before variceal obliteration. One problem with this group of studies is that in only one study was the effect of β-blockers evaluated after obliteration.[248] In the others, the drug was stopped at eradication. There was statistically significant heterogeneity caused by differences

Table 31.11 Randomized controlled trials of sclerotherapy plus drugs versus sclerotherapy for the prevention of re-bleeding

Study	No. of patients S/S + D	Child C (%)	Bleeding S/S + D	Death S/S + D
Westaby et al.[247]	27/26	41	8/7	7/9
Jensen and Krarup[248]	26/25	29	12/3	1/1
Lundell et al.[249]	22/19	51	11/12	NR
Bertoni et al.[255]	14/14	36	4/1	3/1
Gerunda et al.[256]	30/30	NR	7/6	3/1
Villaneuva et al.[257]	35/39	NR	14/7	5/5
Avgerinos et al.[251]	40/45	7	21/14	9/8
Villanueva et al.[257]	18/22	NR	7/12	0/2
Acharya et al.[253]	56/58	NR	12/10	7/5
Vickers et al.[252]	34/39	34	14/17	9/9
Bertoni et al.[258]	37/39		15/4	9/2
Elsayed et al.[254]	87/91		34/13	10/11
POR (95% CI)			0·54 (0·34 to 0·86)[a]	0·65 (0·43 to 0·97)

[a]Der Simonian and Laird method
S, sclerotherapy; S + D, sclerotherapy plus drugs; NR, not reported; POR, pooled odds ratio

between studies both in the direction and in the size of the effect of treatment: three studies were in favor of sclerotherapy alone[249,252,257] while nine were in favor of sclerotherapy plus β-blockers[247,248,250,251,253–256,258] (statistically significant difference reported in three[248,254,258]). POR showed that there was statistically significantly less re-bleeding in the combined treatment arm (Der Simonian and Laird method: POR 0·54, 95% CI 0·34–0·86). There was no statistically significant heterogeneity in the evaluation of survival. There were statistically significantly fewer deaths in the combined treatment arm (POR 0·65, 95% CI 0·43–0·97). Ald

Combination sclerotherapy plus subcutaneous octreotide was also compared with sclerotherapy alone for the prevention of early re-bleeding, as well as for long-term management of patients after variceal hemorrhage.[259] This last study showed significantly less re-bleeding and mortality rates in the combined treatment group. However, the possibility of a severe selection bias was raised due to the exceedingly high re-bleeding rates in the sclerotherapy group. Therefore the clinical efficacy of subcutaneous octreotide in reducing re-bleeding rates remain uncertain, despite the post-prandial increase in portal pressure being blunted by octreotide but not by propranolol.[259]

Sclerotherapy versus variceal ligation

Sclerotherapy does significantly decrease re-bleeding rates and mortality, but it has been associated with serious complications, the most common of which are esophageal stricture and bleeding from treatment-induced ulcers. Variceal ligation was developed with the aim to provide an endoscopic therapy at least as effective as sclerotherapy, but with fewer complications. There are 20 studies[173–186,260–265] (n = 1634)

comparing sclerotherapy to variceal ligation for the prevention of recurrent bleeding: 11 were published as peer-reviewed articles[174,175,177–191,184,261,263,265] and nine as abstracts[173,176,182,183,185,186,260,262,264] (see Table 31.9). Thirteen studies included only cirrhotic patients,[173,174,177–181,260–265] six studies patients with cirrhosis or non-cirrhotic portal hypertension,[175,176,182–185] and one study only patients with hepatic fibrosis due to schistosomiasis.[186] The sclerosing agent used was sodium tetradecyl sulfate (eight trials[173,174,177,178,180,181,261,262]), ethanolamine oleate (four trials[179,183,186,265]), polidocanol (two trials[260,263]), absolute alcohol (one trial[184]) and was not reported in five studies.[175,176,182,185,264] The same ligation equipment (Bard Interventional Products, Tewksbury, Massachusetts, USA) was used in all trials. All treatment sessions were done at intervals of 1–3 weeks. Meta-analysis showed that re-bleeding was significantly less common with variceal ligation than with sclerotherapy (POR 0·53, 95% CI 0·42 to 0·67), without significant heterogeneity amongst trials. The NNT with variceal ligation than with sclerotherapy to prevent one re-bleeding episode is 10 (95% CI 7 to 17). Ald Publication bias assessment showed that 121 null or negative studies would be needed to render the results of the meta-analysis statistically non-significant. Variceal ligation was also associated with significantly lower mortality when compared with sclerotherapy as the result just reached statistical significance (POR 0·77, 95% CI 0·59 to 0·99, P = 0·048). Ald Complications were also less common in patients treated with variceal ligation, in all the studies except one,[179] although the size of the difference varied between studies, causing significant heterogeneity (P = 0·004). Meta-analysis showed that the difference was statistically significant in favor of variceal ligation (Der Simonian and Laird method:

Table 31.12   Randomized controlled trials of variceal ligation versus variceal ligation plus sclerotherapy for the prevention of re-bleeding

Study	No. of patients L/L + S	Child C (%)	Re-bleeding L/L + S	Death L/L + S	Variceal eradication L/L + S	Complications L/L + S
Combined						
Laine *et al.* (1996)[267]	20/21	44	6/6	3/3	12/15	2/6
Argonz *et al.* (2000)[269]	29/30	NR	11/5	9/4	16/24	1/8
Saeed *et al.* (1997)[270]	25/22	28	6/8	4/8	16/12	5/13
Traif *et al.* (1999)[271]	31/29	25	7/5	7/3	NR	7/6
El-Khayat *et al.* (1997)[272]	30/34	NR	2/2	3/4	NR	4/6
Hou *et al.* (2001)[273]	47/47	20	11/13	6/7	40/41	23/31
Bobadilla-Diaz *et al.* (2002)[274]	15/18	NR	1/0	NR	NR	NR
POR (95% CI)			0·86 (0·52 to 1·4)	0·90 (0·52 to 1·56)	1·55 (0·79 to 3·04)	2·71 (1·48 to 4·96)
Sequential						
Bhargava and Pokharna (1997)[275]	25/25	18	4/5	NR	5/20	8/14
Lo *et al.* (1998)[276]	35/37	21	11/3	10/7		

L, variceal ligation; L + S, variceal ligation plus sclerotherapy; NR, not reported; POR, pooled odds ratio

POR 0·29, 95% CI 0·19 to 0·44). In addition the number of treatment sessions needed to achieve variceal obliteration was less with variceal ligation in all the studies (2·7–4·1 sessions with variceal ligation compared with 4–6·5 sessions with sclerotherapy). However, there was no difference between the endoscopic modalities in the number of patients with varices obliterated (POR 1·23, 95% CI 0·93 to 1·61), while the recurrence of varices was more frequent in patients treated with variceal ligation (POR 1·36, 95% CI 0·96 to 1·92). However re-bleeding after initial eradication seems unusual especially if patients are in a regular endoscopic follow up, and varices that recur are re-obliterated.[266]

Variceal ligation versus variceal ligation plus sclerotherapy

In an attempt to further improve the results achieved with variceal ligation, which requires between three and four therapeutic sessions for variceal eradication and 25% of patients would have an episode of recurrent bleeding before completion of therapy, it has been suggested that variceal ligation combined with low-volume sclerotherapy could lead to more rapid eradication of varices than the use of variceal ligation alone. The use of sclerotherapy along with ligation is based on the rationale that sclerotherapy obliterates deeper paraesophageal varices that serve as feeder vessels for the submucosal vessels, whereas ligation can only be applied to submucosal varices. Seven studies,[267–274] involving 398 patients have tested this hypothesis: five were pulished as peer-reviewed articles[267–271,273] and two as abstracts[272,274] (Table 31.12). Meta-analysis showed no significant differences between the two endoscopic treatments in the

number of patients with varices eradicated (POR 1·55, 95% CI 0·79 to 3·04), in re-bleeding (POR 0·86, 95% CI 0·52 to 1·4) or deaths (POR 0·90, 95% CI 0·52 to 1·56). Alc However complications were significantly higher from the combined therapy compared with variceal ligation alone (POR 2·71, 95% CI 1·48 to 4·96). Moreover, the number of sessions required to achieve eradication was greater in the combined therapy arm in all the studies, significantly in one.[267] A detailed meta-analysis has been published.[268]

Two other studies investigated whether there was an additive effect of sclerotherapy in small varices (inaccessible to variceal ligation) after the completion of repeated variceal ligation treatment.[275,276] Bhargava and Pokharna[275] reported that the combined treatment eradicated the varices in a significantly greater number of patients than variceal ligation alone but they did not find any difference in re-bleeding. In contrast Lo *et al.*[276] reported that the combined treatment resulted in significantly less recurrence of esophageal varices and re-bleeding. Ald

Finally, three studies of comparison between combined variceal ligation and sclerotherapy with sclerotherapy alone have been reported.[277–279] There was no difference in re-bleeding and mortality between the two treatment modalities in any of these studies. Moreover, this comparison is not justified since sclerotherapy has been replaced by variceal ligation for the secondary prevention of variceal bleeding.

Variceal ligation versus drug combination (β-blockers plus nitrates)

Four randomized controlled trials[280–283] (one published in abstract form[280]), involving 471 patients, assessed the efficacy

Table 31.13 Randomized controlled trials of variceal ligation versus β-blockers plus nitrates

Study	No. of patients Lig/D	Child C (%)	Re-bleeding Lig/D	Death Lig/D
Villanueva *et al.* (2001)[280]	72/72	22	35/24	30/23
Agrawall *et al.* (2002)[281a]	53/51	NR	10/13	7/7
Lo *et al.* (2002)[282]	60/61	21	12/26	15/8
Patch *et al.* (2002)[283]	51/51	51	27/19	17/17
POR (95% CI)			0·97 (0·66 to 1·41)	0·72 (0·47 to 1·1)

[a]Abstract.
Lig, variceal ligation; D, β-blockers + nitrates; NR, not reported; POR, pooled odds ratio

of variceal ligation versus drug combination of β-blockers (propranolol or nadolol) and nitrates (ISMN) (Table 31.13). In one study[279] the ligation group experienced significantly less re-bleeding while in the other three studies there was no statistically significant difference between the two treatment arms. Meta-analysis showed no difference in re-bleeding rate (POR 0·97, 95% CI 0·66 to 1·41) and survival (POR 0·72, 95% CI 0·47 to 1·1) although in the latter endpoint there was a trend in favor of drug combination. Alc One randomized trial has compared obliteration of *n*-butyl-2-cyanoacrylate versus propranolol, with no difference in re-bleeding rates nor survival, but with more complications with the adhesive injection.[284] Ald

TIPS versus drug therapy

In a recent trial Escorsell *et al.* compared TIPS with drug therapy and found that the 2-year re-bleeding rate was significantly lower in the TIPS group.[285] However, patients who received drug therapy experienced less encephalopathy and more frequent improvement in the Child–Pugh score, with lower associated costs. Ald

TIPS versus sclerotherapy or variceal ligation

Thirteen trials, involving 948 patients, compared TIPS with endoscopic treatment (with or without the addition of propranolol): 9 with sclerotherapy[286–294] and 4 with variceal ligation[295–298]: 12 were published as peer-reviewed articles[287–298] and one in abstract form[286] (Table 31.14). The median range of follow up was from 10 to 32 months. Re-bleeding was significantly less common in patients randomized to TIPS (POR 3·28, 95% CI 2·28 to 4·72). Ald However there was a trend toward fewer deaths in the endoscopic treatment arm,

although the difference was not statistically significant (POR 0·87, 95% CI 0·65 to 1·17). In addition hepatic encephalopathy was statistically significantly more common in patients randomized to TIPS (POR 0·48, 95% CI 0·34 to 0·67). These results are a mirror image of the surgical trials for the secondary prevention of variceal bleeding. However, an important difference is that the mean follow up was less than 2 years in all but two of these trials,[288,298] whereas the surgical shunt trials had a much greater average follow up (3–4 years). As TIPS stenosis occurs in 50–70% of patients within the first year, this approach involves regular monitoring with Doppler/ultrasound, and repeat procedures for recanalization,[299] and it is not a good long-term shunt. A similar conclusion was reached in a recent trial comparing TIPS to propranolol and ISMN in 91 patients with cirrhosis and a Child–Pugh score >7.[300] It was shown that TIPS, although effective in reducing re-bleeding did not improve survival, caused hepatic encephalopathy and had a worse cost–benefit profile than pharmacological treatment. Ald

Surgical shunts

There is still a role for surgical shunting in the modern management of portal hypertension. The ideal patients for a decompressive surgical shunt should be well compensated cirrhotic patients, who have had troublesome bleeding – either who have failed at least one other modality of therapy (drugs or sclerotherapy), have bled from gastric varices despite medical or endoscopic therapy, or live far from suitable medical services. These shunts achieve an overall re-bleeding rate of 14·3% and a survival rate of 86%, but they may cause encephalopathy in 20·6% of patients (severe encephalopathy in 3%). The advent of TIPS has had a major impact on the need for these operations. Today, a common indication for a surgical shunt is in patients who have had a TIPS, without major encephalopathy, but have had recurrent symptomatic TIPS stenosis. In essence, they have had a non-surgical trial of shunting, and have selected themselves as good candidates. Small diameter portacaval H-graft or distal splenorenal shunts are probably the favored surgical option, as the portal vein is then still available should liver transplantation be required.

Randomized controlled trials of surgical therapy

Total portacaval shunt versus selective distal splenorenal shunt

Selective distal splenorenal shunt (DSRS) was designed to reduce the incidence of hepatic encephalopathy and liver failure following total portacaval shunt (PCS) by partially maintaining portal liver perfusion while decreasing portal blood flow to varices. Six trials, including 336 patients,

Table 31.14   Randomized controlled trials of TIPS versus sclerotherapy/variceal ligation for the prevention of re-bleeding

Study	No. of patients TIPS/Scl	Child C (%)	Re-bleeding TIPS/Scl	Death TIPS/Scl	PSE TIPS/Scl
GEAIH (1995)[286]	32/33	100	13/20	16/14	
Cabrera et al. (1996)[287]	31/32	10	7/16	6/5	10/4
Sanyal et al. (1997)[288]	41/39	49	10/9	12/7	12/5
Cello et al. (1997)[289]	24/25	NR	3/12	8/8	12/11
Rossle et al. (1997)[290]	61/65	18	9/29	8/8	18/9
Sauer et al. (1997)[291]	42/41	24	6/21	12/11	14/3
Merli et al. (1998)[292]	38/43	12	7/17	9/8	21/10
Garcia-Villarreal et al. (1999)[293]	22/24	32	2/12	1/8	5/6
Jalan et al. (1997)[295]	31/27	47	3/15	13/10	5/3
Pomier-Layrargues et al. (1997)[296]	41/39	NR	10/22	17/12	13/10
Narahara et al. (2001)[294]	38/40	NR	7/13	11/7	13/6
Gulberg et al. (2002)[297]	28/26	11	7/7	4/4	2/1
Sauer et al. (2002)[298]	43/42	29	7/10	8/7	17/9
POR (95% CI)			3·28 (2·28 to 4·72)	0·87 (0·65 to 1·17)	0·48 (0·34 to 0·67)

Scl, sclerotherapy; NR, not reported; POR, pooled odds ratio; TIPS, transjugular intrahepatic portosystemic shunt; PSE, porto–systemic encephalopathy

compared PCS with DSRS.[301–306] A meta-analysis of these trials has been published.[1] There was no statistical significance in re-bleeding between the two surgical treatments (POR 0·88, 95% CI 0·54 to 1·45). Ald Patients with DSRS showed a trend toward less hepatic encephalopathy (POR 1·29, 95% CI 0·76 to 2·17) and better long-term survival (POR 1·28, 95% CI 0·82 to 2·01), but the differences were not statistically significant. The calibrated small-diameter portacaval H-graft shunt (PCHGS) is effective in the control of variceal hemorrhage and has been associated with reduced hepatic encephalopathy when compared with total PCS.[291]

Surgery versus drugs

A recent randomized controlled trial including 119 patients compared the effectiveness of portal blood flow-preserving procedures (selective shunts and the Sugiura–Futagawa operation), β-blockers and sclerotherapy for secondary prevention of variceal hemorrhage.[308] The re-bleeding rate was significantly lower in the surgical group compared with patients receiving drugs (16·6% v 77·5%, P < 0·0001) and survival was better for Child's A cirrhosis in all groups, but there was no significant difference between treatment groups. Ald

Surgery versus sclerotherapy

DSRS was compared with sclerotherapy in four trials, involving 292 patients[309–312] (Table 31.15). A comprehensive meta-analysis of these studies, using individual patient data

provided by the principal authors, has been previously published.[313] Re-bleeding was statistically significantly reduced by DSRS (pooled relative risk (PRR) 0·16, 95% CI 0·10 to 0·27). There was statistically significant heterogeneity in the evaluation of mortality, as the risk of death was increased in one study[311] and decreased in the other three.[309,310,312] The pooled relative risk was not statistically significant different between the treatment modalities (PRR 0·78, 95% CI 0·47 to 1·29). Alc Chronic hepatic encephalopathy was increased after DSRS but the difference was not statistically significant (PRR 1·86, 95% CI 0·90 to 3·86). The results of this meta-analysis are in accordance with the trial discussed above[308] in which significantly lower re-bleeding rates were documented in the surgical compared with sclerotherapy group (16·7% v 63%, P < 0·0001), but no difference in mortality was observed. However, this study was heavily criticized for the different exclusion criteria that were used in different treatment arms, the lack of information regarding cause of portal hypertension and differences in the surveillance endoscopy program. Finally two trials[314,315] (one an abstract[314]) have compared PCS with sclerotherapy in the elective treatment of variceal hemorrhage. Re-bleeding was significantly less in the portacaval shunt group. Ald However the incidence of hepatic encephalopathy was significantly increased with the surgical treatment and there was no difference in survival.

Surgery versus TIPS

Recently Rosemurgy et al. extended the follow up (median 4 years) of a previously published randomized trial comparing 8-mm prosthetic H-graft portacaval shunts (HGPCS) with

Table 31.15 Randomized controlled trials of DSRS versus sclerotherapy for the prevention of re-bleeding

Study	No. of patients DSRS/Scl	Child C (%)	Re-bleeding DSRS/Scl	Death DSRS/Scl	PSE DSRS/Scl
Henderson *et al.* (1990)[311]	35/37	43	1/22	20/12	5/3
Teres *et al.* (1987)[310]	57/55	7·3[a]	6/18	9/15	8/3
Rikkers *et al.* (1987)[309]	30/30	42	5/18	12/20	6/4
Spina *et al.* (1990)[312]	34/32	0	1/10	4/8	2/2
POR (95% CI)			0·16 (0·10 to 0·27)	0·78 (0·47 to 1·29)	1·86 (0·9 to 3·86)

[a]Child score DSRS, distal splenorenal shunt; Scl, sclerotherapy; NR, not reported; POR, pooled odds ratio; PSE, porto–systemic encephalopathy

TIPS as definitive therapy for bleeding varices who failed non-operative management.[316] The trial included 132 patients and shunting was carried out as an elective, urgent or emergency procedure. Placement of TIPS resulted in more re-bleeding (16% *v* 3%), liver transplantations (7·5% *v* 0%) and late deaths (34% *v* 13·2%). Ald According to a cost–benefit analysis carried out by the same group of investigators, TIPS was associated with much higher costs than HGPCS, due to subsequent occlusion and re-bleeding.[317] DSRS has also been shown to be superior to TIPS in terms of recurrent bleeding (6·25% *v* 25·7%), encephalopathy (18·75% *v* 42·86%) and shunt occlusion (6·25% *v* 68·57%) in a comparative study with 67 patients with Child's A and B cirrhosis.[318] Finally Zachs *et al.* recently showed that in a population of Child's A cirrhosis DSRS is a more cost-effective treatment than TIPS.[319]

Whether the recent introduction of lined stents will significantly improve results of TIPS remains to be proven.

Conclusion

Pharmacological treatment with β-blockers is a safe and effective long-term treatment for the prevention of recurrence of variceal bleeding. The combination of β-blockers with isosorbide-5-mononitrate needs further testing in randomized controlled trials. The use of hemodynamic targets of HVPG response should be further evaluated during pharmacologic therapy for the prevention of re-bleeding. If endoscopic treatment is chosen, variceal ligation is the modality of choice. The combination of simultaneous variceal ligation and sclerotherapy does not offer any benefit. However, the use of additional sclerotherapy for the complete eradication of small varices after variceal ligation should be further addressed in future trials. The results of randomized controlled trials comparing variceal ligation with pharmacologic treatment showed that combination treatment with non-selective β-blockers and nitrates and variceal ligation are equally effective. Finally the use of TIPS for the secondary prevention of variceal bleeding is not supported by the current data, mainly because of its worse cost–benefit profile compared with other treatments. In contrast there is a role for the selective surgical shunts (DSRS or HGPCS) in the modern management of portal hypertension. The ideal patients should be well compensated cirrhotic patients, who have had troublesome bleeding – who have failed at least one other modality of therapy (drugs or ligation) or have bled from gastric varices despite medical or endoscopic therapy or live far from suitable medical services.

Summary

In conclusion this critical review of the studies of treatment in portal hypertension has highlighted several issues with regard to the design of clinical trials and the analysis of the data that should be addressed in future trials. The quality of future trials will also be significantly improved if standardized definitions of critical endpoints (for example bleeding or re-bleeding episodes, treatment failure, etc.), agreed upon in consensus conferences,[12,210] are applied. This will aid the reduction of the heterogeneity that is present in randomized controlled trials in portal hypertension and lead to better evidence for the optimal treatment options.

References

1 D'Amico G, Pagliaro L, Bosch J. The treatment of portal hypertension: a meta-analytic review. *Hepatology* 1995; **22**:332–54.

2 Robbins J. Estimators of the Mantel-Haenszel variance consistent in both sparse data and large strata limiting models. *Biometrics* 1986;**42**:311–23.

3 Der Simonian R, Laird N. Meta-analysis in clinical trials. *Controlled Clin Trials* 1986;**7**:177–88.

4 Garcia-Tsao G, Groszmann RJ, Fisher RL, Conn HO, Atterbury CE, Glickman M. Portal pressure, presence of gastroesophageal varices and variceal bleeding. *Hepatology* 1985;**5**:419–24.

5 Cales P, Desmorat H, Vinel JP *et al.* Incidence of large esophageal varices in patients with cirrhosis – application to prophylaxis of 1st bleeding. *Gut* 1990;**31**:1298–302.

6 Vorobioff J, Groszmann RJ, Picabea E *et al.* Prognostic value of hepatic venous pressure gradient measurements in alcoholic cirrhosis: A 10-year prospective study. *Gastroenterology* 1996;**111**:701–9.

7 Primignani M, Carpinelli L, Preatoni P *et al.* Natural history of portal hypertensive gastropathy in patients with liver cirrhosis. The New Italian Endoscopic Club for the study and treatment of esophageal varices (NIEC). *Gastroenterology* 2000;**119**:181–7.

8 Pagliaro L, D'Amico G, Pasta L *et al.* Portal hypertension in cirrhosis: Natural history. In: Bosch J, Groszmann R (eds). *Portal hypertension. Pathophysiology and treatment.* Cambridge, MA: Blackwell Scientific, 1994.

9 Graham DY, Smith JL. The course of patients after variceal hemorrhage. *Gastroenterology* 1981;**80**:800–9.

10 DeFranchis R. Prediction of the first variceal hemorrhage in patients with cirrhosis of the liver and esophageal varices – a prospective multicenter study. *N Engl J Med* 1988;**319**:983–9.

11 Merli M, Nicolini G, Angeloni S *et al.* Incidence and natural history of small esophageal varices in cirrhotic patients. *J Hepatol* 2003;**38**:266–72.

12 Grace ND, Groszmann RJ, Garcia-Tsao G *et al.* Portal hypertension and variceal bleeding: an AASLD single topic symposium. *Hepatology* 1998;**28**:868–80.

13 Armonis A, Patch D, Burroughs AK. Hepatic venous pressure measurement: An old test as new prognostic marker in cirrhosis? *Hepatology* 1997;**25**:245–8.

14 Merkel C, Gatta A. Can we predict the 1st variceal bleeding in the individual patient with cirrhosis and esophageal varices. *J Hepatol* 1991;**13**:378.

15 Nevens F, Bustami R, Scheys I, Lesaffre E, Fevery J. Variceal pressure is a factor predicting the risk of a first variceal bleeding: A prospective cohort study in cirrhotic patients. *Hepatology* 1998;**27**:15–19.

16 Conn HO, Lindermuth WW, May CJ, Ramsby GR. Prophylactic portacaval anastomosis in cirrhotic patients with esophageal varices. *N Engl J Med* 1965;**272**:1255–63.

17 Jackson FC, Perrin EB, Smith AG, Dagradi AE, Nadal HM. A clinical investigation of the portacaval shunt. II. Survival analysis of the prophylactic operation. *Am J Surg* 1968;**115**:22–42.

18 Resnick RH, Chalmers TC, Ishihara AM *et al.* A controlled study of the prophylactic portacaval shunt. A final report. *Ann Intern Med* 1969;**70**:675–88.

19 Conn HO, Lindenmuth WW, May CJ, Ramsby GR. Prophylactic portacaval anastomosis. *Medicine (Baltimore.)* 1972;**51**:27–40.

20 Inokuchi K. Improved survival after prophylactic portal nondecompression surgery for esophageal varices – a randomized clinical trial. *Hepatology* 1990;**12**:1–6.

21 Paquet KJ. Prophylactic endoscopic sclerosing treatment of the esophageal wall in varices – a prospective controlled randomized trial. *Endoscopy* 1982;**14**:4–5.

22 Witzel L, Wolbergs E, Merki H. Prophylactic endoscopic sclerotherapy of esophageal varices – a prospective controlled study. *Lancet* 1985;**i**:773–5.

23 Koch H, Henning H, Grimm H, Soehendra N. Prophylactic sclerosing of esophageal varices: results of a prospective controlled study. *Endoscopy* 1986;**18**:40–3.

24 Kobe E, Zipprich B, Schentke KU, Nilius R. Prophylactic endoscopic sclerotherapy of esophageal varices – a prospective randomized trial. *Endoscopy* 1990;**22**:245–8.

25 Wordehoff D, Spech HJ. Prophylactic sclerotherapy of esophageal varices – results of a prospective, randomized long-term trial over 7 years. *Deutsche Med Wochenschrift* 1987;**112**:947–51.

26 Santangelo WC, Dueno MI, Estes BL, Krejs GJ. Prophylactic sclerotherapy of large esophageal varices. *N Engl J Med* 1988;**318**:814–18.

27 Sauerbruch T, Wotzka R, Kopcke W *et al.* Prophylactic sclerotherapy before the 1st episode of variceal hemorrhage in patients with cirrhosis. *N Engl J Med* 1988;**319**:8–15.

28 Piai G, Cipolletta L, Claar N *et al.* A prospective controlled randomized study of prophylactic sclerotherapy of esophageal varices prior to 1st hemorrhage. *Int J Gastroenterol* 1986;**18**:223.

29 Potzi R, Bauer P, Reichel W, Kerstan E, Renner F, Gangl A. Prophylactic endoscopic sclerotherapy of esophageal varices in liver- cirrhosis – a multicenter prospective controlled randomized trial in vienna. *Gut* 1989;**30**:873–9.

30 Russo A, Giannone G, Magnano A, Passanisi G, Longo C. Prophylactic sclerotherapy in nonalcoholic liver-cirrhosis – preliminary results of a prospective controlled randomized trial. *World J Surg* 1989;**13**:149–53.

31 Andreani T, Poupon RE, Balkau BJ *et al.* Preventive therapy of 1st gastrointestinal-bleeding in patients with cirrhosis – results of a controlled trial comparing propranolol, endoscopic sclerotherapy and placebo. *Hepatology* 1990;**12**:1413–19.

32 Triger DR, Smart HL, Hosking SW, Johnson AG. Prophylactic sclerotherapy for esophageal varices – long-term results of a single-center trial. *Hepatology* 1991;**13**:117–23.

33 Gregory PB. Prophylactic sclerotherapy for esophageal varices in men with alcoholic liver-disease – a randomized, single-blind, multicenter clinical-trial. *N Engl J Med* 1991;**324**:1779–84.

34 De Franchis R, Primignani M, Arcidiacono PG *et al.* Prophylactic sclerotherapy (St) In high-risk cirrhotics selected by endoscopic criteria. A multicenter randomized controlled trial. *Gastroenterology* 1989;**101**:1087–93.

35 Bendsten F, Christensen E, Hardt F *et al.* Prophylaxis of 1st hemorrhage from esophageal varices by sclerotherapy, propranolol or both in cirrhotic-patients – a randomized multicenter trial. *Hepatology* 1991;**14**:1016–24.

36 Saggioro A, Pallini P, Chiozzini G, Nardin M, Ancilotto F. Prophylactic sclerotherapy – a controlled-study [Abstract]. *Dig Dis Sci* 1986;**31**:S504.

37 Fleig WE, Stange EF, Wordehoff D *et al.* Prophylactic (Ps) Vs therapeutic sclerotherapy (Ts) In cirrhotic patients with large esophageal varices and no previous hemorrhage – a randomized clinical trial [Abstract]. *Hepatology* 1988;**8**:1242.

38 Strauss E, Desa MG, Albano A, Lacet CC, Leite MO, Maffei RA. A randomized controlled trial for the prevention of the 1st upper gastrointestinal-bleeding due to portal-hypertension in cirrhosis – sclerotherapy or

propranolol versus control-groups [Abstract]. *Hepatology* 1988;**8**:1395.

39 Planas R, Boix J, Dominguez M *et al.* Prophylactic sclerosis of esophageal varices (EV). Prospective trial [Abstract]. *J Hepatol* 1989;**9**:S73.

40 Paquet KJ, Kalk JF, Klein CP, Gad HA. Prophylactic sclerotherapy for oesophageal varices in high risk cirrhotic patients selected by endoscopic and haemodynamic criteria: a randomised single centre controlled trial. *Endoscopy* 1994;**26**:743–40.

41 van Buuren HR, Marijke CR, Batenburg PL *et al.* Endoscopic sclerotherapy compared with no specific treatment for the primary prevention of bleeding from esophageal varices. A randomized controlled multicentre trial. *BMC Gastroenterology* 2003;**3**:22.

42 Pagliaro L, D'Amico G, Sorensen TIA *et al.* Prevention of first bleeding in cirrhosis. A meta-analysis of randomized clinical trials of nonsurgical treatment. *Ann Intern Med* 1992;**117**:59–70.

43 Laine L, Cook D. Endoscopic ligation compared with sclerotherapy for treatment of esophageal variceal bleeding. A meta-analysis [See comments]. *Ann Intern Med* 1995;**123**:280–7.

44 Sarin SK, Guptan RC, Jain AK *et al.* A randomized controlled trial of endoscopic variceal band ligation for primary prophylaxis of variceal bleeding. *Eur J Gastroenterol Hepatol* 1996;**8**:337–42.

45 Lay CS, Tsai YT, Teg CY *et al.* Endoscopic variceal ligation in prophylaxis of first variceal bleeding in cirrhotic patients with high-risk esophageal varices. *Hepatology* 1997;**25**:1346–50.

46 Lo GH, Hwu JH, Lai KH. Prophylactic banding ligation of high-risk esophageal varices – an interim report [Abstract]. *Gastroenterology* 1995;**108**:A1112.

47 Chen CY, Chang TT. Prophylactic endoscopic variceal ligation (EVL) for esophageal varices [Abstract]. *Gastroenterology* 1997;**112**:A1240.

48 Svoboda P, Kantorova I, Ochmann J, Kozumplik L, Marsova J. A prospective randomized controlled trial of sclerotherapy versus ligation in the prophylactic treatment of high-risk esophageal varices. *Surg Endosc* 1999;**13**:580–4.

49 Gameel K, Waked I, Saleh S, Sallam S, Abdel-Fattah S. Prophylactic endoscopic variceal band ligation (EVL) versus sclerotherapy (ES) for the prevention of variceal bleeding: an interim report of a prospective randomized controlled trial in schistosomal portal hypertension [Abstract]. *Hepatology* 1995;**22**:251A.

50 Perezayuso RM, Pique JM, Bosch J *et al.* Propranolol in prevention of recurrent bleeding from severe portal hypertensive gastropathy in cirrhosis. *Lancet* 1991;**337**:1431–4.

51 Pascal JP, Cales P. Propranolol in the prevention of first upper gastrointestinal tract haemorrhage in patients with cirrhosis of the liver and esophageal varices. *N Engl J Med* 1987;**317**:856–61.

52 Ideo G, Bellati G, Fesce E, Grimoldi D. Nadolol can prevent the 1st gastrointestinal-bleeding in cirrhotics – a prospective, randomized study. *Hepatology* 1988;**8**:6–9.

53 Lebrec D, Poynard T, Capron JP *et al.* Nadolol for prophylaxis of gastrointestinal-bleeding in patients with cirrhosis – a randomized trial. *J Hepatol* 1988;**7**:118–25.

54 Pasta L. Propranolol prevents 1st gastrointestinal-bleeding in non-ascitic cirrhotic-patients – final report of a multicenter randomized trial. *J Hepatol* 1989;**9**:75–83.

55 Conn HO, Grace ND, Bosch J *et al.* Propranolol in the prevention of the 1st hemorrhage from esophagogastric varices – a multicenter, randomized clinical trial. *Hepatology* 1991;**13**:902–12.

56 Colman J, Jones P, Finch C, Dudley F. Propranolol in the prevention of variceal hemorrhage in alcoholic cirrhotic patients [Abstract]. *Hepatology* 1990;**8**:1395A.

57 Poynard T, Cales P, Pasta L *et al.* Beta-adrenergic antagonist drugs in the prevention of gastrointestinal bleeding in patients with cirrhosis and esophageal varices – an analysis of data and prognostic factors in 589 patients from 4 randomized clinical trials. *N Engl J Med* 1991;**324**:1532–8.

58 Abraczinskas DR, Ookubo R, Grace ND *et al.* Propranolol for the prevention of first esophageal variceal hemorrhage: a lifetime commitment? *Hepatology* 2001;**34**:1096–102.

59 Merkel C, Marin R, Enzo E *et al.* Randomised trial of nadolol alone or with isosorbide mononitrate for primary prophylaxis of variceal bleeding in cirrhosis. Gruppo-Triveneto per L'ipertensione portale (GTIP). *Lancet* 1996;**348**:1677–81.

60 Merkel C, Marin R, Sacerdoti D *et al.* Long-term results of a clinical trial of nadolol with or without isosorbide mononitrate for primary prophylaxis of variceal bleeding in cirrhosis. *Hepatology* 2000;**31**:324–29.

61 Garcia-Pagan JC, Morillas R, Banares R *et al.* Propranolol plus placebo vs. propranolol plus isosorbide mononitrate in the prevention of the first variceal bleed. A double blind RCT. *Hepatology* 2003;**37**:1260–6.

62 Sarin SK, Lamba GS, Kumar M, Mishra A, Murthy NS. Comparison of endoscopic ligation and propranolol for the primary prevention of variceal bleeding. *N Engl J Med* 1999;**340**:988–93.

63 De BK, Ghosal UC, Das T, Santra A, Biswas PK. Endoscopic variceal ligation for primary prophylaxis of oesophageal varices bleed: preliminary report of a randomized controlled trial. *J Gastroenterol Hepatol* 1999;**14**:220–4.

64 de la Mora JG, Farca-Belsaguy AA, Uribe M *et al.* Ligation vs propranolol for primary prophylaxis of variceal bleeding using a multiple band ligator and objective measurements of treatment adequacy: Preliminary results [Abstract]. *Gastroenterology* 2000;**118** (Suppl 2):6512.

65 Jutabha R, Jensen DM, Martin P *et al.* A randomized, prospective study of prophylactic rubber band ligation compared to propranolol for prevention of first variceal hemorrhage in cirrhotics with large esophageal varices [Abstract]. *Gastrointest Endosc* 2001;**53**:568.

66 Psilopoulos DI, Mavrogiannis C, Vafiadis I *et al.* A randomized controlled trial comparing endoscopic variceal ligation (EVL) with propranolol for primary prevention of variceal bleeding (preliminary report) [Abstract]. *Gastrointest Endosc* 2002;**55**:T1897.

67 Lui HF, Stanley AJ, Forrest EH *et al.* Primary prophylaxis of variceal haemorrhage: a randomized controlled trial comparing band ligation, propranolol and isosorbide mononitrate. *Gastroenterology* 2002;**123**:735–44.

68 Schepke M, Goebel C, Nuernberg D *et al.* Endoscopic banding ligation versus propranolol for the primary prevention of variceal bleeding in cirrhosis: a randomized controlled multicenter trial [Abstract]. *Hepatology* 2003; **38**:218A.

69 Svoboda P, Kantorova I, Ochmann J, Kozumplik L, Marsova J. A prospective randomized controlled trial of sclerotherapy versus ligation in the prophylactic treatment of high-risk esophageal varices. *Surg Endosc* 1999;**13**:580–4.

70 Gameel K, Waked I, Saleh S, Sallam S, Abdel-Fattah S. Prophylactic endoscopic variceal band ligation (EVL) versus sclerotherapy (ES) for the prevention of variceal bleeding: an interim report of a prospective randomized controlled trial in schistosomal portal hypertension [Abstract]. *Hepatology* 1995;**22**:251A.

71 Gotoh Y, Iwakiri R, Sakata Y *et al.* Evaluation of endoscopic variceal ligation in prophylactic therapy for bleeding oesophageal varices: a prospective controlled trial compared with endoscopic injection sclerotherapy. *J Gastroenterol Hepatol* 1999;**14**:241–4.

72 Burroughs AK, Mezzanote G, Phillips A, McCormick PA, McIntyre N. Cirrhotics with variceal hemorrhage: the importance of the time interval between admission and the start of analysis for survival and rebleeding rates. *Hepatology* 1989;**9**:801–7.

73 D'Amico G, De Franchis R, Cooperative Study Group upper digestive bleeding in cirrhosis. Post-therapeutic outcome and prognostic indicators. *Hepatology* 2003;**38**:599–612.

74 Goulis J, Armonis A, Patch D, Sabin C, Greenslade L, Burroughs AK. Bacterial infection is independently associated with failure to control bleeding in cirrhotic patients with gastrointestinal hemorrhage. *Hepatology* 1998;**27**:1207–12.

75 Ben-Ari Z, Cardin F, McCormick PA, Wannamethee G, Burroughs AK. A predictive model for failure to control bleeding during acute variceal bleeding. *J Hepatol* 1999; **31**:443–50.

76 Ready JB, Robertson AD, Goff JS, Rector WG. Assessment of the risk of bleeding from esophageal varices by continuous monitoring of portal pressure. *Gastroenterology* 1991;**100**: 1403–10.

77 Moitinho E, Escorsell A, Bandi JC *et al.* Prognostic value of early measurements of portal pressure in acute variceal bleeding. *Gastroenterology* 1999;**117**:626–31.

78 Rimola A, Bory F, Teres J, Perez-Ayuso RM, Arroyo V, Rodes J. Oral, nonabsorbable antibiotics prevent infection in cirrhotics with gastrointestinal hemorrhage. *Hepatology* 1985;**5**:463–7.

79 Soriano G, Guarner C, Tomas A *et al.* Norfloxacin prevents bacterial infection in cirrhotics with gastrointestinal hemorrhage. *Gastroenterology* 1992;**103**:1267–72.

80 Blaise M, Pateron D, Trinchet JC *et al.* Systemic antibiotic therapy prevents bacterial infection in cirrhotic patients with gastrointestinal hemorrhage. *Hepatology* 1994;**20**:34–8.

81 Pauwels A, Mostefa-Kara N, Debenes B, Degoutte E, Levy VG. Systemic antibiotic prophylaxis after gastrointestinal hemorrhage in cirrhotic patients with a high risk of infection. *Hepatology* 1996;**24**:802–6.

82 Hou M-C, Lin H-C, Lee F-Y *et al.* Prophylactic antibiotic prevents rebleeding in patients with acute gastroesophageal variceal bleeding following endoscopic treatment: a randomized trial [Abstract]. *Hepatology* 2003;**38**:292A.

83 Hsieh WJ, Lin HC, Hwang SJ *et al.* The effect of ciprofloxacin in the prevention of bacterial infection in patients with cirrhosis after upper gastrointestinal bleeding. *Am J Gastroenterol* 1998;**96**:962–6.

84 Zacharof A, Petrogiannopoulos C, Soutos D, Katsaros D, Zacharof HJP. Bacterial infection is prevented by ciprofloxacin in cirrhotics with a gastrointestinal hemorrhage [Abstract]. *Gut* 1997;**41**:A189.

85 Rolando N, Gimson A, Philpott-Howard J *et al.* Infectious sequelae after endoscopic sclerotherapy of oesophageal varices: role of antibiotic prophylaxis. *J Hepatol* 1993; **18**:290–4.

86 Selby WS, Norton ID, Pokorny CS *et al.* Bacteremia and bacterascites after endoscopic sclerotherapy for bleeding esophageal varices and prevention by intravenous cefotaxime: a randomized trial. *Gastrointest Endosc* 1994; **40**:680–4.

87 Soares-Weiser K, Brezis M, Tur-Kaspa R, Paul M, Yahav J, Leibovici L. Antibiotic prophylaxis of bacterial infections in cirrhotic inpatients: a meta-analysis of randomized controlled trials. *Scand J Gastroenterol* 2003;**38**:193–200.

88 Goulis J, Patch D, Burroughs AK. The role of bacterial infection in the pathogenesis of variceal bleeding. *Lancet* 1999;**354**:1053–60.

89 Sarin SK. Long-term follow-up of gastric variceal sclerotherapy: an eleven-year experience. *Gastrointest Endosc* 1997;**46**:8–14.

90 Levacher S, Letoumelin P, Pateron D, Blaise M, Lapandry C, Pourriat JL. Early administration of terlipressin plus glyceryl trinitrate to control active upper gastrointestinal bleeding in cirrhotic patients. *Lancet* 1995;**346**:865–8.

91 Conn HO, Ramsby GR, Storer EH *et al.* Intraarterial vasopressin in the treatment of upper gastrointestinal hemorrhage: a prospective, controlled clinical trial. *Gastroenterology* 1975;**68**:211–21.

92 Bosch J, Groszmann RJ, Garcia-Pagan JC *et al.* Association of transdermal nitroglycerin to vasopressin infusion in the treatment of variceal hemorrhage: a placebo-controlled clinical trial. *Hepatology* 1989;**10**:962–8.

93 Sonnenburg GE, Keller U, Perruchud A, Burcharth F. Effect of somatostatin on splanchnic haemodynamics. *Gastroenterology* 1981;**80**:5226–32.

94 Bosch J, Kravetz D, Rodes J. Effects of somatostatin on hepatic and systemic haemodynamics inpatients with cirrhosis of the liver: comparison with vasopressin. *Gastroenterology* 1981;**80**:518–25.

95 Moitinho E, Planas R, Banres R *et al.* Multicenter randomized controlled trial comparing different schedules of somatostatin administration in the treatment of acute variceal bleeding. *J Hepatol* 2001;**35**:712–18.

96 Jenkins SA, Baxter JN, Snowden S. The effects of somatostatin and SMS 201–995 on hepatic haemodynamics inpatients with cirrhosis and portal hypertension. *Fibrinolysis* 1988;**2**:48–50.

97 McCormick PA, Dick R, Siringo S *et al.* Octreotide reduces azygous blood flow in cirrhotic patients with portal hypertension. *Eur J Gastroenterol Hepatol* 1990;**2**: 489–92.

98 Escorsell A, Bandi JC, Andreu V *et al.* Desensitization to the effects of intravenous octreotide in cirrhotic patients with portal hypertension *Gastroenterology* 2001;**120**: 161–9.

99 Merigan TCJ, Poltkin JR, Davidson CS. Effect of intravenously administered posterior pituitary extract on haemorrhage from bleeding esophageal varices. *N Engl J Med* 1962;**266**:134–5.

100 Mallory A, Schaefer JW, Cohen JR, Holt AS, Norton LW. Selective intra-arterial vasopressin infusion for upper gastrointestinal tract hemorrhage. A controlled trial. *Arch Surg* 1980;**115**:30–2.

101 Fogel RM, Knauer CM, Andress LL. Continuous intravenous vasopressin in active upper gastrointestinal bleeding. A placebo controlled trial. *Ann Intern Med* 1982;**96**:565–9.

102 Tsai YT, Lay CS, Lai KH *et al.* Controlled trial of vasopressin plus nitroglycerin vs. vasopressin alone in the treatment of bleeding esophageal varices. *Hepatology* 1986;**6**:406–9.

103 Gimson AE, Westaby D, Hegarty J, Watson A, Williams R. A randomized trial of vasopressin and vasopressin plus nitroglycerin in the control of acute variceal hemorrhage. *Hepatology* 1986;**6**:410–13.

104 Walker S, Stiehl A, Raedsch R, Kommerell B. Terlipressin in bleeding esophageal varices: a placebo-controlled, double-blind study. *Hepatology* 1986;**6**:112–15.

105 Freeman JG, Cobden MD, Record CO. Placebo-controlled trial of terlipressin (glypressin) in the management of acute variceal bleeding. *J Clin Gastroenterol* 1989;**11**:58–60.

106 Soderlund C, Magnusson I, Torngren S, Lundell L. Terlipressin (triglycyl-lysine vasopressin) controls acute bleeding oesophageal varices. A double-blind, randomized, placebo-controlled trial. *Scand J Gastroenterol* 1990;**25**: 622–30.

107 Pawels A, Florent C, Desaint B *et al.* Terlipressin and somatostatin in the treatment of hemorrhages from rupture of esophageal varices [Letter] [French]. *Gastroenterol Clin Biol* 1994;**18**:388–9.

108 Patch D, Caplin M, Greenslade L, Burroughs A. Randomized double blind controlled trial of 5 day terlipressin vs placebo in acute variceal hemorrhage [Abstract]. *J Hepatol* 1999;**30**:55.

109 Valenzuela JE, Schubert T, Fogel RM, Strong RM, Levine J, Mills PR. A multicenter, randomized, double-blind trial of somatostatin in the management of acute hemorrhage from esophageal varices. *Hepatology* 1989;**10**:958–61.

110 Burroughs AK, McCormick PA, Hughes MD, Sprengers S, D'Heygere F, McIntyre N. Randomised, double-blind, placebo-controlled trial of somatostatin for variceal bleeding. *Gastroenterology* 1990;**99**:1388–95.

111 Gotzsche PC. Somatostatin analogues for acute bleeding oesophageal varices (Cochrane Methodology Review). In: Cochrane Collaboration. *Cochrane library*, Issue 4, 2003.

112 Loperfido S, Godena F, Tosolini G *et al.* [Somatostatin in the treatment of bleeding oesophagogastric varices. Controlled clinical trial in comparison with ranitidine] [Italian]. *Recenti Progressi in Medicina* 1987;**78**:82–6.

113 Flati G, Negro P, Flati D *et al.* [Somatostatin. Massive upper digestive hemorrhage in portal hypertension. Results of a controlled study] [Spanish]. *Revista Espanola de Las Enfermedades del Aparato Digestivo* 1986;**70**:411–14.

114 Testoni PA, Masci E, Passaretti S *et al.* Comparison of somatostatin and cimetidine in the treatment of acute esophageal variceal bleeding. *Curr Ther Res* 1986;**39**: 759–66.

115 Burroughs AK, International Octreotide Varices Study Group. Double blind RCT of 5 day octreotide versus placebo, associated with sclerotherapy for trial failures [Abstract]. *Hepatology* 1996;**24**:352A.

116 Primignani M, Andreoni B, Carpinelli L *et al.* Sclerotherapy plus octreotide versus sclerotherapy alone in the prevention of early rebleeding from esophageal varices – a randomized, double-blind, placebo-controlled, multicenter trial. *Hepatology* 1995;**21**:1322–7.

117 D'Amico G, Politi F, Morabito A *et al.* Octreotide compared with placebo in a treatment strategy for early rebleeding in cirrhosis. A double blind, randomized pragmatic trial. *Hepatology* 1998;**28**:1206–14.

118 Colin R, Giuli N, Czernichow P, Ducrotte P, Lerebours E. Prospective comparison of glypressin, tamponade and their association in the treatment of bleeding esophageal varices. In: Lebrec D, Blei AT (eds). *Vasopressin analogs and portal hypertension.* Paris: John Libbey Eurotext, 1987.

119 Fort E, Sauterau D, Silvaine C, Ingrand P, Pillegrand B, Beauchant M. A randomized trial of terlipressin plus nitroglycerin vs balloon tamponade in the control of acute variceal haemorrhage. *Hepatology* 1990;**11**:678–81.

120 Blanc P, Bories J, Desprez D *et al.* Balloon tamponade with Linton-Michel tube versus terlipressin in the treatment of acute oesophageal and gastric variceal bleeding [Abstract]. *J Hepatol* 1994;**21**:133S.

121 Jaramillo JL, de la Mata M, Mino G, Costan G, Gomez-Comacho F. Somatostatin versus Sengstaken tube balloon tamponade for primary haemostasis of bleeding esophageal varices: a randomized pilot study. *J Hepatol* 1991;**12**: 100–5.

122 Avgerinos A, Klonis C, Rekoumis G, Gouma P, Papadimitriou N, Raptis S. A prospective randomized trial comparing somatostatin, baloon tamponade and the combination of both methods in the management of acute variceal haemorrhage. *J Hepatol* 1991;**13**:78–83.

123 McKee R. A study of octreotide in oesophageal varices. *Digestion* 1990;**45** (Suppl 1):60–4.

124 Freeman JG, Cobden MD, Lishaman AH, Record CO. Controlled trial of terlipressin ("glypressin") versus vasopressin in the early treatment of esophageal varices. *Lancet* 1989;**2**:62–8.

125 Desaint B, Florent C, Levy VG. A randomized trial of triglycyl-lysine vasopressin versus lysine vasopressin in

active cirrhotic variceal hemorrhage. In: Lebrec D, Blei AT (eds). *Vasopressin analogs and portal hypertension.* Paris:John Libbey Eurotext, 1987.

126 Lee FY, Tsai YT, Lai KH *et al.* A randomized controlled study of triglycyl-vasopressin and vasopressin plus nitroglycerin in the control of acute esophageal variceal hemorrhage. *Chin J Gastroenterol* 1988;**5**:131–8.

127 Chiu WK, Sheen IS, Liaw YF. A controlled study of glypressin versus vasopressin in the control of bleeding from esophageal varices. *J Gastroenterol Hepatol* 1988;**5**:549–53.

128 D'Amico G, Traina M, Vizzini G *et al.* Teripressin or vasopressin plus transdermal nitroglycerin in a treatment strategy for digestive bleeding in cirrhosis. A randomized clinical trial. *J Hepatol* 1994;**20**:206–12.

129 Kravetz D, Bosch J, Teres J, Bruix J, Rimola A, Rodes J. Comparison of intravenous somatostatin and vasopressin infusion in treatment of acute variceal hemorrhage. *Hepatology* 1984;**4**:442–6.

130 Jenkins SA, Baxter JN, Corbett W, Devitt P, Ware J, Shields R. A prospective randomised controlled clinical trial comparing somatostatin and vasopressin in controlling acute variceal haemorrhage. *BMJ* 1985;**290**:275–8.

131 Bagarani M, Albertini V, Anza M *et al.* Effect of somatostatin in controlling bleeding from esophageal varices. *Ital J Surg Sci* 1987;**17**:21–6.

132 Cardona C, Vida F, Balanzo J, Cusso X, Farre A, Guarner C. Efficacia terapeutica de la somatostatina versus vasopressina mas nitroglicerina en la hemorragia activa por varices esofagogastrica. *Gastroenterol Hepatol* 1989;**12**:30–4.

133 Hsia HC, Lee FY, Tsai YT *et al.* Comparison of somatostatin and vasopressin in the control of acute esophageal variceal hemorrhage. A randomized, controlled study. *Chin J Gastroenterol* 1990;**7**:71–8.

134 Saari A, Klvilaasko E, Inberg M *et al.* Comparison of somatostatin and vasopressin in bleeding esophageal varices. *Am J Gastroenterol* 1990;**85**:804–7.

135 Rodriguez-Moreno F, Santolaria F, Gles-Reimers E *et al.* A randomized trial of somatostatin vs vasopressin plus nitroglycerin in the treatment of acute variceal bleeding [Abstract]. *J Hepatol* 1991;**13**:S162.

136 Feu F, DelArbol LR, Banares R *et al.* Double-blind randomized controlled trial comparing terlipressin and somatostatin for acute variceal hemorrhage. *Gastroenterology* 1996;**111**:1291–9.

137 Walker S, Kreichgauer HP, Bode JC. Terlipressin (glypressin) versus somatostatin in the treatment of bleeding esophageal varices – Final report of a placebo-controlled, double-blind study. *Z Gastroenterol* 1996;**34**:692–8.

138 Hwang SJ, Lin HC, Chang CF *et al.* A randomized controlled trial comparing octreotide and vasopressin in the control of acute esophageal variceal bleeding. *J Hepatol* 1992;**16**:320–5.

139 Huang CC, Sheen IS, Chu SM *et al.* A prospective randomised controlled trial of sandostatin and vasopressin in the management of acute bleeding esophageal varices. *Chang Keng I Hsueh* 1992;**15**:78–83.

140 Silvain C, Carpentier S, Sautereau D *et al.* Terlipressin plus transdermal nitroglycerin vs octreotide in the control of acute bleeding from esophageal varices – a multicenter randomized trial. *Hepatology* 1993;**18**:61–5.

141 Thabut D, De Franchis R, Bendtsen F *et al.* Efficacy of activated recombinant factor VII (RFVIIA) Novoseven (R) in cirrhotic patients with upper gastrointestinal bleeding: a randomized placebo-controlled double blind multicenter trial [Abstract]. *J Hepatology* 2003;**38**:128A.

142 Hartigan PM, Gebhard RL, Gregory PB, for the Veterans Cooperative Variceal Sclerotherapy Group. Sclerotherapy for actively bleeding esophageal varices in male alcoholics with cirrhosis. *Gastrointest Endosc* 1997;**46**:1–7.

143 Prindiville T, Trudeau W. A comparison of immediate versus delayed endoscopic injection sclerosis of bleeding esophageal varices. *Gastrointest Endosc* 1986;**32**:385–8.

144 Shemesh E, Czerniac A, Klein E, Pines A, Bat L. A comparison between emergency and delayed endoscopic injection sclerotherapy of bleeding esophageal varices in non-alcoholic portal hypertension. *J Clin Gastroenterol* 1990;**12**:5–9.

145 Franchis R, Banares R, Silvain C. Emergency endoscopy stratefies for improved outcomes. *Scand J Gastroenterol* 1998;**33** (Suppl 226):25–36.

146 Soderlund C, Ihre T. Endoscopic sclerotherapy v conservative management of bleeding oesophageal varices. A 5-year prospective controlled trial of emergency and long-term treatment. *Acta Chir Scand* 1985;**151**:449–56.

147 Larson AW, Cohen H, Zweiban B *et al.* Acute esophageal variceal sclerotherapy. Results of a prospective randomized controlled trial. *JAMA* 1986;**255**:497–500.

148 Alexandrino P, Alves MM, Fidalgo P *et al.* Is sclerotherapy the first choice treatment for active oesophageal variceal bleeding in cirrhotic patients? Final report of a randomized controlled trial [Abstract]. *J Hepatol* 1990;**11** (Suppl):S1.

149 Novella MT, Villanueva C, Ortiz J *et al.* Octreotide vs sclerotherapy and octreotide for acute variceal bleeding. A pilot study [Abstract]. *Hepatology* 1996;**24**:207A.

150 Villanueva C, Ortiz J, Sabat M *et al.* Somatostatin alone or combined with emergency sclerotherapy in the treatment of acute esophageal variceal bleeding: a prospective randomised trial. *Hepatology* 1999;**30**:384–9.

151 Westaby D, Hayes P, Gimson AES, Polson R, Williams R. Controlled trial of injection sclerotherapy for active variceal bleeding. *Hepatology* 1989;**9**:274–7.

152 Escorsell A, Ruiz del Arbol L, Planas R *et al.* Multicenter randomized controlled trial of terlipressin versus sclerotherapy in the treatment of acute variceal bleeding: The TEST Study: *Hepatology* 2000;**32**:471–6.

153 Shields R, Jenkins SA, Baxter JN *et al.* A prospective randomized controlled trial comparing the efficacy of somatostatin with injection sclerotherapy in the control of bleeding esophageal varices. *J Hepatol* 1992;**16**:128–37.

154 Planas R, Quer JC, Boix J *et al.* A prospective randomized trial comparing somatostatin and sclerotherapy in the treatment of acute variceal bleeding. *Hepatology* 1994;**20**:370–5.

155 Di Febo G, Siringo S, Vacirca M *et al.* Somatostatin (SMS) and urgent sclerotherapy (US) in active oesophageal

variceal bleeding [Abstract]. *Gastroenterology* 1990;
98:583A.

156 Ramires R, Zils C, Mattos A. Escleroterapia versus somatostatina na hemorragia digestiva alta por ruptura de varizes esofagicas. *Arq Gastroenterol* 2000;**37**:148–54.

157 Sung JJ, Chung SS, Lai CW *et al.* Octreotide infusion or emergency sclerotherapy for variceal hemorrhage. *Lancet* 1993;**342**:637–41.

158 Jenkins SA, Shields R, Davies M *et al.* A multicentre randomised trial comparing octreotide and injection sclerotherapy in the management and outcome of acute variceal haemorrhage. *Gut* 1997;**41**:526–33.

159 Poo JL, Bosques F, Garduno R *et al.* Octreotide versus emergency sclerotherapy in acute variceal hemorrhage in liver cirrhosis [Abstract]. *Gastroenterology* 1996;**110**: 1297A.

160 El-Jackie A, Rowaisha I, Waked I, Saleh S, Abdel Ghaffar Y. Octreotide vs. sclerotherapy in the control of acute variceal bleeding in schistosomal portal hypertension: a randomized trial [Abstract]. *Hepatology* 1998;**28**:553A.

161 Lopez F, Vargas, Margarita G, Rizo T, Arguelles D. Octreotide vs sclerotherapy in the treatment of acute variceal bleeding [Abstract]. *Hepatology* 1999;**30**:574A.

162 Bildozola M, Kravetz D, Argonz J *et al.* Efficacy of octreotide and sclerotherapy in the treatment of acute variceal bleeding in cirrhotic patients. A prospective, multicenter and randomised clinical trial. *Scand J Gastroenterol* 2000;**35**:419–25.

163 Freitas CD, Sofia C, Pontes JM *et al.* Octreotide in acute bleeding esophageal varices: a prospective randomised study. *Hepatogastroenterology* 2000;**47**:1310–14.

164 Sivri B, Oksuzoglou G, Bairaktar Y, Kayhan B. A prospective randomized trial from Turkey comparing octreotide versus injection sclerotherapy in acute variceal bleeding. *Hepatogastroenterology* 2000;**47**:166–73.

165 Yousuf MH, Rauf AH, Baig IM, Akram M, Rizwan Z. Initial management of acute variceal haemorrhage. Comparison of octreotide and sclerotherapy. *J Coll Phys Surg Pak* 2000;**10**:95–7.

166 Cales P, Masliah C, Bernard B *et al.* Early administration of vapreotide in variceal bleeding in patients with cirrhosis. *N Engl J Med* 2001;**344**:23–8.

167 Besson I, Ingrand P, Person B *et al.* Sclerotherapy with or without octreotide for acute variceal bleeding. *N Engl J Med* 1995;**333**:555–60.

168 Avgerinos A, Nevens F, Raptis S, Fevery J, and the ABOVE Study Group. Early administration of somatostatin and efficacy of sclerotherapy in acute oesophageal variceal bleeds: the European Acute Bleeding Oesophageal Variceal Episodes (ABOVE) randomised trial. *Lancet* 1997;**350**: 1495–9.

169 Signorelli S, Negrini F, Paris B, Bonelli M, Girola M. Sclerotherapy with or without somatostatin or octreotide in the treatment of acute variceal haemorrhage: our experience [Abstract]. *Gastroenterology* 1996;**110**:1326A.

170 Brunati S, Ceriani R, Curioni R, Brunelli L, Repaci G, Morini L. Sclerotherapy alone vs sclerotherapy plus terlipressin vs sclerotherapy plus octreotide in the treatment of acute variceal haemorrhage [Abstract]. *Hepatology* 1996;**24**:207A.

171 Signorelli S, Paris B, Negrini F, Bonelli M, Auriemma L. Esophageal varices bleeding: comparison between trearment with sclerotherapy alone vs sclerotherapy plus octreotide [Abstract]. *Hepatology* 1997;**26**:137A.

172 Zuberi BF, Baloch Q. Comparison of endoscopic variceal sclerotherapy alone and in combination with octreotide in controlling acute variceal hemorrhage and early rebleeding in patients with low-risk cirrhosis. *Am J Gastroenterol* 2000;**95**:768–771.

173 Jensen DM, Kovacs TOG, Randall GM *et al.* Initial results of a randomized prospective study of emergency banding vs sclerotherapy for bleeding gastric or esophageal varices [Abstract]. *Gastrointest Endosc* 1993;**39**:128A.

174 Lo GH, Lai KH, Cheng JS *et al.* Emergency banding ligation versus sclerotherapy for the control of active bleeding from esophageal varices. *Hepatology* 1997;**25**:1101–4.

175 Shafqat F, Khan AA, Alam A *et al.* Band ligation vs endoscopic sclerotherapy in esophageal varices: a prospective randomised comparison. *J Pak Med Assoc* 1998;**48**:192–6.

176 Salem S, Shiha G. A prospective randomised trial of sclerotherapy versus Saeed six-shooter multiband ligation in the control of acute bleeding from oesophageal varices [Abstract]. *Gut* 1999;**44**:T73.

177 Stiegmann GV, Goff JS, Michaletz-Onody PA *et al.* Endoscopic sclerotherapy as compared with endoscopic ligation for bleeding esophageal varices. *N Engl J Med* 1992;**326**:1527–32.

178 Laine L, El-Newihi HM, Migikovsky B, Sloane R, Garcia F. Endoscopic ligation compared with sclerotherapy for the treatment of bleeding esophageal varices. *Ann Intern Med* 1993;**119**:1–7.

179 Gimson AES, Ramage JK, Panos MZ, Hayllar PM, Williams R, Westaby D. Randomised trial of variceal banding ligation versus injection sclerotherapy for bleeding esophageal varices. *Lancet* 1993;**342**:391–4.

180 Lo GH, Lai KH, Cheng JS *et al.* A prospective, randomized trial of sclerotherapy versus ligation in the management of bleeding esophageal varices. *Hepatology* 1995;**22**:466–71.

181 Hou MC, Lin HC, Kuo BIT, Chen CH, Lee FY, Lee SD. Comparison of endoscopic variceal injection sclerotherapy and ligation for the treatment of esophageal variceal hemorrhage: a prospective randomized trial. *Hepatology* 1995;**21**:1517–22.

182 Jain AK, Ray RP, Gupta JP. Management of acute variceal bleed: randomized trial of variceal ligation and sclerotherapy [Abstract]. *Hepatology* 1996;**23**:138P.

183 Mostafa I, Omar MM, Fakhry S *et al.* Prospective randomized comparative study of injection sclerotherapy and band ligation for bleeding esophageal varices [Abstract]. *Hepatology* 1996;**23**:185P.

184 Sarin SK, Govil A, Jain AK *et al.* Prospective randomized trial of endoscopic sclerotherapy versus variceal band ligation for esophageal varices: influence on gastropathy, gastric varices and variceal recurrence. *J Hepatol* 1997;**26**:826–32.

185 Shiha GE, Farag FM. Endoscopic variceal ligation versus endoscopic sclerotherapy for the management of bleeding varices: a prospective randomized trial [Abstract]. *Hepatology* 1997;**26**:136A.

186 Fakhry S, Omar MM, Mustafa I, El-Behairy N, Hunter S. Endoscopic sclerotherapy versus endoscopic variceal ligation in the management of bleeding esophageal varices: A final report of a prospective randomized study in schistisomal hepatic fibrosis [Abstract]. *Hepatology* 1997;**26**:137A.

187 Cello JP, Crass RA, Trunkey DD. Endoscopic sclerotherapy versus esophageal transection in Child's class C patients with variceal hemorrhage. Comparison with results of portacaval shunt. Preliminary report. *Surgery* 1982; **91**:333–8.

188 Huizinga WKJ, Angorn PA, Baker WW. Oesophageal transection versus injection sclerotherapy in the management of bleeding oesophageal varices in patients at high risk. *Surg Gynecol Obstet* 1985;**160**:539–46.

189 Teres J, Baroni R, Bordas JM, Visa J, Pera C, Rodes J. Randomized trial of portacaval-shunt, stapling transection and endoscopic sclerotherapy in uncontrolled variceal bleeding. *J Hepatol* 1987;**4**:159–67.

190 Burroughs AK, Hamilton G, Phillips A, Mezzanotte G, McIntyre N, Hobbs KEF. A comparison of sclerotherapy with staple transection of the esophagus for the emergency control of bleeding from esophageal- varices. *N Engl J Med* 1989;**321**:857–62.

191 Cello JP, Grendell JH, Crass RA, Weber TE, Trunkey DD. Endoscopic sclerotherapy versus portacaval-shunt in patients with severe cirrhosis and acute variceal hemorrhage – long-term follow-up. *N Engl J Med* 1987;**316**:11–15.

192 Orloff MJ, Bell RH, Orloff MS, Hardison WGM, Greenburg AG. Prospective randomized trial of emergency portacaval-shunt and emergency medical therapy in unselected cirrhotic-patients with bleeding varices. *Hepatology* 1994;**20**:863–72.

193 Soehendra N, Grimm H, Nam VC, Berger B. N-butyl-2-cyanoacrylate: a supplement to endoscopic sclerotherapy. *Endoscopy* 1987;**19**:221–4.

194 Maluf-Filho F, Sakai P, Ishioka S *et al.* Endoscopic sclerosis versus cyanoacrylate endoscopic injection for the first episode of variceal bleeding. A prospective controlled and randomized study in Child–Pugh class C patients. *Endoscopy* 2001;**33**:421–7.

195 Feretis C, Dimopoulos C, Benakis P, Kalliakmanis B, Apostolodis N. n-Butyl-cyanoacrylate (Histoacryl) plus sclerotherapy alone in the treatment of bleeding esophageal varices: a randomized prospective study. *Endoscopy* 1995;**27**:355–7.

196 Thakeb F, Salama Z, Salama H, Abdel R, Abdel K, Abdel H. The value of combined use of n-butyl-2-cyanoacrylate and ethanolamine oleate in the management of bleeding esophagogastric varices. *Endoscopy* 1995;**27**:358–64.

197 Sung JY, Lee YT, Suen R, Chung SCS. Banding is superior to cyanoacrylate for the treatment of esophageal variceal bleeding: a prospective randomized study [Abstract]. *Gastrointest Endosc* 1998;**47**:210.

198 Duvall GA, Haber G, Kortan P *et al.* A prospective randomized trial of cyanoacrylate (CYA) vs endoscopic variceal ligation (EVL) for acute esophagogastric variceal hemorrhage [Abstract]. *Gastrointest Endosc* 1997; **45**:172.

199 Zimmer T, Rucktaschel F, Stolzel U *et al.* Endoscopic sclerotherapy with fibrin glue as compared with polidocanol to prevent early esophageal variceal rebleeding. *J Hepatol* 1998;**28**:292–7.

200 Shim CS, Cho JY, Park YJ *et al.* Mini-detachable snare ligation for the treatment of esophageal varices. *Gastrointest Endosc* 1999;**50**:673–6.

201 Chau TN, Patch D, Chan YW, Nagral A, Dick R, Burroughs AG. "Salvage" transjugular intrahepatic portosystemic shunts: Gastric fundal compared with esophageal variceal bleeding. *Gastroenterology* 1998;**114**:981–7.

202 Sarin SK, Lahoti D, Saxena SP, Murthy NS, Makwana UK. Prevalence, classification and natural-history of gastric varices – a long-term follow-up-study in 568 portal-hypertension patients. *Hepatology* 1992;**16**:1343–9.

203 Ramond MJ, Valla D, Mosnier JF *et al.* Successful endoscopic obturation of gastric varices with butyl cyanoacrylate. *Hepatology* 1989;**10**:488–93.

204 Oho K, Iwao T, Sumino M, Toyonaga A, Tanikawa K. Ethanolamine oleate versus butyl cyanoacrylate for bleeding gastric varices – a nonrandomized study. *Endoscopy* 1995;**27**:349–54.

205 Sarin SK, Jain AK, Jain M, Gupta R. A randomized controlled trial of cyanoacrylate versus alcohol injection in patients with isolated fundic varices. *Am J Gastroenterol* 2002;**97**:1010–15.

206 Williams SGJ, Peters RA, Westaby D. Thrombin – an effective treatment for gastric variceal hemorrhage. *Gut* 1994;**35**:1287–9.

207 Merican I, Burroughs AK. Gastric varices. *Eur J Gastroenterol Hepatol* 1992;**4**:511–20.

208 Matsumoto A, Hamamoto N, Nomura T *et al.* Balloon-occluded retrograde transvenous obliteration of high risk gastric fundal varices. *Am J Gastroenterol* 1999;**94**:643–9.

209 De Franchis R. Developing consensus in portal hypertension. *J Hepatol* 1996;**25**:390–4.

210 Sanyal AJ, Freedman AM, Luketic VA *et al.* Transjugular intrahepatic portosystemic shunts for patients with active variceal hemorrhage unresponsive to sclerotherapy. *Gastroenterology* 1996;**111**:138–46.

211 Groszmann RJ, Bosch J, Grace ND *et al.* Hemodynamic events in a prospective randomized trial of propranolol versus placebo in the prevention of a 1st variceal hemorrhage. *Gastroenterology* 1990;**99**:1401–7.

212 Feu F, Garcia-Pagan JC, Bosch J *et al.* Relation between portal pressure response to pharmacotherapy and risk of recurrent variceal haemorrhage in patients with cirrhosis [See comments]. *Lancet* 1995;**346**:1056–9.

213 McCormick PA, Patch D, Greenslade L, Chin J, McIntyre N, Burroughs AK. Clinical vs haemodynamic response to drugs in portal hypertension. *J Hepatol* 1998;**28**:1015–19.

214 Lebrec D, Poynard T, Bernuau J *et al.* A randomized controlled-study of propranolol for prevention of recurrent

gastrointestinal-bleeding in patients with cirrhosis – a final report. *Hepatology* 1984;**4**:355–8.

215 Burroughs AK, Jenkins WJ, Sherlock S *et al.* Controlled trial of propranolol for the prevention of recurrent variceal hemorrhage in patients with cirrhosis. *N Engl J Med* 1983;**309**:1539–42.

216 Villeneuve JP, PomierLayrargues G, Infanterivard C *et al.* Propranolol for the prevention of recurrent variceal hemorrhage – a controlled trial. *Hepatology* 1986;**6**: 1239–43.

217 Cerbelaud P, Lavignolle A, Perrin D *et al.* Propranolol et prevention des recidives de rupture de varice oesophagienne du cirrhotique [Abstract]. *Gastroenterol Clin Biol* 1986;**18**:A10.

218 Queuniet AM, Czernichow P, Lerebours E, Ducrotte P, Tranvouez JL, Colin R. Controlled trial of propranolol for the prevention of recurrent gastrointestinal-bleeding in patients with cirrhosis. *Gastroenterol Clin Biol* 1987; **11**:41–7.

219 Sheen IS, Chen TY, Liaw YF. Randomized controlled-study of propranolol for prevention of recurrent esophageal varices bleeding in patients with cirrhosis. *Liver* 1989;**9**:1–5.

220 Garden OJ, Mills PR, Birnie GG, Murray GD, Carter DC. Propranolol in the prevention of recurrent variceal hemorrhage in cirrhotic-patients – a controlled trial. *Gastroenterology* 1990;**98**:185–90.

221 Rossi V, Cales P, Burtin P *et al.* Prevention of recurrent variceal bleeding in alcoholic cirrhotic-patients – prospective controlled trial of propranolol and sclerotherapy. *J Hepatol* 1991;**12**:283–9.

222 Gatta A, Merkel C, Sacerdoti D *et al.* Nadolol for prevention of variceal rebleeding in cirrhosis – a controlled clinical-trial. *Digestion* 1987;**37**:22–8.

223 Kobe E, Schentke KU. Unsichere rezidivprophylaxe von osophagusvarizenblutungen durch Propranolol bei Leberzirrhotikern: eine prospektive kontrolliertr studie. *Zeitschrift Fur Klinische Medizin-Zkm* 1987;**42**:507–10.

224 Colombo M, Defranchis R, Tommasini M, Sangiovanni A, Dioguardi N. Beta-blockade prevents recurrent gastrointestinal-bleeding in well-compensated patients with alcoholic cirrhosis – a multicenter randomized controlled trial. *Hepatology* 1989;**9**:433–8.

225 Bernard B, Lebrec D, Mathurin P, Opolon P, Poynard T. Beta-adrenergic antagonists in the prevention of gastrointestinal rebleeding in patients with cirrhosis: a meta-analysis. *Hepatology* 1997;**25**:63–70.

226 Garcia-Pagan JC, Feu F, Bosch J, Rodes J. Propranolol compared with propranolol plus isosorbide-5-mononitrate for portal-hypertension in cirrhosis – a randomized controlled-study. *Ann Intern Med* 1991;**114**:869–73.

227 Gonzalez-Abraldes J, Albillos A *et al.* Randomized comparison of long-term losartan versus propranolol in lowering portal pressure in cirrhosis. *Gastroenterology* 2001;**12**:382–8.

228 Albillos A, Garcia-Pagan JC, Iborra J *et al.* Propranolol plus prazosin compared with propranolol plus isosorbide-5-monitrate in the treatment of portal hypertension. *Gastroenterology* 1998;**115**:116–23.

229 Abecasis R, Kravetz D, Fassio E *et al.* Nadolol plus spironolactone in the prophylaxis of first variceal bleed in nonascitic cirrhotic patients: a preliminary study. *Hepatology* 2003;**37**:359–65.

230 Gournay J, Masliah C, Martin T *et al.* Isosorbide mononitrate and propranolol compared with propranolol alone for the prevention of variceal rebleeding. *Hepatology* 2000;**31**:1239–45.

231 Patti R, D'Amico G, Pasta H *et al.* Isosorbite mononitrate with nadolol compared to nadolol alone for prevention of recurrent bleeding in cirrhosis. Double-blind placebo controlled randomized trial. *J Hepatol* 1999;**30**:81 [Abstract].

232 Terblanche J, Kahn D, Campbell JH *et al.* Failure of repeated injection sclerotherapy to improve long-term survival after esophageal variceal bleeding – a 5-year prospective controlled clinical trial. *Lancet* 1983;**2**:1328–32.

233 The Copenhagen Esophageal Varices Sclerotherapy Project: sclerotherapy after first variceal hemorrhage in cirrhosis. A randomized multicenter trial. *N Engl J Med* 1984;**311**: 1594–600.

234 Westaby D, Macdougall BD, Williams R. Improved survival following injection sclerotherapy for esophageal varices – final analysis of a controlled trial. *Hepatology* 1985; **5**:827–30.

235 Korula J, Balart LA, Radvan G *et al.* A prospective, randomized controlled trial of chronic esophageal variceal sclerotherapy. *Hepatology* 1985;**5**:584–9.

236 Burroughs AK, McCormick PA, Siringo S, Phillips A, McIntyre N. Prospective randomized trial of long term sclerotherapy for variceal rebleeding, using the same protocol to treat rebleeding in all patients. Final report [Abstract]. *J Hepatol* 1989;**9**:S12.

237 Alexandrino PT, Alves MM, Correia JP. Propranolol or endoscopic sclerotherapy in the prevention of recurrence of variceal bleeding – a prospective, randomized controlled trial. *J Hepatol* 1988;**7**:175–85.

238 Dollet JM, Champigneulle B, Patris A, Bigard MA, Gaucher P. Endoscopic sclerotherapy versus oral propranolol after variceal hemorrhage in cirrhosis – results of a 4-year prospective randomized trial. *Gastroenterologie Clinique Et Biologique* 1988;**12**:234–9.

239 Fleig WE, Stange EF, Schonborn W *et al.* Final analysis of a randomized trial of propranolol (P) Vs sclerotherapy (Eps) For the prevention of recurrent variceal hemorrhage [Abstract]. *Hepatology* 1988;**8**:1220.

240 Westaby D, Polson RJ, Gimson AS, Hayes PC, Hayllar K, Williams R. A controlled trial of oral propranolol compared with injection sclerotherapy for the long-term management of variceal bleeding. *Hepatology* 1990;**11**:353–9.

241 Liu JD, Jeng YS, Chen PH, Siauw CP, Lin KY. Endoscopic injection sclerotherapy and propranolol in the prevention of recurrent variceal bleeding [Abstract]. *1990 Gastroenterology World Congress abstract book* 1990;FP 1181.

242 Martin T, Taupignon A, Lavignolle A, Perrin D, Lebodic L. Prevention of recurrent bleeding in patients with cirrhosis – results of a controlled trial of propranolol versus endoscopic sclerotherapy. *Gastroenterol Clin Biol* 1991; **15**:833–7.

243 Andreani T, Poupon RE, Balkau BJ *et al.* Efficacite comparée du propranolol et des scleroses endoscopiques du varices oesophagiennes dans la prevention des recidives d'hemorragies digestives au cours des cirrhoces [Abstract]. Etude controlee. *Gastroenterol Clin Biol* 1991;**15**:A215.

244 Dasarathy S, Dwivedi M, Bhargava DK, Sundaram KR, Ramachandran K. A prospective randomized trial comparing repeated endoscopic sclerotherapy and propranolol in decompensated (Child class b and class c) cirrhotic patients. *Hepatology* 1992;**16**:89–94.

245 Teres J, Bosch J, Bordas JM *et al.* Endoscopic sclerotherapy (Es) Vs propranolol (Pr) In the elective treatment of variceal bleeding – preliminary-results of a randomized controlled clinical-trial [Abstract]. *J Hepatol* 1987;**5**:S210.

246 Villanueva C, Balanzo J, Novella MT *et al.* Nadolol plus isosorbide mononitrate compared with sclerotherapy for the prevention of variceal rebleeding [See comments]. *N Engl J Med* 1996;**334**:1624–9.

247 Westaby D, Melia W, Hegarty J, Gimson AE, Stellon AJ, Williams R. Use of propranolol to reduce the rebleeding rate during injection sclerotherapy prior to variceal obliteration. *Hepatology* 1986;**6**:673–5.

248 Jensen LS, Krarup N. Propranolol in prevention of rebleeding from esophageal varices during the course of endoscopic sclerotherapy. *Scand J Gastroenterol* 1989;**24**:339–45.

249 Lundell L, Leth R, Lind T, Lonroth H, Sjovall M, Olbe L. Evaluation of propranolol for prevention of recurrent bleeding from esophageal varices between sclerotherapy sessions. *Acta Chir Scand* 1990;**156**:711–15.

250 Vinel JP, Lamouliatte H, Cales P *et al.* Propranolol reduces the rebleeding rate during endoscopic sclerotherapy before variceal obliteration. *Gastroenterology* 1992;**102**:1760–3.

251 Avgerinos A, Rekoumis G, Klonis C *et al.* Propranolol in the prevention of recurrent upper gastrointestinal bleeding in patients with cirrhosis undergoing endoscopic sclerotherapy – a randomized controlled trial. *J Hepatol* 1993;**19**:301–11.

252 Vickers C, Rhodes J, Chesner I *et al.* Prevention of rebleeding from esophageal varices – 2-year follow-up of a prospective controlled trial of propranolol in addition to sclerotherapy. *J Hepatol* 1994;**21**:81–7.

253 Acharya SK, Dasarathy S, Saksena S, Pande JN. A prospective randomized study to evaluate propranolol in patients undergoing long-term endoscopic sclerotherapy. *J Hepatol* 1993;**19**:291–300.

254 Elsayed SS, Shiha G, Hamid M, Farag FM, Azzam F, Awad M. Sclerotherapy versus sclerotherapy and propranolol in the prevention of rebleeding from oesophageal varices: a randomised study. *Gut* 1996;**38**:770–4.

255 Bertoni G, Fornaciari G, Beltrami M *et al.* Nadolol for prevention of variceal rebleeding during the course of endoscopic injection sclerotherapy – a randomized pilot-study. *J Clin Gastroenterol* 1990;**12**:364–5.

256 Gerunda GE, Neri D, Zangrandi F *et al.* Nadolol does not reduce early rebleeding in cirrhotics undergoing endoscopic variceal sclerotherapy (Evs) – a multicenter randomized controlled trial [Abstract]. *Hepatology* 1990;**12**:988.

257 Villanueva C, Martinez FJ, Torras X *et al.* [Nadolol as an adjuvant to sclerotherapy of esophageal varices for prevention of recurrent hemorrhaging] [Spanish]. *Revista Espanola de Enfermedades Digestivas* 1994;**86**:499–504.

258 Bertoni G, Sassatelli R, Fornaciari G *et al.* Oral isosorbide-5-mononitrate reduces the rebleeding rate during the course of injection sclerotherapy for esophageal varices. *Scand J Gastroenterol* 1994;**29**:363–70.

259 Vorobioff JD, Gamen M, Kravetz D *et al.* Effects of long-term propranolol and octreotide on postprandial hemodynamics in cirrhosis: a randomized, controlled trial. *Gastroenterology* 2002;**122**:916–22.

260 Mundo F, Mitrani C, Rodriguez G, Farca A. Endoscopic variceal treatment, is band ligation taking over sclerotherapy? [Abstract]. *Am J Gastroenterol* 1993;**88**:1493A.

261 Young HS, Sanowski RA, Rasche R. Comparison and characterization of ulcerations induced by endoscopic ligation of esophageal varices versus endoscopic sclerotherapy. *Gastrointest Endosc* 1993;**39**:119–22.

262 Jensen DM, Kovacs TOG, Jutabha R *et al.* Randomized, blinded prospective study of banding vs. sclerotherapy for preventing recurrent variceal hemorrhage for patients without active bleeding at endoscopy [Abstract]. *Gastrointest Endosc* 1995;**41**:351A.

263 Baroncini D, Milandri GL, Borioni D *et al.* A prospective randomized trial of sclerotherapy versus ligation in the elective treatment of bleeding esophageal varices. *Endoscopy* 1997;**29**:235–40.

264 Masci E, Norberto L, D'Imperio N *et al.* Prospective multicentric randomized trial comparing banding ligation with sclerotherapy of esophageal varices [Abstract]. *Gastrointest Endosc* 1997;**45**:874A.

265 Avgerinos A, Armonis A, Manolakopoulos S *et al.* Endoscopic sclerotherapy versus variceal ligation in the long-term management of patients with cirrhosis after variceal bleeding. A prospective randomized study. *J Hepatol* 1997;**26**:1034–41.

266 de la Pena J, Rivero M, Hernandez ES *et al.* Variceal recurrence after ligation and endoscopic sclerotherapy [Abstract]. *Hepatology* 1998;**28**:1173.

267 Laine L, Stein C, Sharma V. Randomized comparison of ligation versus ligation plus sclerotherapy in patients with bleeding esophageal varices. *Gastroenterology* 1996;**110**:529–33.

268 Singh P, Pooran N, Indaram A, Bank S. Combined ligation and sclerotherapy versus ligation alone for secondary prophylaxis of esophageal variceal bleeding: a meta-analysis. *Am J Gastroenterol* 2002;**97**:623–9.

269 Argonz J, Kravetz D, Suarez A *et al.* Variceal band ligation and variceal band ligation plus sclerotherapy in the prevention of recurrent variceal bleeding in cirrhotic patients:a randomized, prospective and controlled trial. *Gastrointest Endosc* 2000;**51**:157–63.

270 Saeed ZA, Stiegmann GV, Ramirez FC, Reveille RM, Goff JS, Hepps KS. Endoscopic variceal ligation is superior to combined ligation and sclerotherapy for esophageal varices: a muticenter, prospective, randomized trial. *Hepatology* 1997;**25**:71–4.

271 Traif IA, Fachartz FS, Jumah AA *et al.* Randomized trial of ligation vs combined ligation and sclerotherapy for bleeding esophageal varices. *Gastrointest Endosc* 1999; **50**:1–6.

272 El Khayat HR, Omar MM, Moustafa I. Comparative evaluation of combined endoscopic variceal ligation together with low volume sclerotherapy versus ligation alone for bleeding esophageal varices [Abstract]. *Hepatology* 1997;**26**:38.

273 Hou MC, Chen WC, Lin HC *et al.* A new "sandwich" method of combined endoscopic variceal ligation and sclerotherapy versus ligation alone in the treatment of esophageal variceal bleeding: a randomized trial. *Gastrointest Endosc* 2001;**53**:572–8.

274 Bobadilla-Diaz J, Castro-Narro G, Chavez EI *et al.* Prospective study of endoscopic variceal ligation (EVL) plus endoscopic sclerotherapy vs EVL alone for the treatment of esophageal varices [Abstract]. *J Hepatol* 2002;**36**:702A.

275 Bhargava DK, Pokharna R. Endoscopic variceal ligation versus endoscopic variceal ligation and endoscopic sclerotherapy: a prospective randomized study. *Am J Gastroenterol* 1997;**92**:950–3.

276 Lo GH, Lai KH, Cheng JS *et al.* The additive effect of sclerotherapy to patients receiving repeated endoscopic variceal ligation: a prospective, randomized trial. *Hepatology* 1998;**28**:391–5.

277 Jensen DM, Jutabha R, Kovacs TOG *et al.* Final results of a randomized prospective study of combination banding and sclerotherapy versus sclerotherapy alone for hemostasis of bleeding esophageal varices [Abstract]. *Gastrointest Endosc* 1998;**47**:184A.

278 El-Khayat HR, Khamis AA. Comparative evaluation of combined endoscopic variceal ligation (EVL) together with low volume endoscopic sclerotherapy (ES) versus sclerotherapy or band ligation alone for bleeding oesophageal varices [Abstract]. *Gastroenterology* 1995; **108**:A1061.

279 Koutsomanis D. Endoscopic variceal ligation combined with sclerotherapy versus sclerotherapy alone: 5-years follow-up [Abstract]. *Gastroenterology* 1997;**112**:1308A.

280 Villanueva C, Minana J, Ortiz J *et al.* Endoscopic ligation compared with combined treatment with nadolol and isosorbide mononitrate to prevent recurrent variceal bleeding. *N Engl J Med* 2001;**345**:647–55.

281 Agrawall SR, Gupta R, Marthy NS *et al.* Comparable efficacy of propranolol plus isosorbide monitrate and endoscopic variceal ligation in prevention of variceal rebleed [Abstract]. *J Hepatol* 2002;**36**:631A.

282 Lo GH, Chen WC, Chen MH *et al.* Banding ligation versus nadolol and isosorbide mononitrate for the prevention of esophageal variceal rebleeding. *Gastroenterology* 2002;**123**:728–34.

283 Patch D, Sabin C, Goulis J *et al.* A randomized, controlled trial of medical therapy versus endoscopic ligation for the prevention of variceal rebleeding in patients with cirrhosis. *Gastroenterology* 2002;**123**:1013–19.

284 Evrard S, Dumonceau JM, Delhaye M *et al.* Endoscopic histoacryl obliteration vs. propranolol in the prevention of esophagogastric variceal rebleeding: a randomized trial. *Endoscopy* 2003;**35**:729–35.

285 Escorsell A, Banares R, Garcia-Pagan JC *et al.* TIPS versus drug therapy in preventing variceal rebleeding in advanced cirrhosis: a randomized controlled trial. *Hepatology* 2002;**35**:385–92.

286 Groupe d Etude des Anastomoses Intrahepatiques. TIPS vs sclerotherapy plus propranolol in the prevention of variceal rebleeding – preliminary results of a multicenter randomized trial [Abstract]. *Hepatology* 1995;**22**:761.

287 Cabrera J, Maynar M, Granados R *et al.* Transjugular intrahepatic portosystemic shunt versus sclerotherapy in the elective treatment of variceal hemorrhage. *Gastroenterology* 1996;**110**:832–9.

288 Sanyal AJ, Freedman AM, Luketic VA *et al.* Transjugular intrahepatic portosystemic shunts compared with endoscopic sclerotherapy for the prevention of recurrent variceal hemorrhage. A randomized, controlled trial [See comments]. *Ann Intern Med* 1997;**126**:849–57.

289 Cello JP, Ring EJ, Olcott EW *et al.* Endoscopic sclerotherapy compared with percutaneous transjugular intrahepatic portosystemic shunt after initial sclerotherapy in patients with acute variceal hemorrhage. A randomized, controlled trial *Ann Intern Med* 1997;**126**:858–65.

290 Rossle M, Deibert P, Haag K *et al.* Randomised trial of transjugular-intrahepatic-portosystemic shunt versus endoscopy plus propranolol for prevention of variceal rebleeding. *Lancet* 1997;**349**:1043–9.

291 Sauer P, Theilmann L, Stremmel W, Benz C, Richter GM, Stiehl A. Transjugular intrahepatic portosystemic stent shunt versus sclerotherapy plus propranolol for variceal rebleeding. *Gastroenterology* 1997;**113**:1623–31.

292 Merli M, Salerno F, Riggio O *et al.* Transjugular intrahepatic portosystemic shunt versus endoscopic sclerotherapy for the prevention of variceal bleeding in cirrhosis: a randomized multicenter trial. Gruppo Italiano Studio TIPS (GIST). *Hepatology* 1998;**27**:48–53.

293 Garcia-Villarreal L, MartinezLagares F, Sierra A *et al.* Transjugular intrahepatic portosystemic stent shunt (TIPS) versus sclerotherapy for the prevention of variceal rebleeding after recent variceal bleeding. *Hepatology* 1999;**29**:27–32.

294 Narahara Y, Kanazawa H, Kawamata H *et al.* A randomized clinical trial comparing transjugular intrahepatic portosystemic shunt with endoscopic sclerotherapy in the long-term management of patients with cirrhosis after recent variceal hemorrhage. *Hepatol Res* 2001;**21**:189–98.

295 Jalan R, Forrest EH, Stanley AJ *et al.* A randomized trial comparing transjugular intrahepatic portosystemic stent shunt with variceal band ligation in the prevention of rebleeding from esophageal varices. *Hepatology* 1997;**26**:1115–22.

296 Pomier-Layrargues G, Dufresne MP, Bui B *et al.* TIPS versus endoscopic variceal ligation in the prevention of variceal rebleeding in cirrhotic patients: a comparative randomized clinical trial (interim analysis) [Abstract]. *Hepatology* 1997;**26**:35.

297 Gulberg V, Schepke M, Geigenberger G *et al.* Transjugular intrahepatic portosystemic shunting is not superior to endoscopic variceal band ligation for prevention of variceal rebleeding in cirrhotic patients. A randomized controlled trial. *Scand J Gastroenterol* 2002;**37**:338–43.

298 Sauer P, Hansmann J, Richter GM, Stremmel W, Stiehl A. Endoscopic variceal ligation plus propranolol vs transjugular intrahepatic portosystemic stent shunt: a long-term randomised trial. *Endoscopy* 2002;**34**:690–7.

299 Casado M, Bosch J, Garcia-Pagan JC *et al.* Clinical events after transjugular intrahepatic portosystemic shunt: correlation with hemodynamic findings. *Gastroenterology* 1998;**114**:1296–303.

300 Escorsell A, Banares R, Garcia-Pagan JC *et al.* TIPS versus drug therapy in preventing variceal rebleeding in advanced cirrhosis: a randomized controlled trial. *Hepatology* 2002;**35**:385–92.

301 Reichle FA, Fahmy WF, Golsorkhi M. Prospective comparative clinical trial with distal splenorenal and mesocaval shunts. *Am J Surg* 1979;**137**:13–21.

302 Fischer JE, Bower RH, Atamian S, Welling R. Comparison of distal and proximal splenorenal shunts – a randomized prospective trial. *Ann Surg* 1981;**194**:531–44.

303 Langer B, Taylor BR, Mackenzie DR, Gilas T, Stone RM, Blendis L. Further report of a prospective randomized trial comparing distal splenorenal shunt with end-to-side portacaval shunt – an analysis of encephalopathy, survival, and quality of life. *Gastroenterology* 1985;**88**:424–9.

304 Millikan WJ, Warren WD, Henderson JM *et al.* The Emory prospective randomized trial – selective versus nonselective shunt to control variceal bleeding – 10-year follow-up. *Ann Surg* 1985;**201**:712–22.

305 Harley HJ, Morgan T, Redeker AG *et al.* Results of a randomized trial of end-to-side portacaval shunt and distal splenorenal shunt in alcoholic liver-disease and variceal bleeding. *Gastroenterology* 1986;**91**:802–9.

306 Grace ND, Conn HO, Resnick RH *et al.* Distal splenorenal vs portal-systemic shunts after hemorrhage from varices – a randomized controlled trial. *Hepatology* 1988;**8**:1475–81.

307 Sarfeh IJ, Rypins EB. Partial versus total portacaval shunt in alcoholic cirrhosis – results of a prospective, randomized clinical trial. *Ann Surg* 1994;**219**:353–61.

308 Orozco H, Mercado MA, Chan C, Guillen-Navarro E, Lopez-Martinez LM. A comparative study of the elective treatment of variceal hemorrhage with beta-blockers, transendoscopic sclerotherapy, and surgery: a prospective, controlled, and randomized trial during 10 years. *Ann Surg* 2000;**232**:216–19.

309 Rikkers LF, Burnett DA, Volentine GD, Buchi KN, Cormier RA. Shunt surgery versus endoscopic sclerotherapy for long-term treatment of variceal bleeding – early results of a randomized trial. *Ann Surg* 1987;**206**:261–71.

310 Teres J, Bordas JM, Bravo D *et al.* Sclerotherapy vs distal splenorenal shunt in the elective treatment of variceal hemorrhage – a randomized controlled trial. *Hepatology* 1987;**7**:430–6.

311 Henderson JM, Kutner MH, Millikan WJ *et al.* Endoscopic variceal sclerosis compared with distal splenorenal shunt to prevent recurrent variceal bleeding in cirrhosis – a prospective, randomized trial. *Ann Intern Med* 1990;**112**: 262–9.

312 Spina GP, Santambrogio R, Opocher E *et al.* Distal splenorenal shunt versus endoscopic sclerotherapy in the prevention of variceal rebleeding. First stage of a randomized, controlled trial. *Ann Surg* 1990;**211**:178–86.

313 Spina GP, Henderson JM, Rikkers LF *et al.* Distal splenorenal shunt versus endoscopic sclerotherapy in the prevention of variceal rebleeding – a metaanalysis of 4 randomized clinical trials. *J Hepatol* 1992;**16**:338–45.

314 Korula J, Yellin A, Yamada S, Weiner J, Cohen H, Reynolds TB. A prospective randomized controlled comparison of chronic endoscopic variceal sclerotherapy and portalsystemic shunt for variceal hemorrhage in Child's class a cirrhotics [Abstract]. *Hepatology* 1988;**8**:1242.

315 Planas R, Boix J, Broggi M *et al.* Portacaval-shunt versus endoscopic sclerotherapy in the elective treatment of variceal hemorrhage. *Gastroenterology* 1991;**100**:1078–86.

316 Rosemurgy AS, Goode SE, Zwiebel B, Black TJ, Brady PG. A prospective trial of TIPS vs small diameter prosthetic H-graft portacaval shunt in the treatment of bleeding varices. *Ann Surg* 1996;**224**:378–84.

317 Rosemurgy AS, Serafini FM, Zwiebel B *et al.* Transjugular intrahepatic portosystamic shunt versus H-graft portacaval shunt in the management of bleeding varices: a cost-benefit analysis. *Surgery* 1997;**122**:794–9.

318 Khaitiyar JS, Luthra SK, Prasad N, Ratnakar N. Daruwala DK. Transjugular intrahepatic portosystamic shunt versus distal splenorenal shunt – a comparative study. *Hepatogastroenterology* 2000;**47**:492–7.

319 Zacks SL, Sandler RS, Biddle AK, Mauro MA, Brown RS Jr. Decision-analysis of tranjugular intrahepatic portosystamic shunt versus distal splenorenal shunt for portal hypertension. *Hepatology* 1999;**29**:1399–405.

32 Ascites, hepatorenal syndrome, and spontaneous bacterial peritonitis

Pere Ginès, Vicente Arroyo, Juan Rodés

Introduction

Patients with cirrhosis frequently develop disturbances in body fluid regulation that result in an increase in the volume of extracellular fluid, which accumulates in the peritoneal cavity as ascites and in the interstitial tissue as edema.[1,2] Although the pathogenesis of ascites is incompletely understood, most available evidence indicates that fluid retention is the consequence of the homeostatic activation of vasoconstrictor and sodium-retaining systems triggered by marked arterial vasodilation mainly in the splanchnic vascular bed. Marked abnormalities in the splanchnic microcirculation due to portal hypertension facilitate the accumulation of the retained fluid in the peritoneal cavity. Ascites is frequently complicated by abnormalities of renal function such as impaired ability to eliminate water and vasoconstriction of the renal circulation, which may lead to development of dilutional hyponatremia and hepatorenal syndrome, respectively.[1,3] Finally, coexistence of ascites and abnormalities in the host defense mechanisms against infection, which occur frequently in patients with advanced cirrhosis, accounts for the spontaneous infection of ascitic fluid, a condition known as spontaneous bacterial peritonitis.[4,5]

The aim of this chapter is to review, on the basis of available evidence, the efficacy of various therapeutic methods in the management of ascites, hepatorenal syndrome and spontaneous bacterial peritonitis in cirrhosis. The pathogenesis of these complications is briefly discussed to provide the reader with an understanding of the pathophysiological basis of the different therapeutic approaches. A comprehensive review of the pathophysiology of these disorders may be found elsewhere.[1,6]

Ascites

As previously mentioned, a large body of evidence indicates that in cirrhosis sodium retention, with subsequent ascites and edema formation, results from the action of neurohumoral factors on the kidney, which are activated during the homeostatic response to a disturbed systemic circulation (Figure 32.1).[1,2,6,7] The initial abnormality is sinusoidal portal hypertension causing marked arterial vasodilation mainly in the splanchnic circulation. The mechanism of this vasodilation is not known, but may involve the increased synthesis/release of vasodilating substances, including nitric oxide and/or vasodilator peptides.[2,6,8] Arterial vasodilation results in an abnormal distribution of blood volume with reduced effective arterial blood volume (the blood volume in the heart, lungs and central arterial tree) sensed by the arterial receptors with subsequent renal sodium

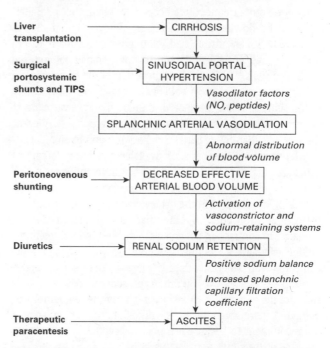

Figure 32.1 Proposed pathogenesis of ascites formation in cirrhosis according to the arterial vasodilatation hypothesis and available therapeutic interventions (in bold). TIPS, transjugular intrahepatic portosystemic shunt; NO, nitric oxide

Sodium restriction

In all diseases associated with generalized edema (cirrhosis, heart failure, renal failure), the amount of exogenous fluid retained depends on the balance between sodium intake and the renal excretion of sodium. Because sodium is retained iso-osmotically in the kidney, 1 l of extracellular fluid is gained for every 130–140 mmol of sodium that is retained. If sodium excretion remains constant, the gain in extracellular fluid volume (and the consequent increase in weight) depends exclusively on sodium intake and increases proportionally to the amount of sodium in the diet. Nevertheless, because sodium excretion may be increased pharmacologically by the administration of diuretics, the sodium balance depends not only on sodium intake but also on the natriuretic response to the diuretics.

With this background, it seems reasonable that a reduction in sodium intake (low salt diet) will favor a negative sodium balance and the elimination of ascites and edema. This was demonstrated in earlier studies[9,10] and is supported by the common clinical observation that the management of ascites is more difficult in patients who do not comply with a low sodium diet. C5, B4 Non-compliant patients usually require higher doses of diuretics to achieve resolution of ascites and are readmitted more frequently to hospital for recurrence of ascites. Surprisingly, however, an advantage of low sodium diet as compared with an unrestricted sodium diet in the management of ascites has not been demonstrated in many randomized controlled trials.[11–13] A1d Nevertheless, it should be pointed out that in these studies most patients had mild sodium retention (urine sodium in the absence of diuretic therapy was close to sodium intake) and showed an excellent response to diuretic therapy (less than 5% of patients did not respond to diuretics).

Therefore, on the basis of available evidence, it can be concluded that in patients with mild sodium retention restriction of dietary sodium is probably not necessary; the hypothetical benefit of low salt diet in the achievement of a negative sodium balance is overridden by the marked natriuretic effect of diuretics. In contrast, in patients with marked sodium retention, who usually have a less intense natriuretic response to diuretics compared with patients with moderate sodium retention, dietary sodium restriction (40–80 mmol of sodium per day) may facilitate the elimination of ascites and delay the reaccumulation of fluid. A more severe restriction of sodium (< 40 mmol/day) is not recommended because it is poorly accepted by patients and may impair their nutritional status. C5

Therapeutic paracentesis

In recent years, therapeutic paracentesis has progressively replaced diuretics as the treatment of choice in the management of patients with cirrhosis and large volume ascites in many centers.[14,15] This change in treatment strategy is based on the results of several randomized controlled trials comparing paracentesis (either removal of all ascitic fluid in a single tap or repeated taps of 4–6 l/day) associated with plasma volume expansion versus diuretics.[16–20] A1d Because paracentesis does not affect renal sodium retention, patients should be given diuretics after paracentesis to avoid reaccumulation of fluid.[21] A1d

Two aspects concerning the use of therapeutic paracentesis in patients with cirrhosis and ascites deserve to be specifically discussed: (i) the population of patients with cirrhosis in whom therapeutic paracentesis should be used; and (ii) the use of plasma expanders to prevent disturbances in circulatory function after paracentesis. While most physicians consider that therapeutic paracentesis is the treatment of choice for all patients with large volume ascites,[14,15] others believe that therapeutic paracentesis should be used only in those patients who show a poor or no response to diuretics.[22] Results of randomized trials indicate that therapeutic paracentesis is faster and in several trials was associated with lower incidence of adverse effects compared with diuretics (Table 32.1).[16–20] A1d Moreover, therapeutic paracentesis may have a better cost–effectiveness profile compared with diuretic treatment that can result in prolonged hospitalization. Therefore, on the basis of the available evidence, it seems clear that the use of therapeutic paracentesis should not be restricted to patients failing to respond to diuretics but should be considered the treatment of choice for all patients with large volume ascites (Box 32.1).

Box 32.1 Recommendations for the management of patients with cirrhosis and large volume ascites[1]

1 Total paracentesis plus intravenous albumin[a] (8 g/l of ascites removed). Patients can be treated as outpatients. Hospitalization is recommended for patients with associated complications (i.e. encephalopathy, bacterial infection, gastrointestinal bleeding)
2 After removal of ascitic fluid, start with moderate sodium restriction (40–80 mmol/day) and diuretics, either aldosterone antagonists alone (i.e. spironolactone 50–400 mg/day) or in combination with loop diuretics (i.e. furosemide 20–160 mg/day). If patients were on diuretics before the development of large volume ascites, check compliance with sodium diet and diuretic therapy. Compliant patients should be given doses of diuretics higher than those given before paracentesis in order to prevent the recurrence of ascites. Non-compliant patients should be instructed to comply with therapy
3 Consider liver transplantation

[a]Although a survival benefit of albumin over other plasma expanders has not been demonstrated, albumin is more effective than other plasma expanders in the prevention of paracentesis-induced circulatory dysfunction when more than 5 l of ascitic fluid are removed.

Table 32.1 Adverse effects in randomized trials comparing the efficacy and safety of diuretics versus therapeutic paracentesis and plasma volume expansion in patients with cirrhosis and large volume ascites[a]

| Adverse effect | Type of plasma expander | No. of patients with adverse effects | | P |
		Diuretics (%)	Paracentesis and plasma volume expansion (%)	
Renal impairment				
Ginès et al.[16]	Albumin	16/59[b] (27)	3/58 (5)	0·003
Salerno et al.[17]	Albumin	1/21 (5)	1/20 (5)	NS
Hagège et al.[18]	Albumin	1/27 (4)	1/26 (4)	NS
Acharya et al.[19]	Dextran-40	1/20 (5)	0/20 (0)	NS
Solà et al.[20]	Dextran-40	5/40 (12)	1/40 (2)	NS
Hyponatremia				
Ginès et al.[16]	Albumin	18/59 (30)	3/58 (5)	0·0009
Salerno et al.[17]	Albumin	–	–	–
Hagège et al.[18]	Albumin	8/27 (30)	2/26 (8)	0·07
Acharya et al.[19]	Dextran-40	1/20 (5)	3/20 (15)	NS
Solà et al.[20]	Dextran-40	8/40 (20)	5/40 (12)	NS
Encephalopathy				
Ginès et al.[16]	Albumin	17/59 (29)	6/58 (10)	0·02
Salerno et al.[17]	Albumin	3/21 (14)	2/20 (10)	NS
Hagège et al.[18]	Albumin	4/27 (15)	1/26 (4)	NS
Acharya et al.[19]	Dextran-40	1/20 (5)	0/20 (0)	NS
Solà et al.[20]	Dextran-40	12/40 (30)	1/40 (2)	0·0015

[a]Differences in the rate of adverse effects among the studies may be due, at least in part, to differences in the populations of patients included.
[b]Figures represent the number of patients developing the adverse effects compared with the total number of patients in each treatment group.

The removal of large volumes of ascitic fluid is associated with circulatory dysfunction characterized by a reduction of effective blood volume.[23–29] Several lines of evidence indicate that this circulatory dysfunction and/or the mechanisms activated to maintain circulatory homeostasis have detrimental effects in cirrhotic patients. First, circulatory dysfunction is associated with rapid reaccumulation of ascites.[29] Secondly, approximately 20% of these patients develop hepatorenal syndrome and/or water retention leading to dilutional hyponatremia.[23] Thirdly, portal pressure increases in patients developing circulatory dysfunction after paracentesis, probably owing to an increased intrahepatic resistance due to the action of vasoconstrictor systems on the hepatic vascular bed.[27] Finally, the development of circulatory dysfunction is associated with shortened survival.[29]

At present, the only effective method to prevent circulatory dysfunction is the administration of plasma expanders. A randomized trial has shown that albumin is more effective than other plasma expanders (dextran-70, polygeline) for the prevention of circulatory dysfunction as estimated by plasma renin activity, probably owing to its persisting longer in the intravascular compartment.[29] Alc When less than 5 l of ascites are removed, dextran-70 or polygeline show efficacy similar to that of albumin. However, albumin is more effective than these two artificial plasma expanders when more than 5 l of ascites are removed.[29] Alc Despite this greater efficacy, randomized trials have not shown differences in survival of patients treated with albumin compared with those treated with other plasma expanders.[29–32] Larger trials would be required to demonstrate a benefit of albumin on survival as well as on renal function, should one exist. Table 32.2 shows the incidence of adverse effects observed in randomized trials comparing therapeutic paracentesis without plasma volume expansion or with three different plasma expanders in patients with cirrhosis and large ascites.

In summary, conclusive results from a randomized trial with adequate power to demonstrate a benefit of albumin administration after therapeutic paracentesis on mortality are not available. However, the currently available data indicate that circulatory dysfunction after removal of large amounts of ascitic fluid is potentially harmful for patients with cirrhosis. Albumin appears to be the plasma expander of choice when more than 5 l of ascites are removed.

Table 32.2 Adverse effects reported in randomized trials assessing the efficacy and safety of therapeutic paracentesis without plasma volume expansion or with different plasma volume expanders in patients with cirrhosis and large ascites

Adverse effect	No. of patients with adverse effects				
	No plasma expander (%)	Polygeline (%)	Dextran-70 (%)	Albumin (%)	*P*
Renal impairment					
Ginès et al.[23]	6/53[a] (11)	–	–	0/52 (0)	0·03
Ginès et al.[29]	–	10/100 (10)	8/93 (9)	7/97 (7)	NS
Planas et al.[30]	–	–	1/42 (2)	1/43 (2)	NS
Salerno et al.[31]	–	1/27 (4)	–	1/27 (4)	NS
Fassio et al.[32]	–	–	1/20 (5)	1/21 (5)	NS
Hyponatremia					
Ginès et al.[23]	9/53 (17)	–	–	1/52 (2)	0·02
Ginès et al.[29]	–	19/100 (19)	23/93 (25)	14/97 (14)	NS
Planas et al.[30]	–	–	4/45 (9)	3/43 (7)	NS
Salerno et al.[31]	–	5/27 (18)	–	4/27 (15)	NS
Fassio et al.[32]	–	–	3/20 (15)	4/21 (19)	NS

[a]Figures represent the number of patients developing the adverse effect compared with the total number of patients in each treatment group.

Diuretics

Diuretics eliminate the excess extracellular fluid presenting as ascites and edema by increasing renal sodium excretion, thus achieving a negative sodium balance.[33] The diuretics most frequently used in patients with cirrhosis and ascites are aldosterone antagonists, mainly spironolactone and potassium canrenoate, drugs that antagonize selectively the sodium-retaining effects of aldosterone in the renal collecting tubules, and loop diuretics, especially furosemide, that inhibit the Na^+-K^+-$2Cl^-$ cotransporter in the loop of Henle.[33,34]

Despite the use of diuretics in clinical practice for more than 30 years, few randomized trials have been reported comparing the efficacy of different diuretic agents in the treatment of ascites.[34–36] In patients without renal failure, the aldosterone antagonist spironolactone in a dose of 150 mg/day (increased to 300 mg/day if there was no response) was shown in one randomized trial to be more effective than the loop diuretic furosemide in a dose of 80 mg/day (increased to 160 mg/day if there was no response).[35] A1 This increased efficacy of aldosterone antagonists has also been suggested in several physiological studies and case series reports.[13,37–40] Based on these findings, aldosterone antagonists are considered the diuretics of choice in the management of cirrhotic ascites.

In clinical practice, aldosterone antagonists are frequently given in combination with loop diuretics. Theoretical advantages of this combination include greater natriuretic potency, earlier onset of diuresis, and less tendency to induce hyperkalemia. Two different regimens of diuretic administration have been proposed. In the first, the dose of

aldosterone antagonists is increased progressively (usually up to 400 mg/day of spironolactone) and loop diuretics (furosemide up to 160 mg/day) are added only if no response is achieved with the highest dose of spironolactone. In the second, the two drugs are given in combination from the start of therapy. Both regimens are similar with respect to efficacy and incidence of complications. The only difference is that when the combination of spironolactone and furosemide is used from the beginning of therapy there is a more frequent need to reduce the dose of the drugs in responsive patients compared with the other stepwise regimen.[41] Ald Diuretic therapy is effective in the elimination of ascites in 80–90% of all patients, a percentage that may increase to 95% when only patients without renal failure are considered.[13,16–20,35–40] Ald, B4 The remaining patients either do not respond to diuretic therapy or develop diuretic-induced adverse effects that prevent the use of high doses of these drugs. This condition is known as refractory ascites.[42] These adverse effects include hepatic encephalopathy, hyponatremia, renal impairment, potassium disturbances, gynecomastia, and muscle cramps.[33,34,40–43] The incidence of renal and electrolyte disorders and encephalopathy vary depending on the population of patients studied, and is higher in patients with marked sodium retention and renal failure (who require higher doses of diuretics) and lower in patients with moderate sodium retention and without renal failure. Although some of these complications may be unrelated to diuretic therapy and may be due to the existence of advanced liver disease,[44] there is no doubt that diuretics are a major cause of these complications because their frequency is markedly lower if ascites is removed by therapeutic paracentesis (see Table 32.1).

Spironolactone-induced gynecomastia is common and may be important enough to lead to the discontinuation of the drug in some patients. An alternative treatment for these patients is amiloride, although its potency is much lower than that of spironolactone.[36] Ald Eplerenone, a new aldosterone antagonist that will be available soon for use in clinical practice, has fewer endocrine adverse effects compared with spironolactone and could be a good alternative to spironolactone in patients with spironolactone-induced gynecomastia.[45] However, its effectiveness in patients with cirrhosis and ascites has not been assessed. Finally, muscle cramps of variable intensity, sometimes severe, may also occur as an adverse effect of diuretics. Effective therapies for muscle cramps include quinine (300 mg/day)[46] or albumin (25 g/week).[43] Zinc sulfate (440 mg/day) was also effective in an uncontrolled study including a small number of patients.[47] B4

Because therapeutic paracentesis has replaced diuretics as the treatment of choice for hospitalized cirrhotic patients with large volume ascites in most centers[14,15] at present the main indications for use of diuretics in cirrhosis are as follows:

- treatment of patients with mild or moderate ascites or those with large volume ascites in whom paracentesis is not effective because of compartmentalization of ascitic fluid due to peritoneal adhesions;
- treatment of patients with edema without ascites;
- prevention of recurrence of ascites after therapeutic paracentesis.

Peritoneovenous shunt

A peritoneovenous shunt is a device designed to transfer ascitic fluid from the abdominal cavity to the systemic circulation via an abdominal tube and a thoracic tube ending in the superior vena cava connected through a one-way valve. This device was used extensively in the 1970s and 1980s for the treatment of refractory ascites in cirrhosis.[48] Although the system was pathophysiologically sound, its use declined progressively during the 1990s due to a high incidence of severe adverse effects, a high rate of obstruction, lack of demonstration of a significant survival benefit, and the development of new procedures, such as the transjugular intrahepatic portosystemic shunt (TIPS).[48–54] For all these reasons, this procedure is rarely used nowadays.

Transjugular intrahepatic portosystemic shunt

TIPS was introduced in clinical practice in the 1990s for the management of refractory variceal bleeding, with the objective of creating a portosystemic shunt, without the need of surgery. The procedure consists of the placement of an intrahepatic stent between one hepatic vein and the portal vein using a transjugular approach.[55] It soon became evident that in patients with variceal bleeding and ascites treated with TIPS there was an increased natriuretic effect of diuretics, leading to the reduction or elimination of ascites in most patients. These beneficial effects of TIPS on ascites are similar to those reported in earlier studies in patients treated with surgical portosystemic shunts, especially side-to-side portacaval shunts.

A large number of uncontrolled studies have shown that TIPS is effective in preventing recurrence of ascites in patients with refractory ascites. This effect is due to reduction in the activity of sodium-retaining mechanisms and amelioration of renal function, which lead to an improvement of the renal response to diuretics.[56–61] B4 The main disadvantages of TIPS include shunt stenosis or obstruction (up to 75% of patients develop stenosis within 6–12 months leading to reaccumulation of ascites in most cases) and a high rate of encephalopathy due to the shunting of blood from the splanchnic to the systemic circulation.[62–64] Other adverse effects include an impairment in liver function, which is usually transient, hemolytic anemia, and heart failure.[65,66] Because of its efficacy and the paucity of good alternative therapies (except for that of repeated large-volume paracentesis with concomitant administration of intravenous albumin), TIPS became a widely used treatment for patients with refractory ascites during the 1990s despite the lack of randomized controlled trials comparing it with medical therapy.

Four randomized trials comparing TIPS and repeated large volume paracentesis with concomitant intravenous albumin in patients with cirrhosis and refractory ascites have been published.[67–70] The main results of these trials are summarized in Table 32.3. Although there are some discrepancies between the results of the trials and a meta-analysis has not been done, the following conclusions may be drawn. A1c

- TIPS is clearly more effective than large volume paracentesis in the prevention of recurrence of ascites.[67–70] However, renal sodium homeostasis is not completely achieved and most patients treated with TIPS still require sodium restriction and diuretics during follow up.[69,70]
- TIPS reduces the risk of developing hepatorenal syndrome type 1.[69]
- TIPS is associated with an increased risk of severe hepatic encephalopathy and does not reduce significantly the risk of other complications of cirrhosis, such as gastrointestinal bleeding or spontaneous bacterial peritonitis.[69,70]
- There is a high rate of TIPS stenosis or obstruction that requires frequent intervention to maintain shunt patency.[67–70]
- Despite better control of ascites and a reduction in the number of hospitalizations for ascites, TIPS does not appear to improve the quality of life compared with repeated large volume paracentesis with concomitant intravenous albumin.[70]

Table 32.3 Complications and survival in randomized trials comparing transjugular intrahepatic portosystemic shunt (TIPS) and large volume paracentesis in patients with cirrhosis and refractory ascites.

Study	TIPS	Paracentesis[a]	P
Recurrent ascites			
Lebrec *et al.*[67]	5/10 (50)[b]	12/12 (100)	<0·05
Rössle *et al.*[68]	3/23 (13)	15/22 (68)	<0·04
Ginès *et al.*[69]	17/35 (49)	29/35 (82)	<0·01
Sanyal *et al.*[70]	22/52 (42)	48/57 (84)	<0·001
Severe hepatic encephalopathy			
Lebrec *et al.*[67]	2/10 (20)	0/12 (0)	NS
Rössle *et al.*[68]	NR	NR	–
Ginès *et al.*[69]	21/35 (60)	12/34 (35)	0·03
Sanyal *et al.*[70]	20/52 (38)	12/57 (21)	0·058
TIPS stenosis/obstruction			
Lebrec *et al.*[67]	3/10 (30)	–	–
Rössle *et al.*[68]	13/29 (45)	–	–
Ginès *et al.*[69]	13/35 (37)	–	–
Sanyal *et al.*[70]	NR	–	–
Hepatorenal syndrome type 1			
Lebrec *et al.*[67]	NR	NR	–
Rössle *et al.*[68]	NR	NR	–
Ginès *et al.*[69]	3/35 (9)	11/35 (31)	0·03
Sanyal *et al.*[70]	NR	NR	–
Mortality during follow up			
Lebrec *et al.*[67]	9/10 (90)	4/12 (33)	<0·05
Rössle *et al.*[68]	15/29 (51)	23/31 (74)	NS
Ginès *et al.*[69]	20/35 (57)	18/35 (51)	NS
Sanyal *et al.*[70]	18/52 (34)	19/57 (33)	NS

[a]In all studies, except that of Rössle *et al.*[68] IV albumin (6–8 g/l ascites removed) was given routinely to all patients treated with paracentesis.
[b](Patients/total number of patients included).
NR, not reported; IV, intravenous

- The cost of TIPS is higher than that of conventional therapy with repeated large volume paracentesis and concomitant intravenous albumin.[69]
- TIPS does not improve either overall or transplant-free survival compared with therapy with repeated large volume paracentesis with intravenous albumin.[67,69,70]

The recommendations for the treatment of refractory ascites based on these conclusions are summarized in Box 32.2.

Liver transplantation

Liver transplantation has become a frequent intervention for patients with advanced cirrhosis. Although randomized trials comparing liver transplantation with conventional medical therapy in patients with ascites are not available for obvious reasons, the 70–80% 5-year probability of survival obtained in adult cirrhotic patients treated with liver transplantation in most centers is markedly greater than the expected 20% in non-transplanted patients with cirrhosis and ascites.[71] B2

Earlier recommendations suggested that ascites *per se* was not an indication for liver transplantation, and patients had to be considered for transplantation only when ascites was refractory to diuretic therapy or was associated with severe complications, such as spontaneous bacterial peritonitis or hepatorenal syndrome. However, with these guidelines a large proportion of these patients die while registered on the transplantation waiting list. This is because of the short survival associated with these conditions. The median survival time is less than 1 year for patients with refractory ascites and those recovering from spontaneous bacterial peritonitis and is even shorter in patients with hepatorenal syndrome, particularly in those with the progressive form of

Box 32.2 Recommendations for the management of patients with cirrhosis and refractory ascites

1 Total paracentesis plus intravenous albumin (8 g/l of ascites removed). Repeat paracentesis during follow up whenever needed. Patients can be treated as outpatients. Consider liver transplantation

2 Patients should be on moderate sodium restriction (40–80 mmol/day) and maximum tolerated doses of diuretics (up to spironolactone 400 mg/day and furosemide 160 mg/day). Check urine sodium under diuretic therapy. If urine sodium is greater than 30 mmol/day, diuretic therapy may be maintained because it may help to delay the recurrence of ascites. If urine sodium is lower than 30 mmol/day or diuretic treatment induces complications, diuretics should be withdrawn

3 Consider the use of transjugular intrahepatic portosystemic shunt (TIPS) in patients with low acceptance of repeated total paracentesis or in those in whom paracentesis is not effective because of the presence of peritoneal adhesions

this syndrome – type 1 – who have a median survival time of less than 1 month.[50,51,72,73]

With the growing knowledge of the natural history of ascites in cirrhosis, it is now known that a number of factors predictive of survival can be used to identify candidates for liver transplantation.[74–76] The most useful predictive factors are related to abnormalities in renal function and systemic hemodynamics and include:

- an impaired ability to excrete a water load (urine volume < 8 ml/min after a water load of 5% dextrose 20 ml/kg intravenous (IV));
- spontaneous dilutional hyponatremia (serum sodium < 130 mmol/l);
- arterial hypotension (mean arterial pressure < 80 mmHg in the absence of diuretic therapy);
- reduced glomerular filtration rate (even moderate reductions, as indicated by serum creatinine levels between 1·2 (106 mmol/l and 1·5 mg/dl (133 mmol/l) in the absence of diuretic therapy);
- marked sodium retention (urine sodium < 10 mmol/day under a moderate sodium-restricted diet and in the absence of diuretic therapy).

Interestingly, in patients with ascites these parameters are better than liver function tests as predictors of prognosis.[74,76] Therefore, patients with one or more of these predictive factors have a poor survival expectancy and should be referred to transplant centers for evaluation.

The recently introduced MELD score (Mayo End-stage Liver Disease score which includes serum bilirubin, international normalized ratio (INR) and serum creatinine)[77] may be suitable for the evaluation of prognosis of patients with cirrhosis and ascites, as it includes a variable that estimates the degree of impairment of renal function. However its accuracy in assessing prognosis in these patients has not been assessed.

Hepatorenal syndrome

Hepatorenal syndrome is at the most severe end of the clinical spectrum of abnormalities of renal function in patients with cirrhosis and ascites.[3,6,42,78] It may occur in two different clinical patterns.[42]

Type 1 hepatorenal syndrome is characterized by rapid and progressive impairment of renal function as defined by a 100% increase of the initial serum creatinine to a level greater than 2·5 mg/dl (221 mmol/l) or a 50% reduction of the initial 24-hour creatinine clearance to a level lower than 20 ml/min in less than 2 weeks; in some patients, this type of hepatorenal syndrome develops spontaneously without any identifiable precipitating factor, while in others it occurs in close chronological relationship with some complicating event, particularly after the resolution of spontaneous bacterial peritonitis.[79]

Type 2 hepatorenal syndrome is characterized by a less severe and non-progressive reduction of glomerular filtration rate (at least in the short term); the main clinical consequence of this type of hepatorenal syndrome is refractory ascites.

Because of the lack of specific diagnostic tests, the diagnosis of hepatorenal syndrome is currently made according to several criteria, as proposed by the International Ascites Club, which are based on demonstration of a marked reduction in glomerular filtration rate (serum creatinine >1·5 mg/dl in the absence of diuretic therapy) and the exclusion of other causes of renal failure that may occur in patients with cirrhosis[42] (Box 32.3).

For many years, no effective therapy existed for patients with hepatorenal syndrome, except for liver transplantation. Recently, several effective, new interventions have been introduced.

Vasoconstrictors

A number of observational studies published in the late 1990s and early 2000s showed that the administration of vasoconstrictor drugs to patients with cirrhosis and hepatorenal syndrome causes a marked improvement of renal function in a large proportion of patients.[80–92] B4, C5 The rationale for the use of vasoconstrictors in patients with hepatorenal syndrome is to improve effective arterial blood volume by causing a vasoconstriction of the extremely dilated splanchnic vascular bed. The improvement in the arterial

Box 32.3   Diagnostic criteria of hepatorenal syndrome[a]

Major criteria

- Low glomerular filtration rate, as indicated by serum creatinine greater than 1·5 mg/dl or 24-hour creatinine clearance lower than 40 ml/min
- Absence of shock, ongoing bacterial infection, fluid losses and current treatment with nephrotoxic drugs
- No sustained improvement in renal function (decrease in serum creatinine to 1·5 mg/dl or less or increase in creatinine clearance to 40 ml/min or more) following diuretic withdrawal and expansion of plasma volume with 1·5 l of a plasma expander
- Proteinuria lower than 500 mg/day and no ultrasonographic evidence of obstructive uropathy or parenchymal renal disease

Additional criteria

- Urine volume lower than 500 ml/day
- Urine sodium lower than 10 mmol/l
- Urine osmolality greater than plasma osmolality
- Urine red blood cells less than 50 per high power field
- Serum sodium concentration lower than 130 mmol/l

[a]All major criteria must be present for the diagnosis of hepatorenal syndrome. Additional criteria are not necessary for the diagnosis, but provide supportive evidence.
Reproduced with permission from Arroyo V *et al. Hepatology* 1996;**23**:164–72.[42]

circulatory function leads to a suppression in the activity of vasoconstrictor systems and a subsequent increase in renal perfusion and glomerular filtration rate.[93]

Two types of vasoconstrictor drugs have been used in patients with hepatorenal syndrome: vasopressin analogs (terlipressin and ornipressin) and α-adrenergic agonists (norepinephrine (noradrenaline) and midodrine), which act on V1 vasopressin receptors and α1-adrenergic receptors, respectively, present in the smooth muscle cells of the vessel wall. The drug most frequently used in published studies is terlipressin, which is marketed in many countries for the indication of acute variceal bleeding in cirrhosis. Ornipressin is no longer available and there is very limited information on the efficacy of α-adrenergic agonists.[85,92] There is only one randomized trial investigating the efficacy and safety of terlipressin in patients with hepatorenal syndrome.[94] Ald The information currently available can be summarized as follows:

1   The administration of terlipressin (0·5–2 mg/4–6 hourly intravenously) is associated with a complete renal response, as defined by a reduction of serum creatinine from pretreatment values to a level below 1·5 mg/dl, in 50–75% of patients treated[86–91] (Table 32.4). Because of

the lack of dose-finding studies, the therapeutic schedule of terlipressin with the best efficacy/safety ratio is unknown.

2   In most studies, treatment with terlipressin is usually maintained until serum creatinine decreases below 1·5 mg/dl (responders) or for a maximum of 15 days. It is unknown whether the continued administration of the drug after the endpoint of 1·5 mg/dl of serum creatinine has been reached may cause a further improvement of renal function.

3   In responding patients, the improvement in urine volume tends to occur immediately after the first doses of terlipressin (within 12–24 hours), while that the improvement of glomerular filtration rate usually occurs slowly over several days. In some, but not all cases, there is also an increased sodium excretion and improvement or normalization of serum sodium concentration.

4   In most studies, intravenous albumin has been given at variable doses for the duration of therapy with terlipressin. The suggestion has been made that intravenous albumin improves the beneficial effects of terlipressin on renal function.[89] However, this remains to be proved conclusively in a randomized trial.

5   A consistent finding in all studies is that the recurrence of hepatorenal syndrome after treatment withdrawal is uncommon (approximately 15% of patients) (Table 32.4). The explanation for this is unknown. Treatment of recurrence is usually effective.

6   The incidence of ischemic adverse effects which require the discontinuation of terlipressin ranges between 5% and 10% of patients. It has to be taken into account that most, if not all, studies excluded high risk patients with ischemic heart disease or other arterial diseases.

7   The possible beneficial effect of terlipressin on survival of patients with hepatorenal syndrome has not been proved. However, the observation of several studies and the single randomized trial that responding patients had a longer survival compared with non-responders, together with the well-known fact that the spontaneous improvement is extremely uncommon, suggests that terlipressin may actually improve survival of patients with hepatorenal syndrome.

8   The above observations refer mainly to type 1 hepatorenal syndrome, as the majority of patients included in the published studies were in this category. Although some reports suggest that vasoconstrictors also improve renal function in patients with type 2 hepatorenal syndrome,[89] their efficacy in this setting remains to be confirmed.

Transjugular intrahepatic portosystemic shunt

There is limited information on the effects of TIPS in patients with type 1 hepatorenal syndrome. Two uncontrolled

Table 32.4 Response rate, recurrence, adverse effects and survival in patients with cirrhosis and hepatorenal syndrome treated with terlipressin

	No. of patients/total no. of patients included (%)
Response[a]	
Uriz et al.[86]	7/9 (77)
Mulkay et al.[87]	11/12 (92)
Moreau et al.[88]	57/99 (58)
Ortega et al.[89]	12/21 (57)
Halimi et al.[90]	13/18 (72)
Colle et al.[91]	11/18 (61)
Recurrence[b]	
Uriz et al.[86]	0/7 (0)
Mulkay et al.[87]	6/11 (55)
Moreau et al.[88]	NR
Ortega et al.[89]	2/12 (17)
Halimi et al.[90]	NR
Colle et al.[91]	7/11 (64)
Adverse effects[c]	
Uriz et al.[86]	0
Mulkay et al.[87]	0
Moreau et al.[88]	16/99 (16) (Ischemia in lower limbs, hypertension, arryhthmia, dyspnea)
Ortega et al.[89]	1/21 (5) (Finger ischemia)
Halimi et al.[90]	3/18 (17) (Skin necrosis)
Colle et al.[91]	1/18 (5) (Finger ischemia)
Mean survival (days)	
Uriz et al.[86]	47
Mulkay et al.[87]	42
Moreau et al.[88]	21
Ortega et al.[89]	32
Halimi et al.[90]	NR
Colle et al.[91]	24

[a]The definition of response varies among studies.
[b]Recurrence of hepatorenal syndrome after treatment withdrawal in responding patients. Definition of recurrence also varies among studies.
[c]Most patients presented self-limited abdominal cramps and/or diarrhea during the administration of the first doses of terlipressin.
NR, not reported

studies reported that TIPS improves renal function in patients with this syndrome.[95,96] B4 There is an important limitation to the use of TIPS in this indication that is the high proportion of patients with very advanced liver disease (Child–Pugh score greater than 12) and/or severe hepatic encephalopathy. No studies have been reported that compared TIPS with vasoconstrictor drugs in patients with type 1 hepatorenal syndrome.

There have been no specific studies assessing the efficacy of TIPS in type 2 hepatorenal syndrome. However, in a subgroup analysis of patients with refractory ascites and type 2 hepatorenal syndrome included in one randomized trial TIPS reduced the recurrence rate of ascites and the risk of progression from type 2 to type 1 hepatorenal syndrome but did not improve survival compared to control patients treated with repeated therapeutic paracentesis with intravenous albumin.[69] A1d

Other therapeutic methods

Hemodialysis is frequently used in the management of type 1 hepatorenal syndrome in many centers, particularly in patients who are candidates for liver transplantation, with the aim of preventing the complications associated with acute renal failure and maintaining patients alive until transplantation is done. However, any beneficial effects of this procedure in type 1 hepatorenal syndrome have not been convincingly demonstrated.[97] Complications during hemodialysis in these patients are common and include arterial hypotension, bleeding and infections. On the other hand, clinical or biochemical features indicating the need for renal replacement therapy, such as heart or respiratory failure, severe acidosis or severe hyperkalemia are uncommon, at least in early stages of type 1 hepatorenal syndrome. In contrast, these features are usually seen in patients with cirrhosis and acute renal failure caused by conditions other than hepatorenal syndrome, especially acute tubular necrosis due to septic or hemorrhagic shock and acute glomerulonephritis. Considering all these facts and the efficacy of measures aimed at improving circulatory function (especially vasoconstrictors), the use of hemodialysis in the management of patients with hepatorenal syndrome needs to be re-evaluated and perhaps used as a second-line therapy for those patients not responding to vasoconstrictors. Recently, a new method of dialysis, the extracorporeal albumin dialysis or molecular adsorbent recirculating system (MARS), a system that uses an albumin-containing dialysate that is used to remove albumin-bound and water-soluble toxic metabolites, has been reported to improve renal function and survival in a small uncontrolled study in patients with hepatorenal syndrome.[98] B4 These promising results, however, require confirmation.

Drugs other than vasoconstrictors have been used for many years in the management of hepatorenal syndrome despite their unproved efficacy. This holds true for drugs with a renal vasodilator effect, such as dopamine or prostaglandins.[99] C5 Several isolated reports suggested a beneficial effect of octreotide, a drug that inhibits the production of several vasodilator peptides of splanchnic origin. However, a recent randomized, controlled trial did not show any benefit.[100] A1d Finally, *N*-acetyl-cysteine was shown to be effective in a small series of patients, but this result requires confirmation in a larger controlled trial.[101] B4

Liver transplantation

Liver transplantation is the only definitive treatment for patients with hepatorenal syndrome without contraindications to the procedure. Even patients showing a complete response to vasoconstrictors or TIPS with normalization of serum creatinine have a poor prognosis, with a median survival time of only 2 months.[88,89] B4 Main causes of death in these patients include liver failure and/or bacterial infections.[88,89] Ideally, patients with hepatorenal syndrome should be prioritized for liver transplantation due to the high mortality rate; otherwise, most patients may die while awaiting liver transplantation. The recently implemented system of organ allocation in USA based on the MELD score may be useful in this respect, because it includes serum creatinine in addition to parameters of liver function (bilirubin and INR).[77,102] Therefore, patients with hepatorenal syndrome usually achieve high values in the MELD score and may receive transplants within a short period of time. In addition to prioritization, these patients should probably be treated with vasoconstrictors, whenever possible, while awaiting transplantation in order to improve renal function and maintain life while they are on the waiting list. A possible additional advantage of pretransplant treatment of hepatorenal syndrome is a reduction of the high morbidity and mortality that has been reported after transplantation in patients with this syndrome.[103,104] A recent study indicates that patients with hepatorenal syndrome treated with vasopressin analogs before transplantation have a complication rate and short-term and long-term survival which are not different from those observed in transplant patients without hepatorenal syndrome.[105]

Dilutional hyponatremia

Patients with advanced cirrhosis often develop spontaneous dilutional hyponatremia due to impairment of the renal excretion of free water. This disorder always occurs in the setting of ascites with severe sodium retention, and most patients have poor or no response to diuretics.[106] B4 The impaired water excretion is due to high circulating levels of vasopressin (antidiuretic hormone) secondary to a hypersecretion of the hormone from the neurohypophysis triggered by a non-osmotic (vasoactive) stimulus.[106] The clinical consequences of dilutional hyponatremia are uncompletely understood, but it has been linked to some neurological and non-neurological symptoms seen frequently in patients with advanced cirrhosis. Dilutional hyponatremia impairs the quality of life of patients with cirrhosis because it requires the restriction of fluid intake to a level similar to that of urine output in order to prevent a positive fluid balance that would lead to a further increase in total body water and impairment of hyponatremia.

There is no effective therapy available in clinical practice to treat spontaneous dilutional hyponatremia. Fluid restriction is effective in preventing further reduction of serum sodium concentration but usually is not followed by an increase in serum sodium.[107] B4 The administration of hypertonic saline solutions does not make much sense from a pathophysiological perspective, because total body sodium and extracellular fluid volume are increased in patients with dilutional hyponatremia. It invariably leads to marked increase in ascites and edema and has only modest effects on serum sodium concentration and therefore is not recommended. There are anecdotal reports of the efficacy of albumin infusions, but this remains to be proved in larger series.[108] B4 In recent years, several orally active drugs that antagonize selectively the vasopressin V2 receptor (the receptor present in collecting duct cells in the kidney responsible for water reabsorption in the distal parts of the nephron), have been developed.[109] C5 The rationale behind the use of these drugs in patients with cirrhosis and dilutional hyponatremia is to antagonize selectively the effects of vasopressin in the kidney so that free water excretion is increased, the abnormal water balance restored, the increased body water reduced, and serum sodium concentration normalized. So far, the results of a few phase II studies in patients with cirrhosis have confirmed the beneficial effects of these drugs. The oral administration of a single dose of a vasopressin receptor antagonist causes a marked increase in urine output and free water clearance, decrease in urine osmolality, and increase in serum sodium concentration.[110–111] B4 These beneficial effects are maintained in patients receiving multiple doses of the drug.[107,112] Normalization of serum sodium concentration is achieved in up to 50% of patients after 7 days of therapy compared with 0% of patients receiving placebo.[107] B4 No major adverse effects were observed in these studies, except for an increase in thirst in patients treated with the highest doses of the drugs. Although a number of issues remain to be answered about the efficacy, clinical usefulness, tolerability, drug interactions (especially with diuretics), and adverse effects of this new family of drugs, they represent a powerful pharmacological tool for the management of patients with advanced cirrhosis and dilutional hyponatremia.

Spontaneous bacterial peritonitis

Spontaneous bacterial peritonitis is a common and severe complication in cirrhotic patients with ascites characterized by infection of ascitic fluid with no apparent intra-abdominal source of infection.[4,5] Spontaneous bacterial peritonitis is generally caused by Gram-negative bacteria from the intestinal flora, especially *Escherichia coli*. However, Gram-positive cocci, particularly *Staphylococcus aureus*, are being isolated with increasing frequency, mainly in hospitalized patients.[113–115] The diagnosis of spontaneous bacterial peritonitis is based on the demonstration of an absolute number of polymorphonuclear cells in ascitic fluid greater than 250/mm[3]. In medical settings in which a cell count of ascitic fluid is not feasible on an emergency basis, the use of reagent strips for leukocyte esterase may be an easy and inexpensive way to diagnose spontaneous bacterial peritonitis.[116] The clinical spectrum is very variable and ranges from complete absence of symptoms to a classic clinical picture of peritonitis.[117] For this reason and because of its high prevalence, spontaneous bacterial peritonitis should be ruled out in patients with cirrhosis admitted to hospital with ascites, outpatients undergoing large volume paracentesis, and hospitalized patients who develop signs and/or symptoms suggestive of peritoneal or systemic infection (i.e. abdominal pain, rebound tenderness, ileus, fever, leukocytosis, shock), hepatic encephalopathy or impairment in renal function.[117,118] Cirrhotic patients with hydrothorax may also develop a spontaneous infection of pleural fluid that is pathogenically similar to spontaneous bacterial peritonitis and should be managed in a similar fashion.[119]

Therapy

Antibiotic therapy should be started whenever the polymorphonuclear count in ascitic fluid is greater than 250/mm[3] and before obtaining microbiological culture results.[117] Third-generation cephalosporins are the antibiotics of choice as initial empiric treatment for spontaneous bacterial peritonitis, because of their broad antibacterial spectrum, high efficacy and safety.[117,120–123] A1c Resolution of infection occurs in up to 90% of patients. Cefotaxime (2 g/8–12 hours) has been the drug most commonly used in randomized trials, but other third-generation cephalosporins have similar efficacy.[124] A1c Cefotaxime has been shown to be more effective than other antibiotics, such as aztreonam or the combination of aminoglycosides plus ampicillin.[120–125] Amoxicillin-clavulinic acid is as effective as third-generation cephalosporins.[126] Quinolones (ofloxacin, ciprofloxacin) administered orally are also effective and may be an alternative to third-generation cephalosporins or amoxicillin-clavulanic acid except in patients who are severely ill (i.e. septic shock, severe renal failure) or with complications that may impair the absorption of the drug (gastrointestinal hemorrhage or ileus).[127] A1c Given the increased frequency of Gram-positive cocci isolates in nosocomial spontaneous bacterial peritonitis,[113–115] the empiric antibiotic treatment for this condition should probably include an antibiotic active against these bacteria, particularly *S. aureus*, until the results of ascitic fluid or blood cultures are available. C5 Antibiotic therapy is maintained until the complete disappearance of all signs of infection and decrease of polymorphonuclear count in

ascitic fluid below the threshold value of 250/mm[3]. In most patients, resolution is achieved in a short period of time, usually less than 6 days.

The development of renal failure, which is one of the most common and severe complications of spontaneous bacterial peritonitis,[79] can be effectively prevented by the administration of albumin together with the antibiotic therapy.[128] B4 The incidence of renal failure is markedly lower in patients receiving albumin plus antibiotics compared with patients receiving antibiotics alone. The prevention of renal failure achieved by administration of albumin improves survival of these patients.[128] B4 This may be particularly important for liver transplant candidates. The beneficial effect of albumin is probably related to its capacity to prevent the reduction in the effective arterial blood volume and subsequent activation of vasoconstrictor systems that occurs during the infection.

Recommendations for the management of spontaneous bacterial peritonitis are summarized in Box 32.4.

Hospital mortality in patients with spontaneous bacterial peritonitis was around 30% in most series published during the 1980s and 1990s. In the series that included patients treated with intravenous albumin, hospital mortality has decreased to 10–15%.[128] Advanced liver failure and associated complications (i.e. gastrointestinal hemorrhage, renal failure) are the main causes of death in these patients. As previously discussed, the most important predictor of survival in patients with spontaneous bacterial peritonitis is the development of renal failure during the infection.[79] Long-term prognosis of patients who have recovered from an episode of spontaneous bacterial peritonitis is poor, and patients should be evaluated for liver transplantation. Recurrent spontaneous bacterial

---

Box 32.4 Recommendations for the management of spontaneous bacterial peritonitis

1 After diagnosis of peritonitis has been made (>250 polymorphonuclear cells/mm[3] in ascitic fluid), start with third-generation cephalosporins (i.e. cefotaxime 2 g/8–12 hourly intravenously or ceftriaxone 1 g/24 hours intravenously) or amoxicillin-clavulinic acid (500 mg/125 mg/8 hourly intravenously). In patients on antibiotic prophylaxis, third-generation cephalosporins are the treatment of choice. In nosocomial spontaneous bacterial peritonitis, consider the addition of an antibiotic active against Gram-positive cocci

2 Give albumin 1·5 g/kg intravenously at the time of diagnosis of the infection and 1 g/kg 48 hours later

3 Maintain antibiotic therapy until disappearance of signs of infection and reduction of polymorphonuclear cells in ascitic fluid below 250/mm[3]

4 After resolution of infection, start long-term norfloxacin 400 mg/day per os (orally)

Table 32.5 Incidence of spontaneous bacterial peritonitis in randomized trials of antibiotic prophylaxis in cirrhosis[a]

Antibiotic regimen	Spontaneous bacterial peritonitis		
	Control	Antibiotic	P
Primary prophylaxis[b]			
Gastrointestinal hemorrhage			
Rimola *et al.*[129] — Non-absorbable antibiotics[c] po	15/72 (21)	6/68 (9)	0·05
Soriano *et al.*[130] — Norfloxacin 400 twice daily po	10/59 (17)	2/60 (3)	0·02
Blaise *et al.*[131] — Ofloxacin 400 mg/day IV	7/45 (16)	3/46 (7)	NS
Pauwels *et al.*[132] — Ciprofloxacin 200 mg IV + amoxicillin and clavulanic acid 1 g/200 mg po thrice daily	7/34 (21)	1/30 (3)	0·05
Ascites			
Soriano *et al.*[137] — Norfloxacin 400 mg/day po	7/31 (23)	0/32 (0)	0·005
Rolanchon *et al.*[138] — Ciprofloxacin 750 mg weekly po	7/32 (22)	1/28 (4)	0·05
Singh *et al.*[139] — Trimethoprim-sulfamethoxazole 160 mg/800 mg 5 days a week po	8/30 (27)	1/30 (3)	0·03
Novella *et al.*[140] — Norfloxacin 400 mg/day po	9/53 (17)[d]	1/56 (2)	0·007
Grange *et al.*[141] — Norfloxacin 400 mg/day po	4/54 (7)	0/53 (0)	NS
Secondary prophylaxis			
Ginès *et al.*[134] — Norfloxacin 400 mg/day po	14/40 (35)	5/40 (12)	0·03

[a]Figures represent the number of patients developing spontaneous bacterial peritonitis during follow up compared with the total number of patients in each treatment group.
[b]Refers to antibiotic prophylaxis given to prevent the first episode of spontaneous bacterial peritonitis.
[c]Combination of gentamicin, vancomycin and nystatin or neomycin, colistin and nystatin.
[d]The control group received norfloxacin only during hospitalizations.
po, per os (orally)

peritonitis is very common in these patients and constitutes a major cause of death.[72]

Prophylaxis

The identification of subsets of patients with an increased risk of developing spontaneous bacterial peritonitis has stimulated the search for interventions to prevent the development of this complication. Conditions associated with an increased risk of spontaneous bacterial peritonitis include: gastrointestinal bleeding, low protein concentration in ascitic fluid, advanced liver failure (high serum bilirubin and/or markedly prolonged prothrombin time), and past history of spontaneous bacterial peritonitis.[4,5,117] Because most episodes are caused by Gram-negative bacteria present in the normal intestinal flora, the rationale for the prophylaxis of spontaneous bacterial peritonitis has been based mainly on the administration of antibiotics that produce a selective decontamination of the gastrointestinal tract, with elimination of aerobic Gram-negative bacteria without affecting aerobic Gram-positive bacteria and anaerobes.

The efficacy of this approach has been demonstrated in patients with gastrointestinal hemorrhage[129–133] and in patients who have recovered from the first spontaneous bacterial peritonitis episode (Table 32.5).[134] A1c In patients with gastrointestinal hemorrhage, the short-term administration of norfloxacin reduces markedly the incidence of spontaneous bacterial peritonitis or bacteremia as compared with patients not receiving prophylactic antibiotics.[130] Other effective approaches consist of the administration of parenteral antibiotics, such as ofloxacin or the combination of ciprofloxacin and amoxicillin-clavulinic acid.[131,132] B4 The absolute risk reduction in four trials of antibiotic prophylaxis in patients with gastrointestinal hemorrhage ranges from 9% to 23%. The results of a meta-analysis indicate that antibiotic prophylaxis in patients with gastrointestinal bleeding not only prevents infection but also improves survival.[133] A1c

Long-term norfloxacin administration is very effective in the prevention of spontaneous bacterial peritonitis recurrence (Table 32.5).[134] The occurrence of episodes caused by Gram-negative bacteria resistant to norfloxacin was very uncommon in the past [134,135] but is now being reported with increasing frequency.[113] However, long-term norfloxacin prophylaxis is still quite effective and is recommended to prevent recurrence in patients who have recovered from an initial episode).[113,117,136–138] A1d

Antibiotic prophylaxis (norfloxacin, ciprofloxacin, or trimethoprim-sulfamethoxazole) also appears to be effective in the prevention of the first episode of spontaneous bacterial peritonitis (primary prophylaxis) in patients with low ascitic fluid protein (< 10–15 g/l), who have a high risk of developing spontaneous bacterial peritonitis (Table 32.5).[138–142] AId However, the published studies summarized in Table 32.5 included only small numbers of patients and were of short duration or were not placebo controlled. Additional randomized controlled trials involving larger numbers of patients with longer periods of followup are needed before primary prophylaxis can be recommended routinely for this patient population.[143] In the mean time, the possible benefit of preventing the first spontaneous bacterial peritonitis episode in these patients has to be weighed against the risk of occurrence of infections by resistant organisms.

References

1 Arroyo V, Ginès P, Planas R *et al.* Pathogenesis, diagnosis and treatment of ascites in cirrhosis. In: McIntyre N, Benhamou JP, Bircher J *et al.* (eds). *Oxford textbook of clinical hepatology, 2nd edn.* Oxford: Oxford University Press, 1999.

2 Ginès P, Fernández-Esparrach G, Arroyo V *et al.* Pathogenesis of ascites in cirrhosis. *Semin Liver Dis* 1997;**17**:175–91.

3 Ginès P, Rodés J. Clinical disorders of renal function in cirrhosis with ascites. In: Arroyo V, Ginès P, Rodés J *et al* (eds). *Ascites and renal dysfunction in liver disease. Pathogenesis, diagnosis and treatment.* Malden: Blackwell Science, 1999.

4 Rimola A, Navasa M. Infections in liver diseases. In: McIntyre N, Benhamou JP, Bircher J *et al.* (eds). *Oxford textbook of clinical hepatology, 2nd edn.* Oxford: Oxford University Press, 1999.

5 Guarner C, Soriano G. Spontaneous bacterial peritonitis. *Semin Liver Dis* 1997;**17**:203–18.

6 Arroyo V, Ginès P, Jiménez W *et al.* Renal dysfunction in cirrhosis. In: McIntyre N, Benhamou JP, Bircher J *et al.* (eds). *Oxford textbook of clinical hepatology, 2nd edn.* Oxford: Oxford University Press, 1999.

7 Schrier RW, Arroyo V, Bernardi M *et al.* Peripheral arterial vasodilation hypothesis: a proposal for the initiation of renal sodium and water retention in cirrhosis. *Hepatology* 1988;**8**:1151–7.

8 Martin PY, Ginès P, Schrier RW. Role of nitric oxide as mediator of hemodynamic abnormalities and sodium and water retention in cirrhosis. *N Engl J Med* 1998;**339**:533–41.

9 Farnsworth EB, Krakusin JS. Electrolyte partition in patients with edema of various origins. *J Lab Clin Med* 1948;**33**:1545–54.

10 Eisenmenger WJ, Blondheim SH, Bongiovanni AM *et al.* Electrolyte studies on patients with cirrhosis of the liver. *J Clin Invest* 1950;**29**:1491–9.

11 Reynolds TB, Lieberman FL, Goodman AR. Advantages of treatment of ascites without sodium restriction and without complete removal of excess fluid. *Gut* 1978;**19**:549–53.

12 Gauthier A, Levy VG, Quinton A *et al.* Salt or no salt in the treatment of cirrhotic ascites: a randomised study. *Gut* 1986;**27**:705–9.

13 Bernardi M, Laffi G, Salvagnini M *et al.* Efficacy and safety of the stepped care medical treatment of ascites in liver cirrhosis: a randomized controlled clinical trial comparing two diets with different sodium content. *Liver* 1993;**13**:156–62.

14 Ascione A, Burroughs AK. Paracentesis for ascites in cirrhotic patients. *Gastroenterol Int* 1990;**3**:120–3.

15 Arroyo V, Ginès A, Saló J. A European survey on the treatment of ascites in cirrhosis. *J Hepatol* 1994;**21**:667–72.

16 Ginès P, Arroyo V, Quintero E *et al.* Comparison of paracentesis and diuretics in the treatment of cirrhotics with tense ascites. Results of a randomized study. *Gastroenterology* 1987;**93**:234–41.

17 Salerno F, Badalamenti S, Incerti P *et al.* Repeated paracentesis and iv albumin infusion to treat "tense" ascites in cirrhotic patients: A safe alternative therapy. *J Hepatol* 1987;**5**:102–8.

18 Hagège H, Ink O, Ducreux M *et al.* Traitement de l'ascite chez les malades atteints de cirrhose sans hyponatrémie ni insuffisance rénale. Résultats d'une étude randomisée comparant les diurétiques et les ponctions compensées par l'albumine. *Gastroenterol Clin Biol* 1992;**16**:751–5.

19 Acharya SK, Balwinder S, Padhee AK *et al.* Large-volume paracentesis and intravenous dextran to treat tense ascites. *J Clin Gastroenterol* 1992;**14**:31–5.

20 Solà R, Vila MC, Andreu M *et al.* Total paracentesis with dextran 40 vs diuretics in the treatment of ascites in cirrhosis: a randomized controlled study. *J Hepatol* 1994;**20**:282–8.

21 Fernádez-Esparrach G, Guevara M, Sort P *et al.* Diuretic requirements after therapeutic paracentesis in non-azotemic patients with cirrhosis. A randomized double-blind trial of spironolactone versus placebo. *J Hepatol* 1997;**26**:614–20.

22 Runyon BA. Treatment of patients with cirrhosis and ascites. *Semin Liver Dis* 1997;**17**:249–60.

23 Ginès P, Titó Ll, Arroyo V *et al.* Randomized comparative study of therapeutic paracentesis with and without intravenous albumin in cirrhosis. *Gastroenterology* 1988;**94**:1493–502.

24 Pozzi M, Osculati G, Boari G *et al.* Time course of circulatory and humoral effects of rapid total paracentesis in cirrhotic patients with tense, refractory ascites. *Gastroenterology* 1994;**106**:709–19.

25 Luca A, Garcia-Pagan JC, Bosch J *et al.* Beneficial effects of intravenous albumin infusion on the hemodynamic and humoral changes after total paracentesis. *Hepatology* 1995;**22**:753–8.

26 Saló J, Ginès A, Ginès P *et al.* Effect of therapeutic paracentesis on plasma volume and trans-vascular escape rate of albumin in patients with cirrhosis. *J Hepatol* 1997;**27**:645–53.

27 Ruiz del Arbol L, Monescillo A, Jiménez W *et al.* Paracentesis-induced circulatory dysfunction: mechanism and effect on hepatic hemodynamics in cirrhosis. *Gastroenterology* 1997;**113**:579–86.

28 Vila MC, Solà R, Molina L *et al.* Hemodynamic changes in patients developing effective hypovolemia after total paracentesis. *J Hepatol* 1998;**28**:639–45.

29 Ginès A, Fernández-Esparrach G, Monescillo A *et al.* Randomized trial comparing albumin, dextran-70 and polygelin in cirrhotic patients with ascites treated by paracentesis. *Gastroenterology* 1996;**111**:1002–10.

30 Planas R, Ginès P, Arroyo V *et al.* Dextran 70 vs albumin as plasma expanders in cirrhotic patients with tense ascites treated with total paracentesis. Results of a randomized study. *Gastroenterology* 1990;**99**:1736–44.

31 Salerno F, Badalamenti S, Lorenzano E *et al.* Randomized comparative study of Hemaccel vs albumin infusion after total paracentesis in cirrhotic patients with refractory ascites. *Hepatology* 1991;**13**:707–13.

32 Fassio E, Terg R, Landeira G *et al.* Paracentesis with dextran 70 vs paracentesis with albumin in cirrhosis with tense ascites: results of a randomized study. *J Hepatol* 1992;**14**:310–16.

33 Bataller R, Ginès P, Arroyo V. Practical recommendations for the treatment of ascites and its complications. *Drugs* 1997; **54**:571–80.

34 Angeli P, Gatta A. Medical treatment of ascites in cirrhosis. In Arroyo V, Ginès P, Rodés J *et al* (eds). *Ascites and renal dysfunction in liver disease. Pathogenesis, diagnosis and treatment.* Malden: Blackwell Science, 1999.

35 Pérez-Ayuso RM, Arroyo V, Planas R *et al.* Randomized comparative study of efficacy of furosemide versus spironolactone in nonazotemic cirrhosis with ascites. Relationship between the diuretic response and the activity of the renin–aldosterone system. *Gastroenterology* 1983; **84**:961–8.

36 Angeli P, Pria MD, De Bei E *et al.* Randomized clinical study of the efficacy of amiloride and potassium canreonate in nonazotemic cirrhotic patients with ascites. *Hepatology* 1994;**19**:72–9.

37 Campra JL, Reynolds TB. Effectiveness of high-dose spironolactone therapy in patients with chronic liver disease and relatively refractory ascites. *Dig Dis Sci* 1978;**23**: 1025–30.

38 Eggert RC. Spironolactone diuresis in patients with cirrhosis and ascites. *BMJ* 1970;**4**:401–3.

39 Strauss E, De SaMF, Lacet CM *et al.* Standardization of a therapeutic approach for ascites due to chronic liver disease. A prospective study of 100 patients. *Gastrointest Endosc Digest* 1985;**4**:79–86.

40 Gatta A, Angeli P, Caregaro L *et al.* A pathophysiological interpretation of unresponsiveness to spironolactone in a stepped care approach to the diuretic treatment of ascites in nonazotemic cirrhotic patients. *Hepatology* 1991;**14**: 231–6.

41 Santos J, Planas R, Pardo A *et al.* Spironolactone alone or in combination with furosemide in the treatment of moderate ascites in nonazotemic cirrhosis. A randomized comparative study of efficacy and safety. *J Hepatol* 2003;**39**:187–92.

42 Arroyo V, Ginès P, Gerbes A *et al.* Definition and diagnostic criteria of refractory ascites and hepatorenal syndrome in cirrhosis. *Hepatology* 1996;**23**:164–76.

43 Angeli P, Albino G, Carraro P *et al.* Cirrhosis and muscle cramps: evidence of a causal relationship. *Hepatology* 1996;**23**:264–73.

44 Gregory PB, Broekelschen PH, Hill MD *et al.* Complications of diuresis in the alcoholic patient with ascites: a controlled trial. *Gastroenterology* 1977;**73**:534–8.

45 Pitt B, Remme W, Zannad F *et al.* Eplerenone Post-Acute Myocardial Infarction Heart Failure. A selective aldosterone blocker, in patients with left ventricular dysfunction after myocardial infarction. Efficacy and Survival Study Investigators. *N Engl J Med* 2003;**348**:1309–21.

46 Lee FY, Lee SD, Tsai YT *et al.* A randomized controlled trial of quinidine in the treatment of cirrhotic patients with muscle cramps. *J Hepatol* 1991;**12**:236–40.

47 Kugelmas M. Preliminary observation: oral zinc sulfate replacement is effective in treating muscle cramps in cirrhotic patients. *J Am Coll Nutr* 2000;**19**:13–15.

48 Blendis LM, Greig PD, Langer B *et al.* Renal and hemodynamic effect of the peritoneovenous shunt for intractable hepatic ascites. *Gastroenterology* 1979;**77**: 250–7.

49 Greig PD, Blendis LM, Langer B *et al.* Renal and hemodynamic effect of the peritoneovenous shunt. II. Long-term effect. *Gastroenterology* 1981;**80**:119–25.

50 Ginès P, Arroyo V, Vargas V *et al.* Paracentesis with intravenous infusion of albumin as compared with peritoneovenous shunting in cirrhosis with refractory ascites. *N Engl J Med* 1991;**325**:829–35.

51 Ginès A, Planas R, Angeli P *et al.* Treatment of patients with cirrhosis and refractory ascites by LeVeen shunt with titanium tip. Comparison with therapeutic paracentesis. *Hepatology* 1995;**22**:124–31.

52 Epstein M. Peritoneovenous shunt in the management of ascites and hepatorenal syndrome. In: Epstein M (ed). *The kidney in liver disease, 4th edn.* Philadelphia: Hanley and Belfus, 1996.

53 Ring-Larsen H. Treatment of refractory ascites. In: Arroyo V, Ginès P, Rodés J, Schrier RW (eds). *Ascites and renal dysfunction in liver disease. Pathogenesis, diagnosis and treatment.* Malden: Blackwell Science, 1999.

54 LeVeen HH, Vujic I, D'Ovidio N *et al.* Peritoneovenous shunt occlusion. Etiology, diagnosis, therapy. *Ann Surg* 1984;**200**:212–23.

55 Rossle M, Deibert P, Haag K *et al.* Randomised trial of transjugular-intrahepatic-portosystemic shunt versus endoscopy plus propranolol for prevention of variceal rebleeding. *Lancet* 1997;**349**:1043–9.

56 Shiffman ML, Jeffers L, Hoofnagle JH *et al.* The role of transjugular intrahepatic portosystemic shunt for treatment of portal hypertension and its complications: a conference sponsored by the National Digestive Disease advisory board. *Hepatology* 1995;**25**:1591–7.

57 Ferral H, Bjarnason H, Wegryn SA *et al.* Refractory ascites: early experience in treatment with transjugular intrahepatic portosystemic shunt. *Radiology* 1993;**189**:7905–801.

58 Somberg KA, Lake JR, Tomlanovich SJ *et al.* Transjugular intrahepatic portosystemic shunt for refractory ascites: assessment of clinical and humoral response and renal function. *Hepatology* 1995;**21**:709–16.

59 Quiroga J, Sangro B, Nuñez M *et al.* Transjugular intrahepatic portal-systemic shunt in the management of refractory ascites: effect on clinical, renal, humoral and hemodynamic parameters. *Hepatology* 1995;**21**:986–94.

60 Wong F, Sniderman K, Liu P *et al.* Transjugular intrahepatic portosystemic stent shunt: effects on hemodynamics and sodium homeostasis in cirrhosis and refractory ascites. *Ann Intern Med* 1995;**122**:816–22.

61 Ochs A, Rössle M, Haag K *et al.* The transjugular intrahepatic portosystemic stent shunt procedure for refractory ascites. *N Engl J Med* 1995;**332**:1192–7.

62 Sanyal AJ, Freedman AM, Shiffman ML *et al.* Porto systemic encephalopathy after transjugular intrahepatic portosystemic shunt: results of a prospective controlled study. *Hepatology* 1994;**20**:46–55.

63 Blei AT. Hepatic encephalopathy in the age of TIPS. *Hepatology* 1994;**20**:249–52.

64 Casado M, Bosch J, Garcia-Pagan JC *et al.* Clinical events after transjugular intrahepatic portosystemic shunt: correlation with hemodynamic findings. *Gastroenterology* 1998;**114**: 1296–303.

65 Braverman AC, Steiner MA, Picus D *et al.* High-output congestive heart failure following transjugular intrahepatic portal-systemic shunting. *Chest* 1995;**107**:1467–9.

66 Sanyal AJ, Freedman AM, Purdum PP *et al.* The hematologic consequences of transjugular intrahepatic portosystemic shunts. *Hepatology* 1996;**23**:32–9.

67 Lebrec D, Giuily N, Hadengue A *et al.* Transjugular intrahepatic portosystemic shunts: comparison with paracentesis in patients with cirrhosis and refractory ascites: a randomized trial. *J Hepatol* 1996;**25**:135–44.

68 Rössle M, Ochs A, Gulberg V *et al.* A comparison of paracentesis and transjugular intrahepatic portosystemic shunting in patients with ascites. *N Engl J Med* 2000; **342**:1701–7.

69 Ginès P, Uriz J, Calahorra B *et al.* Transjugular intrahepatic portosystemic shunting versus paracentesis plus albumin for refractory ascites in cirrhosis. *Gastroenterology* 2002;**123**: 1839–47.

70 Sanyal AJ, Genning C, Reddy KR *et al.* The North American Study for the Treatment of Refractory Ascites. *Gastroenterology* 2003;**124**:634–41.

71 Rimola A, Navasa M, Grande L. Liver transplantation in cirrhotic patients with ascites. In: Arroyo V, Ginès P, Rodés J *et al.* (eds). *Ascites and renal dysfunction in liver disease. Pathogenesis, diagnosis and treatment.* Malden: Blackwell Science, 1999.

72 Titó L, Rimola A, Ginès P *et al.* Recurrence of spontaneous bacterial peritonitis in cirrhosis. Frequency and predictive factors. *Hepatology* 1988;**8**:27–31.

73 Ginès A, Escorsell A, Ginès P *et al.* Incidence, predictive factors, and prognosis of the hepatorenal syndrome in cirrhosis with ascites. *Gastroenterology* 1993;**105**: 229–36.

74 Llach J, Ginès P, Arroyo V *et al.* Prognostic value of arterial pressure, endogenous vasoactive systems, and renal function in cirrhotic patients admitted to the hospital for the treatment of ascites. *Gastroenterology* 1988;**94**:482–7.

75 Ginès P, Fernández-Esparrach G. Prognosis of cirrhosis with ascites. In: Arroyo V, Ginès P, Rodés J *et al.* (eds). *Ascites and renal dysfunction in liver disease. Pathogenesis, diagnosis and treatment.* Malden: Blackwell Science, 1999.

76 Fernandez-Esparrach G, Sanchez-Fueyo A, Gines P *et al.* A prognostic model for predicting survival in cirrhosis with ascites. *J Hepatol* 2001;**34**:46–52.

77 Malinchoc M, Kamath PS, Gordon FD *et al.* A model to predict poor survival in patients undergoing transjugular intrahepatic portosystemic shunts. *Hepatology* 2000;**31**: 864–71.

78 Schrier RW, Niederberger M, Weigert A *et al.* Peripheral arterial vasodilation: determinant of functional spectrum of cirrhosis. *Semin Liver Dis* 1994;**14**:14–22.

79 Follo A, Llovet JM, Navasa M *et al.* Renal impairment after spontaneous bacterial peritonitis in cirrhosis: incidence, clinical course, predictive factors and prognosis. *Hepatology* 1994;**20**:495–501.

80 Guevara M, Ginès P, Fernández-Esparrach G *et al.* Reversibility of hepatorenal syndrome by prolonged administration of ornipressin and plasma volume expansion. *Hepatology* 1998;**27**:35–41.

81 Ganne–Carrié N, Hadengue A, Mathurin P *et al.* Hepatorenal syndrome. Long-term treatment with terlipressin as a bridge to liver transplantation. *Dig Dis Sci* 1996;**41**:1054–6.

82 Hadengue A, Gadano A, Moreau R *et al.* Beneficial effects of the 2-day administration of terlipressin in patients with cirrhosis and hepatorenal syndrome. *J Hepatol* 1998; **29**:565–70.

83 Le Moine O, el Nawar A, Jagodzinski R *et al.* Treatment with terlipressin as a bridge to liver transplantation in a patient with hepatorenal syndrome. *Acta Gastroenterol Belg* 1998;**61**:268–70.

84 Gülberg V, Bilzer M, Gerbes AL. Long-term therapy and retreatment of hepatorenal syndrome type 1 with ornipressin and dopamine. *Hepatology* 1999;**30**:870–5.

85 Angeli P, Volpin R, Gerunda G *et al.* Reversal of type 1 hepatorenal syndrome with the administration of midodrine and octreotide. *Hepatology* 1999;**29**:1690–7.

86 Uriz J, Ginés P, Cardenas A *et al.* Terlipressin plus albumin infusion is an effective and safe therapy of hepatorenal syndrome. *J Hepatol* 2000;**33**:43–8.

87 Mulkay JP, Louis H, Donckter V *et al.* Long-term terlipressin administration improves renal function in cirrhotic patients with type 1 hepatorenal syndrome: a pilot study. *Acta Gastroenterol Belg* 2001;**64**:15–19.

88 Moreau R, Durand F, Poynard T *et al.* Terlipressin in patients with cirrhosis and type 1 hepatorenal syndrome: A restrospective multicenter study. *Gastroenterology* 2002; **122**:923–30.

89 Ortega R, Ginès P, Uriz J *et al.* Terlipressin therapy with and without albumin for patients with hepatorenal syndrome. Results of a prospective, non-randomized study. *Hepatology* 2002;**36**:941–8.

90 Halimi C, Bonnard P, Bernard B *et al.* Effect of terlipressin (Glypressin) on hepatorenal syndrome in cirrhotic patients: results of a multicentre pilot study. *Eur J Gastroenterol Hepatol* 2002;**14**:153–8.

91 Colle I, Durand F, Pessione F *et al.* Clinical course, predictive factors and prognosis in patients with cirrosis and type 1 hepatorenal syndrome treated with terlipressin: a retrospective analysis. *J Gastroenterol Hepatol* 2002;**17**:882–8.

92 Duvoux C, Zanditenas D, Hezode C *et al.* Effects of noradrenalin and albumin in patients with type I hepatorenal syndrome: a pilot study. *Hepatology* 2002;**36**:374–80.

93 Ginès P, Guevara M. Good news for hepatorenal syndrome. *Hepatology* 2002;**36**:374–80.

94 Solanki P, Chawla A, Garg R, Gupta R, Jain M, Sarin SK. Beneficial effects of terlipressin in hepatorenal syndrome: a prospective randomized placebo controlled clinical trial. *J Gastroenterol Hepatology* 2003;**18**:152–6.

95 Guevara M, Ginès P, Bandi JC *et al.* Transjugular intrahepatic portosystemic shunt in hepatorenal syndrome: effects on renal function and vasoactive systems. *Hepatology* 1998;**28**:416–22.

96 Brensing KA, Textor J, Perz J *et al.* Long-term outcome after transjugular intrahepatic portosystemic stent-shunt in non-transplant patients with hepatorenal syndrome: a phase II study. *Gut* 2000;**47**:288–95.

97 Perez GO, Golper TA, Epstein M, Oster JR. Dialysis hemofiltration, and other extracorporeal techniques in the treatment of renal complications of liver disease. In: Epstein M (ed). *The kidney in liver disease, 4th edn.* Philadelphia: Hanley and Belfus, 1996.

98 Mitzner SR, Stange J, Klammt S *et al.* Improvement of hepatorenal syndrome with extracorporeal albumin dialysis MARS: results of a prospective, randomized controlled clinical trial. *Liver Transpl* 2000;**6**:277–86.

99 Arroyo V, Bataller R, Guevara M. Treatment of hepatorenal syndrome in cirrhosis. In: Arroyo V, Ginès P, Rodés J *et al.* (eds). *Ascites and renal dysfunction in liver disease. Pathogenesis, diagnosis and treatment.* Malden: Blackwell Science, 1999.

100 Pomier-Layraigues G, Paquin SC, Hassoun Z *et al.* Octreotide in hepatorenal syndrome: a randomised double blind placebo-controlled cross-over study in cirrhotic patients. *Hepatology* 2003;**38**:238–43..

101 Holt S, Goodier D, Marley R *et al.* Improvement in renal function in hepatorenal syndrome with *N*-acetylcysteine. *Lancet* 1999;**353**:294–5.

102 Wiesner R, Edwards E, Freeman R *et al.* Model for end-stage liver disease (MELD) and allocation of donor livers. *Gastroenterology* 2003;**124**:91–6.

103 Gonwa TA, Morris CA, Goldstein RM *et al.* Long-term survival and renal function following liver transplantation in patients with and without hepatorenal syndrome – experience in 300 patients. *Transplantation* 1991;**51**:428–30.

104 Nair S, Verma S, Thuluvath PJ. Pretransplant renal function predicts survival in patients undergoing orthotopic liver transplantation. *Hepatology* 2002;**35**:1179–85.

105 Restuccia T, Guevara M, Ginès P, *et al.* Impact of pretransplant treatment of hepatorenal syndrome (hrs) with vasopressin analogues on outcome after liver transplantation (ltx). A case–control study. *J Hepatol* 2004;**40**:140–46.

106 Ginès P, Berl T, Bernardi M *et al.* Hyponatremia in cirrhosis: from pathogenesis to treatment. *Hepatology* 1998;**28**:851–64.

107 Gerbes AL, Gulberg V, Ginès P *et al.* Therapy of hyponatremia in cirrhosis with a vasopressin receptor antagonist: a randomized double-blind multicenter trial. *Gastroenterology* 2003;**124**:933–9.

108 McCormick PA, Mistry P, Kaye G *et al.* Intravenous albumin infusion is an effective therapy for hyponatraemia in cirrhotic patients with ascites. *Gut* 1990;**31**:204–7.

109 Ginès P, Jiménez W. Aquaretic agents: a new potential treatment of dilutional hyponatremia in cirrhosis. *J Hepatol* 1996;**24**:506–12.

110 Inoue T, Ohnishi A, Matsuo A *et al.* Therapeutic and diagnostic potential of a vasopressin-2 antagonist for impaired water handling in cirrhosis. *Clin Pharmacol Ther* 1998;**63**:561–70.

111 Guyader D, Patat A, Ellis-Grosse EJ *et al.* Pharmacodynamic effects of a nonpeptide antidiuretic hormone V2 antagonist in cirrhotic patients with ascites. *Hepatology* 2002;**36**:1197–205.

112 Wong F, Blei AT, Blendis LM *et al.* A vasopressin receptor antagonist (VPA-985) improves serum sodium concentration in patients with hyponatremia: a multicenter, randomized, placebo-controlled trial. *Hepatology* 2003;**37**:182–91.

113 Fernández J, Navasa M, Gómez J *et al.* Bacterial infections in cirrhosis: epidemiological changes with invasive procedures and norfloxacin prophylaxis. *Hepatology* 2002;**35**:140–8.

114 Campillo B, Richardet JP, Kheo T, Dupeyron C. Nosocomial spontaneous bacterial peritonitis and bacteremia in cirrhotic patients: impact of isolate type on prognosis and characteristics of infection. *Clin Infect Dis* 2002;**35**:1–10.

115 Bert F, Andreu M, Durand F *et al.* Nosocomial and community-acquired spontaneous bacterial peritonitis: comparative microbiology and therapeutic implications. *Eur J Clin Microbiol Infect Dis* 2003;**22**:10–15.

116 Castellote J, Lopez C, Gornals J *et al.* Rapid diagnosis of spontaneous bacterial peritonitis by use of reagent strips.*Hepatology* 2003;**37**:893–6.

117 Rimola A, Garcia-Tsao G, Navasa M *et al.* Diagnosis, treatment and prophylaxis of spontaneous bacterial peritonitis: a consensus document. International Ascites Club. *J Hepatol* 2000;**32**:142–53.

118 Evans LT, Kim WR, Poterucha JJ, Kamath PS. Spontaneous bacterial peritonitis in asymptomatic outpatients with cirrhotic ascites. *Hepatology* 2003;**37**:745–7.

119 Castellvì JM, Guardiola J, Sesé E *et al.* Spontaneous bacterial empyema of cirrhotic patients: a prospective study. *Hepatology* 1996;**23**:719–24.

120 Felisart J, Rimola A, Arroyo V *et al.* Cefotaxime is more effective than is ampicillin-tobramycin in cirrhotics with severe infections. *Hepatology* 1985;**5**:457–62.

121 Toledo C, Salmerón JM, Rimola A *et al.* Spontaneous bacterial peritonitis in cirrhosis: predictive factors of infection resolution and survival in patients treated with cefotaxime. *Hepatology* 1993;**17**:251–7.

122 Rimola A, Salmerón JM, Clemente G *et al.* Two different dosages of cefotaxime in the treatment of spontaneous bacterial peritonitis in cirrhosis: results of a prospective, randomized, multicenter study. *Hepatology* 1995;**21**: 674–9.

123 Runyon BA, McHutchinson JG, Antillon MR. Short-course versus long-course antibiotic treatment of spontaneous bacterial peritonitis: a randomized, controlled study of 100 patients. *Gastroenterology* 1991;**100**:1737–42.

124 Gómez-Jimènez J, Ribera E, Gasser I *et al.* Randomized trial comparing ceftriaxone with cefonicid for treatment of spontaneous bacterial peritonitis in cirrhotic patients. *Antimicrob Agents Chemother* 1993;**37**:1587–92.

125 Ariza J, Xiol X, Esteve M *et al.* Aztreonam vs Cefotaxime in the treatment of Gram-negative spontaneous peritonitis in cirrhotic patients. *Hepatology* 1991;**14**:91–8.

126 Ricart E, Soriano G, Novella MT *et al.* Amoxicillin-clavulanic acid versus cefotaxime in the therapy of bacterial infections in cirrhotic patients. *J Hepatol* 2000; **32**:596–602.

127 Navasa M, Follo A, Llovet JM *et al.* Randomized, comparative study of oral ofloxacin versus intravenous cefotaxime in spontaneous bacterial peritonitis. *Gastroenterology* 1996;**111**:1011–17.

128 Sort P, Navasa M, Arroyo V *et al.* Effect of intravenous albumin on renal impairment and mortality in patients with cirrhosis and spontaneous bacterial peritonitis. *N Engl J Med* 1999;**341**:403–9.

129 Rimola A, Bory F, Terés J *et al.* Oral non-absorbable antibiotics prevent infection in cirrhosis with gastrointestinal hemorrhage. *Hepatology* 1985;**5**:463–7.

130 Soriano G, Guarner C Tomás A *et al.* Norfloxacin prevents bacterial infection in cirrhotics with gastrointestinal hemorrhage. *Gastroenterology* 1992;**103**:1267–72.

131 Blaise M, Pateron D, Trinchet JC *et al.* Systemic antibiotic therapy prevents bacterial infections in cirrhotic patients with gastrointestinal hemorrhage. *Hepatology* 1994;**20**: 34–8.

132 Pauwels A, Mostefa-Kara N, Debenes B *et al.* Systemic antibiotic prophylaxis after gastrointestinal hemorrhage in cirrhotic patients with a high risk of infection. *Hepatology* 1996;**24**:802–6.

133 Bernard B, Grangé JD, Khac NE *et al.* Antibiotic prophylaxis for the prevention of bacterial infections in cirrhotic patients with gastrointestinal bleeding: a meta-analysis. *Hepatology* 1999;**29**:1655–61.

134 Ginès P, Rimola A, Planas R *et al.* Norfloxacin prevents spontaneous bacterial peritonitis recurrence in cirrhosis: results of a double blind, placebo-controlled trial. *Hepatology* 1990;**12**:716–24.

135 Llovet J, Rodrìguez-Iglesias P, Moitinho E *et al.* Spontaneous bacterial peritonitis in patients with cirrhosis undergoing selective intestinal decontamination. A retrospective study of 229 spontaneous bacterial peritonititis episodes. *J Hepatol* 1997;**26**:88–95.

136 Bauer TM, Follo A, Navasa M *et al.* Daily norfloxacin is more effective than weekly rufloxacin in prevention of spontaneous bacterial peritonitis recurrence. *Dig Dis Sci* 2002;**47**:1356–61.

137 Soriano G, Guarner C, Teixidó M *et al.* Selective intestinal decontamination prevents spontaneous bacterial peritonitis. *Gastroenterology* 1991;**100**:77–81.

138 Rolanchon A, Cordier L, Bacq Y *et al.* Ciprofloxacin and long-term prevention of spontaneous bacterial peritonitis: results of a prospective controlled trial. *Hepatology* 1995;**22**:1171–4.

139 Singh N, Gayowski T, Yu VL *et al.* Trimethoprim-sulfamethoxazole for the prevention of spontaneous bacterial peritonitis in cirrhosis: a randomized trial. *Ann Intern Med* 1995;**122**:595–8.

140 Novella M, Solá R, Soriano G *et al.* Continuous versus inpatient prophylaxis of the first spontaneous bacterial peritonitis with norfloxacin. *Hepatology* 1997;**25**:532–6.

141 Grange JD, Roulot D, Pelletier G *et al.* Norfloxacin primary prophylaxis of bacterial infections in cirrhotic patients with ascites: a double-blind randomized trial. *J Hepatol* 1998; **29**:430–6.

142 Bernard B, Grange JD, Kbac EN *et al.* Antibiotic prophylaxis for the prevention of bacterial infections in cirrhotic patients with ascites: a metaanalysis. *Digestion* 1998;**59**:54–7.

143 Ginès P, Navasa M. Antibiotic prophylaxis for spontaneous bacterial peritonitis: how and whom? *J Hepatol* 1998;**29**: 490–4.

33 Hepatic encephalopathy

Peter Ferenci, Christian Müller

Introduction

Because the pathogenesis of hepatic encephalopathy is unknown,[1] no truly "specific" treatment exists. Nevertheless, a variety of compounds have been introduced for its treatment (Table 33.1). Some of these treatments are based on clinical observations, and some on extrapolation of experimental data obtained from animal models of hepatic encephalopathy. Research is hampered by the imprecise definition of this disabling complication of liver disease. In this light, the Organisation Mondiale de Gastroentérologie commissioned a working party to reach a consensus in this area, which was presented at the 11th World Congress of Gastroenterology in Vienna (1998). The working party continued its work thereafter and published its final report recently.[2] In summary, the working party has suggested a modification of current nomenclature for clinical diagnosis of hepatic encephalopathy and proposed guidelines for future clinical trials in hepatic encephalopathy. It indicated also the need for a large study to redefine neuropsychiatric abnormalities in liver disease, which would allow the diagnosis of minimal (i.e. subclinical) encephalopathy to be made on firm statistical grounds.[2] These new definitions will be the basis to improve the design of clinical studies but cannot be applied to already published trials. Nevertheless, the new nomenclature was used in this analysis.

Design of clinical trials in hepatic encephalopathy

A large spectrum of clinical conditions comes under the term "hepatic encephalopathy" and includes a variety of neuropsychiatric symptoms, ranging from minor, not readily discernible signs of altered brain function, overt psychiatric and/or neurological symptoms to deep coma.[3] Accordingly, the methods to quantify treatment effects and treatment endpoints are highly variable. Another variable is the selection of a control intervention. Most studies compare a new drug to "standard treatment" (which by itself may be highly effective) such as oral lactulose, for which efficacy has not been demonstrated in a randomized controlled trial for

Table 33.1   Interventions for hepatic encephalopathy

	Controlled studies	
	v Lactulose	*v* Placebo
Decrease of ammoniagenic substrates		
Enemas with lactulose		+
Reduction of dietary protein		?
Inhibition of ammonia production		
Antibiotics		
Neomycin	=	=
Rifaximin	=	*v* neomycin =
Vancomycin	= / +	not done
Disaccharides		
Lactulose		? =
Lactitol	=	not done
Lactose in lactase deficiency		+
Modification of colonic flora		
Lactobacillus SF 68	=	not done
Metabolic ammonia removal		
Ornithine aspartate IV		+
Benzoate	=	not done
BCAA supplementation		
Modified AA solutions ("FO80" type)	=	±
Dietary BCAA supplementation		+
Neuroactive drugs		
Flumazenil IV		+
L-Dopa, bromocriptine		=

+ Superior to control treatment; = equal to control treatment; ± conflicting results
BCAA, branched chain amino acids, IV; intravenous

ethical reasons. However, in view of the natural history of hepatic encephalopathy, the inclusion of a placebo control group in trials of new agents is highly desirable. In studies comparing a new drug with effective "standard treatment" demonstration of effectiveness of the new drug

Table 33.2   Methods to assess treatment in various groups of patients with hepatic encephalopathy

Study group	Treatment endpoint	Assessment of treatment effects	Natural history	Problems
Episodic HE type C	Clinical improvement	Clinical grading, EEG, SEP	Well documented	High mortality, precipitating factors
Persistent HE type C	Clinical improvement	Clinical grading, PSE index[a]	Well documented	
Episodic HE type C, recurrent	Recurrence	PSE index, MDF	Variable	Compliance
TIPS or portocaval shunts (surgical)	Prevention of HE	Psychometry, MDF, PSE index[a]	Well documented	
Minimal HE	Psychometry EEG	Psychometry, MDF, P300	Unknown	Clinical meaning of certain tests

[a] PSE index according to Conn and Lieberthal.[4] (The use of this index was not recommended by the WCOG-working party[2]). SEP, somatosensory evoked potentials; MDF, mean dominant frequency; P300, event-related acoustic evoked responses; HE, hepatic encephalopathy; TIPS, transjugular intrahepatic portosystemic shunt; EEG, electroencephalogram

may require a very large sample size. Table 33.2 summarizes the appropriate study endpoints in various patient groups.

Natural history of hepatic encephalopathy

The natural history of hepatic encephalopathy is not well studied. However, examination of the outcomes in the placebo groups in nine randomized controlled trials (Table 33.3) reveals that patients with grades III and IV hepatic encephalopathy may have recovery rates from 22% to greater than 90%. Therefore, in studies of new agents which lack controls, high response rates may be anticipated, and trials of new agents may require quite large numbers of patients to demonstrate benefits. Short-term mortality of patients with hepatic encephalopathy appears to be low if unstable patients are excluded. The course of patients with *subclinical* hepatic encephalopathy is unknown, and it is by definition impossible to detect clinical improvement in such cases. Studies of new agents with subclinical illness should focus on progression to more severe levels of hepatic encephalopathy. The grade of encephalopathy of patients selected for clinical trials may be expected to have a substantial influence on results.

Methods to quantify hepatic encephalopathy

Clinical assessment

The simplest assessment of hepatic encephalopathy is a description of the mental state according to Conn and Lieberthal,[4] which grades hepatic encephalopathy in stages I–IV based on changes in consciousness, intellectual function and behavior. It does not include neurological changes or asterixis. The Glasgow Coma scale is useful in stages III and IV.

Portal–systemic encephalopathy index

In 1977 the portal–systemic encephalopathy (PSE) index[5] was introduced in a trial comparing neomycin with lactulose and has been subsequently used by other investigators. The main problem with this index is the inclusion of arterial ammonia estimations. Hyperammonemia is possibly a cause, but not a symptom or effect of hepatic encephalopathy. Measurements of arterial ammonia concentration require serial arterial punctures. The scoring of actual arterial ammonia concentration is arbitrary and not based on a sound statistical analysis. Furthermore, the other parameters of the PSE index – mental state, electroencephalogram (EEG), and number connection test (NCT) – are also graded by arbitrary units. No age-dependent normal values are used for NCT.[15] Finally, the PSE index does not discriminate between overt, mild or subclinical hepatic encephalopathy and has not been validated prospectively. In clinically overt hepatic encephalopathy the PSE index does not appear to be superior to simple clinical grading.

Psychometric tests

Grading of hepatic encephalopathy does not allow the documentation of subtle changes. Several psychometric tests have been evaluated to quantify the impairment of mental function in mild stages of hepatic encephalopathy.[16–18] Detailed psychometric testing is more sensitive in the detection of minor deficits of mental function than either conventional clinical assessment or the EEG.[19] However, the tests are cumbersome, and when applied repeatedly the reliability of most of them is adversely affected by the learning effect. Few are useful in routine practice. The most frequently applied test is the NCT.[18] This test is easily administered and the results can be quickly quantified. One important

Table 33.3 Survival rates and improvement of hepatic encephalopathy in placebo-treated patients in randomized controlled trials

Study	Test drug	HE grade	No. of patients	Observation time	Exclusion criteria	% Survival (on placebo)	% HE better (on placebo)
Barbaro et al.[a] (1998)[6]	Flumazenil	III	265	6 days	HR, RF, acidosis	97·3	> 90
		IV	262			91·3	> 90
Kircheis et al. (1997)[7]	Ornithine aspartate	MHE	27	7 days	GI bleed, HR, RF	100	0
		I	19			100	22
		II	27			100	44
Stauch et al. (1998)[8]	Ornithine asparate	MHE		14 days	Unstable patients	100	0
		I+II	20			100	40
Marchesini et al. (1990)[9]	BCAA oral	I	34	3 months	Unstable patients	100	38
Michel et al. (1980)[10]	L-Dopa	I–III	38	7 days	None	61	37
Michel et al. (1984)[11]	BCAA IV	I–III	24	5 days	Unstable patients	74	26
Wahren et al. (1983)[12]	BCAA IV	II–IV	25	5 days	None	80	48
Blanc et al. (1994)[13]	Neomycin + lactulose	II–IV	40	5 days	?	85	70
Strauss et al. (1992)[14]	Neomycin	II–IV	19	5 days	MOF	89·5	89·5

[a]All patients were on neomycin.
HR, hepatorenal syndrome; RF, respiratory failure; MOF, multiorgan failure; BCAA, branched chain amino acids; MHE, minimal hepatic encephalopathy; HE, hepatic encephalopathy, IV, intravenous

consequence of the application of psychometric tests in cirrhotic patients was the finding that even patients with apparently normal mental status have a measurable deficit in their intellectual performance.[16] These patients are usually referred to as suffering from "minimal hepatic encephalopathy" or "stage 0 hepatic encephalopathy". However, psychometric tests may overdiagnose minimal hepatic encephalopathy, because scores are usually not corrected for age.[15,19] Furthermore, it is unknown whether abnormalities of test results correlate with impaired quality of life or performance in daily life.[20] On the contrary, the driving ability of patients with test results classifying them as "unable to drive a car"[16] was not different from that of healthy controls.[21] A quality-of-life questionnaire (sickness impact profile – SIP) detects the extent and frequency of deficits in daily functioning in patients without clinically apparent hepatic encephalopathy. From the 136 statements, five were selected as predictive of minimal hepatic encephalopathy.[20]

A standardized prospectively developed test battery that includes the NCT A and B, the line tracing test, the serial dotting test and the digit symbol test was recommended by the working party to be used in future studies.[2] This test can be applied at the bedside and performed within 10–20 minutes and examines visual perception, visuospatial orientation, visual construction, motor speed and accuracy, and is also sensitive against disturbances of concentration, attention and working memory. Each individual test and the whole battery has been standardized on a large group of healthy controls (including all ages). A composite score of the single test results was calculated. Each individual test result was scored 0 points in the ±1 SD range from the mean. Thereby, subjects can achieve between +6 and −8 points. When a cut-off between normal and pathological results was set at −4 points, only 0·9% (1) of the controls, 25% of cirrhotic patients without clinical evidence of hepatic encephalopathy but all patients with grade 1 hepatic encephalopathy achieved pathological results. The test has a high specificity for hepatic encephalopathy as compared with other metabolic encephalopathies.[3]

Electrophysiological tests

The simplest EEG assessment of hepatic encephalopathy is to grade the degree of abnormality of the conventional EEG

Table 33.4 Medline search, 1966–2003

Search parameter	No. of articles
Hepatic encephalopathy (HE)	7085
Treatment of HE	4116
Placebo and HE	92
Randomized controlled trial and HE	223
Double blind and HE	90
HE and publication type = RCT	203
HE and treatment and publication type = RCT	198
RCTs with the endpoint "improvement of HE" and more than 10 patients per study group	41

RCT, randomized controlled trial

trace. A more refined assessment by computer-assisted techniques allow variables in the EEG such as the mean dominant EEG frequency and the power of a particular EEG rhythm to be quantified. Evoked responses (by visual, somatosensory, or acoustic stimuli) or event-related responses, like the P300 peak after auditory stimuli, are sensitive to detect subtle changes of brain function and can be used for diagnosis of minimal hepatic encephalopathy.[22]

Evidence-based medicine and hepatic encephalopathy

Evidence-based medicine is a process of systematically finding, appraising and using research findings as the basis for clinical decisions[23] following the formulation of relevant questions concerning the patient's problems.

The answer to the question "Does treatment with specific drugs, compared with placebo, improve hepatic encephalopathy?" should be addressed separately for overt and subclinical hepatic encephalopathy. In the following sections we have identified the studies that attempt to answer this question and critically appraised the evidence for the most important treatment regimens. The magnitude of the treatment effect of various interventions has been assessed. This assessment is difficult in hepatic encephalopathy because of the use of different methods which are not readily comparable for quantifying the severity of this disease. The question of the clinical applicability and generalizability of the findings of randomized controlled studies in hepatic encephalopathy must be addressed in the context of the treatment and the grade of encephalopathy studied.

Database

To identify all randomized controlled trials in hepatic encephalopathy, a Medline search was conducted using several terms (Table 33.4). Of a total of 1320 papers that dealt with treatment of hepatic encephalopathy, less than a hundred were reports of controlled trials. In this group, 34 randomized trials had the endpoint "improvement of hepatic encephalopathy" and included more than 10 patients per study group (Table 33.5). In addition, two meta-analyses have been published.[24,25]

Treatment of hepatic encephalopathy

Clinically overt hepatic encephalopathy (grades I–IV) in patients with cirrhosis

Supportive care and treatment of precipitating causes of hepatic encephalopathy

It is important to recognize that hepatic encephalopathy, acute and chronic, is reversible and that a precipitating cause rather than worsening of hepatocellular function can be identified in the majority of patients.[1,4] These causes include gastrointestinal bleeding, increased protein intake, hypokalemic alkalosis, infection, and constipation (all of which increase arterial ammonia levels), hypoxia, and the use of sedatives and tranquilizers. Patients with advanced cirrhosis may be particularly sensitive to benzodiazepines.

Treatment of these precipitating events is typically associated with a prompt and permanent improvement of hepatic encephalopathy. As a result, every attempt should be made to identify and to treat such precipitating events. This approach has never been tested formally but is based on common clinical experience. As judged from the outcomes observed in placebo groups of controlled trials (see Table 33.3) standard medical care is highly effective. AId

Enemas

Cleansing of the colon by enemas is a rapid and effective procedure to remove ammoniagenic substrates. The efficacy of enemas of 1–3 l of 20% lactulose or lactitol solutions was proved in randomized controlled trials; a favorable response was noted in 78–86% of patients (absolute risk reduction (ARR) 0·4, numbers needed to treat (NNT) = 3).[26,27] AId Interestingly, enemas with tap water were ineffective, raising the possibility that colonic acidification rather than bowel cleansing was the effective therapeutic mechanism.

Nutrition

Patients with grades III–IV hepatic encephalopathy usually do not receive oral nutrition. In general, there is no need for parenteral nutrition, if patients improve within 2 days.

Table 33.5 Randomized trials with endpoint "improvement of HE"

Test drug	Placebo	Standard therapy[a]	Lactulose/lactitol	Neomycin	Total
Flumazenil	7				7
BCAA IV	4	2			6
BCAA oral	2				2
Lactulose	5			3	8
Lactitol				3	3
Neomycin	1				1
Lactulose + neomycin	1				1
Lactulose/lactose enemas	1			1	2
Zinc		2			2
Benzoate			1		1
L-Dopa	1				1
Rifaximine			2	2	4 + 1 dose finding study
SF-68			1		1
AO 128	1				1
Total	23	4	4	9	40 + 1

[a]Usually includes lactulose or neomycin.

Based on the "false neurotransmitter hypothesis", total parenteral nutrition with specific amino acid solutions has been proposed. C5 A number of randomized controlled studies have evaluated the use of solutions with a high content of branched chain amino acids (BCAA) and a low content of aromatic amino acids (AAA). These studies differ with respect to the amino acid solutions used, the study protocols, patient selection, and the duration of treatment, and are difficult to compare. The results have been conflicting, but most studies did not find any improvement in hepatic encephalopathy or any reduction in mortality in patients treated with BCAA.[28,29] A1d Although a meta-analysis revealed a significant trend toward improvement in these outcomes, it was concluded that further randomized controlled trials are needed.[24] A1c At present, infusions of modified amino acid solutions should not be used in the standard treatment of patients with hepatic encephalopathy.

There is no proven need for a specific diet for patients with hepatic encephalopathy. Although mentioned in all textbooks, the recommendation of a low protein diet in patients with advanced liver disease is not supported by good clinical or experimental evidence. On the contrary, in patients with alcoholic hepatitis, low protein intake is associated with worsening hepatic encephalopathy while a higher protein intake correlates with improvement in hepatic encephalopathy.[30] The recommendations of the European Society of Parenteral and Enteral Nutrition (ESPEN) are that oral protein intake should not exceed 70 g/day in a patient with a history of hepatic encephalopathy; a level below 70 g/day is rarely necessary and

minimum intake should not be lower than 40 g/day to avoid negative nitrogen balance.[31] C5

Pharmacotherapy

Flumazenil

Based upon the GABA-benzodiazepine hypothesis of the pathogenesis of hepatic encephalopathy, the benzodiazepine receptor antagonist flumazenil has been tested for treatment of hepatic encephalopathy in five randomized placebo controlled trials involving over 600 patients. Four were crossover trials, and one used a parallel group design. Flumazenil was superior to placebo in four of these studies (Table 33.6). In the only large double blind, placebo-controlled crossover trial[6] 527 cirrhotic patients with grade III (265 patients) or IVa (262 patients) hepatic encephalopathy were randomized to receive intravenous flumazenil or a placebo over a 3–5-minute period. Patients subsequently received the other study medication if they were still in grade III or IVa encephalopathy after the first study period. Treatment was begun within 15 minutes of randomization. Outcome measures included both a neurological score and a grading derived from continuous EEG recordings. Table 33.6 shows the results obtained by combining the scores from the initial and crossover period. Improvement of the neurological score was documented in 46 of grade III and in 39 of grade IVa patients during the combined flumazenil treatment periods and in 10 (Grade III) and 3 (Grade IVa) of the patients

Table 33.6 Randomized controlled trials of flumazenil for hepatic encephalopathy

						No. improved/No. of treatment periods (%)			
						Flumazenil		Placebo	
Study	Study design	No. of patients	Dose (mg)	Outcome measure	HE grade	Clinical	EEG	Clinical	EEG
Barbaro *et al.* (1998)[6]	Crossover RCT	527	1	Neurological EEG and score	III	46/262* (17·6)	73/262* (27·9)	10/262 (3·8)	13/262 (5)
					IV	39/265* (14·7)	57/265* (21·5)	3/265 (1·1)	9/265 (3·4)
Gyr *et al.* (1996)[32]	RCT	49[a]	1/hour ×3hour	PSE score dependent on neurologic symptoms	II–IV	5/14* (35) (28)[b]*	0/11 (0) (0)		
Pomier-Layrargues *et al.* (1994)[33]	Crossover RCT	21	2	HE grade EEG	II–IV	6/13* (46)	4/12 (33)	0/15 (0)	2/13 (15)
Cadranel (1995)[34]	Crossover RCT	14[c]	1	HE grade EEG	II–IV	[d]	12/18* (67)	0/8 (17)	
Van der Rijt *et al.* (1995)[35]	Crossover RCT	18	0·25/hour for 3 days	HE grade EEG	0–IV	6/18** (34)	0/18	2/18 (12)	0/18
Lacetti *et al.* (2000)[36]	RCT[e]	54	2	Glasgow coma scale	III–IV	22/28* (79)		16/26 (61)	

[a]24 patients excluded from analysis (see text).
[b]Intent to treat analysis.
[c]18 episodes of HE in 14 patients.
[d]"Modest improvement".
[e]All patients received BCAA, IV fluids and lactulose.
*$P < 0·05$.
**$P = 0·06$.
See Tables 33.1–33.5 for abbreviations

during placebo treatment periods. Improvement of the EEG score occurred in 73 (Grade III) and 57 (Grade IVa) patients during flumazenil treatment and 13 (Grade III) and 9 (Grade IVa) patients during placebo treatment. The effects of flumazenil were statistically significant ($P < 0·01$). Ald In the second study,[32] 24 of 49 randomized patients were excluded from the final analysis, mainly due to inadequate benzodiazepine screening. However, flumazenil was superior to placebo even when the data were evaluated by intention to treat analysis; among the 25 patients who were not excluded, clinically relevant improvement was seen in 35% compared with 0% in patients given placebo. Ald In the Canadian trial,[33] very strict exclusion criteria resulted in the rejection of 56 of 77 potential patients. Improvement in neurological symptoms was observed in six of 11 flumazenil treatment periods compared with zero of 10 placebo periods; a few patients showed improvement in the EEG during both treatments. The beneficial effect of flumazenil was not related to the presence of identifiable benzodiazepines in the blood. Ald In the fourth positive study,[34] drug effects were evaluated on continuous EEG recordings obtained before, during, and 10 minutes after a bolus dose of the drug. No patient improved on placebo; on flumazenil the EEG recording improved in 12 out of 18 cases (66%) and was associated with a shortlasting modest clinical improvement. Ald In the fifth study the response rate with flumazenil was greater than that observed with placebo, but the result was not statistically significant.[35]

A recent meta-analysis of all published trials involving a total of 641 patients showed that flumazenil induces clinical and electroencephalographic improvement of hepatic encephalopathy in patients with cirrhosis.[37] Ald Taken together, these studies suggest that some patients with severe hepatic encephalopathy will experience clinical improvement when flumazenil is added to standard treatment.

Antibiotics

Neomycin has been used as standard treatment of hepatic encephalopathy for almost 40 years. Surprisingly, there is no evidence that neomycin is effective. The only randomized placebo-controlled trial found no benefit of neomycin compared to standard treatment alone.[14] Ald Based on this negative study and the potential for serious adverse effects of this drug, neomycin should not be prescribed for this condition. The combination of neomycin with lactulose was not superior to placebo.[25] Other antibiotics including paromomycin, metronidazole, vancomycin[38] and rifaximin[39,40] are better tolerated, but there is no evidence supporting their efficacy. Ald Two doses of rifaximin were compared for treatment of hepatic encephalopathy, but this prospective trial unfortunately did not include a control group. A dose of 1200 mg/day appeared to be most effective.[41] B4 Rifaximin was then compared with lactitol in a prospective randomized double blind, "double-dummy", controlled trial. The overall efficacy of both drugs in episodic hepatic encephalopathy type was similar (81·6% and 80·4% improved on rifaximin and lactitol, respectively) but rifaximin was associated with a more profound decrease of serum ammonia levels.[42] Ald Rifaximin was well tolerated but further placebo-controlled studies are needed to determine its efficacy.

Disaccharides

Synthetic disaccharides (lactulose, lactitol, lactose in lactase deficiency) are currently the mainstay of therapy of hepatic encephalopathy. The dose of lactulose (45–90 g/day) should be titrated in every patient to achieve two to three soft stools with a pH below 6 per day. Lactitol has been evaluated in a number of clinical trials. It appears to be as effective as lactulose, is more palatable, and may have fewer adverse effects.[25,43] Ald In patients with lactase deficiency, lactose has most of the same effects as the synthetic disaccharides in the colon.[44]

Although a properly conducted placebo-controlled trial has not been done, the efficacy of these disaccharides is considered to be beyond doubt.[43] B4, C5 Approximately 70–80% of patients with hepatic encephalopathy improve on lactulose treatment, a response rate comparable with that observed in patients treated with neomycin.[5,45] Treatment is usually well tolerated, and the principal toxicity is abdominal cramping, diarrhea and flatulence. Nevertheless, in view of the questionable efficacy of neomycin, the efficacy of oral lactulose or lactitol for treatment of clinically overt hepatic encephalopathy has to be questioned. Since most new treatments are considered to be effective if improvement rates are not different from a group treated with lactulose, a randomized placebo-controlled study of lactulose for treatment of overt hepatic encephalopathy would be desirable. The first placebo-controlled trial (with a crossover design) involved just seven patients, of whom[46] only two had clinical symptoms. One patient improved on lactulose. This result is clearly not significant, and the trial lacked adequate power. The second trial reported only the outcome of 14 of the 26 randomized patients.[47] The interpretation of three studies[48–50] is difficult due to the definitions used to document the effect of therapy. In contrast with oral lactulose administration, the efficacy of lactulose or lactose enemas is beyond any doubt (see above).

Theoretically, the inhibition of intestinal disaccharidases should induce malabsorption of disaccharides and increase delivery of undigested carbohydrates to the colon. AO-128 is an N-substituted derivative of valiolamine, an aminocyclitol that selectively inhibits intestinal disaccharidases. A double blind randomized controlled trial was carried out in 35 cirrhotic patients with PSE. Patients were given a 2-week treatment of AO-128 (2 mg three times daily) or an identical placebo. Efficacy of treatment was assessed by the PSE index at weekly intervals. More patients receiving AO-128 than patients receiving placebo showed > 40% improvement in the PSE index (83% v 35%; $P < 0.05$). Ald The mean stool pH decreased from 5·8 ± 0·3 to 5·5 ± 0·3 ($P < 0.004$) after AO-128 treatment, whereas no changes were observed in the placebo group. The EEG and nitrogen balance did not change in either group. Improvement in the NCT performance was seen after AO-128 treatment (from grade 2·0 ± 1·04 to grade 1·25 ± 0·87; $P < 0.05$). Ald Seven patients treated with AO-128 developed diarrhea compared with none in the placebo group ($P < 0.05$).[51]

Ornithine aspartate

Ornithine and aspartate increase ammonia removal. In cirrhotic patients, ornithine aspartate infusions prevented hyperammonemia after an oral protein load in a dose-dependent fashion.[52] In a randomized placebo-controlled trial in patients with hepatic encephalopathy, ornithine aspartate (20 g/day given intravenously over 4 hours for 7 days) improved fasting and postprandial blood ammonia levels compared with placebo-treated patients.[7] Ald There was also symptomatic improvement (assessed by psychometric tests and the PSE index) in patients with grade I or II hepatic encephalopathy, but no effect was observed in those with minimal hepatic encephalopathy. The results of this study are encouraging, and a confirmatory trial is needed.

Benzoate

A different approach to elimination of ammonia is the use of benzoate. Benzoate reacts with glycine to form hippurate. For each mole of benzoate, one mole of waste nitrogen is excreted into the urine. Sodium benzoate (5 g twice daily) was compared with lactulose in a randomized double blind

Table 33.7   Randomized controlled trials (RCT) of lactulose (L) for hepatic encephalopathy (HE)

Study	No. of patients	Design	Lactulose (g/day)	Control	Standard treatment	Outcome measures	Baseline characteristics	Result
Elkington *et al.* (1969)[46]	7	Crossover	67	Sorbitol	40 g protein	NH$_3$, PSE, EEG	Not given, 2 patients overt HE	No difference
Simmons *et al.* (1970)[47]	26	RCT	60	Glucose	40 g protein	HE grade	Not given, all overt HE	? No difference, data for 12 patients not given
Dhiman *et al.* (2000)[48]	26	RCT	30–60	–		No. of abnormal psychometric tests	Only MHE control group worse	L Better than control, but no difference from baseline
Watanabe *et al.* (1997)[49]	36	RCT	27	–	40 g protein	No. of abnormal psychometric tests	Only MHE	?
Horsmans *et al.* (1997)[50]	14	RCT	60	Lactose	60 g protein	No. of abnormal psychometric tests	Only MHE control group worse	L better than control, but no difference from baseline

MHE, minimal HE; PSE, portal–systemic encephalopathy index; NH$_3$ ammonia; EEG, electoencephalogram

trial in 74 patients with acute hepatic encephalopathy.[53] Outcome measures included the PSE index, visual, auditory and somatosensory evoked potentials, and a battery of psychometric tests. The improvement in encephalopathic parameters and the incidence of adverse effects were similar in the two treatment groups. Ald In view of the unknown efficacy of lactulose, a confirmatory placebo-controlled trial is needed.

Persistent hepatic encephalopathy type C

Patients with hepatic encephalopathy that is refractory to standard therapy are rare. Most have surgical shunts or a large diameter transjugular intrahepatic portosystemic shunt (TIPS). Due to the small number of such patients, there are no controlled trials. Case reports on individual patients describe successful approaches by narrowing or closure of the shunt, protein restriction together with BCAA supplementation, supplementation of zinc and thiamin, and the use of bromocriptin and oral flumazenil. The only controlled study was carried out in 37 hospitalized patients with documented severe protein intolerance.[54] Addition of BCAA to the diet enabled the daily protein intake to be increased to up to 80 g without worsening of cerebral function. Ald Many control patients who received casein as a protein source deteriorated after increasing dietary protein intake. No benefit of BCAA-supplementation was observed in protein-tolerant patients.

In protein-intolerant patients vegetable proteins appear to be better tolerated than proteins derived from fish, milk or meat. In three controlled trials a vegetable diet was better tolerated then a diet that also included meat.[55,56] Ald Other studies did not show these favorable effects.[57] The beneficial effects of a vegetable diet on the protein tolerance of patients with hepatic encephalopathy cannot be explained by the amino acid compositions of the proteins alone.[58]

Minimal hepatic encephalopathy

Although the number of patients with minimal hepatic encephalopathy is large, good clinical studies are rare. Even among experts, there is no agreement on how to define minimal hepatic encephalopathy or whether minimal hepatic encephalopathy even exists. Efficacy of treatment is judged by the improvement of psychometric tests or of electrophysiological measurements (see Table 33.7). The clinical relevance of these outcomes is uncertain. Substances that improved responses in psychometric tests in randomized trials include lactulose[49,50] modification of colonic flora to increase lactobacilli,[59] ornithine aspartate,[7] and oral BCAA.[8,60,61] Ald

Prevention of hepatic encephalopathy

The occurrence of hepatic encephalopathy is a problem after TIPS insertion.[62] Although most clinicians administer prophylactic treatments after TIPS placement, the frequency of episodes of overt hepatic encephalopathy is about 10% per month. The manifestation of hepatic encephalopathy before TIPS and/or reduced liver function were identified as independent risk factors. Refractory encephalopathy can be managed with a reduced size shunt.[63] B4

Summary of recommended treatment of hepatic encephalopathy in clinical practice

Treatment of episodic hepatic encephalopathy type C

Treatment of episodic hepatic encephalopathy type C involves two steps. The first is to identify and correct precipitating causes:

- gastrointestinal bleeding
- sedatives or tranquilizers
- infections
- hypovolemia, hypoxia, electrolyte imbalance, hypoglycemia.

The second step is initiation of measures to lower blood ammonia concentrations with:

- lactulose enemas
- intravenous ornithine aspartate
- parenteral or enteral nutrition, if patient is unable to eat
- flumazenil if the patient has been given benzodiazepines.

Chronic therapy

Chronic management of the patient with recurrent episodic hepatic encephalopathy type C requires individual adjustment of treatment. The titration of protein tolerance after an episode of hepatic encephalopathy should permit the design of an individual diet for each patient. Limitation of protein intake is reasonable in some patients, but protein restriction should be avoided if possible, since it will lead to negative nitrogen balance. In protein-intolerant patients, vegetable proteins are better tolerated than proteins derived from fish, milk, or meat. The supplementation of a low protein diet with BCAA should be considered. Additionally, patients may benefit from zinc and thiamin supplementation. The long term benefit of all other treatments (including lactulose and neomycin) is uncertain. The need for treatment of minimal hepatic encephalopathy is not established, and unproved therapy should be administered in the context of randomized controlled clinical trials.

References

1 Ferenci P, Püspök A, Steindl P. Current concepts in the pathophysiology of hepatic encephalopathy. *Eur J Clin Invest* 1992;**22**:573–81.
2 Ferenci P, Lockwood A, Mullen K, Tarter R, Weissenborn K, Blei AT Hepatic encephalopathy: definition, nomenclature, diagnosis and quantification. Final report of the Working Party at the 11th World Congresses of Gastroenterology, Vienna 1998. *Hepatology* 2002;**35**:716–21.
3 Weissenborn K, Ennen JC, Schomerus H,Rückert N, Hecker H. Neuropsychological characterization of hepatic encephalopathy. *J Hepatol* 2001;**34**:768–773.
4 Conn HO, Lieberthal MM. *The hepatic coma syndromes and lactulose*. Baltimore, Maryland: Williams & Wilkins, 1979.
5 Conn HO, Leevy CM, Vlahcevic ZR *et al.* Comparison of lactulose and neomycin in the treatment of chronic portal-systemic encephalopathy. *Gastroenterology* 1977;**72**:573–83.
6 Barbaro G, Di Lorenzo G, Soldini M *et al.* Flumazenil for hepatic encephalopathy grade III and IVa in patients with cirrhosis: an Italian multicenter double-blind, placebo-controlled, cross-over study. *Hepatology* 1998;**28**:374–8.
7 Kircheis G, Nilius R, Held C *et al.* Therapeutic efficacy of l-ornithine-l-aspartate infusions in patients with cirrhosis and hepatic encephalopathy: results of a placebo-controlled, double-blind study. *Hepatology* 1997;**25**:1351–60.
8 Stauch S, Kircheis G, Adler G *et al.* Oral l-ornithine-l-aspartate therapy of chronic hepatic encephalopathy: results of a placebo-controlled double-blind study. *J Hepatol* 1998;**28**:856–64.
9 Marchesini G, Dioguardi FS, Bianchi GP *et al.* Long-term oral branched-chain amino acid treatment in chronic hepatic encephalopathy. A randomized double-blind casein-controlled trial. The Italian Multicenter Study Group. *J Hepatol* 1990;**11**:92–101.
10 Michel H, Solere M, Granier P *et al.* Treatment of cirrhotic hepatic encephalopathy with L-dopa. A controlled trial. *Gastroenterology* 1980;**79**:207–11.
11 Michel H, Pomier-Layrargues G, Aubin JP *et al.* Treatment of hepatic encephalopathy by infusion of a modified amino acid solution: results of a study in 47 cirrhotic patients. In: Capocaccia L, Fischer JE, Rossi-Fanelli F (eds). *Hepatic encephalopathy and chronic liver failure*. New York: Plenum Press, 1984.
12 Wahren J, Denis J, Desurmont P *et al.* Is intravenous administration of branched chain amino acids effective in the treatment of hepatic encephalopathy? A multicenter study. *Hepatology* 1983;**3**:475–80.
13 Blanc P, Daures JP, Liautard J *et al.* Lactulose-neomycin combination versus placebo in the treatment of acute hepatic encephalopathy. Results of a randomized controlled trial. *Gastroenterol Clin Biol* 1994;**18**:1063–8.
14 Strauss E, Tramote R, Silva EP *et al.* Double-blind randomized clinical trial comparing neomycin and placebo in the treatment of exogenous hepatic encephalopathy. *Hepatogastroenterology* 1992;**39**:542–5.
15 Weissenborn K, Ruckert N, Hecker H *et al.* The number connection tests A and B: interindividual variability and use for the assessment of early hepatic encephalopathy. *J Hepatol* 1998;**28**:646–53.
16 Schomerus H, Hamster W, Blunck H *et al.* Latent portosystemic encephalopathy I. Nature of cerebral functional defects and fitness to drive. *Dig Dis Sci* 1981;**26**:622–30.
17 Rikkers L, Jenko P, Rudman D *et al.* Subclinical hepatic encephalopathy: detection, prevalence and relationship to nitrogen metabolism. *Gastroenterology* 1978;**75**:462–9.

18 Conn HO. Trailmaking and number connection tests in the assessment of mental state in portal systemic encephalopathy. *Am J Dig Dis* 1977;**22**:541–50.

19 Quero JC, Hartmann IJ, Meulstee J *et al.* The diagnosis of subclinical hepatic encephalopathy in patients with cirrhosis using neuropsychological tests and automated electroencephalogram analysis. *Hepatology* 1996;**24**:556–60.

20 Groeneweg M, Quero JC, De Bruijn I *et al.* Subclinical hepatic encephalopathy impairs daily functioning. *Hepatology* 1998;**28**:45–9.

21 Srivastava A, Mehta R, Rothke SP *et al.* Fitness to drive in patients with cirrhosis and portal systemic shunting: a pilot study evaluating driving performance. *J Hepatol* 1994;**21**:1023–8.

22 Kullmann F, Hollerbach S, Holstege A *et al.* Subclinical hepatic encephalopathy: the diagnostic value of evoked potentials. *J Hepatol* 1995;**22**:101–10.

23 Rosenberg W, Donald A. Evidence based medicine: an approach to clinical problem-solving. *BMJ* 1995;**310**:1122–6.

24 Naylor CD, O'Rourkee K, Detsky AS *et al.* Parenteral nutrition with branched-chain amino acids in hepatic encephalopathy. A meta-analysis. *Gastroenterology* 1989;**97**:1033–42.

25 Blanc P, Daures JP, Rouillon JM *et al.* Lactitol or lactulose in the treatment of chronic hepatic encephalopathy: results of a meta-analysis. *Hepatology* 1992;**15**:222–8.

26 Uribe M, Berthier J, Lewis H *et al.* Lactose enemas plus placebo tablets vs. neomycin tablets plus starch enemas in acute portal systemic encephalopathy. A double-blind randomized controlled study. *Gastroenterology* 1981;**81**:101–6.

27 Uribe M, Campollo O, Vargas-F *et al.* Acidifying enemas (lactitol and lactose) vs. nonacidifying enemas (tap water) to treat acute portal-systemic encephalopathy: a double-blind, randomized clinical trial. *Hepatology* 1987;**7**:639–43.

28 Ferenci P. Critical evaluation of the role of branched chain amino acids in liver disease. In: Thomas JC, Jones EA (eds). *Recent advances in hepatology 2*. New York: Churchill Livingstone, 1986.

29 Fabbri A, Magrini N, Bianchi G *et al.* Overview of randomized clinical trials of oral branched-chain amino acid treatment in chronic hepatic encephalopathy. *J Parent Ent Nutr* 1996;**20**:159–64.

30 Morgan TR, Moritz TE, Mendenhall CL *et al.* Protein consumption and hepatic encephalopathy in alcoholic hepatitis. VA Cooperative Study Group 275. *J Am Coll Nutr* 1995;**14**:152–8.

31 Plauth M, Merli M, Kondrup J *et al.* ESPEN Guidelines for nutrition in liver disease and transplantation. *Clin Nutr* 1997;**16**:43–55.

32 Gyr K, Meier R, Haussler J *et al.* Evaluation of the efficacy and safety of flumazenil in the treatment of portal systemic encephalopathy: a double blind, randomized, placebo controlled multicenter study. *Gut* 1996;**39**:319–25.

33 Pomier-Layrargues G, Giguere JF, Lavoie J *et al.* Flumazenil in cirrhotic patients in hepatic coma: a randomized double-blind placebo-controlled crossover trial. *Hepatology* 1994;**19**:32–7.

34 Cadranel JF, el Younsi M, Pidoux B *et al.* Flumazenil therapy for hepatic encephalopathy in cirrhotic patients: a double-blind pragmatic randomized, placebo study. *Eur J Gastroenterol Hepatol* 1995;**7**:325–9.

35 Van der Rijt CC, Schalm SW, Meulstee J *et al.* Flumazenil therapy for hepatic encephalopathy. A double-blind cross over study. *Gastroenterol Clin Biol* 1995;**19**:572–80.

36 Laccetti M, Manes G, Uomo G, Lioniello M, Rabitti PG, Balzano A. Flumazenil in the treatment of acute hepatic encephalopathy in cirrhotic patients: a double blind randomized placebo controlled study. *Dig Liver Dis* 2000;**32**:335–8.

37 Goulenok C, Bernard B, Cadranel JF *et al.* Flumazenil vs. placebo in hepatic encephalopathy in patients with cirrhosis: a meta-analysis. *Aliment Pharmacol Ther* 2002;**16**:361–72.

38 Tarao K, Ikeda T, Hayashi K *et al.* Successful use of vancomycin hydrochloride in the treatment of lactulose resistant chronic hepatic encephalopathy. *Gut* 1990;**31**:702–6.

39 Bucci L, Palmieri GC. Double-blind, double-dummy comparison between treatment with rifaximin and lactulose in patients with medium to severe degree hepatic encephalopathy. *Curr Med Res Opin* 1993;**13**:109–18.

40 Miglio F, Valpiani D, Rossellini SR, Ferrieri A. Rifaximin, a non-absorbable rifamycin, for the treatment of hepatic encephalopathy. A double-blind, randomised trial. *Curr Med Res Opin* 1997;**13**:593–601.

41 Williams R, James OF, Warnes TW, Morgan MY. Evaluation of the efficacy and safety of rifaximin in the treatment of hepatic encephalopathy: a double-blind, randomized, dose-finding multi-centre study. *Eur J Gastroenterol Hepatol* 2000;**12**:203–8.

42 Mas A, Rodes J, Sunyer L *et al.* Comparison of rifaximin and lactitol in the treatment of acute hepatic encephalopathy: results of a randomized, double-blind, double-dummy, controlled clinical trial. *J Hepatol* 2003;**38**:51–8.

43 Morgan MY, Hawley KE. Lactitol vs lactulose in the treatment of acute hepatic encephalopathy in cirrhotic patients: a double blind, randomized trial. *Hepatology* 1987;**7**:1278–84.

44 Uribe-Esquivel M, Moran S, Poo JL *et al. In vitro* and *in vivo* lactose and lactulose effects on colonic fermentation and portal-systemic encephalopathy parameters. *Scand J Gastroenterol* 1997;**222** (Suppl):49.

45 Orlandi F, Freddara U, Candelaresi MT *et al.* Comparison between neomycin and lactulose in 173 patients with hepatic encephalopathy: a randomized clinical study. *Dig Dis Sci* 1981;**26**:408–506.

46 Elkington SG, Floch MH, Conn HO. Lactulose in the treatment of chronic portal-systemic encephalopathy. A double-blind clinical trial. *N Engl J Med* 1969;**281**:498–12.

47 Simmons F, Goldstein H, Boyle JD. A controlled clinical trial of lactulose in hepatic encephalopathy. *Gastroenterology* 1970;**59**:827–32.

48 Dhiman RK, Sawhney MS, Chawla YK, Das G, Ram S, Dilawari JB. Efficacy of lactulose in cirrhotic patients with

subclinical hepatic encephalopathy. *Dig Dis Sci* 2000;**45**: 1549–52.

49 Watanabe A, Sakai T, Sato S *et al.* Clinical efficacy of lactulose in cirrhotic patients with and without subclinical hepatic encephalopathy. *Hepatology* 1997;**26**:1410–14.

50 Horsmans Y, Solbreux PM, Daenens C *et al.* Lactulose improves psychometric testing in cirrhotic patients with subclinical encephalopathy. *Aliment Pharmacol Ther* 1997;**11**:165–70.

51 Uribe M, Moran S, Poo JL, Mendez-Sanchez N, Guevara L, Garcia-Ramos G. Beneficial effect of carbohydrate maldigestion induced by a disaccharidase inhibitor (AO-128) in the treatment of chronic portal-systemic encephalopathy. A double-blind, randomized, controlled trial. *Scand J Gastroenterol* 1998;**33**:1099–106.

52 Staedt U, Leweling H, Gladisch R *et al.* Effects of ornithine aspartate on plasma ammonia and plasma amino acids in patients with cirrhosis. A double-blind, randomized study using a four-fold crossover design. *J Hepatol* 1993;**19**: 424–30.

53 Sushma S, Dasarathy S, Tandon RK *et al.* Sodium benzoate in the treatment of acute hepatic encephalopathy: a double-blind randomized trial. *Hepatology* 1992;**16**:138–44.

54 Horst D, Grace ND, Conn HO *et al.* Comparison of dietary protein with an oral, branched chain-enriched amino acid supplement in chronic portal-systemic encephalopathy: a randomized controlled trial. *Hepatology* 1984;**4**:279–87.

55 Uribe M, Marquez MA, Ramos GG *et al.* Treatment of chronic portal-systemic encephalopathy with vegetable and animal protein diets. *Dig Dis Sci* 1982;**27**:1109–16.

56 Bianchi GP, Marchesini G, Fabbri A *et al.* Vegetable versus animal protein diet in cirrhotic patients with chronic encephalopathy. A randomized cross-over comparison. *J Intern Med* 1993;**233**:385–92.

57 Greenberger NJ, Carley J, Schenker S *et al.* Effect of vegetable and animal protein diets in chronic hepatic encephalopathy. *Dig Dis Sci* 1977;**22**:845–55.

58 Keshavarzian A, Meek J, Sutton C *et al.* Dietary protein supplementation from vegetable sources in the management of chronic portal systemic encephalopathy. *Am J Gastroenterol* 1984;**79**:945–9.

59 Loguercio C, Abbiati R, Rinaldi M *et al.* Long-term effects of *Enterococcus faecium* SF68 versus lactulose in the treatment of patients with cirrhosis and grade 1–2 hepatic encephalopathy. *J Hepatol* 1995;**23**:39–46.

60 Egberts EH, Schomerus H, Hamster W *et al.* Branched chain amino acids in the treatment of latent portosystemic encephalopathy. A double-blind placebo-controlled crossover study. *Gastroenterology* 1985;**88**:887–95.

61 Plauth M, Egberts EH, Hamster W *et al.* Long-term treatment of latent portosystemic encephalopathy with branched-chain amino acids. A double-blind placebo-controlled crossover study. *J Hepatol* 1993;**17**:308–14.

62 Nolte W, Wiltfang J, Schindler C *et al.* Portosystemic hepatic encephalopathy after transjugular intrahepatic portosystemic shunt in patients with cirrhosis: clinical, laboratory, psychometric, and electroencephalographic investigations. *Hepatology* 1998;**28**:1215–25.

63 Madoff D, Perez-Young IV, Wallace MJ, Stolkin MD, Toombs BD. Management of TIPS-related refractory hepatic encephalopathy with Wallgraft prostheses. *J Vasc Interv Radiol* 2003;**14**:369–374.

34 Hepatocellular carcinoma

Massimo Colombo

Introduction

Since the widespread adoption of ultrasound (US) scan for screening high risk patients, the number of patients identified with a small, potentially treatable hepatocellular carcinoma (HCC) has more than doubled.[1,2] However, due to the lack of randomized controlled trials, it is not clear whether mortality for HCC has reduced in parallel. Features of the natural history of HCC such as the long-lasting subclinical period observed in many patients, as well as the large number of tumors that grow as a solitary mass to a size which can be detected by US, seem to favor screening programs. Conversely, in many patients aspects of HCC such as multinodal onset of the tumor and great variations in the growth rates of single nodes, with doubling volume times from 1 to 20 months, may hinder the effectiveness of screening.[3]

Target population

HCC is linked to environmental, dietary and lifestyle factors. Not surprisingly, therefore, epidemiological surveys were instrumental in identifying groups of individuals who are at risk for HCC. In two consensus conferences, held in Milan (Italy),[4] and Barcelona (Spain)[5] patients with cirrhosis, chronic carriers of HBsAg, and patients with rare metabolic liver diseases were identified as populations at risk for HCC. The cost effectiveness of screening would certainly be improved if we could assess an individual's cancer risk. However, this assessment is difficult because of individual variations in the metabolism of carcinogens, DNA repair capacities, genomic stability and inherited cancer predisposition.

Patients with cirrhosis

Three to four percent of all patients with cirrhosis due to chronic viral hepatitis or alcohol abuse develop HCC each year.[6-8] Patients with chronic viral hepatitis without histological evidence of cirrhosis also develop HCC, but at a lower incidence rate (1%).[9] HCC risk is particularly high in patients with cirrhosis and histological markers of increased liver cell proliferation. In a cohort study of 307 Italian patients with viral cirrhosis followed up for 4 years, HCC developed in 60% of 27 patients with liver cell dysplasia compared with 18% of 40 patients without it.[10] HCC risk was also high in cirrhotic patients with either fluctuating or persistently elevated serum levels of α-fetoprotein (AFP)[7,11] as well as in cirrhotic patients presenting with more than one risk factor for liver cell damage and regeneration (for example hepatitis B and C).[12] Liver cell regeneration is thought to be the crucial oncogenic event promoting selection and clonal expansion of committed hepatocytes after damage caused by genotoxic agents.

Chronic carriers of HBsAg

More than 250 million persons worldwide are persistently infected with HBV.[13] Epidemiological, clinical and experimental studies have established a strong link between chronic infection with this virus and HCC. HBV is responsible for both genotoxic lesions of the liver cells and tumor promotion through increased liver cell proliferation associated with persisting hepatitis. HBV does not necessarily require the step to cirrhosis to be oncogenic.[14] In a prospective cohort study in Taiwan, the risk of HCC in 3454 HBsAg carriers was 102 times greater than in 19 253 non-carriers.[15] However, the carriers at especially high risk for developing HCC were those with actively replicating HBV (HBeAg$^+$/HBV-DNA$^+$) and those with cirrhosis. Healthy carriers may develop HCC, but are at substantially lower risk.[16] Often, distinguishing between clinical subsets of HBsAg carriers may be difficult, unless the patients are periodically assessed with laboratory or histological investigations. The strong link between HBV and HCC has been further confirmed by the decrease of HCC that has been observed among Taiwanese children since the start of mass vaccination of all newborns against HBV.[17] B2

Table 34.1   Prospective cohort studies of patients with compensated cirrhosis undergoing surveillance by ultrasound examination

Study	Screening interval (month)	No. of patients with cirrhosis	Hepatocellular carcinoma				
			No.	Annual rate (%)	Single node (%)	< 3 cm (%)	AFP(−) (%)
Sato *et al.* (1993)[11]	3	361	33	3·0	88	64	41
Cottone *et al.* (1994)[8]	6	157	30	4·4	87	53	60
Colombo *et al.* (2004)[73]	12	417	88	3·4	54	27	38

Patients with rare metabolic diseases

Patients with porphyria cutanea tarda, genetic hemochromatosis, α-1-antitrypsin deficiency, tyrosinemia, and hypercitrullinemia are also at high risk for HCC. Patients with glycogenosis types I and III, Wilson disease and hereditary fructose intolerance may also develop HCC, but are at substantially lower risk.[3] HCC has developed also in patients with primary biliary cirrhosis, probably reflecting treatment-related improvement in patient survival. HCC was also found in 64% of 160 Japanese patients and in 48% of 101 South African blacks with Budd–Chiari syndrome.[18,19] However, in these studies the possible role of other unidentified carcinogens could not be excluded.

Screening tests

Serum AFP

AFP is a normal serum protein synthesized by fetal liver cells and by yolk sac cells. The normal range for serum AFP is 0–20 ng/ml (< 7 µg/l) in healthy adults. Serum levels of 400 ng/ml are very suggestive of HCC. However, two-thirds of patients with small HCCs have less than 200 ng/ml and more than 30% of patients with HCC do not have abnormal circulating levels of AFP, even in advanced stages.[6–8,20] Moreover, in the range of 20–200 ng/ml, patients with chronic liver disease and false positive results due to hepatitis flares outnumber those with HCC.

In patients with borderline elevations of serum AFP, the microheterogeneity of the sugar component of AFP can be assessed by lectin affinity electrophoresis coupled with antibody affinity blotting. Serum AFP in patients with HCC has greater proportions of this atypical AFP than serum AFP of patients with cirrhosis. In a prospective study of 361 cirrhotic patients, 33 showed elevated atypical AFP 3–18 months before HCC was detected by imaging techniques.[11]

Abdominal ultrasound

To minimize the false results of AFP determinations, cirrhotic patients are undergoing surveillance by means of real-time US. As a general rule, a lesion seen as a discrete node in the liver should be presumed to be a preneoplastic lesion or HCC, and should be investigated accordingly. Most HCCs can be detected as a hypodysechoic mass.[21] Tumors may escape detection when located in the upper and posterior portion of the right lobe, an area that is technically difficult to assess by US, or because HCC nodes are present as isoechoic masses or are too small to be detected. One major problem in US screening of cirrhotic patients is false diagnosis due to regenerative macronodules smaller than 2 cm and small hyperechoic hemangiomas. In a 12-year prospective cohort study of 447 cirrhotic patients, we found that 83 had had an initial diagnosis of benign node that later turned out to be HCC in seven patients (8%) (Colombo *et al* unpublished data).

Screening strategies

In population-based studies, most individuals are asymptomatic, and therefore the screening intervals can be easily standardized. Serum AFP is the method of choice for screening in such studies because these include thousands of healthy persons and relatively few patients with liver disease who are at risk of false positive results with AFP. Between 1982 and 1992, 18 299 AFP determinations were carried out on 2230 symptomless Alaskan Natives who were HBsAg carriers.[22] At least one AFP determination was elevated (> 25 ng/ml or < 7 µg/l) for 371 persons, including 292 pregnant women, 24 patients with hepatitis-related events, and 16 patients with HCC. Because of the high risk of false results, AFP is not appropriate for screening cirrhotic patients. Abdominal US is the method of choice for screening and surveillance. In fact, in 25–60% of the cirrhotic patients studied by US, HCC would have gone undetected if the patients had been screened by AFP only (Table 34.1).[7,8,11] In a prospective cohort study of 447 cirrhotic patients in Milan, the negative predictive value of US was 92% and the positive predictive value was 66%.[7] At the Milan Conference,[5] it was recommended that patients with cirrhosis or with certain congenital conditions known to be risk factors for HCC should be screened by US and AFP twice a year, whereas HBsAg carriers should be screened for HCC by determinations of serum AFP levels once a year.

Recently prospective surveillance studies[23,24] have suggested that the proportion of cirrhotic patients diagnosed with HCC who fulfill liver transplantation criteria is increased, and thus survival is increased through this route.[25]

Treatment

Treatment options are selected according to the presence or absence of cirrhosis, number and size of tumors, and degree of hepatic deterioration. Staging is a crucial variable in treatment outcome, since many therapeutic failures have resulted from incorrect patient selection. When patients are scanned by biphasic spiral computed tomography (CT) during the arterial phase (about 20 seconds after the start of injection), highly vascularized tumors appear against a background of relatively unenhanced liver that is primarily enhanced during the late portal vein phase.[26] However, most tumors smaller than 2 cm are hypovascular and therefore escape detection with such gold standard staging techniques as biphasic spiral CT.[27] For staging clinical status, the Child–Pugh scoring system provides accurate estimates of patient survival. The 3-year survival of untreated patients with a small tumor and well compensated cirrhosis was approximately 25%.[28]

A review of treatments offered for this disease encounters a number of difficulties. First, few controlled trials have been done comparing the efficacy of the available surgical or locoregional ablative treatments. Secondly, there is substantial heterogeneity of survival between control groups in various trials, making it even riskier than usual to compare the results of small individual trials.[29] Some trials have not been analyzed on the basis of intention to treat and probably yield exaggerated estimates of treatment effects.

Patients with normal livers

Hepatic resection is the primary option for the few patients with HCC who present with normal livers and well preserved hepatic function. In two case series,[30,31] the cumulative 5-year survival for 128 such patients in two centers treated with hepatic resection was approximately 45%, compared with 12–26% for the 51 treated with orthotopic liver transplantation (OLT). B2 The good results with hepatic resection probably depended on the absence of cirrhosis, which allowed for extensive resection of the liver without affecting survival. The poor results with OLT probably reflected bias in patient selection, for example transplantation may have been done in patients with advanced HCC who were judged to be unsuitable candidates for resection.

Patients with cirrhosis and a small tumor

The functional capacity of the liver not involved by HCC is the major factor in these patients' prognosis. Thus, starting in 1950, surgical resection of the tumor for treating HCC in cirrhotic livers was frequently done in China and Japan, with substantial benefit for patients with small tumors and well preserved hepatic function. More recently, in the wake of substantial improvements in transplantation technology and better understanding of the natural history of HCC, liver transplantation has gained further popularity as curative treatment for patients with HCC and cirrhosis.

Orthotopic liver transplantation

Transplants eliminate both detectable and undetectable tumor nodes and all the preneoplastic lesions in the cirrhotic liver. Removal of the diseased liver also reduces the risk of morbidity and mortality from portal hypertension. Opposing these "pros" for OLT are several important "cons" – for example, shortage of donated organs, high costs of the procedure, the need for stringent criteria for selection of patients, high risk of early tumor recurrence due to faulty staging of the disease and immunosuppression, and recurrence of hepatitis.

Overall survival after OLT has improved markedly since the introduction of cyclosporine and more accurate criteria for patient selection. One major obstacle to the interpretation of OLT results is the large differences between transplantation centers in terms of time lag between candidacy and operation. The best long-term survivors (90% at 5 years) were patients for whom HCC was not the primary indication for OLT but was discovered by chance as a minute nodule during examination of the explanted liver.[31] B4 Between January 1988 and June 1994, the 5-year survival of 834 patients with HCC (7% of total) who were given transplants in 82 European Centers was 39%. B4 This included the 54·5% survival of 176 patients in whom cirrhosis was the primary indication for OLT and 45·5% of 361 cirrhotic patients in whom HCC was the primary indication. Transplantation of accurately selected patients with a single, less than 5-cm tumor or with a maximum of three less than 3 cm nodes, resulted in significantly extended survival (Table 34.2).

Although survival of transplant patients seems to be largely influenced by tumor size and number, there is no general agreement on the ideal tumor size that entails the least risk of recurrence, mostly because small tumor volume does not mean an early biological stage for all cases. Indeed, vascular invasion by the tumor and perihepatic lymph nodes can occur even in patients with small HCCs.[30,31] Unfortunately, vascular invasion can be assessed only during the operation and lymph nodes can be precisely assessed only during laparoscopy or laparotomy. The most common cause of early death, within 3 months of OLT, was graft failure. In all studies, the most

Table 34.2 Outcomes of liver transplantation in cirrhotic patients with a single small tumor or less than three small tumors

Center	Selection	Cases	Survival (%)		Reference
			1-year	5-year	
Milan	Single ≤ 5 cm ≤ three ≤ 3 cm	48	84	74	Mazzaferro *et al.* (1996)[32]
Barcelona	Single ≤ 5 cm	58	84	74	Llovet *et al.* (1998)[33]
Paris	three ≤ 3 cm	28	82	74	Bismuth *et al.* (1999)[34]
Berlin	Single ≤ 5 cm three ≤ 3 cm	120	90	71	Jonas *et al.* (2001)[35]

common cause of late death, from 3 months after OLT, was recurrence of the original tumor. The outcome of OLT may be influenced by recurrence of viral hepatitis, since infection of the graft may facilitate rejection and re-establish the oncogenic potential of the liver. The efficacy of interferon and the nucleoside analog ribavirin against hepatitis C is under evaluation. For hepatitis B, hyperimmune γ-globulins and the nucleoside analog lamivudine are protective but costly.[36,37] B4 There has been an evolution of selection criteria over the years, which has generated renewed interest with the possibility of live related donors to optimize timing and maybe extend the criteria for transplantation.

Hepatic resection

Liver transplantation cannot be offered to all patients with cirrhosis who are found to harbor a small HCC. Thus, in many countries, hepatic resection remains the primary therapeutic option for these patients. Since the functional capacity of the remaining liver is a major factor affecting prognosis for patients undergoing hepatic resection, limited hepatic resection (segmentectomy and subsegmentectomy) is the technical procedure of choice. Since 1983 the widespread adoption of intraoperative US has changed the outlook of this treatment. The best results in terms of both short-term and long-term survival were for patients with single tumors less than 2 cm in diameter and well preserved hepatic function. In 347 Japanese patients, the 5-year survival rate was as high as 60·5%,[39] with very low mortality (0–5%). Considering all patients in Japan treated with hepatic resection, the most powerful predictor of survival was a combination of the three factors: AFP, tumor size, and number of tumors.[40] Portal invasion by the tumor and metachronous multifocal tumorigenesis are the mechanisms by which HCC may recur after resection. In a series of 102 patients with tumors smaller than 3 cm, without portal vein invasion or intrahepatic metastases, recurrence 5 years after resection was recorded as 68%,[41] with the highest recurrence rates being observed in patients with more

Table 34.3 Five-year survival of 77 Spanish patients with Child–Pugh A cirrhosis and a less than 5-cm tumor treated by resection

Overall 5-year survival	50%	
Median survival (months)	(a) 91 < 1 mg bilirubin	*P* = 0·03
	(b) 30 ≥ 1 mg	
	(c) 80 < 10 mmHg HVPG	*P* = 0·02
	(d) 69 ≥ 10	
5-year survival	74% a + c	
	50% a + d	
	15% b + d	

From Bruix J *et al. Gastroenterology* 1996;**111**:1018–23.[44]
HVPG, hepatic venous pressure gradient

compromised hepatic function, for example high ALT and low albumin values. In fact, survival of patients undergoing hepatic resection is influenced not only by the tumor size and invasiveness, but also by the functional status of the liver expressed as the Child–Pugh score and degree of portal hypertension. The 3-year cumulative survival was 50% for 78 Japanese patients with single tumors and Child's A status, 35% for 26 with Child's B status and 0 for three with Child's C status.[42] B4 For 72 patients in Paris, these figures were 51% for Child's A and 12% for Child's B–C.[43] B4 In patients with Child–Pugh A cirrhosis, portal hypertension is the most reliable predictor of survival after resection. In Barcelona none of the 14 operated patients with less than 10 mmHg hepatic venous pressure gradient had had unresolved hepatic decompensation, compared with 11 of the 15 patients with higher gradients (Table 34.3).[44] Thus, resection is definitely contraindicated for patients with deteriorated cirrhosis or severe portal hypertension in view of the high operative risk and short life expectancy. There are no controlled data demonstrating that chemotherapy improves the survival of resected patients by eradicating occult nests of tumor cells.[45] Also, there are no controlled trials comparing

OLT and resection. In Barcelona, the 5-year "intention to treat" survival was greater for transplant patients than for resected patients (69% *v* 51%).[46] However, after stratification for liver impairment and portal hypertension, the 5-year survival of the best candidates treated by resection was 74% compared with the 54% 2-year survival after OLT for the worst candidates. B2 The shortened survival of the latter patients related to the excess risk of dropout while waiting for a liver donation.

Patients with cirrhosis not eligible for surgery

Patients may be refused surgery because of advanced age, deteriorated liver function, large tumors, tumors localized in strategic positions or associated clinical conditions that contraindicate surgery.

Percutaneous interstitial treatments

US-guided interstitial treatments include tumor injection with absolute ethanol, 50% acetic acid or hot saline, or tumor thermoablation with radiofrequency, microwaves or laser. Most treatments were carried out with intratumor percutaneous ethanol injection (PEI), which causes extensive coagulative necrosis of the tumor cells, and thrombosis of the tumor vessels, and is well tolerated. Up to 73% of the lesions treated with PEI underwent complete coagulative necrosis. Once more, survival was largely influenced by liver function, size, and number of tumors.[47-50] B4 The 5-year survival of 293 Italian patients with Child's A cirrhosis was 47%, compared with 29% for 149 with Child's B cirrhosis (Table 34.4).[47] Life expectancy of Child's A patients with a small tumor treated by PEI appeared to be as good as that of similar patients treated with hepatic resection, and associated with a low risk of severe complications (1·7%) and mortality (0·1%). In the Italian multicenter PEI study, the 5-year survival of 28 patients with larger than 5 cm HCC was 30% compared with 47% for the 392 patients with smaller than 5 cm tumors and compensated cirrhosis. B4 The 5-year survival of 121 patients with two or three tumor nodes and compensated cirrhosis was 36%. PEI is thought to be successful for small HCCs because these tumors are often hypovascular, and therefore trap the injected ethanol better. In fact, patients with smaller than 2-cm tumors that were hypovascular by US–CO2 scan survived longer than similar patients with hypervascular tumors (5-year survival rate: 86% *v* 37%, *P* = 0·02).[27]

Tumor disease recurred in virtually all treated patients, more often in those with high levels of serum AFP and those without peritumoral capsule or with cirrhosis.[48,49] Up to 26% of the patients had locoregional metastases of HCC; in the remaining cases, recurrence was due to development of second primary HCCs.[30,50] In 60 randomly selected patients with tumors smaller than 3 cm and compensated cirrhosis,

Table 34.4 Five-year survival of patients with cirrhosis and tumors smaller than 5 cm treated by percutaneous ethanol injection

Liver stage (Child–Pugh)	No. of patients	% alive
A	293	47
B	149	29
C	20	0

From Livraghi T *et al. Radiology* 1995;**197**:101–8.[47]

injection with 50% acetic acid was superior to ethanol in terms of 2-year cancer-free survival (acetic acid 92%, alcohol 63%, *P* = 0·02, number needed to treat (NNT) = 3). A1d The benefits of acetic acid injection appeared to be most marked in patients with hypervascular tumors.[51] However, this study may have a problem of patient selection, since the 3-year survival of patients treated with PEI was half that reported in previous studies of patients who appeared to be comparable with respect to tumor size and liver function. Re-treatment of patients with tumor recurrence is thought to prolong patient survival.

Radiofrequency thermoablation is safe and convenient in patients with compensated cirrhosis and a small HCC. An 8-minute course of thermoablation results in complete necrosis of a 3-cm tumor. However, radiofrequency may cause complications in patients with strategically located tumors and usually requires general anesthesia.[52] In a randomized trial of 86 patients with compensated cirrhosis and small HCC, radiofrequency thermoablation was superior to PEI in terms of complete tumor necrosis (90% *v* 80%), and numbers of treatments (1·2 *v* 4·8), but it caused more complications (9·5% *v* 0).[53] A1c

There are no guidelines on how to prevent tumor recurrence after percutaneous interstitial therapy. In a single randomized trial, the risk of second primary tumors in 44 patients who were successfully treated with hepatic resection or PEI was reduced by 12 months administration of polyprenoic acid.[54] The incidence of recurrent or new hepatomas at 38 months of follow up was 49% in the placebo group and 22% in the treatment group (*P* = 0·04, NNT = 5). A1d

Transcatheter arterial chemoembolization

Transcatheter arterial chemoembolization (TACE) of HCC is possible because the liver has a dual blood supply, while HCC is supplied virtually only from the hepatic artery. TACE through the femoral artery leads to ischemic necrosis of the tumor and makes hepatic arterial injection of antitumor agents possible, giving higher local concentrations of drugs with fewer systemic adverse effects. TACE of the proximal hepatic artery (conventional TACE) has been widely employed in Eastern and Western countries as an alternative

Table 34.5 Outcomes of randomized controlled studies of transarterial embolization therapy in patients with inoperable HCC

Authors	Treatment	No. of patients	2-year survival Treated (%)	Controls (%)	P value
Trinchet *et al.* (1995)[56]	TACE	96	38	26	NS
Bruix *et al.* (1998)[57]	TAE	80	49	50	NS
Pelletier *et al.* (1998)[58]	TACE	73	24	25	NS
Lo *et al.* (2002)[60]	TACE	80	31	11	0·002
Llovet *et al.* (2002)[61]	TACE	75	63	27	0·009

TACE, transcatheter arterial chemoembolization; TAE, transarterial embolization (without chemotherapy); NS not significant

to hepatic resection and has now been improved, as segmental or subsegmental TACE. The procedure is contraindicated for patients with venous tumor supply (hypovascular tumors), advanced liver deterioration, complete thrombosis of the portal vein trunk, renal failure or extrahepatic metastases. In the past decade, three randomized controlled trials of TACE and one randomized controlled trial of transarterial embolization (TAE, without chemotherapy) treatment of patients with unresectable HCC have been conducted.[55–58] One trial[56] showed a significant reduction of tumor growth in the treated patients. A meta-analysis of 18 randomized controlled trials carried out between 1988 and 2000 to assess the anti-HCC effectiveness of TAE and TACE, indicates that chemoembolization significantly reduces the overall 2-year mortality rate (odds ratio (OR) 0·54, 95% CI 0·33 to 0·89, $P = 0·015$) compared with inactive treatment[59] and that the two treatments were of comparable activity. A1a Recently, two randomized controlled trials in Hong Kong[60] and in Barcelona[61] demonstrated that chemoembolization significantly improved survival of selected patients with unresectable HCC (Table 34.5). A1a Uncontrolled studies of segmental TACE in 63 Japanese patients with Child–Pugh A cirrhosis and a small HCC reported 4-year survival comparable with that for similar patients treated with resection or PEI.[62] B4 Thus, TACE should be compared with these interventions in a randomized trial in patients with compensated cirrhosis and a small vascularized HCC.

Other treatments

Systemic chemotherapy has been widely used to treat inoperable HCC, but the response rate is very low (20%). In the only randomized controlled trial[63] doxorubicin not only failed to prolong survival of 60 patients with inoperable HCC but also caused fatal complications in 15 (25%) due to cardiotoxicity. A1d The possible sex hormone dependence of HCC and the presence of tumor hormone receptors have

suggested a potential for hormonal manipulation of tumor growth, particularly using anti-estrogens. Initially, three small randomized controlled trials in patients considered to be unsuitable for any treatment because of advanced tumors or impaired hepatic function showed improved survival.[64–66] A1d However, in two large randomized trials of 120 and 477 patients with inoperable HCC, but less deteriorated liver function, treatment with the anti-estrogen tamoxifen did not improve survival or quality of life, compared with controls.[67,68] A1a Differences in patient selection reflected in large differences in survival between control groups may explain the contrasting results. The 1-year survival of control groups in the two studies which showed a benefit with tamoxifen was 5% and 9% compared with 43% and 56% for the two studies with negative results. A meta-analysis[68] of the five randomized studies comparing tamoxifen alone versus no active treatment yielded a pooled odds ratio of being alive at 1 year of 1·19 (95% CI 0·88 to 1·61). A1a

Perhaps hormonal treatment of patients with inoperable HCC could be refined on the basis of the type of estrogen receptor expressed by tumor cells as indicated by the high response rate in patients with the wild-type estrogen receptor.[69] In a randomized trial of 58 patients with advanced HCC, treatment with subcutaneous octreotide 250 micrograms twice daily increased survival from 13% to 56% at 12 months.[70] A1d

The conventional method of external irradiation is not effective against HCC. Using three-dimensional radiation planning (conformal radiotherapy) the beam scatter can be minimized to deliver the therapeutic dose, making selective irradiation of the liver possible. Local radiation was carried out safely in patients with Child A cirrhosis and smaller than 8-cm tumor, with a partial response rate of 64%.[71] B4 With proton radiation therapy, a large amount of radiation is focused only on the lesion, and the exposure of surrounding non-tumoral liver can be limited. Of 83 patients thus treated only 19% had a complete response without any appreciable effect on survival.[72] B4

The maxim in therapy for HCC is 'the smaller the HCC the more effective the treatment.' Recently a surveillance study for HCC in cirrhotics has shown increased patient survival.

Acknowledgement

This work was supported by a grant from Fondazione Italiana Ricerca Cancro.

References

1 Collier J, Sherman M. Screening for hepatocellular carcinoma. *Hepatology* 1998;**27**:273–8.

2 Sallie R. Screening for hepatocellular carcinoma in patients with chronic viral hepatitis: can the result justify the effort? *Viral Hep Rev* 1995;**1**:77–95.

3 Colombo M. Hepatocellular carcinoma in cirrhotics. *Semin Liv Dis* 1993;**13**:374–83.

4 Colombo M. Early diagnosis of hepatocellular carcinoma in Italy. A summary of a Consensus Development Conference held in Milan, 16 November 1990 by the Italian Association for the Study of the Liver (AISF). *J Hepatol* 1992;**14**:401–3.

5 Bruix J, Sherman M, Llovet JM *et al.* Clinical management of hepatocellular carcinoma. Conclusions of the Barcelona–2000 EASL Conference, Barcelona, September 15–17, 2000. *J Hepatol* 2001;**35**:421–30.

6 Oka H, Kurioka N, Kim K *et al.* Prospective study of early detection of hepatocellular carcinoma in patients with cirrhosis. *Hepatology* 1990;**12**:680–7.

7 Colombo M, de Franchis R, Del Ninno E *et al.* Hepatocellular carcinoma in Italian patients with cirrhosis. *N Engl J Med* 1991;**325**:675–80.

8 Cottone M, Turri M, Caltagirone M *et al.* Screening for hepatocellular carcinoma in patients with Child's A cirrhosis: a 8 year prospective study by ultrasound and alphafetoprotein. *J Hepatol* 1994;**21**:1029–34.

9 Tsukuma H, Hiyama T, Tanaka S *et al.* Risk factors for hepatocellular carcinoma among patients with chronic liver disease. *N Engl J Med* 1993;**328**:1797–801.

10 Borzio M, Bruno S, Roncalli M *et al.* Liver cell dysplasia is a major risk factor for hepatocellular carcinoma in cirrhosis: a prospective study. *Gastroenterology* 1995;**108**:812–17.

11 Sato Y, Nakata K, Kato Y *et al.* Early recognition of hepatocellular carcinoma based on altered profiles of alpha-fetoprotein. *N Engl J Med* 1993;**328**:1802–6.

12 Donato F, Boffetta P, Puoti M. A meta-analysis of epidemiological studies on the combined effect of hepatitis B and C virus infections in causing hepatocellular carcinoma. *Int J Cancer* 1998;**30**:347–54.

13 Maynard JE. Hepatitis B: global importance and need for control. *Vaccine* 1990;**8**:S18–20.

14 Rogler CE. Cellular and molecular mechanisms of hepatocarcinogenesis associated with hepadnavirus infection. In: Mason WS, Seager C (eds). *Hepadnavirus molecular biology and pathogenesis*. Berlin: Springer-Verlag, 1991.

15 Beasley RP. Hepatitis B virus. The major etiology of hepatocellular carcinoma. *Cancer* 1988;**61**:1842–56.

16 de Franchis R, Meucci G, Vecchi M *et al.* The natural history of asymptomatic hepatitis B surface antigen carriers. *Ann Intern Med* 1993;**118**:191–4.

17 Chang MH, Chen CJ, Lai MS *et al.* Universal hepatitis B vaccination in Taiwan and the incidence of hepatocellular carcinoma in children. *N Engl J Med* 1997;**336**:1855–9.

18 Nakamura T, Nakamura S, Aikawa T *et al.* Obstruction of the inferior vena cava in the hepatic portion and the hepatic vein: report of eight cases and review of the Japanese literature. *Angiology* 1968;**19**:479–98.

19 Kew MC, McKnight A, Hodkingson H *et al.* The role of membranous obstruction of the inferior vena cava in the etiology of hepatocellular carcinoma in Southern African Blacks. *Hepatology* 1989;**9**:121–5.

20 Okuda K. Early recognition of hepatocellular carcinoma. *Hepatology* 1986;**6**:729–38.

21 Okuda K. Hepatocellular carcinoma: recent progress. *Hepatology* 1992;**5**:948–63.

22 McMahon BJ, Alberts SR, Wainwright RB *et al.* Hepatitis B sequelae: prospective study in 1400 hepatitis B surface antigen-positive Alaska Native carriers. *Arch Intern Med* 1990;**150**:1051–4.

23 Bolondi L, Sofia S, Siringo S *et al.* Surveillance programme of cirrhotic patients for early diagnosis and treatment of hepatocellular carcinoma: a cost-effective analysis. *Gut* 2001;**48**:251–9.

24 Trevisani F, De Notariis S, Rapaccini G *et al.* Semiannual and annual surveillance of cirrhotic patients for hepatocellular carcinoma: effects on cancer stage and patient survival (Italian experience). *Am J Gastroenterol* 2002;**97**:734–44.

25 Bolondi L. Screening for hepatocellular carcinoma in cirrhosis. *J Hepatol* 2003;**39**:1076–84.

26 Ros PR, Davis GL. The incidental focal liver lesion: photon, proton or needle? *Hepatology* 1998;**27**:1183–90.

27 Toyoda H, Kumuda T, Nakano S *et al.* The significance of tumor vascularity as a predictor of long-term prognosis in patients with small hepatocellular carcinoma treated by percutaneous ethanol injection. *J Hepatol* 1997;**26**:1055–62.

28 Livraghi T, Bolondi L, Buscarini L *et al.* No treatment, resection and ethanol injection in hepatocellular carcinoma: a retrospective analysis of survival in 391 patients with cirrhosis. *J Hepatol* 1995;**22**:522–6.

29 Llovet JM, Burroughs A, Bruix J. Hepatocellular carcinoma. *Lancet* 2003;**362**:1907–17.

30 Ringe B, Pichlmayr R, Wittekind C *et al.* Surgical treatment of hepatocellular carcinoma: experience with liver resection and transplantation in 198 patients. *World J Surg* 1991;**15**:270–85.

31 Iwatsuki S, Starzl TE, Sheahan DG *et al.* Hepatic resection versus transplantation for hepatocellular carcinoma. *Ann Surg* 1991;**214**:221–9.

32 Mazzaferro V, Regalia E, Doci R *et al.* Liver transplantation for the treatment of small hepatocellular carcinomas in patients with cirrhosis. *N Engl J Med* 1996;**334**:693–9.

33 Llovet JM, Bruix J, Fuster J *et al.* Liver transplantation for small hepatocellular carcinoma: the tumor-node-metastasis

classification does not have prognostic power. *Hepatology* 1998;**27**:1572–7.

34 Bismuth H, Majno PE, Adam R. Liver transplantation for hepatocellular carcinoma. *Semin Liv Dis* 1999;**19**:311–22.

35 Jonas S, Bechstein WO, Steinmüller T et al. Vascular invasion and histopathologic grading determine outcome after liver transplantation for hepatocellular carcinoma in cirrhosis. *Hepatology* 2001;**33**:1080–6.

36 Samuel D, Muller R, Alexander G et al. Liver transplantation in European patients with the hepatitis B surface antigen. *N Engl J Med* 1993;**329**:1842–7.

37 Bain VG, Kneteman NM, Ma MM et al. Efficacy of lamivudine in chronic hepatitis B patients with active viral replication and decompensated cirrhosis undergoing liver transplantation. *Transplantation* 1996;**62**:1456–62.

38 Adam R, Del Gaudio M. Evolution of liver transplantation for hepatocellular carcinoma. *J Hepatol* 2003;**39**:888–95.

39 Tobe T, Arii S. Improving survival after resection of hepatocellular carcinoma: characteristics and current status of surgical treatment of primary liver cancer in Japan. In: Tobe T, Kameda H, Okudaira M et al (eds). *Primary liver cancer in Japan*. Tokyo/Berlin: Springer, 1992.

40 The Liver Cancer Study Group of Japan. Predictive factors for long term prognosis after partial hepatectomy for patients with hepatocellular carcinoma in Japan. *Cancer* 1994;**74**: 2772–80.

41 Adachi E, Maeda T, Matsumata T et al. Risk factors for intrahepatic recurrence in human small hepatocellular carcinoma. *Gastroenterology* 1995;**108**:768–75.

42 Nagasue N, Yukaya H. Liver resection for hepatocellular carcinoma: results from 150 consecutive patients. *Cancer Chemother Pharmacol* 1989;**23**:S78–S82.

43 Franco D, Capussotti L, Smadja C et al. Resection of hepatocellular carcinomas. Results in 72 European patients with cirrhosis. *Gastroenterology* 1990;**98**:733–8.

44 Bruix J, Castells A, Bosch J et al. Surgical resection of hepatocellular carcinoma in cirrhotic patients: prognostic value of preoperative portal pressure. *Gastroenterology* 1996;**111**:1018–23.

45 Harada T, Shigemura T, Kodama S et al. Hepatic resection is not enough for hepatocellular carcinoma. A follow-up study of 92 patients. *Am J Gastroenterol* 1992;**14**:245–50.

46 Llovet JM, Fuster J, Bruix J for the Barcelona Clinic Liver Cancer (BCLC) Group. Intention-to-treat analysis of surgical treatment for early hepatocellular carcinoma: resection versus transplantation. *Hepatology* 1999;**30**:1434–40.

47 Livraghi T, Giorgio T, Marin G et al. Hepatocellular carcinoma in cirrhosis in 746 patients: long-term results of percutaneous ethanol injection. *Radiology* 1995;**197**:101–8.

48 Castellano L, Calandra M, Del Vecchio Blanco et al. Predictive factors of survival and intrahepatic recurrence of hepatocellular carcinoma in cirrhosis after percutaneous ethanol injection: analysis of 71 patients. *J Hepatol* 1997;**27**:862–70.

49 Pompili M, Rapaccini GL, de Luca F et al. Risk factors for intrahepatic recurrence of hepatocellular carcinoma in cirrhotic patients treated by percutaneous ethanol injection. *Cancer* 1997;**79**:1501–8.

50 Ebara M, Otho M, Sugiura N et al. Percutaneous ethanol injection for the treatment of small hepatocellular carcinoma. Study of 95 patients. *J Gastroenterol Hepatol* 1990;**5**:616–26.

51 Ohnishi K, Yoshioka H, Ito S et al. Prospective randomized controlled trial comparing percutaneous acetic acid injection and percutaneous ethanol injection for small hepatocellular carcinoma. *Hepatology* 1998;**27**:67–72.

52 Nagata Y, Abe M, Hiroada M et al. Radiofrequency hyperthermia and radiotherapy for hepatocellular carcinoma. In: Tobe T, Kameda H, Okudaira M et al. (eds), *Primary liver cancer in Japan*. Tokyo/Berlin: Springer, 1992.

53 Livraghi T, Goldberg SN, Lazzaroni S et al. Small hepatocellular carcinoma treatment with radio-frequency ablation versus ethanol injection. *Radiology* 1999;**210**: 655–61.

54 Muto Y, Moriwaki H, Ninomiya M et al. Prevention of second primary tumors by an acyclic retinoid, polyprenoic acid, in patients with hepatocellular carcinoma. *N Engl J Med* 1996;**334**:1561–7.

55 Pelletier G, Roche A, Ink O et al. A randomized trial of hepatic arterial chemoembolization in patients with unresectable hepatocellular carcinoma. *J Hepatol* 1990;**11**:181–4.

56 Groupe d'Etude et de Traitement du Carcinome Hépatocellulaire. A comparison of lipiodol chemoembolization and conservative treatment for unresectable hepatocellular carcinoma. *N Engl J Med* 1995;**332**:1256–61.

57 Bruix J, Llovet JM, Castells A et al. Transarterial embolization versus symptomatic treatment in patients with advanced hepatocellular carcinoma: results of a randomized controlled trial in a single institution. *Hepatology* 1998;**27**: 1578–83.

58 Pelletier G, Ducreux M, Gay F et al. Treatment of unresectable hepatocellular carcinoma with lipiodol chemoembolization: a multicenter randomized trial. *J Hepatol* 1998;**28**:129–34.

59 Cammà C, Schepis F, Orlando A et al. Transarterial chemoembolization for unresectable hepatocellular carcinoma: meta-analysis of randomized controlled trials. *Radiology* 2002;**224**:47–54.

60 Lo CM, Ngan H, Tso WK et al. Randomized controlled trial of transarterial lipiodol chemoembolization for unresectable hepatocellular carcinoma. *Hepatology* 2002;**35**:1164–71.

61 Llovet JM, Real MI, Montana X et al. Arterial embolisation or chemoembolisation versus symptomatic treatment in patients with unresectable hepatocellular carcinoma: a randomised controlled trial. *Lancet* 2002;**359**:1734–9.

62 Matsui O, Kodoya M, Yoshikawa J et al. Small hepatocellular carcinoma: treatment with subsegmental transcatheter arterial embolization. *Radiology* 1993;**188**:79–83.

63 Lai CL, Wu PC, Chan GCB et al. Doxorubicin versus no antitumor therapy in inoperable hepatocellular carcinoma. A prospective randomized trial. *Cancer* 1988;**62**:479–83.

64 Farinati F, Salvagnini M, De Maria N et al. Unresectable hepatocellular carcinoma: a prospective controlled trial with tamoxifen. *J Hepatol* 1990;**11**:297–301.

65 Martinez Cerezo FJ, Tomas A, Donoso L et al. Controlled trial of tamoxifen in patients with advanced hepatocellular carcinoma. *J Hepatol* 1994;**20**:702–6.

66 Elba S, Giannuzzi V, Misciagna G *et al.* Randomized controlled trial of tamoxifen versus placebo in inoperable hepatocellular carcinoma. *Ital J Gastroenterol* 1994;**26**: 66–8.

67 Castells A, Bruix J, Bru C *et al.* Treatment of hepatocellular carcinoma with tamoxifen: a double-blind placebo-controlled trial in 120 patients. *Gastroenterology* 1995;**109**: 917–22.

68 CLIP Group. Tamoxifen in treatment of hepatocellular carcinoma: a randomised controlled trial. *Lancet* 1998;**352**: 17–20.

69 Villa E, Camellini L, Dugani A *et al.* Variant estrogen receptor messenger RNA species detected in human primary hepato-cellular carcinoma. *Cancer Res* 1995;**55**:498–500.

70 Kouroumalis E, Skordilis P, Thermos K *et al.* Treatment of hepatocellular carcinoma with octreotide: a randomised controlled study. *Gut* 1998;**42**:442–7.

71 Lawrence TS, Tesser RJ, Tam Haken RK. An application of dose volume histograms to the treatment of intrahepatic malignancies with radiation therapy. *Int J Radiat Oncol Biol Phys* 1991;**20**:555–61.

72 Matsuzaki Y, Osuga T, Saito Y *et al.* A new, effective and safe therapeutic option using proton irradiation for hepatocellular carcinoma. *Gastroenterology* 1994;**106**:1032–41.

73 Sangiovanni A, Del Ninno E, Fasani P *et al.* Increased survival of cirrhotic patients with a hepatocellular carcinoma detected during surveillance. *Gastroenterology* 2004: in press.

35 Fulminant hepatic failure

Nick Murphy, Julia Wendon

Introduction

Intensive care medicine has developed over the past 40 years in response to the need to support failing organ systems in critically ill patients. The majority of methods used have been introduced without the prior benefit of controlled clinical trials.

The small numbers of patients and their heterogeneity within general intensive care units (ICUs) have hampered the search for proved remedies. This lack of evidence of benefit in intensive care medicine is also present in the treatment of patients with fulminant hepatic failure (FHF) who require the full spectrum of organ support in the ICU.

The management of FHF can be considered in two divisions: (i) general supportive care and (ii) therapies aimed at managing the failing liver and its complications.

Definition

In 1970 Trey and Davidson[1] introduced the term "fulminant hepatic failure" to describe a syndrome of rapidly progressing liver failure in which encephalopathy follows the onset of symptoms within 8 weeks in someone without previous liver disease. This definition is still used today; however, it has become clear that this definition is too broad and that subgroups exist. Both etiology and speed of progression to encephalopathy from the onset of jaundice can be used to define subgroups. This is important, as both factors have been shown to be independent predictors of prognosis (Figure 35.1).[2] Interestingly, it is the hyperacute group that has the best chance for spontaneous recovery, although it also carries the highest risk of cerebral edema.[2,3]

Etiology

FHF has many causes. Worldwide, viral hepatitis is by far the most common cause. Within the UK, acetaminophen (paracetamol) self-poisoning has been the most frequent cause of FHF over the past 15 years, however recent epidemiological data from the major UK liver units suggest that the incidence of acetaminophen-induced FHF is falling. In 1998 legislation was introduced in the UK limiting the

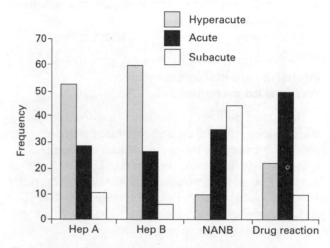

Figure 35.1 Speed of onset according to etiology. (Note that the majority of acetaminophen (paracetamol) poisonings would appear in the hyperacute group[2])

amount of acetaminophen that could be sold over the counter. This appears to have reduced the morbidity and mortality associated with acetaminophen self-poisoning in some parts of the UK.[4] However, the effect has not been shown across the whole country and there appears to be regional variation.[5]

The fall in numbers presenting with acetaminophen hepatotoxicity in the UK is at odds with recent data from the USA, which show that there has been an increase in the presentation of acute liver failure secondary to acetaminophen poisoning. The authors suggest that the majority are due to therapeutic misadventure rather than suicidal intent.[6]

In both the UK and the USA the second most common cause of FHF is seronegative or FHF of indeterminate cause. Despite intensive research in this area the cause or causes in this group, as the name suggests, remain elusive.

Pathogenesis

FHF is not a disease but a syndrome whose severity is proportional to the degree of hepatic necrosis. FHF causes profound physiological derangement characterized by encephalopathy, vasoparesis,[7] and coagulopathy. As the syndrome progresses, cerebral edema[8] and renal failure are prominent and there is impaired immunity with increased susceptibility to infection.[9]

The rate of progression of FHF can be unpredictable in the hyperacute group. The syndrome typically evolves over several days, but deep coma can occur within hours. The mainstay of treatment in FHF is supportive management while the decision to proceed to hepatic transplantation is being considered.

The causes of death in FHF can split the patients with FHF into two main groups: those with cerebral edema who die of brain ischemia or brain stem compression, and those who succumb to sepsis and multiple organ failure.[10]

Intensive care management versus ward management

There have been no controlled clinical trials comparing intensive care with ward management, but considering the almost 100% mortality before the adoption of modern ICUs[11] it seems likely that intensive care management improves survival. B4 Patients with grades III and IV encephalopathy should be intubated, ventilated and managed within an ICU. High dependency areas for patients with liver failure and lower levels of coma are to be encouraged.[12]

Management in a liver unit

Again, management of FHF in a liver unit has not been subjected to a controlled clinical trial but the access to a liver transplant program has obvious advantages. Survival rates for FHF with medical therapy alone in cases that progress to grade III or IV encephalopathy are poor, varying between 10% and 40%. With the introduction of orthotopic liver transplantation (OLT) as a therapeutic option for patients with FHF, survival rates have increased to 60–80% (Figure 35.2).[13] B4

Criteria have been developed to help advise peripheral hospitals when patients should be transferred to a liver unit (Box 35.1).[14] These criteria are based on clinical judgment and have not been subjected to a controlled clinical trial.

General supportive management

Fluid resuscitation and circulatory management

Patients with FHF develop marked hemodynamic changes. Vasodilatation can be profound and is invariably accompanied by a compensatory increase in cardiac output.[15] This distributive shock, with relative hypovolemia, causes hypotension despite the increased cardiac output. Prognostic

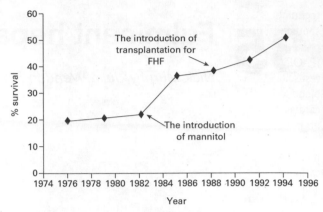

Figure 35.2   Improving survival in FHF

Box 35.1   Criteria for when patients should be transferred to liver unit

- International normalized ratio (INR) > 3·0
- Prothrombin time in seconds greater than the time in hours since the overdose (for acetaminophen (paracetamol) poisoning)
- Any evidence of encephalopathy
- Hypotension following fluid resuscitation
- Evidence of a metabolic acidosis

criteria such as acidosis and renal function should only be assessed following adequate resuscitation, as there can be marked improvement in these following fluid intake.

The choice of resuscitation fluid in FHF is not clear. Despite 30 years of investigation in various patient groups the optimal fluid is unknown. There have not been any controlled clinical trials comparing fluid regimens in FHF. Recent systematic reviews comparing the use of crystalloids and colloids in fluid resuscitation[16,17] have not produced clarity. The choice of colloid solution is as unclear as the comparison of crystalloid and colloid. The most recent systemic review from the Cochrane Injury Group concluded that there is no evidence that one colloid solution is more effective or safer than any other.[18] The authors go on to state that the confidence intervals are wide and do not rule out clinically significant differences between the colloids that a sufficiently large and well run trial may find.[18] A1c

The hemodynamic changes associated with FHF are fairly predictable. As stated above, profound systemic vasodilatation is followed by a compensatory increase in cardiac output. Blood pressure is often low despite aggressive fluid resuscitation. Endpoints in resuscitation are difficult to define and so the use of some sort of monitor of both cardiac preload and cardiac output can be used to observe response to interventions. There is little evidence to suggest any technique is superior to any other and so local experience should dictate which techniques are used. Central venous pressure (CVP) and pulmonary artery occlusion pressure (PAOP) are often used to assess preload and the adequacy of resuscitation but the correlation between CVP, PAOP and blood volume is poor.[19] The use of trends in preload and cardiac output and the response to a series of fluid challenges improve their usefulness. C5

There remains some controversy about the use of invasive monitoring in general and the use of pulmonary artery (PA) catheters in particular. The observational study by Conners and colleagues demonstrated an increased mortality associated with the use of the pulmonary artery catheter in critically ill patients during the first 24 hours of intensive care compared with case-matched control individuals.[20] B4 The calls for a moratorium on the use of PA catheters following publication of this paper have not stopped their use. The results of current ongoing prospective trials into the therapeutic use of PA catheter-directed therapy are eagerly awaited.

During the early 1970s it was first suggested that during critical illness a pathological supply–dependency line is seen (See Figure 35.2).[21] This was proposed because of markedly increased resting oxygen consumption noted in critical illness associated with systemic inflammation. Oxygen delivery increases to meet the demand. It was noted that survivors had higher oxygen transport parameters than non-survivors. It was also noted that if oxygen delivery was increased, by fluid resuscitation and or inotropic drugs, oxygen consumption increased, suggesting that there was covert tissue hypoxia and that this may be the cause of multiple organ failure.

Work by Bihari *et al.* in the 1980s suggested the presence of a pathological supply–dependency for oxygen in patients with FHF. The patients with FHF who failed to survive had both a lower baseline VO_2 than survivors and greater increases in VO_2 following infusion of epoprostenol, suggesting a greater oxygen debt.[22] However, since then the whole premise of this argument – that there exists a pathological supply–dependency in critical illness – has been questioned because of the inevitable increase in calculated oxygen consumption when delivery is increased due to mathematical coupling.[23]

Patients who fail to achieve normal or supra-normal oxygen transport parameters despite fluid resuscitation in the face of critical illness have a poor prognosis. Investigators have proposed that the targeting of survivor parameters may improve outcome in critically ill patients. However studies investigating the augmentation of oxygen delivery have not shown any advantage when applied indiscriminately to all patients. In fact, an increase in mortality was shown in a group of patients achieving supra-normal goals with the aid of inotropes.[24] A European consensus conference concluded

that the continued aggressive attempts to increase oxygen transport in all critically ill patients is unwarranted, although timely resuscitation and achievement of normal hemodynamics is essential.[25] B4 C5

Epinephrine and norepinephrine are effective agents and are frequently employed to improve MAP in FHF, commencing at 0·1 micrograms/kg per minute. Both of these agents have been shown to improve MAP; the addition of epoprostenol (a microcirculatory vasodilator) to norepinephrine increases oxygen delivery while maintaining MAP.[26] Epinephrine, like other β-agonists has deleterious effects on intermediary metabolism if used over an extended period of time. These effects include hyperlactemia and hyperglycemia and are related partly to the effect of epinephrine on glycolysis within skeletal muscles.[27] Norepinephrine does not have these effects and so is recommended on the basis of current evidence. C5

Blood pressure is important in maintaining flow to essential organs but what value or threshold pressure is acceptable in FHF is unknown. However, cerebral autoregulation is disturbed in FHF making cerebral blood flow directly proportional to cerebral perfusion pressure (CPP).[28] This implies that hypotension will result in cerebral ischemia, which may be a factor precipitating brain swelling in FHF,[29] and that hypertension will result in cerebral hyperemia and increased intracranial pressure (ICP). However, as discussed later, targeting a specific blood pressure to maintain cerebral perfusion in the face of cerebral edema is often futile and probably unnecessary.[30]

Mechanical ventilation

Intubation of the trachea and mechanical ventilation is indicated for several reasons in FHF but not usually for hypoxemia.[15] As patients progress from grade II to grade III encephalopathy, decreasing consciousness can lead to compromising the airway with the risk of aspiration. Grade III encephalopathy is often characterized by agitation and aggressive behavior. Sedation in these patients is required to allow appropriate monitoring and treatment but requires intubation and ventilation.

As opposed to other causes of systemic inflammatory response syndrome, the lungs are relatively spared early in the course of FHF. However, a proportion of patients progress to multiple organ dysfunction in which lung disease is prominent.[31]

The normal lung can tolerate "conventional" ventilation with physiological tidal volumes and low levels of positive end expiratory pressure (PEEP) for extended periods without apparent harm. The situation is different for damaged lungs and particularly so in patients with acute respiratory distress syndrome (ARDS). There is increasing evidence that mechanical ventilation in the setting of ARDS can increase lung injury and negatively impact on outcome. Ventilator-induced lung injury (VILI) encompasses a wide spectrum of damage, consisting of conventional barotrauma, pneumothorax, pneumomediastinum, and alveolar damage increasing pulmonary edema.[32] Recent controlled clinical trials have shown improvements in mortality with a protective ventilatory strategy[33,34] and a consensus conference has recommended certain steps to minimize damage to the lungs during mechanical ventilation.[35] A1c

1   Minimize the inspired oxygen level and take aggressive steps to do this if the inspired fraction is greater than 0·65.
2   Recruit alveoli by increasing PEEP. The amount of PEEP necessary to prevent cyclic opening and closure of alveoli is approximately 7·4–11 mmHg (10–15 cmH$_2$O).
3   Minimize high airway pressures. Transalveolar pressures should not exceed 18·4–22 mmHg (25–30 cmH$_2$O). This corresponds to an end inspiratory static (plateau) pressure of 22–29·4 mmHg (30–40 cmH$_2$O).
4   Prevent atelectasis by employing larger breaths periodically to re-expand collapsed units during tidal ventilation with small tidal volumes.

Sedation and paralysis

Patients with acute hepatic failure requiring mechanical ventilation are deeply encephalopathic. The need for sedation varies between patients and should be tailored individually. Sedation scoring with, for example, the six-point Ramsay scale[36] have not been validated in FHF and are difficult to interpret in the setting of hepatic encephalopathy. Mechanical ventilation is usually tolerated with minimum amounts of opiate and little if any hypnotic agent. Deep sedation is unnecessary and will only add to cardiovascular depression and prolong recovery in patients with impaired liver function. These considerations, however, have to be contrasted with the need to prevent surges in ICP during routine nursing care and supplemental sedation or small doses of a non-depolarizing neuromuscular blocker may be useful during suctioning of the patient's trachea. The issue of paralysis in FHF should be considered. It had been common practice to paralyze all ventilated patients with FHF whilst at risk from cerebral edema. However, there have not been any controlled clinical trials comparing paralysis or not in FHF in any other branch of intensive care medicine. A retrospective review of 1030 patients with acute traumatic brain injury showed that ICU stay and infectious complications were higher in the group who received routine paralysis.[37] B4 Anecdotal reports have also suggested an association between long-term paralysis and a necrotizing myopathy, in patients with asthma, that may prolong ICU stay and impinge adversely on outcome.[38,39] Thus, there is no indication for routine paralysis in FHF.

Nutrition in fulminant hepatic failure: enteral versus parenteral nutrition

It seems obvious that nutrition is of benefit in critically ill patients but proving it with controlled clinical trials is more difficult. Starvation is not an option! Data from the hunger strikes in Northern Ireland and from Nazi Germany confirm death is inevitable within 60–80 days without nutrition when fluids and electrolytes are given. B2

There are few data in the literature from which to draw conclusions regarding feeding in FHF but in common with other forms of critical illness, FHF is associated with an increased metabolic rate and catabolism.[40] Depending on the severity of the injury and the duration of the disease, weight loss associated with the loss of body fat and skeletal muscle mass may vary from being relatively insignificant to being life-threatening, primarily through the development of immunosuppression and a reduction or delay in wound healing and tissue repair.[41,42] The loss of body protein cannot be prevented by nutrition but the rate of loss can be slowed. It is the treatment of the underlying problem that eventually reverses the catabolic phase of the illness and it is at that time that anabolism can be promoted by nutrition.[43]

The route used in supplying nutrition is more easily compared and, where possible, enteral nutrition is the preferred method. Intestinal stimulation from enteral nutrition tract helps to maintain the gastrointestinal integrity and results in reduced infection rates when compared with total parenteral nutrition (TPN).[44] B4 Recent interest has been shown in the supplementation of both enteral nutrition and TPN. Immuno-enhanced enteral feeds containing arginine, purine nucleotides and ω-3 fatty acids have been compared with standard enteral nutrition in ICUs. There appears to be a reduction in the number of infectious complications and other adverse events including length of hospital stay and the number of days on ventilation.[45] A1c This reduction in morbidity has not yet translated into a decrease in mortality.[45,46]

TPN when given to well nourished elective surgical patients preoperatively results in an increase in postoperative infectious complications.[47] The risk of coagulase negative staphylococcal bacteremia in neonates is increased six times by the administration of lipid emulsions. The question is which patients, if any, should receive TPN. The Veterans Affairs group found that a group of severely malnourished patients benefited from 10 days perioperative TPN.[47] However, TPN has not been shown to benefit patients with FHF or other critically ill patients.

Glutamine is a non-essential amino acid in health. However, during critical illness, because of its central role in protein metabolism, glutamine deficiency is common. Original TPN formulations did not contain glutamine because of problems with its stability in solution and standard enteral feed preparations contain minimal amounts. There is evidence that glutamine-enriched TPN can reduce gut atrophy, infectious complications and 6-month mortality in critically ill patients.[48] Meta-analysis of controlled trials suggests that glutamine supplementation in critical illness results in a reduction in infectious complications.[49] Alc

Stress ulcer prophylaxis

Many small randomized controlled clinical trials over the past 20 years have looked at the prevention of stress ulceration. While the incidence of stress ulcer has fallen over this period, the cause of this decline is unclear. It is probably the result of both improved resuscitation and the widespread use of stress ulcer prophylaxis.

H_2-blockers are effective in the prevention of stress ulceration in FHF. Macdougall *et al.*[50] investigated the effects of H_2-blockers and antacid solutions in two small controlled trials. They found a significant decrease in the incidence of stress ulceration and blood transfusions with the use of H_2-blockers, but not with antacids. There was a trend toward an improved survival in the treated patients but this was not statistically significant.[50] Alc

Stress ulceration is probably the result of ischemic injury to the gastric mucosa, and adequate resuscitation is the single most important factor in its prevention. Apart from good general ICU care there have been two broad approaches to reducing the incidence of stress ulceration: decreasing the acidity of the stomach with the use of antacids, H_2-blockers, or proton pump inhibitors, and the use of sucralfate, a cytoprotective agent. The role of acid suppression in encouraging an increase in bacterial overgrowth and the ensuing microaspiration of colonized pharyngeal fluid thus promoting the development of hospital-acquired pneumonia, has led to the comparison of the ulcer and pneumonia rates, and mortality between the two methods.

Several meta-analyses have attempted to resolve the uncertainty regarding the efficacy on the one hand and adverse effects of the drugs on the other.[51,52] After combining their efforts, the two main groups of investigators published a meta-analysis which included all relevant published and unpublished randomized clinical trials.[52] The meta-analysis demonstrated similar efficacy for H_2-blockers and sucralfate for the outcome of reduction in stress ulceration bleeding, but an increase in the incidence of pneumonia and an excess mortality in the H_2-blocker group. A more recent trial conducted by some of the same authors suggests a significantly higher rate of stress ulceration with sucralfate compared to ranitidine without any difference in pneumonia rates or mortality.[53] Ala

FHF was excluded in most of the trials comparing sucralfate to pH-altering drugs and was not included in the meta-analysis. It is therefore difficult to draw firm conclusions. Patients with FHF tend to fall into the high risk group by virtue of both being ventilated and having a

coagulopathy. The balance of evidence suggests that pH-altering drugs such as H_2-blockers or proton pump inhibitors provide the best defense against stress ulceration, but that this may be offset by an increased incidence of pneumonia.

Prophylactic antibiotics and selective decontamination of the digestive tract

Patients with acute liver failure have increased susceptibility to infections, principally as a result of impaired phagocytic function, reduced complement levels, and the need for invasive procedures.[54] Bacteriologically proved infection is recorded in up to 80% of patients with FHF, and fungal infection (predominantly candidiasis) in 32%. Clinical signs such as fever and elevated white blood cell count are absent in 30% of the cases. Pneumonia accounts for 50% of infective episodes.[9] Risk factors for infection that have been identified are a high peak international normalized ratio (INR), grade III or IV encephalopathy, and intubation of the trachea.[54,55]

Because of the high incidence of infection the use of prophylactic anti-microbial agents has been investigated. Both parenteral antibiotics and the use of selective decontamination of the digestive tract (SDD), in combination and individually, have been studied.

Intravenous antibiotics if given prophylactically will reduce the incidence of infection in patients with FHF to approximately 20%.[54,55] Alc However, prophylactic antibiotics have not been shown to improve outcome or reduce the length of stay in patients with FHF.[54] Alc The role of SDD is less clear and has not been evaluated in controlled trials compared with placebo or intravenous antibiotics alone in FHF. Rolando *et al.* reported that SDD used in combination with intravenous antibiotics provided no additional benefit.[54–56]

The most recent systematic review of randomized controlled trials of antibiotic prophylaxis in ICUs was published in the Cochrane database of systematic reviews.[57] This systematic review evaluated 32 randomized controlled trials, which included 5639 unselected general ICU patients. Selected groups, for example patients with FHF, were excluded from the review. Pooled estimates of the 16 randomized controlled trials testing the effect of the SDD and systemic antibiotic combination indicate a significant reduction of both respiratory tract infections (odds ratio (OR) 0·35, 95% (confidence interval) CI 0·29 to 0·41) and total mortality (OR 0·80, 95% CI 0·68 to 0·93) (Figure 35.3). The number of patients needed to treat (NNT) to prevent one infection is 5, and the NNT to prevent one death is 23. Ala When the data on the effect of SDD alone compared with the control groups were pooled from the 16 available trials a marked reduction in respiratory tract infections was demonstrated (OR 0·56, 95% CI 0·46 to 0·68) but no

Review: Antibiotics for preventing respiratory tract infection in adults receiving intensive care
Comparison: topical plus systemic vs no prophylaxis
Outcome: RTIs

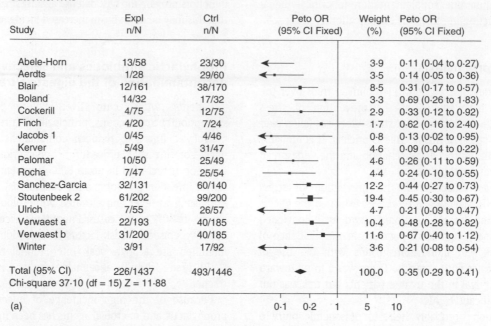

Study	Expl n/N	Ctrl n/N	Peto OR (95% CI Fixed)	Weight (%)	Peto OR (95% CI Fixed)
Abele-Horn	13/58	23/30		3·9	0·11 (0·04 to 0·27)
Aerdts	1/28	29/60		3·5	0·14 (0·05 to 0·36)
Blair	12/161	38/170		8·5	0·31 (0·17 to 0·57)
Boland	14/32	17/32		3·3	0·69 (0·26 to 1·83)
Cockerill	4/75	12/75		2·9	0·33 (0·12 to 0·92)
Finch	4/20	7/24		1·7	0·62 (0·16 to 2·40)
Jacobs 1	0/45	4/46		0·8	0·13 (0·02 to 0·95)
Kerver	5/49	31/47		4·6	0·09 (0·04 to 0·22)
Palomar	10/50	25/49		4·6	0·26 (0·11 to 0·59)
Rocha	7/47	25/54		4·4	0·24 (0·10 to 0·55)
Sanchez-Garcia	32/131	60/140		12·2	0·44 (0·27 to 0·73)
Stoutenbeek 2	61/202	99/200		19·4	0·45 (0·30 to 0·67)
Ulrich	7/55	26/57		4·7	0·21 (0·09 to 0·47)
Verwaest a	22/193	40/185		10·4	0·48 (0·28 to 0·82)
Verwaest b	31/200	40/185		11·6	0·67 (0·40 to 1·12)
Winter	3/91	17/92		3·6	0·21 (0·08 to 0·54)
Total (95% CI)	226/1437	493/1446		100·0	0·35 (0·29 to 0·41)

Chi-square 37·10 (df = 15) Z = 11·88

(a)

0·1   0·2   1   5   10

Review: Antibiotics for preventing respiratory tract infection in adults receiving intensive care
Comparison: Topical plus systemic vs no prophylaxis
Outcome: Overall mortality

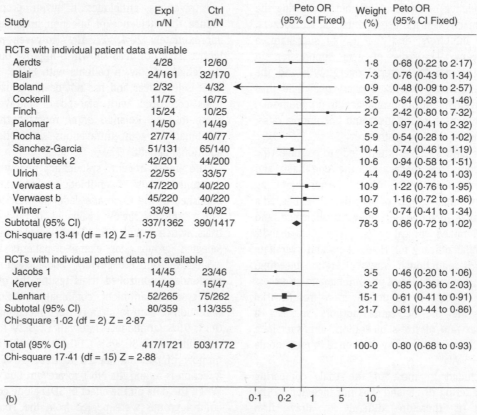

Study	Expl n/N	Ctrl n/N	Peto OR (95% CI Fixed)	Weight (%)	Peto OR (95% CI Fixed)
RCTs with individual patient data available					
Aerdts	4/28	12/60		1·8	0·68 (0·22 to 2·17)
Blair	24/161	32/170		7·3	0·76 (0·43 to 1·34)
Boland	2/32	4/32		0·9	0·48 (0·09 to 2·57)
Cockerill	11/75	16/75		3·5	0·64 (0·28 to 1·46)
Finch	15/24	10/25		2·0	2·42 (0·80 to 7·32)
Palomar	14/50	14/49		3·2	0·97 (0·41 to 2·32)
Rocha	27/74	40/77		5·9	0·54 (0·28 to 1·02)
Sanchez-Garcia	51/131	65/140		10·4	0·74 (0·46 to 1·19)
Stoutenbeek 2	42/201	44/200		10·6	0·94 (0·58 to 1·51)
Ulrich	22/55	33/57		4·4	0·49 (0·24 to 1·03)
Verwaest a	47/220	40/220		10·9	1·22 (0·76 to 1·95)
Verwaest b	45/220	40/220		10·7	1·16 (0·72 to 1·86)
Winter	33/91	40/92		6·9	0·74 (0·41 to 1·34)
Subtotal (95% CI)	337/1362	390/1417		78·3	0·86 (0·72 to 1·02)
Chi-square 13·41 (df = 12) Z = 1·75					
RCTs with individual patient data not available					
Jacobs 1	14/45	23/46		3·5	0·46 (0·20 to 1·06)
Kerver	14/49	15/47		3·2	0·85 (0·36 to 2·03)
Lenhart	52/265	75/262		15·1	0·61 (0·41 to 0·91)
Subtotal (95% CI)	80/359	113/355		21·7	0·61 (0·44 to 0·86)
Chi-square 1·02 (df = 2) Z = 2·87					
Total (95% CI)	417/1721	503/1772		100·0	0·80 (0·68 to 0·93)

Chi-square 17·41 (df = 15) Z = 2·88

(b)

0·1   0·2   1   5   10

Figure 35.3   (a, b) Antibiotic prophylaxis in intensive care units. (Source: *Cochrane Library*, issue 2. Oxford: Update Software, 1999)

corresponding effect on overall mortality (OR 1·01, 95% CI 0·84 to 1·22) was found (Figure 35.4). A1a A recent study[58] in a low prevalence setting for vancomycin-resistant enterococci and methicillin-resistant staphylococci has shown reduced mortality, but the applicability to all types of ICU patients is still questioned.[59]

Although prophylactic intravenous antibiotics have been shown to reduce the number of proved infections in FHF, improvements in outcome have not been demonstrated. SDD on its own has not been shown to reduce infection or improve outcome in FHF. There is also a risk of promoting the emergence of multiply resistant organisms within ICUs by the blanket use of broad-spectrum antimicrobials. SDD selects for an increase in Gram-positive organisms, especially methicillin-resistant *Staphylococcus aureus* (MRSA) and vancomycin-resistant *Enterococcus* (VRE). Future research should be aimed at determining the cost-effectiveness of SDD, with inclusion of estimates of the effects of the emergence of resistant microorganisms. However, for the individual patient the evidence in favor of the use of prophylactic anti-microbials is compelling.[59]

Management of cerebral edema

The etiology of cerebral edema in acute liver failure is an area of active research. The link with increasing grade of encephalopathy, the relative absence of cerebral edema in encephalopathic patients with chronic liver disease and the increased incidence in those with hyperacute FHF, continue to be debated.

Although not completely understood two main pathological processes are thought to contribute to intracranial hypertension in acute liver failure. These are brain swelling due to water influx into astrocytes down an osmotic gradient and cerebrovascular vasodilation resulting in an increase in cerebral blood volume.[60] Under normal conditions, ammonia produced mainly in the gut, kidney and pancreas, is metabolized in the liver to both urea and glutamine. When the liver fails there is an increase in circulating ammonia. Both skeletal muscle and brain are alternative sites for metabolism and their activity is increased in liver failure.[61] Within the brain ammonia is detoxified to produce glutamine within astrocytes. The ammonium load associated with liver failure fuels this reaction and the glutamine produced increases the osmotic potential in the cells. Indeed inhibition of glutamine synthetase ameliorates brain edema and improves the survival in animal models of acute liver failure.[62] The rapid onset of acute liver failure reduces the time for cellular adaptation. This is in contrast to chronic liver disease where there is time for the astrocytes to adapt to the increase in circulating ammonia.[63] A partial breakdown of the blood–brain barrier has been demonstrated in experimental animals, although it has never been proved to occur in humans.[64] Osmotherapy plays a large part in the treatment of intracranial hypertension in FHF, and it appears that the blood–brain barrier is not damaged to a great extent, at least in the initial stages of brain swelling.

As well as the accumulation of water, changes in cerebral hemodynamics may lead to an increase in cerebral blood volume. Vascular autoregulation within the brain is defective in patients with acute liver failure, with uncoupling of blood flow and cerebral metabolic rate.[28,65] Cerebral hyperemia has been shown to contribute to an increase in ICP in animal models based on portocaval anastomosis and ammonia infusions[66] and an increase in cerebral blood flow has been shown in some human studies in acute liver failure[65] but not in others.[29,68] Indeed, studies have shown a wide variation in cerebral blood flow in patients with acute liver failure, but also an increase in cerebral lactate production has been shown suggesting the possibility that ischemia may induce cerebral swelling.[29] These conflicting results could be reconciled because of the observation that cerebral blood flow in acute liver failure is not uniform, with areas of decreased blood flow and areas of hyperemia.[69]

Intracranial pressure monitoring

The use of ICP monitors in FHF has not been subjected to a randomized controlled trial. As with any monitor used in critical illness, finding a positive outcome related to their use is difficult. At best, studies have suggested they may help with the management of patients with raised ICP. One study using historical controls suggested greater interventions associated with their use, and assuming the interventions were appropriate, this may be of benefit. The duration of survival from the onset of grade IV encephalopathy was significantly greater in the ICP monitored group (median 60 *v* 10 hours, $P < 0.01$), although overall survival was unchanged.[70] B4 Blei *et al.* carried out a postal survey of complications in 262 patients from liver transplant centers across the USA.[71] Epidural transducers were the most commonly used devices and had the lowest complication rate (3·8%); subdural bolts and parenchymal monitors (fiberoptic pressure transducers in direct contact with brain parenchyma and intraventricular catheters) were associated with complication rates of 20% and 22%, respectively. Fatal hemorrhage occurred in 1% of patients undergoing epidural ICP monitoring, whereas subdural and intraparenchymal devices had fatal hemorrhage rates of 5% and 4%, respectively. They concluded that epidural transducers were the safest form of monitoring even if not the most accurate.[71] B4

Their use may help in the decision as whether to list a patient for transplantation or not. A CCP (mean arterial pressure minus ICP) of less than 50 mmHg has in the past been considered a contraindication for OLT.[72] This was

Review: Antibiotics for preventing respiratory tract infection in adults receiving intensive care
Comparison: topical vs. control
Outcome: RTIs

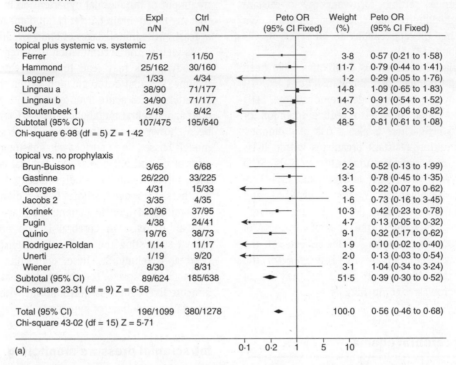

Study	Expl n/N	Ctrl n/N	Peto OR (95% CI Fixed)	Weight (%)	Peto OR (95% CI Fixed)
topical plus systemic vs. systemic					
Ferrer	7/51	11/50		3·8	0·57 (0·21 to 1·58)
Hammond	25/162	30/160		11·7	0·79 (0·44 to 1·41)
Laggner	1/33	4/34		1·2	0·29 (0·05 to 1·76)
Lingnau a	38/90	71/177		14·8	1·09 (0·65 to 1·83)
Lingnau b	34/90	71/177		14·7	0·91 (0·54 to 1·52)
Stoutenbeek 1	2/49	8/42		2·3	0·22 (0·06 to 0·82)
Subtotal (95% CI)	107/475	195/640		48·5	0·81 (0·61 to 1·08)
Chi-square 6·98 (df = 5) Z = 1·42					
topical vs. no prophylaxis					
Brun-Buisson	3/65	6/68		2·2	0·52 (0·13 to 1·99)
Gastinne	26/220	33/225		13·1	0·78 (0·45 to 1·35)
Georges	4/31	15/33		3·5	0·22 (0·07 to 0·62)
Jacobs 2	3/35	4/35		1·6	0·73 (0·16 to 3·45)
Korinek	20/96	37/95		10·3	0·42 (0·23 to 0·78)
Pugin	4/38	24/41		4·7	0·13 (0·05 to 0·32)
Quinio	19/76	38/73		9·1	0·32 (0·17 to 0·62)
Rodriguez-Roldan	1/14	11/17		1·9	0·10 (0·02 to 0·40)
Unerti	1/19	9/20		2·0	0·13 (0·03 to 0·54)
Wiener	8/30	8/31		3·1	1·04 (0·34 to 3·24)
Subtotal (95% CI)	89/624	185/638		51·5	0·39 (0·30 to 0·52)
Chi-square 23·31 (df = 9) Z = 6·58					
Total (95% CI)	196/1099	380/1278		100·0	0·56 (0·46 to 0·68)
Chi-square 43·02 (df = 15) Z = 5·71					

(a)

Review: Antibiotics for preventing respiratory tract infection in adults receiving intensive care
Comparison: topical vs. control
Outcome: overall mortality

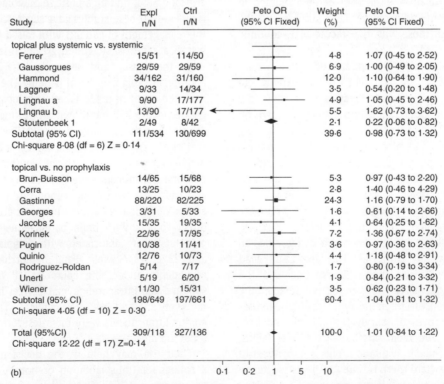

Study	Expl n/N	Ctrl n/N	Peto OR (95% CI Fixed)	Weight (%)	Peto OR (95% CI Fixed)
topical plus systemic vs. systemic					
Ferrer	15/51	114/50		4·8	1·07 (0·45 to 2·52)
Gaussorgues	29/59	29/59		6·9	1·00 (0·49 to 2·05)
Hammond	34/162	31/160		12·0	1·10 (0·64 to 1·90)
Laggner	9/33	14/34		3·5	0·54 (0·20 to 1·48)
Lingnau a	9/90	17/177		4·9	1·05 (0·45 to 2·46)
Lingnau b	13/90	17/177		5·5	1·62 (0·73 to 3·62)
Stoutenbeek 1	2/49	8/42		2·1	0·22 (0·06 to 0·82)
Subtotal (95% CI)	111/534	130/699		39·6	0·98 (0·73 to 1·32)
Chi-square 8·08 (df = 6) Z = 0·14					
topical vs. no prophylaxis					
Brun-Buisson	14/65	15/68		5·3	0·97 (0·43 to 2·20)
Cerra	13/25	10/23		2·8	1·40 (0·46 to 4·29)
Gastinne	88/220	82/225		24·3	1·16 (0·79 to 1·70)
Georges	3/31	5/33		1·6	0·61 (0·14 to 2·66)
Jacobs 2	15/35	19/35		4·1	0·64 (0·25 to 1·62)
Korinek	22/96	17/95		7·2	1·36 (0·67 to 2·74)
Pugin	10/38	11/41		3·6	0·97 (0·36 to 2·63)
Quinio	12/76	10/73		4·4	1·18 (0·48 to 2·91)
Rodriguez-Roldan	5/14	7/17		1·7	0·80 (0·19 to 3·34)
Unerti	5/19	6/20		1·9	0·84 (0·21 to 3·32)
Wiener	11/30	15/31		3·5	0·62 (0·23 to 1·71)
Subtotal (95% CI)	198/649	197/661		60·4	1·04 (0·81 to 1·32)
Chi-square 4·05 (df = 10) Z = 0·30					
Total (95%CI)	309/118	327/136		100·0	1·01 (0·84 to 1·22)
Chi-square 12·22 (df = 17) Z=0·14					

(b)

Figure 35.4 (a, b) Antibiotic prophylaxis in intensive care units (topical versus control). (Source: *Cochrane Library,* issue 2. Oxford: Update Software, 1999)

because of concern regarding cerebral ischemia resulting in poor neurological outcome. Recent reports of patients with CCPs of less than 50 mmHg in which full neurological recovery has taken place have called this practice into question. Davies *et al.*[30] reported four patients with FHF who developed prolonged intracranial hypertension (> 35 mmHg for 24–38 hours) that was refractory to standard therapy and associated with impaired CCP (< 50 mmHg for 2–72 hours). All survived with complete neurological recovery.

Radiological assessment

Computed tomography (CT) scanning, since its introduction into routine clinical practice, has become a standard investigation in any patient with suspected intracranial pathology. In FHF correlation between ICP measurements and pressures predicted by CT imaging have been generally poor.[73] As little information is gained in relation to the difficulty associated with transporting these very sick patients to the CT scanner, a decision regarding the need for a CT must be carefully considered. CT may be of help if there is any diagnostic difficulty as to the cause of the coma or if a complication of ICP bolt insertion is suspected.

Functional radiology – single photon emission tomography (SPECT) scanning – has been used to assess regional cerebral blood flow in patients with FHF but it is difficult to see this being used clinically.[69]

Monitoring of cerebral oxygenation

ICP and CCP monitoring are used to infer the adequacy of cerebral perfusion and oxygenation. The direct monitoring of cerebral oxygenation and blood flow are appealing. Instead of inferring the adequacy of cerebral perfusion and oxygenation from clinical signs and pressure measurements they provide direct evidence for the ongoing viability of the brain.

Methods used for the estimation of cerebral oxygenation include the sampling of jugular venous blood for oxygen saturation and products of metabolism such as lactate. A brain that is affected by limitation of supply will extract more oxygen from the arterial blood. This will result in a reduction in venous oxygen saturation. Jugular venous saturation of less than 55% suggests an ischemic brain and steps can be made to improve the blood flow to the brain, either by increasing blood flow, decreasing ICP or reducing the metabolic demands of the brain. High jugular venous saturation, > 85%, may represent a hyperemic brain and steps can be made to reduce cerebral blood volume if ICP is raised. Very high jugular venous saturation is often seen as a terminal event and may represent a complete loss of oxygen extraction by the brain.

Direct estimates of cerebral oxygenation can be achieved by the insertion of a probe into the brain parenchyma to either measure the partial pressure of oxygen or if a microdialysis is used, to measure extracellular metabolic products.[74] Non-invasive methods of measuring cerebral oxygenation and blood flow include near infrared spectroscopy, transcranial Doppler and SPECT scanning. All of these techniques are being evaluated in the investigation of cerebral pathophysiology in FHF.

Validation of non-invasive methods of monitoring cerebral function are ongoing but there is a lack of controlled trials showing improvement in outcome.

Treatment of intracranial hypertension

Osmotherapy initially with urea and then mannitol has been used for many years to treat cerebral edema associated with traumatic brain injury. Canalase *et al.*[75] showed that 1 g/kg of mannitol was an effective treatment for established intracranial hypertension in FHF and that dexamethasone was ineffective for prevention. Since then, the same workers have shown that 0·5 g/kg of mannitol is as effective.[76] Alc They suggest that boluses should be delivered rapidly to achieve maximum effect.

Hyperventilation decreases ICP by inducing cerebro-vascular vasoconstriction – this reduces cerebral blood volume. It has not been shown to be of any advantage in the long term in controlling ICP in FHF.[77] A short-term period of hyperventilation in patients with raised ICP unresponsive to osmotherapy may be tried while monitoring jugular venous saturation to assess cerebral oxygenation.

Barbiturates decrease cerebral metabolic rate via their anesthetic action and cause cerebral vasoconstriction. They have been used as agents to prevent secondary brain damage in traumatic brain injury. However, myocardial depression and hypotension with a possible compromise in CCP have limited the enthusiasm for routine use. There have not been any randomized controlled clinical trials evaluating barbiturate infusions in FHF. Forbes *et al.*[78] B4 investigated the role of thiopentone infusions in 13 patients with FHF in an uncontrolled study. The overall survival rate of five out of 13 was claimed to be better than expected, but it is difficult to come to any conclusions from these data.[78] Prolonged recovery and hypotension limit the use of thiopentone in FHF, although it may be tried when all else fails. A study in traumatic brain injury found barbiturate infusion to be of no additional benefit to acute hyperventilation.[79]

Hypothermia has been investigated extensively in patients with traumatic brain injury. Initial enthusiasm for the technique in small trials were tempered with the publication of a large multicenter trial that failed to show an improved outcome but also demonstrated an increase in complications including bleeding and infections.[80] Alc This is in contrast to ischemic injury following cardiac arrest where improved survival has been shown.[81,82] In FHF small case series have suggested a reduction in ICP and an improvement in systemic hemodynamics but as yet there are no controlled data to base a change in management.[83] B4

N-acetylcysteine (NAC) has been shown to reduce clinical signs of intracranial hypertension in patients with FHF following acetaminophen hepatotoxicity.[84] NAC-treated patients had a lower incidence of cerebral edema (10/25, 40%) than that observed in control patients (17/25, 68%; $P = 0.047$; 95% CI for difference in incidence 2 to 54).[84]

Anticonvulsant therapy

The incidence of clinical seizure activity in FHF has not been reported but it is likely that sedative and paralyzing agents mask it during mechanical ventilation. Ellis and colleagues recently reported the incidence of subclinical seizure activity and the effect of the anticonvulsant phenytoin in FHF.[85] With a cerebral function monitor they found an incidence of 32% in the control group. Alc The occurrence of seizure activity likely increases the risk of developing cerebral edema. The use of phenytoin reduced the incidence of subclinical seizure activity although not significantly. The incidence of cerebral edema, in the patients that received an autopsy was significantly higher in the control group.[85]

Renal failure

The incidence of acute renal failure associated with FHF is high; up to 70% of all patients develop renal failure (defined as urine output of less than 300 ml/24 hours and a serum creatinine of greater than 300 μmol/l in the presence of adequate intravascular filling).[8] The etiology of renal failure in FHF is multifactorial with both prerenal and renal components. Relative hypovolemia and hypotension contribute to prerenal causes. Disordered renal vascular autoregulation, present in sepsis, may also exist in the hyperdynamic circulatory failure of FHF, making renal blood flow directly dependent on blood pressure. Direct renal toxicity in patients with FHF secondary to acetaminophen poisoning contributes to the very high incidence of renal failure in this group of patients.[8] The contribution of the hepatorenal syndrome, or functional renal failure in the presence of FHF, is difficult to quantify and it probably represents one end of a continuum of disordered renal function from the hepatorenal syndrome to acute tubular necrosis.[86]

Renal protection

There is no proved preventive strategy against the development of renal failure, or treatment that will shorten the duration of established renal dysfunction in FHF.

Dopamine has agonist activity at all adrenergic receptors depending on concentration. Dopamine at a so-called "renal dose" (< 5 μg/kg per minute) augments renal blood flow and increases urine volume and sodium excretion in animals and healthy humans. In FHF and other forms of distributive circulatory failure an increase in renal blood flow has been difficult to show.[87] There is now good evidence that dopamine does not prevent renal failure in critically ill patients[88] Alc and it has been suggested that dopamine may exacerbate renal dysfunction by delivering a sodium load to an already ischemic renal medulla.[89] C5 The term "low dose" dopamine has been questioned because of the wide variation in plasma concentration in critically ill patients[90] and because of significant effects on other organ systems, specifically anterior pituitary and immune function.[91]

Other strategies including furosemide, aminophylline and fenoldopam infusions have not been shown to prevent renal failure in the critically ill. Atrial natriuretic peptide showed promise in animal models but early human trials have not been shown to be useful in the clinical setting.[92]

The magic bullet for preventing renal failure in FHF remains elusive and so therapy is directed at the maintenance of intravascular volume and an adequate perfusion pressure. Despite this the need for extracorporeal support is common.

Renal replacement therapy

While the incidence of renal failure in FHF remains high and attempts to prevent or treat it remain poor, renal replacement therapy has become a major part of the routine management. Proving that renal replacement therapy improves outcome is difficult as no randomized controlled trials have been done, but it can be assumed that it has contributed in part to the improvement in mortality figures over the past 30 years.

The type of renal replacement has been investigated in critically ill patients. Intermittent forms of therapy cause more hemodynamic compromise than continuous forms of therapy. This has been examined in FHF. Davenport *et al.*[93] investigated the effect of various modes of renal replacement therapy in 30 consecutive patients referred with both FHF and acute renal failure. Continuous forms of therapy were associated with more hemodynamic stability during the first hour of treatment and ICP remained stable during the continuous modes, but increased significantly during intermittent hemofiltration.[93] B4 The adequacy of renal replacement must be considered. Patients with FHF often have severe metabolic acidosis and rapidly progress to anuria. They are markedly catabolic and serum concentrations of creatinine rise rapidly. Urea is notably low in FHF. The rate of ultrafiltration in critically ill patients has been investigated recently. It has been shown that in general modest increases in ultrafiltration rates are associated with an improved outcome overall.[94] B4

Adrenal function

The hemodynamic changes associated with FHF have been mentioned previously. Cardiovascular collapse is characterized by systemic vasoparesis with vasopressor-resistant hypotension prominent in severe cases. In many ways these changes are similar to those seen in septic shock and other forms of systemic inflammatory response syndrome. Patients with inadequate adrenal function can develop similar cardiovascular changes. Inadequate adrenal function, as defined by response to the short synacthen test (SST), can worsen the severity of the cardiovascular collapse and response to vasopressors in septic shock.[95] Recently Harry and colleagues[96] investigated the serum cortisol levels and the response to SST in 45 patients with acute hepatic dysfunction. Abnormal tests were common, occurring in 62% of patients. Those who required norepinephrine for blood pressure support had a significantly lower increment (median 161 v 540 nmol/l; $P < 0.001$) following synacthen compared with patients who did not. Increment was significantly lower in those who fulfilled liver transplant criteria compared with those who did not. There was an inverse correlation between increment and severity of illness (Sequential Organ Failure Assessment, $r = 0.63$; $P < 0.01$).[96] In patients with septic shock who fail to mount a response to synacthen, the replacement of supra-physiological doses of steroids (50 mg hydrocortisone 6 hourly and 50 micrograms fludrocortisone once daily) is associated with a reduction in mortality and duration of vasopressor therapy.[95] Ala It remains to be seen if there will be any benefit from the replacement of steroids in patients with FHF.

Specific therapies

N-acetylcysteine in acetaminophen poisoning and other etiologies

Acetaminophen poisoning is the single largest cause of FHF in the UK, accounting for between 50% and 60% of cases seen.[97] NAC can prevent hepatic damage following acetaminophen poisoning. Smilkstein *et al.*[98] evaluated the time interval from poisoning to treatment with NAC in relation to the incidence of hepatic damage as defined by increased transaminase values. NAC was found to be most effective when given during the first 8 hours following ingestion.[98] More recent data suggest that NAC is effective when given up to 72 hours after ingestion with a decrease in the occurrence of grade III/IV encephalopathy, cerebral edema, hypotension requiring inotropic support, and mortality when compared with untreated controls.[84,99] B4

The mechanism of action of NAC in patients with established hepatic necrosis is unclear. Improvements in oxygen transport parameters have been shown with NAC use in patients with FHF due to acetaminophen poisoning and FHF due to other causes.[100] This, however, has been questioned.[101] Although NAC has not been shown to reduce mortality with FHF due to causes other than acetaminophen, a hemodynamic effect of this agent is seen when it is used in conjunction with epoprostenol. The beneficial effects may be attributable to a repletion of glutathione status and/or the antioxidant properties of NAC. NAC is also a sulfhydryl donor and this may be beneficial in patients in whom sulfhydryl groups may be oxidized, impairing microcirculatory function. Infusion of NAC has been shown to increase serum cGMP with no change in atrial natriuretic peptide, suggesting it may indeed have a role in the nitric oxide pathway in patients with acute liver failure.[102]

Blood purification: dialysis, plasmapheresis, hemofiltration, sorbant hemoperfusion and artificial hepatic support

To effectively support the acutely failing liver there needs to be a thorough understanding of the functional role of the liver in whole body homeostasis. The liver is a complex organ with many functions in addition to the metabolic functions of the hepatocyte which make up two-thirds of its mass. The remaining third is made up of other cell types including the Kupffer cells and endothelial cells. These other cells are important in many of its functions including the immunological activity of the liver.

There are two main components to the pathophysiology of FHF. The metabolic mass theory, which states that there is a decrease in the functioning mass of hepatocytes leading to end-organ dysfunction and the manifestations of FHF and ultimately death. The toxic liver hypothesis states that it is the toxins produced by the failing liver itself that are the cause of the syndrome of FHF. The truth probably lies somewhere in between and so any extracorporeal system has to both clear the serum of any toxins produced by the failing liver and to maintain the metabolic and, if possible, the other functions of the native liver. Established FHF will lead inexorably to multiple organ failure and ultimately death in the majority of patients managed with medical therapy alone, and so some kind of liver support, to maintain organ function, is very attractive while waiting for definitive surgical treatment or regeneration and recovery. There are two main types of blood purification system available: biological or non-biological.

Experience with extracorporeal systems designed to clear the blood through physiochemical means alone consist of dialysis, sorbant hemoperfusion, hemofiltration and plasmapheresis and combinations of the above. More recently, extracorporeal dialysis against 20% albumin has been employed with the commercially available MARS (molecular adsorbent recirculation system).[103]

Early work with hemodialysis showed improved coma scores in patients with chronic liver disease. With increasing pore size and improving biocompatibility with polyacrylonitrile (PAN) membranes the hope was to improve middle-molecule clearance. No improvement in mortality in FHF was shown.[104]

B4 Hemoperfusion involves the adsorption of lipophilic chemicals onto activated charcoal or synthetic resins. Again early studies suggested an improvement in coma scores,[105] but controlled studies failed to show an improved outcome with treatment.[8] A1c Plasmapheresis or the exchange of plasma by fresh frozen plasma (FFP) has theoretical advantages over other forms of blood cleansing regimens in that it removes both low molecular weight molecules and the higher molecular weight middle-molecules whether bound or unbound. The Copenhagen group have been studying high volume plasmapheresis with exchanges of 1 l/hour for 3 consecutive days.[106] Their studies suggest an improvement in hemodynamics and improved CPP but no reduction in ICP. They also noted a decrease in Glasgow coma score, INR and serum bilirubin.[106] Improvement in mortality has yet to be shown with the technique. B4

The MARS system is an extracorporeal circuit in which 20% human albumin solution is dialyzed against the patient's blood. The albumin within the circuit binds protein-bound molecules, including bilirubin and bile acids, from the patient.[103] MARS therapy has been proposed as a liver support device in the management of FHF. The evidence for effect is limited to case reports and small case series with heterogeneous patients but some success has been reported including the improvement of coma scores.[107]

Bioreactors containing hepatocytes have been the basis for biological extracorporeal support systems. These remain experimental and confined to clinical trials. Experience with the systems so far suggest few problems with biocompatibility but there are few data to suggest an improvement in clearance or synthesis by the artificial liver. The systems at the present time are divided into those using porcine hepatocytes or immortalized hepatoblastoma cell lines. The ELAD system comprises a continuous system using a hepatoblastoma cell line. A randomized study using this system, assessing biocompatibility, showed an improvement in galactose clearance at 6 hours, but no other measured variables were significantly different between the treatment and control groups.[108] The system of Demetriou uses plasma separation and passage of the plasma over charcoal and thence over pig hepatocytes on a daily basis for 6 hours. The system has not been subjected to a randomized controlled trial but has been reported to demonstrate improved level of consciousness and improvements in mean arterial pressure, ICP and CCP. A systematic review could find no evidence of benefit of artificial or bio-artificial devices in FHF.[109] A1c

Temporizing hepatectomy

The toxic liver theory of FHF has led to the introduction of temporizing hepatectomy in an attempt to regain haemodynamic control or a reduction in ICP in patients on the super-urgent transplant list. There have been several published case reports of successful liver transplantation following a prolonged anhepatic state. Ringe *et al.*[110] presented the results of 30 patients who underwent hepatectomy (and temporary portacaval shunting to provide an outflow of the transected portal vein) between 1986 and 1993. Improvement in hemodynamic parameters was seen in 17 of the 30 patients following hepatectomy, with liver transplantation occurring 6–41 hours later (the effect on ICP was not stated). It is impossible to draw conclusions from these anecdotal data. Temporizing hepatectomy has been criticized because of removing the option to perform an auxiliary transplant. Temporizing hepatectomy may have a role in severe liver trauma, with uncontrollable bleeding and primary graft non-function where there is no hope of recovery. C5

Liver transplantation

Prognostic factors in fulminant hepatic failure and orthotopic liver transplantation

Hepatic transplantation in FHF has not been and never will be subjected to a controlled clinical trial. However, patients with FHF due to causes other than acetaminophen poisoning who undergo transplantation have a 65% 2-month survival rate[13] compared with 20–25% for patients managed with maximal medical therapy alone.[111] The survival without transplantation after acetaminophen poisoning is higher than with FHF from other causes.

The task for the medical staff looking after patients with FHF is to decide which of these patients will not survive without liver transplantation. The decision needs to be made as early as possible because there is a "window" during which a successful outcome can be expected.[112] Following acetaminophen poisoning, time from ingestion to transplant was significantly longer in non-survivors following transplantation.[13]

In order to make an informed decision regarding the likelihood of spontaneous recovery from FHF an understanding of the natural history of the disease is necessary. Because FHF is a rare syndrome these data have only become available over the past 20 years, since the introduction of liver failure units around the world.

Poor prognostic markers developed from analysis of large databases from these liver units have been refined into clinically usable indications for transplantation. O'Grady *et al.* developed criteria from a database of 588 patients presenting to King's College Hospital liver unit (see Box 35.2).[97] The time course of the illness is important. It has been known for many years that the time to encephalopathy from the onset of symptoms is important prognostically, the "hyperacute" patients having a better prognosis than the "sub-acute".

Etiology and age are important in that different criteria were developed for FHF caused by acetaminophen poisoning. The extremes of age are associated with a poor prognosis. A high serum creatinine and bilirubin were associated with a poor prognosis, as was prolongation of coagulation parameters.[97] Following acetaminophen poisoning no particular prognostic cut-off level of INR has been found, but it has been noted that a rise of the INR from day 3 to day 4 is associated with a 7% survival as compared to a 79% survival in those whose INR fell from day 3 to 4.[99] Metabolic acidosis following fluid resuscitation was found to be highly specific for a poor outcome in acetaminophen poisoning. A serum pH persistently less than 7·3 has become an independent transplant criterion regardless of grade of encephalopathy.[97] The metabolic acidosis seen in FHF is often associated with a raised whole blood lactate concentration. This hyperlactatemia is caused by both an increased production but also by decreased clearance by the liver.[113,114] Prolonged high blood lactate concentration in critical illness other than FHF is associated with poor prognosis. The relationship between whole blood lactate and prognosis in FHF has been investigated recently. Bernal and colleagues[115] showed that a post-resuscitation lactate concentration of greater than 3·0 mmol/l can predict death with similar accuracy to the King's criteria but earlier in the course of the illness. The addition of post-resuscitation lactate concentration to the King's criteria increased sensitivity from 76% to 91% and lowered the negative likelihood ratio from 0·25 to 0·10.[115]

A French group carried out multivariate analysis of data from 115 patients with fulminant hepatitis B and found that a low factor V following the onset of grade III encephalopathy was the strongest predictor of a poor outcome (see Box 35.3).[116]

Both the King's and the Clichy criteria are in common use around the world. Following the publication of the King's College Hospital data the criteria were evaluated retrospectively in a French liver unit. Eighty-one non-transplant patients with non-acetaminophen-induced acute liver failure were studied. The mortality rate was 0·81. The predictive accuracies, respectively on admission and 48 hours before death, were 0·80 and 0·79 for the King's criteria and 0·60 and 0·73 for the Clichy criteria. The positive and negative predictive values, 48 hours before death, were 0·89 and 0·47 for the King's criteria and 0·89 and 0·36 for the Clichy criteria, respectively. The low negative predictive values (0·36 and 0·47) indicated that neither of these could identify a subgroup with a low risk of death.[117] The additions to the King's criteria have yet to be subjected to external validation but studies are ongoing.

While the above study compared prognostic criteria in non-acetaminophen-induced FHF, two studies compared general ICU scoring systems, the Acute Physiology and Chronic Health Evaluation (APACHE) scores, and the King's criteria for urgent liver transplantation.[13,118] Mitchell *et al.* prospectively evaluated the APACHE II system in patients with FHF due to

---

Box 35.2 King's College Hospital prognostic criteria for fulminant hepatic failure

In non-acetaminophen (paracetamol)-induced liver failure
- Prothombin time >100 seconds (international normalized ratio (INR) >6·5)

or

- pH < 7·3

or any three of the following:

- age < 10 years
- age > 40 years
- Seronegative hepatitis (non-A,B,C,E,F), halothane or other drug reaction
- Duration of jaundice >7 days before encephalopathy
- Prothrombin time >50 seconds (INR >3·5)
- Bilirubin >300 µmol/l

In acetaminophen (paracetamol)-induced fulminant hepatic failure
- pH < 7·3 (following fluid resuscitation)

or the coexistence of:

- prothrombin time >100 (INR >6·5), creatinine >300 µmol/l and grade III or worse encephalopathy

---

Box 35.3 The Clichy criteria for prognosis of viral fulminant hepatic failure

- Coma or confusion

and

- Factor V < 20% if under 30 years of age

or

- Factor V < 30% if over 30 years of age

---

acetaminophen poisoning. The aim of the study was to see whether the APACHE system is able to provide an accurate risk of hospital death in patients with acetaminophen-induced FHF or identify those patients needing transfer for possible hepatic transplantation and compared this with the King's College Hospital transplant criteria. A total of 102 patients were studied. An APACHE II score of > 15 had the ability to predict death which was similar to that of the King's criteria (sensitivity 82% and 65%, respectively; specificity 98% and 99%, respectively) when evaluating those patients who were transplanted as "deaths". An APACHE II score of > 15 was able to identify four more patients than the King's criteria on the first day of admission. The calculated risk of death according to the APACHE II score, using the original drug overdose coefficient, was poorly calibrated. This is probably due to the lower incidence of potentially life-threatening drug overdoses in the original calibration population. From these data the crude APACHE II score may be able to identify non-survivors at an earlier stage than the King's College Hospital criteria.[118]

Delays in listing patients for transplantation and in organ procurement result in further patient deterioration. This altered status results in the withdrawal of patients from the urgent list. Withdrawal of patients is based on clinical experience. However, several authors have analyzed the outcome from transplantation in FHF to help define contraindications to transplantation on the basis of poor outcome after transplantation. Devlin *et al.*[13] used APACHE III data to look at 100 patients transplanted for FHF. They found that in the acetaminophen group at the time of transplantation APACHE III scores and serum bilirubin were significantly higher in the non-survivors. In the non-acetaminophen group serum creatinine, organ system failure scores, and APACHE III scores were significantly higher in the non-survivors.[13] Bernal *et al.*[119] studied liver transplantation and the application of King's College Hospital transplant criteria in 548 patients presenting to the liver failure unit with severe acetaminophen poisoning. Of 424 patients who did not fulfill the criteria, 28 (7%) died. Of 124 who fulfilled the criteria, 68 (55%) were listed for transplantation and 44 underwent transplantation. Thirty-three of the transplanted patients left hospital. Of the 80 patients who satisfied the criteria but did not undergo transplantation, nine survived to leave hospital. The reasons why patients who satisfied criteria were not listed were multiple organ failure and cerebral edema.[119] These reasons also applied to the patients listed but withdrawn before a graft was available. In contrast to the report of Devlin *et al.*[13] the authors were unable to identify any preoperative factors predictive of death in the transplant group. This suggests that patients unlikely to survive with a transplant are recognized and subsequently removed from the list. However, graft factors (identified by early markers of graft function, INR and aspartate aminotransferase) were also significantly worse in the non-survivors.

Auxiliary orthotopic liver transplantation and regeneration

Auxiliary partial OLT holds potential advantages over conventional OLT in the setting of FHF. It has been known for many years that survivors from FHF often return to full health with normal or only slightly abnormal livers. The liver has great powers of regeneration and this has led to the introduction of partial liver transplantation in the hope of native liver regeneration and the eventual withdrawal of immunosuppression. A multicenter European observational study reported the results of 30 patients who underwent auxiliary transplantation for FHF.[120] After 3 months, 19 of the 30 patients survived; 13 had resumed normal native liver function with interruption of immunosuppression. B4 The indications are not well defined, but the survivors off immunosuppression were aged less than 40 years and had FHF secondary to viral hepatitis and acetaminophen poisoning.[120]

References

1 Trey C, Davidson LS. The management of fulminant hepatic failure. In: Popper H, Schaffner F, eds. *Progress in Liver Disease.* New York: Grune and Stratton, 1970.
2 O'Grady J, Schalm SW, Williams R. Acute liver failure: redefining the syndromes. *Lancet* 1993;**342**:273–5.
3 Gimson AES *et al.* Late-onset hepatic failure: clinical, serological and histological features. *Hepatology* 1986;**6**:288–94.
4 Hawton K *et al.* Effects of legislation restricting pack sizes of paracetamol and salicylate on self poisoning in the United Kingdom: before and after study. *BMJ* 2001;**322**:1–7.
5 Newsome PN *et al.* Referal patterns and social deprivation in paracetamol-induced liver injury in Scotland. *Lancet* 2001;**358**:1612–13.
6 Ostapowicz G *et al.* Results of a prospective study of acute liver failure at 17 tertiary care centers in the United States. *Ann Intern Med* 2002;**137**:947–56.
7 Trewby P, Williams R. Pathophysiology of hypotension in patients with fulminant hepatic failure. *Gut* 1977;**18**:1021–6.
8 O'Grady J, *et al.* Controlled trials of charcoal hemoperfusion and prognostic factors in fulminant hepatic failure. *Gastroenterology* 1988;**94**:1186–92.
9 Rolando N, *et al.* Prospective study of bacterial infections in acute liver failure: an analysis of fifty patients. *Hepatology* 1990;**11**:49–53.
10 Makin AJ, Wendon J, Williams R. A 7-year experience of severe acetominophen-induced hepatotoxicity (1987–1993). *Gastroenterology* 1995;**109**:1907–16.
11 Lucke B, Mallory T. Fulminant form of epidemic hepititis. *Am J Pathol* 1946;**22**:867–945.
12 McQuillan P, *et al.* Confidential enquiry into quality of care before admission to intensive care. *BMJ* 1998;**316**:1853–8.
13 Devlin J, *et al.* Pretransplantation clinical status and outcome of emergency transplantation for acute liver failure. *Hepatology* 1995;**21**:1018–24.
14 O'Grady J. Acute liver failure. *J R Coll Phys Lond* 1997;**31**:603–7.
15 Bihari DJ, Gimson ASE, Williams R. Disturbances in cardiovascular and pulmonary function in fulminant hepatic failure. In: Williams R ed. *Liver Failure.* Edinburgh: Churchill Livingstone, 1986.
16 Schierhout G, Roberts I. Fluid resuscitation with colloid or crystalloid solution in critically ill patients: a systematic review if randomised trials. *BMJ* 1998;**316**:961–4.
17 Choi P, *et al.* Crystalloid vs. colloid in fluid resuscitation. *Crit Care Med* 1999;**27**:200–10.
18 Bunn F, Alderson P, Hawkins V. Colloid solutions for fluid resuscitation (Cochrane Review). *Cochrane Database Syst Rev* 2003(1): CD001319.
19 Shippy BR, Appel PL, Shoemaker WC. Reliability of clinical monitoring to assess blood volume in critically ill patients. *Crit Care Med* 1984;**12**:107–12.
20 Conners AF *et al.* The effectiveness of right heart catheterisation in the intitial care of critically ill patients. *JAMA* 1996;**276**:889–97.

21 Powers SR *et al.* Physiologic consequences of positive end expiratory pressure (PEEP) ventilation. *Ann Surg* 1973; **178**:265–72.

22 Bihari DJ, Gimson AE, Williams R. Cardiovascular, pulmonary and renal complications of fulminant hepatic failure. *Semin Liver Dis* 1986;**6**:119–28.

23 Gasman JD, *et al.* Hazards with both determining and utilizing oxygen consumption measurements in the management of critically ill patients. *Crti Care Med* 1996; **24**:6–9.

24 Durham RM *et al.* The use of oxygen consumption and delivery as endpoints for resuscitation in critically ill patients. *J Trauma* 1996;**41**:32–40.

25 Medicine TEC .C.o.IC Tissue hypoxia: how to detect, how to correct, how to prevent? *Am J Resp Crit Care Med* 1996;**154**:1573–1578.

26 Wendon J, *et al.* Effects of systemic hemodynamics on oxygen transport variables in patients with fulminant hepatic failure. *Hepatology* 1992;**15**:1067–71.

27 James JH, *et al.* Lactate is an unreliable indicator of tissue hypoxia in injury or sepsis. *Lancet* 1999;**354**:505–8.

28 Larson FS, *et al.* Functional loss of cerebral blood flow autoregulation in patients with fulminant hepatic failure. *J Hepatol* 1995;**23**:212–17.

29 Wendon JA *et al.* Cerebral blood flow and metabolism in fulminant liver failure. *Hepatology* 1994;**19**:1407–13.

30 Davis MA, *et al.* Recovery despite impaired cerebral perfusion in fulminant hepatic failure. *Lancet* 1994;**343**:1329–30.

31 Baudouin SV *et al.* Acute lung injury in fulminant hepatic failure following paracetamol poisoning. *Thorax,* 1995;**50**: 399–402.

32 Dreyfuss DG. Saumon ventilator-induced lung injury. *Am J Respir Crti Care Med* 1998;**157**:294–323.

33 Amato MBP *et al.* Effects of a protective-ventilation stratergy on mortality in the acute respiratory distress syndrome. *N Engl J Med* 1998;**338**:347–54.

34 Network TARDS. Ventilation with lower tidal volumes as compared with traditional tidal volumes for acute lung injury and the acute respiratory distress syndrome. *N Engl J Med* 2000;**342**:1301–8.

35 Artigas A, *et al.* The American-European Consensus Conference on ARDS Part 2 Ventilatory pharmacologic supportive therapy study design strategies and issues related to recovery and remodeling. *Intensive Care Med* 1998; **28**:378–98.

36 Ramsay MAE *et al.* Controlled sedation with alphaxalone-alphadone. *BMJ* 1974;**2**:656–9.

37 Hsiang JK *et al.* Early, routine paralysis for intracranial pressure control in severe head injury: Is it necessary? *Crit Care Med* 1994;**22**:1471–6.

38 Road J. Reversible paralysis with status asthmaticus, steroids, and pancuronium: clinical electrophysiological correlates. *Muscle Nerve* 1997;**20**:1587–90.

39 Douglass JA, *et al.* Myopathy in severe asthma. *Am Rev Respir Dis* 1992;**146**:517–19.

40 Walsh TS, *et al.* Energy expenditure in acetaminophen-induced fulminant hepatic failure. *Crit Care Med* 2000;**28**: 649–54.

41 Chandra RK. Nutrition, infection and immunity: present knowledge and future directions. *Lancet* 1983;**1**:688–91.

42 Shukla VK *et al.* Correlation of immune and nutritional status with wound complications in patients undergoing abdominal surgery. *Ann Surg* 1985;**51**:442–5.

43 Baudouin S, Evans TW. Nutrition in the critically ill. In: Hall JB, Schmidt GA, Wood LDH eds. *Principles of critical care.* New York: McGraw Hill, 1998.

44 Heyland D, *et al.* Enteral nutrition in the critically ill patient: A prospective survey. *Crit Care Med* 1995;**23**: 1055–60.

45 Atkinson S, Sieffert E, Bihari D. A prospective, randomised, double-blind, controlled clinical trial of enteral immunonutrition in the critically ill. Guy's Hospital Intensive Care Group. *Crit Care Med* 1998;**26**:1164–72.

46 Kudsk KA *et al.* A randomised trial of isonitrogenous enteral diets after severe trauma. An immune-enhancing diet reduces septic complications. *Ann Surg* 1996;**224**:531–40.

47 Group TVATPNCS. Perioperative total parenteral nutrition in surgical patients. *N Engl J Med* 1991;**325**:525–32.

48 Griffiths RD, Jones C, Palmer TE. Six month outcome of critically ill patients given glutamine-supplemented parenteral nutrition. *Nutrition* 1997;**13**:295–302.

49 Novak F, *et al.* Glutamine supplementation in serious illness: a systematic reveiw of the evidence. *Crit Care Med* 2002;**30**:2022–9.

50 Macdougall BRD, Bailey RJ, Williams R. H_2-Receptor antagonists and antacids in the prevention of acute gastrointestinal haemorrhage in fulminant hepatic failure. *Lancet* 1977;**1**:617–19.

51 Tryba M. Prophylaxis of stress ulcer bleeding. *J Clin Gastroenterology* 1991;**13(Suppl 2)**:S44–55.

52 Cook DJ *et al.* Stress ulcer prophylaxis in critically ill patients. Resolving discordant meta-analysis. *JAMA* 1996; **275**:308–14.

53 Cook D, *et al.* A comparison of sucralfate and ranitidine for the prevention of upper gastrointestinal bleeding in patients requiring mechanical ventilation. Canadian Critical Trials Group. *N Engl J Med* 1998;**338**:791–7.

54 Rolando N, Philpott-Howard J, Williams R. Bacterial and fungal infection in acute liver failure. *Semin Liver Dis* 1996; **16**:389–402.

55 Rolando N, *et al.* Prospective controlled trial of selective parenteral and enteral antimicrobial regimen in fulminant hepatic failure. *Hepatology* 1993;**17**:196–201.

56 Rolando N, *et al.* Prospective study comparing the efficacy of prophylactic parenteral antimicrobials, with or without enteral decontamination, in patients with acute liver failure. *Liver Transpl Surg* 1996;**2**:8–13.

57 Liberati A, *et al.* Anti-biotic prophylaxis for respiratory tract infections in adult patients in intensive care units. Cochrane Database 1997.

58 Jonge E *et al.* Effects of selective decontamination of digestive tract on mortality and acquisition of resistant bacteria in intensive care – a randomised controlled trial. *Lancet* 2003;**362**:1011–16.

59 Vincent J-L. Selective digestive decontamination: for everyone, everywhere. *Lancet* 2003;**362**:1006–7.

60 Blei AT, F Larsen S. Pathophysiology of cerebral edema in fulminant hepatic failure. *J Hepatol* 1999;**31**:771–6.

61 Clemmesen JO, *et al.* Cerebral herniation in patients with acute liver failure is correlated with arterial ammonia concentrations. *Hepatology* 1999;**29**:648–53.

62 Blei AT, *et al.* Ammonia-induced brain edema and intracranial hypertension in rats after portacaval anastomosis. *Hepatology* 1994;**19**:1437–4.

63 Cordoba J, Gottstein J, Blei AT. Chronic hyponatremia exacerbates ammonia-induced brain edema in rats after portacaval anastomosis. *J Hepatol* 1998;**29**:589–94.

64 Gove CD, *et al.* Regional cerebral edema and chloride space in galactosamine-induced liver failure in rats. *Hepatology* 1997;**25**:295–301.

65 Strauss G, *et al.* Liver function, cerebral blood flow autoregulation, and hepatic encephalopathy in fulminant hepatic failure. *Hepatology* 1997;**25**:837–9.

66 Larson FS, Gottstein J, Blei AT. Cerebral hyperemia and nitric oxide synthase in rats with ammonia-induced brain edema. *J Hepatol* 2001;**34**:548–54.

67 Aggarwal S, *et al.* Cerebral hemodynamic and metabolic changes in fulminant hepatic failure: a retrospective study. *Hepatology* 1994;**19**:80–7.

68 Almdal T, Schroeder T, Ranek L. Cerebral blood flow and liver function in patients with encephalopathy due to acute and chronic liver disease. *Scand J Gastroenterol* 1989;**24**:299–303.

69 Strauss GI, *et al.* Regional cerebral blood flow during mechanical hyperventilation in patients with fulminant hepatic failure. *Hepatology* 1999;**30**:1368–73.

70 Keays RT, Alexander GL, Williams R. The safety and value of extradural intracranial pressure monitors in fulminant hepatic failure. *J Hepatol* 1993;**18**:205–9.

71 Blei AT, *et al.* Complications of intracranial pressure monitoring in fulminant hepatic failure. *Lancet* 1993;**341**: 157–8.

72 Donovan JP *et al.* Brain water and acute liver failure: the emerging role of intracranial pressure monitoring. *Hepatology* 1992;**16**:267–8.

73 Munoz SJ *et al.* Elevated intracranial pressure and computed tomography of the brain in fulminant hepatocellular failure. *Hepatology* 1991;**13**:209–12.

74 Tofteng F, *et al.* Cerebral microdialysis in patients with fulminant hepatic failure. *Hepatology* 2002;**36**:1333–40.

75 Canalase J, *et al.* Controlled trial of dexamethasone and mannitol for the cerebral oedema of fulminant

76 Ede RJ, Williams R. Hepatic encephalopathy and cerebral oedema. *Semin Liver Dis* 1986;**6**:107–18.

77 Ede RJ *et al.* Controlled hyperventilation in the prevention of cerebral oedema in fulminant hepatic failure. *J Hepatol* 1986;**2**:43–51.

78 Forbes AG, Alexander JM, O'Grady JG. Thiopental infusion in the treatment of intracranial hypertension complicating fulminant hepatic failure. *Hepatology* 1989;**10**:549–55.

79 Louis PT *et al.* Barbiturates and hyperventilation during intracranial hypertension. *Crit Care Med* 1993;**21**:1200–6.

80 Clifton GL *et al.* Lack of effect of induction of hypothermia after acute brain injury. *N Engl J Med* 2001;**344**:556–63.

81 Bernard SA, *et al.* Treatment of comatose survivors of out-of-hospital cardiac arrest with induced hypothermia. *N Engl J Med* 2002;**346**:557–63.

82 Group TH .a.CAS Mild therapeutic hypothermia to improve the neurological outcome after cardiac arrest. *N Engl J Med* 2002;**346**:549–6.

83 Jalan R, *et al.* Moderate hypothermia for uncontrolled intracranial hypertension in acute liver failure. *Lancet* 1999;**354**:2082.

84 Keays R, *et al.* Intravenous acetylcysteine in paracetamol induced fulminant hepatic failure: a prospective controlled trial. *BMJ* 1991;**303**:1026–9.

85 Ellis AJ, Wendon JA, Williams R. Subclinical seizure activity and prophylactic phenytoin infusion in acute liver failure: a controlled clinical trial. *Hepatology* 2000;**32**: 536–41.

86 Arroyo V, *et al.* Definition and diagnostic criteria of refractory ascites and hepatorenal syndrome in cirrhosis. International Ascites Club. *J Hepatol* 1996;**23**:164–76.

87 Bersten AD, Holt AW. Vasoactive drugs and the importance of renal perfusion pressure. *New Horizons* 1995;**3**:650–61.

88 Bellomo R, *et al.* Low-dose dopamine in patients with early renal dysfunction: a placebo-controlled randomised trial. Australian and New Zealand Intensive Care Society (ANZICS). *Lancet* 2000;**356**:2139–43.

89 Weisberg LS, Kurnik PB, Kurnik BRC. Risk of radiocontrast nephropathy in patients with and without diabetes mellitus. *Kidney Int* 1994;**45**:259–65.

90 Juste RN *et al.* Dopamine clearance in critically ill patients. *Intensive Care Med* 1998;**24**:1217–20.

91 Van den Berghe G, de Zegher F. Anterior pituitary function during critical illness and dopamine treatment. *Crit Care Med* 1996;**24**:1580–90.

92 Brenner RM, Chertow GM. The rise and fall of atrial natriuretic peptide for acute renal failure. *Curr Opin Nephrol Hypertens,* 1997;**6**:474–6.

93 Davenport AE, Will J, Davison AM. Effect of renal replacement therapy on patients with combined acute renal and fulminant hepatic failure. *Kidney Int Suppl* 1993;**41**: S245–S251.

94 Ronco C, *et al.* Effects of different doses in continuous veno-venous haemofiltration on outcomes of acute renal failure: a prospective randomised trial. *Lancet* 2000;**356**:26–30.

95 Annane D, *et al.* Effect of treatment with low doses of hydrocortisone and fludrocortisone on mortality in patients with septic shock. *JAMA* 2002;**288**:862–71.

96 Harry R, Auzinger G, Wendon J. The clinical importance of adrenal insufficiency in acute hepatic dysfunction. *Hepatology* 2002;**36**:395–402.

97 O'Grady JG *et al.* Early indicators of prognosis in fulminant hepatic failure. *Gastroenterology* 1989;**97**:439–45.

98 Smilkstein MJ *et al.* Efficacy of oral *N*-acetylcysteine in the treatment of acetaminophen overdose: analysis of the national multicenter study (1976–1985). *N Engl J Med* 1988;**319**:1557–62.

99 Harrison P, *et al.* Serial prothrombin times: a prognostic indicator in acetaminophen-induced fulminant hepatic failure. *BMJ* 1990;**301**:964–6.

100 Harrison PM *et al.* Improvement by acetylcysteine of hemodynamics and oxygen transport in fulminant hepatic failure. *N Engl J Med* 1991;**324**:1852–7.

101 Walsh TS, Philips HPBJ, Mackenzie SJ, Lee A. The effect of *N*-acetylcysteine on oxygen transport and uptake in patients with fulminant hepatic failure. *Hepatology* 1998; **27**:1332–40.

102 Harrison P, Wendon J, Williams R. Evidence of increased guanylate cyclase activation by acetylcysteine in fulminant hepatic failure. *Hepatology* 1996;**23**:1067–72.

103 Stange J, *et al.* The molecular adsorbents recycling system as a liver support system based on albumin dialysis: a summary of preclinical investigations prospective randomized controlled clinical trial, and clinical experience from 19 centers. *Artificial Organs* 2002;**26**:103–10.

104 Losgen H, *et al.* Correction of increased plasma amino acid levels by dialysis with amino-acid-electrolyte-glucose solutions. In: Brunner G, Schmidt FW, eds. *Artificial Liver Support* New York: Springer-Verlag, 1981.

105 Gimson AE *et al.* Earlier charcoal haemoperfusion in fulminant hepatic failure. *Lancet* 1982;**2**:681–3.

106 Tygstrup N, Larson FS, Hansen BA. Treatment of acute liver failure by high volume plasmapheresis. In: Lee WM, Williams R, eds. *Acute Liver Failure.* Cambridge: Cambridge University Press, 1997.

107 Novelli G, *et al.* MARS (Molecular Adsorbent recirculating System): experience in 34 cases of acute liver failure. *Liver* 2002;**22(Suppl. 2)**:43–7.

108 Ellis AJ *et al.* Pilot-controlled trial of the extracorporeal liver assist device in acute liver failure. *Hepatology* 1996;**24**:1446–51.

109 Kjaergard I.I., *et al.* Artificial and bioartificial support systems for acute and acute on chronic liver failure. *JAMA* 2003;**289**:217–22.

110 Ringe B, *et al.* Management of emergencies before and after liver transplantation by early total hepatectomy. *Transpl Proc* 1993;**235**:1090.

111 Benhamou JP. Fulminant and sub-fulminant hepatic failure: definitions and causes. In: Williams R, Hughes RD, eds. *Acute liver failure: improved understanding and better therapy.* London: Mitre Press, 1991.

112 O'Grady JG *et al.* Liver transplantation after paracetamol overdose [See comments]. *BMJ* 1991;**303**:221–3.

113 Walsh TS *et al.* Hyperlactatemia and pulmonary lactate production in patients with fulminant hepatic failure. *Chest* 1999;**116**:471–6.

114 Murphy ND *et al.* Liver and intestinal lactate metabolism in patients with acute hepatic failure undergoing liver transplantation. *Crit Care Med* 2001;**29**:2111–18.

115 Bernal W, *et al.* Blood lactate as an early predictor of outcome in paracetamol-induced acute liver failure: a cohort study. *Lancet* 2002;**359**:558–63.

116 Bernuau J, *et al.* Multivariate analysis of prognostic factors in fulminant hepatitis B. *Hepatology* 1986;**6**:648–51.

117 Pauwels A, *et al.* Emergency liver transplantation for acute liver failure. Evaluation of London and Clichy criteria. *J Hepatol* 1993;**17**:124–7.

118 Mitchell I, *et al.* Earlier identification of patients at risk from acetaminophen-induced acute liver failure. *Crit Care Med* 1998;**26**:279–84.

119 Bernal W, *et al.* Use and outcome of liver transplantation in acetaminophen-induced acute liver failure. *Hepatology* 1998;**27**:1050–5.

120 Chenard-Neu MP *et al.* Auxillary liver transplantation: regeneration of the native liver and outcome in 30 patients with fulminant hepatic failure – a multicenter European study. *Hepatology* 1996;**23**:1119–27.

36 Liver transplantation: prevention and treatment of rejection

Laura Cecilioni, Lucy Dagher, Andrew Burroughs

Introduction

Liver transplantation has been one of the most rapidly evolving clinical specialties in medicine over the past three decades. It may seem logical to consider liver transplant recipients as a homogeneous group of patients who should be managed using universally applicable protocols, but they are a heterogeneous group of individuals, with different predisposing factors and co-factors for the development of rejection.[1] However, appropriate therapeutic approaches should be generated on the basis of evidence. In this chapter we attempt to elucidate the following:

- Do the severity, timing and number of episodes of acute cellular rejection affect prognosis?
- Is it possible to predict which patients will develop clinically significant acute rejection?
- Can immunosuppression be tailored to the individual patient?
- What is the evidence from randomized controlled trials that supports the choice of an immunosuppressive agent?
- Is it possible to withdraw immunosuppression or to change to less toxic immunosuppression?
- What is the influence of immunosuppression on HCV (hepatitis C virus) recurrence after transplantation?

During the past two decades orthotopic liver transplantation has become the standard therapy for acute and chronic liver failure of all etiologies. Nowadays most patients and liver grafts survive beyond the perioperative period, achieving 1-year and 10-year survival rates of 62% and 70–90%, respectively.[2] In addition to longer survival, many liver transplant recipients are now experiencing improved quality of life, including resumption of active employment and reproductive capacity.[3–6] Despite these advances, liver transplantation faces several major challenges. Long-term outcome of patients is becoming the main concern for clinicians who have to deal with the side effects of immunosuppressant drugs in the long term. These include opportunistic infections that affect up to 50% of recipients, contributing to mortality in approximately 10%, and an increased incidence of *de novo* malignancy as a consequence of immunosuppression. In addition, complications arise from direct drug toxicity such as nodular regenerative hyperplasia in the liver, which is a rare complication in patients receiving azathioprine[7] and hypertension, renal dysfunction, induction of diabetes and dyslipidemias.[8–11] The most dramatic example is the development of nephrotoxicity due to cyclosporin. In a series reported from Birmingham 4% of patients surviving 1 year or more developed severe chronic renal failure, with a mortality of 44% in this group.[12] Moreover, the nephrotoxic effects, hypertension and hyperlipidemia of some immunosuppressive agents have been implicated in the pathogenesis of chronic allograft loss.[13] These problems have stimulated the re-evaluation of the ability of some patients to tolerate their liver graft without the need for long-term immunosuppression, or with greatly reduced immunosuppression with the benefits derived from the return of natural immunity and reduction in drug-related toxicity.[14–16]

However, at present the "manipulation" of the immune system to induce tolerance and thus significantly reduce or eliminate immunosuppression is yet not clinically viable.[17] Therefore, the vast majority of liver transplant recipients need to take lifelong immunosuppressive therapy and this situation will not change until more reliable methods for predicting tolerance in individual patients are developed.

Definition of rejection

Viewed from a biological perspective, the recipient's immune system is activated after transplantation[18] but, because of the baseline immunosuppressive therapy, only some recipients will have clinical manifestations of this. An important distinction has to be made between histological changes of cellular rejection, which are seen in the absence of any significant clinical or biochemical abnormalities (biological rejection), and those accompanied by clinical signs of graft dysfunction (clinical rejection). However, abnormalities of liver function tests are almost universally present, and symptoms absent, so in the vast majority of the cases, the distinction between clinical and biological rejection, as defined above, can rarely be made in clinical practice.

Acute cellular rejection

Cellular rejection was defined in 1995, by an international panel of experts, as "inflammation of the allograft elicited by genetic disparity between the donor and recipient, primarily affecting interlobular bile ducts and vascular endothelia, including portal veins and hepatic venules and occasionally the hepatic artery and its branches".[18]

Clinical and laboratory findings

Most cases occur in the early postoperative period within 30 days. Late cases are usually associated with non-compliance of immunosuppressive therapy. A major problem is that the incidence varies according to whether rejection is defined on the basis of *clinically significant* rejection or simply on the basis of *histological abnormalities* or a *combination* of the two.

Clinically significant rejection occurs in approximately 50% of patients, whereas histological abnormalities can be seen in up to 80% of protocol biopsies performed at the end of the first week following transplantation.[19]

Several reports have clearly indicated that standard liver tests, when elevated, have a low sensitivity and specificity for rejection and show only a weak correlation with the severity of histopathological findings.[20,21] Various markers have been studied in an attempt to seek a specific indicator of graft rejection.[22] Although markers of immune activation, such as peripheral eosinophilia, serum intercellular adhesion molecule (ICAM)-1 and interleukin (IL)-2 receptor are elevated, there is considerable overlap with other conditions (including sepsis and reperfusion injury) and none of these markers has been adopted into routine clinical practice.

Graft eosinophilia has been identified as an independently associated feature of acute cellular rejection in liver transplantation.[23] The absence of peripheral eosinophilia predicted the absence of moderate/severe histological rejection in one study.[24] However, as yet this has not been validated in other centers. Eosinophilia cannot be used to predict or to assess the response to corticosteroids for the treatment of acute rejection.[24] Therefore, liver histology remains the gold standard for the diagnosis of acute rejection.[25–27]

Histopathological features

The three main histopathological features are:

- a predominantly mononuclear but mixed portal inflammation, containing blast-like or activated lymphocytes, neutrophils and eosinophils (graded 1 to 3)

Table 36.1 Banff schema for grading of acute liver allograft rejection[31]

Overall grade[a]	Criterion
Indeterminate	Portal inflammatory infiltrate that fails to meet the criteria for the diagnosis of acute rejection
Mild	Rejection infiltrate in a minority of the triads that is generally mild and confined within the portal spaces
Moderate	Rejection infiltrate that expands most or all of the triads
Severe	As for "moderate" but with spillover into periportal areas and moderate to severe perivenular inflammation that extends into the hepatic parenchyma and is associated with perivenular hepatocyte necrosis

[a]Verbal descriptions of mild, moderate and severe acute rejection could also be labeled as grades 1, 2 and 3 respectively.

- subendothelial inflammation of portal or terminal hepatic veins (or both) (graded 1 to 3)
- bile duct inflammation and damage (graded 1 to 3).

In general, at least two of the above histopathological findings and biochemical evidence of liver damage constitutes the minimal diagnostic criterion for hepatic rejection. The diagnosis is strengthened if > 50% of the ducts are damaged or if unequivocal endothelitis of the portal vein branches or terminal hepatic venules can be identified.

Grading and staging

In 1997, a worldwide consensus on a common grading system for acute allograft rejection was achieved and subsequently it has been prospectively tested and proved to be simple, reliable, and clinically relevant.[28–30]

According to this Banff schema, which represents a merger and simplification of many previously published studies (Table 36.1), there are two main components: the first is a global assessment of the overall rejection grade (indeterminate, mild, moderate, severe), the second involves scoring the three specific features of rejection semiquantitatively to produce an overall Rejection Activity Index (RAI).[31]

Datta-Gupta *et al.* from our center[23] showed that graft eosinophilia was an independent diagnostic marker of acute cellular rejection and it was included in the scoring system developed at the Royal Free Hospital.

Role of liver biopsy and indication for treatment

The use of liver biopsy in the early post-transplant setting depends on each center's policy. Nowadays there is less uniformity regarding the use of protocol liver biopsies. This is mainly for two reasons: risks associated with the procedure[32] and doubts about the usefulness of these biopsies to guide therapy, particularly amongst patients with normalizing transaminase values and other biochemical values. However, to date, no large series has described a substantial risk associated with percutaneous liver biopsies in transplant recipients,[32–34] and greater use of transjugular liver biopsies will lessen the small complication rate of percutaneous biopsies.[35]

Whereas most transplant centers agree that liver histology is the gold standard and is essential for the diagnosis of acute cellular rejection, controversy continues to arise over the indications for treatment of rejection. The implication of this is that if treatment is not going to be given, why do a liver biopsy? Specifically there is the question of the patient who has histological features of acute cellular rejection on protocol liver biopsy, with static or improving graft dysfunction. Some studies suggest that there is spontaneous resolution of mild rejection without biochemical dysfunction.[36,37] However abnormal liver function is usually the norm, and normal liver function tests are rare at 5–7 days post-transplantation when protocol biopsies are usually done.

Recently, Bartlett *et al.* presented a review of the literature of the natural history of acute cellular rejection.[38] They included 1566 patients, all of whom had protocol biopsies: 331 (21%) patients had evidence of acute histologic rejection with "normal or normalizing liver function tests". The majority (91%) of these patients did not receive adjuvant immunosuppression, and only 4% developed chronic rejection. B Given these results, the authors concluded that withholding adjuvant immunosuppression from patients with histologic acute cellular rejection with "normal or normalizing liver function tests" is safe, thus not supporting the practice of protocol liver biopsies. However, the study has some limitations: the retrospective nature of the analysis of a heterogeneous group of studies, the lack of definition of "normal or normalizing liver function tests" and the lack of evaluation of histological severity of acute cellular rejection in patients without "biochemical graft dysfunction". Before abandoning protocol biopsies, a hard look needs to be given to the evidence supporting this approach, and well designed prospective studies are necessary.[39]

A further issue is that even severe histological rejection, and not only mild rejection, may resolve spontaneously[40] and only on occasion this leads to graft loss.[1] There is now evidence that the development of early rejection which responds to treatment has no negative long-term effects and may even be associated with lower risk for later immunological complications.[41]

Prognostic factors

Do the severity, timing and number of episodes of acute cellular rejection affect prognosis?

Number of episodes

In an abstract, Wiesner *et al.* evaluating a liver transplant database with 870 patients followed for a median of 3 years, showed that the number of episodes of acute rejection and the histological severity were significantly associated with chronic rejection ($P < 0.001$).[42] Dousset *et al.*,[43] in a prospective study with 170 liver transplant patients, showed that there was no difference in graft function between patients with a single episode of acute rejection ($n = 56$) and those without rejection ($n = 84$). Among patients treated for a single episode of acute rejection, late hepatic function was not influenced by the severity of acute rejection, and the response to corticosteroids. In contrast, patients with more than one acute rejection episode ($n = 30$) had significant impairment of liver function tests (aspartate aminotransferase (AST) $P < 0.05$; alanine aminotransferase, $P < 0.001$; alkaline phosphatase, $P < 0.01$), lower dye clearances ($P < 0.01$), and more severe histological damage ($P < 0.001$). The authors concluded that a single episode of acute rejection does not impair long-term hepatic function, whereas recurrent episodes can lead to damage to the liver allograft.

Severity

McVicar *et al.* describe a group of patients who had focal rejection in the hepatic allograft biopsy defined as lymphocytic infiltration involving less than 20% of portal tracts.[44] In the follow up of patients showing focal or mild rejection, only six (15%) patients subsequently developed abnormal liver function tests and required treatment with additional immunosuppression for acute cellular rejection.[41] The authors concluded that patients showing focal or mild rejection do not necessarily need additional immunosuppression and can be followed closely without immediate treatment.

In Birmingham, during follow up of 151 patients to assess the effect of not treating mild acute rejection (protocol 7-day biopsies), 97 had histologically mild rejection: 50 had biochemical dysfunction and received prednisone for 3 days, while the remaining 47 cases with stable biochemistry had no additional treatment. Fifty-four patients with no rejection were included for comparison. The outcome at 3 months in all three groups was similar.[19] B4

Wiesner *et al.* using the Liver Transplantation Database in a cohort study of 762 consecutive adult liver transplant recipients, examined the association of histological severity of acute rejection and overall patient outcome.[30] They showed, using univariate analysis, that acute rejection overall, including mostly the milder grades, was significantly associated with an increased patient survival (relative risk (RR) 0·71, $P = 0·05$) and a trend toward improved graft survival. Moreover, adjusting for other risk factors such as age and renal insufficiency revealed no significant decrease in survival among patients who had rejection. These findings were similar to those of Fisher *et al.* who analyzed nine studies (comprising a total of 1473 patients), and found that there was no correlation between mortality and incidence of treated acute cellular rejection.[45]

These findings in liver transplantation are in contrast to renal transplantation in which acute rejection is significantly associated with decreased patient and graft survival. Why acute cellular rejection in liver transplant recipients is not associated with decreased patient and graft survival remains unexplained. It is possible that acute rejection in the setting of controlled alloreactivity exerts a tolerizing effect, making the graft less susceptible to further immunological attack. However, it should be noted that successful treatment for cellular rejection occurs in nearly all cases. Thus the correct interpretation of the finding reported above is that the occurrence and successful treatment of acute cellular rejection does not influence survival in liver transplant patients, but it does imply that abolishing early cellular rejection need not, and indeed, should not be a goal of initial immunosuppression.

Timing

As regards timing of acute cellular rejection, there is no firm consensus to define what is early or late rejection. In three different studies the timing and the outcome vary according to the definition of each center.

In a retrospective multicenter analysis[42] of 623 liver transplants, the cumulative incidence of biopsy proved rejection was 59% for early episodes (< 6 months) and 21% for late episodes (≥ 6 months). Patient and graft survival did not differ significantly between those who experienced an early acute rejection episode and those who did not ($P = 0·49$ and $P = 0·13$, respectively). Furthermore, these parameters did not differ significantly between recipients who experienced a late acute rejection episode and those who did not (patient survival $P = 0·18$ and graft survival $P = 0·20$).

Wiesner *et al.* analyzed 762 consecutive adult liver transplant recipients (Liver Transplantation Database) and found 367 (48%) who developed at least one acute cellular rejection episode within the first 6 weeks post-transplantation (occurring at a median time of 8 days).[30] Multivariate analysis indicated that acute cellular rejection was not significantly associated with survival although there was a trend to better survival (RR 0·78, $P = 0·25$) and re-transplantation free survival (RR 0·86, $P = 0·44$). However, severe rejection doubled the risk of death or re-transplantation compared to mild rejection. Using proportional hazards modeling, in the same study, seven factors were identified that were independently associated with an increased incidence of early acute hepatic allograft rejection: younger recipient age, lack of renal impairment, lack of edema, higher AST levels, fewer human leukocyte antigen (HLA) DR matches, longer cold ischemic times and older donors.

Mor *et al.* retrospectively reviewed 375 liver transplants, and defined late onset acute cellular rejection as that which occurred after 6 months.[46] There were 315 episodes of early acute cellular rejection in 226 patients and 31 episodes of late acute cellular rejection in 26 patients. Low cyclosporin levels appeared to account for 58% of these late episodes. Most episodes of rejection responded to pulse corticosteroids, and chronic ductopenic rejection arose in only two patients. There was no difference in survival between patients experiencing early and late rejection.

Anand *et al.* reviewed late onset acute cellular rejection, defining it as rejection recognized after the first 30 days post-transplantation.[47] They evaluated 717 patients who had undergone transplantation in Birmingham between 1982 and 1994: 59 (8%) patients had 71 episodes of late rejection. They too found that the most common precipitating event was low levels of calcineurin antagonists, and that most acute episodes of rejection in this timeframe were responsive to standard therapy. However, in contrast to Mor *et al.*[46] Anand found that 16 (27%) of 59 patients developing late onset rejection progressed to chronic ductopenic rejection and graft loss. Delayed response to an earlier episode of acute rejection, and centrilobular necrosis or bile duct loss at the time of diagnosis of late rejection, were associated with high risk of progression to chronic rejection and graft loss.

These results regarding timing, severity and number of episodes of early acute cellular rejection lead one to question whether an attempt to further reduce the incidence of early acute rejection in liver transplantation is either necessary or appropriate. This is especially questionable because increased immunosuppression theoretically could inhibit the development of donor-specific tolerance, increase the incidence of immunosuppressive-related complications, and result in poorer outcome. Indeed, it may be better not to treat certain mild acute or other rejection episodes. However, randomized controlled trials are needed to provide evidence supporting the latter approach.

Prediction of acute rejection

Is it possible to predict which patients will develop clinically significant acute rejection?

Data from Birmingham[1,48] suggest that there is a lower incidence of acute rejection when there is no evidence of immune involvement in the pathogenesis of the original liver disease, for example fulminant hepatic failure from paracetamol. In contrast, in patients transplanted for primary biliary cirrhosis and sclerosing cholangitis, in which immune-mediated damage of bile ducts is a feature of the original disease, acute rejection occurs more frequently and there is more frequent progression to ductopenic rejection. Wiesner *et al.* in a study of 870 consecutive primary liver transplant recipients found that autoimmune liver disease was an independent risk factor for developing chronic rejection.[49] A similar conclusion was obtained in a second small series of 63 patients reported by Hayashi *et al.*[50]; patients with autoimmune hepatitis had a higher incidence of acute rejection than patients with alcoholic cirrhosis (81% *v* 46·8%, *P* < 0·001) regardless of the type of immunosuppression. In addition, steroid-resistant rejection occurred slightly more frequently in patients transplanted for autoimmune liver disease (13·1% *v* 12·8%; *P* = 0·003). There was also a trend toward a higher incidence of chronic rejection. However, there was no difference in allograft or patient survival at 1 and 3 years. Berlakovich *et al.* reported data from a group of 252 liver transplant patients that showed that patients who had undergone transplantation for alcoholic cirrhosis (*n* = 60), hepatoma (*n* = 91) and post-hepatitic cirrhosis (*n* = 59) had a lower risk for acute rejection and the need to receive rescue therapy than patients who had received transplants for cholestatic disease (*n* = 42).[51] The cumulative rates of acute rejection episodes per patient per month at 6 months, when 94% of all acute rejection episodes occurred, were: 0·45 for alcoholic cirrhosis, 0·55 for post-hepatitic cirrhosis, 0·65 for hepatoma and 1·0 for cholestatic disease.

The group which has been consistently shown to have a lower incidence of acute and chronic rejection is chronic hepatitis B. It has been proposed that the reduced incidence of rejection in these patients might reflect the underlying defect in cell-mediated immunity, which allowed the patients to become chronically infected with the virus in the first place.[52,53]

Farges *et al.*[52] in a retrospective analysis of the data obtained from 330 patients who were transplant recipients for chronic liver disease, found that the incidence of acute rejection (48% at 1 year) and chronic rejection (10% at 3 years) was comparable in patients who had undergone transplantation for primary biliary cirrhosis, sclerosing cholangitis, autoimmune cirrhosis and hepatitis C cirrhosis. However, the incidence of acute (but not chronic) rejection was significantly lower in patients who had undergone transplantation or alcoholic cirrhosis (29% at 1 year). In patients who had undergone transplantation for hepatitis B virus (HBV) cirrhosis, the incidence of both acute (21% at 1 year) and chronic (0% at 3 years) rejection was significantly lower. They suggest that patients who undergo transplantation for alcoholic liver cirrhosis, because they are at high risk of sepsis and low risk of acute rejection, would probably benefit from a reduction in the level of immunosuppression. Because HBV replication is potentiated by immunosuppression, it could also prove beneficial to reduce the level of immunosuppression in these patients. However, Wiesner *et al.*, using multivariate analysis, showed that the 6-week incidence of acute rejection in a cohort of 762 consecutive adult liver transplant recipients was not dependent on the underlying disease.[30]

Although it is difficult to draw firm recommendations from these studies, it should be possible to test the hypothesis that patients undergoing transplantation for HBV, HCV cirrhosis, alcoholic liver disease or hepatoma can be treated safely with early steroid withdrawal, or less intense immunosuppression, such as monotherapy, from the outset. Conversely, patients with autoimmune hepatitis, primary biliary cirrhosis, or primary sclerosing cholangitis may need steroid maintenance and heavier initial immunosuppression.

Gomez-Manero *et al.* reviewed 133 transplanted recipients to identify predisposing factors for early acute rejection (within the first 45 days post-liver transplantation).[54] No protocol liver biopsies were performed. They found that the younger recipient, those with a better hepatocellular liver function (Child A) and those who underwent transplantation for liver disease other than alcoholic cirrhosis, had a greater risk for early acute rejection. Combining these three variables, they developed a mathematical model to allow prediction of the individual risk of each patient. In our center we have recently retrospectively analyzed a cohort of 470 transplant patients who received protocol biopsies, looking at the presence of predictive factors for the absence of acute cellular rejection, during the first three months after transplantation. We found that the absence of rejection was associated with pretransplant need of renal support, higher INR (International Normalized Ratio) level and a "healthy" appearance of the graft.[55]

In summary, different studies have aimed to identify patients with a greater risk for developing acute rejection, but with some exceptions, they have been limited to a small number of patients and focused on a limited number of risk factors, and the results have been frequently contradictory. For this reason there is no consensus about the majority of factors predisposing to the occurrence of acute rejection after liver transplantation.

Weaning immunosuppression

Steroid withdrawal

In the past decade there has been an evolution of immunosuppressive protocols driven by a deeper understanding of immunological events after transplantation, and due to the necessity to reduce long-term drug-related morbidity and mortality.

The first step has been a change in the use of steroids. The use of long-term corticosteroids hàs been questioned because of their adverse effect profile. The trend during the past 15 years has been to use fewer steroids for maintenance therapy. In 1988, 20 mg of prednisone per day was suggested[56] and by 1995, this recommendation had decreased to 5–10 mg daily.[57] B4 The first report of steroid withdrawal in liver transplantation was published in 1989 by Margarit *et al.* in which 73% of 18 children were successfully withdrawn from steroids.[58] In the first years after the development of liver transplantation, steroids were withdrawn only when the risk of further rejection was considered less. Following this, studies documented withdrawal in two different settings: early withdrawal (3 months)[59–61] and late withdrawal (> 1 year).[62–66]

The bulk of evidence in studies with more than 10 patients (Table 36.2) shows that steroid withdrawal does not increase patient or graft loss, but on the other hand reduces the rates of long-term complications including hypertension, development of diabetes and hypercholesterolemia. B4, AId

Long-term steroid-free regimens are therefore now widely used.[40,60,67–69] Recently the safety and efficacy of early steroid withdrawal (at 3 months) were determined in a multicenter prospective trial[70] in which 143 patients were randomized to tacrolimus (target levels 10–20 ng/ml first month then 5–15 ng/ml) or microemulsion cyclosporin (microCyA, adjusted according to therapeutic levels changing over time), together with azathioprine (1 mg/kg per day) and corticosteroids (tapering dose from 20 mg/day to 10 mg/day for the first 3 months, then discontinued). No protocol biopsies were done. The incidence of biopsy-proven rejection within the first 3 months and during the first year after transplantation was: 30% and 35% in the tacrolimus group and 40% and 43% in the microCyA group, respectively. AId Steroid-resistant rejection occurred in 5·6% of the tacrolimus and 9·7% of the microCyA group. Chronic rejection was not observed in either group during the first follow up year and the incidence of adverse events was similar between the two groups. Following the introduction of new immunosuppressive drugs, several centers have developed new "steroid-free" protocols, but have substituted steroids for the new agents (for example mycophenolate mofetil, antithymocyte globulin or anti-IL-2 agents) so that overall immunosuppressive potency is not necessarily reduced.

Samuel *et al.* had reported the result of 1-year comparative, double blind, placebo-controlled study to evaluate the efficacy and safety of early steroid withdrawal (fourteenth day post-liver transplantation).[71] Peritransplant immunosuppression in the 174 randomized patients consisted of basiliximab (two doses of 20 mg day 0–day 4), cyclosporin (trough levels of 200–400 ng/ml day 0–month 3, and 150–300 ng/ml thereafter) and intravenous methylprednisolone. Early steroid withdrawal strategy at day 14 was associated with higher incidence of acute rejection – biopsy proven (but not protocol biopsies) and a trend to more severe rejection, only balanced by a trend of needing less antidiabetic treatment. AIa However an opposite conclusion comes from the study by Llado *et al.*, in which 72 patients were randomized to immunosuppression with basiliximab and cyclosporin, with or without prednisone, and protocol biopsies were done.[72] The rate of acute rejection was similar between the groups, with less infectious and metabolic complications without steroids. AIc

Results from a multicenter randomized trial of 708 recipients, comparing a tacrolimus plus steroids regimen with tacrolimus plus daclizumab (Tac/Dac), showed no difference in acute rejection rates, with a lower incidence of steroid-resistant acute rejection, diabetes and viral infections in the Tac/Dac regimen.[73] AIa

The divergent results of these new "steroid-free" trials could be in part explained by the lack of uniformity in performing biopsies, with a higher incidence of acute rejection and complications when protocol biopsies are done. Moreover, the real benefit of steroid withdrawal cannot be evaluated if new and potent immunosuppressants agents are substituted as replacement therapy.

The only deleterious effect of steroid withdrawal reported to date is a possible worsening of the recurrence of primary biliary cirrhosis,[74] although Levitsky[75] had recently reported no difference in frequency of rejection episodes or duration of corticosteroid therapy between those who did and did not have recurrent primary biliary cirrhosis. B4

However, it is difficult to establish the real impact of an *ab initio* steroid-free protocol on chronic rejection, graft and patient survival, mainly due to the short-term follow up period and the use of steroid boluses during surgery in many of the reported trials.

Pirenne *et al.* conducted a prospective single-center pilot study to determine the influence of a completely steroid-free tacrolimus-based immunosuppression on early and late graft function and rejection.[76] Induction and maintenance immunosuppression of the 21 liver recipients consisted of tacrolimus (trough level 8–10 ng/ml) and azathioprine (1–2 mg/kg), and 52% of recipients never received steroids throughout the whole study period. Steroids were transiently needed to treat biopsy proven acute rejection in 23·5% of recipients and for tacrolimus or azathioprine toxicity or other reasons in 28% of patients. Of those who received steroids,

Table 36.2 Studies of steroid withdrawal in liver transplantation

Study	Immuno-suppression	Interval at withdrawal	No. of patients	Follow up (months)	Steroid restarted	Acute rejection	Chronic rejection	Deaths	Graft loss
Late withdrawal									
(a) Uncontrolled studies; prospective evaluation									
Punch et al. (1995)[64]	CyA+AZA	>1 year	51	13.8	6	2	0	0	0
Tchervenkov et al. (1996)[66]	CyA+AZA	1 year	42 (33)[a]	12	1	3 (9%)	0	0	1
Stegall et al. (1997)[65]	CyA	>2 year	28	12	5	2 (7.1%)	0	0	0
	CyA+S		24			1 (4.2%)	0	0	
Gomez et al. (1998)[62]	CyA	>1 year	72	23±8	0	0	0	0	
	CyA+AZA+S		14		0	0	0	0	
(b) Randomized trial									
McDiarmid, et al. (1995)[63]	CyA+AZA	>1 year	33	19·7	2 (6%)	0	0	0	
	CyA+AZA+S		31	17·6	2 (6·5%)	0	0	0	
Early withdrawal									
(a) Uncontrolled studies; retrospective evaluation									
Padbury et al. (1993)[61]	CyA+AZA	≥3 months	168	28	14	7 (4.2%)	6 (3.6%)	20	17
Fraser et al. (1996)[60]	CyA+AZA	>3 months	96	24·3±1	0	8 (8.3%)	3 (3%)	14 (14.5%)	4 (4%)
	CyA+AZA+S		18		0	7 (39.9%)		8 (44%)	2 (22%)
(b) Randomized trial									
Belli et al. (1998)[59]	CYA+S	>3 months	37[b]	41±16	1	3 (8%)	1		
	CYA		51[b]		1	2 (4%)	0		

[a]Only 33 of 42 patients were evaluated for steroid weaning.
[b]Only 37 of 50 and 51 of 54 patients were evaluated for acute rejection.
CyA, cyclosporin; S, steroids; AZA, azathioprine

the majority (70%) was eventually taken off steroids. No patients developed chronic rejection. The 3-year graft and patient survival was 95% and 100%, respectively. B4 Conclusions from the study were that steroids are not necessary in more than 50% of liver transplantations and result in no changes in acute and chronic rejection, graft and patient survival rates.

Total withdrawal and "subtherapeutic doses" of immunosuppression

Today the main aspiration of transplant clinicians is the acceptance of the graft by the recipient without any long-term pharmacological help. Long-term surviving liver transplant recipients are often systematically and excessively immunosuppressed. Consequently, drug weaning is an important management strategy providing it is done gradually under careful physician surveillance.

Although there have been small series of human liver grafts not requiring lifelong immunosuppression[14,15] it is impossible to predict who these individuals will be and the consequences of late rejection are more serious than those of early cellular rejection, including reports of fatalities.

Takatsuki *et al.* described a cohort of 63 living donor liver transplant recipients receiving tacrolimus[77]: 26 of them were entered in a elective program of withdrawal, while in the remaining 37 the choice was mainly due to serious complications of immunosuppression (mostly Epstein-Barr-associated post-transplant lymphoproliferative disease in 30 patients). Criteria for elective withdrawal were an interval of more than 2 years after the transplant with good graft function and no episodes of rejection in the previous 12 months. Tacrolimus was gradually weaned. In 24 patients (38·1%, six of them from the elective cohort) tacrolimus could be stopped with a median drug-free period of 23·5 months; 23 patients (36·5%) were still undergoing the weaning process. Rejection occurred in 16 patients (25·4%) after a median interval of 9·5 months (with a range of 1–63 months), but all the episodes could be treated by reintroducing tacrolimus or with short courses of steroids. B4

Devlin *et al.*, in 18 patients, showed that it was possible to either completely withdraw (five of 18 patients) or significantly reduce (nine of 18 patients) maintenance immunosuppression to levels previously considered subtherapeutic.[14] Parameters associated with successful drug withdrawal were transplantation for non-immune-mediated liver disorders, fewer donor–recipient HLA A, B and DR mismatches, and low incidence of early rejection. B4

In a series of 95 patients from the University of Pittsburgh,[14–16] there were 18 (19%) patients who had been drug free from 10 months to 4·8 years. Thirty-seven (39%) patients were in an uninterrupted process of drug weaning, 28 (29%) patients had weaning interrupted because of rejection, and 12 (13%) were withdrawn from the protocol, eight of them because of non-compliance, two because of

recurrent primary biliary cirrhosis, one for pregnancy, and one for renal failure necessitating kidney transplant. There were also five patients who had "self weaned" and three of the five remained well after a drug-free interval of 14–17 years. A fourth patient died in a road traffic accident after 11 years off immunosuppression, and the fifth underwent re-transplantation because of hepatitis C infection after 9 drug-free years. Although recurrence of autoimmune hepatitis has not yet been observed, two (15%) of 13 patients with primary biliary cirrhosis developed recurrence. In this study no patients were diagnosed with chronic rejection. B4

Taking all reports into account the data on empirical withdrawal does not make this a current nor viable management strategy, as individual response cannot be predicted. No data are available as to whether HLA matching or lymphotoxicity assays might help in identifying those who remain well without immunosuppression.

The optimal regimen of drug withdrawal is unknown. Criteria that can be used to select appropriate patients are required. Disorders with a well characterized immunological or viral basis appear to experience graft dysfunction after withdrawal.[78,79] B4

Single drug therapy

Further improvement in clinical transplantation might be obtained by modification of the timing, dosage, and type of immunosuppression to achieve tolerogenic immuno-suppression using the minimal effective level of therapy to allow or induce tolerance, and to reduce long-term complications. This means trying to find the lowest effective dose and safest combination of drugs, and to develop agents that are more specific to the prevention of organ rejection and less likely to cause global immunosuppression.

The potential advantages of less potent but still "safe" immunosuppressive regimens has led several transplant centers worldwide, to use regimens which end up using a single drug, usually reported in carefully studied cohorts of patients in whom steroids were withdrawn some months after transplantation. Patients with stable graft function can be easily maintained using a single drug (usually calcineurin inhibitor) after 6 or 12 months. The more evolved step of using monotherapy *ab initio* has also proved to be effective in a few studies. There is only one prospective randomized trial from our center[69] which included 64 recipients, reporting the safe use of monotherapy with either cyclosporin or tacrolimus *ab initio*, avoiding steroids and other immunosuppressive agents for induction or maintenance. With both drugs, there was adequate immunosuppression, no increased risk of biopsy proven severe rejection (17% tacrolimus *v* 11% cyclosporin) and no chronic rejection episodes were seen. A1c

Further evidence supporting the safe use of monotherapy comes from trials of steroid withdrawal in which the comparison group was on a single drug, usually a standard dose of a calcineurin inhibitor. In the largest study, Belli *et al.* described the long-term follow up of a cohort of 104 patients, 54 of whom were randomized 6 months after transplantation to CyA monotherapy, while the remaining 50 were maintained on CyA + steroids.[59] Alc Only two patients in the CyA group experienced acute rejection (due to drug malabsorption) resolved with steroid boluses but without the need for long-term treatment. At 5 years patient survival rates did not significantly differ between the two groups (77% CyA *v* 82% CyA + steroids) while the prevalence of hypertension and diabetes at 12 months was significantly reduced in the monotherapy group. Gomez *et al.* described steroid withdrawal in 86 recipients with stable graft function and no rejection 1 year after the transplant[62]: 72 patients were maintained on CyA monotherapy and 14 required azathioprine to allow calcineurin inhibitor dose reduction due to nephrotoxicity. After a mean follow up of 23 months there had been no episode of rejection or need to resume steroid treatment. B4

In a Canadian cohort[66] of patients with a mean follow up of 12 months, 39 of 42 patients could be maintained on CyA monotherapy, stopping azathioprine and steroids; only three of 33 patients with a follow up > 3 months and subtherapeutic CyA levels experienced an episode of acute rejection, which was successfully treated. B4

Another small report includes 28 patients on CyA monotherapy after steroid withdrawal with a mean follow up of 12 months: four (14.2%) were treated with steroid boluses for rejection (biopsy proven in two cases) and three (10.7%) needed to resume long-term steroid treatment because of generalized symptoms and colitis. A series from Denver (which was reported within another study) included patients treated with steroids only within the first 14 days after orthotopic liver transplantation and left on calcineurin inhibitor monotherapy (CyA or tacrolimus) from that point onward. One-year patient and graft survival were[80] 94% and 89%, respectively.[81] B4

Long-term follow up of patients treated with tacrolimus-based protocols in Pittsburgh showed that nearly 70% of liver recipients were stable on monotherapy, while 26% needed steroids or azathioprine (8/82 patients, 9.7%) at 84 months after orthotopic liver transplantation.[82] B4 Similarly, in a clinical trial[83] in 84 patients of low dose tacrolimus (0.1 mg/kg per day) which is now the dose commonly used, 74% remained on tacrolimus monotherapy without the need for steroids at 1 year. B4

Choice of an immunosuppressive agent

What evidence is there from randomized controlled trials to support the choice of an immunosuppressive agent?

Calcineurin inhibitors

Calcineurin inhibitors are still the keystones of most immunosuppressive regimens used in clinical organ transplantation. Both cyclosporin and tacrolimus bind to cytoplasmic receptors (cyclophilin and FK-binding protein (FK BP-12), respectively) and resulting complexes inactivate calcineurin, a pivotal enzyme in T cell receptor signaling. Calcineurin inhibition prevents IL-2 gene transcription, thereby inhibiting T cell IL production.[84]

Three separate randomized trials have been conducted to compare the efficacy of tacrolimus and cyclosporin (Sandimmune) in primary liver transplant patients (Table 36.3).

1   European Multicentre Tacrolimus Trial (8 centers, 545 patients)[85]
2   US Multicenter Tacrolimus Liver Study Group (12 centers, 529 patients)[86]
3   University of Pittsburgh (single center, 154 patients)[87]

In all these trials tacrolimus was administered with corticosteroids, but no azathioprine. However, in the two large trials, the cyclosporin group received corticosteroids and azathioprine and, in some cases, antilymphocyte globulin. Moreover, the adjunctive immunosuppression was not the same in all centers that participated in the studies. These protocols of double therapy with tacrolimus versus triple or quadruple therapy with cyclosporin have been noted as being unbalanced and therefore not representing a comparison of tacrolimus versus cyclosporin.[88] However, the net non-specific immunosuppression in both arms seems to have been similar, since the frequency of cytomegalovirus infection in both arms did not differ.[89] Interpretation of the relative benefit of tacrolimus and cyclosporin is difficult in the framework of these studies.

Patient and graft survival

In the multicenter studies the tacrolimus-based regimen produced 1-year graft and patient survival rates similar to the cyclosporin-based regimen. Ala In the Pittsburgh trial, the 1-year patient and graft survival were not different when data were analyzed on an intention to treat basis, although as in the other two studies a trend was shown for a better survival in the tacrolimus group. Moreover, a recent long-term follow up of the US tacrolimus study group[90] has shown that cumulative 5-year patient and graft survival were comparable for the tacrolimus-based regimen (79%, 71.8%) and cyclosporin based regimens (73.1%, 66.4%) but median patient survival was longer for tacrolimus-treated patients (tacrolimus 25.1 ± 5.1 years, cyclosporin 15.2 ± 2.5 years). Ala In the 3-year follow up of the European multicenter trial[89,91] the analysis according to intention to treat at 3 years showed a significant difference in patient survival in favor of

Table 36.3 Randomized trials of tacrolimus versus cyclosporin (Sandimmune) with cumulative number or actuarial proportion of events at yearly follow up intervals

Study	Patients	Initial dosage regimen (mg/kg per day)	Time of assessment (years)	Results (% of patients)					Crossover for intractable rejection (n)
				Graft survival (%)	Patient survival (%)	ACR	Refractory rejection	Chronic rejection	
European FK506 Multicentre	264	TAC 0.075 mg/kg IV then 0·30 mg/kg oral +S (0·164 mg/kg)	1 2 3	77·5[a] 74·5[a] 70·6[a]	82·9[a] 80·6[a] 77·0[a]	107 (41%) 45·4%[f] 45·4%[f]	2 (1%) 3 (1%) 1·2%[f]	4 (1·5%) 4 (1·5%) 2%[f]	NA NA
Tacrolimus Trial[85]	265	CyA 1–6 mg/kg IV then 8–15 mg/kg oral + AZA + S, Oral (0·168 mg/kg) +ATG days 1–7[b]	1 2 3	72·6[a] 70[a] 65·2[a]	77·5[a] 74·8[a] 69·7[a]	132 (50%) 56%[f] 55%[f]	14 (5%) 16 (6%) 5·9%[f]	14 (5%) 14 (5%) 7%[f]	14 27 NA
US Multicentre FK506	263	TAC 0.075 mg/kg IV reduced to 0·05 mg/kg then 0·15 mg/kg oral +S (90+65 mg/kg)	1 3	82[a] 77	88[a] 84[a]	154 (58%) 17%	6 (3%) NA	5 (2%) NA	3 NA
Liver Study Group[86]	266	CyA 1–2 mg/kg IV, then 5 mg/kg oral + AZA + S (131+61 mg/kg) ±ATG[c]	5 1 3 5	71·8 79[a] 72 66·4	79[a] 88[a] 79[a] 73[a]	4·9% 173 (65%) 13% 6%	0 32 (12%) NA 0	0 4 (1·5%) NA 0	6 22 (8%) NA 22
Fung et al.[87]	79	TAC 0·1 mg/kg[d] IV + S 20 mg/day	4	78%[e]	84	50 (64%)	1 (1·2%)	NA	NA
	75	CyA 4 mg/kg IV then 8 mg/kg[d] + S 20 mg/day	4	70%[e]	84	62 (83%)	1 (1·3%)	13	47[g]

[a] Actuarial rates of survival.
[b] ATG was administered at dose of 5 mg/kg per day for a week induction period post-transplant in three centers.
[c] Regimen varied among centers.
[d] Ad hoc dose adjustments according to levels.
[e] Estimated from a graph.
[f] Kaplan–Meier estimates.
[g] 47 patients crossed over to tacrolimus: seven before and 40 after rejection (one tacrolimus crossed into cyclosporin group).
TAC, tacrolimus; CyA, cyclosporin; AZA, azathioprine; S, steroids; ATG, antithymocyte globulin; ACR, acute cellular rejection IV, intravenous

the tacrolimus-based regimen[91] (tacrolimus 75·7%, cyclosporin 67·5%, $P = 0·036$).

Rejection

In the randomized trials a notable difference between tacrolimus and cyclosporin-based regimens was the lower incidence of acute rejection with tacrolimus. In the European study acute rejection was less frequent in the tacrolimus-based group (tacrolimus 40·5%, cyclosporin 49·8% $P = 0·004$). Refractory rejection (tacrolimus 0·8%, cyclosporin 5·6%, $P = 0·005$) and chronic rejection (tacrolimus 1·5%, cyclosporin 5·3%, $P = 0·032$) were also less common with the tacrolimus regimen. These differences were observed despite higher concomitant use of corticosteroids or azathioprine in the cyclosporin group. Ala

Data from the US multicenter study also showed less frequent rejection with tacrolimus – acute rejection: tacrolimus 154 (68%), cyclosporin 173 (76%), $P < 0·002$; corticosteroid-resistant rejection: tacrolimus 42 (16·3%) and cyclosporin 82 (30·8%), $P < 0·001$; refractory rejection: tacrolimus 6 (3%), cyclosporin 32 (15%), $P < 0·001$. Ala The Pittsburgh group obtained similar results. In all three trials a large percentage of patients (see Table 36.3) were switched from cyclosporin to tacrolimus, mainly because of persistent rejection (European $n = 14$, US $n = 22$, Pittsburgh $n = 47$).

Ninety-one patients with chronic rejection that developed during cyclosporin-based immunosuppression were converted to tacrolimus in an open label multicenter study[92] involving 17 liver transplant centers in the USA. Sixty four (70·3%) were alive with their initial hepatic allograft after a mean follow up of 251 days. In this study patients with total bilirubin of ≤ 10 mg/dl at the time of conversion had a significantly better graft and patient survival than patients with total bilirubin > 10 mg/dl. The time between liver transplantation and conversion to tacrolimus therapy also affected graft and patient survival. Patients who converted to tacrolimus ≤ 90 days after transplantation had 1-year actuarial graft and patient survival of 51·9% and 65·9% respectively, compared with 73·2% ($P = 0·002$) and 87·7% ($P = 0·02$) for those who converted > 90 days after transplantation. B4

Steroid-sparing effect

In the US trial the cumulative dose of steroids for both prophylaxis and rejection was significantly less with tacrolimus than with the cyclosporin-based regimen (90 mg/kg *v* 131 mg/kg, $P < 0·001$).[86] Ala Similarly, lower intravenous (but not oral) corticosteroid doses were required during maintenance therapy with tacrolimus versus cyclosporin in the European study at 1 year, and both oral and intravenous doses were lower with tacrolimus after 3 years

($P < 0·05$). At 3 years steroid therapy had been successfully withdrawn in 80% of tacrolimus and 68% of cyclosporin-treated patients ($P = 0·025$). Ala

Microemulsified cyclosporin

Microemulsified formulation of cyclosporin (Neoral) has addressed the major limitation of the previous oil-based drug preparations, i.e. the highly variable partial and bile-dependent gastrointestinal absorption process.[93–98] In two randomized controlled trials comparing Neoral with Sandimmune,[99,100] the Neoral group experienced less rejection, fewer episodes of steroid-resistant rejection, and a lower incidence of moderate/severe histological rejection. Ala Indeed the microemulsion formulation may remove or reduce the discrepancy in outcomes between cyclosporin and tacrolimus-based regimens seen in the randomized trials described above. In a randomized trial involving 71 patients, Stegall observed a similar incidence of acute rejection episodes whether mycophenolate mofetil was combined with Neoral or with tacrolimus.[101] Fisher *et al.*[102] in a similar trial of mycophenolate mofetil combined with Neoral or tacrolimus, also found similar rates of acute rejection (Neoral 46%, tacrolimus 42·3%), and there were no differences observed between treatment groups with respect to the incidence of diabetes mellitus, hypertension or hyperglycemia. Ala

However, the superiority of tacrolimus versus cyclosporin has been strengthened by the results of a large recent trial in the UK[103] in which 606 transplant recipients were randomly assigned to receive open-label tacrolimus or microemulsified cyclosporin. Of the tacrolimus-treated patients 52% were alive with their original graft and free of rejection at 12 months compared with 41% of the cyclosporin-treated group (monitored with trough levels). The incidence at 12 months of more than two episodes of acute rejection and chronic rejection in the tacrolimus-group was 3% and 0·3% respectively compared to the 8% and 2% of the cyclosporin group. On the basis of these data, tacrolimus should be the first choice of calcineurin inhibitors for patients receiving their first liver graft.[103] Ala

Therapeutic drug monitoring of cyclosporin

Therapeutic monitoring of calcineurin inhibitors is recommended. Cyclosporin has a narrow therapeutic index, and an extremely variable pharmacokinetic profile and a strong pharmacodynamic linkage between desired and adverse effects. There is currently some debate as to whether the dose of cyclosporin should be monitored by the trough or 2-hour post-dose levels.

A multicenter prospective study involving 307 *de novo* liver transplant recipients,[104] compared the clinical usefulness of monitoring 2-hour post-dose cyclosporin levels (C2) with conventional trough cyclosporin blood levels (pre-dose) (C0).

No protocol biopsies were done. The overall incidence of acute cellular rejection was lower (23·6% v 31·6%) and the histological severity was significantly milder for the C2 group. [Ala] Villamil *et al.* have recently reported the results of the planned 3 month interim analysis of the first 300 *de novo* liver transplant patients,[105] randomized to either cyclosporin (target C-2-hour levels 800–1200 ng/ml) or tacrolimus (target C-0-hour levels 5–15 ng/ml) in addition to steroids with or without azathioprine. Although protocol biopsies were not done, the incidence and severity of biopsy proven episodes of acute cellular rejection were similar and infrequent, regardless of whether patients received dual or triple immunosuppressive therapy. [Ala]

Conversion from twice to once daily dosing of cyclosporin (100 ± 25 ng/ml, C2 level 748 ± 105 ng/ml) utilizing C2 monitoring in maintenance of 68 liver transplant patients with abnormal renal function, at 4 ± 1·3 year after transplantation, has been reported to be safe, with no rejection episodes noted (although protocol biopsies were not done) and with improvement in renal function. [B4] The Consensus on Neoral C2: Expert Review in Transplantation (CONCERT) Conference[106] suggested that C2 monitoring is the optimal method to monitor cyclosporin both in adults *de novo* and in maintenance liver transplant patients, but no controlled trials comparing C2 with C0 monitoring have been carried out.

The possible, but as yet unproved, benefit of C2 monitoring must be weighed against its practical disadvantages. Once a day dosing of cyclosporin is already current practice in many centers.

Tacrolimus rescue for acute cellular rejection

Several studies[107,108] have demonstrated that tacrolimus (at blood levels of 15–20 mg/dl) is effective as rescue therapy for steroid-resistant acute rejection in patients on cyclosporin-based therapy. Moreover, a pilot study suggested that increasing tacrolimus dosage (increments of 1–2 mg every 1 or 2 days with trough tacrolimus blood levels of 15–20 ng/ml), and continued low doses of steroids could be considered as treatment for early acute rejection episodes (biopsy proven) including severe grades of rejection.[109] [B4]

Therapeutic drug monitoring of tacrolimus

Trough whole blood concentration monitoring is the common method used to monitor tacrolimus therapy. The relationships between the dose of tacrolimus, trough tacrolimus blood concentration (enzyme linked immunosorbent assay, ELISA) and selected clinical endpoints (acute rejection, nephrotoxicity and other toxicities) were examined in a prospective multicenter study. The study confirmed the poor correlation between the daily dose (mg/kg per day) and the steady-state whole-blood concentration achieved and showed that to minimize nephrotoxicity without increasing the risk of rejection, it is necessary to maintain trough tacrolimus blood concentration below 15 ng/ml.[110] Recently it has been reported that HCV transplant recipients require significantly lower oral doses of tacrolimus to achieve the same trough blood levels compared with non-HCV patients, probably due to a decreased hepatic clearance of tacrolimus caused by mild hepatic injury from recurrent HCV.[111]

Mycophenolate mofetil

In many centers, mycophenolate mofetil is now replacing azathioprine in standard immunosuppression protocols. The rationale for this switch is that mycophenolate mofetil is a selective inhibitor of the *de novo* pathway of purine biosynthesis, thereby providing more specific and potent inhibition of T cell and B cell proliferation. [C5] It has been used for both treatment and prevention of rejection in combination with calcineurin inhibitors.[112] Compared with azathioprine, mycophenolate mofetil appears to have fewer myelotoxic and hepatotoxic adverse effects.[113] [B4]

The most common adverse effects at the standard dose of 2 g/day are nausea, abdominal pain, anorexia, gastritis and diarrhea. The latter affects 30% of patients but usually responds to a decreased dose. Neutropenia affects 3% of patients and usually requires dose reduction. This effect is potentiated by azathioprine, and the two agents should never be used together. Opportunistic infections do not appear to be significantly increased in comparison to azathioprine treatment. Blood levels are not clinically monitored with mycophenolate mofetil. An enteric-coated formulation of mycophenolate sodium (EC-MPS) has been developed to reduce the gastrointestinal side effects. Single dose pharmacokinetic studies have revealed bioequivalent exposure when compared with orally administered conventional mycophenolate mofetil and clinical trials are underway with this agent.[114]

Mycophenolate mofetil may be a safe and potentially adjuvant immunosuppressive agent for initiation and maintenance therapy, but to date there is no evidence that combined with calcineurin inhibitor, it is superior to tacrolimus and steroid immunosuppression.

However its role may be more as a renal-sparing agent. Mycophenolate mofetil has been administered to reduce the calcineurin inhibitor dose in patients with impaired renal function, and rarely also as monotherapy. Two recent randomized trials of mycophenolate mofetil monotherapy (started at 1 year[115] and at 6 months[116] after transplantation) in patients with chronic renal dysfunction due to calcineurin inhibitor nephrotoxicity recorded an increased risk of rejection, both acute and chronic, (60% in the first study[115] and 50% in the second[116]) but only 11 patients received monotherapy and all for less than 1 year. [Alc]

Table 36.4 Sirolimus primary immunosuppression liver transplantation protocols

Author	No.	Regimen	SRL level	ACR (%)	SRR (%)	Patient/graft survival (%)
Watson, *et al.* (1999)[122]	15	SRL (3·5–7 mg/day)+CyA+S	–	0	0	Overall 66
		SRL (7–21 mg/day)+S	–	28	0	
		SRL (7–21 mg/day)+S	–	75	0	
McAlister, *et al.* (2001)[123]	56	SRL (mean, 3·5 mg/day)+TAC+S	6·5–8·5 ng/ml	14	0	93/91
Pridohl, *et al.* (2001)[124]	22	SRL (6 mg/day loading dose, 2 mg/day maintenance)+TAC+S	6–8 ng/ml	14	0	91/78
Trotter, *et al.* (2001)[81]	39	SRL (6 mg loading dose, 2mg/day maintenance) + TAC or CyA+S	5–8 ng/ml	36	3	92/89

SRL, sirolimus; S, steroids; SRR, steroid-resistant rejection; ACR, acute cellular rejection

We reported a retrospective review[117] of 45 patients with renal dysfunction who were treated at a median of 45 months after transplantation, either with mycophenolate mofetil as monotherapy ($n = 16$), or in combination with low dose of calcineurin inhibitor, i.e. deliberately kept below therapeutic trough levels < 5 ng/ml or cyclosporin < 50 ng/ml. The incidence of acute cellular rejection in the mycophenolate mofetil monotherapy group was only 6%, and the serum creatinine values decreased, more so in the monotherapy group compared with the low dose calcineurin inhibitor group. B4 Mycophenolate mofetil can help reduce the dose of calcineurin inhibitor and decrease nephrotoxicity, but a randomized trial is needed to provide stronger evidence, particularly given the high rate of discontinuation due to side effects.

Sirolimus

Sirolimus (rapamycin) is a macrocyclic lactone with a structure similar to tacrolimus. However, the mechanism and adverse effect profiles of the two drugs are quite different. Sirolimus blocks signal transduction in T lymphocytes and inhibits cell-cycle progression from G1 to S phase.[118,119] The adverse effect profile of sirolimus includes dose-dependent hyperlipidemia, thrombocytopenia, anemia, leukopenia, with the absence of neurotoxicity, nephrotoxicity and diabetogenesis, but it has adverse effects on wound healing.[120] Recently, the risk of oligospermia in young male patients has been reported.[121]

Randomized controlled trials comparing sirolimus with conventional immunosuppression have not been completed. Currently the published data are derived from four open-label studies (Table 36.4).

The first report to demonstrate the safety of sirolimus as primary immunosuppression was published by Watson *et al.*[122] Fifteen patients were treated with sirolimus in three different regimens and by 3 months after transplantation were maintained on sirolimus monotherapy. None of the patients on triple therapy experienced rejection, while 28% and 75% of patients had rejection with dual and monotherapy, respectively. B4

Trotter *et al.*[81] reported that low dose sirolimus with minimal corticosteroids (3-day taper), with either tacrolimus or cyclosporin, (compared with cyclosporin or tacrolimus plus 14-day tapered dose of prednisone) was associated with 30% incidence of acute rejection, which was significantly less than historical controls (70%; $P < 0.01$) and 90% decreased incidence of steroid-resistant rejection. No protocol biopsies were done. B4 Similar efficacy was reported by McAlister *et al.*[123] in a open label report of 56 patients who received low-dose tacrolimus and sirolimus (target trough levels, ng/ml and 7 ng/ml, respectively) with prednisone up to 6 months after transplantation. The acute cellular rejection rate was 14%, which was approximately 50% lower than the historical rejection rate, and no patients had steroid-resistant rejection. B4

Other studies have suggested that the best use of sirolimus should be in combination with low dose tacrolimus in order to minimize adverse effects from either drug.[124,125] In the study by Pridohl *et al.*, patients undergoing transplantation for acute liver failure received triple immunosuppression.[124] The rate of acute rejection and steroid-resistant rejection were 14% and 0%, respectively. Dunkelberg *et al.* have recently reported the largest series of liver transplant recipients treated with sirolimus (2 mg/day) as part of primary immunosuppression.[126] One-year patient (93%) and graft survival rates (92%) in sirolimus-treated patients were not different from those for historical controls (95% and 89%, respectively) and the incidence of acute rejection and use of OKT3 (monoclonal antibody against CD3, muromonabCD3) was significantly lower in sirolimus-treated patients (14%) versus controls (39%) as reported previously.[81] B4 However, the percentage needing OKT3 is high, both in the controls and sirolimus-treated groups. Importantly, the prevalence of hepatic artery and wound complications in sirolimus-treated patients was similar to that in historic controls. These results are in contrast with a recent international trial studying sirolimus in liver transplantation, which was halted because of a greater incidence of hepatic artery thrombosis in patients given tacrolimus with sirolimus.[127] B4

Further studies are needed to assess the value of sirolimus, as a single agent or in combination with other agents.

Sirolimus conversion therapy in liver transplantation

A number of centers have reported outcomes in patients converted from calcineurin inhibitor to sirolimus following liver transplantation. The indications for conversion or addition of sirolimus to the immunosuppressive regimen (with reduction of calcineurin inhibitor) include: nephrotoxicity or neurotoxicity of the calcineurin inhibitor and severe chronic rejection.

One small study reported the addition of sirolimus (4 mg/day) to maintenance immunosuppression with tacrolimus after 3·3 years from transplantation, in 27 patients with chronic renal insufficiency (creatinine > 1·5 mg/dl).[128] Rejection occurred in 29% of patients and in 37% sirolimus had to be discontinued, with minimal improvement in renal function. B4 Chang et al.[129] reported the use of sirolimus either as a primary immunosuppressive agent (3·1 days after transplantation) or as conversion therapy for renal dysfunction, with improvement of serum creatinine in all patients and normalization in most. Nishida et al. reported the introduction of sirolimus after 995 days from liver transplantation in a diverse group of 16 recipients with severe chronic rejection.[130] The authors concluded that sirolimus may be successfully used as a "rescue treatment" for these patients. B4

Nair et al. retrospectively reviewed 16 transplant patients who were more than 3 years post-transplantation, who had chronic renal dysfunction (creatinine clearance < 70 ml/min).[131] The conversion to sirolimus (2 mg/day) allowed safe cyclosporin withdrawal and a significant recovery of renal function, without developing cellular rejection or other graft-related complications. B4

Fairbanks et al. reported the safety of the use of sirolimus monotherapy in transplant patients with renal insufficiency caused by calcineurin inhibitors.[132] Eighteen patients were converted to sirolimus monotherapy and three patients were switched to sirolimus and low dose steroid therapy after 310 weeks from transplantation. Renal function improved significantly in the majority of recipients (15/21, 71%), and only one patients developed biopsy proven acute cellular rejection, which was treated with sirolimus and mycophenolate mofetil. Adverse events were mostly mild and self-limited. B4

In summary, the current published data on the outcomes in recipients converted from calcineurin inhibitor to sirolimus following liver transplantation are on small numbers of patients, with conversion occurring at disparate intervals and different dosages and immunosuppression regimens. Thus, the data are insufficient to permit specific recommendations for patient selection and dosing regimens for sirolimus conversion to be made.

Antithymocyte and antilymphocyte globulins

Another advance has been the introduction and incorporation of antilymphocyte and antithymocyte globulins into cyclosporin-based immunosuppressive protocols, used for both prophylaxis and treatment of acute cellular rejection. Thymoglobulin is a polyclonal rabbit antithymocyte globulin (RATG) previously shown to be an effective immunosuppressive agent in liver transplantation.[44,133] B4 In conjunction with steroids, it has been shown to effectively reduce the incidence of rejection without an increased incidence of infectious complications or malignancy.[133,134] Eason and colleagues[135] reported the first study of 71 transplant patients, treated with two doses of RATG as induction therapy in conjunction with tacrolimus on its own at 3 months from transplantation, in a completely steroid-free regimen. The rate of biopsy proven rejection was similar to standard triple-drug regimens that included steroids (20·5% v 32%), without an increased incidence of complications, in particular cytomegalovirus infection, diabetes and HCV recurrence. Recently, the same authors have published the follow up on these patients and also data on additional patients who were randomized to receive RATG in a regimen of tacrolimus monotherapy at 2 weeks from transplantation.[136] A1d Steroid-free liver transplantation with two doses of RATG induction and early tacrolimus monotherapy is achievable in most of the transplant patients, with effective prevention and therapy for rejection. However the preliminary data of tacrolimus monotherapy versus triple therapy in HCV patients[137] and the previous experience of calcineurin inhibitor monotherapy[69] suggest that added antithymocyte regimens may increase immunosuppression, suppressing the possibility of tolerance. Long-term follow up is needed.

Recently Starzl et al. have reported the use of RATG (5 mg/kg) as pre-treatment therapy in 82 solid organ transplant recipients (17 with liver transplantation) followed by minimum use of post-transplant immunosuppression (tacrolimus monotherapy during the first 4 months, then spaced tacrolimus therapy).[138] No liver grafts were lost to biopsy proven rejection, and from the fourth month onward, between 10 and 12 recipients needed only spaced monotherapy. B4

Interleukin-2 receptor blockers

T lymphocytes play a central role in the initiation and progression of the rejection response. Activated T lymphocytes secrete IL-2 that acts in an autocrine and paracrine fashion to drive the response forward, and produces more IL-2 receptors (IL-2R). As only activated T lymphocytes express IL-2R, it was suggested that blocking this receptor with a monoclonal antibody could allow for an even more highly selective approach to prevent rejection.[139]

IL-2R blockers, for example daclizumab and basiliximab are chimeric and humanized antibodies that act on a receptorial subunit which is expressed only on activated T lymphocytes, thus selectively inhibiting their proliferation. Considering the sequence of events in graft rejection in liver transplantation, immunosuppression with IL-2R blockers could play a role at the very beginning, leaving the introduction of calcineurin inhibitor when these agents can be introduced without excessive risk of infection or renal dysfunction, i.e. monotherapy with IL-2R blockade for the first to second week and then monotherapy with calcineurin inhibitors.

Daclizumab has been reported only in a few small uncontrolled studies of induction therapy particularly in patients with pre-operative renal failure or at risk of developing postoperative renal dysfunction, but always in combination with other immunosuppressants. There are contrasting results.[140–144] These pilot studies all suggest that induction therapy with daclizumab in combination with non-calcineurin inhibitor drugs followed by calcineurin inhibitor administration was safe B4 . However one study[143] was stopped because of a very high rate of acute cellular rejection (7/7 enrolled patients, with 4 of 7 patients experiencing steroid-resistant rejection requiring OKT3 treatment). B4 Nelson et al. used adjuvant daclizumab (three doses of 1 mg/kg, days 0, 4, 21) in combination with mycophenolate mofetil (1 g twice daily) in the early post-transplantation period in HCV transplant recipients.[145] They found early onset of hepatitis, greater histological activity and more rapid progression to advanced recurrent HCV disease (by 1 year, 45% v 26%). The incidence of biopsy-proven acute rejection was similar between HCV positive and negative group. B4

Calmus et al.[146] evaluated a single-arm, open label, multicenter trial, with historical control data (derived from Multicentre International Study in Liver Transplantation of Neoral (MILTON) study[147]), in which 101 patients were given basiliximab (two 20 mg doses day 0 and 4) in conjunction with cyclosporin (adjusted according to therapeutic levels changing over time), azathioprine (1·5 mg/kg per day), and corticosteroids (tapering dose from 200 mg/day to 5 mg/day until the end of the study). One-year patient and graft survival rates were 90·1% and 88·1% with a reduction of the overall biopsy-proven rejection rate compared with historic controls (22·8% at 6 months v 49·9% at 1 year), without increased incidence of malignancies, infections or other adverse effects. Rejection episodes were more frequent in the HCV positive than HCV negative subgroup (29% v 20%) but this was not statistically significant. B4

Neuhaus et al. reported a large, multicenter randomized trial of 381 patients (placebo or basiliximab 20 mg on day 0 and 4 in addition to cyclosporin and corticosteroids).[148] Primary outcomes were acute rejection and a composite endpoint, including death or graft loss, assessed at 6 and 12 months and by HCV cohort. There were no protocol

biopsies, and clinically suspected rejection episodes were confirmed by liver biopsy. The biopsy proven rejection rates after 6 months from transplantation were 35·1% in the basiliximab-treated group and 43·5% in the placebo group but this was not statistically significant. Rejection rates for the HCV positive patients were slightly greater in the basiliximab versus the placebo arm (39·1% v 36·2%) and again this was not statistically significant. The incidence of complications, including infections, was similar in the two groups. A1a

In both studies, the slightly greater rejection rates in the HCV positive group might result from false positive reporting linked to histological similarities between recurrent hepatitis C and acute rejection.[149] However, caution may be needed in HCV infection as suggested by the report of Nelson et al.[145] in which the use of adjuvant IL-2R antibodies in combination with mycophenolate mofetil in the early peritransplantation period was associated with early recurrence of hepatitis C and more rapid histological progression of disease.

Data from Garcia-Retordillo et al.[150] provide a strong indication that the use of induction anti-IL-2R monoclonals combined in a protocol without steroids, might avoid the early expansion of circulating HCV RNA. C5 However, at present, the published data from seven studies[140,143,146,148,147,151–153] do not allow a consensus on the impact of induction monoclonals or polyclonals on HCV (Table 36.5). Limitations of these studies include small numbers, use of a variety of induction agents, lack of controls in the study design and variable endpoints. B4

Recently, Yan et al.[151] have reported that induction therapy with single dose of daclizumab is safe and effective and appears to reduce the rate of acute rejection. B4

Use of anti-IL-2R monoclonal antibodies in liver transplantation, suggests that the drugs have good early safety, at least in patients with non-HCV cirrhosis and are well tolerated, but more randomized trials are needed to better elucidate the ideal regimens and indications for these promising drugs. Long-term studies are needed to assess potential effects on *de novo* malignancies as well as progression of HCV.

New protocols of tolerogenic preconditioning have been developed using alentuzumab (Campath-1H) and low doses of calcineurin inhibitors. Alentuzumab is a humanized monoclonal antibody directed against the CD52 antigen, a pan T, B, and natural killer cell, and monocyte markers. It rapidly depletes lymphocytes, monocytes, and other cells without affecting neutrophils and hematopoietic stem cells. The depleted cells begin to re-emerge gradually during a period of 6 months without returning to baseline levels. This activity is believed to prevent an aggressive lymphocytic immune response after transplantation and allow a more gradual engagement of the host immune system under low conventional immunosuppression. This regimen of host conditioning prior to transplantation followed by minimum post-transplant immunosuppression could increase the chance of developing tolerance.[154] Encouraging results have

Table 36.5 Studies of induction therapy in liver transplantation

Authors	Monoclonal	Immunosuppression	Patients	Impact on HCV
Yan *et al.*[151]	Daclizumab	CyA, S, MMF	23 (31 controls)	Possible benefit
Neuhaus *et al.*[148]	Basiliximab	CyA, S	381	Possible benefit
Calmus *et al.*[146]	Basiliximab	CyA, S, AZA	101 (31 HCV+)	No obvious harm
Eckhoff *et al.*[140]	Daclizumab	CyA, S, MMF	39 (58 controls)	Not specifically examined
Hirose *et al.*[143]	Daclizumab	MMF, S	32	Not specifically examined
Washburn *et al.*[152]	Daclizumab	TAC, MMF, S	30	No obvious harm
Eason *et al.*[136]	RATG	TAC, MMF, S	35 (35 controls)	No obvious harm

RATG, rabbit antithymocyte globulin; CyA, cyclosporin; MMF, mycophenolate mofetil; TAC, tacrolimus; HCV, hepatitis C virus; AZA, azathioprine; S, steroid

been reported in 31 kidney recipients treated with alentuzumab and half dose cyclosporin,[155] and in 14 intestinal and nine multivisceral transplantations treated with Campath-1H and low dose of tacrolimus.[156] Tzakis *et al.* reported their experience of 19 liver transplant patients (HCV patients were excluded) treated with Campath-1H and half the usual dose of tacrolimus in a steroid-free maintenance regimen.[157] Over a follow up period of 4 months, opportunistic infections were not frequent and only four patients presented clinical evidence of mild acute rejection. These are preliminary results and larger series and longer follow up are needed. B4

In summary, available data on the use of anti-IL-2R monoclonal antibodies in liver transplantation suggest that the drugs have good early safety, at least in patients with non-HCV cirrhosis and are well tolerated, but more randomized trials are needed to elucidate the ideal dose and indications for these promising drugs. Then long-term studies are needed to assess potential effects on *de novo* malignancies.

Trials of ursodeoxycholic acid

Ursodeoxycholic acid (UDCA) is a hydrophilic bile acid that has been shown to protect the liver parenchyma in cholestatic states and possibly to slow the progression of primary biliary cirrhosis.[158,159] Additionally, UDCA has been shown to reduce the expression of major histocompatibility complex (MHC) class I antigens in patients with primary biliary cirrhosis and therefore may have immunomodulatory effects on T cell-dependent liver damage.[158–160] During acute cellular rejection, there is an expression of MHC class I and II antigens on hepatocytes, although these are not primary target cells. Cholestasis itself may induce an increased expression of MHC class I antigens on hepatocytes, which can lead to lymphocyte CD8 $^+$ -dependent cytotoxicity.[161] Based on these theoretical considerations, UDCA could be used as adjuvant therapy to decrease acute cellular rejection episodes in liver transplant patients. C5

There are five randomized controlled trials evaluating UDCA (10–15 mg/kg) for prevention of acute allograft rejection in liver transplant patients.

1 The Nordic Multicenter double blind randomized controlled trial of prophylactic UDCA in liver transplant patients (54 UDCA, 48 placebo)[162]
2 Fleckenstein *et al.* (14 UDCA, 16 placebo)[163]
3 Pageaux *et al.* (26 UDCA, 24 placebo)[164]
4 Barnes *et al.* (28 UDCA, 24 placebo)[165]
5 Angelico *et al.* (16 UDCA, 17 placebo)[166]

Four randomized controlled trials[162–164,166] showed that UDCA was not effective for prevention of acute rejection in liver transplant patients. Although Barnes *et al.*[165] found that there were significantly fewer patients in the UDCA treatment group who had multiple episodes of acute rejection (0 *v* 6), the severity of rejection was not described. There is no good evidence to recommend UDCA as therapy to prevent rejection (Table 36.6). A1d

Granulocyte-colony stimulating factor

Studies in animal models as well as clinical trials have demonstrated significant benefits of human recombinant granulocyte-colony stimulating factor (G-CSF) for the treatment of infections in bone marrow recipients, while the experience in solid organ transplantation is more limited. However G-CSF is useful in reversing leukopenia in solid organ transplant recipients and is safe. Only one study has suggested an association with a worsening of renal graft function,[167] but in most series renal function was not affected and no increase in rejection episodes was seen. Indeed in one study, G-CSF used for the first 7–10 days was associated with a lower incidence of acute rejection in 37 liver transplant recipients, as compared with historical controls ($n = 49$) receiving the same immunosuppressive protocol (22% *v* 51%).[168] B4 A proposed mechanism to account for a lower rate of rejection with G-CSF, is the significant reduction in serum TNF levels, which may be a key factor in allograft rejection.[169,170] C5 However, a subsequent

Table 36.6 Randomized controlled trials of ursodeoxycholic acid (UDCA) for prevention of liver transplant rejection

Study	Dose (duration)	Days after transplant	Acute rejection (%)
Pageaux *et al.* (1995)[164]			
26 UDCA	600 mg/day	3–5	34
24 placebo	(2 months)		37
Nordic Multicentre (1997)[162]		1	65
58 UDCA	15 mg/kg per day		68
48 placebo	(3 months)		
Barnes *et al.* (1997)[165]			
28 UDCA	10–15 mg/kg per day	3–5	61
24 placebo	(3 months)		71
Fleckenstein *et al.* (1998)[163]			
14 UDCA	15 mg/kg per day	1	79
Angelico *et al.* (1999)[166]			
16 UDCA	250 mg twice daily	5	57
17 placebo	(12 months)		67

multicenter randomized placebo-controlled trial comprising 194 patients[171] did not confirm the previous report, showing that the prophylactic administration of G-CSF (100 or 300 micrograms/day for a maximum of 21 days) had no beneficial effects on infection rates. Ala Moreover the incidence of biopsy proven rejection was more common in the G-CSF treated group compared with placebo (30% *v* 19%). Additional studies are needed to determine the optimal use of G-CSF to prevent or treat acute rejection.

Future immunosuppressive drugs: non-biological agents in preclinical and clinical studies

The future immunosuppressive strategies will be designed to help the development of tolerance of the allograft, selectively stimulating instead of suppressing the recipient's immune reaction. Studies of the current immunosuppressive agents suggest two ways in which this goal might be attained: first, the use of calcineurin inhibitors could be avoided in the first few days after transplantation, allowing initial allorecognition and potential tolerizing interactions to take place; or second, newer immunosuppressive agents that do not block tolerance induction in experimental models could be used instead.[172,173]

Everolimus is a rapamycin derivate with improved bioavailability, currently in multiple phase III clinical trials. Everolimus has been studied in large randomized trials designed to evaluate efficacy equivalency with mycophenolate mofetil. These ongoing studies show that everolimus (1·5 mg and 3 mg/day) and mycophenolate mofetil (2 mg/day) produce similar low rates of acute renal rejection in renal transplant recipients receiving triple immunosuppression therapy with cyclosporin and corticosteroids. Lower incidence of cytomegalovirus infection was also reported.[174] Ald

It has been reported that it inhibits the growth of human Epstein-Barr virus-transformed B lymphocytes *in vitro* and *in vivo*, suggesting that it may be effective in prevention and treatment of post-transplant lymphoproliferative diseases.[175] Studies of everolimus in liver transplantation are currently being carried out.

Leflunomide, a member of malononitrilamide family, targets the *de novo* pathway of pyrimidine biosynthesis and thus inhibits T and B cell proliferation. It has been approved for use in patients with active rheumatoid arthritis. A retrospective review of the use of leflunomide was carried out in 53 liver and kidney transplant recipients. In 12 of 18 renal patients treated with leflunomide for 200 days or more the dose of calcineurin inhibitors was reduced by a mean of 38·5%, and stopped in one patient. The prednisone dose was reduced by a mean of 25% in these same 13 patients. Calcineurin inhibitors were stopped completely in four liver recipients and reduced by 65% in another patient. No evidence of acute rejection developed in any of these liver or kidney transplant patients.[176] B4

FK778, a synthetic derived of leflunomide, has been developed to reduce the extended half-life of leflunomide, while maintaining similar therapeutic efficacy and with a more favorable pharmacokinetic profile.[177]

FTY 720 is a unique immunosuppressive agent that not only inhibits lymphocyte proliferation, but also results in a redistribution of lymphocytes into lymph nodes and out of circulation. This ability of FTY 720 to impair effector T cell homing is achieved without affecting induction or expansion of memory responses, suggesting that it may leave tolerizing interactions intact.[178] C5 In animal models its use prolonged allograft survival with remarkable potency.[179]

C5 In stable renal transplanted recipients, a single oral dose of FTY 720 (0·25–3·5 mg) was well tolerated and caused reversible selective lymphopenia within 6 hours.[180] B4

Immunosuppression in HCV recipients

HCV reinfection after liver transplantation seems to have a much more rapid and aggressive course. Thus, modulation of immunosuppression may be a clinical approach to prevent rapid progression of HCV infection after liver transplantation. The exact role of the immune system in the pathogenesis of HCV-related chronic liver injury and progression of fibrosis has not been clarified.[181] Collier and Heathcote[182] reviewed the behavior of HCV infection in patients with impaired B cell or CD4 T helper 1 cell immunity, confirming that in these patients, HCV-related disease has a more rapid progression than in immunocompetent patients and the rate of progression seems to correlate with the degree of immunosuppression. The association between HCV recurrence and immunosuppression, as cause and effect seems logical, but as yet has not been clearly defined.[183] Global immunosuppression, and not a single immunosuppressive agent, influences the severity of recurrence of HCV.

Steroids massively increase serum HCV-RNA levels and high total cumulative dose and/or high number of steroid boluses have been associated with worse outcome.[184] B4 The link of steroid treatment and anti-rejection therapy to the worsening of hepatitis C recurrence has prompted many centers to advocate steroid therapy withdrawal.[59,185–187] Despite widespread acceptance of the principle of steroid withdrawal in patients with chronic hepatitis C, data are limited on the efficacy of this approach. Rapid withdrawal of steroids,[188] or even no steroids at all,[80] and also a slow tapering of steroids over a prolonged period[189] have all been suggested to prevent aggressive post-orthotopic liver transplantation HCV recurrence. Recently, Fasola *et al.*[190] have retrospectively evaluated the effect of steroids on HCV recurrence (assessed by the degree of fibrosis) at 24 months from transplantation, during recent years. The authors concluded that the shorter intervals and reduced doses of steroids used in recent years, could explain the more aggressive HCV recurrence after transplantation. Our experience is completely the opposite. Randomized controlled trials of steroid withdrawal or of steroid avoidance in HCV-positive transplanted recipients, are needed to fully address these issues.

Existing data show no consistent differences between cyclosporin and tacrolimus-based immunosuppressive regimens in the incidence and severity of post-orthotopic liver transplantation recurrent hepatitis C.[191,192] There does not seem to be any association between the type of triple or double immunosuppressive therapy and the outcome of post-transplant HCV infection. In one study, however, azathioprine

containing regimens were suggested to reduce histological HCV recurrence and delay post-transplant hepatitis C progression.[191] Moreover, in a retrospective analysis of 59 HCV transplant patients who survived at least 12 months, single immunosuppressive therapy *ab initio* (cyclosporin or tacrolimus) was found to be associated with less fibrosis compared with triple or double immunosuppressive regimens.[80] B4 In particular, severe fibrosis or cirrhosis at a median follow up of 24–36 months developed in 17 (37%) of 46 patients treated with triple or double immunosuppressive regimens and in only 1 (6%) of 17 patients treated with a single agent (*P* = 0·01).[80] In an ongoing randomized trial in our center patients transplanted for HCV-related cirrhosis are being treated with tacrolimus monotherapy *ab initio* with no increase in the frequency or severity of histological or treated rejection compared with a triple regimen of tacrolimus azathioprine and prednisolone.[137] Single-agent immunosuppression is possible in liver transplantation.[193]

The influence of azathioprine on the recurrence of hepatitis C has been reported in a few studies. In a retrospective review[194] histological hepatitis C recurrence was seen in 43 of 65 patients, with progression in 19 (fibrosis, = grade 2 at last follow up). Those patients who received azathioprine-containing immunosuppressive regimens experienced less frequent recurrence (6/17 *v* 37/48, *P* < 0·005) and progression (1/17 *v* 18/48, *P* = 0·014) than those who did not receive azathioprine. B4

In a recent review of current advances and potential future therapies for hepatitis C, mycophenolate mofetil was mentioned as a possible antiviral agent because of its ribavirin-like effects.[195] C5

Yet, the impact of mycophenolate mofetil therapy in HCV-positive transplant recipients remains unclear. Jain *et al.*[196] in a randomized controlled trial of 106 HCV-positive patients, using mycophenolate mofetil in conjunction with tacrolimus plus prednisolone found no benefit in term of HCV recurrence rates, graft loss and death. A large controlled trial comparing mycophenolate mofetil with azathioprine in patients given cyclosporin plus prednisolone found a lower prevalence of clinical and histological recurrence of chronic hepatitis C at 6 and 12 months after transplantation (18·5% with mycophenolate mofetil *v* 29·1% with azathioprine).[112] A1a However, another report suggested that mycophenolate mofetil was detrimental, resulting in greater than a three-fold increase in risk of graft failure.[197] Reasons for the potential beneficial effect of mycophenolate mofetil could include a direct effect on HCV versus better suppression of rejection and reduced need of anti-rejection treatment. To evaluate the antiviral effect of mycophenolate mofetil on HCV replication, 30 patients with chronic hepatitis C who had not undergone transplantation, were randomized to treatment with mycophenolate mofetil (2 g/day, 1 g/day, 0·5 g/day or placebo) for 8 weeks. HCV RNA levels and serum transaminase did not change during the study.[198] A1d

Recently, Berenguer *et al.*,[199] in a retrospective evaluation of 554 liver recipients in more than one center, had developed a model based on pre and/or early post-transplantation variables, which may predict severe HCV recurrence. Amongst the evaluated variables, they found that use of OKT3, induction with mycophenolate mofetil and short duration of prednisone (12 months) and azathioprine (< 6 months) therapy had an adverse effect on HCV-related disease progression. B4

Induction immunosuppression (with monoclonal or polyclonal antibody) is not a common practice in liver transplantation, except in recipients with compromised renal function. This therapy given in the perioperative period, allows depletion of circulating lymphocytes and permits the withholding of calcineurin inhibitors. Data from Garcia-Retordillo *et al.*[150] suggest that the use of induction with anti IL-2R monoclonals combined in a protocol without steroids, avoids the early expansion of circulating HCV RNA.

However, at present, the published data from seven studies[140,143,146,148,151–153] do not allow a consensus on the impact of induction monoclonals or polyclonals on HCV recurrence or its severity (see Table 36.5). Limitations of these studies include small numbers, use of a variety of induction agents, lack of comparative study design and variable endpoints.

Thus, further data are needed before definite conclusions for the role of induction on post-transplant HCV recurrence can be drawn. Given that increased immunosuppression is associated with more severe recurrent hepatitis C, and rejection may not need to be treated as aggressively as once believed, the inverse maxim of "less is more" should be followed.

There is no conclusive evidence, but less intense immunosuppression in general appears to be beneficial to patients. This probably applies even more to transplanted HCV-cirrhotic patients than transplanted non-HCV cirrhotic patients.

Chronic ductopenic rejection

Definition

Chronic or ductopenic rejection is mainly an immunologic injury to the allograft and can result in irreversible damage to the bile ducts, arteries and veins. The pathogenetic mechanism is obscure and the role of histocompatibility and viral agents is unclear. Mast cells seem to be important effector cells.[200]

Its incidence at 5 years after transplantation has decreased from 10–15% in the 1980s to 3–5% in current recipients.[201] This may be due to a better recognition and control of acute and early phases of chronic rejection,[202,203] but there may be other reasons such as improvements in preservation solutions.

Clinical and laboratory findings

The natural history is poorly understood. Many cases occur following unresolved acute cellular rejection episodes. Chronic rejection in liver allografts shares risk factors and morphological characteristics with chronic rejection seen in other solid organ transplants but there are also substantial differences. It has a relatively rapid onset, usually within several months, but it can be weeks after transplantation, often following a progressive course. The peak incidence of graft failure from chronic rejection is 2–6 months post-transplantation[204] and it progressively decreases with time. Most cases require re-transplantation within the first year. Chronic rejection presenting after 1 year post-transplantation is "late onset chronic rejection" which presents more insidiously and may have different histological features.[205]

However, despite its progressive course, in most cases it is potentially reversible, a quality that has been attributed to apparently unique immunologic properties and remarkable regenerative capabilities of the liver.[206]

The diagnosis is clinically suspected when a patient develops progressive cholestasis and an increase in canalicular enzymes.[18] The early transition from acute to chronic rejection may be associated with an elevation in AST levels, which along with bilirubin concentrations, are associated with graft failure from chronic rejection. As with acute rejection, the clinical and biochemical manifestations of chronic rejection are non-specific and therefore the diagnosis also requires histological confirmation.

In the study by Theruvath *et al.*, evaluating 924 liver transplants with a median follow up of 66 months, the overall incidence of histologically proved chronic rejection was 2·1%. Primary sclerosing cholangitis and a history of acute rejection were variables associated with an increased risk for development of chronic rejection.[207]

Histopathological features

Two main histologic features are considered diagnostic: damage or loss of small ducts (less than $60 < \mu m$ in diameter) in more than 50% of the portal tracts, and foam cell obliterative arteriopathy of large and medium sized arteries.[18] Recently it as been recognized that distinct early histopathological changes presage disappearance of bile ducts in the form of a parenchymal inflammatory reaction. The early recognition of this "hepatitic" phase[208] may be of fundamental importance. It could indicate the need for increased or altered immunosuppressive therapy. In the past it may have been mistakenly diagnosed as superimposed hepatitis leading to an inappropriate reduction of immunosuppression, which could exacerbate the chronic rejection.

Bile duct loss in more than 50% of portal tracts and absence of necroinflammatory activity, represent late histopathologic changes, the classic textbook description, but

Box 36.1 NIDDK definitions of grades for chronic rejection, and for rejection uncertain for chronicity (indefinite for bile duct loss)[18]

Rejection, uncertain for chronicity (indefinite bile duct loss)

No complicating lobular changes

Lobular changes, including one of the three findings:

- Centrilobular cholestasis, perivenular sclerosis, or hepatocellular ballooning or necrosis or dropout

Chronic rejection[a]

Bile duct loss, without centrilobular cholestasis, perivenular sclerosis, or hepatocyte ballooning or necrosis and dropout

Bile duct loss, with one of the following four findings:

- Centrilobular cholestasis, perivenular sclerosis or hepatocellular ballooning or necrosis and dropout

Bile duct loss, with at least two of the four following findings:

- Centrilobular cholestasis; perivenular sclerosis or hepatocellular ballooning or centrilobular necrosis and dropout

[a]Bile duct loss > 50% of triads.

NIDDK, National Institute of Diabetes, Digestive, and Kidney disease

these changes are late in the evolution of the process and are likely to be irreversible. Diagnosis at this stage may be useful in deciding when to list a patient for re-transplantation; additional immunosuppressive therapy is unlikely to be of any benefit and may do harm by increasing the risk of infection prior to transplantation.

Grading and staging

There is a tentative scheme for grading chronic rejection proposed by the National Institute of Diabetes, Digestive, and Kidney disease[209] (Box 36.1).

Treatment

Treatment is dependent on the stage at which the process is diagnosed. Cases of early chronic rejection may respond to increased dosage of tacrolimus which is the only effective rescue therapy, documented by different centers, resulting in a 70% graft survival at 1-year follow up. Patients who have a serum bilirubin level less than 10 mg/dl at the time of conversion to tacrolimus and who develop chronic rejection more than 90 days after transplantation, have the best response.[94] B4 The combination of mycophenolate mofetil with sirolimus has also been reported in an animal model to be effective in chronic rejection. Sirolimus may help to reduce arterial intimal thickening which is believed to be a pathophysiological root cause of chronic rejection.[210] C5 However, the safety and benefit of sirolimus alone for chronic rejection is currently unknown.

Neff *et al.* in a retrospective review of 21 transplant recipients with clinical and histological diagnosis of chronic rejection treated with sirolimus (0·07 mg/kg) and tacrolimus (serum level 8–10 ng/dl), showed an improvement in the bile duct to hepatic artery ratio and total bilirubin levels. However, a large number of patients experienced drug-related side effects and were unable to tolerate therapy.[211] B4

Re-transplantation remains the best treatment for chronic rejection associated with severe biochemical cholestasis and advanced bile duct loss which is usually unresponsive to immunosuppression. The recurrence rate of chronic rejection is as high as 90%,[212] although it is not clear if some characteristics, for example early re-transplantation are predictive factors for recurrence.

Recently it has been recognized that some cases of advanced chronic rejection have recovered spontaneously, or with the use of additional immunosuppression. In some of these cases, follow up liver biopsies have shown a persistent paucity of bile ducts without other histological features of chronic rejection. Ductopenia has also been noted as an incidental finding in protocol biopsies taken at annual review from patients who are clinically well, with no previous biopsies suggesting chronic rejection. These findings suggest that some patients may suffer permanent duct loss as a result of rejection, but that sufficient ducts remain to allow the graft to function normally. Because of these observations and the risks associated and logistical difficulties with a second transplantation, the decision to re-transplant should only be made when a confident diagnosis of irreversible and progressive graft damage is established.

Acknowledgements

Dr Laura Cecilioni is supported by Hospital S. Orsola-Malpighi, Department of Internal Medicine, University of Bologna, Italy. Dr Lucy Dagher is supported by Fundagastro (Hospital General del Oeste) and Fundayacucho, and Fundacion Vollmer, Caracas-Venezuela.

References

1 Neuberger J, Adams DH. What is the significance of acute liver allograft rejection? *J Hepatol* 1998;**29**:143–50.

2 Abbasoglu O, Levy MF, Brkic BB *et al.* Ten years of liver transplantation: an evolving understanding of late graft loss. *Transplantation* 1997;**64**:1801–7.

3 Gross CR, Malinchoc M, Kim WR *et al.* Quality of life before and after liver transplantation for cholestatic liver disease. *Hepatology* 1999;**29**:356–64.

4 Jain AB, Reyes J, Marcos A *et al.* Pregnancy after liver transplantation with tacrolimus immunosuppression: a single center's experience update at 13 years. *Transplantation* 2003; **76**:827–32.

5   Ratcliffe J, Longworth L, Young T, Bryan S, Burroughs A, Buxton M. Assessing health-related quality of life pre- and post-liver transplantation: a prospective multicenter study. *Liver Transpl* 2002;**8**:263–270.

6   United Network for Organ Sharing. Allocation of livers. 13 October 2000. www.unos.org

7   Gane E, Portmann B, Saxena R, Wong P, Ramage J, Williams R. Nodular regenerative hyperplasia of the liver graft after liver transplantation. *Hepatology* 1994;**20**(1 Pt 1): 88–94.

8   Abouljoud MS, Levy MF, Klintmalm GB. Hyperlipidemia after liver transplantation: long-term results of the FK506/cyclosporine a US Multicenter trial. US Multicenter Study Group. *Transplant Proc* 1995;**27**:1121–1123.

9   Jindal RM, Sidner RA, Milgrom ML. Post-transplant diabetes mellitus. The role of immunosuppression. *Drug Saf* 1997;**16**:242–57.

10 Mor E, Facklam D, Hasse J *et al.* Weight gain and lipid profile changes in liver transplant recipients: long-term results of the American FK506 Multicenter Study. *Transplant Proc* 1995;**27**:1126.

11 Pham H, Lemoine A, Salvucci M *et al.* Occurrence of gammopathies and lymphoproliferative disorders in liver transplant recipients randomized to tacrolimus (FK506)- or cyclosporine-based immunosuppression. *Liver Transpl Surg* 1998;**4**:146–51.

12 Fisher NC, Nightingale PG, Gunson BK, Lipkin GW, Neuberger JM. Chronic renal failure following liver transplantation: a retrospective analysis. *Transplantation* 1998;**66**:59–66.

13 Pelletier RP, Orosz CG, Cosio FG, Ferguson RM. Risk factors in chronic rejection. *Curr Opin Organ Transpl* 1998;**4**: 28–40.

14 Devlin J, Doherty D, Thomson L *et al.* Defining the outcome of immunosuppression withdrawal after liver transplantation. *Hepatology* 1998;**27**:926–33.

15 Mazariegos GV, Reyes J, Marino IR *et al.* Weaning of immunosuppression in liver transplant recipients. *Transplantation* 1997;**63**:243–9.

16 Ramos HC, Reyes J, Abu-Elmagd K *et al.* Weaning of immunosuppression in long-term liver transplant recipients. *Transplantation* 1995;**59**:212–17.

17 Adams DH, Neuberger JM. Patterns of graft rejection following liver transplantation. *J Hepatol* 1990;**10**:113–19.

18 International Working Party. Terminology for hepatic allograft rejection. *Hepatology* 1995;**22**:648–54.

19 Hubscher S. Diagnosis and grading of liver allograft rejection: a European perspective. *Transplant Proc* 1996; **28**:504–7.

20 Prieto M, Berenguer M, Rayon JM *et al.* High incidence of allograft cirrhosis in hepatitis C virus genotype 1b infection following transplantation: relationship with rejection episodes. *Hepatology* 1999;**29**:250–6.

21 Slapak GI, Saxena R, Portmann B *et al.* Graft and systemic disease in long-term survivors of liver transplantation. *Hepatology* 1997;**25**:195–202.

22 Neuberger J. Liver allograft rejection – current concepts on diagnosis and treatment. *J Hepatol* 1995;**23**(Suppl 1): 54–61.

23 Datta GS, Hudson M, Burroughs AK *et al.* Grading of cellular rejection after orthotopic liver transplantation. *Hepatology* 1995;**21**:46–57.

24 Barnes EJ, Abdel-Rehim MM, Goulis Y *et al.* Applications and limitations of blood eosinophilia for the diagnosis of acute cellular rejection in liver transplantation. *Am J Transplant* 2003;**3**:432–8.

25 Aran PP, Bissel MG, Whitington PF, Bostwick DG, Adamac T, Baker AL. Diagnosis of hepatic allograft rejection: role of liver biopsy. *Clin Transplant* 1993;**7**:475–81.

26 Neuberger J, Wilson P, Adams D. Protocol liver biopsies: the case in favour. *Transplant Proc* 1998;**30**:1497–9.

27 Wiesner RH. Is hepatic histology the true gold standard in diagnosing acute hepatic allograft rejection? *Liver Transpl Surg* 1996;**2**:165–7.

28 Demetris AJ, Ruppert K, Dvorchik I *et al.* Real-time monitoring of acute liver-allograft rejection using the Banff schema. *Transplantation* 2002;**74**:1290–6.

29 Ormonde DG, de Boer WB, Kierath A *et al.* Banff schema for grading liver allograft rejection: utility in clinical practice. *Liver Transpl Surg* 1999;**5**:261–8.

30 Wiesner RH, Demetris AJ, Belle SH *et al.* Acute hepatic allograft rejection: incidence, risk factors, and impact on outcome. *Hepatology* 1998;**28**:638–45.

31 Banff schema for grading liver allograft rejection: an international consensus document. *Hepatology* 1997;**25**: 658–63.

32 Bubak ME, Porayko MK, Krom RA, Wiesner RH. Complications of liver biopsy in liver transplant patients: increased sepsis associated with choledochojejunostomy. *Hepatology* 1991;**14**:1063–5.

33 Garcia-Tsao G, Boyer JL. Outpatient liver biopsy: how safe is it? *Ann Intern Med* 1993;**118**:150–3.

34 Larson AM, Chan GC, Wartelle CF *et al.* Infection complicating percutaneous liver biopsy in liver transplant recipients. *Hepatology* 1997;**26**:1406–9.

35 Papatheodoridis GV, Patch D, Watkinson A, Tibballs J, Burroughs AK. Transjugular liver biopsy in the 1990s: a 2-year audit. *Aliment Pharmacol Ther* 1999;**13**:603–8.

36 Klintmalm GB, Nery JR, Husberg BS, Gonwa TA, Tillery GW. Rejection in liver transplantation. *Hepatology* 1989; **10**:978–85.

37 Williams JW, Peters TG, Vera SR, Britt LG, van Voorst SJ, Haggitt RC. Biopsy-directed immunosuppression following hepatic transplantation in man. *Transplantation* 1985;**39**: 589–96.

38 Bartlett AS, Ramadas R, Furness S, Gane E, McCall JL. The natural history of acute histologic rejection without biochemical graft dysfunction in orthotopic liver transplantation: A systematic review. *Liver Transpl* 2002; **8**:1147–53.

39 Burroughs AK, Patch DW, Stigliano R, Cecilioni L. Protocol liver biopsy in liver transplantation. *Liver Transpl* 2003; **9**:780–1.

40 Tisone G, Orlando G, Vennarecci G *et al.* Spontaneous resolution of severe acute rejection in liver transplantation. *Transplant Proc* 1999;**31**:3164–6.

41 Tippner C, Nashan B, Hoshino K *et al.* Clinical and subclinical acute rejection early after liver transplantation:

contributing factors and relevance for the long-term course. *Transplantation* 2001;**72**:1122–8.

42 Wiesner RH, Goldstein RM, Donovan JP, Miller CM, Lake JR, Lucey MR. The impact of cyclosporine dose and level on acute rejection and patient and graft survival in liver transplant recipients. *Liver Transpl Surg* 1998;**4**:34–41.

43 Dousset B, Conti F, Cherruau B *et al.* Is acute rejection deleterious to long-term liver allograft function? *J Hepatol* 1998;**29**:660–8.

44 McVicar JP, Kowdley KV, Bacchi CE *et al.* The natural history of untreated focal allograft rejection in liver transplant recipients. *Liver Transpl Surg* 1996;**2**: 154–60.

45 Fisher LR, Henley KS, Lucey MR. Acute cellular rejection after liver transplantation: variability, morbidity, and mortality. *Liver Transpl Surg* 1995;**1**:10–15.

46 Mor E, Gonwa TA, Husberg BS, Goldstein RM, Klintmalm GB. Late-onset acute rejection in orthotopic liver transplantation – associated risk factors and outcome. *Transplantation* 1992;**54**:821–4.

47 Anand AC, Hubscher SG, Gunson BK, McMaster P, Neuberger JM. Timing, significance, and prognosis of late acute liver allograft rejection. *Transplantation* 1995;**60**: 1098–103.

48 Neuberger J. Incidence, timing, and risk factors for acute and chronic rejection. *Liver Transpl Surg* 1999;**5**(4 Suppl 1): S30–S36.

49 Wiesner R, Demetris A, Seabera E. Chronic allograft rejection: defining clinical risk factors and assessing impact on graft outcome [Abstract]. *Hepatology* 1998;(4 Pt 2): 314A.

50 Hayashi M, Keeffe EB, Krams SM *et al.* Allograft rejection after liver transplantation for autoimmune liver diseases. *Liver Transpl Surg* 1998;**4**:208–14.

51 Berlakovich GA, Rockenschaub S, Taucher S, Kaserer K, Muhlbacher F, Steiniger R. Underlying disease as a predictor for rejection after liver transplantation. *Arch Surg* 1998;**133**: 167–72.

52 Farges O, Saliba F, Farhamant H *et al.* Incidence of rejection and infection after liver transplantation as a function of the primary disease: possible influence of alcohol and polyclonal immunoglobulins. *Hepatology* 1996;**23**:240–8.

53 Adams DH, Hubscher SG, Neuberger JM, McMaster P, Elias E, Buckels JA. Reduced incidence of rejection in patients undergoing liver transplantation for chronic hepatitis B. *Transplant Proc* 1991;**23**(1 Pt 2):1436–7.

54 Gomez-Manero N, Herrero JI, Quiroga J *et al.* Prognostic model for early acute rejection after liver transplantation. *Liver Transpl* 2001;**7**:246–54.

55 Cecilioni L, Stigliano R, Patch D, Quaglia A, Burroughs A. Predictive factors for the absence of cellular rejection after liver transplantation in a protocol biopsy population [Abstract]. American Association for the Study of Liver Diseases (54th Meeting) *Hepatology* 2003;**38**(Suppl 1): 379A.

56 Van Thiel Dh. Past, present and future in liver transplantation. In: Maddrey WC (ed). *Transplantation of the liver.* New York: 1998.

57 Ascher N. Rejection of the transplanted liver. In: *Transplantation of the liver, 2nd edn.* Norwalk: Appleton and Lange, 1995.

58 Margarit C, Martinez IV, Tormo R, Infante D, Iglesias H. Maintenance immunosuppression without steroids in pediatric liver transplantation. *Transplant Proc* 1989;**21** (1 Pt 2):2230–1.

59 Belli LS, de Carlis L, Rondinara G *et al.* Early cyclosporine monotherapy in liver transplantation: a 5-year follow-up of a prospective, randomized trial. *Hepatology* 1998;**27**: 1524–9.

60 Fraser GM, Grammoustianos K, Reddy J, Rolles K, Davidson B, Burroughs AK. Long-term immunosuppression without corticosteroids after orthotopic liver transplantation: a positive therapeutic aim. *Liver Transpl Surg* 1996;**2**:411–17.

61 Padbury RT, Gunson BK, Dousset B *et al.* Steroid withdrawal from long-term immunosuppression in liver allograft recipients. *Transplantation* 1993;**55**:789–94.

62 Gomez R, Moreno E, Colina F *et al.* Steroid withdrawal is safe and beneficial in stable cyclosporine-treated liver transplant patients. *J Hepatol* 1998;**28**:150–6.

63 McDiarmid SV, Farmer DA, Goldstein LI *et al.* A randomized prospective trial of steroid withdrawal after liver transplantation. *Transplantation* 1995;**60**(12): 1443–50.

64 Punch JD, Shieck VL, Campbell DA, Bromberg JS, Turcotte JG, Merion RM. Corticosteroid withdrawal after liver transplantation. *Surgery* 1995;**118**:783–6.

65 Stegall MD, Everson GT, Schroter G *et al.* Prednisone withdrawal late after adult liver transplantation reduces diabetes, hypertension, and hypercholesterolemia without causing graft loss. *Hepatology* 1997;**25**:173–7.

66 Tchervenkov JI, Tector AJ, Cantarovich M *et al.* Maintenance immunosuppression using cyclosporine monotherapy in adult orthotopic liver transplant recipients. *Transplant Proc* 1996;**28**:2247–9.

67 Belli LS, Alberti AB, Rondinara GF *et al.* Early ribavirin treatment and avoidance of corticosteroids in hepatitis C virus (HCV)-positive liver transplant recipients: interim report of a prospective randomized trial. *Transplant Proc* 2001;**33**(1–2):1353–4.

68 Ringe B, Braun F, Schutz E *et al.* A novel management strategy of steroid-free immunosuppression after liver transplantation: efficacy and safety of tacrolimus and mycophenolate mofetil. *Transplantation* 2001;**71**:508–15.

69 Rolles K, Davidson BR, Burroughs AK. A pilot study of immunosuppressive monotherapy in liver transplantation: tacrolimus versus microemulsified cyclosporin. *Transplantation* 1999;**68**:1195–8.

70 Greig P, Lilly L, Scudamore C *et al.* Early steroid withdrawal after liver transplantation: The Canadian tacrolimus versus microemulsion cyclosporin a trial: 1-year follow-up. *Liver Transpl* 2003;**9**:587–95.

71 Samuel D, Boillot O, Calmus Y *et al.* Steroid withdrawal at day 14 is not satisfactory after liver transplantation: a placebo controlled study [Abstract]. 9th Congress of the International Liver Transplantation Society (ILTS), Barcelona, 2003.

72 Llado L, Figueras J, Torras J *et al.* Immunosuppression without steroids in liver transplantation is safe and reduces infectious and metabolic complications [Abstract]. 9th Congress of the International Liver Transplantation Society (ILTS), Barcelona, 2003.

73 Boillot O, Mayer AD, Boudjema K. Effective and safe steroid-free immunosuppression with a tacrolimus/ daclizumab regimen after liver transplantation [Abstract]. *Am J Transplant* 2003;**3**(Suppl 5):324.

74 Neuberger J. Recurrent primary biliary cirrhosis. *Liver Transpl* 2003;**9**:539–46.

75 Levitsky J, Hart J, Cohen SM, Te HS. The effect of immunosuppressive regimens on the recurrence of primary biliary cirrhosis after liver transplantation. *Liver Transpl* 2003; **9**:733–6.

76 Pirenne J, Aerts R, Koshiba T *et al.* Steroid-free immunosuppression during and after liver transplantation – a 3-yr follow-up report. *Clin Transplant* 2003;**17**:177–82.

77 Takatsuki M, Uemoto S, Inomata Y *et al.* Weaning of immunosuppression in living donor liver transplant recipients. *Transplantation* 2001;**72**:449–54.

78 Bird GL, Smith H, Portmann B, Alexander GJ, Williams R. Acute liver decompensation on withdrawal of cytotoxic chemotherapy and immunosuppressive therapy in hepatitis B carriers. *Q J Med* 1989;**73**:895–902.

79 Cakaloglu Y, Devlin J, O'Grady J *et al.* Importance of concomitant viral infection during late acute liver allograft rejection. *Transplantation* 1995;**59**:40–5.

80 Papatheodoridis GV, Davies S, Dhillon AP *et al.* The role of different immunosuppression in the long-term histological outcome of HCV reinfection after liver transplantation for HCV cirrhosis. *Transplantation* 2001;**72**:412–18.

81 Trotter JF, Wachs M, Bak T *et al.* Liver transplantation using sirolimus and minimal corticosteroids (3-day taper). *Liver Transpl* 2001;**7**:343–51.

82 Jain AB, Kashyap R, Rakela J, Starzl TE, Fung JJ. Primary adult liver transplantation under tacrolimus: more than 90 months actual follow-up survival and adverse events. *Liver Transpl Surg* 1999;**5**:144–50.

83 Denton MD, Magee CC, Sayegh MH. Immunosuppressive strategies in transplantation. *Lancet* 1999;**353**:1083–91.

84 Margarit C, Rimola A, Gonzalez-Pinto I *et al.* Efficacy and safety of oral low-dose tacrolimus treatment in liver transplantation. *Transpl Int* 1998;**11**(Suppl 1): S260–S266.

85 European FK. Randomised trial comparing tacrolimus (FK506) and cyclosporin in prevention of liver allograft rejection. *Lancet* 1994;**344**:423–8.

86 The US Multicenter FK506 Liver Study Group. A comparison of tacrolimus (FK 506) and cyclosporine for immunosuppression in liver transplantation. *N Engl J Med* 1994;**331**:1110–15.

87 Fung JJ, Eliasziw M, Todo S *et al.* The Pittsburgh randomized trial of tacrolimus compared to cyclosporine for hepatic transplantation. *J Am Coll Surg* 1996;**183**:117–25.

88 Starzl TE, Donner A, Eliasziw M *et al.* Randomised trialomania? The multicentre liver transplant trials of tacrolimus. *Lancet* 1995;**346**:1346–50.

89 Morris RE, Brown BW Jr. Tacrolimus for prevention of liver allograft rejection: clinical trials and tribulations. *Lancet* 1995;**346**:1310–11.

90 Wiesner RH. A long-term comparison of tacrolimus (FK506) versus cyclosporine in liver transplantation: a report of the United States FK506 Study Group. *Transplantation* 1998;**66**:493–9.

91 Pichlmayr R, Winkler M, Neuhaus P *et al.* Three-year follow-up of the European Multicenter Tacrolimus (FK506) Liver Study. *Transplant Proc* 1997;**29**:2499–502.

92 Williams R, Neuhaus P, Bismuth H *et al.* Two-year data from the European multicentre tacrolimus (FK506) liver study. *Transpl Int* 1996;**9**(Suppl 1):S144–S150.

93 Trull AK, Tan KK, Tan L, Alexander GJ, Jamieson NV. Absorption of cyclosporin from conventional and new microemulsion oral formulations in liver transplant recipients with external biliary diversion. *Br J Clin Pharmacol* 1995;**39**:627–31.

94 Sher LS, Cosenza CA, Michel J *et al.* Efficacy of tacrolimus as rescue therapy for chronic rejection in orthotopic liver transplantation: a report of the US Multicenter Liver Study Group. *Transplantation* 1997;**64**: 258–63.

95 Perico N, Remuzzi G. Prevention of transplant rejection: current treatment guidelines and future developments. *Drugs* 1997;**54**:533–70.

96 Noble S, Markham A. Cyclosporin. A review of the pharmacokinetic properties, clinical efficacy and tolerability of a microemulsion-based formulation (Neoral). *Drugs* 1995;**50**:924–41.

97 Holt DW, Johnston A. Monitoring new immunosuppressive agents. Are the methods adequate? *Drug Metabol Drug Interact* 1997;**14**:5–15.

98 Hemming AW, Greig PD, Cattral MS *et al.* A microemulsion of cyclosporine without intravenous cyclosporine in liver transplantation. *Transplantation* 1996;**62**:1798–802.

99 Graziadei IW, Wiesner RH, Marotta PJ *et al.* Long-term results of patients undergoing liver transplantation for primary sclerosing cholangitis. *Hepatology* 1999;**30**: 1121–7.

100 Freise CE, Galbraith CA, Nikolai BJ *et al.* Risks associated with conversion of stable patients after liver transplantation to the microemulsion formulation of cyclosporine. *Transplantation* 1998;**65**:995–7.

101 Stegall MD, Wachs ME, Everson G *et al.* Prednisone withdrawal 14 days after liver transplantation with mycophenolate: a prospective trial of cyclosporine and tacrolimus. *Transplantation* 1997;**64**:1755–60.

102 Fisher RA, Ham JM, Marcos A *et al.* A prospective randomized trial of mycophenolate mofetil with Neoral or tacrolimus after orthotopic liver transplantation. *Transplantation* 1998;**66**:1616–21.

103 O'Grady JG, Burroughs A, Hardy P, Elbourne D, Truesdale A. Tacrolimus versus microemulsified cyclosporin in liver transplantation: the TMC randomised controlled trial. *Lancet* 2002;**360**:1119–25.

104 Levy G, Burra P, Cavallari A *et al.* Improved clinical outcomes for liver transplant recipients using cyclosporine

monitoring based on 2-hr post-dose levels (C2). *Transplantation* 2002;**73**:953–9.

105 Villamil F, Ericzon BG, Risaliti A *et al.* Efficacy and safety of cyclosporine microemulsion with C2 monitoring versus tacrolimus in de novo liver transplant recipients [Abstract]. 9th Congress of the International Liver Transplantation Society (ILTS), Barcelona, 2003.

106 Levy GA, Lilly L, Grant D *et al.* Once daily dosing with Neoral C2 monitoring in maintenance liver transplant patients [Abstract]. *Am J Transplant* 2003;**3**(Suppl 5): 422–3.

107 Levy G, Thervet E, Lake J, Uchida K. Patient management by Neoral C monitoring: an international consensus statement. *Transplantation* 2002;**73**(9 Suppl):S12–S18.

108 Klintmalm GB, Gibbs JF, McMillan R *et al.* Rejection: FK 506 for rescue or maintenance. *Transplant Proc* 1993; **25**:1914–15.

109 Millis JM, Woodle ES, Piper JB *et al.* Tacrolimus for primary treatment of steroid-resistant hepatic allograft rejection. *Transplantation* 1996;**61**:1365–9.

110 Venkataramanan R, Shaw LM, Sarkozi L *et al.* Clinical utility of monitoring tacrolimus blood concentrations in liver transplant patients. *J Clin Pharmacol* 2001;**41**:542–51.

111 Osborne J, Heller M, Forman L. Tacrolimus level/dose ratio is significantly higher in hepatitis C liver transplant recipient: impact on cost [Abstract]. *Hepatology* 2003;**38** (4 Suppl 1):228A.

112 Wiesner R, Rabkin J, Klintmalm G *et al.* A randomized double-blind comparative study of mycophenolate mofetil and azathioprine in combination with cyclosporine and corticosteroids in primary liver transplant recipients. *Liver Transpl* 2001;**7**:442–50.

113 Fulton B, Markham A. Mycophenolate mofetil. A review of its pharmacodynamic and pharmacokinetic properties and clinical efficacy in renal transplantation. *Drugs* 1996;**51**: 278–98.

114 Schmouder RL. Immunosuppressive therapies for the twenty-first century. *Transplant Proc* 2000;**32**:1463–7.

115 Stewart SF, Hudson M, Talbot D, Manas D, Day CP. Mycophenolate mofetil monotherapy in liver transplantation. *Lancet* 2001;**357**:609–10.

116 Schlitt HJ, Barkmann A, Boker KH *et al.* Replacement of calcineurin inhibitors with mycophenolate mofetil in liver-transplant patients with renal dysfunction: a randomised controlled study. *Lancet* 2001;**357**:587–91.

117 Raimondo ML, Dagher L, Papatheodoridis GV *et al.* Long-term mycophenolate mofetil monotherapy in combination with calcineurin inhibitors for chronic renal dysfunction after liver transplantation. *Transplantation* 2003;**75**: 186–90.

118 Neuhaus P, Klupp J, Langrehr JM. mTOR inhibitors: an overview. *Liver Transpl* 2001;**7**:473–84.

119 Sehgal SN. Rapamune (RAPA, rapamycin, sirolimus): mechanism of action immunosuppressive effect results from blockade of signal transduction and inhibition of cell cycle progression. *Clin Biochem* 1998;**31**:335–40.

120 Murgia MG, Jordan S, Kahan BD. The side effect profile of sirolimus: a phase I study in quiescent cyclosporine-prednisone-treated renal transplant patients. *Kidney Int* 1996;**49**:209–16.

121 Bererhi L, Flamant M, Martinez F, Karras A, Thervet E, Legendre C. Rapamycin-induced oligospermia. *Transplantation* 2003;**76**:885–6.

122 Watson CJ, Friend PJ, Jamieson NV *et al.* Sirolimus: a potent new immunosuppressant for liver transplantation. *Transplantation* 1999;**67**:505–9.

123 McAlister VC, Peltekian KM, Malatjalian DA *et al.* Orthotopic liver transplantation using low-dose tacrolimus and sirolimus. *Liver Transpl* 2001;**7**:701–8.

124 Pridohl O, Heinemann K, Hartwig T *et al.* Low-dose immunosuppression with FK 506 and sirolimus after liver transplantation: 1-year results. *Transplant Proc* 2001;**33**: 3229–31.

125 McAlister VC, Gao Z, Peltekian K, Domingues J, Mahalati K, MacDonald AS. Sirolimus-tacrolimus combination immunosuppression. *Lancet* 2000;**355**:376–7.

126 Dunkelberg JC, Trotter JF, Wachs M *et al.* Sirolimus as primary immunosuppression in liver transplantation is not associated with hepatic artery or wound complications. *Liver Transpl* 2003;**9**:463–8.

127 Wyeth Ayerst Pharmaceuticals. Data File, 2002.

128 Heffron TG, Smallwood GA, Davis L, Martinez E, Stieber AC. Sirolimus-based immunosuppressive protocol for calcineurin sparing in liver transplantation. *Transplant Proc* 2002;**34**:1522–3.

129 Chang GJ, Mahanty HD, Quan D *et al.* Experience with the use of sirolimus in liver transplantation – use in patients for whom calcineurin inhibitors are contraindicated. *Liver Transpl* 2000;**6**:734–40.

130 Nishida S, Pinna A, Verzaro R *et al.* Sirolimus (rapamycin)-based rescue treatment following chronic rejection after liver transplantation. *Transplant Proc* 2001;**33**:1495.

131 Nair S, Eason J, Loss G. Sirolimus monotherapy in nephrotoxicity due to calcineurin inhibitors in liver transplant recipients. *Liver Transpl* 2003;**9**:126–9.

132 Fairbanks KD, Eustace JA, Fine D, Thuluvath PJ. Renal function improves in liver transplant recipients when switched from a calcineurin inhibitor to sirolimus. *Liver Transpl* 2003;**9**:1079–85.

133 Wall WJ. Use of antilymphocyte induction therapy in liver transplantation. *Liver Transpl Surg* 1999;**5**(4 Suppl 1): S64–S70.

134 Langrehr JM, Nussler NC, Neumann U *et al.* A prospective randomized trial comparing interleukin-2 receptor antibody versus antithymocyte globulin as part of a quadruple immunosuppressive induction therapy following orthotopic liver transplantation. *Transplantation* 1997;**63**: 1772–81.

135 Eason JD, Nair S, Cohen AJ, Blazek JL, Loss GE Jr. Steroid-free liver transplantation using rabbit antithymocyte globulin and early tacrolimus monotherapy. *Transplantation* 2003;**75**:1396–9.

136 Eason JD, Nair S, Cohen AJ, Blazek JL, Loss GE Jr. Steroid-free liver transplantation using rabbit antithymocyte globulin induction: results of a prospective randomized trial. *Liver Transpl* 2001;**7**:693–7.

137 Mela M, Raimondo ML, Quaglia A *et al.* Randomised trial of tacrolimus monotherapy versus tacrolimus/prednisolone/azathioprine in liver transplantation for HCV cirrhosis: early rejection rates [Abstract]. *J Hepatol* 2003; **38**(S2):44.

138 Starzl TE, Murase N, Abu-Elmagd K *et al.* Tolerogenic immunosuppression for organ transplantation. *Lancet* 2003;**361**:1502–10.

139 Kupiec-Weglinski JW, Diamantstein T, Tilney NL. Interleukin 2 receptor-targeted therapy – rationale and applications in organ transplantation. *Transplantation* 1988;**46**:785–92.

140 Eckhoff DE, McGuire B, Sellers M *et al.* The safety and efficacy of a two-dose daclizumab (zenapax) induction therapy in liver transplant recipients. *Transplantation* 2000;**69**:1867–72.

141 Emre S, Gondolesi G, Polat K *et al.* Use of daclizumab as initial immunosuppression in liver transplant recipients with impaired renal function. *Liver Transpl* 2001;**7**:220–5.

142 Heffron TG, Smallwood GA, de Vera ME, Davis L, Martinez E, Stieber AC. Daclizumab induction in liver transplant recipients. *Transplant Proc* 2001;**33**:1527.

143 Hirose R, Roberts JP, Quan D *et al.* Experience with daclizumab in liver transplantation: renal transplant dosing without calcineurin inhibitors is insufficient to prevent acute rejection in liver transplantation. *Transplantation* 2000;**69**:307–11.

144 Markus BH, Weber S, Allers C, Hauser I, Encke A. Daclizumab induction therapy in combination with tacrolimus. *Transplant Proc* 2001;**33**:1418–19.

145 Nelson DR, Soldevila-Pico C, Reed A *et al.* Anti-interleukin-2 receptor therapy in combination with mycophenolate mofetil is associated with more severe hepatitis C recurrence after liver transplantation. *Liver Transpl* 2001;**7**:1064–70.

146 Calmus Y, Scheele JR, Gonzalez-Pinto I *et al.* Immunoprophylaxis with basiliximab, a chimeric anti-interleukin-2 receptor monoclonal antibody, in combination with azathioprine-containing triple therapy in liver transplant recipients. *Liver Transpl* 2002;**8**:123–31.

147 Otto MG, Mayer AD, Clavien PA, Cavallari A, Gunawardena KA, Mueller EA. Randomized trial of cyclosporine microemulsion (neoral) versus conventional cyclosporine in liver transplantation: MILTON study. Multicentre International Study in Liver Transplantation of Neoral. *Transplantation* 1998;**66**:1632–40.

148 Neuhaus P, Clavien PA, Kittur D *et al.* Improved treatment response with basiliximab immunoprophylaxis after liver transplantation: results from a double-blind randomized placebo-controlled trial. *Liver Transpl* 2002; **8**:132–42.

149 Petrovic LM, Villamil FG, Vierling JM, Makowka L, Geller SA. Comparison of histopathology in acute allograft rejection and recurrent hepatitis C infection after liver transplantation. *Liver Transpl Surg* 1997;**3**:398–406.

150 Garcia R, Forns X, Feliu A *et al.* Hepatitis C virus kinetics during and immediately after liver transplantation. *Hepatology* 2002;**35**:680–7.

151 Yan LN, Wang W, Li B *et al.* Single-dose daclizumab induction therapy in patients with liver transplantation. *World J Gastroenterol* 2003;**9**:1881–3.

152 Washburn K, Speeg KV, Esterl R *et al.* Steroid elimination 24 hours after liver transplantation using daclizumab, tacrolimus, and mycophenolate mofetil. *Transplantation* 2001;**72**:1675–9.

153 Eason JD, Nair S, Cohen AJ, Blazek JL, Loss GE Jr. Steroid-free liver transplantation using rabbit antithymocyte globulin and early tacrolimus monotherapy. *Transplantation* 2003;**75**:1396–9.

154 Calne R. "Almost tolerance" in the clinic. *Transplant Proc* 1998;**30**:3846–8.

155 Calne R, Friend P, Moffatt S *et al.* Prope tolerance, perioperative campath 1H, and low-dose cyclosporin monotherapy in renal allograft recipients. *Lancet* 1998; **351**:1701–2.

156 Tzakis AG, Kato T, Nishida S *et al.* Alemtuzumab (Campath-1H) combined with tacrolimus in intestinal and multivisceral transplantation. *Transplantation* 2003;**75**: 1512–17.

157 Tzakis A, Madariaga JR, Tryphonopoulos P, Nishida S, Levi DM, DeFaria W. Campath 1H with tacrolimus immunosuppression in adult liver allotransplantation: our experience with 19 cases [Abstract]. *Am J Transplant* 2003;**3**(Suppl 5):326.

158 Angulo P, Batts KP, Therneau TM, Jorgensen RA, Dickson ER, Lindor KD. Long-term ursodeoxycholic acid delays histological progression in primary biliary cirrhosis. *Hepatology* 1999;**29**:644–7.

159 Lindor KD, Therneau TM, Jorgensen RA, Malinchoc M, Dickson ER. Effects of ursodeoxycholic acid on survival in patients with primary biliary cirrhosis. *Gastroenterology* 1996;**110**:1515–18.

160 Calmus Y, Gane P, Rouger P, Poupon R. Hepatic expression of class I and class II major histocompatibility complex molecules in primary biliary cirrhosis: effect of ursodeoxycholic acid. *Hepatology* 1990;**11**:12–15.

161 Calmus Y, Arvieux C, Gane P *et al.* Cholestasis induces major histocompatibility complex class I expression in hepatocytes. *Gastroenterology* 1992;**102**(4 Pt 1):1371–7.

162 Keiding S, Hockerstedt K, Bjoro K *et al.* The Nordic multicenter double-blind randomized controlled trial of prophylactic ursodeoxycholic acid in liver transplant patients. *Transplantation* 1997;**63**:1591–4.

163 Fleckenstein JF, Paredes M, Thuluvath PJ. A prospective, randomized, double-blind trial evaluating the efficacy of ursodeoxycholic acid in prevention of liver transplant rejection. *Liver Transpl Surg* 1998;**4**:276–9.

164 Pageaux GP, Blanc P, Perrigault PF *et al.* Failure of ursodeoxycholic acid to prevent acute cellular rejection after liver transplantation. *J Hepatol* 1995;**23**:119–22.

165 Barnes D, Talenti D, Cammell G *et al.* A randomized clinical trial of ursodeoxycholic acid as adjuvant treatment to prevent liver transplant rejection. *Hepatology* 1997;**26**:853–7.

166 Angelico M, Tisone G, Baiocchi L *et al.* One-year pilot study on tauroursodeoxycholic acid as an adjuvant

treatment after liver transplantation. *Ital J Gastroenterol Hepatol* 1999;**31**:462–8.

167 Minguez C, Mazuecos A, Ceballos M, Tejuca F, Rivero M. Worsening of renal function in a renal transplant patient treated with granulocyte colony-stimulating factor. *Nephrol Dial Transplant* 1995;**10**:2166–7.

168 Foster PF, Mital D, Sankary HN *et al.* The use of granulocyte colony-stimulating factor after liver transplantation. *Transplantation* 1995;**59**:1557–63.

169 Foster PF, Kociss K, Shen J *et al.* Granulocyte colony-stimulating factor immunomodulation in the rat cardiac transplantation model. *Transplantation* 1996;**61**:1122–5.

170 Imagawa DK, Millis JM, Olthoff KM *et al.* The role of tumor necrosis factor in allograft rejection. I. Evidence that elevated levels of tumor necrosis factor-alpha predict rejection following orthotopic liver transplantation. *Transplantation* 1990;**50**:219–25.

171 Winston DJ, Foster PF, Somberg KA *et al.* Randomized, placebo-controlled, double-blind, multicenter trial of efficacy and safety of granulocyte colony-stimulating factor in liver transplant recipients. *Transplantation* 1999;**68**: 1298–304.

172 Brazelton TR, Morris RE. Molecular mechanisms of action of new xenobiotic immunosuppressive drugs: tacrolimus (FK506), sirolimus (rapamycin), mycophenolate mofetil and leflunomide. *Curr Opin Immunol* 1996;**8**:710–20.

173 Smiley ST, Csizmadia V, Gao W, Turka LA, Hancock WW. Differential effects of cyclosporine A, methylprednisolone, mycophenolate, and rapamycin on CD154 induction and requirement for NFkappaB: implications for tolerance induction. *Transplantation* 2000;**70**:415–19.

174 Nashan B. Early clinical experience with a novel rapamycin derivative. *Ther Drug Monit* 2002;**24**:53–8.

175 Majewski M, Korecka M, Kossev P *et al.* The immunosuppressive macrolide RAD inhibits growth of human Epstein-Barr virus-transformed B lymphocytes in vitro and in vivo: A potential approach to prevention and treatment of posttransplant lymphoproliferative disorders. *Proc Natl Acad Sci USA* 2000;**97**:4285–90.

176 Williams JW, Mital D, Chong A *et al.* Experiences with leflunomide in solid organ transplantation. *Transplantation* 2002;**73**:358–66.

177 Jin MB, Nakayama M, Ogata T *et al.* A novel leflunomide derivative, FK778, for immunosuppression after kidney transplantation in dogs. *Surgery* 2002;**132**:72–9.

178 Pinschewer DD, Ochsenbein AF, Odermatt B, Brinkmann V, Hengartner H, Zinkernagel RM. FTY720 immunosuppression impairs effector T cell peripheral homing without affecting induction, expansion, and memory. *J Immunol* 2000;**164**:5761–70.

179 Vincenti F. What's in the pipeline? New immunosuppressive drugs in transplantation. *Am J Transplant* 2002;**2**:898–903.

180 Budde K, Schmouder RL, Brunkhorst R *et al.* First human trial of FTY720, a novel immunomodulator, in stable renal transplant patients. *J Am Soc Nephrol* 2002;**13**:1073–83.

181 Papatheodoridis GV, Patch D, Dusheiko GM, Burroughs AK. The outcome of hepatitis C virus infection after liver transplantation – is it influenced by the type of immunosuppression? *J Hepatol* 1999;**30**:731–8.

182 Collier J, Heathcote J. Hepatitis C viral infection in the immunosuppressed patient. *Hepatology* 1998;**27**:2–6.

183 Teixeira R, Papatheodoridis GV, Burroughs AK. Management of recurrent hepatitis C after liver transplantation. *J Viral Hepat* 2001;**8**:159–68.

184 Berenguer M, Ferrell L, Watson J *et al.* HCV-related fibrosis progression following liver transplantation: increase in recent years. *J Hepatol* 2000;**32**:673–84.

185 Burroughs AK. Posttransplantation prevention and treatment of recurrent hepatitis C. *Liver Transpl* 2000;**6** (6 Suppl 2):S35–S40.

186 Everson GT, Trouillot T, Wachs M *et al.* Early steroid withdrawal in liver transplantation is safe and beneficial. *Liver Transpl Surg* 1999;**5**(4 Suppl 1):S48–S57.

187 Gane EJ, Naoumov NV, Qian KP *et al.* A longitudinal analysis of hepatitis C virus replication following liver transplantation. *Gastroenterology* 1996;**110**:167–77.

188 Mueller AR, Platz K, Willimski C *et al.* Influence of immunosuppression on patient survival after liver transplantation for hepatitis C. *Transplant Proc* 2001;**33**: 1347–9.

189 Brillanti S, Vivarelli M, De Ruvo N *et al.* Slowly tapering off steroids protects the graft against hepatitis C recurrence after liver transplantation. *Liver Transpl* 2002;**8**:884–8.

190 Fasola CG, Netto GJ, Onaca N *et al.* A more severe hepatitis C recurrence (HCVR) post liver transplantation (OLT) observed in recent years may be explained by the use of lower-dose corticosteroid (CS) maintenance protocols [Abstract]. *Hepatology* 2003;**38**(4 Suppl 1):226A.

191 Zervos XA, Weppler D, Fragulidis GP *et al.* Comparison of tacrolimus with microemulsion cyclosporine as primary immunosuppression in hepatitis C patients after liver transplantation. *Transplantation* 1998;**65**:1044–6.

192 Feray C, Shouval D, Samuel D. Will transplantation of an hepatitis C-infected graft improve the outcome of liver transplantation in HCV patients? *Gastroenterology* 1999; **117**:263–5.

193 Raimondo ML, Burroughs AK. Single-agent immunosuppression after liver transplantation: what is possible? *Drugs* 2002;**62**:1587–97.

194 Hunt J, Gordon FD, Lewis WD *et al.* Histological recurrence and progression of hepatitis C after orthotopic liver transplantation: influence of immunosuppressive regimens. *Liver Transpl* 2001;**7**:1056–63.

195 Di Bisceglie AM, McHutchison J, Rice CM. New therapeutic strategies for hepatitis C. *Hepatology* 2002; **35**:224–31.

196 Jain A, Kashyap R, Demetris AJ, Eghstesad B, Pokharna R, Fung JJ. A prospective randomized trial of mycophenolate mofetil in liver transplant recipients with hepatitis C. *Liver Transpl* 2002;**8**:40–6.

197 Burak KW, Kremers WK, Batts KP *et al.* Impact of cytomegalovirus infection, year of transplantation, and donor age on outcomes after liver transplantation for hepatitis C. *Liver Transpl* 2002;**8**:362–9.

198 Firpi RJ, Nelson DR, Davis GL. Lack of antiviral effect of a short course of mycophenolate mofetil in patients with chronic hepatitis C virus infection. *Liver Transpl* 2003;**9**:57–61.

199 Berenguer M, Crippin J, Gish R *et al.* A model to predict severe HCV-related disease following liver transplantation. *Hepatology* 2003;**38**:34–41.

200 O'Keeffe C, Baird AW, Nolan N, McCormick PA. Mast cell hyperplasia in chronic rejection after liver transplantation. *Liver Transpl* 2002;**8**:50–7.

201 Demetris AJ, Murase N, Lee RG *et al.* Chronic rejection. A general overview of histopathology and pathophysiology with emphasis on liver, heart and intestinal allografts. *Ann Transplant* 1997;**2**:27–44.

202 Freese DK, Snover DC, Sharp HL, Gross CR, Savick SK, Payne WD. Chronic rejection after liver transplantation: a study of clinical, histopathological and immunological features. *Hepatology* 1991;**13**:882–91.

203 Hubscher SG, Buckels JA, Elias E, McMaster P, Neuberger J. Vanishing bile-duct syndrome following liver transplantation – is it reversible? *Transplantation* 1991;**51**: 1004–10.

204 Lowes JR, Hubscher SG, Neuberger JM. Chronic rejection of the liver allograft. *Gastroenterol Clin North Am* 1993; **22**:401–20.

205 Kemnitz J, Gubernatis G, Bunzendahl H, Ringe B, Pichlmayr R, Georgii A. Criteria for the histopathological classification of liver allograft rejection and their clinical relevance. *Transplant Proc* 1989;**21**(1 Pt 2):2208–10.

206 Blakolmer K, Seaberg EC, Batts K *et al.* Analysis of the reversibility of chronic liver allograft rejection implications for a staging schema. *Am J Surg Pathol* 1999;**23**:1328–39.

207 Theruvath T, Neumann U, Langrehr JM, Tullius SG, Neuhaus P. Risk factors for chronic rejection after liver transplantation [Abstract]. 9th Congress of the International Liver Transplantation Society (ILTS), Barcelona, 2003.

208 Quaglia AF, Del Vecchio BG, Greaves R, Burroughs AK, Dhillon AP. Development of ductopaenic liver allograft rejection includes a "hepatitic" phase prior to duct loss. *J Hepatol* 2000;**33**:773–80.

209 Demetris AJ, Seaberg EC, Batts KP *et al.* Reliability and predictive value of the National Institute of Diabetes and Digestive and Kidney Diseases Liver Transplantation Database nomenclature and grading system for cellular rejection of liver allografts. *Hepatology* 1995;**21**:408–16.

210 Gregory CR, Huang X, Pratt RE *et al.* Treatment with rapamycin and mycophenolic acid reduces arterial intimal thickening produced by mechanical injury and allows endothelial replacement. *Transplantation* 1995;**59**: 655–61.

211 Neff GW, Montalbano M, Slapak-Green G *et al.* A retrospective review of sirolimus (Rapamune) therapy in orthotopic liver transplant recipients diagnosed with chronic rejection. *Liver Transpl* 2003;**9**:477–83.

212 van Hoek B, Wiesner RH, Ludwig J, Gores GJ, Moore B, Krom RA. Combination immunosuppression with azathioprine reduces the incidence of ductopenic rejection and vanishing bile duct syndrome after liver transplantation. *Transplant Proc* 1991;**23**(1 Pt 2):1403–5.

37 Liver transplantation: prevention and treatment of infection

Nancy Rolando, Jim J Wade

Introduction

Rejection and infection – including post-transplant lymphoproliferative disease – are now the major barriers to successful orthotopic liver transplantation (OLT). The interplay of rejection and infection is complex.[1] Infection dominates the early postoperative period with bacterial sepsis the leading cause of death in several series,[2–4] and an independent risk factor for mortality[5]; increasingly these infections are due to multiply resistant bacteria, some of which have become significant pathogens in liver transplant centers. These "hospital pathogens" include glycopeptide-resistant enterococci, methicillin-resistant *Staphylococcus aureus* (MRSA), extended-spectrum β-lactamase (ESBL) producing "coliforms" and non-fermentative bacteria such as *Stenotrophomonas maltophilia* and *Acinetobacter baumannii*.[6] There is evidence that bacterial infection is a risk factor for fungal infection[7–9]; that cytomegalovirus (CMV) exerts an immunomodulatory effect, and that CMV and hepatitis C virus are risk factors for fungal[10] and bacterial infection, respectively.[11]

Bacterial infection

The overall rate of bacterial infections following OLT is between 5% and 60%,[2,4,12–21] and related mortality between 4.6% and 81%.[3,13] Comparing infection rates from different centers is hindered by variable duration of follow up,[22–25] inconsistent inclusion or exclusion of second or subsequent OLTs,[21,22,25] and the use of a variety of regimens for immunosuppression.[11,27–29] Some OLT series include data from both adult and pediatric patients[16,26,30,31] and from living related donors.[19,32] Further, lack of definitions of infection sometimes makes meaningful interpretation difficult.[2,14,25,33–36] This variability also complicates interpretation of the efficacy of different regimens for prophylaxis.

Risk factors for bacterial infection

Identifying those patients most at risk for infection should allow more rational decisions concerning prophylaxis and treatment. Multivariate analysis has identified risk factors for bacterial infection (Table 37.1). These include elevated serum bilirubin pre-OLT, although the reported cut-off values differ.[2,37] In the perioperative period the only surgical variable identified in more than one study as a risk factor is prolonged duration of surgery.[31,37] Following OLT, one or more episodes of cellular rejection[21,24] and additional immunosuppression[24,38] are interrelated risk factors for bacterial infection demonstrated in more than one study.[24,38] Other risk factors include acute renal failure.[39]

Perioperative antibacterial prophylaxis

Based on local experience and observational studies, there is a consensus that antibacterial prophylaxis should be used in the perioperative period. For a long surgical procedure requiring an extensive incision and both biliary and vascular anastomoses, this approach seems reasonable. However, there are no randomized controlled trials of perioperative prophylaxis. Most OLT centers use a regimen comprising a cephalosporin (cefotaxime, cefoxitin, ceftriaxone or ceftazidime) with either ampicillin or tobramycin, with various combinations advocated for penicillin-allergic patients.[2,4,14,22,23,25,27,34,35,40,41] Cefotaxime has been described as "the antibiotic of choice", as its spectrum of activity encompasses many of the Gram-negative and Gram-positive bacteria implicated, without affecting the anaerobic intestinal flora. Cefotaxime is also used in centers employing selective bowel decontamination (SBD). Some centers use the extremely broad spectrum carbapenem, imipenem.[42,43] Gaps in the spectrum of the carbapenems may encourage superinfection with enterococci (including glycopeptide-resistant *Enterococcus faecium*), or the intrinsically

Table 37.1 Risk factors for bacterial infection following orthotopic liver transplantation (OLT) determined by multivariate analyses

Study	No. of patients	Risk factors
Cuervas-Mons et al., Pittsburgh (1986)[2]	93	Pre-creatinine ≥ 1·52 mg/%; pre-PMN ≥ 4847 cell/mm; pre-IgG ≥ 1546 mg/dl; pre-bilirubin ≥ 18·28 mg/dl; pre-WBC ≥ 7211 cell/mm^3
Murcia et al., Madrid (1990)[31]	30	Previous surgery; prolonged surgery; arterial thrombosis
George et al., Chicago (1991)[37]	79	Pre-OLT bilirubin ≥ 12·28 mg/dl; duration of surgery ≥ 8 hours
Wade et al., London (1994)[21]	284	One or more episodes of acute cellular rejection; prolonged hospital admission
Saliba et al., Paris (1994)[39]	304	Pre-transplant thrombocytopenia; post-OLT acute renal failure; diabetes mellitus
Arnow et al., Chicago (1996)[30]	69	Pediatric; surgical complications
Gotzinger et al., Vienna (1996)[24]	248	Increased immunosuppression; prolonged cold ischemia time, one or more rejection episodes; high blood replacement
Singh et al., Pittsburgh (1997)[11]	130	Early infections; portal vein thrombosis (100 days); late infections; hepatitis C virus recurrence
Whiting et al., Cincinnati (1997)[28]	102	Re-transplantation
Gayowski et al., Pittsburgh (1998)[38]	130	Length of ICU stay; additional immunosuppression

PMN ; ICU, intensive care unit

carbapenem-resistant *S. maltophilia.* Similarly, third-generation cephalosporin use can select for multiply resistant Gram-negative bacilli such as *Acinetobacter* spp. and ESBL-producing *Enterobacter* spp. Generally, the choice of regimen for perioperative antibacterial prophylaxis does not appear to determine subsequent infection rates. Local experience and microbiology results should dictate the agents used. It may be appropriate to use a narrow spectrum agent for elective OLTs whilst reserving broader spectrum regimens for re-transplants or for patients with complex pre-OLT hospital admissions.

Depending on the local incidence of infection, consideration should be given to the use of nasal mupirocin ointment pre-OLT to eradicate carriage of methicillin-sensitive *S. aureus* or MRSA; for the latter preoperative skin decontamination may be appropriate, though there are no controlled trials in OLT to support either approach.[44–47] C5 No interventions are available for eradicating other multiply resistant bacteria. Isoniazid chemoprophylaxis to prevent reactivation of *Mycobacterium tuberculosis* may be warranted for OLT patients with a previous history, a family history or tuberculin skin test reactivity, though in an endemic area the latter may not be a sensitive indicator of those most at risk.[48–50]

Prophylaxis in the post-transplant period

For post-OLT prophylaxis of bacterial infection, the major difference between centers is in the use of SBD. The concept of SBD evolved from data suggesting that elimination of enteric aerobic Gram negatives, whilst preserving the gut anaerobic flora, limits colonization or overgrowth by aerobic Gram-negative bacilli,[51–53] which are major nosocomial pathogens. The topical, non-absorbable antibiotics of SBD regimens usually eradicate aerobic Gram-negative bacilli from the mouth in 2–3 days, but eradication from the gut may take from 7 to 10 days[54]; intravenous antibacterials may be used to cover this period. The rationale for SBD in OLT is the predominance of infections caused by Gram-negative bacilli,[4,34,37] and yeasts,[55] both of which are "targeted" by SBD. Gram-negative bacillus infections may follow enterotomy,[33] or occur via translocation from the gut,[56] or aspiration of pharyngeal secretions as a prelude to pneumonia.[57]

The Mayo Clinic group were the first to adopt SBD routinely for all OLT patients. The regimen is administered from 2 to 3 days pretransplant and continued until discharge (21 days); a topical antibacterial paste is applied while the patient is ventilated.[9,14,58] Although the uncontrolled Mayo Clinic data consistently suggest that SBD reduces peri-operative Gram-negative infections,[9,14,22,23] not all centers using this regimen (Table 37.2) have achieved similarly low infection rates.[40,59,60] The optimal timing,[9,14,23,26,58] duration, and composition of the SBD regimen have not been established. A regimen of gentamicin, nystatin, and polymyxin E is used at the Mayo Clinic,[9,14,22] while tobramycin replaces gentamicin at other centers. At the Mayo Clinic the SBD is initiated 3 days before transplantation. Initiating SBD in patients on a waiting list, when the time to transplantation is unknown, is difficult. Adverse effects on the gastrointestinal tract, especially diarrhea, have been reported in up to a third of patients,[26,30,58] and poor compliance has been reported in up to 18% of patients.[30] The economic

Table 37.2 Infection rate in centers employing selective bowel decontamination (SBD) in orthotopic liver transplantation (OLT)

Study	No. of patients	Antibiotic regimen	Timing of SBD	Total % infections
Wiesner *et al.*, Mayo Clinic (1987)[58]	145	Polymyxin E, gentamicin, and nystatin	$-3 \rightarrow 21$ days	24·1 early
Busuttil *et al.*, UCLA (1987)[40]	100	Neomycin, erythromycin, and nystatin	Not stated	51
Paya *et al.*, Mayo Clinic (1989)[14]	100	Polymyxin E, gentamicin, and nystatin	$-3 \rightarrow 21$ days	25·5
Rosman *et al.*, Groningen, the Netherlands (1990)[59]	39	Polymyxin E, tobramycin, amphotericin B	-6 hours $\rightarrow$ ~36 days	45
Kuo *et al.*, Baltimore (1997)[60]	18	Ciprofloxacin, nystatin	High risk patients, admission to OLT ~23 days	55

implications of SBD have been evaluated; regimens containing amphotericin B are the most expensive.[30]

Results from six randomized controlled trials of SBD are given in Table 37.3. An initial report from Birmingham[25] demonstrated a significant reduction in episodes of infection during an observation period of 15 days, but the final report did not show a significant effect on the incidence of infection, the occurrence of endotoxemia, the development of organ system failure, or mortality.[61] A study from Chicago showed no statistically significant benefit of SBD on infection rates during a 28-day period of observation.[30] This study also highlighted the practical problems associated with the administration of SBD: adverse effects, poor compliance and the difficulty of predicting the time of transplantation if SBD is initiated whilst the patient is on a waiting list. A study of 36 pediatric patients in Pittsburgh which used a short period of SBD did not show a statistically significant reduction in either the number of total episodes of infection or mortality,[26] although it did show a significant reduction in the number of patients experiencing Gram-negative infections. Two recent studies[62,63] reported that SBD did not affect the incidences of total infections, or any specific infection (though there was a reduction in pneumonia in the Mayo Clinic study[63]); that the infection-related mortality was not reduced, and that SBD was not cost-effective. In the Mayo Clinic study the SBD was microbiologically monitored and the authors did not encounter an increase in resistant bacteria. The study from Rotterdam[62] revealed a reduction in the proportion of infections due to Gram-negative yeasts, an effect of SBD described elsewhere.[60,64] Other studies from Rotterdam conclude that SBD does not prevent endotoxemia in OLT[65] and is not a cost effective intervention for this group.[66] A meta-analysis of 22 randomized controlled trials involving 4142 patients in intensive care units showed that SBD reduces infection-related morbidity (number needed to treat (NNT) to avoid one respiratory tract infection = 6; range 6–9).[67] However, no significant effect on mortality was demonstrated, except by subgroup analysis of those trials that employed combined topical and systemic antibiotics. A1d

An alternative approach employed by some centers in the USA is the use of oral quinolones to eliminate the gut "pool" of aerobic Gram-negative bacilli.[60,68] The Cleveland group used quinolones in the interval between listing for transplantation and 28 days post transplant and reported a decrease in infection rates compared with historical controls.[68] B4

Although some centers consider SBD to be of benefit,[69] available data from controlled trials is insufficient to recommend SBD for all OLT patients: prophylactic regimens should target those patients identified as being at high risk of infection (see Table 37.1). Administration of SBD for 3 or more days *before* transplantation may be beneficial but there is only comparatively weak evidence to support this view.

Treatment of bacterial infections

The global increase in multiply resistant bacteria[6] dictates that bacterial infections should be treated not only according to the site of infection and the confirmed or most likely pathogen, but also taking in to account local susceptibility patterns and antimicrobial policy.

Fungal infection

The incidence of systemic fungal infection in OLT patients varies from 2·9% to 31%, and fungal infection has a major impact on morbidity and mortality.[9,10,21,42,43,55,64,70–74] Difficulties in the clinical or laboratory confirmation of fungal infection make comparisons of infection rates problematical. Reports that only include cases confirmed by isolation of the

Table 37.3   Randomized controlled trials of elective bowel decontamination (SBD) in orthotopic liver transplantation

Study	No. of patients	Control	SBD antibiotic regimen	Infection rate controls	Infection rate SBD	P
[a]Badger et al., Birmingham, UK (1991)[25]	30	Nystatin	Polymyxin E, tobramycin, amphotericin B5 → 15 days	8/16	2/14	<0·05
[a]Bion et al., Birmingham, UK (1994)[61]	52	Nystatin	Polymyxin E, tobramycin, amphotericin B5 → 15 days	12/31	3/21	NS
Arnow et al., Chicago (1996)[30]	69	Nystatin	Polymyxin E, gentamicin, nystatin, −3 → 21 days	14/33	14/36	NS
Smith et al., Pittsburgh (1993)[26] (pediatrics)	36	Perioperative parenteral antibiotics only	Polymyxin E, tobramycin, amphotericin B6 ± 4 days	19 episodes in 18 patients	32 episodes in 18 patients	NS
Zwavelling et al., Rotterdam (2002)[62]	53	Placebo Drugs	Colistin, tobramycin Amphotericin B → 30 days	25/29	22/26	NS
Hellinger et al., Jacksonville (2002)[63]	80	Nystatin	Polymyxin E, gentamicin Nystatin −3 to 21 days	12/43	12/37	NS

[a]Interim and final analyses of this series.
NS, not significant

organism, or serological detection of antigens or antibodies, without histopathological confirmation of invasion, may overestimate the true incidence of fungal infection. In addition, as the diversity of interventions for prophylaxis increases, so does the difficulty in making meaningful comparisons between centers.

Fungal infections in OLT usually occur within the first month after transplantation, and are associated with mortality rates between 5·3% and 80%.[29,34,42,43,64,75,76] There is some evidence that invasive aspergillosis is occurring later in the post-transplant course with a lower mortality (60%).[77] The majority of fungal infections in OLT recipients are caused by *Candida* spp.; mold infections, including *Aspergillus* spp., may be encountered in patients receiving transplants for fulminant hepatic failure, severely immunosuppressed patients or those with CMV infection. The proportion caused by *Candida* spp. was reported to be 87% in Boston,[10] 78% in Pittsburgh,[78] and approximately 50% in other centers.[9,21,74] *Aspergillus* spp. and the agents of mucormycosis are far less often implicated, but these infections are associated with mortality ranging from 60% to 100%.[5,55,78-80]

Risk factors for fungal infection

Problems with diagnosing and attributing mortality to fungal infection have prompted attempts to identify those patients most at risk.[9,10,14,21,29,43,75,76] Multivariate analyses have identified risk factors related to the severity or complexity of the patient's pretransplant status (Table 37.4). Prolonged duration of surgery and an increase in transfusion

requirements have been identified as risk factors by two or more centers.[10,14,29,55,76] It is impossible to ascertain whether these associations reflect severity of underlying illness, complexity of surgery or are markers for other unidentified variables. In the post-transplant period, re-transplantation,[10,75] bacterial infection,[14,75] and return to the operating room[10,21] have been identified as risk factors (see Table 37.4). Other risk factors associated with enhanced immunosuppression identified by multivariate analysis include corticosteroid use and CMV infection.[10,29,75,81-83] An association between CMV infection and fungal infection has also been reported[82,84] (see below).

Prophylaxis against fungal infection

Due to the potentially high mortality of fungal infection, all liver transplant centers employ some form of antifungal prophylaxis, often empirical use of the oral non-absorbable polyenes, nystatin and amphotericin B, or clotrimazole. A total of 1233 patients from six case series (Table 37.5) received nystatin. The average incidence of fungal infection with this intervention ranges from 11% to 34%,[7,8,19,54,55-58,68] and appears not to correlate with duration of antifungal prophylaxis.[9,10,21,85] When oral amphotericin B was used for prophylaxis in two case series, the observed incidence of fungal infection was 7%[21] and 16·5%.[43] The combination of low dose intravenous amphotericin B with nystatin did not prevent disseminated fungal infections in high risk patients.[11,86] The value of topical polyenes for preventing

Table 37.4   Risk factors for fungal infection following OLT – multivariate analyses

Study	No. of patients	Pre-OLT variables	OLT variables	Post-OLT variables
Tollemar *et al.*, Sweden (1990)[70]	29	Sex: male	Prolonged surgery; ↑ transfusions	
Castaldo *et al.*, Omaha (1991)[75]	303	Urgent status, RISK score	↑ Transfusions	Re-transplantation; reintubation; bacterial infection; ↑ steroids; vascular complications; ↑ antibiotic use
Collins *et al.*, NEDH, Boston (1994)[10]	158		↑ Operative time; renal failure	Re-transplantation; reoperation; CMV infection
Briegel *et al.*, Munich (1995)[43]	152			Hemofiltration or hemodialysis; ↑ FFP transfusion
Hadley *et al.*, Boston (1995)[29]	118	CMV infection	Choledochojejunostomy; ↑ transfusions	CMV infection ICU duration
Wade *et al.*, London (1994)[21]	284	↑ Hemoglobin ↑ Bilirubin		Return to surgery; prolonged therapy with ciprofloxacin
Patel *et al.*, Mayo Clinic (1996)[9]	405	Class II HLA partial or complete match	↑ Cryoprecipitates	Bacterial infection
Fortun *et al.*, Madrid (2002)[83a]	260			Dialysis re-transplantation CMV

[a]Invasive aspergillosis only.
OLT, orthotopic liver transplantation; CMV, cytomegalovirus; HLA, human leukocyte antigen; ICU, intensive care unit; FFP, fresh frozen plasma.

fungal infection is unproved, although the use of these non-toxic agents to prevent oropharyngeal or esophageal candidiasis seems logical. B4 C5

A randomized controlled trial compared the safety and efficacy of fluconazole (100 mg/day) and nystatin[73] (Table 37.6). Fluconazole was safe in OLT patients and there was no evidence of interaction with cyclosporin. Fluconazole resulted in fewer superficial fungal infections (fluconazole 13%, nystatin 34%, $P = 0.022$, absolute risk reduction (ARR) = 21%, NNT = 5). However, no statistically significant difference in systemic infection (fluconazole 2·6%, nystatin 9·0%, $P = 0.12$) or mortality was demonstrated. A1c However, in a study using a higher dose of fluconazole (400 mg daily) there was a reduction in superficial and invasive fungal infection, as well as infection-related mortality.[88] In a randomized controlled trial, the incidence of fungal infections in patients receiving fluconazole (400 mg twice daily) or itraconazole solution (200 mg twice daily) – from day of OLT to 10 weeks – was comparable.[89] A1c The emergence of azole-resistant yeasts has been reported in patients undergoing bone marrow transplantation,[90] and in AIDS patients, this was not a significant problem in these trials, although as expected, *Candida glabrata* infections were

not prevented. Fluconazole resistance has not been a problem in other studies where this agent has been used as short-term prophylaxis.[91]

The randomized trial reported by Tollemar *et al.*[92] in 86 OLT patients (Table 37.6) demonstrated that liposomal amphotericin B (1 mg/kg per day for 5 days) significantly decreased early invasive fungal infections (amphotericin 0%, nystatin 16%, ARR = 16%, NNT = 6), but not invasive *Aspergillus* spp. infections. A1c Although liposomal amphotericin B is expensive, this approach to prophylaxis may still be cost effective given the cost of treating fungal infection. There are no controlled trials identifying interventions to reduce *Aspergillus* infections in OLT recipients, presumably because of the low incidence. In a retrospective study, Singh *et al.*, showed that prophylaxis with a lipid preparation of amphotericin B in patients requiring renal replacement therapy post-OLT reduced the incidence of invasive fungal infections.[93] B4 Further trials of pre-emptive prophylaxis with standard (for example amphotericin B, itraconazole) and novel (for example voriconazole, caspofungin) anti-fungals in OLT patients at high risk of *Aspergillus* spp. are needed. Recent data suggest that prophylaxis for CMV infection may also reduce the incidence of fungal infections (see below).[84]

Table 37.5 Incidence of fungal infection following orthotopic liver transplantation in case series employing antifungal prophylaxis

Study	No. of patients	Antifungal prophylaxis regimen	Fungal infection (%)
Mora *et al.*, Dallas (1992)[42]	150	In high risk patients: oral nystatin plus IV amphotericin B → 10–14 days	7·5
Collins *et al.*, Boston (1994)[10]	158	Nystatin oral → 3–6 months	21
Castaldo *et al.*, Omaha (1991)[55]	307	Nystatin oral → 3 months	23·8
Steffen *et al.*, Germany (1994)[64]	206	Nystatin, SBD	27·8
Briegel *et al.*, Munich (1995)[43]	152	Amphotericin B SBD	16·5
Wade *et al.*, London (1995)[21]	33	No prophylaxis	12
	198	Amphotericin B oral	7
	36	Nystatin	19
Patel *et al.*, Mayo Clinic (1996)[9]	405	Nystatin, SBD	11
Rabkin *et al.*, Portland (2000)[87]	96	Clotrimazole	38

SBD, selective bowel decontamination

Table 37.6 Randomized trials of interventions for prophylaxis against invasive fungal infection in orthotopic liver transplant patients

Study	No. of patients	Experimental antifungal therapy	Control antifungal therapy	Fungal infection/total (%)		*P*
				Experimental	Control	
Tollemar *et al.*, Sweden (1995)[92]	86	Liposomal amphotericin B and nystatin until discharge	Nystatin	0/40 (0)	6/37 (16)	<0·01
Lumbreras *et al.*, Madrid (1996)[73]	143	Fluconazole → 28 days	Nystatin	2/76 (3)	6/67 (9)	0·12
Winston *et al.*, Los Angeles (1999)[88]	212	Fluconazole 400 mg/day → 10 weeks	Placebo	10/108 (9)	45/104 (43)	<0·001
Winston and Busuttil, Los Angeles (2002)[89]	188	Itraconazole solution (200 mg twice daily) → 10 weeks	Fluconazole (400 mg once daily)	9/97 (9)	4/91 (4)	NS

NS, not significant

The value of routine prophylaxis for *Pneumocystis jiroveci* (formerly *Pneumocystis carinii*) has not been proved. In the absence of prophylaxis, the incidence of pneumocystis pneumonia (PCP) has been reported to be between 3% and 11%.[5,14,42,94,95] Low dose co-trimoxazole appeared to be effective in reducing the incidence of PCP in a center with an incidence of 30% prior to its introduction, but the evidence for this benefit rests only on case series before and after the intervention.[96] B4

Treatment of fungal infection

There are no controlled trials of therapy for fungal infection in OLT patients. Although superficial yeast infections may respond to topical agents (nystatin, amphotericin B) or azoles, resistance is a possibility and may take time to confirm. At most centers the standard therapy for proved or suspected invasive fungal infection is amphotericin B – or a lipid preparation of amphotericin B – sometimes in low dose combined with 5-flucytosine.[76] Some retrospective studies suggest that lipid preparations of amphotericin B may be more effective than amphotericin B deoxycholate.[97,98] B4 However, the major benefits of the three lipid preparations of amphotericin B are reduced allergic reactions and, more importantly, reduced nephrotoxicity allowing administration of considerably larger doses. Early diagnosis of *Aspergillus* spp. infection is essential and currently depends heavily on clinical acumen and high-resolution radiology; eventually molecular diagnostics will improve early diagnosis reliably. Other potential but unproved interventions include the use of granulocyte-colony stimulating factor (G-CSF) or granulocyte macrophage-colony stimulating factor (GM-CSF); interferon-γ; surgical excision,[99] and reducing immunosuppression.[85] C5 Novel agents (for example voriconazole, caspofungin, micafungin) require evaluation in randomized controlled trials. It is hoped that regimens combining polymerase chain reaction (PCR)-based diagnostics with prompt, appropriate and non-toxic anti-fungals – perhaps reflecting the "pre-emptive therapy" approaches evaluated for CMV disease (see below) – will result in optimum care.

Viral infection

Cytomegalovirus (CMV) is the most important and most studied opportunist infection following OLT. Infection may manifest as a syndrome of fever, leukopenia and thrombo-cytopenia, and result in disseminated infection with hepatitis, pneumonitis or gastrointestinal tract infection, usually within 3 months of transplantation. CMV infection is also implicated in acute and chronic rejection and, via its immunosuppressive effect, is a risk factor for bacterial and fungal infection. The serological status of donor and recipient are important factors: post-transplant CMV infection may be acquired from the graft or, less often, blood products, or result from reactivation of latent virus or superinfection with a new strain. Primary infections are more severe than reactivation infection or superinfection. Seronegative recipients of seropositive grafts (D+/R–) are at highest risk of CMV infection. Up to 80% of these graft recipients become infected and 60% develop CMV disease. Protective matching of the graft reduces the risk of CMV infection for seronegative recipients but the scarcity of donor organs makes this approach impractical. Re-transplantation and the use of antilymphocyte globulin or OKT3 are also risk factors for CMV disease. Preventing CMV disease, especially in D+/R– patients, would be a major advance in liver transplantation.[100–102] The value of active immunization against CMV is being evaluated in various clinical settings.

Interpretation of trials that compare different interventions for CMV prevention (Table 37.7) is complicated by variation with respect to patient population, immunosuppressive regimens, outcome measures, and even by variability among batches in human normal immunoglobulin (HN Ig) and CMV hyperimmune globulins (CMV Ig). Some studies evaluated interventions in all OLT recipients, while others studied pre-emptive therapy for those with known risk factors for disease such as use of OKT3, D+/R– status or evidence of CMV shedding or viremia.

Passive immunization: immunoglobulin

HN Ig was shown to be ineffective for preventing CMV disease in a randomized double blind trial comparing HN Ig with albumen in 50 patients.[103] In contrast, the small randomized trial of CMV Ig conducted by Saliba *et al.*,[104] found that 4 of 15 (26·6%) D+/R– patients receiving CMV Ig post-OLT developed severe CMV disease, compared to 6 of 7 (85·7%) D+/R– control patients ($P = 0·01$). In a subsequent randomized, double-blind, placebo controlled trial Snydman *et al.* showed that CMV Ig decreased the incidence of severe CMV-associated disease (including invasive fungal disease with CMV infection) following OLT. Although subgroup analysis did not show a reduction in CMV disease or severe CMV-associated disease in D+/R– patients, there were only 19 such patients in each treatment arm and OKT3 was used more often in the CMV Ig arm.[82] In a further *post hoc* analysis of this trial, which also included patients from a further open label trial who received less OKT3, it appeared that the same CMV Ig regimen reduced severe CMV disease in the D+/R– subgroup.[105] A meta-analysis of 18 studies of HN Ig or CMV Ig prophylaxis in transplantation did not show benefit of CMV Ig over HN Ig. However, this analysis included patients with various solid organ transplants, as well as bone marrow transplants.[106] A1c In summary there is evidence that CMV Ig but not HN Ig can prevent CMV disease in OLT patients other than in the high risk (D+/R–) group.

Antiviral prophylaxis: acyclovir and ganciclovir

Saliba *et al.*,[107] in a randomized controlled trial which included 120 CMV seropositive OLT recipients, showed that acyclovir was well tolerated and was effective for prophylaxis against CMV reactivation, reinfection, and CMV disease. No differences in acute rejection, chronic rejection or mortality were demonstrated.[107] A1a The randomized trial of Green *et al.*[108] in 29 children undergoing OLT did not show any reduction in CMV infection from 1 year of acyclovir therapy following an initial 2 weeks of ganciclovir post-OLT. A1c

Nakazato *et al.*,[109] randomized 104 patients to receive HN Ig plus either acyclovir or ganciclovir whilst hospitalized. After discharge all patients received oral acyclovir. Ganciclovir reduced the incidence of CMV disease (ganciclovir 3·8%, acyclovir 15%, $P < 0·05$) and rejection and the duration of hospitalization after OLT. A1a Subgroup analysis of 16 D+/R– patients did not show

Table 37.7 Randomized trials of interventions for prevention of CMV disease in OLT

Study	No. of patients	Patient selection	Experimental intervention	Control intervention	CMV disease		P
					Experimental	Control	
Cofer et al., Dallas (1991)[103]	50	No	HN Ig	Albumen	8/25	5/25	NS
Saliba et al., France (1989)[104]	22	D+/R−	CMV Ig	Nil	4/15	6/7	0·01
Snydman et al., Massachusetts (1993)[82]	141	No	CMV Ig	Albumen	21/169	41/72	NS
Saliba et al., France (1993)[107]	120	No	ACV × 3 months	Nil	4/60	14/60	0·01
Green et al., Pittsburg (1994)[108]	29	No	GCV × 2 weeks plus ACV × 1 year	GCV × 2 weeks	2/10	1/19	NS
Nakazato et al., San Francisco (1993)[109]	104	No	HN Ig plus GCV in hospital plus ACV after discharge	HN Ig plus ACV in hospital then ACV after discharge	2/52	8/52	0·046
Martin et al., Pittsburg (1994)[110]	139	No	GCV × 2 weeks then ACV × 10 weeks	ACV × 12 weeks	6/68	20/71	0·0001
Cohen et al., London (1993)[111]	65	No	GCV for weeks 3–4	GCV for therapy of established disease	9/33	11/32	NS
Winston et al., Los Angeles (1995)[112]	250	No	GCV × 100 days	ACV × 100 days	1/124	12/126	0·002
King et al., USA, Canada (1997)[114]	56	D+/R−	GCV × 30 days plus HN Ig	Saline plus HN Ig	5/29	7/27	NS
Badley et al., USA (1997)[115]	167	No	GCV × 14 days then ACV × 106 days	ACV × 120 days	9/83	19/84	0·003
Stratta et al., Nebraska (1992)[118]	100	OKT3 treatment	HN Ig plus ACV × 3 months	Nil	18/50	21/50	NS
Barkholt et al., Stockholm (1999)[116]	55	No	ACV 800 mg four times daily × 12 weeks	Placebo	7/28	14/27	0·013
Winston et al., UCLA (2003)[117]	219	CMVAb (+) and IV GCV × 14 day	GCV oral 1 g three times daily until 100 days	ACV oral 800 mg four times daily until 100 days	1/110	8/109	0·019

CMV, cytomegalovirus; OLT, orthotopic liver transplantation; UCLA, University of California at Los Angeles; HN Ig, human normal immunoglobulin; ACV, acyclovir; GCV, ganciclovir; IV, intravenous; NS, not significant; OKT3

any benefit of ganciclovir.[109] In a randomized trial in which sequential ganciclovir (14 days) and high dose acyclovir (10 weeks) was compared with high dose acyclovir alone for 12 weeks,[110] ganciclovir delayed the onset and decreased the incidence of overall CMV infection, but neither regimen was shown to prevent primary CMV infection. Cohen *et al.*[111] randomized 65 patients to receive ganciclovir prophylaxis given during weeks 3 and 4 post-transplant or ganciclovir only as a therapeutic intervention. They did not find a difference in the incidence of CMV disease, although ganciclovir prophylaxis was associated with a lower incidence of serologically diagnosed secondary infection.[111] Winston *et al.*[112] compared 100 days of therapy with ganciclovir and acyclovir for prophylaxis and reported that ganciclovir produced a highly significant reduction in CMV infection (ganciclovir 5%, acyclovir 38%, $P < 0.0001$, ARR = 33%, NNT = 3) and disease (ganciclovir 0.8%, acyclovir 10%, $P = 0.002$, ARR = 9.2%, NNT = 11). Ala Subgroup analysis suggested that the benefit of ganciclovir over acyclovir was observed in the R– patients (ganciclovir 42%, acyclovir 11%, $P = 0.06$, ARR = 31 % NNT = 3), although not in the D+/R– patients.[112] In a subsequent uncontrolled study, the same group later followed 37 D+/R– OLT patients following administration of intravenous ganciclovir for a mean of 15 months (range 5–38 months). None of these high risk patients developed CMV disease, while four of 10 D+/R– patients who received less than 7 weeks of ganciclovir (mean duration 3 weeks) developed disease.[113] King *et al.*[114] randomized 56 D+/R– children to receive ganciclovir plus HN Ig or placebo plus HN Ig and found a delay in the onset of CMV disease in the ganciclovir group, but did not show a statistically significant decrease in incidence (ganciclovir 17%, placebo 26%, $P = 0.429$).

Badley *et al.*[115] randomized 167 OLT patients to receive either acyclovir for 120 days or ganciclovir followed by oral acyclovir for 106 days. Ganciclovir was effective for reducing CMV infection (acyclovir 57%, ganciclovir 37%, $P = 0.001$) and CMV disease (acyclovir 23%, ganciclovir 11%, $P = 0.03$). The NNT – the number of patients needed to be treated with ganciclovir rather than acyclovir to prevent one infection – was 5 and to prevent one occurrence of CMV disease, 8. The ganciclovir regimen was effective even in D+/R– patients.[87] Ala

Barkholt *et al.*[116] randomized 55 OLT patients to receive either placebo or high dose acyclovir prophylaxis, 800 mg four times a day for 12 weeks. Although there was no difference in the incidence of CMV infection, acyclovir reduced the incidence of CMV disease (7/28 *v* 14/27; $P = 0.013$) and the time to CMV disease from the start of "prophylaxis" was longer for acyclovir recipients than recipients of placebo ($P = 0.013$). Acyclovir delayed approximately 32% of CMV infections that would have occurred in the placebo group, and prevented or delayed 59% of cases of CMV disease.

Winston *et al.*[117] randomized 219 CMV seropositive patients to receive prophylaxis with either ganciclovir ($n = 110$) or acyclovir ($n = 109$), after an initial period of prophylaxis with intravenous ganciclovir through a central venous catheter at 6 mg/kg once daily for the first 14 days. After this period patients received oral ganciclovir (1 g every 8 hours), or oral acyclovir (800 mg every 6 hours) until day 100 after OLT. The authors reported the development of CMV disease in 8/109 (7.3%) in the acyclovir group compared with only 1/110 (0.9%) in the ganciclovir group, and concluded that ganciclovir is superior to acyclovir for CMV prophylaxis, after an initial period of intravenous ganciclovir. Ala The main adverse effect of the use of ganciclovir was myelosuppression.

Pre-emptive therapy for cytomegalovirus disease

The purpose of pre-emptive therapy is to prevent disease in those patients with known risk factors, viral shedding, viremia or antigenemia which place them at risk of subsequent CMV disease (Table 37.8). This approach avoids administration of a prophylactic regimen to all OLT patients. It is recognized that some patients develop CMV disease without preceding detectable viremia or CMV shedding. More sensitive methods of CMV detection, such as PCR, will improve the identification of patients at risk and the effectiveness of pre-emptive therapy.

Stratta *et al.* randomized 100 patients receiving OKT3 to receive HN Ig plus oral acyclovir for 3 months after OKT3 therapy or no intervention and did not demonstrate any reduction in incidence or severity of CMV infections.[118] Ala Lumbreras *et al.* found that CMV disease occurred less frequently in a group of patients who received ganciclovir prophylaxis than in a historical control group.[119] In a randomized controlled trial of 47 patients, Singh *et al.* showed that short course ganciclovir therapy, administered only if CMV shedding occurred, was more effective than a prophylactic regimen of high dose acyclovir for the prevention of CMV disease.[120] This approach has been adopted in several transplant centers. Alc

Paya *et al.*[121] conducted a placebo-controlled randomized trial to assess the role of pre-emptive therapy with oral ganciclovir for preventing CMV infection and disease after the detection of CMV by PCR in the first 8 weeks after OLT. In this study 69/168 OLT patients became CMV positive by PCR (with no concomitant CMV disease) and were randomized to placebo ($n = 34$) or ganciclovir ($n = 35$). CMV infection developed in 21% in the placebo group versus 3% in the ganciclovir group ($P = 0.02$), and CMV disease in 12% of the placebo group versus none in the ganciclovir group ($P = 0.03$). Alc This study addressed the clinical usefulness of PCR for guiding pre-emptive therapy with ganciclovir: when given at the first PCR positive test, oral ganciclovir

Table 37.8   Randomized trials of pre-emptive antiviral therapy for prevention of CMV disease in OLT patients

Study	No. of patients	Patient selection	Experimental intervention	Control intervention	CMV disease Experimental	Control	P
Singh *et al.*, Pittsburgh (1994)[120]	47	CMV antigenemia	GCV 2×5 mg/kg per day×7 days	Oral ACV 4×800/d	1/23	7/24	P=0·05
Singh *et al.*, Pittsburgh (2000)[123]	72	CMV antigenemia	GCV oral 3×2 g×6 weeks +3×1 g× 4 weeks	GCV IV 2×5 mg/kg× 7 days	0/11	1/11	NS
Paya *et al.*, Mayo Clinic (2002)[121]	69	CMV PCR positive but no disease	Oral GCV× 8 weeks *n*=35	Placebo× 8 weeks *n*=34	0% CMV disease	CMV disease in 12%	P=0·003
Rayes *et al.*, Berlin, Germany (2001)[124]	60		Oral GCV 3×1 g/day× 14 days	Nil	3/30	6/30	P=NS

PCR, polymerase chain reaction. For other abbreviations see Table 37.7

effectively reduced both CMV infection and disease. This was true for both low (R+) and high (D+/R–) risk patients (R+).[121]

Torre-Cisneros *et al.*[122] conducted a small non-randomized sequential study of pre-emptive ganciclovir in patients monitored by qualitative PCR; 25 patients received no prophylaxis and the subsequent 40 consecutive patients received pre-emptive oral ganciclovir (1 g three times a day) if D+/R– or PCR positive in 2 consecutive weeks (*n* = 11 high risk patients). The overall rate of CMV disease at 6 months was 20% in the no prophylaxis group and 2·5% in the high risk pre-emptive ganciclovir group (*P* = 0·04). B4 Singh *et al.*[123] compared the efficacy of pre-emptive oral ganciclovir with that of intravenous ganciclovir for prevention of CMV disease in patients with CMV pp65 antigenemia, and sought to determine whether withholding prophylaxis in the absence of CMV antigenemia could reliably identify those in whom prophylaxis is not required. Seventy-two OLT patients were enrolled in this randomized controlled trial, and CMV antigenemia developed in 22 (31%). Of these 22, one group (*n* = 11) received oral ganciclovir for 6 weeks (2 g three times daily for 2 weeks, then 1 g three times daily for 4 weeks) and the second group (*n* = 11) received intravenous ganciclovir (5 mg/kg twice daily) for 7 days. CMV disease occurred in 1/11 in the oral group and none in the intravenous group. None of the study patients (including the 50 without antigenemia) developed CMV disease. Both regimens – and this approach to pre-emptive therapy for CMV – appeared effective for preventing CMV disease. Rayes *et al.*,[124] randomized 60 asymptomatic pp65 anti-gen positive patients to receive pre-emptive therapy with oral ganciclovir (1 g three times daily, or adjusted for creatinine clearance) for 14 days (*n* = 30) or no pre-emptive therapy (*n* = 30). Patients who subsequently developed CMV disease received intravenous

ganciclovir for 14 days or until recovery. CMV disease developed in 3/30 (10%) receiving oral ganciclovir pre-emptive therapy, compared with 6/30 (20%) of those with no antiviral therapy. Alc The authors concluded that the positive predictive value of pp65 antigenemia for CMV disease was low, and that the pre-emptive strategy was not superior to conventional treatment. Daly *et al.*,[125] conducted a study evaluating the efficacy, including cost efficacy, of a strategy of pre-emptive ganciclovir therapy for OLT patients with "CMV activity": CMV antigenemia, or serological or PCR positivity. They found that their strategy resulted in a low incidence of symptomatic CMV disease, with no organ-invasive disease, whilst minimizing ganciclovir use and, presumably, the potential for resistance, toxicity and costs.

Some benefits of pre-emptive strategies for preventing CMV disease are clear. Targeted antiviral therapy can avoid toxicity, may reduce the emergence of resistance and can be more cost effective. Further studies are required to identify the optimum combination of: high risk patient subgroups, markers of CMV activity (for example CMV copy number), sampling schedules and timing of antiviral intervention. The role of the novel oral antiviral, valacyclovir, for CMV in OLT patients requires evaluation.

References

1 Cainelli F, Vento S. Infections and solid organ transplant rejection: a cause-and-effect relationship. *Lancet Infect Dis* 2002;**2**:539–47.

2 Cuervas-Mons V, Millan J, Gavaler S *et al.* Prognostic value of preoperatively obtained clinical and laboratory data in predicting survival following orthotopic liver transplantation. *Hepatology* 1986;**6**:922–7.

3 Cuervas-Mons V, Martinez AJ, Dekker A *et al.* Adult liver transplantation: an analysis of the early causes of death in 40 consecutive cases. *Hepatology* 1986;**6**: 495–501.

4 Kusne S, Dummer JS, Singh N *et al.* Infections after liver transplantation. An analysis of 101 consecutive cases. *Medicine* 1988;**67**:132–43.

5 Martin M, Kusne M, Alessiani R *et al.* Infection after liver transplantation: risk factors and prevention. *Transplant Proc* 1991;**23**:1929–30.

6 Singh N, Gayowski T, Rihs JD, Wagener MM, Marino IR. Evolving trends in multiple-antibiotic-resistant bacteria in liver transplant recipients: a longitudinal study of antimicrobial susceptibility patterns. *Liv Transpl* 2001;**7**:22–6.

7 Castaldo P, Stratta RJ, Wood RP *et al.* Clinical spectrum of fungal infections after orthotopic liver transplantation. *Arch Surg* 1991;**126**:149–56.

8 Patel R, Paya C. Infections in solid-organ transplant recipients. *Clin Microbiol Rev* 1997;**10**:86–124.

9 Patel R, Portela D, Badley AD *et al.* Risk factors of invasive *Candida* and non-*Candida* fungal infections after liver transplantation. *Transplantation* 1996;**62**:926–34.

10 Collins LA, Samore MH, Roberts MS *et al.* Risk factors for early invasive fungal infection complicating orthotopic liver transplantation. *J Infect Dis* 1994;**170**:644–52.

11 Singh N, Gayowski T, Wagener M *et al.* Predictors and outcome of early versus late onset major bacterial infections in liver transplant recipients receiving tacrolimus (FK506) as primary immuno-suppression. *Eur J Clin Microbiol Infect Dis* 1997;**16**:821–6.

12 Kirby RM, McMaster P, Clements D *et al.* Orthotopic liver transplantation: postoperative complications and their management. *Br J Surg* 1987;**74**:3–11.

13 Moulin D, Clement de Clety S, Reynaert M *et al.* Intensive care for children after orthotopic liver transplantation. *Intensive Care Med* 1989;**15**:S71–2.

14 Paya CV, Hermans PE, Washington JA *et al.* Incidence distribution and outcome of episodes of infection in 100 orthotopic liver transplantations. *Mayo Clin Proc* 1989;**64**: 554–64.

15 Lumbreras C, Lizasoain M, Moreno E *et al.* Major bacterial infections following liver transplantation: a prospective study. *Hepatogastroenterology* 1992;**39**:362–5.

16 Martinez-Ibañez V, Iglesias J, Llorret J *et al.* Experiencia de siete años en el transplante hepático pediátrico. *Cir Pediatr* 1993;**6**:7–10.

17 Barkholt L, Ericzon BG, Tollemar J *et al.* Infections in human liver recipients: different patterns early and late. *Transplant Int* 1993;**6**:77–84.

18 Kizilisik TA, Larsen IM, Bain VG *et al.* Liver transplantation at the University of Alberta Hospitals: a review of the first three years. *Transplant Proc* 1993;**25**:2203–5.

19 Uemoto S, Tanaka K, Fujita S *et al.* Infection complication in living related liver transplantation. *J Pediatr Surg* 1994;**29**: 514–17.

20 Singh N, Gayowski T, Wagener M *et al.* Pulmonary infections in liver transplant recipients receiving tacrolimus. *Transplantation* 1996;**61**:396–401.

21 Wade J, Rolando N, Hayllar K *et al.* Bacterial and fungal infection after liver transplantation: an analysis of 284 patients. *Hepatology* 1995;**21**:1328–36.

22 Wiesner RH. The incidence of Gram-negative bacterial and fungal infections in liver transplant patients treated with selective decontamination. *Infection* 1990;**18**: S19–S21.

23 Wiesner RH. Selective bowel decontamination for infection prophylaxis in liver transplantation patients. *Transplant Proc* 1991;**23**:1927–8.

24 Gotzinger P, Sautner T, Wamser P *et al.* Early post operative infections after liver transplantation, pathogen spectrum and risk factors. *Wien Klin Wochenschr* 1996;**108**: 795–801.

25 Badger IL, Crosby HA, Kong KL *et al.* Is selective decontamination of the digestive tract beneficial in liver transplant patients? Interim result of a prospective, randomised trial. *Transplant Proc* 1991;**23**:1460–1.

26 Smith S, Jackson J, Hannakan CJ *et al.* Selective decontamination in paediatric liver transplants. *Transplantation* 1993;**55**:1306–9.

27 Kusne S, Fung J, Alessiani M *et al.* Infections during a randomised trial comparing cyclosporine to FK506 immunosuppression in liver transplantation. *Transplant Proc* 1992;**24**:429.

28 Whiting JF, Rossi SJ, Hanto DW. Infectious complications after OKT3 induction in liver transplantation. *Liver Transplant Surg* 1997;**3**:563–70.

29 Hadley S, Samore MH, Lewis WD *et al.* Major infectious complications after orthotopic liver transplantation and comparison of outcomes in patients receiving cyclosporine or FK506 as primary immunosuppression. *Transplantation* 1995;**59**:851–9.

30 Arnow PM, Carandang GC, Zabner R *et al.* Randomized controlled trial of selective bowel decontamination for prevention of infections following liver transplantation. *Clin Infect Dis* 1996;**22**:997–1003.

31 Murcia J, Vasquez J, Hierro L *et al.* La infección como complicación del transplante hepático. *Cir Pediatr* 1990;**3**: 121–4.

32 Hasegawa S, Mori K, Inomata Y *et al.* Factors associated with post operative respiratory complications in paediatric liver transplantation from living-related donors. *Transplantation* 1996;**62**:943–7.

33 Ascher NL, Stock PG, Bumgardner GL *et al.* Infection and rejection of primary hepatic transplant in 93 consecutive patients treated with triple immunosuppressive therapy. *Surg Gynecol Obstet* 1988;**167**:474–8.

34 Colonna JO, Winston DJ, Brill JE *et al.* Infectious complications in liver transplantation. *Arch Surg* 1988;**123**;360–4.

35 Jacobs F, van de Stadt J, Burgeois N *et al.* Severe infections early after liver transplantation. *Transplant Proc* 1989;**21**:2271–3.

36 Raakow R, Steffen R, Lefebre B *et al.* Selective bowel decontamination effectively prevents Gram-negative bacterial infections after liver transplantation. *Transplant Proc* 1990;**22**:1556–7.

37 George DL, Arnow PM, Fox AS *et al.* Bacterial infection as a complication of liver transplantation: epidemiology and risk factors. *Rev Infect Dis* 1991;**13**:387–96.

38 Gayowski T, Marino IR, Singh N *et al.* Orthotopic liver transplantation: in high risk patients; risk factors associated with mortality and infectious morbidity. *Transplantation* 1998;**27**:499–504.

39 Saliba F, Ephraim R, Mathieu D *et al.* Risk factors for bacterial infection after liver transplantation. *Transplant Proc* 1994;**26**:266.

40 Busuttil RW, Colonna JO, Hiatt JR *et al.* The first 100 liver transplants at UCLA. *Ann Surg* 1987;**206**:387–402.

41 Grazi GL, Mazziotti A, Fisichella S, Scalzi E, Cavallari A. Antimicrobial prophylaxis with ceftraixone for prevention of early postoperative infections after 49 liver transplantations. *J Chemother* 2000;**12(Suppl3)**:10–16.

42 Mora NP, Klintmalm GB, Solomon H *et al.* Selective amphotericin B prophylaxis in the reduction of fungal infections after liver transplant. *Transplant Proc* 1992;**24**:154–5.

43 Briegel J, Forst H, Spill B *et al.* Risk factors for systemic fungal infections in liver transplant recipients. *Eur J Clin Microbiol Infect Dis* 1995;**14**:375–82.

44 Bert F, Galbart J-O, Zarrouk V *et al.* Association between nasal carriage of *Staphylococcus aureus* and infections in liver transplant recipients. *Clin Infect Dis* 2000;**31**:1295–9.

45 Torre-Cisneros J, Herrero C, Canas E *et al.* High mortality related with *Staphylococcus aureus* bacteremia after liver transplantation. *Eur J Clin Microbiol Infect Dis* 2002;**21**:385–8.

46 Singh N, Paterson DL, Chang FY *et al.* Methicillin-resistant *Staphylococcus aureus*: the other emerging resistant Gram-positive coccus among liver transplant recipients. *Clin Infect Dis* 2000;**30**:322–7.

47 Patel R. Association between nasal methicillin-resistant *Staphylococcus aureus* carriage and infection in liver transplant recipients. *Liver Transpl* 2001;**7**:752–4.

48 Verma A, Dhawan A, Wade JJ *et al. Mycobacterium tuberculosis* infection in pediatric liver transplant recipients. *Pediatr Infect Dis J* 2000;**19**:625–30.

49 Singh N, Wagener MM, Gayowski T. Safety and efficacy of isoniazid chemoprophylaxis administered during liver transplant candidacy for the prevention of posttransplant tuberculosis. *Transplantation* 2002;**74**:892–5.

50 Benito N, Sued O, Moreno A *et al.* Diagnosis and treatment of latent tuberculosis infection in liver transplant recipeints in an endemic area. *Transplantation* 2002;**74**:1381–6.

51 van der Waaij D, Berghuis-de Vries JM, Lekkerkerk-van der Wees JEC. Colonisation resistance of the digestive tract in conventional antibiotic-treated mice. *J Hygiene* 1971;**69**:405–11.

52 van der Waaij D, de Vries-Hospers HG, Welling GW. The influence of antibiotics on gut colonisation. *J Antimicrob Chemother* 1986;**18(Suppl C)**:155–8.

53 Vollard RJ, Clasener HAL, van Griethuysen AJA *et al.* Influence of cefaclor, phenethicillin, cotrimoxazole and doxycycline on colonisation resistance in healthy volunteers. *J Antimicrob Chemother* 1988;**22**:747–58.

54 Stoutenbeek CP, van Saene HKF, Miranda DR *et al.* The prevention of superinfection in multiple trauma patients. *J Antimicrob Chemother* 1984;**14(Suppl B)**:203–11.

55 Castaldo P, Stratta RJ, Wood RP *et al.* Clinical spectrum of fungal infections after orthotopic liver transplantation. *Arch Surg* 1991;**126**:149–56.

56 Wells CL, Maddaus MA, Simmons RL. Proposed mechanism for the translocation of intestinal bacteria. *Rev Infect Dis* 1988;**10**:958–9.

57 Vallés J, Artigas A, Rello J *et al.* Continuous aspiration of subglotic secretions in preventing ventilator associated pneumonia. *Ann Intern Med* 1995;**122**:179–86.

58 Wiesner RH, Hermans P, Rakela J *et al.* Selective bowel decontamination to prevent Gram-negative bacterial and fungal infection following orthotopic liver transplantation. *Transplant Proc* 1987;**19**:2420–3.

59 Rosman C, Klompmaker IJ, Bonsel GJ *et al.* The efficacy of selective bowel decontamination as infection prevention after liver transplantation. *Transplant Proc* 1990;**22**:2554–5.

60 Kuo PC, Bartlett ST, Lim JW *et al.* Selective bowel decontamination in hospitalised patients awaiting liver transplantation. *Am J Surg* 1997;**174**:745–8.

61 Bion JF, Badger I, Crosby HA *et al.* Selective decontamination of the digestive tract reduces Gram-negative pulmonary colonization but not systemic endotoxemia in patients undergoing elective liver transplantation. *Crit Care Med* 1994;**22**:40–9.

62 Zwavelling JH, Maring JK, Klompmaker IJ *et al.* Selective decontamination of the digestive tract to prevent postoperative infection: a randomized placebo-controlled trial in liver transplant patients. *Crit Care Med* 2002;**30**:12–49.

63 Hellinger WC, Yao JD, Alvarez S *et al.* A randomized, prospective, double-blinded evaluation of selective bowel decontamination in liver transplantation. *Transplantation* 2002;**73**:1904–9.

64 Steffen R, Reinhartz O, Blumhardt G *et al.* Bacterial and fungal colonization and infections using oral selective bowel decontamination in orthotopic liver transplantation. *Transpl Int* 1994;**7**:101–8.

65 Maring JK, Zwaveling JH, Klompmaker IJ, Meer J, Slooff MJH. Selective bowel decontamination in elective liver transplantation: no improvement in endotoxaemia, initial graft function and post-operative morbidity. *Transpl Int* 2002;**15**:329–34.

66 van Enckevort PJ, Zwaveling JH, Bottema JT *et al.* Cost effectiveness of selective decontamination of the digestive tract in liver transplant patients. *Pharmacoeconomics* 2001;**19**:523–30.

67 Selective Decontamination of the Digestive Tract Trialists' Collaborative Group. Meta analysis of randomised controlled trials of selective decontamination of the digestive tract. *BMJ* 1993;**307**:525–32.

68 Gorensek MJ, Carey WD, Washington JA *et al.* Selective bowel decontamination with quinolones and nystatin reduces Gram negative and fungal infections in orthotopic liver transplant recipients. *Cleve Clin J Med* 1993;**60**:139–44.

69 Emre S, Sebastian A, Chodoff L *et al.* Selective decontamination of the digestive tract helps prevent bacterial infections in the early postoperative period after liver transplant. *Mt Sinai J Med* 1999;**66**:310–13.

70 Tollemar J, Ericzon BG, Holmberg K *et al.* The incidence and diagnosis of invasive fungal infection in liver transplant recipients. *Transplant Proc* 1990;**22**:242–4.

71 Ruskin JD, Wood RP, Bailey MR *et al.* Comparative trial of oral clotrimazole and nystatin for oropharyngeal candidiasis prophylaxis in orthotopic liver transplant patients. *Oral Surg Oral Med Oral Pathol* 1992;**74**:567–71.

72 Viviami MA, Tortorano AM, Malaspina C *et al.* Surveillance and treatment of liver transplant recipients for candidiasis and aspergillosis. *Eur J Epidemiol* 1992;**8**:433–6.

73 Lumbreras C, Cuervas-Mons V, Jara P *et al.* Randomized trial of fluconazole versus nystatin for the prophylaxis of *Candida* infection following liver transplantation. *J Infect Dis* 1996;**174**:583–8.

74 Grauhan O, Lohmann R, Lemmens P *et al.* Fungal infection in liver transplant recipients. *Langenbecks Arch Chir* 1994;**379**:372–5.

75 Castaldo P, Stratta RJ, Wood RP *et al.* Fungal disease in liver transplant recipients: a multivariate analysis of risk factors. *Transplant Proc* 1991;**23**:1517–19.

76 Tollemar J, Ericzon BG, Barkholt L *et al.* Risk factors for deep fungal infections in liver transplant recipients. *Transplant Proc* 1990;**22**:1826–7.

77 Singh N, Avery RK, Munoz P *et al.* Trends in risk profiles and mortality associated with invasive aspergillosis among liver transplant recipients. *Clin Infect Dis* 2003;**36**:46–52.

78 Wajszczuk CP, Dummer JS, Ho M *et al.* Fungal infections in liver transplant recipients. *Transplantation* 1985;**40**: 347–53.

79 Plá MP, Berenguer J, Arzuaga FA *et al.* Surgical wound infection by *Aspergillus fumigatus* in liver transplant recipients. *Diagn Microbiol Infect Dis* 1992;**15**:703–6.

80 Rossi G, Tortorano AM, Viviani MA *et al. Aspergillus fumigatus* infections in liver transplant patients. *Transplant Proc* 1989;**21**:2268.

81 Kusne S, Torre-Cisneros J, Mañes R *et al.* Factors associated with invasive lung aspergillosis and the significance of positive *Aspergillus* culture after liver transplantation. *J Infect Dis* 1992;**16**:1379–83.

82 Snydman DR, Werner BG, Dougherty NN *et al.* Cytomegalovirus immune globulin prophylaxis in liver transplantation: a randomized, double-blind, placebo-controlled trial. *Ann Intern Med* 1993;**119**:984–91.

83 Fortun J, Martin-Davila P, Moreno S *et al.* Risk factors for invasive aspergillosis in liver transplant recipients. *Liver Transpl* 2002;**8**:1065–70.

84 Snydman DR, Werner BG, Heinze-Lacey B *et al.* Use of cytomegalovirus immune globulin to prevent cytomegalovirus disease in renal transplant recipients. *N Engl J Med* 1987; **217**:1049–54.

85 Castaldo P, Stratta RJ, Wood RP *et al.* Fungal infection in liver allograft recipients. *Transplant Proc* 1991;**23**:1967.

86 Mora NP, Cofer JB, Solomon H *et al.* Analysis of severe infections (INF) after 180 consecutive liver transplants: the impact of amphotericin B prophylaxis for reducing the incidence and severity of fungal infections. *Transplant Proc* 1991;**23**:1528–30.

87 Rabkin JM, Oroloff SL, Corless CL *et al.* Association of fungal infection and increased mortality in liver transplant recipients. *Am J Surg* 2000;**179**:426–9.

88 Winston DJ, Pakrasi A, Busuttil RW. Prophylactic fluconazole in liver transplant recipients. A randomized, double-blind, placebo-controlled trial. *Ann Intern Med* 1999;**131**:729–37.

89 Winston DJ, Busuttil RW. Randomized controlled trial of oral itraconazole solution versus intravenous/oral fluconazole for prevention of fungal infections in liver transplant recipients. *Transplantation* 2002;**74**:688–95.

90 Wingard JR, Merz WG, Rinaldi MG *et al.* Increase in *Candida krusei* infection among patients with bone marrow transplantation and neutropenia treated prophylactically with fluconazole. *N Engl J Med* 1991;**325**: 1274–7.

91 Fisher NC, Cooper MA, Hastings JGM, Mutimer DJ. Fungal colonization and fluconazole therapy in acute liver disease. *Liver* 1998;**18**:320–5.

92 Tollemar J, Hickerstedt K, Ericzon BG *et al.* Liposomal amphotericin B prevents invasive fungal infections in liver transplant recipients. A randomised, placebo-controlled study. *Transplantation* 1995;**59**:45–50.

93 Singh N, Paterson DL, Gayowski T, Wagener MM, Marino GR. Preemptive prophylaxis with a lipid preparation of amphotericin B for invasive fungal infections in liver transplant recipients requiring renal replacement therapy. *Transplantation* 2001;**7**:910–13.

94 Hayes MJ, Torzillo PJ, Sheil AGR *et al. Pneumocystis carinii* pneumonia after liver transplantation in adults. *Clin Transplant* 1994;**8**:499–503.

95 Colombo JL, Sammut PH, Langnas AN *et al.* The spectrum of *Pneumocystis carinii* infection after liver transplantation in children. *Transplantation* 1992;**316**:621–4.

96 Torres-Cisneros J, de la Mata M, Lopez-Cillero P *et al.* Effectiveness of daily low-dose cotrimoxazole prophylaxis for *Pneumocystis carinii* pneumonia in liver transplantation. *Transplantation* 1996;**62**:1519–21.

97 Linden P, Coley K, Kramer D *et al.* Invasive aspergillosis in liver transplant recipients: comparison of outcome with amphotericin B lipid complex and conventional amphotericin B therapy. *Transplantation* 1999;**67**:S232.

98 Tollemar J, Klingspor L, Ringden O. Liposomal amphotericin B (AmBisome) for fungal infections in immunocompromised adults and children. *Clin Microbiol Infect* 2001;**7(Suppl 2)**:68–79.

99 Duchini A, Redfgield DC, McHutchinson JG, Brunson ME, Pockros PJ. Aspergillosis in liver transplant recipients: successful treatment and improved survival using a multistep approach. *Southern Med J* 2002;**95**:897–9.

100 Patel R, Paya CV. Infections in solid-organ transplant recipients. *Clin Microbiol Rev* 1997;**10**:86–124.

101 Patel R, Snydman DR, Rubin RH *et al.* Cytomegalovirus prophylaxis in solid organ transplant recipients. *Transplantation* 1996;**61**:1279–89.

102 Kanj SS, Sharara AI, Clavien P-A *et al.* Cytomegalovirus infection following liver transplantation: review of the literature. *Clin Infect Dis* 1996;**22**:537–49.

103 Cofer JB, Morris CA, Sutker WL *et al.* A randomized double-blind study of the effect of prophylactic immune globulin on the incidence and severity of CMV infection in the liver transplant recipient. *Transplant Proc* 1991;**23**:1525–7.

104 Saliba F, Arulnaden JL, Gugenheim J *et al.* CMV hyperimmune globulin prophylaxis after liver transplantation: a prospective randomized controlled study. *Transplant Proc* 1989;**21**:2260–2.

105 Snydman DR, Werner BG, Dougherty NN *et al* and the Boston Center for liver transplantation CMVIG Study Group. A further analysis of the use of cytomegalovirus immune globulin in orthotopic liver transplant patients at risk for primary infection. *Transplant Proc* 1994;**26**:23–7.

106 Glowacki LS, Smaill FM. Use of immune globulin to prevent symptomatic cytomegalovirus disease in transplant recipients – a meta-analysis. *Clin Transplantation* 1994;**8**:10–18.

107 Saliba F, Eyraud D, Samuel D *et al.* Randomized controlled trial of acyclovir for the prevention of cytomegalovirus infection and disease in liver transplant recipients. *Transplant Proc* 1993;**25**:1444–5.

108 Green M, Reyes J, Nour B *et al.* Randomized trial of ganciclovir followed by high-dose oral acyclovir vs ganciclovir alone in prevention of cytomegalovirus disease in paediatric liver transplant recipients: preliminary analysis. *Transplant Proc* 1994;**26**:173–4.

109 Nakazato PZ, Burns W, Moore P *et al.* Viral prophylaxis in hepatic transplantation: preliminary report of a randomized trial of acyclovir and ganciclovir. *Transplant Proc* 1993;**2**:1935–7.

110 Martin M, Manez R, Linden P *et al.* A prospective randomized trial comparing sequential ganciclovir-high dose acyclovir for prevention of cytomegalovirus disease in adult liver transplant recipients. *Transplantation* 1994;**58**:779–85.

111 Cohen AT, O'Grady J, Sutherland S *et al.* Controlled trial of prophylactic versus therapeutic use of ganciclovir after liver transplantation in adults. *J Med Virol* 1993;**40**:5–9.

112 Winston DW, Wirin D, Shaked A *et al.* Randomised comparison of ganciclovir and high-dose acyclovir for long-term cytomegalovirus prophylaxis in liver-transplant recipients. *Lancet* 1995;**346**:69–74.

113 Seu P, Winston DJ, Holt CD *et al.* Long-term ganciclovir prophylaxis for successful prevention of primary cytomegalovirus (CMV) disease in CMV-seronegative liver transplant recipients with CMV-seropositive donors. *Transplantation* 1997;**64**:1614–17.

114 King SM, Superina R, Andrews W *et al.* Randomized comparison of ganciclovir plus intravenous immune globulin (IVIG) with IVIG alone for prevention of primary cytomegalovirus disease in children receiving liver transplants. *Clin Infect Dis* 1997;**25**:1173–9.

115 Badley AD, Seaberg EC, Porayko MK *et al.* Prophylaxis of cytomegalovirus infection in liver transplantation. A randomized trial comparing a combination of ganciclovir and acyclovir to acyclovir. *Transplantation* 1997;**64**:66–73.

116 Barkholt, Lewensohn-Fuchs I, Ericzon B G, *et al.* High-dose acyclovir prophylaxis reduces cytomegalovirus disease in liver transplant patients. *Transplant Infect Dis* 1999;**1**:89–97.

117 Winston DJ, Busutil RW. Randomized controlled trial of oral ganciclovir versus oral acyclovir after induction with intravenous ganciclovir for long-term prophylaxis of cytomegalovirus disease in cytomegalovirus seropositive liver transplant patients. *Transplantation* 2003;**75**:229–33.

118 Stratta RJ, Shaefer MS, Cushing KA *et al.* A randomized prospective trial of acyclovir and immune globulin prophylaxis in liver transplant recipients receiving OKT3 therapy. *Arch Surg* 1992;**127**:55–63.

119 Lumbreras C, Otero JR, Herrero JA *et al.* Ganciclovir prophylaxis decreases frequency and severity of cytomegalovirus disease in seropositive liver transplant recipients treated with OKT3 monoclonal antibodies. *Antimicrob Agents Chemother* 1993;**37**:2490–2.

120 Singh N, Yu VL, Mieles L *et al.* High-dose aciclovir compared with short-course pre-emptive ganciclovir therapy to prevent cytomegalovirus disease in liver transplant recipients. *Ann Intern Med* 1994;**120**:375–81.

121 Paya CV, Wilson JA, Espy MJ *et al.* Preemptive use of oral ganciclovir to prevent cytomegalovirus infection in liver transplant patients: a randomized, placebo-controlled trial. *J Infect Dis* 2002;**185**:854–60.

122 Torre-Cisneros J, Madueno JA, Herrero C *et al.* Pre-emptive oral gancyclovir can reduce the risk of cytomegalovirus disease in liver transplant recipients. *Clin Microbiol Infect* 2002;**8**:773–80.

123 Singh N, Paterson D, Gayowski T *et al.* Cytomegalovirus antigenemia directed pre-emptive prophylaxis with oral versus IV gancyclovir for the prevention of cytomegalovirus disease in liver transplant recipients. *Transplantation* 2000;**70**:717–22.

124 Rayes N, Seehofer D, Schmidt CA *et al.* Prospective randomised trial to asses the value of preemptive oral therapy for CMV infection following liver transplantation. *Transplantation* 2001;**72**:881–5.

125 Daly JS, Kopasz A, Anandakrishnan R *et al.* Preemptive strategy for ganciclovir administration against cytomegalovirus in liver transplantation recipients. *Am J Transplant* 2002;**2**:955–8.

38 Management of hepatitis B and C after liver transplantation

George V Papatheodoridis, Rosângela Teixeira

Introduction

Hepatitis C virus (HCV)-related chronic liver disease represents the most common indication for orthotopic liver transplantation (OLT) worldwide, while hepatitis B virus (HBV)-related chronic liver disease is a frequent indication for OLT in the Far East and the Mediterranean countries. Post-transplant HBV recurrence, which was almost universal in the era of no or short-term immunoprophylaxis, usually has an aggressive course resulting in graft loss, if left untreated.[1–3] Recurrence of HCV infection after OLT is still universal and is associated with a more rapid progression of liver disease than has been observed in immunocompetent patients.[4] Therefore, the management of both hepatitis B and C is crucial for a satisfactory long-term outcome of HBV or HCV transplant patients.

Management of hepatitis B in transplant patients

HBV-related liver disease was considered to be a relative or even absolute contraindication to OLT in many centers, until the introduction of long-term hepatitis B immune globulin (HBIG) use in the early nineties, which significantly decreased the post-transplant HBV recurrence rate and improved the prognosis in this setting.[5] During the last 4–5 years, new antiviral agents, mainly nucleos(t)ide analogs, have been used or evaluated, either as monotherapy or in combination with HBIG, in an effort to further improve the outcome, treat HBIG failures, and/or reduce the need for the use of the expensive HBIG preparations.[6] The management of hepatitis B in HBV transplant patients can be divided into the pretransplant, the prophylactic post-transplant and the therapeutic post-transplant approaches.[6]

Pretransplant approach

The pretransplant approach consists of antiviral therapy during the pretransplant period to lower or clear the viral load at the time of OLT and thus prevent post-transplant HBV recurrence.[6] The pretransplant approach is usually combined with prophylactic post-transplant therapy.[6]

Lamivudine, a cytosine analog with quite potent anti-HBV activity, was the first therapeutic agent that could be widely used in the pretransplant period. It is generally well tolerated even in severely ill cirrhotic patients and has an extremely good safety profile with rare and generally mild adverse effects. In contrast, interferon-alpha (IFN-α), which was the only available anti-HBV therapeutic option until the late nineties, is usually contraindicated or poorly tolerated and therefore could not be used in patients with decompensated cirrhosis.[7] Lamivudine monotherapy, at a daily dose of 100 mg, has been shown to stabilize or even improve liver function[8–10] sometimes resulting in withdrawal of the patients from transplant lists. B4 Unfortunately, the improvement or stabilization of liver function is not often sustained, since the prolongation of lamivudine therapy is associated with progressively increasing rates of virologic and biochemical breakthroughs due to selection of lamivudine-resistant YMDD mutant HBV strains[8,9,11,12] (common YMDD mutations: rtM204V or rtM204I and rtL180M[13,14]).

Breakthroughs during lamivudine therapy are associated with a risk of severe exacerbation of liver disease[12,15] and perhaps with an increased probability of post-transplant HBV recurrence.[16] In fact, the post-transplant outcome of patients with pretransplant HBV viremia due to YMDD mutants is currently unclear. Post-transplant HBV recurrence was not observed during the first 32–35 months post-transplantation in 10 patients with pretransplant YMDD mutants, who received high dose HBIG and lamivudine.[17,18] B4 However, two patients with pretransplant YMDD mutants were reported to rapidly develop post-transplant HBV recurrence despite combined prophylaxis with low dose HBIG and lamivudine.[19] Whether the dose of HBIG is an important factor determining post-transplant HBV recurrence in patients with resistance to lamivudine pretransplantation, and the precise risk of HBV recurrence in such patients is currently unknown. However, transplant centers may be reluctant to perform OLT in patients with HBV cirrhosis and detectable serum HBV-DNA irrespective of the type of HBV strains.[20]

The recent availability of adefovir dipivoxil, a nucleotide analog of adenosine esterified with two pivalic acid molecules, which is effective against both wild and lamivudine-resistant HBV strains,[21,22] is expected to ameliorate the consequences of lamivudine resistance. In fact, the addition of adefovir dipivoxil, at a daily dose of 10 mg, has been shown to result in biochemical, virologic and liver function improvement in HBV patients with decompensated cirrhosis and resistance to lamivudine.[23] B4 Thus, it seems reasonable to suggest that all HBV transplant candidates with detectable serum HBV-DNA should be treated with lamivudine and followed up closely for viral resistance. Adefovir dipivoxil should be started immediately if evidence of viral resistance develops. The long-term safety and efficacy of adefovir therapy, the need for continuing lamivudine after development of resistance, and the cost effectiveness of *ab initio* use of adefovir alone or in combination of lamivudine are unknown.

Prophylactic post-transplant approach

Passive immunoprophylaxis alone

The efficacy of HBIG is related to the pretransplant type of liver disease and viremic status as well as to the dose of HBIG and duration of the treatment, while the most widely accepted recommendations for HBIG prophylaxis depend mainly on the pretransplant viremic status.[24] Patients with detectable serum HBV-DNA by conventional hybridization assays, who may be transplanted only after clearance of HBV-DNA by lamivudine, are treated with more aggressive HBIG protocols compared with non-viremic patients.[24] However, several practical questions, mainly about the ideal duration of therapy, and also about dosage, frequency and mode of HBIG administration remain to be answered.[6]

HBIG may only rarely lead to eradication of HBV and therefore is needed for indefinite HBIG prophylaxis, which is an extremely expensive approach. The most cost effective approach seems to be the individual tailoring of HBIG administration according to serum anti-HBs levels.[6,24] Cheaper HBIG preparations for intramuscular administration have also been tried,[25–27] but no evidence from long-term studies of such an approach is currently available. Another reported strategy to reduce cost is the substitution of HBIG by anti-HBV vaccination.[28,29] C5 However, data on the efficacy of vaccination are rather conflicting[28–30] and therefore greater numbers of patients and longer follow up periods are required before the long-term efficacy of this strategy can be determined.

Besides the high cost, long-term HBIG administration has also been associated with emergence of escape mutant HBV strains, which seem to progressively accumulate over time and to be associated with increasing rates of graft failure.[14,24,31–33] B4 Since the clinical significance of such HBV escape mutants has not been clarified, there is no consensus about whether

HBIG therapy should be continued after their emergence.[24] Most centers probably stop HBIG administration.[6]

Prophylactic post-transplant monotherapy with lamivudine

Lamivudine was first tried as monotherapy administered before and prophylactically after OLT and had promising short-term results in initial reports.[34] However, it was subsequently shown that the efficacy of such a strategy declines over time with very frequent development of virologic breakthroughs and HBV recurrence in 40–50% of cases at 2 years post transplantation, and serious adverse clinical outcomes in some patients.[35–39] B4 This approach should be abandoned.

Prophylactic post-transplant combined approach

Post-transplant prophylactic combined administration of HBIG and lamivudine was tried in HBV transplant patients in an effort to improve the efficacy of post-transplant prophylaxis and/or reduce cost. The overall efficacy of such a combined regimen appears to be superior to the efficacy of either of the two agents alone. In particular, in 17 recent studies of prophylactic therapy with HBIG and lamivudine, post-transplant HBV recurrence was observed in only 20 (4%) of 481 patients during a mean follow up of 13–30 months (Table 38.1).[19,25,26,40–53] B4 This combined prophylactic therapy post-transplantation is usually preceded by pretransplant lamivudine monotherapy in pretransplant viremic patients.[19,25,26,40–42,44,45,47,48,51–53] It should be also noted that five of the 20 patients with post-transplant HBV recurrence had developed YMDD mutants during the pretransplant lamivudine therapy,[19,42,52] while HBIG had been discontinued when HBV recurrence occurred in another two patients.[52] However, a potentially important finding in one study was that serum HBV-DNA could be detected by polymerase chain reaction (PCR) in 16 of 26 (61·5%) cases.[48] Thus, longer follow up is required before definite conclusions can be drawn about the efficacy of the prophylactic combination of HBIG and lamivudine.

One particularly important aspect in favor of the combination of HBIG and lamivudine for prophylaxis is that this approach was used in patients with high pretransplant serum HBV-DNA levels (> 50% of cases had HBV-DNA detectable by hybridization assays) and achieved low HBV reinfection rates at a reduced cost. A relatively low HBIG dosage,[19,25,26,40,43,48,50] similar to that currently recommended for non-viremic HBV transplant patients[24] and/or intramuscular HBIG preparations were usually used.[25,26,43,50,51] HBIG was even discontinued after a certain period.[52,53] Moreover, conversion from intravenous to low dose intramuscular HBIG administration in combination with lamivudine has been suggested to be a safe, effective, and cost effective approach

Table 38.1 Published studies of combination therapy with hepatitis B immune globulin (HBIG) and lamivudine (LAM) for prevention of hepatitis B virus (HBV) recurrence after orthotopic liver transplantation (OLT) for HBV-related chronic liver disease

Study	No.	Patients with HBV-DNA (+)[a]: baseline/at OLT	Pre-OLT, LAM (mg)	Post-OLT HBIG dose (IU), (cumulative within 1st month) – after the 1st month	Post-OLT LAM (mg)	Mean follow-up (months)	No. of HBV recurrences (%)	Survival (%)
Markowitz et al. (1998)[40]	14	5/1	150	(80 000)–10 000/month IV	150	13	0	93
Yao et al. (1999)[25]	10	9/2	150	(5555[b])–1111/3 weeks IM	150	16	1 (10)	90
Yoshida, et al. (1999)[26]	7	4/0	100	(34 720)–2170/1–4 weeks IM	100	18	1 (14)	86
McCaughan et al. (1999)[41]	9	6[c]/c[c]	0	Low dose (no details)	NA	17	0	89
Roche et al. (1999)[42]	15	15/4	100	No details – anti-HBs > 500 IU/l	100	16	1 (7)	93
Angus et al. (2000)[43]	32	NA	100	(3200–6400) – 400 or 800/month IM	100	18	1 (3)	100[i]
Han et al. (2000)[44]	59	20/16	150	(80 000)–10 000/month IV	150	15	0	98
Lee et al. (2000)[45]	5	1/0	100	(26 000)–2000/month IV[d]	100	11	0	80
Andreone et al. (2000)[46]	19	NA	100	(45 000)–5000/month IV	100	17	1 (5)	95
Buti et al. (2000)[47]	12	9/0	100	(62 000)–2000/month IV–IM[e]	100	12	0	100
Marzano et al. (2001)[48]	26	9/0[f]	100	(60 000)–5000/month IV	100	30	1[h] (4)	92
Rosenau et al. (2001)[19]	21	12/5[g]	100–150	(40 000 – anti-HBs > 500 IU/l) – anti-HBs > 100 IU/l IV	100–150	20	2 (10)	90
Machicao et al. (2001)[49]	30	NA	NA	High dose	NA	22	0	97
Choi et al. (2002)[50]	56	38/NA	–	(10 000)–10 000/month IV × 6 months[j]–2000/2 months IM	100	26	4 (7)	NA
Gane et al. (2002)[51]	107	74/35	100	(3200–6400)–400 or 800/month IM	100	27	4 (4)	87
Kim et al. (2002)[52]	51	30/NA	100–150	(80 000)–10 000/month IV × 6 or 12 months	100–150	21	4 (8)	NA
Chu et al. (2002)[53]	8	NA	100	(10 000)–10 000/month IV × 43 months –1000/month IM × 12 months	100[k]	16[k]	0	100

[a]Serum HBV-DNA detectable by hybridization assays.

[b]Plus 10 000 IU during anhepatic phase in all patients and another 70 000 IU during the first 7 days in two HBV-DNA positive patients.

[c]Another three patients had detectable serum HBV-DNA by a polymerase chain reaction (PCR) assay.

[d]One patient received 80 000 IU of HBIG during the first month, while another patient received only 2000 IU of HBIG during the anhepatic phase and four IM injections of 650 IU each within the first 6 months after OLT.

[e]IV for the first 4 weeks and IM thereafter; five of the 12 patients received HBIG only for the first 4 weeks after OLT.

[f]Seven patients had detectable serum HBV-DNA by a PCR assay.

[g]Two out of four patients tested had YMDD mutant strains, while another three patients had detectable serum HBV-DNA by a PCR assay.

[h]Serum HBV-DNA was detected by PCR in another 61·5% (16 patients).

[i]Five patients, who died within one month after OLT from unrelated to HBV causes, were not included in this survival estimation.

[j]Thirteen patients received higher HBIG dosage (10 000 IU IV daily for 7 days, 10 000 IU IV weekly for 1 month, and then 10 000 IU IV monthly for several years before conversion to IM HBIG.

[k]Post-transplant LAM was added when HBIG administration changed from IV to IM; 16 months median follow up after the onset of LAM.

Reproduced with permission from Papatheodoridis GV et al. Am J Transplant 2003;3:250–8.[6]

NA, not available; IV intravenous; IM intramuscular

for the prevention of post-OLT HBV recurrence.[44,54] Thus, the prophylactic post-transplant combination of HBIG and lamivudine preceded by short-term pretransplant lamivudine therapy appears to be the current strategy of choice in high risk viremic HBV transplant patients, since it is associated with the lowest post-transplant HBV recurrence rate and probably has reduced costs due to low HBIG dosage.[6] B4

Another strategy using combination therapy for prophylaxis has been the withdrawal of HBIG administration after a certain period, followed by maintenance lamivudine alone,[55] but good evidence supporting this approach is still lacking. In a recent small randomized trial in 24 HBV transplant patients with low risk of recurrence (no pretransplant viremia and no HBV recurrence on ≥ 6 months of post-transplant HBIG prophylaxis), there was no difference in the 12-month recurrence rates between patients remaining on HBIG and those receiving lamivudine alone.[56] A1d Similarly, HBV recurrence was not observed in any of 16 HBV transplant patients who continuously received HBIG for 2 years and then switched over to lamivudine monotherapy for an additional period of up to 27 months.[57] B4 Thus, it seems that post-transplant HBIG prophylaxis might be replaced by lamivudine after ≥ 6 months post-transplant in selected HBV transplant patients with low risk of HBV recurrence, but data on the long-term efficacy of such a strategy are still needed.

Therapeutic post-transplant approach

Therapeutic post-transplant approach in patients without resistance to lamivudine

The therapeutic post-transplant approach is usually used in cases with HBV recurrence despite previous post-transplant prophylaxis. The primary targets of treatment of post-transplant HBV recurrence are the control of liver disease and stabilization of graft function.[6] Lamivudine is currently the most frequently used agent in patients with recurrence in spite of HBIG prophylaxis (Table 38.2), but it may be inactive in patients receiving lamivudine-based prophylactic regimens who may exhibit resistance to lamivudine. In eight studies including about 200 patients with post-transplant HBV infection despite HBIG prophylaxis, a 12–25 month course of lamivudine resulted in significant reduction of serum HBV-DNA levels and no significant clinical manifestations developed.[37,58–64] B4 Lamivudine has also shown promising results in the treatment of fibrosing cholestatic hepatitis.[65,66]

Similarly to the results described in the pre-transplant approach, the main disadvantage of long-term lamivudine monotherapy is the progressively increasing rates of viral resistance, exceeding 50% at 3 years of therapy in the transplant setting.[60,64,67–69] The clinical significance of resistance to lamivudine is not clear. In both transplant and non-transplant patients and lamivudine-resistant post-transplant reinfection cases it appears that the clinical course

is relatively milder than is observed in cases with wild HBV recurrence.[70] However, the emergence of such HBV mutants has been associated with rapid development of advanced histologic lesions and even liver failure and death in some HBV transplant patients.[68,71,72] Thus, all HBV transplant patients with resistance to lamivudine are candidates for treatment with new antiviral agents effective against such mutant HBV strains.

Besides lamivudine, several other nucleos(t)ide analogs have been tried or are currently being evaluated for the treatment of subgroups of patients with HBV infection, including those with post-transplant HBV recurrence. Adefovir dipivoxil has now been approved in several countries for the treatment of HBV-related chronic liver disease. It is well tolerated without evidence of nephrotoxicity in the currently recommended daily dose of 10 mg.[22,73,74] Relatively higher doses (30–120 mg daily) have been associated with an increased risk of nephrotoxicity after ≥ 20 weeks of therapy[75] and the dose should be reduced to 5 mg daily if creatinine clearance is < 50 ml/min. A significant advantage of adefovir is that it seems to be associated with rather rare and slow development of viral resistance (< 2% of cases treated for 96-weeks developed N236T mutation[76]). B4

Entecavir, a carboxylic analog of guanosine, has been found to suppress HBV replication satisfactorily in chronic hepatitis B patients.[77] B4 Famciclovir, a guanosine analog with cross resistance with lamivudine,[78,79] was inferior to lamivudine and has never been used widely.[67,69,80] Ganciclovir, another guanosine analog, was found to have some biochemical, virologic and histological benefit,[81,82] but the need for intravenous use restricts its use. B4 The safety and effectiveness of adefovir and entecavir as well as of other newer nucleos(t)ide analogues are currently under evaluation in clinical trials in transplant or non-transplant patients infected with wild or lamivudine resistant HBV strains.

In the pre-lamivudine era, IFN-α was a common therapeutic option for patients with post-transplant HBV recurrence. The role of IFN-α as first line treatment in this setting has currently almost disappeared due to both its low efficacy[83,84] and a low but possible theoretical risk of graft rejection.[83,84] B4, C5

Therapeutic post-transplant approach in patients with resistance to lamivudine

Since lamivudine is currently widely used in HBV transplant patients as pretransplant or prophylactic post-transplant therapy or as treatment for HBV recurrence, the number of transplant patients with HBV strains resistant to lamivudine is expected to increase.[6] Several antiviral agents are currently being evaluated as candidates for the treatment of patients with such HBV strains.

Adefovir dipivoxil has been shown to be effective in HBV transplant patients with resistance to lamivudine for

Table 38.2   Published studies of lamivudine (LAM) therapy for hepatitis B virus (HBV) recurrence or *de novo* HBV infection after orthotopic liver transplantation (OLT)

Study	No.	Baseline serum HBV-DNA (+)[a]: n (%)	Baseline HBeAg (+): n (%)	Mean duration of LAM (months)	Clearance of serum HBV-DNA. n (%) (Hybridization–PCR)	Clearance of HBeAg: n (%)	Clearance of HBsAg: n (%)	YMDD mutants: n (%)
Andreone *et al.* (1998)[58]	11[b]	11 (100)	2 (18)	16	8 (73)–5 (45)	2/2 (100)	5 (45)	3 (27)
Nery *et al.* (1998)[59]	11[c]	10 (91)	NA	25	8 (73)–NA	NA	NA	2 (18)
Perrillo *et al.* (1999)[60]	52	52 (100)	45 (87)	12	31 (60)–NA	14/45 (31)	3 (6)	14 (27)
Roche *et al.* (1999)[61]	16	16 (100)	10 (63)	16	7 (44)–NA	3/10 (30)	3 (19)	6/12 (50)
Balan *et al.* (1999)[62]	24	NA	NA	25	9 (37)	NA	NA	15 (63)
Malkan *et al.* (2000)[37]	15[d]	14 (93)	6 (40)	23	13 (87)–NA	NA	4 (27)	2 (13)
Seehofer *et al.* (2000)[63]	41[e]	41 (100)	NA	≥12	31 (76)–NA	NA	9 (22)	14 (34)
Fontana *et al.* (2001)[64]	31	29 (94)	23 (74)	20	11 (36)–NA	3/23 (13)	0	13/29 (45)
Ben-Ari *et al.* (2001)[68]	8[f]	8 (100)	5 (63)	36	3 (38)–NA	1/5 (20)	0	5 (63)

[a]Serum HBV-DNA detectable by hybridization assays.
[b]All patients had acute HBV recurrence.
[c]Three patients had *de novo* HBV recurrence and another two patients had been treated with famciclovir before start of LAM.
[d]Four patients had *de novo* HBV recurrence.
[e]Twenty-two patients had been treated with famciclovir therapy before start of LAM.
[f]Two patients had *de novo* HBV recurrence.
Reproduced with permission from Papatheodoridis GV *et al. Am J Transplant* 2003;**3**:250–8.[6]
NA, not available; PCR, polymerase chain reaction

improving serum HBV-DNA and transaminase levels.[22,73,74,85] B4 In addition to clinical trials, protocols of compassionate use of adefovir dipivoxil in HBV transplant or pretransplant patients are currently running in many centers. Recent case reports suggested that adefovir dipivoxil is effective against lamivudine-resistant HBV strains and for prevention of HBV recurrence after OLT for fulminant liver failure in a renal transplant recipient,[72] for treatment of post-transplant fibrosing cholestatic hepatitis,[86,87] and for treatment of acute liver graft failure.[88]

Entecavir appears also to be effective against lamivudine-resistant HBV strains in non-transplant[89,90] and transplant patients.[91] B4 Although IFN-α has been almost abandoned as first line therapy for post-transplant HBV recurrence, it may still have a role, alone or in combination with other antiviral agents, as a second choice therapeutic option for patients who develop resistance to lamivudine or other nucleoside analogs.[92] The addition of IFN-α to lamivudine therapy has been used for the treatment of a few transplant and non-transplant patients with lamivudine-resistant HBV mutant strains with promising initial results.[93] However, more studies

with greater patient numbers are needed before any conclusion can be drawn about the effectiveness of IFN-α for lamivudine-resistant HBV strains.

Management of hepatitis C in transplant patients

The course of post-transplant hepatitis C appears to be accelerated compared with that seen in non-transplant immunocompetent patients with chronic hepatitis C.[4] It is estimated that histological recurrence occurs in the majority of patients within the first year after OLT[94,95] and that approximately 15–30% develop cirrhosis within the first 5 years with subsequent reduced graft and patient survival.[95–98] Although 2–5% of HCV transplant patients may develop severe cholestatic hepatitis and early graft failure,[99] a large proportion of them may have a rather benign course with mild to moderate histological lesions.[95,96] Since not all HCV transplant patients progress to advanced fibrosis, at least in the medium term, many studies have tried to identify significant

Table 38.3 Parameters suggested to be associated with the outcome of hepatitis C virus (HCV) recurrence after liver transplantation.[97,98,100–112]

Pretransplantation	Peritransplantation	Post-transplantation
Sex and race	Time of surgery	Type and doses of immunosuppressive drugs
Age at HCV infection	Number of blood transfusions	Use of monoclonal antibodies
Route of infection	Time of cold ischemia	Number of acute rejection episodes
Concomitant hepatocellular carcinoma	Time of ischemic rewarming	Number of prednisolone bolus
Child's class at transplantation	Histocompatibility	Duration of steroids
Alcohol disease	Year of transplant	Time of acute hepatitis C
HCV-RNA viral load pretransplant	Donor age	HCV RNA viral load post-transplant
HCV genotype		Evolution of HCV quasi-species
Coinfection with HBV or HDV		Antiviral therapy
Iron overload		Immune response
Steatosis		CMV hepatitis

factors associated with rapid progression of disease. Several viral, host, donor and transplant-related factors have been suggested to be associated with the severity of HCV recurrence (Table 38.3),[97,98,100–112] but as yet no factor has been repeatedly shown to be a strong predictor of the outcome of these patients.[113–116] Recently, several centers have reported worsening progression of recurrent HCV disease with more recently transplanted patients.[98,108,114,115] It is unclear, however, if this is due to changes in immunosuppression with time, increasing donor age or other factors.

The management of hepatitis C in transplant patients can be based on two distinct therapeutic strategies: antiviral therapy and/or modification of immunosuppression. Antiviral therapy may be tried before OLT in an effort to lower HCV-RNA levels. Both antiviral therapy and modification of immunosuppression may be applied separately or in combination after OLT in two situations (i) pre-emptively in the early post-transplant phase, or (ii) if and when moderate or severe HCV recurrence develops. The primary targets of any therapeutic strategy in HCV transplant patients should be eradication or permanent suppression of HCV or at least prevention of liver disease progression.[113,114,117]

Antiviral therapy

IFN-α, and recently, pegylated IFN-α (PEG-IFN-α) and ribavirin are the currently available agents for the treatment of HCV.[118] Recent large randomized trials have shown that the combination of PEG-IFN-α and ribavirin is the most potent therapeutic option for non-transplant chronic hepatitis C patients.[119,120] In the HCV transplant setting, however, information on the safety and efficacy of most antiviral regimens is based on limited data from relatively small, usually uncontrolled studies. Moreover, data from the non-transplant setting cannot be extrapolated to the HCV transplant setting, since HCV transplant patients are difficult to treat effectively, and the therapy is less applicable. In

particular, they often have several factors that reduce the probability of response to therapy, such as high proportion of HCV genotype 1b, extremely high serum HCV-RNA levels (10 to 100-fold higher after OLT[102,103]), and failure to respond to previous therapies,[118] treatment with immunosuppressive drugs and contraindications to the use of full doses or even any dose of the antiviral agents that include low hemoglobin, platelet and/or neutrophil counts early after transplant and renal failure.

Pre-transplant antiviral therapy

On the basis of some reports – that high pre-transplant HCV-RNA levels are strongly associated with significantly worse 5-year survival[104] – it might be anticipated that a decrease of pretransplant viremia may improve the course of recurrent disease after transplantation. In patients with decompensated cirrhosis, however, IFN-α is associated with frequent and potentially severe adverse events and is often limited by thrombocytopenia and/or neutropenia and thus its applicability is rather limited. Thus, IFN-α as pretransplant treatment may only be appropriate for patients with Child's class A and perhaps early B cirrhosis who may be listed because of hepatocellular carcinoma.[121] B4, C5 If new antiviral agents effective for inhibiting HCV replication, which are safe and well tolerated even in patients with decompensated cirrhosis become available, they will be a major advance in the treatment of such patients and pretransplant antiviral therapy may be widely applied to all HCV-RNA positive patients.[122]

Pre-emptive post-transplant antiviral therapy

The aim of antiviral therapy starting soon after OLT is to prevent significant HCV-related liver disease by rendering patients HCV-RNA negative or sufficiently reducing HCV replication. This time may be "optimal" because: (i) the antiviral therapy will start before the peak of viremia and the acute HCV reinfection; (ii) immunosuppression has just started; and (iii) cellular rejection occurs more frequently in this period, necessitating large bolus doses of corticosteroids, that will increase viremia.[117] However, anti-viral therapy should not start until about 10–14 days post-OLT because of frequent thrombocytopenia and intercurrent bacterial infections in this period.[117] The safety and efficacy of pre-emptive post-transplant therapy with IFN-α monotherapy or combination therapy with IFN-α and ribavirin have been evaluated in only a few, relatively small, studies.

In an initial uncontrolled trial, only four of 48 patients had no hepatitis at 1-year liver biopsy after 1-year therapy with IFN-α started within 1 week post OLT.[123] Subsequently, three controlled trials evaluated pre-emptive 6 and 12-month courses of IFN-α monotherapy starting within the first 4 weeks post OLT.[124-126] Acute hepatitis C was delayed in one (408 and 188 days in the treated and untreated group),[124] but not in the other (194 and 220 days in the treated and untreated group),[125] while sustained virologic responses were observed in 33% of patients treated with the combination of IFN-α and ribavirin and in only 13% of those treated with either IFN-α monotherapy or untreated controls.[126] There was no difference in graft and patient survival or cellular rejection rate between treated and untreated patients in any of these trials. Alc

PEG-IFN-α monotherapy has also begun to be evaluated in this setting. Preliminary results at 24 weeks from a recent randomized trial[127] showed that PEG-IFNa-2α (180 micrograms once weekly), starting after 2 weeks post-OLT, achieved a 2-log decrease in viremia levels in 57% and clearance of serum HCV-RNA in 29% of treated patients compared with none from the untreated controls. PEG-IFN-2α was well tolerated and it was associated with a lower incidence of adverse effects compared with controls and no increase in the incidence of rejection.[127] Ald

In a pilot study,[128] a 12-month course of combination therapy with IFN-α (3 MU thrice weekly) and ribavirin (10 mg/kg daily), starting at a median of 18 days post-OLT, achieved sustained virologic response in 12 (33%) of 36 patients. Moreover, histological chronic hepatitis developed in only 7 (19%) and chronic graft damage in only 4 (11%) patients during a median follow up of 4.5 years without any adjustment in immunosuppression. No patient experienced chronic rejection or cholestatic hepatitis.[128] However, in a subsequent randomized, placebo-controlled trial of IFN-α plus ribavirin sustained virologic response was observed in only 3/21 (14%) treated patients compared with 0/11 controls ($P = 0.53$).[129] Ald

Although several preliminary results may appear to be encouraging, well-designed randomized trials are needed to provide definitive evidence for the safety and efficacy of PEG-IFN-α-based regimens as HCV pre-emptive post-transplant therapy. The key question is whether pre-emptive antiviral therapy can improve the long-term outcome of HCV transplant patients, since causing a delay of an inevitable HCV

recurrence with similar severity and progression of liver disease may not be cost effective.[117]

Anti-HCV immunoglobulin has also been tried as an alternative pre-emptive approach. Repeated doses of immunoglobulin have been found to reduce viremia levels in chimpanzees with chronic HCV infection.[130] However, in a small pilot randomized controlled trial, high or low doses of anti-HCV human immunoglobulins (prepared by fractionation of solvent/detergent-treated plasma pools from anti-HCV positive plasma donors), administered intravenously during the anhepatic phase and every 2 weeks for 48 weeks after OLT, had no benefit on clinical or virologic HCV recurrence in 16 patients transplanted for HCV cirrhosis.[131] Ald Thus, to date, there are no data to support the efficacy of immunoglobulins for the prevention of post-OLT HCV recurrence.

Post-transplant antiviral therapy

In HCV transplant patients with established histological recurrence of chronic hepatitis C, the targets of therapy are to achieve clearance of serum HCV-RNA, or, alternatively, to prevent or even delay progression of fibrosis and liver disease. Persistently elevated serum transaminases and at least moderate graft fibrosis during the first 12 months after OLT are associated with an increased risk of progression to cirrhosis and have been adopted as indications for therapy.[121] IFN-α, or recently PEG-IFN-α, based regimens are usually tried in this setting.

IFN-α monotherapy is less effective in transplant than non-transplant HCV patients and therefore it probably should be abandoned. Short (6-month) courses of IFN-α are rather ineffective,[83,132-134] while long (12-month) courses of IFN-α have been reported to achieve conflicting results.[135-137] IFN-α therapy in post-transplant patients has also been associated with possible increased risk of graft rejection. In HCV liver transplant patients, however an increase in the incidence of rejection was only observed in one[133] of several studies.[83,124,125,132,134-137] B4

PEG-IFN-α monotherapy has also been used in HCV transplant patients. In a preliminary randomized trial, PEG-IFN-2-α achieved virologic response at 24-weeks in 31% of 16 treated compared with none of 11 untreated patients with post-OLT recurrent hepatitis C. The therapy was well tolerated with only 7% withdrawals.[138] Ald In another recent study in post-OLT recurrent hepatitis C, daily IFN-α therapy was well tolerated and was associated with histological benefit,[128] thus providing a rationale for investigation of the potential efficacy of maintenance therapy with low doses of daily standard IFN-α or, more likely, of PEG-IFN-α.

Ribavirin monotherapy may transiently reduce the aminotransferase activity in HCV transplant patients, but has no effect on viremia,[139-141] and therefore it should not be used for the treatment of post-OLT recurrent hepatitis C. C5 As

Table 38.4 Efficacy of the combination of interferon-alpha (IFNα) and ribavirin (RIB) in the treatment of post-transplant recurrent hepatitis C

Study	Duration of therapy (months)	No.	ETR (%)	SVR (%)
Bizollon et al. (1997)[143]	6[a]	21	48	24
Gotz et al. (1998)[144]	12	10	10	–
Bellati et al. (1999)[147]	12	122	35	18
Wietzke et al. (2000)[148]	6[a]	7	–	29
Ben-Ari et al. (2000)[149]	6	5	0	0
Alberti et al. (2001)[146]	12	18	44	27
Ahmad et al. (2001)[151]	12	20	40	20
de Vera et al. (2001)[153]	12	32	9	9
Gopal et al. (2001)[152]	12	12	50	8
Andreone et al. (2001)[150b]	12	9	–	11
Lavezzo et al. (2002)[156]	12	30	23	17
Shakil et al. (2002)[157]	12	22	13	5
Menon et al. (2002)[158]	12	26	35	31
Kornberg et al. (2001)[154]	12	20	66	50
Firpi et al. (2002)[159]	12	54	38	30
Bizollon et al. (2003)[160]	12	54	–	26
Samuel et al. (2003)[161]	12	28	32	21

[a]Followed by 6 months of RIB monotherapy
[b]IFNα + RIB + Amantadine
ETR, end-of-therapy virologic response; SVR, sustained virologic response

occurs in the non-transplant setting, ribavirin may be associated with dose-related hemolytic anemia. Moreover, as ribavirin undergoes renal clearance and is generally contraindicated in patients with renal failure, dose adjustment or even discontinuation may be required in transplant patients who frequently have reduced glomerular filtration rate usually due to nephrotoxic immunosuppressive agents.[142]

There are several studies on the safety and efficacy of IFN-α plus ribavirin therapy in patients with post-OLT recurrent hepatitis C (Table 38.4).[143] However, patient numbers are always rather small, the inclusion criteria and the design differ from study to study, and response rates are reported only for the end-of-therapy and not for the longer term in some of these studies. Thus, end-of-therapy virologic response rates have been reported to range widely from 0% to 66% and sustained response rates from 0% to 50%.[143–161] B4 Therefore, no reliable estimate of the probability of sustained virologic response in patients with post-transplant hepatitis C treated with IFN-α and ribavirin can be made. Moreover, the combination of IFN-α and ribavirin is associated with frequent and potentially severe adverse effects, which may often require reduction of drug dosage or even withdrawal of therapy.

The effect of IFN-α and ribavirin therapy on liver histology in HCV transplant patients has not been clarified. Marked histologic improvement was reported in 86% of 14 patients in one study,[162] but little or no impact on fibrosis progression was reported by others.[161] B4 Moreover, the addition of an anti-interleukin (IL)-2 receptor anti-body to the combination of IFN-α and ribavirin was reported to improve lobular inflammation and reduce HCV viremia, but to have no effect on liver fibrosis.[163] B4

The combination of PEG-IFN-α and ribavirin is the treatment of choice for non-transplant patients with chronic hepatitis C, particularly those infected with genotype 1.[118] However, there are very few preliminary data, and only in abstract form, for transplant patients.[164–172] Given the superiority of this combination in non-transplant patients, the guidelines for treatment of non-transplant patients may also be used for patients with post-OLT recurrent hepatitis C, at least until data from appropriate studies in this population become available.[121] B4, C5 However, the safety and efficacy of the combination of PEG-IFN-α and ribavirin as well as the optimal dose and duration of therapy have not been established in the transplant population, and increased toxicity is recognized.

Modification of immunosuppression

The exact role of the immune system in the pathogenesis of HCV-related chronic liver injury and progression of fibrosis remains unclarified.[113] However, it is well accepted that immunosuppressive therapy favors HCV replication and is associated with a more accelerated course of HCV-related liver disease.[4] Calcineurin inhibitors, tacrolimus or cyclosporin, which inhibit early T-cell signal pathways and IL-2 production and release, are the mainstays of current immunosuppressive regimens. Azathioprine and mycophenolate mofetil may be used to enhance immunosuppression or allow dose reductions of cyclosporin or tacrolimus, while corticosteroids are usually used only during the first post-transplant period and to treat acute cellular rejection.

Existing data show no consistent difference between cyclosporin and tacrolimus-based immunosuppressive regimens in the incidence and severity of post-OLT recurrent hepatitis C.[173,174] B4 There does not seem to be any association between the type of triple or double maintenance immunosuppressive therapy and the outcome of post-transplant HCV infection. In one study, however, azathioprine-containing regimens appeared to reduce histological HCV recurrence and delay post-transplant hepatitis C progression.[175] Moreover, in a retrospective analysis of 59 HCV transplant patients who survived at least 12 months, single immunosuppressive therapy *ab initio* (cyclosporin or tacrolimus) was found to be associated with histological benefit compared with triple or double immunosuppressive regimens.[106] B4 In particular, severe fibrosis or cirrhosis at a median follow up of 24–36 months developed in 37% (17/46) of patients treated with triple or double immunosuppressive regimens and in only 8% (1/13) of patients treated with a single agent ($P = 0.01$).[106] Thus, further data are needed before any definite conclusion can be drawn concerning the role of immunosuppression in post-transplant HCV recurrence.

Steroids are usually withdrawn within the first 3–6 months after OLT, but doses and duration of steroid therapy may vary considerably between transplant centers. Steroids massively increase serum HCV-RNA levels and high total cumulative dose and/or high number of steroid boluses have been associated with worse outcomes.[176] However, data on the effect of steroids appear also to be conflicting. Rapid withdrawal of steroids,[177] complete avoidance of steroids[106] and a slow tapering of steroids over a prolonged period[178] have all been suggested to prevent aggressive post-OLT HCV recurrence. C5

Mycophenolate mofetil was suggested to have a beneficial effect on HCV recurrence, since it appeared to have some antiviral activity. However, data from preliminary studies did not show any beneficial effect of mycophenolate mofetil on serum HCV-RNA levels,[179,180] the timing of HCV recurrence, or the response rate to therapy with IFN-α and ribavirin,[181] although a delay of hepatitis C recurrence in HCV transplant patients treated with mycophenolate mofetil was reported in one study.[182] In a recent randomized trial, mycophenolate mofetil therapy was not found to have any effect on patient and graft survival, rejection or HCV recurrence rate.[183] A1d Thus, no benefit of mycophenolate mofetil on post-OLT recurrent hepatitis C has been shown. Therefore, its use should be based on the usual indications for mycophenolate mofetil in HCV transplanted patients.

References

1 Todo S, Demetris AJ, Van Thiel D, Teperman L, Fung JJ, Starzl TE. Orthotopic liver transplantation for patients with hepatitis B virus-related liver disease. *Hepatology* 1991;**13**: 619–26.

2 O'Grady JG, Smith HM, Davies SE *et al.* Hepatitis B virus reinfection after orthotopic liver transplantation. Serological and clinical implications. *J Hepatol* 1992;**14**:104–11.

3 Davies SE, Portmann BC, O'Grady JG *et al.* Hepatic histological findings after transplantation for chronic hepatitis B virus infection, including a unique pattern of fibrosing cholestatic hepatitis. *Hepatology* 1991;**13**:150–7.

4 Collier J, Heathcote J. Hepatitis C viral infection in the immunosuppressed patient. *Hepatology* 1998;**27**:2–6.

5 Samuel D, Muller R, Alexander G *et al.* Liver transplantation in European patients with the hepatitis B surface antigen. *N Engl J Med* 1993;**329**:1842–7.

6 Papatheodoridis GV, Sevastianos V, Burroughs AK. Prevention of and treatment for hepatitis B virus infection after liver transplantation in the nucleoside analogs era. *Am J Transplant* 2003;**3**:250–8.

7 Hoofnagle JH, Di Bisceglie AM, Waggoner JG, Park Y. Interferon alfa for patients with clinically apparent cirrhosis due to chronic hepatitis B. *Gastroenterology* 1993;**104**: 1116–21.

8 Villeneuve JP, Condreay LD, Willems B *et al.* Lamivudine treatment for decompensated cirrhosis resulting from chronic hepatitis B. *Hepatology* 2000;**31**:207–10.

9 Kapoor D, Guptan RC, Wakil SM *et al.* Beneficial effects of lamivudine in hepatitis B virus-related decompensated cirrhosis. *J Hepatol* 2000;**33**:308–12.

10 Kitay-Cohen Y, Ben-Ari Z, Tur-Kaspa R, Fainguelernt H, Lishner M. Extension of transplantation free time by lamivudine in patients with hepatitis B-induced decompensated cirrhosis. *Transplantation* 2000;**69**:2382–3.

11 Liaw Y-F, Leung NWY, Chang T-T *et al.* Effects of extended lamivudine therapy in Asian patients with chronic hepatitis B. *Gastroenterology* 2000;**119**:172–80.

12 Papatheodoridis GV, Dimou E, Laras A, Papadimitropoulos V, Hadziyannis SJ. Course of virologic breakthroughs under long-term lamivudine in HBeAg-negative precore mutant HBV liver disease. *Hepatology* 2002;**36**: 219–26.

13 Allen MI, DesLauriers M, Andrews CW *et al.* Identification and characterization of mutations in hepatitis B virus-resistant to lamivudine. *Hepatology* 1998;**27**:1670–7.

14 Hunt CM, McGill JM, Allen ML, Condreay LD. Clinical relevance of hepatitis B virus mutations. *Hepatology* 2000;**31**:1037–44.

15 Liaw YF, Chien RN, Yeh CT, Tsai SL, Chu CM. Acute exacerbation and hepatitis B virus clearance after emergence of YMDD motif mutation during lamivudine therapy. *Hepatology* 1999;**30**:567–72.

16 Merle P, Trepo C. Therapeutic management of hepatitis B-related cirrhosis. *J Viral Hepat* 2001;**8**:391–9.

17 Saab S, Kim M, Wright TL, Han SH, Martin P, Busuttil RW. Successful orthotopic liver transplantation for lamivudine-associated YMDD mutant hepatitis B virus. *Gastroenterology* 2000;**119**:1382–4.

18 Romeo R, Caccamo L, Rossi G, Facchetti F, Fassati LR, Colombo M. Low rate of S gene mutants in transplanted patients is associated to a maintained HBIG response even in the presence of YMDD mutants. *Hepatology* 2002;**36**: 185A.

19 Rosenau J, Bahr MJ, Tillmann HL *et al.* Lamivudine and low-dose hepatitis B immune globulin for prophylaxis of hepatitis B reinfection after liver transplantation possible role of mutations in the YMDD motif prior to transplantation as a risk factor for reinfection. *J Hepatol* 2001;**34**: 895–902.

20 Samuel D. Liver transplantation and hepatitis B virus infection: the situation seems to be under control, but the virus is still there. *J Hepatol* 2001;**34**:943–5.

21 Ono-Nita SK, Kato N, Shiratori Y *et al.* Susceptibility of lamivudine-resistant hepatitis B virus to other reverse transcriptase inhibitors. *J Clin Invest* 1999;**103**:1635–40.

22 Perrillo R, Schiff E, Yoshida E *et al.* Adefovir dipivoxil for the treatment of lamivudine-resistant hepatitis B mutants. *Hepatology* 2000;**32**:129–34.

23 Perrillo R, Schiff E, Hann H-WL *et al.* The addition of adefovir dipivoxil to lamivudine in decompensated chronic hepatitis B patients with YMDD variant HBV and reduced response to lamivudine – preliminary 24 week results. *Hepatology* 2001;**34**:349A.

24 Shouval D, Samuel D. Hepatitis B immune globulin to prevent hepatitis B virus graft reinfection following liver transplantation: a concise review. *Hepatology* 2000;**32**: 1189–95.

25 Yao FY, Osorio RW, Roberts JP *et al.* Intramuscular hepatitis B immune globulin combined with lamivudine for prophylaxis against hepatitis B recurrence after liver transplantation. *Liver Transpl Surg* 1999;**5**:491–6.

26 Yoshida EM, Erb SR, Partovi N *et al.* Liver transplantation for chronic hepatitis B infection with the use of combination lamivudine and low-dose hepatitis B immune globulin. *Liver Transpl Surg* 1999;**5**:520–5.

27 van Hoek B, Kroes AC, Ringers J, Veenendaal RA, Terpstra OT, Lamers CB. Switching intravenous to out-of-hospital fixed-dose intramuscular hepatitis B immunoglobulin after liver transplantation for HBsAg-positive HBV-DNA negative cirrhosis is feasible and reduces cost. *Hepatology* 2000;**32**:242A.

28 Sanchez-Fueyo A, Rimola A, Grande L *et al.* Hepatitis B immunoglobulin discontinuation followed by hepatitis B virus vaccination: a new strategy in the prophylaxis of hepatitis B virus recurrence after liver transplantation. *Hepatology* 2000;**31**:496–501.

29 Angelico M, Di Paolo D, Trinito MO *et al.* Failure of a reinforced triple course of hepatitis B vaccination in patients transplanted for HBV-related cirrhosis. *Hepatology* 2002; **35**:176–81.

30 Bienzle U, Gunther M, Neuhaus R, Neuhaus P. Successful hepatitis B vaccination in patients who underwent transplantation for hepatitis B virus-related cirrhosis: preliminary results. *Liver Transpl* 2002;**8**:562–4.

31 Carman WF, Trautwein C, van Deursen FJ *et al.* Hepatitis B virus envelope variation after transplantation with and without hepatitis B immune globulin prophylaxis. *Hepatology* 1996;**24**:489–93.

32 Ghany MG, Ayola B, Villamil FG *et al.* Hepatitis B virus S mutants in liver transplant recipients who were reinfected despite hepatitis B immune globulin prophylaxis. *Hepatology* 1998;**27**:213–22.

33 Terrault NA, Zhou S, McCory RW *et al.* Incidence and clinical consequences of surface and polymerase gene mutations in liver transplant recipients on hepatitis B immunoglobulin. *Hepatology* 1998;**28**:555–61.

34 Grellier L, Mutimer D, Ahmed M *et al.* Lamivudine prophylaxis against reinfection in liver transplantation for hepatitis B cirrhosis. *Lancet* 1996;**348**:1212–15.

35 Mutimer D, Pillay D, Dragon E *et al.* High pre-treatment serum hepatitis B virus titre predicts failure of lamivudine prophylaxis and graft re-infection after liver transplantation. *J Hepatol* 1999;**30**:715–21.

36 Mutimer D, Dusheiko G, Barrett C *et al.* Lamivudine without HBIg for prevention of graft reinfection by hepatitis B: long-term follow up. *Transplantation* 2000;**70**:809–15.

37 Malkan G, Cattral MS, Humar A *et al.* Lamivudine for hepatitis B in liver transplantation: a single-center experience. *Transplantation* 2000;**69**:1403–7.

38 Wai CT, Lim SG, Tan KC. Outcome of lamivudine-resistant hepatitis B virus infection in liver transplant recipients in Singapore. *Gut* 2001;**48**:581.

39 Fontana RJ, Keefe EB, Han S *et al.* Prevention of recurrent hepatitis B infection following liver transplantation: experience in 112 North American patients. *Hepatology* 1999;**30**:301A.

40 Markowitz JS, Martin P, Conrad AJ *et al.* Prophylaxis against hepatitis B recurrence following liver transplantation using combination lamivudine and hepatitis B immune globulin. *Hepatology* 1998;**28**:585–9.

41 McCaughan GW, Spencer J, Koorey D *et al.* Lamivudine therapy in patients undergoing liver transplantation for hepatitis B virus precore mutant-associated infection: high resistance rates in treatment of recurrence but universal prevention if used as prophylaxis with very low dose hepatitis B immune globulin. *Liver Transpl Surg* 1999;**5**: 512–19.

42 Roche B, Samuel D, Roque AM *et al.* Intravenous anti- HBs Ig combined with oral lamivudine for prophylaxis against HBV recurrence after liver transplantation. *J Hepatol* 1999;**30(Suppl 1)**:80.

43 Angus PW, McCaughan GW, Gane EJ, Crawford DH, Harley H. Combination low-dose hepatitis B immune globulin and lamivudine therapy provides effective prophylaxis against posttransplantation hepatitis B. *Liver Transpl* 2000;**6**: 429–33.

44 Han SH, Ofman J, Holt C *et al.* An efficacy and cost-effectiveness analysis of combination hepatitis B immune globulin and lamivudine to prevent recurrent hepatitis B after orthotopic liver transplantation compared with hepatitis B immune globulin monotherapy. *Liver Transpl* 2000;**6**:741–8.

45 Lee PH, Hu RH, Tsai MK *et al.* Liver transplantation for patients with hepatitis B: prevention of hepatitis B recurrence by intravenous antihepatitis B immunoglobulin and lamivudine. *Transplant Proc* 2000;**32**:2245–7.

46 Andreone P, Grazi GL, Gramenzi A *et al.* Lamivudine (LAM) plus HBIg combination therapy compared to HBIg or no therapy in preventing hepatitis B (HBV) recurrence after liver transplantation (LT). *J Hepatol* 2000;**32(Suppl 2)**:51.

47 Buti M, Mass A, Prieto M *et al.* Randomized clinical trial of lamivudine vs lamivudine + hepatitis B gammaglobulin in the prevention of HBV recurrence after liver transplant – preliminary results. *Hepatology* 2000;**32**:217A.

48 Marzano A, Salizzoni M, Debernardi-Venon W *et al.* Prevention of hepatitis B virus recurrence after liver transplantation in cirrhotic patients treated with lamivudine and passive immunoprophylaxis. *J Hepatol* 2001;**34**:903–10.

49 Machicao VI, Soldevilla-Pico C, Devarbhavi HC, Lukens FJ, Ishitani MB, Dickson RC. Hepatitis B liver transplant patients on combination of lamivudine and high dose IV immune globulin have less significant histological progression than hepatitis C transplanted patients. *Hepatology* 2001;**34**:411A.

50 Choi J, Bae S, Yoon S *et al.* Intramuscular hepatitis B immune globulin and lamivudine for prophylaxis against hepatitis B recurrence after liver transplantation. *Hepatology* 2002;**36**:184A.

51 Gane EJ, McCaughan G, Strasser S *et al.* Combination lamivudine plus low dose intramuscular hepatitis B immunoglobulin prevents recurrent hepatitis B and may eradicate residual graft infection. *Hepatology* 2002;**36**:221A.

52 Kim DD, Heffernan DJ, Bass NM, Roberts JP, Ascher NL, Terrault NA. Comparison of 6 versus 12 months hepatitis B immune globulin in combination with lamivudine as prophylaxis in liver transplant recipients with hepatitis B. *Hepatology* 2002;**36**:221A.

53 Chu C-J, Fontana RJ, Moore C *et al.* Efficacy of HBIG weaning in the long-term prophylaxis of HBV reinfection following liver transplantation. *Hepatology* 2002;**36**:221A.

54 Han SH, Martin P, Edelstein M *et al.* Conversion from intravenous to intramuscular hepatitis B immune globulin in combination with lamivudine is safe and cost-effective in patients receiving long-term prophylaxis to prevent hepatitis B recurrence after liver transplantation. *Liver Transpl* 2003; **9**:182–7.

55 Terrault NA, Wright TL. Combined short-term hepatitis B immunoglobulin (HBIG) and long-term lamivudine (LAM) versus HBIG monotherapy as hepatitis B virus (HBV) prophylaxis in liver transplant recipients. *Hepatology* 1998;**28**:389A.

56 Naoumov NV, Lopes AR, Burra P *et al.* Randomized trial of lamivudine versus hepatitis B immunoglobulin for long-term prophylaxis of hepatitis B recurrence after liver transplantation. *J Hepatol* 2001;**34**:888–94.

57 Dodson SF, de Vera ME, Bonham CA, Geller DA, Rakela J, Fung JJ. Lamivudine after hepatitis B immune globulin is effective in preventing hepatitis B recurrence after liver transplantation. *Liver Transpl* 2000;**6**:434–9.

58 Andreone P, Caraceni P, Grazi GL *et al.* Lamivudine treatment for acute hepatitis B after liver transplantation. *J Hepatol* 1998;**29**:985–9.

59 Nery JR, Weppler D, Rodriguez M, Ruiz P, Schiff ER, Tzakis AG. Efficacy of lamivudine in controlling hepatitis B virus recurrence after liver transplantation. *Transplantation* 1998;**65**:1615–21.

60 Perrillo R, Rakela J, Dienstag J *et al.* Multicenter study of lamivudine therapy for hepatitis B after liver transplantation. Lamivudine Transplant Group. *Hepatology* 1999;**29**:1581–6.

61 Roche B, Samuel D, Roque AM *et al.* Lamivudine therapy for HBV infection after liver transplantation. *J Hepatol* 1999;**30(Suppl 1)**:78.

62 Balan V, Dodson FS, Vargas HE *et al.* long-term follow up of lamivudine therapy for hepatitis B before and after liver transplantation; clinical implication of development of the YMDD mutant. *Hepatology* 1999;**30**:346A.

63 Seehofer D, Rayes N, Berg T *et al.* Lamivudine as first- and second-line treatment of hepatitis B infection after liver transplantation. *Transpl Int* 2000;**13**:290–6.

64 Fontana RJ, Hann HW, Wright T *et al.* A multicenter study of lamivudine treatment in 33 patients with hepatitis B after liver transplantation. *Liver Transpl* 2001;**7**:504–10.

65 Brind AM, Bennett MK, Bassendine MF. Nucleoside analog therapy in fibrosing cholestatic hepatitis – a case report in an HBsAg positive renal transplant recipient. *Liver* 1998;**18**: 134–9.

66 Chan TM, Wu PC, Li FK, Lai CL, Cheng IK, Lai KN. Treatment of fibrosing cholestatic hepatitis with lamivudine. *Gastroenterology* 1998;**115**:177–81.

67 Seehofer D, Rayes N, Bechstein WO *et al.* Therapy of recurrent hepatitis B infection after liver transplantation. A retrospective analysis of 200 liver transplantations based on hepatitis B associated liver diseases. *Z Gastroenterol* 2000;**38**:773–83.

68 Ben-Ari Z, Mor E, Shapira Z, Tur-Kaspa R. Long-term experience with lamivudine therapy for hepatitis B virus infection after liver transplantation. *Liver Transpl* 2001;**7**: 113–17.

69 Rayes N, Seehofer D, Hopf U *et al.* Comparison of famciclovir and lamivudine in the long-term treatment of hepatitis B infection after liver transplantation. *Transplantation* 2001;**71**:96–101.

70 Seehofer D, Rayes N, Steinmuller T *et al.* Occurrence and clinical outcome of lamivudine-resistant hepatitis B infection after liver transplantation. *Liver Transpl* 2001;**7**: 976–82.

71 Ben-Ari Z, Pappo O, Zemel R, Mor E, Tur-Kaspa R. Association of lamivudine resistance in recurrent hepatitis B after liver transplantation with advanced hepatic fibrosis. *Transplantation* 1999;**68**:232–6.

72 Peters MG, Singer G, Howard T *et al.* Fulminant hepatic failure resulting from lamivudine resistant hepatitis B virus in a renal transplant recipient: durable response after orthotopic liver transplantation on adefovir dipivoxil and hepatitis B immune globulin. *Transplantation* 1999;**68**:1912–14.

73 Ahmad J, Dodson SF, Balan V *et al.* Adefovir dipivoxil suppresses lamivudine resistant hepatitis B virus in liver transplant recipients. *Hepatology* 2000;**32**:292A.

74 Schiff E, Neuhaus P, Tillmann H *et al.* Adefovir dipivoxil (ADV) for the treatment of lamivudine resistant HBV (LAM-R) in patients post liver transplant (post-OLT) patients. *J Hepatol* 2002;**36(Suppl 1)**:32

75 Deeks SG, Collier A, Larezra J *et al.* The safety and efficacy of adefovir dipivoxil, a novel anti-human immunodeficiency virus (HIV) therapy in HIV-infected adults: a randomised, double-blind, placebo-controlled trial. *J Infect Dis* 1997; **176**:1517–23.

76 Xiong S, Yang H, Westland CE *et al.* Resistance surveillance of HBeAg- chronic hepatitis B (CHB) patients treated for two years with adefovir dipivoxil (ADV). *J Hepatol* 2003; **38(Suppl 2)**:182.

77 Nevens F, de Man RA, Chua D *et al.* Effectiveness of a low dose of entecavir in treating recurrent viremia in chronic hepatitis B. *Hepatology* 2000;**32**:377A.

78 Mutimer D, Pillay D, Cook P *et al.* Selection of multiresistant hepatitis B virus during sequential nucleoside-analog therapy. *J Infect Dis* 2000;**181**:713–16.

79 Tillmann HL, Trautwein C, Bock T *et al.* Mutational pattern of hepatitis B virus on sequential therapy with famciclovir and lamivudine in patients with hepatitis B virus reinfection occurring under HBIg immunoglobulin after liver transplantation. *Hepatology* 1999;**30**:244–56.

80 Singh N, Gayowski T, Wannstedt CF, Waggener MM, Marino IM. Pretransplant famciclovir as prophylaxis for hepatitis B virus recurrence after liver transplantation. *Transplantation* 1997;**63**:1415–19.

81 Gish RG, Lau JY, Brooks L *et al.* Ganciclovir treatment of hepatitis B virus infection in liver transplant recipients. *Hepatology* 1996;**23**:1–7.

82 Roche B, Samuel D, Gigou M *et al.* Long-term ganciclovir therapy for hepatitis B virus infection after liver transplantation. *J Hepatol* 1999;**31**:584–92.

83 Wright H, Gavaler J, Van Thiel D. Preliminary experience with a-2b-interferon therapy in viral hepatitis in allograft recipients. *Transplantation* 1992;**53**:121–4.

84 Terrault NA, Holland CC, Ferrell L *et al.* Interferon alfa for recurrent hepatitis B infection after liver transplantation. *Liver Transpl Surg* 1996;**2**:132–8.

85 Schiff E, Lai C-L, Neuhaus P *et al.* Adefovir dipivoxil (ADV) for the treatment of chronic hepatitis B in patients pre- and post-liver transplantation (OLT) with lamivudine-resistant HBV (LAM-R) hepatitis B virus. *Hepatology* 2002;**36**:371A.

86 Walsh KM, Woodall T, Lamy P, Wight DG, Bloor S, Alexander GJ. Successful treatment with adefovir dipivoxil in a patient with fibrosing cholestatic hepatitis and lamivudine-resistant hepatitis B virus. *Gut* 2001;**49**:436–40.

87 Tillmann HL, Bock T, Bleck JS *et al.* Successful treatment of fibrosing cholestatic hepatitis using adefovir dipivoxil in a patient with cirrhosis and renal insufficiency. *Liver Transpl* 2003;**9**:191–6.

88 Mutimer D, Feraz-Neto BH, Harrison R *et al.* Acute liver graft failure due to emergence of lamivudine resistant hepatitis B virus: rapid resolution during treatment with adefovir. *Gut* 2001;**49**:860–3.

89 de Man RA, Wolters L, Nevens F *et al.* A study of oral entecavir given for 28 days in both treatment-naive and pre-treatment subjects with chronic hepatitis. *Hepatology* 2000;**32**:376A.

90 Tassopoulos N, Hadziyannis S, Cianciara J *et al.* Entecavir is effective in treating patients with chronic hepatitis B who have failed lamivudine therapy. *Hepatology* 2001;**34**:340A.

91 Shakil OA, Lilly L, Angus P *et al.* Entecavir signifcantly reduces viral load in liver transplant recipients failing lamivudine therapy for chronic hepatitis B infection. *J Hepatol* 2002;**36(Suppl 1)**:122.

92 Terrault NA. Hepatitis B virus and liver transplantation. *Clin Liver Dis* 1999;**3**:389–415.

93 Seehofer D, Rayes N, Berg T *et al.* Additional interferon alpha for lamivudine resistant hepatitis B infection after liver transplantation: a preliminary report. *Transplantation* 2000;**69**:1739–42.

94 Wright TL, Donegan E, Hsu HH *et al.* Recurrent and acquired hepatitis C viral infection in liver transplant recipients. *Gastroenterology* 1992;**103**:317–22.

95 Gane EJ, Portmann BC, Naoumov NV *et al.* Long-term outcome of hepatitis C infection after liver transplantation. *N Engl J Med* 1996;**334**:815–20.

96 Feray C, Gigou M, Samuel D *et al.* The course of hepatitis C virus infection after liver transplantation. *Hepatology* 1994;**20**:1137–43.

97 Prieto M, Berenguer M, Rayon JM *et al.* High incidence of allograft cirrhosis in hepatitis C virus genotype 1b infection following transplantation: relationship with rejection episodes. *Hepatology* 1999;**29**:250–6.

98 Berenguer M, Ferrell L, Watson J *et al.* HCV-related fibrosis progression following liver transplantation: increase in recent years. *J Hepatol* 2000;**32**:673–84.

99 Schluger LK, Sheiner PA, Thung SN *et al.* Severe recurrent cholestatic hepatitis C following orthotopic liver transplantation. *Hepatology* 1996;**23**:971–6.

100 Feray C, Gigou M, Samuel D *et al.* Influence of the genotypes of hepatitis C virus on the severity of recurrent liver disease after liver transplantation. *Gastroenterology* 1995;**108**:1088–96.

101 Zhou S, Terrault NA, Ferrell L *et al.* Severity of liver disease in liver transplantation recipients with hepatitis C virus infection: relationship to genotype and level of viremia. *Hepatology* 1996;**24**:1041–6.

102 Papatheodoridis GV, Barton SG, Andrew D *et al.* Longitudinal variation in hepatitis C virus (HCV) viraemia and early course of HCV infection after liver transplantation for HCV cirrhosis: the role of different immunosuppressive regimens. *Gut* 1999;**45**:427–34.

103 Gane EJ, Naoumov NV, Qian K-P *et al.* A longitudinal analysis of hepatitis C virus replication following liver transplantation. *Gastroenterology* 1996;**110**:167–77.

104 Charlton M, Seaberg E, Wiesner R *et al.* Predictors of patient and graft survival following liver transplantation for hepatitis C. *Hepatology* 1998;**28**:823–30.

105 Charlton M, Seaberg E. Impact of immunosuppression and acute rejection on recurrence of hepatitis C: results of the National Institute of Diabetes and Digestive and Kidney Diseases Liver Transplantation Database. *Liver Transpl Surg* 1999;**5**:S107–S114.

106 Papatheodoridis GV, Davies S, Dhillon AP *et al.* The role of different immunosuppression in the long-term histological outcome of HCV reinfection after liver transplantation for HCV cirrhosis. *Transplantation* 2001;**72**:412–18.

107 Berenguer M, Prieto M, Cordoba J *et al.* Early development of chronic active hepatitis in recurrent hepatitis C after liver transplantation: association with treatment of rejection. *J Hepatol* 1998;**28**:756–63.

108 Berenguer M, Prieto M, San Juan F *et al.* Contribution of donor age to the recent decrease in patient survival among HCV-infected liver transplant recipients. *Hepatology* 2002;**36**:202–10.

109 Rosen HR, Lentz JJ, Rose SL *et al.* Donor polymorphism of tumor necrosis factor gene: relationship with variable severity of hepatitis C recurrence after liver transplantation. *Transplantation* 1999;**68**:1898–902.

110 Rosen HR, Shackleton CR, Higa L *et al.* Use of OKT3 is associated with early and severe recurrence of hepatitis C after liver transplantation. *Am J Gastroenterol* 1997;**92**: 1453–7.

111 Rosen HR, Gretch DR, Oehlke M *et al.* Timing and severity of initial hepatitis C recurrence as predictors of long-term liver allograft injury. *Transplantation* 1998;**65**:1178–82.

112 Burak KW, Kremers WK, Batts KP *et al.* Impact of cytomegalovirus infection, year of transplantation, and donor age on outcomes after liver transplantation for hepatitis C. *Liver Transpl* 2002;**8**:362–9.

113 Papatheodoridis GV, Patch D, Dusheiko GM, Burroughs AK. The outcome of hepatitis C virus infection after liver transplantation – is it influenced by the type of immunosuppression? *J Hepatol* 1999;**30**:731–8.

114 Teixeira R, Pastacaldi S, Papatheodoridis GV, Burroughs AK. Recurrent hepatitis C after liver transplantation. *J Med Virol* 2000;**61**:443–54.

115 Berenguer M. Natural history of recurrent hepatitis C. *Liver Transpl* 2002;**8(Suppl 1)**:S14–S18.

116 Berenguer M. Outcome of posttransplantation hepatitis C virus disease – is it the host, the virus, or how we modify the host and/or the virus? *Liver Transpl* 2002;**8**:889–91.

117 Burroughs AK. Postransplantation prevention and treatment of recurrent hepatitis C. *Liver Transpl* 2000; **6(Suppl 2)**:S35–S40.

118 National Institute of Health Consensus Development Conference Statement: Management of hepatitis C: June 10–12, 2002. *Hepatology* 2002;**36(Suppl 1)**:S3–S20.

119 Manns MP, McHutchison JG, Gordon SC *et al.* Peginterferon alfa-2b plus ribavirin compared with interferon alfa-2b plus ribavirin for initial treatment of chronic hepatitis C: a randomised trial. *Lancet* 2001; **358**:958–65.

120 Fried MW, Shiffman ML, Reddy KR *et al.* Peginterferon alfa-2a plus ribavirin for chronic hepatitis C virus infection. *N Engl J Med* 2002;**347**:975–82.

121 Gane E. Treatment of recurrent hepatitis C. *Liver Transpl* 2002;**8(Suppl 1)**:S28–S37.

122 Di Bisceglie AM, McHutchison J, Rice CM. New therapeutic strategies for hepatitis C. *Hepatology* 2002;**35**:224–31.

123 Reddy KR, Weppler D, Zervos XA *et al.* Recurrent HCV infection following liver transplantation: the role of early post transplant interferon treatment. *Hepatology* 1996;**24**:295A.

124 Singh N, Gayowski T, Wannstedt CF *et al.* Interferon-α for prophylaxis of recurrent viral hepatitis C in liver transplant recipients. A prospective, randomized, controlled trial. *Transplantation* 1998;**65**:82–6.

125 Sheiner PA, Boros P, Klion FM *et al.* The efficacy of prophylactic interferon alfa-2b in preventing recurrent hepatitis C after liver transplantation. *Hepatology* 1998; **28**:831–8.

126 Mazzaferro V, Schiavo M, Caccamo L *et al.* Prospective randomized trial of early treatment of HCV infection after

liver transplantation in HCVRNA positive patients. *Liver Transpl* 2003;**9**:C-36.

127 Manzarbeitia C, Tepermann L, Chalasani N *et al.* 40 kDa Peginterferon as prophylaxis against HCV recurrence after liver transplantation; preliminary results of a randomized multicenter trial. *Hepatology* 2001;**34**:406A.

128 Cotler SJ, Ganger DR, Kaur S *et al.* Daily interferon therapy for hepatitis C virus infection in liver transplant recipients. *Transplantation* 2001;**71**:261–6.

129 Reddy R, Fried M, Dickson R *et al.* Interferon alfa-2b and ribavirin vs placebo as early treatment in patients transplanted for hepatitis C endstage liver disease: results of multicenter, randomized trial. *Gastroenterology* 2002; **122(Suppl)**: A-632.

130 Krawczynski K, Alter M, Tankersley D *et al.* Effect of immune globulin on prevention of experimental HCV infection. *J Infect Dis* 1996;**173**:822–8.

131 Willems B, Ede M, Marotta P *et al.* Anti-HCV human immunoglobulins for the prevention of graft infection in HCV-related liver transplantation. A pilot study. *J Hepatol* 2002;**36(Suppl 1)**:32.

132 Wright TL, Combs C, Kim M *et al.* Interferon-a therapy for hepatitis C virus infection after liver transplantation. *Hepatology* 1994;**20**:773–9.

133 Feray C, Samuel D, Gigou M *et al.* An open trial of interferon alfa recombinant for hepatitis C after liver transplantation: antiviral effects and risk of rejection. *Hepatology* 1995;**22**:1084–9.

134 Vargas V, Charco R, Castells L *et al.* Alpha interferon for acute hepatitis C in liver transplant recipients. *Transplant Proc* 1995;**27**:1222–3.

135 Boillot O, Berger E, Rasolofo E *et al.* Effectiveness of early alpha interferon therapy for hepatitis C virus infection recurrence after liver transplantation. *Transplant Int* 1996; **9**:S202–S203.

136 Singh N, Gayowski T, Wannstedt CF, Marino IR, Wagener MM. Interferon-alpha therapy for hepatitis C virus recurrence after liver transplantation: long term response with maintenance therapy. *Clin Transpl* 1996;**10**: 348–51.

137 Firpi J, Abdemlakek MF, Nelson DR, Laurwers GY, Sodevila Pico C, Davis GL. Outcome of liver transplant recipients treated with interferon alpha monotherapy for recurrent hepatitis C. *Hepatology* 1999;**30**:214A.

138 Ferenci P, Peck-Radosavljevic M, Vogel W *et al.* 40kDa Peginterferon alfa-2a (Pegasys) in post-liver transplant recipients with established recurrent hepatitis C: preliminary results of a randomized multicenter trial. *Hepatology* 2001;**34**:406A.

139 Gane EJ, Tibbs CJ, Ramage JK, Portmann BC, Williams R. Ribavirin therapy for hepatitis C infection following transplantation. *Transpl Int* 1995;**8**:61–4.

140 Cattral MS, Krajden M, Wanless IR *et al.* A pilot study of ribavirin therapy for recurrent hepatitis C virus infection after liver transplantation. *Transplantation* 1996;**61**: 1483–8.

141 Cattral MS, Hemming AW, Wanless IR *et al.* Outcome of long-term ribavirin therapy for recurrent hepatitis C after liver transplantation. *Transplantation* 1999;**67**:1277–80.

142 Jain AB, Eghtesad B, Venkataramanan R *et al.* Ribavirin dose modification based on renal function is necessary to reduce hemolysis in liver transplant patients with hepatitis C virus infection. *Liver Transpl* 2002;**8**:1007–13.

143 Bizollon T, Palazzo U, Ducerf C *et al.* Pilot study of the combination of interferon alfa and ribavirin as therapy of recurrent hepatitis C after liver transplantation. *Hepatology* 1997;**26**:500–4.

144 Gotz G, Schon MR, Haefker A *et al.* Treatment of recurrent hepatitis C virus infection after liver transplantation with IFN and ribavirin. *Transplant Proc* 1998;**30**:2104–6.

145 Fischer L, Sterneck M, Valentin-Gamazo C, Feucht HH, Malago M, Broelsch CE. Treatment of severe recurrent hepatitis C after liver transplantation with ribavirin plus interferon alpha. *Transplant Proc* 1999;**31**:494–5.

146 Alberti AB, Belli LS, Airoldi A *et al.* Combined therapy with interferon and low-dose ribavirin in posttransplantation recurrent hepatitis C: a pragmatic study. *Liver Transpl* 2001;**7**:870–6.

147 Bellati G, Alberti AB, Belli LS *et al.* Therapy of chronic hepatitis C after liver transplantation: multicenter Italian experience. *J Hepatol* 1999;**30(Suppl 1)**:51.

148 Wietzke P, Braun F, Ringe B, Ramadori G. Interferon alfa-2a and ribavirin therapy for hepatitis C recurrence after liver transplantation. *Transplant Proc* 2000;**32**:2539–42.

149 Ben-Ari Z, Mor E, Shaharabani E, Bar-Nathan N, Shapira Z, Tur-Kaspa R. Combination of interferon-alpha and ribavirin therapy for recurrent hepatitis C virus infection after liver transplantation. *Transplant Proc* 2000;**32**:714–16.

150 Andreone P, Gramenzi A, Cursaro C *et al.* Interferon-alpha plus ribavirin and amantadine in patients with post-transplant hepatitis C: results of a pilot study. *Dig Liver Dis* 2001;**33**:693–7.

151 Ahmad J, Dodson SF, Demetris AJ, Fung JJ, Shakil AO. Recurrent hepatitis C after liver transplantation: a non-randomized trial of interferon alfa alone versus interferon alfa and ribavirin. *Liver Transpl* 2001;**7**:863–9.

152 Gopal DV, Rabkin JM, Berk BS *et al.* Treatment of progressive hepatitis C recurrence after liver transplantation with combination interferon plus ribavirin. *Liver Transpl* 2001;**7**:181–90.

153 de Vera ME, Smallwood GA, Rosado K *et al.* Interferon-alpha and ribavirin for the treatment of recurrent hepatitis C after liver transplantation. *Transplantation* 2001;**71**:678–86.

154 Kornberg A, Hommann M, Tannapfel A *et al.* Long-term combination of interferon alfa-2b and ribavirin for hepatitis C recurrence in liver transplant patients. *Am J Transplant* 2001;**1**:350–5.

155 Israeli E, Galun E, Eid A *et al.* Combination therapy for hepatitis C virus reinfection after orthotopic liver transplantation. *Transplant Proc* 2001;**33**:2929.

156 Lavezzo B, Franchello A, Smedile A *et al.* Treatment of recurrent hepatitis C in liver transplants: efficacy of a six versus a twelve month course of interferon alfa 2b with ribavirin. *J Hepatol* 2002;**37**:247–52.

157 Shakil AO, McGuire B, Crippin J *et al.* A pilot study of interferon alfa and ribavirin combination in liver transplant recipients with recurrent hepatitis C. *Hepatology* 2002;**36**:1253–8.

158 Menon KVN, Poterucha JJ, El-Amin OM *et al.* Treatment of post transplantation recurrence of hepatitis C with interferon and ribavirin: lessons on tolerability and efficacy. *Liver Transpl* 2002;**8**:623–9.

159 Firpi RJ, Abdelmalek MF, Soldevila-Pico C *et al.* Combination of interferon alfa-2b and ribavirin in liver transplant recipients with histological recurrent hepatitis C. *Liver Transpl* 2002;**8**:1000–6.

160 Bizollon T, Ahmed SN, Radenne S *et al.* Long term histological improvement and clearance of intrahepatic hepatitis C virus RNA following sustained response to interferon-ribavirin combination therapy in liver transplanted patients with hepatitis C virus recurrence. *Gut* 2003;**52**:283–7.

161 Samuel D, Bizollon T, Feray C *et al.* Interferon-alpha 2b plus ribavirin in patients with chronic hepatitis C after liver transplantation: a randomized study. *Gastroenterology* 2003;**124**:642–50.

162 Bizollon T, Trepo C. Ribavirin and interferon combination for recurrent post-transplant hepatitis C: which benefit beyond 6 months? *J Hepatol* 2002;**37**:274–6.

163 Pinna AD, Ricordi C, Weppler D, Ruiz P, Tzakis AG. Treatment of recurrent hepatitis C after liver transplantation with IL-2r Ab. *Transplant Proc* 2001;**33**:1087–9.

164 Levitsky J, Cohen SM, Dasgupta KA, Faust TW, Te HS. Pegylated interferon therapy with/without ribavirin in liver transplant recipients with recurrent hepatitis C infection. *Hepatology* 2002;**36**:182A.

165 Khatib MA, Arenas JI, Carey E *et al.* Treatment with combination of PEG IFNa-2b and ribavirin suppresses viral replication in liver transplantation recipients with recurrent HCV hepatitis. *Hepatology* 2002;**36**:182A.

166 Mukherjee S, Gilroy RK, McCashland TM, Schafer DF, Zetterman RK, Sorrell MF. Pegylated-interferon and ribavirin for recurrent hepatitis C after liver transplantation. A preliminary analysis. *Hepatology* 2002;**36**:184A.

167 Vogel W, Ferenci P, Fontana R *et al.* Peginterferon alfa-2a (40KD) (Pegasys) in liver transplant recipients with established recurrent hepatitis C: interim results of an ongoing randomized multicenter trial. *Hepatology* 2002;**36**:312A.

168 Lavezzo B, Franchello A, Smedile A *et al.* Preliminary results of naive combination therapy with 12KDa PEG-IFNa-2b and ribavirin in recurrent hepatitis C after liver transplantation (LT). *J Hepatol* 2003;**38(Suppl 2)**:42.

169 Rodriguez-Luna H, Khatib A, Sharma P *et al.* Treatment of recurrent hepatitis C infection after liver transplantation with combination of PEG-IFNa2b and ribavirin: an open label series. *Liver Transpl* 2003;**9**:C-6.

170 Roche B, Roque-Alfonso AM, Sebagh M *et al.* Pilot study of treatment with pegylated interferon and ribavirin in liver transplant recipients with hepatitis C infection. *Liver Transpl* 2003;**9**:C-6.

171 Neumann UP, Berg T, Bahra M, Langrehr JM, Neuhaus P. Effectiveness of peginterferon alfa-2b plus ribavirin in

patients with hepatitis C recurrence after OLT. *Liver Transpl* 2003;**9**:C-7.

172 Gordon FD, Morin D, Keaveny A *et al.* Peg-interferon a-2b (PEG) and ribavirin is effective and safe after liver transplantation (LT). *Am J Transplant* 2003;**3(Suppl 5)**:518.

173 Feray C, Caccamo L, Alexander GJ *et al.* European collaborative study on factors influencing outcome after liver transplantation for hepatitis C. *Gastroenterology* 1999;**117**:619–25.

174 Zervos XA, Weppler D, Fragulidis GP *et al.* Comparison of tacrolimus with microemulsion cyclosporine as primary immunosuppression in hepatitis C patients after liver transplantation. *Transplantation* 1998;**65**:1044–6.

175 Hunt J, Gordon FD, Lewis WD *et al.* Histological recurrence and progression of hepatitis C after orthotopic liver transplantation: influence of immunosuppressive regimens. *Liver Transpl* 2001;**7**:1056–63.

176 Berenguer M, Lopez-Labrador FX, Wright TL. Hepatitis C and liver transplantation. *J Hepatol* 2001;**35**:666–78.

177 Mueller AR, Platz K, Willimski C *et al.* Influence of immunosuppression on patient survival after liver transplantation for hepatitis C. *Transplant Proc* 2001;**33**:1347–9.

178 Brillanti S, Vivarelli M, De Ruvo N *et al.* Slowly tapering off steroids protects the graft against hepatitis C recurrence after liver transplantation. *Liver Transpl* 2002;**8**:884–8.

179 Fasola CG, Netto GJ, Jennings LW *et al.* Recurrence of hepatitis C in liver transplant recipients treated with mycophenolate mofetil. *Transplant Proc* 2002;**34**:1563–4.

180 Firpi RJ, Nelson DR, Davis GL. Lack of antiviral effect of a short course of mycophenolate mofetil in patients with chronic hepatitis C virus infection. *Liver Transpl* 2003;**9**:57–61.

181 Smallwood GA, Davis L, Martinez E, Stieber AC, Heffron TG. Mycophenolate's influence in the treatment of recurrent hepatitis c following liver transplantation. *Transplant Proc* 2002;**34**:1559–60.

182 Fasola CG, Netto GJ, Christensen LL *et al.* Delay of hepatitis C recurrence in liver transplant recipients: impact of mycophenolate mofetil on transplant recipients with severe acute rejection or with renal dysfunction. *Transplant Proc* 2002;**34**:1561–2.

183 Jain A, Kashyap R, Demetris AJ, Eghstesad B, Pokharna R, Fung JJ. A prospective randomized trial of mycophenolate mofetil in liver transplant recipients with hepatitis C. *Liver Transpl* 2002;**8**:40–6.

Index

Note: page numbers in *italics* refer to figures, those in **bold** refer to tables and boxes.